Hugo and Russell's Pharmaceutical Microbiology

Hugo and Russell's Pharmaceutical Microbiology

Ninth Edition

Edited by

Brendan F. Gilmore, BSc, PhD, FRSC, FRSB
Professor of Pharmaceutical Microbiology
School of Pharmacy
Queen's University Belfast
Belfast, UK

Stephen P. Denyer, B. Pharm, PhD, FRPharmS
Emeritus Professor of Pharmacy
Universities of Brighton and Sussex
Brighton, UK

WILEY Blackwell

This edition first published 2023

Registered Offices
John Wiley & Sons, Inc., 111 River Street, Hoboken, NJ 07030, USA
John Wiley & Sons Ltd, The Atrium, Southern Gate, Chichester, West Sussex, PO19 8SQ, UK

Editorial Office
9600 Garsington Road, Oxford, OX4 2DQ, UK

For details of our global editorial offices, customer services and more information about Wiley products, visit us at www.wiley.com.

Wiley also publishes its books in a variety of electronic formats and by print-on-demand. Some content that appears in standard print versions of this book may not be available in other formats.

Library of Congress Cataloging-in-Publication Data applied for
[PB ISBN: 9781119434498]

Cover Design: Wiley
Cover Image: © CNRI/Getty Images

Set in 9.5/12.5pt STIXTwoText by Straive, Pondicherry, India

Printed in Singapore
M081591_191222

Contents

Notes on Contributors

David Allison
Reader in Pharmacy Education, Division of Pharmacy and Optometry, School of Health Sciences, The University of Manchester, Manchester, UK

Rosamund M. Baird
Former Visiting Senior Lecturer, School of Pharmacy and Pharmacology, University of Bath, Bath, UK
Now Sherborne, Dorset, UK

James C. Birchall
Professor of Pharmaceutical Sciences, School of Pharmacy and Pharmaceutical Sciences, Cardiff University, Cardiff, UK

Alistair K. Brown
Lecturer in Molecular Microbiology, Institute of Biosciences, Newcastle University, Newcastle upon Tyne, UK

Miguel Cámara
Professor of Molecular Microbiology and Co-Director of the National Biofilms Innovation Centre, School of Life Sciences, Biodiscovery Institute, University of Nottingham, Nottingham, UK

Elaine Cloutman-Green
Consultant Clinical Scientist, Great Ormond Street Hospital, London, UK

Sion A. Coulman
Senior Lecturer, School of Pharmacy and Pharmaceutical Sciences, Cardiff University, Cardiff, UK

Rebecca Craig
Senior Lecturer (Education), School of Pharmacy, Queen's University Belfast, Belfast, UK

Stephen P. Denyer
Emeritus Professor of Pharmacy, Universities of Brighton and Sussex, Brighton, UK

Brendan F. Gilmore
Professor of Pharmaceutical Microbiology, School of Pharmacy, Queen's University Belfast, Belfast, UK

Sean P. Gorman
Emeritus Professor of Pharmaceutical Microbiology, Queen's University Belfast, Belfast, UK

Mark Gumbleton
Professor of Experimental Therapeutics, School of Pharmacy and Pharmaceutical Sciences, Cardiff University, Cardiff, UK

Stephan Heeb
Assistant Professor in Molecular Microbiology, School of Life Sciences, University of Nottingham, Nottingham, UK

Norman Hodges
Former Principal Lecturer, University of Brighton, Brighton, UK
Now Lewes, East Sussex, UK

Gavin J. Humphreys
Lecturer in Medical Microbiology, Division of Pharmacy and Optometry, School of Health Sciences, The University of Manchester, Manchester, UK

Conor Jamieson
Regional Antimicrobial Stewardship Lead (Midlands Region), NHS England, Birmingham, UK

Kevin Kavanagh
Professor of Microbiology, Department of Biology, Maynooth University, Maynooth, Co. Kildare, Ireland

Peter Lambert
Emeritus Professor of Microbial Chemistry, Aston University, Birmingham, UK

Jean-Yves Maillard
Professor of Pharmaceutical Microbiology, School of Pharmacy and Pharmaceutical Sciences, Cardiff University, Cardiff, UK

Andrew J. McBain
Professor of Microbiology, Division of Pharmacy and Optometry, School of Health Sciences, The University of Manchester, Manchester, UK

Tim Paget
Professor of Medical Microbiology, School of Medicine, University of Sunderland, UK

Tim Sandle
Head of Compliance and Quality Risk Management, Bio Products Laboratory, Elstree, UK

Timofey Skvortsov
Lecturer in Microbial Biotechnology and Bioinformatics, School of Pharmacy, Queen's University Belfast, Belfast, UK

Mathew W. Smith
Reader, School of Pharmacy and Pharmaceutical Sciences, Cardiff University, Cardiff, UK

Hayley Wickens
Consultant Pharmacist Genomic Medicine, NHS Central and South Genomic Medicine Service Alliance, Southampton, UK

Preface to the First Edition

When we were first approached by the publishers to write a textbook on pharmaceutical microbiology to appear in the spring of 1977, it was felt that such a task could not be accomplished satisfactorily in the time available.

However, by a process of combined editorship and by invitation to experts to contribute to the various chapters, this task has been accomplished thanks to the cooperation of our collaborators.

Pharmaceutical microbiology may be defined as that part of microbiology which has a special bearing on pharmacy in all its aspects. This will range from the manufacture and quality control of pharmaceutical products to an understanding of the mode of action of antibiotics. The full extent of microbiology on the pharmaceutical area may be judged from the chapter contents.

As this book is aimed at undergraduate pharmacy students (as well as microbiologists entering the pharmaceutical industry), we were under constraint to limit the length of the book to retain it in a defined price range. The result is to be found in the following pages. The editors must bear responsibility for any omissions, a point which has most concerned us. Length and depth of treatment were determined by the dictate of our publishers. It is hoped that the book will provide a concise reading for pharmacy students (who, at the moment, lack a textbook in this subject) and help to highlight those parts of a general microbiological training which impinge on the pharmaceutical industry.

In conclusion, the editors thank most sincerely the contributors to this book, both for complying with our strictures as to the length of their contribution and for providing their material on time, and our publishers for their friendly courtesy and efficiency during the production of this book. We also wish to thank Dr. H. J. Smith for his advice on various chemical aspects, Dr. M. I. Barnett for useful comments on reverse osmosis, and Mr. A. Keall who helped with the table on sterilisation methods.

W. B. Hugo
A. D. Russell

Preface to the Ninth Edition

When we first started planning for this edition in 2017, we could not have foreseen how many aspects of microbiology, particularly pharmaceutical microbiology, would come to prominence in the following pandemic years. Now, as we are slowly emerging from COVID-19, we have first-hand experience of the vital importance of antisepsis, infection prevention and control measures, epidemiology, immunology, vaccine development and an understanding of viral pathogenicity. The power of the pandemic to mobilise individual, national, international and commercial effort to combat infection and research new measures of treatment and immunisation has been inspiring. It is against this backdrop that many of our authors have been preparing their chapters, sometimes in the most demanding of circumstances; we thank them for their willing contribution and for their perseverance. Throughout this time, the understanding and patience of our publishers have been much appreciated.

While the structure of this edition draws much from the previous one, all chapters are revised, some with new authors, and they incorporate many significant developments in the discipline. These include: the gathering momentum of antibiotic resistance; the risk of microbicide cross-resistance; emerging pathogens; healthcare-associated infection; new vaccine technologies; advances in pharmaceutical production; and alternative strategies to antibiosis. Inevitably COVID-19 features, and while our understandings and conclusions may change with long-term analysis, our authors have attempted to draw as many reliable insights as possible while the pandemic progresses.

For this edition, we would like to acknowledge the contribution of past editors, Sean Gorman and Norman Hodges (who both remain as authors), and Barry Hugo and Denver Russell who were instrumental in recognising and building the discipline of pharmaceutical microbiology. They would not have been surprised at the contribution it now makes to safeguarding society.

S. P. Denyer
B. F. Gilmore

About the Companion Website

This book is accompanied by a companion website.

https://www.wiley.com/go/HugoandRussells9e

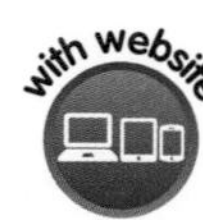

This website includes:

- Figures from the book available to download in PowerPoint.

Part 1

Introducing Pharmaceutical Microbiology

1

Introduction to Pharmaceutical Microbiology

Brendan F. Gilmore[1] and Stephen P. Denyer[2]

[1] Professor of Pharmaceutical Microbiology, School of Pharmacy, Queen's University Belfast, Belfast, UK
[2] Emeritus Professor of Pharmacy, Universities of Brighton and Sussex, Brighton, UK

CONTENTS

1.1 Pharmaceutical Microbiology: Microorganisms and Medicines

1.1.1 The Discipline of Pharmaceutical Microbiology

In its most literal sense, pharmaceutical microbiology is the study of microorganisms relevant to pharmacy and the pharmaceutical sciences. As a branch of the much wider discipline of applied microbiology, however, it is also concerned with understanding the fundamental importance of microorganisms in global health and disease. Pharmaceutical microbiology therefore includes an understanding of: the fundamentals of microbial physiology and pathogenicity, including host interactions; immunological products; the design, manufacture and appropriate use of antibiotics and other antimicrobial agents; strategies to prevent the emergence of resistance; practices in public health designed to control infectious disease; environmental design for the manufacture of medicinal products and medical devices; microbiological control in the preparation of pharmaceutical products and their preservation during use; the beneficial exploitation of microorganisms, including pharmaceutical biotechnology; and advances in molecular microbiology.

1.1.2 Microorganisms and Medicines

The observed steady improvement in global public health and the increasing trajectory of human life expectancy owes much to improved sanitation and healthcare, alongside better nutrition and a wider availability and access to effective medicines for the treatment and control of human and animal diseases. Indeed, the opening comments in previous editions of *Hugo & Russell's Pharmaceutical Microbiology* have reflected positively on global trends in controlling infectious disease, whilst recognising that still microbial infections and diarrhoeal diseases remain the leading causes of death in low- and low-middle-income countries (LMICs). Two infectious diseases, smallpox and rinderpest, the high-mortality cattle disease, have been declared eradicated by the World Health Organisation (WHO). At the time of writing, polio, once a global epidemic, remains endemic in only two countries, Afghanistan and Pakistan, with Africa having been declared free of wild-type polio in 2020. It is now expected that polio, and parasitic infection by the guinea worm *Dracunculus medinensis*, will be eradicated in the next few years. These and other significant advances in public health are major achievements, but a new threat has emerged, antibiotic

Hugo and Russell's Pharmaceutical Microbiology, Ninth Edition. Edited by Brendan F. Gilmore and Stephen P. Denyer.

Companion website: https://www.wiley.com/go/HugoandRussells9e

resistance, which has been referred to as the silent pandemic. Antibiotics have been estimated to extend human lifespan by 23 years on average, yet the emergence of antibiotic resistance to all current classes of antibiotics has been reported, and no major new class of antibiotic drug has been brought to the market in over 35 years. In 2019, the Institute and Faculty of Actuaries (UK) published their antibiotic resistance working party report on the impact of antimicrobial resistance (AMR) on mortality and morbidity, which predicted for the first time a reduction in UK life expectancy attributable to AMR. A recent analysis of the global burden of antimicrobial resistance estimated that in 2019, 1.27 million deaths were attributable to antibiotic-resistant bacteria, greater than from either human immunodeficiency virus/acquired immunodeficiency syndrome (HIV/AIDS) or malaria. Antibiotic resistance is a problem not of the future, but of the present.

The development of the many vaccines and medicines that have been crucial to the improvement in world health has been the result of the large investment in research and development made by the major international pharmaceutical companies and also by national governments investing in research infrastructure and training. As a result, the research, development and production of pharmaceuticals has become one of the most successful, profitable and important industries in many countries worldwide. The global pharmaceutical market has experienced unprecedented growth in the past two decades, from $390 billion in 2001 to $1.27 trillion by the end of 2020. In the UK, the pharmaceutical industry is a major contributor to the national economy, with 2 of the top 15 global pharmaceutical companies headquartered there, representing a 2.5% share of the global pharmaceutical sector. The UK industry generates a turnover of £36.7 billion, with an export market value of £23.4 billion and an import value of £21.4 billion. It employs more than 63,000 people, and whilst 41% of pharmaceutical products are exported, 30% are for the domestic UK market and the remainder are substances used in the manufacture of other pharmaceutical products. Overall, the UK pharmaceutical industry contributes £14 billion (gross value added, GVA) to the UK economy. During the coronavirus disease (COVID)-19 global pandemic, the UK pharmaceutical industry supported 68 commercial COVID-19 clinical trials in 2020 alone.

The growth in the pharmaceutical industry in recent decades has been paralleled by the development and implementation of increasingly rigorous and stringent standards and regulations for pharmaceutical product manufacture and quality. Manufacture or assembly of a pharmaceutical product must be conducted under license from the appropriate authority (e.g., the Medicines and Healthcare Products Regulatory Agency [MHRA] in the UK, or the Food and Drug Administration [FDA] in the USA), and manufacturers must demonstrate compliance with current good manufacturing practice (GMP) guidelines, the minimum standards that a medicines manufacturer must meet in their production process. The final product must meet all current standards for quality, safety and efficacy; many of these standards are harmonised across national bodies. Most medicines or pharmaceutical products are complex formulations containing the active ingredient formulated with inactive excipients which ensure the stability, safety and efficacy of the final product. Whilst the efficacy and safety of the active agent or drug fall within the domain of the pharmacologist and the toxicologist, respectively, ensuring the quality of the final pharmaceutical product requires a multidisciplinary approach. Analytical chemists and pharmacists/pharmaceutical scientists take lead responsibility for ensuring that the components of the final formulation are present in the correct physical form and concentration; however, quality is not established solely on the physicochemical properties of the product but also through stringent microbiological quality control to ensure formulation efficacy and safety.

Whilst not yet a feature of this book, the appearance of three-dimensional (3D) printed pharmaceuticals will be a matter for consideration in the future. This technology signals a potential shift from the traditional centralised mass production of medicines to the point-of-care manufacture of discrete batches of highly personalised dosage forms for particular patient and clinical circumstances. Thus, GMP approaches towards quality and safety that have been designed around conventional medicine manufacture will need to be adjusted to include real-time quality-assurance mechanisms, GMP-compliant 3D printer validation and new requirements to accommodate multiple manufacturing sites. The first 3D printed oral antiepileptic drug, levetiracetam, was approved for human use by the FDA in 2015.

It is obvious that medicines contaminated with potentially pathogenic microorganisms pose a significant risk of harm to the end-user, especially in vulnerable patients. Indeed, medicines to be administered to patients parenterally, that is, other than via the gastrointestinal tract, which include intravenous, intramuscular, subcutaneous and intraspinal injections, and ocular, otic and intranasal products, must be sterile and are marketed as sterile products. They must also be free from microbially derived toxins and pyrogens, including lipopolysaccharides, which can lead to anaphylactic reactions. Perhaps less predictable, although still self-evident, the presence of microorganisms in pharmaceutical products can cause physical and chemical spoilage, which may lead to changes in the formulation itself or to degradation or decomposition of the active drug and/or excipients. This can result in sub-therapeutic concentrations of the active drug in the contaminated formulation or impaired delivery characteristics, both leading to therapeutic failure, or the presence of toxic drug metabolites. Physical and chemical changes to the formulation may be obvious, such as changes to odour, flavour or elegance of the product, which would lead to lack of patient acceptance. Thus, it is clear that pharmaceutical microbiology must encompass the practices of sterilisation and preservation of often complex formulations capable of supporting the growth or survival of contaminating microorganisms. The pharmacist or pharmaceutical scientist with responsibility for the safe manufacture of medicines must appreciate the factors which predispose to product spoilage and how these might be managed by effective product design, and also the sources of potential contaminants and their control by good manufacturing practices. In these respects, the pharmaceutical microbiologist has much in common with microbiologists in the food and cosmetic industries, and many practices have been successfully shared.

The properties of antimicrobial chemicals used as disinfectants, preservatives and antiseptics (often termed microbicides) have direct relevance to the pharmacist and pharmaceutical scientist responsible for preserving formulated products and for managing microbiological risks in the manufacturing environment, and also because antiseptics and disinfectants are pharmaceutical products in their own right. However, they are not the only antimicrobial agents with which the pharmaceutical microbiologist must be familiar; antibiotic medicines are one of the most important and frequently prescribed pharmaceutical products, and are a major focus of several chapters of this book. The term antibiotic was originally used to refer to a naturally occurring substance, produced by one microorganism which inhibits the growth of, or kills, another microorganism. This strict definition of an antibiotic as a microbial metabolite did not, however, allow for the many generations of semi-synthetic compounds based on naturally occurring antibiotic templates and wholly synthetic agents (although significantly fewer in number) arising from high-throughput synthetic compound library screening efforts. The manufacture, quality control, formulation and, of particular relevance given the global crisis of antibiotic resistance, the appropriate use of antibiotics are important areas of knowledge which contribute significantly to the discipline of pharmaceutical microbiology.

The study of microorganisms continues to be important in both drug discovery and pharmaceutical manufacture. Screening of microorganisms for the production of bioactive agents has led not only to the discovery of almost all of the classes of antibiotics which are clinically used, but also to a number of important antifungal (such as nystatin, griseofulvin and amphotericin B), anti-cancer (including actinomycin, bleomycin, taxol and doxorubicin) and immunosuppressant (sirolimus and tacrolimus) agents in current clinical use. Following the discovery of penicillin in 1928, commercial antibiotic production began in the 1940s with the large-scale fermentation of *Penicillium chrysogenum* for production of benzylpenicillin (penicillin G). For many years, antibiotics were the only significant example of an active drug that was manufactured using microorganisms. However, exploitation of microorganisms for the manufacture and modification of steroids in the 1950s, and the development of recombinant DNA technologies in the last three decades of the twentieth century, has given significant momentum to the use of microorganisms in the production of pharmaceuticals and has supported a burgeoning biotechnology sector. The global market for recombinant DNA technology is forecast to reach $844.6 billion by 2025, with medical products dominating the market in terms of revenue generation. Biopharmaceuticals, or biological medical products (sometimes shortened to 'biologics' or 'biologicals'), broadly defined as pharmaceuticals inherently biological in nature and manufactured using biotechnology or bioprocesses (including fermentation and recombinant DNA technology/heterologous expression in *Escherichia coli*), represent a major proportion of all drugs under clinical development with an anticipation that biologics will account for 50% of drugs under development in the coming decade. Whilst a traditional focus for pharmaceutical interest in microorganisms has been their control, the more recent exploitation of microbial metabolism for the manufacture of drugs and the particular regulatory and quality control challenges of products arising through biotechnological and bioprocessing pipelines is now an area of knowledge which is of central importance to the discipline of pharmaceutical microbiology. This will be of increasing significance not only in the pharmacy and pharmaceutical sciences curricula, but also those of disciplines employed in the pharmaceutical industry. Table 1.1 summarises the benefits and uses of microorganisms in pharmaceutical manufacture, alongside more widely recognised hazards and problems they present.

Looking ahead, an understanding of microbial physiology and genetics will be increasingly important within the discipline of pharmaceutical microbiology, both in terms of the production of new therapeutic agents and in the understanding of infection microbiology, where host–pathogen interactions and the impact of the human microbiome on drug metabolism and its role in health and disease are becoming increasingly clear. The accessibility of pharmacists to the public often leads to them being called upon to explain the terminology and concepts of genetics and the biological sciences to patients. This has been evident during the global COVID-19 pandemic, which has been characterised by multiple genetic variants of the severe acute respiratory syndrome (SARS)-CoV-2 virus, rapid development of novel mRNA vaccine

Table 1.1 Microorganisms in pharmacy: benefits and problems.

Benefits or uses	Related study topics	Harmful effects	Related study topics
The manufacture of: Antibiotics Steroids Therapeutic enzymes Polysaccharides Products of recombinant DNA technology	Good manufacturing practice Industrial 'fermentation' technology Microbial genetics	May contaminate non-sterile and sterile medicines with a risk of infection	Non-sterile medicines: Enumeration of microorganisms in the manufacturing environment (environmental monitoring) and in raw materials and manufactured products Identification and detection of specific organisms
Use in the production of vaccines	Quality control of immunological products		Sterile medicines: Sterilisation methods Sterilisation monitoring and validation procedures Sterility testing Assessment and calculation of sterility assurance Aseptic manufacture
As assay organisms to determine antibiotic, vitamin and amino acid concentrations	Assay methods		
To detect mutagenic or carcinogenic activity	Ames mutagenicity test		
As adjuncts or alternatives to antibiotics	Bacteriophage, lysins and probiotic therapy		
		May contaminate non-sterile and sterile medicines with a risk of product deterioration	Enumeration, identification and detection as above, plus: Characteristics, selection and testing of antimicrobial preservatives
		Cause infectious and other diseases	Immunology and infectious diseases Microbial biofilms Microbiome Characteristics, selection and use of vaccines and antibiotics Infection and contamination control Control of antibiotic resistance Alternative strategies for antimicrobial chemotherapy
		Cause pyrogenic reactions (fever) when introduced into the body even in the absence of infection	Bacterial structure Pyrogen and endotoxin testing
		Provide a reservoir of antibiotic resistance genes	Microbial genetics

technologies and delivery of a vaccination programme in part through community pharmacies. Unfortunately, at the time of writing, the UK measles, mumps and rubella (MMR) vaccination rates are at their lowest in 10 years, which has been attributed to lack of parental knowledge of the significant risks associated with infections such as measles in children, and misinformation regarding potential adverse effects. The pharmacist's scientific training in pharmaceutical microbiology is critically important in advancing public health through patient understanding of the underpinning scientific concepts. The re-emergence of bacterial infections which were once associated with high mortality rates, such as tuberculosis and diphtheria, as antibiotic-resistant infections is posing an additional threat to public health, alongside threats from new pathogens; this latter has been illustrated in particular by SARS-CoV-2 and the global COVID-19 pandemic, estimated in October 2022 to have caused more than 634 million infections and over 6.62 million deaths globally.

The ability of microorganisms to adapt to new environments and exploit changes in modern clinical practices are also considerations within the discipline of pharmaceutical microbiology. The ability to conduct a wider range of routine and life-saving surgeries, and the demographic trend towards ageing populations, has led to an increased reliance on implantable medical devices, made from a variety of materials and used to support normal physiological functions. These include urinary catheters, ureteral stents, endotracheal tubes, central venous catheters, intraocular lenses, prosthetic joints and heart valves. Undoubtedly, such devices have saved countless lives and improved the quality of life for many millions of patients, but they come with the inherent risk of infectious complications. Many bacteria, including commensal bacteria, and fungi are capable of adhering to implantable medical device surfaces and, through production of extensive extracellular polymeric substances, can form biofilms which are often characterised by a uniquely high tolerance to antimicrobial challenge and resistance to clearance by the host's immune system. Biofilms are a source of chronic, recurrent infection which are typically only resolved on removal and replacement of the colonised device, which may lead to discomfort or extended morbidity for the patient, increased risk of mortality and increased attendant care costs to healthcare providers. The development of strategies for the accurate assessment of antimicrobial susceptibility in, and antimicrobial selection for, device-associated biofilm infections and strategies for the prevention and elimination of these infections is a challenge for pharmacy practitioners and other healthcare professionals.

The participation of microorganisms in human disease other than by clear-cut infection is becoming increasingly recognised. This is no more obvious than in the role of a healthy microbiome, where the dysbiosis caused by antibiotic therapy can have a dramatic effect on chronic diseases, with growing evidence that perturbations in the gut microbiome are not only associated with intestinal disorders (inflammatory bowel and coeliac disease) but also extra-intestinal disorders including cardiovascular disease, type-2 diabetes, allergy, asthma, obesity and central nervous system disorders (the impact of the so-called 'gut–brain axis'). Further examples include: the finding that *Helicobacter pylori* is implicated not only in peptic ulceration but also stomach cancers; the oncogenic nature of certain viruses (e.g., the association of human papilloma virus [HPV] and cervical cancer); and recent findings that suggest the Epstein–Barr virus may cause multiple sclerosis. Such discoveries offer the possibility that in situations where microbial infection has a clear link to the development of chronic disease, vaccination programmes could have a preventative role to play. This is best evidenced in the recent widespread school-based immunisation programme against HPV aimed at the prevention of cervical cancer, rather than the infection itself. Whilst not all chronic diseases will be found to have an association with infection, advances in genomic sequencing technologies now permit further examination of the interplay between infectious agents, microbiota, and chronic disease, and it is likely that more relationships will be discovered in the future.

Clearly, a knowledge of the mechanisms whereby microorganisms are able to resist antibiotics, colonise medical devices and cause or predispose humans to other disease states is essential in the development not only of new antibiotics, but of other medicines and healthcare practices, including protection of the host biome, which will minimise the risks of these adverse situations developing.

1.2 Scope and Content of the Book

In the manufacture of medicines, the criteria and standards for microbiological quality are governed primarily by the intended route of administration. The vast majority of medicines intended for oral administration or application to the skin are not required to be sterile. Non-sterile pharmaceuticals, such as creams, ointments, oral suspensions and so on, may contain some microorganisms, within strict acceptance criteria as to the number and type, whereas all parenteral formulations, for example, injections and ophthalmic preparations, must be sterile, that is, free from all living microorganisms. Products for administration at various other sites (nose, ear, vagina and bladder, for instance) are usually sterile formulations but not invariably so (Chapter 22). The microbiological quality of non-sterile pharmaceuticals is controlled by specifications (typically defined in the relevant pharmacopoeial standards) defining the number of organisms that may be present, and requiring the absence of specific, potentially pathogenic microorganisms (also called *objectionable* organisms). To fulfil these stringent requirements, the ability to isolate and identify the microorganisms present, to detect those that are prohibited from particular categories of pharmaceutical product and to enumerate microbial contaminants in the manufacturing environment, raw materials and the finished product are essential for the pharmaceutical microbiologist (Chapters 2–6). Knowledge of the characteristics of antimicrobial preservatives, included in formulations to restrain growth of microorganisms and prevent product spoilage during storage and use by the patient, and the means of assessment of preservative efficacy within complex formulations are also critical for demonstration that a product conforms to the relevant microbiological quality standards (Chapters 17–19).

For sterile products, quality criteria are simple: there should be no detectable microorganisms whatsoever. The product must be able to pass a sterility test, and a knowledge of the experimental design and procedures, and interpretation of results of these tests alongside understanding concepts of sterility assurance levels and process validation are important aspects of pharmaceutical microbiology (Chapter 21). In addition to stringent requirements for sterility, parenteral products for injection are also required to be free from pyrogens; these are substances which cause a rise in body temperature when administered to the patient. Strictly, any compound capable of causing fever following administration is classified as a pyrogen; however, with respect to pharmaceutical formulation, the vast majority of pyrogens are of bacterial origin, with thermally stable lipopolysaccharides from Gram-negative bacteria a particular issue (Chapter 3). Therefore, the detection, assay and removal of bacterial pyrogens (endotoxins) fall within the realm of pharmaceutical microbiology (Chapter 22).

There are two main strategies for the manufacture of sterile medicines. The first, and most straightforward, is to make the product, package it in its final market container and sterilise it by heat, radiation or other means. This approach, known as terminal sterilisation (Chapter 21), is the preferred option, as samples of the batch may be assessed for sterility to provide an assurance of sterility of the population of sterile items. The alternative is to formulate the product using sterile ingredients under conditions that do not permit entry of contaminating microorganisms (aseptic manufacture, Chapters 17 and 22). This strategy is usually adopted when the ingredients or physical form of the product render it unstable, or heat- or radiation-sensitive. It is a suitable approach for the manufacture of sterile products which have a short shelf- or half-life. Those responsible for the manufacture of sterile products must be familiar with both aseptic manufacturing techniques and sterilisation procedures for different product types, and assessment of the microbiological quality of those formulations. Those who have caused to open, use or dispense sterile products should be aware of the aseptic manipulation procedures to be adopted to minimise the risk of product contamination.

The microbial spoilage of medicines has as its main consequence financial loss rather than harm to patients, since microbial spoilage is often detected, through change of odour, appearance and so on, before the formulation is used. However, the other major problem associated with microbial contamination of medicines, that of patient harm through initiation of infection, although uncommon, is far more important in terms of risk of morbidity and mortality in the patient (Chapters 7 and 17).

The range of antimicrobial drugs to treat infections is large, despite being restricted to a relatively small number of mechanistic classes, thanks to the discovery of antibiotic scaffolds which are amenable to modification and optimisation using medicinal chemistry approaches. This has given rise to multiple generations of antibiotics from the same class, for example, penicillins and cephalosporins. Whilst approval of new antibiotics used to depend on the demonstration of superiority to currently available drugs, the crisis in the antibiotic discovery pipeline means that the need to find new antibiotics to treat infections that were once manageable with available agents has become critical. Therefore, there has been some focus not only on developing narrow-spectrum antibiotics for specific difficult-to-treat infections caused by antibiotic-resistant pathogens, including the ESKAPE pathogens (Chapter 13), but also away from finding superior drugs with the intention instead of identifying safe and effective antibiotics which are 'non-inferior' rather than 'superior' to treat those infections where therapeutic options are limited. As a result of this range and diversity of drugs, and the emergence of antibiotic resistance to current antibiotics, pharmacists are required to advise on the relative merits and appropriateness of certain antibiotics, and on the development of formularies and prescribing guidelines to ensure compliance with the principles of good antimicrobial stewardship (Chapters 11, 12, 14, and 15). In addition to knowledge of the drugs in question, this also requires an understanding of the factors which might influence the success of a given antibiotic therapy, including the likelihood of microbial growth as a biofilm, where antibiotic tolerance is significantly elevated (Chapters 7 and 8).

Whilst cardiovascular, pulmonary and malignant diseases are more frequent causes of death in the most developed high-income countries, infectious diseases still remain of paramount importance in countries of low to middle income, with lower respiratory infections and diarrhoeal diseases ranking above malaria, tuberculosis and HIV/AIDS. In 2019, over 12% of the 55.4 million deaths worldwide were caused by these five communicable diseases; the WHO estimates that overall 1 in 5 global deaths can be attributed to sepsis, the life-threatening reaction to infection caused by disease or injury. Infectious diseases, although showing significant reductions in mortality over the last 20 years, still rank amongst the top 10 leading causes of death globally, despite the significant advances in their treatment through the introduction of safe and effective antibiotics and vaccines. Worryingly too, the reservoir of antibiotic resistance is growing and the WHO estimates that 1.27 million people died worldwide in 2019 from antibiotic-resistant infections. Confidence that the antibiotic pipeline would continue to deliver antibiotics for the treatment of the vast majority of bacterial infectious diseases indefinitely has now been replaced by the realisation that the widespread emergence of resistance, and diminishing returns in antibiotic discovery programmes, has left the antibiotic pipeline critically depleted and unable to keep pace with antibiotic resistance (Chapter 13). Resistance to antibiotics has been reported for all major classes of antibiotics, and across virtually all pathogenic bacteria. As mentioned above, antibiotic-resistant infections have imposed a significant, and increasing, burden of mortality globally. It is clear that the number of infections, particularly healthcare-acquired infections, for which there is no effective antibiotic (and none in development), is on the rise. This worrying scenario leads to an increasing reliance on effective infection control measures designed to minimise the risk of transmission of infection from one patient to another within the healthcare setting (Chapter 16). The importance of such infection-control measures in reducing the transmission of SARS-CoV-2 during the global COVID-19 pandemic has brought this important aspect of global public health microbiology squarely into the public arena. As a key component of infection-control measures, the properties of microbicides (disinfectants and antiseptics), the assessment of their antimicrobial activity in real-world scenarios and the factors which influence their selection for use in infection-control strategies, or for contamination control in pharmaceutical manufacturing, are topics with which pharmacists, pharmaceutical scientists and industrial microbiologists should be familiar (Chapters 18–20). Furthermore, as antibiotic resistance threatens to curtail the 'antibiotic era', significant interest is now focused on potential alternatives, such as bacteriophage therapy, endolysins, novel vaccines and biological drugs, and antimicrobial peptides, bringing diversification to the available therapeutic options for treatment of infection (Chapter 26).

The beneficial biotechnological applications of microorganisms in the production of antibiotics, steroids and other medicines, including recombinant proteins from heterologous expression systems, have revolutionised the pharmaceutical world, giving rise to a burgeoning biopharmaceuticals and biological pharmaceuticals industry. The application of microorganisms and their enzymes (biocatalysts) has driven down the manufacturing cost of active pharmaceutical ingredients by improving yield, streamlining synthetic pathways by circumvention of multiple synthetic steps and by providing cheap and accessible starting materials for semi-synthetic compounds. Recombinant DNA technologies have supported the growth of a pharmaceutical sector worth hundreds of billions of pounds, and recombinant proteins (such as insulin and growth hormone), recombinant monoclonal antibodies and recombinant enzymes and vaccines are available for the treatment of a diverse range of diseases, including infections (Chapters 10, 23, and 24).

All of these developments, alongside miscellaneous applications in the detection of mutagenic and carcinogenic activity in drugs and chemicals, and in the assay of vitamins, amino acids and antibiotics (Chapter 25), have cemented the role of microorganisms in the production of human and animal medicines, and a basic knowledge of immunology (Chapter 9), gene cloning and expression and other biotechnological approaches (Chapter 24) form an integral part of pharmaceutical microbiology.

Part 2

Biology of Microorganisms

2

Fundamental Features of Microbiology

Norman Hodges[1] *and Stephen P. Denyer*[2]

[1] *Former Principal Lecturer, University of Brighton, Brighton, UK. Now Lewes, East Sussex, UK*
[2] *Emeritus Professor of Pharmacy, Universities of Brighton and Sussex, Brighton, UK*

CONTENTS

2.1 Introduction

Microorganisms differ enormously in terms of their shape, size and appearance and in their genetic and metabolic characteristics. All these properties are used in classifying microorganisms into the major groups with which many people are familiar, for example, bacteria, fungi, protozoa and viruses, and into the less well-known categories such as chlamydia, rickettsia and mycoplasmas. The major groups are the subject of individual chapters immediately following this, so the purpose here is not to describe any of them in great detail but to summarise their features so that the reader may better understand the distinctions between them. A further aim of this chapter is to avoid undue repetition of information in the early part of the book by considering such aspects of microbiology as cultivation, enumeration and genetics that are common to some, and sometimes all, of the various types of microorganism.

2.1.1 Viruses, Viroids and Prions

Viruses do not have a cellular structure. They are particles composed of nucleic acid surrounded by protein; some possess a lipid envelope and associated glycoproteins, but recognisable chromosomes, cytoplasm and cell membranes are invariably absent. Viruses are incapable of independent replication, as they do not contain the enzymes necessary to copy their own nucleic acids; as a consequence, all viruses are intracellular parasites and are

Hugo and Russell's Pharmaceutical Microbiology, Ninth Edition. Edited by Brendan F. Gilmore and Stephen P. Denyer.

Companion website: https://www.wiley.com/go/HugoandRussells9e

reproduced using the metabolic capabilities of the host cell. Viruses, and virus-like entities such as viroids, are sometimes known as mobile genetic elements; these are considered selfish genetic elements that move between hosts and/or change their integration in host genes. A great deal of variation is observed in the shape of viruses (helical, linear or spherical), size (20–1500 nm) and nucleic-acid composition (single- or double-stranded, linear or circular RNA or DNA), but almost all are smaller than bacteria and they cannot be seen with a normal light microscope; instead they may be viewed using an electron microscope which affords much greater magnification.

Viroids (virusoids) are even simpler than viruses, being infectious particles comprising single-stranded RNA without any associated protein. Those that have been described are plant pathogens, sometimes of considerable economic importance; so far, there are no known human pathogens in this category, although human hepatitis D virus shares some features in common with viroids, and may have originated from them.

Prions are unique as infectious agents in that they contain no nucleic acid. A prion is an atypical form of a mammalian protein that can interact with a normal protein molecule and cause it to undergo a conformational change so that it, in turn, becomes a prion and ceases its normal function. Prions are the agents responsible for transmissible spongiform encephalopathies, for example, Creutzfeldt–Jakob disease (CJD) and bovine spongiform encephalopathy (BSE). They are the simplest and most recently recognised agents of infectious disease, and are important in a pharmaceutical context owing to their extreme resistance to conventional sterilising agents such as steam, gamma radiation and disinfectants (see Chapter 21).

2.1.2 Prokaryotes and Eukaryotes

The most fundamental distinction between the various microorganisms having a cellular structure (i.e., all except those described in Section 2.1.1 above) is their classification into two groups – the prokaryotes and eukaryotes – based primarily on their structural characteristics and mode of reproduction. Expressed in the simplest possible terms, prokaryotes are the bacteria and archaea (see Section 2.1.2.1), and eukaryotes are all other cellular microorganisms, for example, fungi, protozoa and algae. The crucial difference between these two types of cell is the possession by the eukaryotes of a true cell nucleus in which the chromosomes are separated from the cytoplasm by a nuclear membrane. The prokaryotes have no true nucleus; they normally possess just a single chromosome that is not separated from the other cell contents by a membrane. Other major distinguishing features of the two groups are that prokaryotes are normally haploid (possess only one copy of the set of genes in the cell) and reproduce asexually; eukaryotes, by contrast, are usually diploid (possess two copies of their genes) and normally have the potential to reproduce sexually. The capacity for sexual reproduction confers the major advantage of creating new combinations of genes, which increases the scope for selection and evolutionary development. The restriction to an asexual mode of reproduction means that the organism in question is heavily reliant on mutation as a means of creating genetic variety and new strains with advantageous characteristics, although many bacteria are able to receive new genes from other strains or species (see Section 2.6.1 and Chapter 3). Table 2.1 lists some distinguishing features of the prokaryotes and eukaryotes.

2.1.2.1 Bacteria and Archaea

Bacteria are essentially unicellular, although some species arise as sheathed chains of cells. They possess the properties listed under prokaryotes in Table 2.1, but, like viruses and other categories of microorganisms, exhibit great diversity of form, habitat, metabolism, pathogenicity and other characteristics. The bacteria of interest in pharmacy and medicine belong to the group known as the eubacteria. The other subdivision of prokaryotes, the archaea, while formerly considered largely to comprise organisms capable of living in extreme environments (e.g., high temperatures, extreme salinity or pH) or organisms exhibiting specialised modes of metabolism (e.g., by deriving energy from sulphur or iron oxidation or the production of methane), are now known to occur in a wide variety of habitats. This recognised tolerance to extremes has led to consideration of the archaea as biocatalysts for industrial processes; as a source of extremely stable enzymes, they are well suited to biotechnological applications, some of which are of potential pharmaceutical importance.

The eubacteria are typically rod-shaped (bacillus, see Figure 2.1a), spherical (cocci), curved or spiral cells of approximately 0.5–5.0 μm (longest dimension) and are divided into two groups designated Gram-positive and Gram-negative according to their reaction to a staining procedure developed in 1884 by Christian Gram (see Chapter 3). Although all the pathogenic species are included within this category, there are very many other eubacteria that are harmless or positively beneficial. Some of the bacteria that contaminate or cause spoilage of pharmaceutical materials are saprophytes, that is, they obtain their energy by decomposition of animal and vegetable material, while many could also be described as parasites (benefiting from growth on or in other living organisms without causing detrimental effects) or pathogens (parasites damaging the host). Rickettsia and chlamydia are

Table 2.1 Distinguishing features of prokaryotes and eukaryotes.

Characteristic	Eukaryotes	Prokaryotes
Size	Normally >10 μm	Typically, 1–5 μm
Location of chromosomes	Within a true nucleus separated from the cytoplasm by a nuclear membrane	In the cytoplasm, usually attached to the cell membrane
Nuclear division	Exhibit mitosis and meiosis	Mitosis and meiosis are absent
Nucleolus	Present	Absent
Reproduction	Asexual or sexual reproduction	Normally asexual reproduction
Chromosome number	>1	1
Mitochondria and chloroplasts	May be present	Absent
Cell membrane composition	Sterols present	Sterols absent
Cell wall composition	Cell walls (when present) usually contain cellulose or chitin but not peptidoglycan	Walls usually contain peptidoglycan
Ribosomes	Cytoplasmic ribosomes are 80S	Ribosomes are smaller, usually 70S
Endoplasmic reticulum	Present	Absent
Extracellular capsule/slime	Absent	Often present
Flagella	Structurally complex	Structurally simple
Pili	Absent	Present
Fimbriae	Cilia	Present
Storage compounds	Poly-β-hydroxybutyrate absent	Poly-β-hydroxybutyrate often present

types of bacteria that are obligate intracellular parasites, that is, they are incapable of growing outside a host cell and so cannot easily be cultivated in the laboratory. Most bacteria of pharmaceutical and medical importance possess rigid cell walls (and are therefore relatively resistant to osmotic stress), grow well at temperatures between ambient and human body temperature and exhibit wide variations in their requirement for, or tolerance of, oxygen. Strict aerobes require atmospheric oxygen, but for strict anaerobes oxygen is toxic. Many other bacteria would be described as facultative anaerobes (normally growing best in air but can grow without it) or microaerophiles (preferring oxygen concentrations lower than those in normal air).

2.1.2.2 Fungi

Fungi are structurally more complex and varied in appearance than bacteria, and, being eukaryotes, differ from them in the ways described in Table 2.1. Fungi are considered to be non-photosynthesising plants, and the term *fungus* covers both yeasts and moulds, although the distinction between these two groups is not always clear. Yeasts are normally unicellular organisms that are larger than bacteria (typically 5–10 μm) and divide either by a process of binary fission (see Section 2.4.2) or budding (whereby a daughter cell arises as a swelling or protrusion from the parent that eventually separates to lead an independent existence, Figure 2.1b). *Mould* is an imprecise term used to describe fungi that do not form fruiting bodies visible to the naked eye, thus excluding toadstools and mushrooms. Most moulds consist of a tangled mass (mycelium) of filaments or threads (hyphae) which vary between 1 and over 50 μm wide (Figure 2.1c); they may be differentiated for specialised functions, for example, absorption of nutrients or reproduction. Some fungi may exhibit a unicellular (yeast-like) or mycelial (mould-like) appearance depending upon cultivation conditions. Although fungi are eukaryotes that should, in theory, be capable of sexual reproduction, there are some species in which this has never been observed. Most fungi are saprophytes with relatively few having pathogenic potential, although this view is changing in the case of immunocompromised patients. The ability of fungi to form spores that are resistant to drying makes them important as contaminants of pharmaceutical raw materials, particularly materials of vegetable origin.

2.1.2.3 Protozoa

Protozoa are eukaryotic, predominantly unicellular microorganisms that have been regarded in the past as animals rather than plants ('protozoa' means 'first animals'), although the distinction between protozoa and fungi is not always clear. Many protozoa are free-living motile organisms that occur in water and soil, although some are

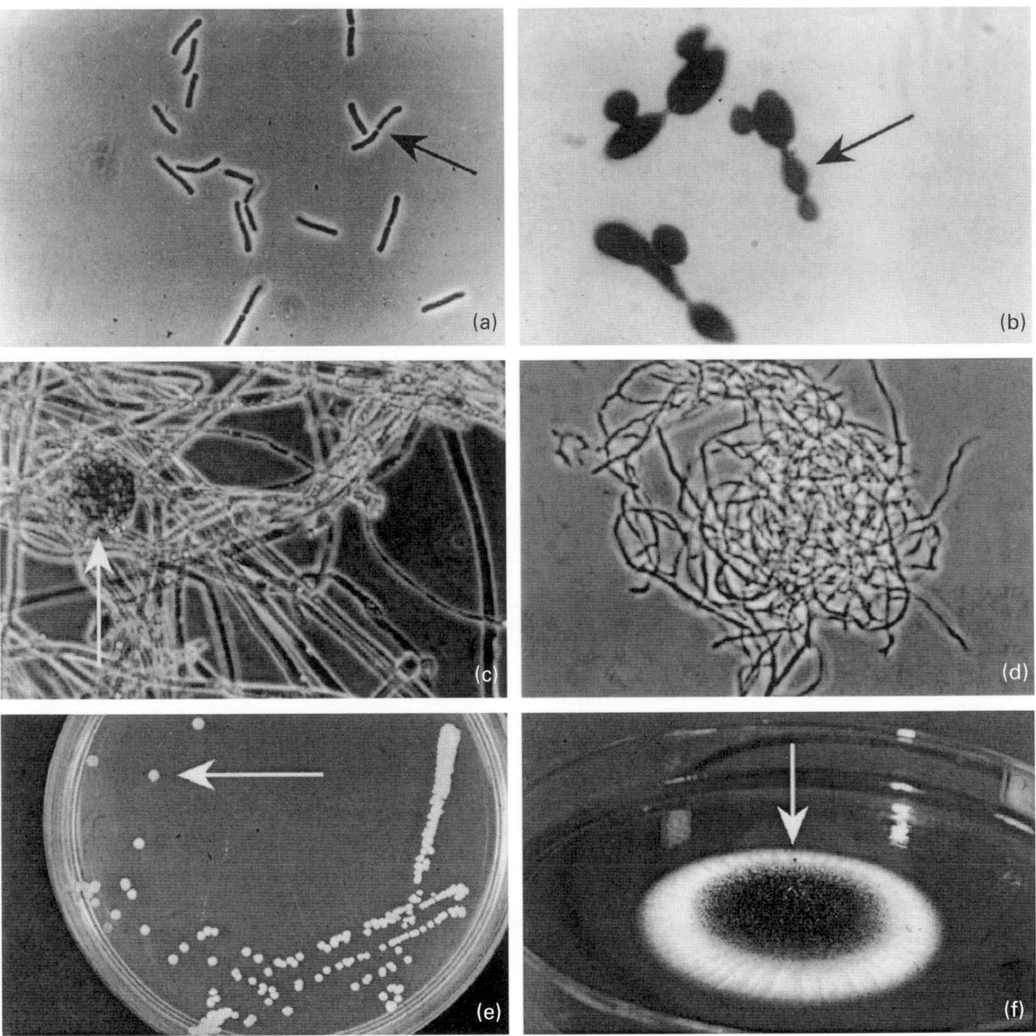

Figure 2.1 (a) A growing culture of *Bacillus megaterium* in which cells about to divide by binary fission display constrictions (arrowed) prior to separation. (b) A growing culture of the yeast *Saccharomyces cerevisiae* displaying budding (arrowed). (c) The mould *Mucor plumbeus* exhibiting the typical appearance of a mycelium in which masses of asexual zygospores (arrowed) are formed on specialised hyphae. (d) The bacterium *Streptomyces rimosus* displaying the branched network of filaments that superficially resembles a mould mycelium. (e) The typical appearance of an overnight agar culture of *Micrococcus luteus* inoculated to produce isolated colonies (arrowed). (f) A single colony of the mould *Aspergillus niger* in which the actively growing periphery of the colony (arrowed) contrasts with the mature central region where pigmented asexual spores have developed.

parasites of plants and animals, including humans, for example, the organisms responsible for malaria and amoebic dysentery. Protozoa are not normally found as contaminants of raw materials or manufactured medicines and the relatively few that are of pharmaceutical interest owe that status primarily to their potential to cause disease.

2.2 Naming of Microorganisms

Microorganisms, just like other organisms, are normally known by two names: that of the genus (plural = genera) and that of the species. The former is normally written with an uppercase initial letter and the latter with a lowercase initial letter, for example, *Staphylococcus aureus* or *Escherichia coli*. These may be abbreviated by shortening the name of the genus provided that the shortened form is unambiguous, for example, *S. aureus* or *E. coli*. Both the full and the shortened names are printed in *italics* to designate their status as proper names (in old books, theses or manuscripts, they might be in roman type but underlined). The species within a genus are sometimes referred to by a collective name, for example, staphylococci or pseudomonads, and neither these names nor names describing groups of organisms from different genera, for example, coliforms, are italicised or spelt with an uppercase initial letter.

Viruses are generally classified by phenotypic characteristics (see Chapter 5) such as morphology, nucleic-acid composition and the nature of the disease they cause. By convention, the name of the family to which the virus belongs ends with the suffix *viridae*, for example, *Adenoviridae*, and the genus ends with *virus*, for example, *Adenovirus*; these are italicised. Species names often take the form [*disease*] *virus*, for example, *influenza virus*. Viral nomenclature has yet to find a standardised form under the authority of the International Committee on Taxonomy of Viruses.

2.3 Microbial Metabolism

As in most other aspects of their physiology, microorganisms exhibit marked differences in their metabolism. While some species can obtain carbon from carbon dioxide and energy from sunlight or the oxidation of inorganic materials such as sulphides, the vast majority of organisms of interest in pharmacy and medicine are described as chemoheterotrophs – they obtain carbon, nitrogen and energy by breaking down organic compounds. The chemical reactions by which energy is liberated by digestion of food materials are termed catabolic reactions, while those that use the liberated energy to make complex cellular polymers, proteins, carbohydrates and nucleic acids are called anabolic reactions.

Food materials are oxidised in order to break them down and release energy from them. The term oxidation is defined as the removal or loss of electrons, but oxidation does not invariably involve oxygen, as a wide variety of other molecules can accept electrons and thus act as oxidising agents. As the oxidising molecule accepts the electrons, the other molecule in the reaction that provides them is simultaneously reduced. Consequently, oxidation and reduction are invariably linked and such reactions are often termed redox reactions. The term redox potential is also used, and this indicates whether oxidising or reducing conditions prevail in a particular situation, for example, in a body fluid or a culture medium. Anaerobic organisms prefer low redox potentials (typically 0 to −200 mV or less), while aerobes thrive in high redox potential environments (e.g., 0 to +200 mV or more).

There are marked similarities in the metabolic pathways used by pathogenic bacteria and by mammals. Many bacteria use the same process of glycolysis that is used by humans to begin the breakdown of glucose and the release of energy from it. Glycolysis describes the conversion of glucose, through a series of reactions, to pyruvic acid, and it is a process for which oxygen is not required, although glycolysis is undertaken by both aerobic and anaerobic organisms. The process releases only a relatively small amount of the energy stored in a sugar molecule, and aerobic microorganisms, in common with mammals, release much more of the energy by aerobic respiration. Oxygen is the molecule at the end of the sequence of respiratory reactions that finally accepts the electrons and allows the whole process to proceed, but it is worth noting that many organisms can also undertake *anaerobic* respiration, which uses other final electron acceptors, for example, nitrate or fumarate.

As an alternative to respiration, many microorganisms use fermentation as a means of releasing more energy from sugar; fermentation is, by definition, a process in which the final electron acceptor is an organic molecule. The term is widely understood to mean the production by yeast of ethanol and carbon dioxide from sugar, but in fact many organisms apart from yeasts can undertake fermentation and the process is not restricted to common sugar (sucrose) as a starting material or to ethanol and carbon dioxide as metabolic products. Many pathogenic bacteria are capable of fermenting several different sugars and other organic materials to give a range of metabolic products that includes acids (e.g., lactic, acetic and propionic), alcohols (e.g., ethanol, propanol and butanediol) and other commercially important materials such as the solvents, acetone and butanol. Fermentation is, like glycolysis, an anaerobic process, although the term is commonly used in the pharmaceutical and biotechnology industries to describe the manufacture of a wide range of substances by microorganisms where the biochemical process is neither fermentative nor even anaerobic, for example, many textbooks refer to antibiotic fermentation, but the production vessels are usually vigorously aerated.

Microorganisms are far more versatile than mammals with respect to the materials that they can use as foods and the means by which those foods are broken down. Some pathogenic organisms can grow on dilute solutions of mineral salts and sugar (or other simple molecules such as glycerol, lactic acid or pyruvic acid), while others can obtain energy from rarely encountered carbohydrates or by the digestion of proteins or other non-carbohydrate foods. In addition to accepting a wide variety of food materials, many microorganisms can use alternative metabolic pathways to break the food down depending on the environmental conditions, for example, facultative anaerobes can switch from respiration to fermentation if oxygen supplies are depleted. It is partly this ability to switch to different metabolic pathways that explains why none of the major antibiotics work by interfering with the chemical processes microorganisms use to metabolise their food. It is a fundamental principle of antibiotic action that the drug must exploit a difference in metabolism between the organism to be killed and the human host; without such a difference, the antibiotic would be very toxic to the patient too. However, not only do bacteria use metabolic pathways for food digestion that are similar to our own, many of them would have the ability to switch to an alternative energy-producing pathway if an antibiotic were developed that interfered with a reaction that is unique to bacteria.

The metabolic products that arise during the period when a microbial culture is actually growing are termed primary metabolites, while those that are produced after cell multiplication has slowed or stopped, that is, in the 'stationary phase' (see Chapter 3), are termed secondary metabolites. Ethanol is a primary metabolite of major commercial importance, although it is produced in large quantities only by some species of yeast. More common than ethanol as primary metabolites are organic acids, so it is a common observation that the pH of a culture progressively falls during growth, and many organisms further metabolise the acids so the pH often rises after cell growth has ceased. The metabolites that are found during secondary metabolism are diverse, and many of them have commercial or therapeutic importance (see Chapter 25). They include antibiotics, enzymes (e.g., amylases that digest starch and proteolytic enzymes used in biological washing powders), toxins (responsible for many of the symptoms of infection but some also of therapeutic value, for example, botox, the toxin of *Clostridium botulinum*) and carbohydrates (e.g., dextran, used as a plasma expander and for molecular separations by gel filtration).

2.4 Microbial Cultivation

The vast majority of microorganisms of interest in pharmacy and medicine can be cultivated in the laboratory and most of them require relatively simple techniques and facilities. Some organisms are parasites and so can only be grown inside the cells of a host species – which often necessitates mammalian cell culture facilities – and there are a few (e.g., the organism responsible for leprosy) that are not cultivated outside the living animal. Viral culture is covered in Chapter 5.

2.4.1 Culture Media

A significant number of common microorganisms are capable of synthesising all the materials they need for growth (e.g., amino acids, nucleotides and vitamins) from simple carbon and nitrogen sources and mineral salts. Such organisms can grow on truly synthetic (chemically defined) media, but many organisms do not have this capability and need a medium that already contains these biochemicals. Such media are far more commonly used than synthetic ones, and several terms have been used to describe them, for example, routine laboratory media, general purpose media and complex media. They are complex in the sense that their precise chemical composition is unknown and likely to vary slightly from batch to batch. In general, they are aqueous solutions of animal or plant extracts that contain hydrolysed proteins, B-group vitamins and carbohydrates.

Readily available and relatively inexpensive sources of protein include meat extracts (from those parts of animal carcasses that are not used for human or domestic animal consumption), milk and soya. The protein is hydrolysed to varying degrees to give peptones (by definition not coagulable by heat or ammonium sulphate) or amino acids. Trypsin or other proteolytic enzymes are preferred to acids as a means of hydrolysis because acids cause more amino acid destruction; the term 'tryptic' denotes the use of the enzyme. Many microorganisms require B-group vitamins (but not the other water- or fat-soluble vitamins required by mammals) and this requirement is satisfied by yeast extract. Carbohydrates are used in the form of starch or sugars, but glucose (dextrose) is the only sugar regularly employed as a nutrient. Microorganisms differ in terms of their ability to ferment various sugars, and their fermentation patterns may be used as an aid in identification. Thus, other sugars included in culture media are normally present for these diagnostic purposes rather than as carbon and energy sources. Sophisticated biochemical profiling using different carbohydrate sources and indicator dyes can establish metabolic patterns applicable to genus and species level; these phenotypic methods are often miniaturised and automated in commercial kits. Sodium chloride may be incorporated in culture media to adjust osmotic pressure, and occasionally buffers are added to neutralise acids that result from sugar metabolism. Routine culture media may be enriched by the addition of materials such as milk, blood or serum, and organisms that need such supplements in order to grow are described as 'exacting' in their nutritional requirements.

Culture media may be either liquid or solid; the latter term describes liquid media that have been gelled by the addition of agar, which is a carbohydrate extracted from certain seaweeds. Agar at a concentration of about 1–1.5% w/v will provide a firm gel that cannot be liquefied by the enzymes normally produced during bacterial growth (which is one reason it is used in preference to gelatin). Agar is unusual in that the melting and setting temperatures for its gels are quite dissimilar. Fluid agar solutions set at approximately 40 °C, but do not re-liquefy on heating until the temperature is in excess of 90 °C. Thus, agar forms a firm gel at 37 °C which is the normal incubation temperature for many pathogenic organisms (whereas gelatin does not) and when used as a liquid at 45 °C is at a sufficiently low temperature to avoid killing microorganisms – this property is important in pour plate counting methods (see Section 2.5).

In contrast to medium ingredients designed to support microbial growth, there are many materials commonly added to selective or diagnostic media whose function is to restrict the growth of certain types of microorganism while permitting or enhancing the growth of others. Examples include antibacterial antibiotics added to fungal media to suppress bacterial contaminants, and bile to suppress organisms from anatomical sites other than the gastrointestinal tract. Many such additives are used in media for organism identification purposes, and these are considered further in subsequent chapters. The term enrichment sometimes causes confusion in this context. It is occasionally used in the sense of making a medium nutritionally richer to achieve more rapid or profuse growth. Alternatively, and more commonly, an enrichment medium is one designed to permit a particular type of organism to grow while restricting others, so the one that grows increases in relative numbers and is 'enriched' in a mixed culture.

Solid media designed for the growth of anaerobic organisms usually contain non-toxic reducing agents, for example, sodium thioglycolate or sulphur-containing amino acids; these compounds create redox potentials of −200 mV or less and so diminish or eliminate the inhibitory effects of oxygen or oxidising molecules on anaerobic growth. The inclusion of such compounds is less important in liquid media where a sufficiently low redox potential may be achieved simply by boiling; this expels dissolved oxygen, which in unstirred liquids only slowly resaturates the upper few millimetres of liquid. Redox indicators such as methylene blue or resazurin may be incorporated in anaerobic media to confirm that a sufficiently low redox potential has been achieved.

Media for yeasts and moulds often have a lower pH (5.5–6.0) than bacterial culture media (7.0–7.4). Lactic acid may be used to impart a low pH because it is not, itself, inhibitory to fungi at the concentrations used. Some fungal media that are intended for use with specimens that may also contain bacteria may be supplemented with antibacterial antibiotics, for example, chloramphenicol or tetracyclines.

2.4.2 Cultivation Methods

Most bacteria and some yeasts divide by a process of binary fission whereby the cell enlarges or elongates, then forms a cross-wall (septum) that separates the cell into two more or less equal compartments each containing a copy of the genetic material. Septum formation is often followed by constriction such that the connection between the two cell compartments is progressively reduced (see Figure 2.1a) until finally it is broken and the daughter cells separate. In bacteria, this pattern of division may take place every 25–30 minutes under optimal conditions of laboratory cultivation, although growth at infection sites in the body is normally much slower owing to the effects of the immune system and scarcity of essential nutrients, particularly iron. Growth continues until one or more nutrients is exhausted, or toxic metabolites (often organic acids) accumulate and inhibit enzyme systems. Starting from a single cell, many bacteria can achieve concentrations of the order of 10^9 cells ml^{-1} or more following overnight incubation in common liquid media. At concentrations below about 10^7 cells ml^{-1}, culture media are clear, but the liquid becomes progressively more cloudy (turbid) as the concentration increases above this value; turbidity is, therefore, an indirect means of monitoring culture growth. Some bacteria produce chains of cells, and some produce elongated cells (filaments) that may exhibit branching to create a tangled mass resembling a mould mycelium (Figure 2.1d). Many yeasts divide by budding (see Section 2.1.2.3 and Figure 2.1b), but they, too, would normally grow in liquid media to produce a turbid culture. Moulds, however, grow by extension and branching of hyphae to produce a mycelium (Figure 2.1c) or, in agitated liquid cultures, pellet growth may arise.

When growing on solid media in Petri dishes (often referred to as 'plates'), individual bacterial cells can give rise to colonies following overnight incubation under optimal conditions. A colony is simply a collection of cells arising by multiplication of a single original cell or a small cluster of them (called a colony-forming unit or CFU). The term 'colony' does not, strictly speaking, imply any particular number of cells, but it is usually taken to mean a number sufficiently large to be visible by eye. Thus, macroscopic bacterial colonies usually comprise hundreds of thousands, millions or tens of millions of cells in an area on a Petri dish that is typically 1–10 mm in diameter (Figure 2.1e). Colony size is limited by nutrient availability and/or waste product accumulation in just the same way as cell concentration is in liquid media. Colonies vary between bacterial species, and their shapes, sizes, opacities, surface markings and pigmentation may all be characteristic of the species in question, so these properties may be an aid in identification procedures (see Chapter 3).

Anaerobic organisms may be grown on Petri dishes provided that they are incubated in an anaerobic jar. Such jars are usually made of rigid plastic with airtight lids, and Petri dishes are placed in them together with a low-temperature catalyst. The catalyst, consisting of palladium-coated pellets or wire, causes the oxygen inside the jar to be combined with hydrogen that is generated by the addition of water to sodium borohydride; this is usually contained in a foil sachet that is also placed in the jar; alternatively, oxygen may be removed by combination with ascorbic acid. After its removal, an anaerobic atmosphere is achieved and this is monitored by an oxidation– reduction (redox) indicator; resazurin is frequently used as a solution soaking a fabric strip.

Yeast colonies often look similar to those of bacteria, although they may be larger and more frequently coloured. The appearance of moulds growing on solid microbiological media is similar to their appearance when growing on common foods. The mould colony consists of a mycelium that may be loosely or densely entangled depending on the species, often with the central area (the oldest, most mature region of the colony) showing pigmentation associated with spore production (Figure 2.1f). The periphery of the colony is that part which is actively growing and it is usually non-pigmented.

2.4.3 Planktonic and Sessile (Biofilm) Growth

Bacteria growing in liquid culture in the laboratory usually exist as individual cells or small aggregates of cells suspended in the culture medium; the term planktonic is used to describe such freely suspended cells. In recent years, however, it has become recognised that planktonic growth is not thc normal situation for bacteria growing in their natural habitats. In fact, bacteria in their natural state far more commonly grow attached to a surface which, for many species, may be solid, for example, soil particles, stone, metal or glass, or for pathogens, an epithelial surface in the body, for example, lung or intestinal mucosa. Bacteria attached to a substrate in this way are described as sessile, and are said to exhibit the biofilm or microcolony mode of growth.

Planktonic cells are routinely used for almost all the testing procedures that have been designed to assess the activity of antimicrobial chemicals and processes, but the recognition that planktonic growth is not the natural state for many organisms prompted investigations of the relative susceptibilities of planktonic- and biofilm-grown cells to antibiotics, disinfectants and decontamination or sterilisation procedures. In many cases, it has been found that planktonic and sessile bacteria exhibit markedly different susceptibilities to these lethal agents, and this has prompted a reappraisal of the appropriateness of some of the procedures used (see Chapters 8, 13, and 19).

2.5 Enumeration of Microorganisms

In a pharmaceutical context, there are several situations where it is necessary to measure the number of microbial cells in a culture, sample or specimen:

- when measuring the levels of microbial contamination in a raw material or manufactured medicine;
- when evaluating the effects of an antimicrobial chemical or decontamination process;
- when using microorganisms in the manufacture of therapeutic agents;
- when assessing the nutrient capability of a growth medium.

In some cases, it is necessary to know the total number of microbial cells present, that is, both living and dead: for example, in vaccine manufacture, dead and living cells may both produce an immune response, and in pyrogen testing, both dead and living cells induce fever when injected into the body. However, in many cases, it is the number or concentration of *living* cells that is required. The terminology in microbial counting sometimes causes confusion. A *total count* is a counting procedure enumerating both living and dead cells, whereas a *viable count*, which is far more common, records the living cells alone. However, the term *total viable count* (TVC) is used in most pharmacopoeias and by many regulatory agencies to mean a viable count that records all the different species or types of microorganism that might be present in a sample (e.g., bacteria plus fungi).

Table 2.2 lists some of the more common counting methods available. The first three traditional methods of viable counting all operate on the basis that a living cell (or a CFU) will give rise to a visible colony when introduced into or onto the surface of a suitable medium and incubated. Thus, the procedure for pour plating (Figure 2.2a) usually involves the addition of a small volume (typically 1.0 ml) of sample (or a suitable dilution thereof) into molten agar at 45 °C which is then poured into empty sterile Petri dishes. After incubation, the resultant colonies are counted and the total is multiplied by the dilution factor (if any) to give the concentration in the original sample. In a surface spread plate technique (Figure 2.2b), the sample (usually 0.1–0.25 ml) is spread over the surface of agar which has previously been dried to permit absorption of the added liquid. The Miles–Misra (surface drop) method (Figure 2.2c)

Table 2.2 Examples of traditional and rapid methods for enumerating cells.

Traditional methods		Rapid methods
Viable counts	**Total counts**	**Indirect viable counts**
1 Pour plate (counting colonies *in* agar)	**1** Direct microscopic counting (using Helber or haemocytometer counting chambers)	**1** Epifluorescence (uses dyes that give characteristic fluorescence only in living cells) often coupled to image analysis
2 Surface spread or surface drop (Miles–Misra) methods (counting colonies *on* agar surface)	**2** Turbidity methods (measure turbidity [opacity] in suspensions or cultures)	**2** ATP methods (measure ATP production in living cells using bioluminescence)
3 Membrane filter methods (colonies growing on membranes *on* agar surface)	**3** Dry weight determinations	**3** Impedance (measures changes in resistance, capacitance or impedance in growing cultures)
4 MPN[a] (counts based on the proportion of liquid cultures growing after receiving low inocula)	**4** Nitrogen, protein or nucleic-acid determinations	**4** Detection of respiring cells either by following changes in gas pressure or by colourimetric dye reduction

[a] MPN = most probable number.

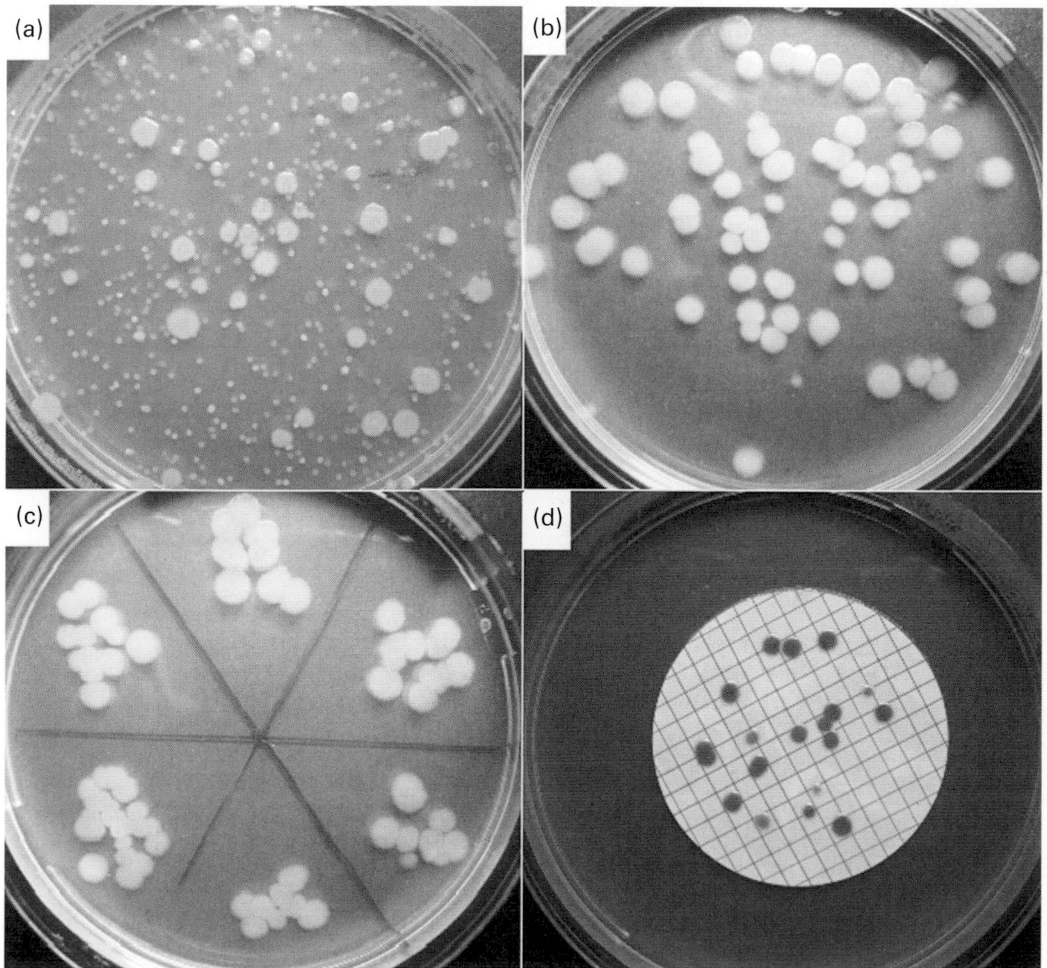

Figure 2.2 Viable counts of bacteria: (a) Pour plate method using *Bacillus subtilis*; the colonies on the surface of the agar are growing larger than those within the agar due to greater oxygen availability. (b) Surface spread and (c) surface drop (Miles–Misra) methods using *B. subtilis*. (d) Membrane filtration method showing *Serratia marcescens* colonies growing on a 47-mm diameter membrane.

is similar in principle, but several individual drops of culture are allowed to spread over discrete areas of about 1 cm diameter on the agar surface. These procedures are suitable for samples that are expected to contain concentrations exceeding approximately 100 CFU ml^{-1} so that the number of colonies arising on the plate is sufficiently large to be statistically reliable. If there are no clear indications of the order of magnitude of the concentration in the sample, it is necessary to plate out the sample at each of two, three or more (decimal, i.e., tenfold) dilutions so as to obtain Petri dishes with conveniently countable numbers of colonies (usually taken to be 30–300 colonies).

If 30 colonies are accepted as the lowest reliable number to count and a pour plate method uses a 1.0 ml sample, it follows that the procedures described above are unsuitable for any sample that is expected to contain <30 CFU ml^{-1}, for example, water samples where the count may be 1 CFU ml^{-1} or less. Here, membrane filter methods are used (Figure 2.2d) in which a large, known volume of sample is passed through the membrane which is placed, without inversion, on the agar surface. Nutrients then diffuse up through the membrane and allow the retained cells to grow into colonies on it just as they would on the agar itself. Some of the relative merits of these colony-counting procedures are described in Table 2.3.

Most probable number (MPN) counts may be used when the anticipated count is relatively low, that is, from <1 up to 100 microorganisms ml^{-1}. The procedure involves inoculating multiple tubes of culture medium (usually three or five) with three different volumes of sample, for example, three tubes each inoculated with 0.1 ml, three with 0.01 ml and three with 0.001 ml. If the concentration in the sample is in the range indicated above, there should be a proportion of the tubes receiving inocula in which no microorganisms are present; these will remain sterile after incubation, while others that received inocula actually containing one or more CFU show signs of growth. The proportions of positive tubes are recorded for each sample volume and the results are compared with standard tables showing the MPN of organisms per millilitre (or per 100 ml) of original sample. The procedure is more commonly used in the water, food and dairy industries than in the pharmaceutical industry; nevertheless, it is a valid technique described in pharmacopoeias and appropriate for pharmaceutical materials, particularly water. The poor accuracy and precision associated with MPN counts usually means that the method is one of last resort – to be considered only when other counting methods are inappropriate.

Turbidity measurements are the most common means of estimating the total numbers of bacteria present in a sample. Measuring the turbidity using a spectrophotometer or colourimeter and reading the concentration from a calibration plot are the simple means of standardising cell suspensions for use as inocula in antibiotic assays or other tests of antimicrobial chemicals. Fungi cannot readily be handled in this way because the suspension may not be uniform or may sediment in a spectrophotometer cuvette. Consequently, dry weight determinations on dried centrifuged pellets or evaporated distilled water suspensions from known volumes of culture are an alternative means of estimating fungal biomass. Direct microscopic counting may be an appropriate method for bacteria, yeasts and fungal spores but not for moulds, and indirect measures of biomass such as assays of insoluble nitrogen, protein or nucleic acids are possible for all cell types, but rarely used outside the research laboratory.

Table 2.3 Relative merits of the common viable counting procedures.

Counting method	Advantages	Disadvantages
Pour plate	Requires no pre-drying of the agar surface	Very small colonies of strict aerobes at the base of the agar may be missed
	Will detect lower concentrations than surface spread/surface drop methods	Colonies of different species within the agar appear similar – so it is difficult to detect contaminants
Surface spread and surface drop methods	Surface spread often gives larger colonies than pour plates – thus they are easier to count	Agar surface requires pre-drying to absorb sample
	Easier to identify contaminants by appearance of the colonies	Possibility of confluent growth, particularly with moulds, masking individual colonies
Membrane filtration	If necessary, will detect lower concentrations than other methods	Viscous samples will not go through the membrane and particulate samples may block the membrane thereby restricting filtration capacity
	Antimicrobial chemicals in the sample can be physically removed from the cells	

The traditional methods of viable counting all suffer from the same limitations:

- relatively labour-intensive;
- not easy to automate;
- slow, because they require an incubation period for colonies to develop or liquid cultures to become turbid;
- and, may require relatively large volumes of culture media, many Petri dishes and a lot of incubator space.

For these reasons, much interest and investigative effort have been invested over recent years in the use of so-called 'rapid' methods of detecting and counting microorganisms (see also Chapter 3). These methods enumerate viable organisms – usually bacteria and yeasts rather than moulds – in a matter of hours and eliminate the 24–48 hour (or longer) incubation periods that are typical of traditional procedures. These alternative methods employ various means of indirect detection of living cells, but the following operating principles are the most common.

- Epifluorescent techniques use fluorescent dyes that either exhibit different colours in living and dead cells (e.g., acridine orange) or appear colourless outside the cell but become fluorescent when absorbed and subjected to cellular metabolism (e.g., fluorescein diacetate which, when cleaved by intracellular esterase, accumulates as fluorescein in the intact cell and fluoresces under ultraviolet light). This technique is aided by automated epifluorescent microscopy and by laser scanning methodologies.
- Living cells generate adenosine triphosphate (ATP) that can be readily released and then detected by enzyme assays, for example, luciferin emits light when exposed to firefly luciferase in the presence of ATP, a process called bioluminescence. To ensure there is sufficient ATP for detection, an enrichment step is often used; light emission can then be measured and related to bacterial concentration. When cells are captured on a membrane filter, samples can be assayed with the assistance of image analysis software.
- The resistance, capacitance or impedance of a culture medium changes as a result of bacterial or yeast growth and metabolism, and these electrical properties vary in proportion to cell concentration.
- Respirometry techniques are appropriate for monitoring the growth of organisms that consume oxygen or produce significant quantities of carbon dioxide during their metabolism, where changes in gas pressure may be measured by pressure transducers (in a closed vessel) or by manometry. Carbon dioxide accumulation in the growth medium can also lead to a pH decrease, which may be detected by an appropriate colourimetric indicator. While successfully detecting viable microbial presence, there is no direct relationship between the original bioburden and the detectable endpoint.
- Metabolically active respiring cells can be detected by colourimetric assay using, for example, tetrazolium salts which are reduced to form a coloured formazan product, the colour change being proportional to the number of viable respiring organisms; this technique can be adapted for use with a microtitre plate reader.

These methods are fast, readily automated and eliminate the need for numerous Petri dishes and incubators. On the other hand, they often require expensive equipment, have limitations in terms of detection limits and may be less readily adapted to certain types of sample than traditional methods. Furthermore, there are problems in some cases with reconciling the counts obtained by alternative methods and by traditional means. The newer techniques may detect organisms that are metabolising but not capable of reproducing to give visible colonies (viable but non-culturable [VBNC] organisms), so may give values many times higher than traditional methods; this has contributed to the caution with which regulatory authorities have accepted the data generated by rapid methods. Nevertheless, they are becoming more widely accepted, and now feature in pharmacopoeial monographs; favoured methods are likely to become an integral part of enumeration procedures in pharmaceutical microbiology in the foreseeable future.

2.6 Microbial Genetics

The nature of the genetic material possessed by a microbial cell and the manner in which that genetic material may be transferred to other cells depend largely upon whether the organism is a prokaryote or a eukaryote (see Section 2.1.2).

2.6.1 Bacteria

The genes essential for growth and metabolism of bacteria are normally contained on a chromosome of double-stranded (ds) DNA, which is in the form of a covalently closed circle (ccc) (and so designated ccc ds DNA). Additional genes that usually just confer upon the cell a survival advantage under certain circumstances may also be contained upon plasmids; these are usually similar in structure to chromosomes but much smaller and replicate independently (see Chapters 3 and 13). The total complement of genes possessed by a cell, that is, those in the chromosome, plasmid(s) and any received from other sources, for example, bacteriophages (bacterial viruses), is referred to as the genome of the cell.

Typically, bacterial chromosomes are 1 mm or more in length and contain about 1000–3000 genes. As many bacterial cells are approximately 1 μm long, it is clear that the chromosome has to be tightly coiled in order to fit in the available volume. Although all the genes are contained on a single chromosome (rather than being distributed over two or more), it is possible for a cell to contain several *copies* of that chromosome at any one time. Usually there are multiple copies during periods of rapid cell division, but some species seem to have many copies all the time. The mechanisms by which bacterial genes may be transferred from one organism to another are described in Chapter 3.

The nucleic-acid sequences in the bacterial genome are usually highly conserved, particularly in the case of ribosomes, and are independent of culture conditions; they are therefore ideal for identification purposes. Genotypic bacterial identification methods have therefore evolved which include DNA–DNA probe hybridisation, 16s and 23s ribosomal RNA gene sequencing and analytical ribotyping following DNA digestion with specific restriction enzymes. Targeted DNA can be amplified by the polymerase chain reaction technique (see Chapter 24). These genotyping methods are technically demanding and are generally not employed for routine characterisation of microflora but for critical identification of contaminants.

Plasmids usually resemble chromosomes except that they are approximately 0.1–1.0% of the size of a bacterial chromosome, and there are a few that are linear rather than circular. Plasmid genes are not essential for the normal functioning of the cell, but may code for a property that affords a survival advantage in certain environmental conditions; bacteria possessing the plasmid in question would therefore be selected when such conditions prevail. Properties which can be coded by plasmids include the ability to utilise unusual sugars or food sources, toxin production, production of pili that facilitate the attachment of a cell to a substrate (e.g., intestinal epithelium) and antibiotic resistance. A cell may contain multiple copies of any one plasmid and may contain two or more different plasmids. However, some plasmid combinations cannot coexist inside the same cell and are said to be incompatible; this phenomenon enables plasmids to be classified into incompatibility groups.

Plasmids replicate independently of the chromosome within the cell, so that both daughter cells contain a copy of the plasmid after binary fission. Plasmids may also be passed from one cell to another by various means (see Chapter 3). Some plasmids exhibit a marked degree of host specificity and may only be transmitted between different strains of the same species, although others, particularly those commonly found in Gram-negative intestinal bacteria, may cross between different species within a genus or between different genera. Conjugative (self-transmissible) plasmids code for genes that facilitate their own transmission from one cell to another by the production of pili. These sex pili initially establish contact between the two cells and then retract, drawing the donor and recipient cells together until membrane fusion occurs.

2.6.2 Eukaryotes

Eukaryotic microorganisms (yeasts, moulds, algae and protozoa) possess a nucleus that normally contains one or more pairs of linear chromosomes, in which the ds DNA is complexed with protein. The cells may divide asexually and the nucleus undergoes mitosis – a sequence of events by which the nucleus and the chromosomes within it are replicated to give copies identical to the originals. Most eukaryotes also have the potential for sexual reproduction during which the nucleus undergoes meiosis, that is, a more specialised form of nuclear and chromosome division creating new gene combinations, so the offspring differ from the parents. Despite this potential, there are some eukaryotic cells, particularly fungi, in which a sexual stage in the life cycle has never been observed. Many eukaryotic microorganisms possess plasmids, and some fungal plasmids are based on RNA instead of DNA.

2.6.3 Genetic Variation and Gene Expression

Microorganisms may adapt rapidly to new environments and devise strategies to avoid or negate stressful or potentially harmful circumstances. Their ability to survive adverse conditions may result from the organism using genes it already possesses, or by the acquisition of new genetic information. The term 'genotype' describes the genetic composition of an organism, that is, it refers to the genes that the organism possesses, regardless of whether they are expressed or not. It is not uncommon for a microbial cell to possess a particular gene but not to express it, that is, not to manufacture the protein or enzyme that is the product of that gene, unless or until the product is actually required; this is simply a mechanism to avoid wasting energy. For example, many bacteria possess the genes that code for β-lactamases; these enzymes hydrolyse and inactivate β-lactam antibiotics (e.g., penicillins). In many organisms, β-lactamases are only produced in response to the presence of the antibiotic. This form of non-genetic adaptation is termed *phenotypic* adaptation, and there are many situations in which bacteria adopt a phenotypic change to counter environmental stress. But microorganisms may also use an alternative strategy of *genetic* adaptation, by which they acquire new genes either by mutation or by conjugation (see Chapter 3); subsequently, a process of selection ensures that the mutant organisms that are better suited to the new environment become numerically dominant.

In bacteria, mutation is an important mechanism by which resistance to antibiotics and other antimicrobial chemicals is achieved, although the receipt of entirely new genes directly from other bacteria is also clinically very important. Spontaneous mutation rates (rates not influenced by mutagenic chemicals or ionising radiation) vary substantially depending on the gene and the organism in question, but rates of 10^{-5}–10^{-7} are typical. These values mean that, on average, a mutant arises once in every 100,000 to every 10 million cell divisions. Although these figures might suggest that mutation is a relatively rare event, the speed with which microorganisms can multiply means, for example, that mutants exhibiting increased antibiotic resistance can arise quite quickly during the course of therapy.

2.7 Pharmaceutical Importance of the Major Categories of Microorganisms

Table 2.4 indicates the ways in which the different types of microorganism are considered relevant in pharmacy. The importance of viruses derives almost exclusively from their pathogenic potential, and because of their lack of intrinsic metabolism they are not susceptible to antibiotics. Partly for these reasons, viral infections are among the most dangerous and difficult to cure, and of all the categories of microorganism, only viruses appear in (the most serious) Hazard Category 4 as classified by the Advisory Committee on Dangerous Pathogens. Because they are not free-living, viruses are incapable of growing on manufactured medicines or raw materials, so they do not cause product spoilage, and they have no synthetic capabilities that can be exploited in medicines manufacture. Viruses are relatively easy to destroy by heat, radiation or toxic chemicals, so they do not represent a problem from this perspective. In this, they contrast with prions; although some authorities would question the categorisation of these infectious agents as microorganisms, they are included here because of their undoubted ability to cause, as yet incurable, fatal disease, and their extreme resistance to lethal agents. Pharmacists and healthcare personnel in general should be aware of the ability of prions to easily withstand sterilising conditions that would be satisfactory for the destruction of all other categories of infectious agent.

There are examples of bacteria that are important in each of the different ways indicated by the column headings of Table 2.4. Many of the medically and pharmaceutically important bacteria are pathogens, and some of these pathogens are of long-standing notoriety as a result of their ability to resist the activity of antibiotics and microbicides (disinfectants, antiseptics and preservatives). In addition to these long-established resistant organisms, other bacteria have given more recent cause for concern including methicillin-resistant *S. aureus* (MRSA), vancomycin-resistant enterococci (VSE) and multiply resistant *Mycobacterium tuberculosis* (see Chapter 13). While penicillin and cephalosporin antibiotics are produced by fungal species, the majority of the other categories of clinically important antibiotics are produced by species of bacteria, notably streptomycetes. In addition, a variety of bacteria are

Table 2.4 Pharmaceutical importance of the major categories of microorganisms.

	Pharmaceutical relevance				
Type of organism	**Contamination or spoilage of raw materials and medicines**	**Pathogens**	**Resistance to antibiotics and microbicides**	**Resistance to sterilising agents and processes**	**Used in the manufacture of therapeutic agents**
Viruses	+	+			+ (vaccines)
Prions	+	+		+	
Bacteria					
Gram-negative	+	+	+		+
Gram-positive	+	+	+	+ (spores)	+
Deinococcus				+ (*D. radiodurans*)	
Mycobacteria		+	+		
Streptomycetes		+			+
Chlamydia		+			
Rickettsia		+			
Mycoplasma		+			
Fungi					
Yeasts	+	+	+		+
Moulds	+	+	+		+
Protozoa		+			

exploited commercially in the manufacture of other medicines including steroids, enzymes and carbohydrates. The ability of bacteria to grow on diverse substrates ensures that their potential as agents of spoilage in manufactured medicines and raw materials is well recognised, and the ability of many species to survive drying means that they survive well in dust and so become important as contaminants of manufactured medicines. The ability to survive not only in dry conditions but in other adverse environments (heat, radiation, toxic chemicals, etc.) is well exemplified by bacterial spores, and their pre-eminence at or near the top of the 'league table' of resistance to lethal agents has resulted in spores acting as the indicator organisms that have to be eliminated in most sterilisation processes (see Chapter 21).

Like bacteria, fungi are able to form spores that survive drying, so they too arise commonly as contaminants of manufactured medicines. However, the degree of resistance presented by the spores is usually less than that exhibited by bacteria, and fungi do not represent a sterilisation problem. Fungi do not generally create a significant infection hazard either; relatively few fungal species are considered major pathogens for animals that possess a fully functional immune system. There are, however, several fungi which, while representing little threat to immunocompetent individuals, are nevertheless capable of initiating an infection in persons with impaired immune function; the term 'opportunist pathogens' is used to describe microorganisms (of all types) possessing this characteristic. In this context, it is worth noting that the immunocompromised represent an increasingly large group of patients, and this is not just because of human immunodeficiency virus/acquired immunodeficiency syndrome (HIV/AIDS). Several other conditions or drug treatments impair immune function, for example, congenital immunodeficiency, cancer (particularly leukaemia), radiotherapy and chemotherapy, the use of systemic corticosteroids and immunosuppressive drugs (often following tissue or organ transplants), severe burns and malnutrition.

Protozoa are of significance largely owing to the pathogenic potential of a few species. Because protozoa do not possess cell walls they do not survive drying well (unless in the form of cysts), so they are not a problem in the manufacturing environment – and even the encysted forms do not display resistance to sterilising processes to match that of bacterial spores. It should be noted that protozoal infections are not currently a major problem to human health in temperate climates, although they are significantly more troublesome in veterinary medicine and in the tropics. There are concerns that the geographical ranges of protozoal infections such as malaria may extend substantially if current fears about global warming translate into reality.

2.8 Preservation of Microorganisms

In addition to their uses in the manufacture of medicines, microorganisms are employed in a variety of tests and assays, particularly those to measure the activity of antimicrobial chemicals (see Chapter 19). Useful organisms, therefore, need to be correctly preserved in order to ensure that their desirable properties are not changed during storage or, worse, the culture dies completely and is irreplaceable. Many bacteria and fungi can conveniently be stored for a few days, or possibly weeks, in the form of liquid cultures in tubes, or as colonies on Petri dishes. Organisms that readily form spores – *Bacillus* and *Clostridium* species of bacteria and most fungi – can be stored for months or even years in this way provided that the culture medium does not evaporate to dryness, but non-sporing organisms vary substantially in their survival capacities. Gram-positive bacteria generally tend to survive better than Gram-negative ones: species such as *Pseudomonas aeruginosa*, for example, may die within a few weeks, even at refrigeration temperatures, if maintained as colonies on unsealed Petri dishes. Even if a culture that is to be preserved does not die completely when stored in the refrigerator, there is a risk that the cells that *do* survive are not typical of the population as a whole; they may, for example, be mutants that have increased resistance to adverse conditions in general, and so fail to give the expected results when used in tests on antibiotic activity. The dual aims of a culture preservation procedure therefore are to maintain the viability of the highest possible percentage of cells and to minimise the risk of selecting atypical mutants.

The most common procedures for long-term storage are by freezing at −80 °C (or lower) in refrigerators, by storage in liquid nitrogen at −196 °C in special vessels or by freeze-drying (also called lyophilisation). In each case, cryoprotectant chemicals – compounds like glycerol or dimethyl sulphoxide – are incorporated at a concentration of about 10% v/v in the liquid culture of the organism in order to minimise both the formation of damaging ice crystals and osmotic stresses that can accelerate cell death during freezing and thawing.

Reference cultures, those with well-defined biosynthetic capabilities or resistance properties, can be obtained in a freeze-dried form from internationally accessible culture collections such as the American Type Culture Collection (cultures having the designation ATCC before a reference number) or the UK National Collection of Industrial, Food and Marine Bacteria (NICMB). Increasingly, pharmacopoeias and regulatory agencies are requiring tests that employ microorganisms to be conducted with cultures or test suspensions of cells that are no more than five subcultures from the reference material obtained from the designated culture collection.

3

Bacteria

David Allison

Reader in Pharmacy Education, Division of Pharmacy and Optometry, School of Health Sciences, The University of Manchester, Manchester, UK

CONTENTS

Hugo and Russell's Pharmaceutical Microbiology, Ninth Edition. Edited by Brendan F. Gilmore and Stephen P. Denyer.

Companion website: https://www.wiley.com/go/HugoandRussells9e

3.1 Introduction

The smallest free-living microorganisms are the prokaryotes, comprising bacteria and archaea (see Chapter 2). Prokaryote is a term used to define cells that lack a true nuclear membrane; they contrast with eukaryotic cells (e.g., plants, animals and fungi) that possess a nuclear membrane and internal compartmentalisation. Indeed, a major feature of eukaryotic cells, absent from prokaryotic cells, is the presence in the cytoplasm of membrane-enclosed organelles. These and other criteria differentiating eukaryotes and prokaryotes are shown in Table 2.1 of Chapter 2.

Bacteria and archaea share many traits and it was not until the early 1980s that differences first became evident from analyses of gene sequences. One major difference is the composition of cell walls. A more striking contrast is in the structure of the lipids that make up their cytoplasmic membranes. Differences also exist in their respective patterns of metabolism: most archaea are anaerobes, and are often found inhabiting extreme environments. It is possible that their unusual membrane structure gives archaeal cells greater stability under extreme conditions. Of notable interest is the observation that no disease-causing archaea have yet been identified; the vast majority of prokaryotes of medical and pharmaceutical significance are bacteria.

Bacteria represent a large and diverse group of microorganisms that can exist as single cells or as cell clusters. Moreover, they are generally able to carry out their life processes of growth, energy generation and reproduction independently of other cells. In these respects, they are very different from the cells of animals and plants, which are unable to live alone in nature and can exist only as part of a multicellular organism. Bacteria are capable of growing in a range of different environments and can not only cause contamination and spoilage of many pharmaceutical products but also a range of different diseases.

3.1.1 Bacterial Diversity and Ubiquity

Bacterial diversity can be seen in terms of variation in cell size and shape (morphology), adaptation to environmental extremes, survival strategies and metabolic capabilities. Such diversity allows bacteria to grow in a multiplicity of environments ranging from hot sulphur springs (65 °C) to deep freezers (−20 °C), from high (pH 1) to low (pH 13) acidity and high (0.7 m) to low osmolarity (water). In addition, they can grow in both nutritionally rich (compost) and nutritionally poor (distilled water) situations. Hence, although each organism is uniquely suited to its own particular environmental niche and rarely grows out of it, the presence of bacteria may be considered ubiquitous. Indeed, there is no natural environment that is free from bacteria. This ubiquity is often demonstrated by the terms used to describe organisms that grow and/or survive in particular environments. An example of such descriptive terminology is shown in Table 3.1.

3.2 Bacterial Ultrastructure

3.2.1 Cell Size and Shape

Bacteria are the smallest free-living organisms, their size being measured in micrometres (microns). Because of this small size, a microscope affording a considerable degree of magnification (×400–1000) is necessary to observe them. Bacteria vary in size from a cell as small as 0.1–0.2 μm in diameter to those that are >5 μm in diameter. Bacteria

Table 3.1 Descriptive terms used to characterise bacteria.

Descriptive term	Adaptive feature
Psychrophile	Growth range −40 °C to +20 °C
Mesophile	Growth range +20 °C to +40 °C
Thermophile	Growth range +40 °C to +85 °C
Thermoduric	Endure high temperatures
Halophile	Salt-tolerant
Acidophile	Acid-tolerant
Aerobe	Air (oxygen)-requiring
Obligate anaerobe	Air (oxygen)-poisoned
Autotroph	Utilises inorganic material
Heterotroph	Requires organic material

this large, such as *Thiomargarita namibiensis*, are extremely rare: the majority of bacteria are 1–5 μm long and 1–2 μm in diameter. By comparison, eukaryotic cells may be 2 μm to >200 μm in diameter. The small size of bacteria has a number of implications with regard to their biological properties, most notably increased and more efficient transport rates. This advantage allows bacteria far more rapid growth rates than eukaryotic cells.

While the classification of bacteria is complex, nowadays relying very much on 16S ribosomal DNA sequencing data, a more simplistic approach is to divide them into major groups on purely morphological grounds. The majority of bacteria are unicellular and possess simple shapes, for example, round (cocci), cylindrical (rod, also called bacillus, spelt with a lowercase initial letter to distinguish from *Bacillus*, the genus) or ovoid (a cross between a coccus and a rod). Some rods are curved (vibrios), while longer rigid curved organisms with multiple spirals are known as spirochaetes. Rarer morphological forms include: the actinomycetes which are rigid bacteria resembling fungi that may grow as lengthy branched filaments; the mycoplasmas which lack a conventional peptidoglycan (murein) cell wall and are highly pleomorphic organisms of indefinite shape; and some miscellaneous bacteria comprising stalked, sheathed, budded and slime-producing forms often associated with aquatic and soil environments.

The shape of an organism is determined by heredity. Genetically, most bacteria are monomorphic; that is, they maintain a single shape. However, a number of environmental conditions can cause that shape to alter, including exposure to sub-lethal concentrations of antibiotics. Moreover, a few bacteria such as *Corynebacterium* species are genetically pleomorphic; that is, they can adopt more than one shape depending on environmental conditions.

Often bacteria remain together in specific arrangements after cell division. These arrangements are usually characteristic of different organisms and can be used as part of a preliminary identification. Examples of such cellular arrangements include chains of rods or cocci, paired cells (diplococci), tetrads and clusters.

3.2.2 Cellular Components

Compared with eukaryotic cells, bacteria possess a fairly simple base cell structure, comprising cell wall, cytoplasmic membrane, nucleoid, ribosomes and occasionally inclusion granules (Figure 3.1). Nevertheless, it is important for several reasons to have a good knowledge of these structures and their functions. First, the study of bacteria provides an excellent route for probing the nature of biological processes, many of which are shared by multicellular organisms. Secondly, at an applied level, normal bacterial processes can be customised to benefit society on a mass scale. Here, an obvious example is the large-scale industrial production (fermentation) of antibiotics. Thirdly, and from a pharmaceutical and healthcare perspective, it is important to be able to know how to kill bacterial contaminants and disease-causing organisms. To treat infections, antimicrobial agents are used to inhibit the growth of bacteria, a process known as antimicrobial chemotherapy. The essence of antimicrobial chemotherapy is selective toxicity (see Chapters 11, 12, and 14), which is achieved by exploiting differences between the structure and metabolism of

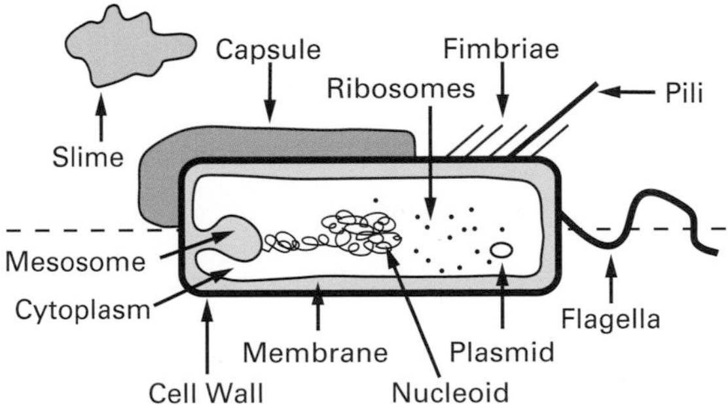

Figure 3.1 Diagram of a bacterial cell. Features represented above the dotted line are only found in some bacteria, whereas those below the line are common to all bacteria.

bacteria and host cells. Selective toxicity is, therefore, most efficient when a similar target does not exist in the host. Examples of such targets will be noted in the following sections.

3.2.2.1 Cell Wall

The bacterial cell wall is an extremely important structure, being essential for the maintenance of the shape and integrity of the bacterial cell. It is also chemically unlike any structure present in eukaryotic cells and is therefore an obvious target for antibiotics that can attack and kill bacteria without harm to the host (see Chapter 12).

The primary function of the cell wall is to provide a strong, rigid structural component that can withstand the osmotic pressures caused by high chemical concentrations of inorganic ions in the cell. Most bacterial cell walls have in common a unique structural component called peptidoglycan (also called murein or glycopeptide); exceptions include the mycoplasmas, extreme halophiles and the archaea. Peptidoglycan is a large macromolecule containing glycan (polysaccharide) chains that are cross-linked by short peptide bridges. The glycan chain acts as a backbone to peptidoglycan, and is composed of alternating residues of *N*-acetyl muramic acid (NAM) and *N*- acetyl glucosamine (NAG). To each molecule of NAM is attached a tetrapeptide consisting of the amino acids L-alanine, D-alanine, D-glutamic acid and either lysine or diaminopimelic acid (DAP). This glycan tetrapeptide repeat unit is cross-linked to adjacent glycan chains, either through a direct peptide linkage or a peptide interbridge (Figure 3.2). The types and numbers of cross-linking amino acids vary from organism to organism. Other unusual features of the cell wall that provide potential antimicrobial targets are DAP and the presence of two amino acids that have the D-configuration.

Bacteria can be divided into two large groups, Gram-positive and Gram-negative, on the basis of a differential staining technique called the Gram stain. Essentially, the

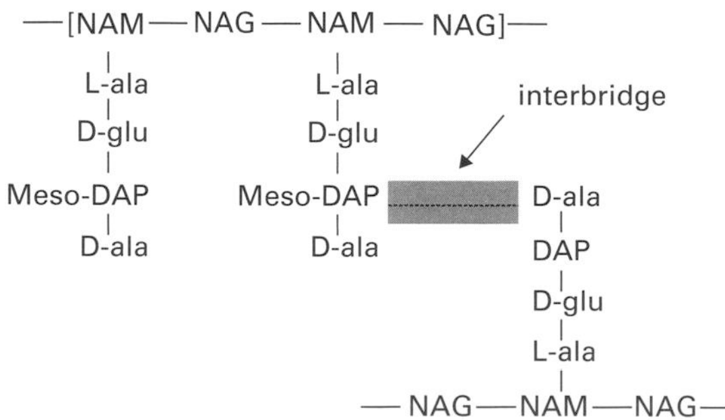

Figure 3.2 Structure of *Escherichia coli* peptidoglycan.

Gram stain consists of treating a film of bacteria dried on a microscope slide with a solution of crystal violet, followed by a solution of iodine; these are then washed with an alcohol solution. In Gram-negative organisms, the cells lose the crystal violet–iodine complex and are rendered colourless, whereas Gram-positive cells retain the dye. Regardless, both cell types are counter-stained with a different coloured dye, for example, carbolfuchsin, which is red. Hence, under the light microscope, Gram-negative cells appear red, while Gram-positive cells are purple. These marked differences in response reflect differences in cell wall structure. The Gram-positive cell wall consists primarily of a single type of molecule, whereas the Gram-negative cell wall is a multilayered structure and quite complex.

The cell walls of Gram-positive bacteria are quite thick (20–80 nm) and consist of between 60 and 80% peptidoglycan, which is extensively cross-linked in three dimensions to form a thick polymeric mesh (Figure 3.3). Gram-positive walls frequently contain acidic polysaccharides called teichoic acids; these are either ribitol phosphate or glycerol phosphate molecules that are connected by phosphodiester bridges. Because they are negatively charged, teichoic acids are partially responsible for the negative charge of the cell surface as a whole. Although they do not confer any extra rigidity to the cell wall, their function may be to effect passage of metal cations through the cell wall. In some Gram-positive bacteria, glycerol–teichoic acids are bound to membrane lipids and are termed lipoteichoic acids. During an infection, lipoteichoic acid molecules released by killed bacteria trigger an inflammatory response. Cell wall proteins, if present, are generally found on the outer surface of the peptidoglycan.

The wall, or more correctly, envelope of Gram-negative cells is a far more complicated structure (Figure 3.4). Although it contains less peptidoglycan (10–20% of wall), a second membrane structure is found outside the peptidoglycan layer. This outer membrane is asymmetrical, composed of proteins, lipoproteins, phospholipids and a component unique to Gram-negative bacteria, lipopolysaccharide (LPS). Essentially, the outer membrane is attached to the peptidoglycan by a lipoprotein, one end of which is covalently attached to peptidoglycan and the other end is embedded in the outer membrane. The outer membrane is not a phospholipid bilayer, although it does contain phospholipids in the inner leaf, and its outer layer is composed of LPS, a polysaccharide–lipid molecule. Proteins are also found in the outer membrane, some of which form trimers that traverse the whole membrane and in so doing form water-filled channels or porins through which small molecules can pass. Other proteins are found at either the inner or outer face of the membrane.

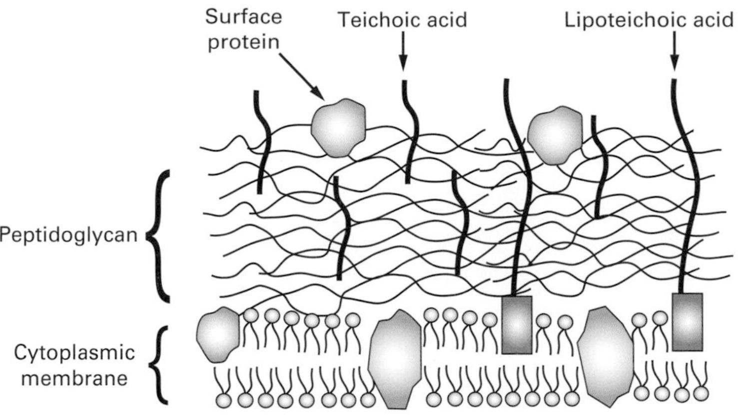

Figure 3.3 Structure of the Gram-positive cell wall.

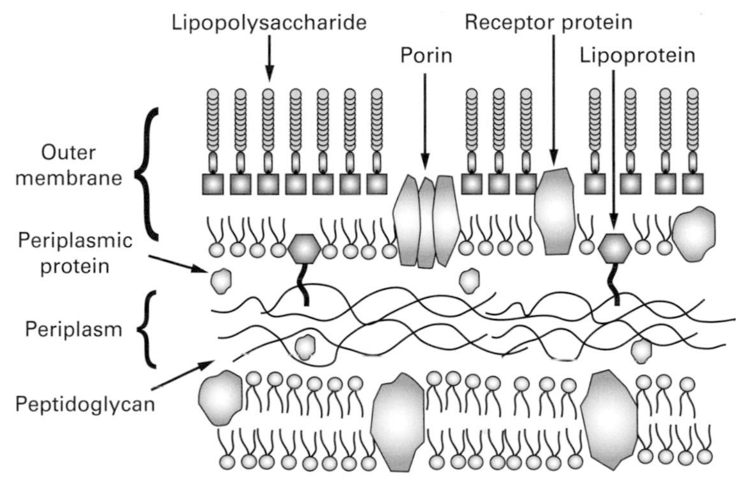

Figure 3.4 Structure of the Gram-negative cell envelope.

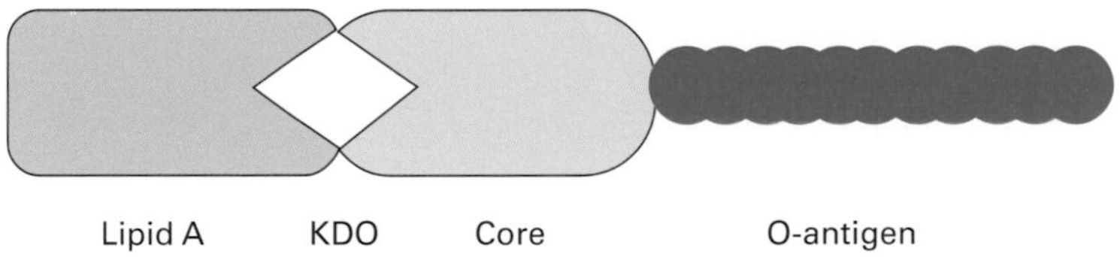

Figure 3.5 Schematic representation of lipopolysaccharide (LPS). KDO, ketodeoxyoctonate.

The LPS (Figure 3.5) is an important molecule because it determines the antigenicity of the Gram-negative cell and it is extremely toxic, if not lethal, to animal cells. For example, if a sterile solution of killed Gram-negative cells were to be injected into a patient, high fever, circulatory collapse and death may occur. This is due to the (endo) toxicity associated with the LPS. It is important, therefore, that injections are not only sterile (free from viable microorganisms) but also free from the LPS endotoxin (see Chapter 22).

Sometimes the LPS endotoxin is referred to as a pyrogen due to its fever-causing properties. The molecule consists of three regions, namely lipid A, core polysaccharide and O-specific polysaccharide. The lipid A portion is composed of a disaccharide of glucosamine phosphate bound to fatty acids and forms the outer leaflet of the membrane. It is the lipid A component that is responsible for the toxic and pyrogenic properties of Gram-negative bacteria. Lipid A is linked to the core polysaccharide by the unique molecule ketodeoxyoctonate (KDO), and at the other end of the core is the O-polysaccharide (O-antigen), which usually contains six-carbon sugars as well as one or more unusual deoxy sugars such as abequose.

Although the outer membrane is relatively permeable to small molecules, it is not permeable to enzymes or macromolecules. Indeed, one of the major functions of the outer membrane may be to keep certain enzymes that are present outside the cytoplasmic membrane from diffusing away from the cell. Moreover, the outer membrane is not readily

Table 3.2 Gram-positive and Gram-negative cell wall composition.

Feature	Gram-positive cells	Gram-negative cells
Peptidoglycan	60–80%	10–20%
Teichoic acid	Present	Absent
Lipoteichoic acid	Present	Absent
Lipoprotein	Absent	Present
Lipopolysaccharide	Absent	Present
Protein	Approximately 15%	Approximately 60%
Lipid	Approximately 2%	Approximately 20%

penetrated by hydrophobic compounds and is, therefore, resistant to dissolution by detergents.

The region between the outer surface of the cytoplasmic membrane and the inner surface of the outer membrane is called the periplasm. This occupies a thickness of about 12–15 nm, is gel-like in consistency and, in addition to the peptidoglycan, contains sugars and an abundance of proteins including hydrolytic enzymes and transport proteins. Table 3.2 summarises the major differences in wall composition between Gram-positive and Gram-negative cells.

Some bacteria have no cell walls or have very little wall material. These include members of the *Mycoplasma* genus. Mycoplasmas are the smallest known bacteria that can grow and reproduce outside living host cells; the majority are parasites of plants and animals with some, such as *Mycoplasma pneumoniae*, causing human disease. Due to the absence of a cell wall, these organisms can change their shape and are pleomorphic. All bacteria of the genus *Mycobacterium* (e.g., *Mycobacterium tuberculosis*, causative agent of TB) have high concentrations of a hydrophobic waxy lipid called mycolic acid in their cell walls, forming a layer outside of a thin layer of peptidoglycan. The waxy nature of the mycolic acid prevents the uptake of dyes, including those of the Gram-stain. These bacteria can only be stained by gently heating the cells with carbolfuchsin. The carbolfuchsin penetrates the cell walls, binds to the cytoplasm and resists removal by rinsing with acid alcohol. These acid-fast bacteria retain the red colour of carbolfuchsin.

3.2.2.2 Cytoplasmic Membrane

Biochemically, the cytoplasmic membrane is a fragile, phospholipid bilayer (20–30%) with proteins (60–70%) distributed randomly throughout. These proteins are involved in the various transport and enzyme functions associated with the membrane. A major difference in chemical composition between prokaryotic and eukaryotic cells is that eukaryotes have sterols in their membranes (e.g., cholesterol) providing rigidity, whereas prokaryotes do not. The cytoplasmic membrane serves many functions, including transport of nutrients, energy generation and electron transport; it is the location for regulatory proteins and biosynthetic proteins, and it acts as a semipermeable selectivity barrier between the cytoplasm and the cell environment.

Invaginations of the cytoplasmic membrane are referred to as *mesosomes*. Those that form near the septum of Gram-positive cells serve as organs of attachment for the bacterial chromosome.

3.2.2.3 Cytoplasm

The cytoplasm consists of approximately 80% water and contains enzymes that generate adenosine triphosphate (ATP) directly by oxidising glucose and other carbon sources. The cytoplasm also contains some of the enzymes involved in the synthesis of peptidoglycan subunits. Ribosomes, the DNA genome (nucleoid) and inclusion granules are also found in the cytoplasm.

3.2.2.4 Nucleoid

The bacterial chromosome exists as a singular, covalently closed circular molecule of double-stranded DNA comprising approximately 4600 kilobase pairs. It is complexed with small amounts of proteins and RNA, but unlike eukaryotic DNA, is not associated with histones. The DNA, if linearised, would be about 1 mm in length. In order to package this amount of material, the cell requires that the DNA is supercoiled into a number of domains (approximately 50) and that the domains are associated with each other and stabilised by specific proteins into an aggregated mass or nucleoid. The enzymes, topoisomerases, that control topological changes in DNA architecture are different from their eukaryotic counterparts (which act on linear chromosomes) and therefore provide a unique biochemical target for antibiotic action.

3.2.2.5 Plasmids

Plasmids are relatively small, circular pieces of double-stranded extrachromosomal DNA. They are capable of autonomous replication and encode for many auxiliary functions that are not usually necessary for bacterial growth but can provide a competitive advantage to the cell. These include production of toxins, pili and siderophores (iron-chelating molecules). One function of great significance is that of antibiotic resistance (see Chapter 13). Plasmids replicate faster than the chromosome, so cells usually contain multiple copies. Plasmids may also transfer readily from one organism to another, and between species (e.g., between a harmless, intrinsic species and a pathogenic species), thereby increasing the spread of resistance.

3.2.2.6 Ribosomes

The cytoplasm is densely packed with ribosomes. Unlike eukaryotic cells, these are not associated with a membranous structure; the endoplasmic reticulum is not a component of prokaryotic cells. Bacterial ribosomes are 70S in size, made up of two subunits of 30S and 50S. This is smaller than eukaryotic ribosomes, which are 80S in size (40S and 60S subunits). Differences will therefore exist in the size and geometry of RNA-binding sites.

3.2.2.7 Inclusion Granules

Bacteria occasionally contain inclusion granules within their cytoplasm. These consist of storage material composed of carbon, nitrogen, sulphur or phosphorus, and are formed when these materials are replete in the environment to act as repositories for these nutrients when shortages occur. Some inclusions are common to a wide variety of bacteria, whereas others are limited to a small number of species. Examples include polysaccharide granules, glycogen, polyphosphate and lipid inclusions, in particular one unique to bacteria, poly-β-hydroxybutyrate.

3.2.3 Cell Surface Components

The surface of the bacterial cell is the portion of the organism that interacts with the external environment most directly. As a consequence, many bacteria deploy components on their surfaces in a variety of ways that allow them to withstand and survive fluctuations in the growth environment. The following sections describe a few of these components that are commonly found, although not universally, that allow bacteria to move, sense their environment, attach to surfaces and provide protection from harsh conditions.

3.2.3.1 Flagella

Active bacterial motility is commonly provided by flagella, long (approximately 12 µm) helical-shaped structures that project from the surface of the cell. The filament of the flagellum is built up from multiple copies of the protein flagellin. Where the filament enters the surface of the bacterium, there is a hook in the flagellum, which is attached to the cell surface by a series of complex proteins comprising the flagellar motor. This rotates the flagellum, causing the bacterium to move through its environment. The numbers and distribution of flagella vary with bacterial species. Some have a single, polar flagellum, whereas others are flagellate over their entire surface (peritrichous); intermediate forms also exist. The direction of rotation of the flagella can be changed in response to changing external chemical stimuli, prompting the bacterial cell to move towards beneficial environments such as nutrient-rich areas and away from harmful locations, a process called chemotaxis.

3.2.3.2 Fimbriae

Fimbriae are structurally similar to flagella, but are not involved in motility. Although they are straighter, more numerous and considerably thinner and shorter (3 µm) than flagella, they do consist of protein and project from the cell surface. Fimbriae are more commonly found on Gram-negative bacteria than on Gram-positive bacteria. There is strong evidence to suggest that fimbriae act primarily as adhesins, allowing organisms to attach to surfaces, including animal tissues in the case of some pathogenic bacteria, and to initiate biofilm formation. Fimbriae are also responsible for haemagglutination and cell clumping in bacteria. Among the best characterised fimbriae are the type I fimbriae of enteric (intestinal) bacteria (e.g., *E. coli* and *Salmonella* species), helping these organisms to colonise the large intestine.

3.2.3.3 Pili

Pili are morphologically and chemically similar to fimbriae, but they are present in much smaller numbers (<10) and are usually longer. They are involved in the genetic exchange process of conjugation (see Section 3.6.3).

3.2.3.4 Capsules and Slime Layers

Many bacteria secrete extracellular polysaccharides (EPS) that are associated with the exterior of the bacterial cell. The EPS is composed primarily of approximately 2% carbohydrate and 98% water, and provides a gummy exterior to the cell. Morphologically, two extreme forms exist: *capsules*, which form a tight, fairly rigid layer closely associated with the cell, and *slimes*, which are loosely associated with the cell. Both forms function similarly, to offer protection against desiccation, to provide a protective barrier against the penetration of biocides, disinfectants and positively charged antibiotics, to protect against engulfment by phagocytes and protozoa and to act as a cement binding cells to each other and to the substratum in biofilms (see below). One such polymer that performs all of these functions is alginate, produced by *Pseudomonas aeruginosa*; dextran, produced by *Leuconostoc mesenteroides*, is another. Both polymers may be harvested and used variously as pharmaceutical aids, surgical dressings and drug delivery systems, although the preferred source of alginate is seaweed rather than bacteria.

3.2.3.5 S-layers

S-layers are the most common cell wall type among the archaea. These consist of a two-dimensional paracrystalline array of proteins or glycoproteins which show various ordered symmetries when viewed under the electron microscope. In many species of bacteria, S-layers are present on their outer surfaces in addition to other cell wall components such as polysaccharides. In such arrangements, the S-layer is always the outermost layer. In addition to increasing the structural robustness of the cell, S-layers can act to a certain extent as an external permeability barrier.

3.3 Biofilms

Any surface, whether it is animate or inanimate, is of considerable importance as a microbial habitat owing to the adsorption of nutrients. A nutrient-rich microenvironment is thus produced in a nutrient-poor macroenvironment whenever a surface–liquid interface exists. Consequently, microbial numbers and activity are usually much greater on a surface than in suspension. Hence, in many natural, medical and industrial settings, bacteria attach to surfaces and form multilayered communities called *biofilms*. These commonly contain more than one species of bacteria, which exist cooperatively together as a functional, dynamic consortium. Moreover, biofilms commonly possess unique properties that are distinct from unattached cells. Biofilm formation usually begins with pioneer cells attaching to a surface, either through the use of specific adhesins such as fimbriae, or non-specifically by EPS. Once established, these cells grow and divide to produce microcolonies, which, with time, eventually coalesce to produce a biofilm. A key characteristic of biofilms is the enveloping of the attached cells in a matrix of EPS and other macromolecules. This helps to cement cells to the surface and to each other, and protects the bacteria from hazardous materials such as antibiotics and biocides, from desiccation and from engulfment by macrophages and phagocytes in much the same way as the capsules and slime layers mentioned above. In addition, strands of EPS hold the bacterial cells at a distance from one another, enabling small water channels to form in the biofilm. These channels act as a primitive circulatory system carrying trapped nutrients and oxygen to the enclosed cells and take waste products away.

Biofilms have a number of significant implications in medicine and industry. In the human body, the resident cells within the biofilm are not exposed to attack by the immune system and in some instances can exacerbate the inflammatory response. An example of this is shown by the growth of *P. aeruginosa* as an alginate-enclosed biofilm in the lungs of cystic fibrosis patients. Bacterial biofilms are also profoundly less susceptible to antimicrobial agents than their free-living, planktonic counterparts. As a consequence, bacterial biofilms that form on contaminated medical implants and prosthetic devices, manufacturing surfaces or fluid conduit systems are virtually impossible to eliminate with antibiotics or biocides. In these situations, antimicrobial resistance occurs as a population or community response. Biofilms are considered in more detail in Chapter 8.

3.4 Bacterial Sporulation

In a few bacterial genera, most notably *Bacillus* and *Clostridium*, a unique process takes place in which the vegetative cell undergoes a profound biochemical change to give rise to a specialised structure called an endospore or spore (Figure 3.6). This process of sporulation is not part of a reproductive cycle, but the spore is a highly resistant cell that enables the producing organism to survive in adverse environmental conditions such as lack of moisture or essential nutrients, or exposure to toxic chemicals, radiation or high temperatures. Because of their extreme resistance to radiation, ethylene oxide and heat, all sterilisation processes for pharmaceutical products have been designed to destroy the bacterial spore (see Chapter 21). Removal of the environmental stress may lead to germination of the spore back to the vegetative cell form.

3.4.1 Endospore Structure

Endospores are differentiated cells that possess a grossly different structure to that of the parent vegetative cell in which they are formed. The structure of the spore is much more complex than that of the vegetative cell in that it has many layers surrounding a central core (Figure 3.7). The outermost layer is the exosporium composed of protein; within this are the spore coats, which are also proteinaceous but

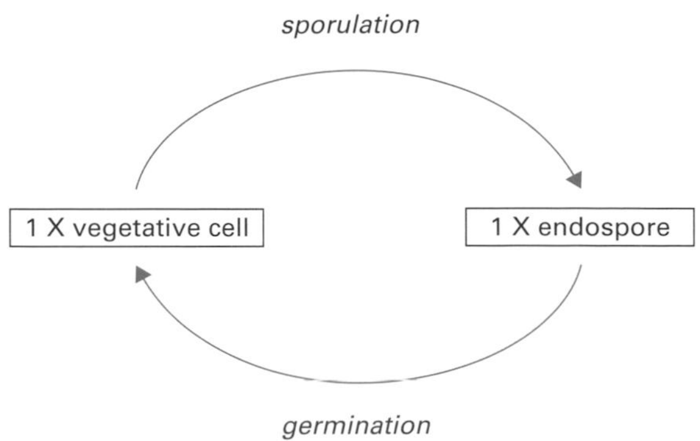

Figure 3.6 Bacterial sporulation and germination.

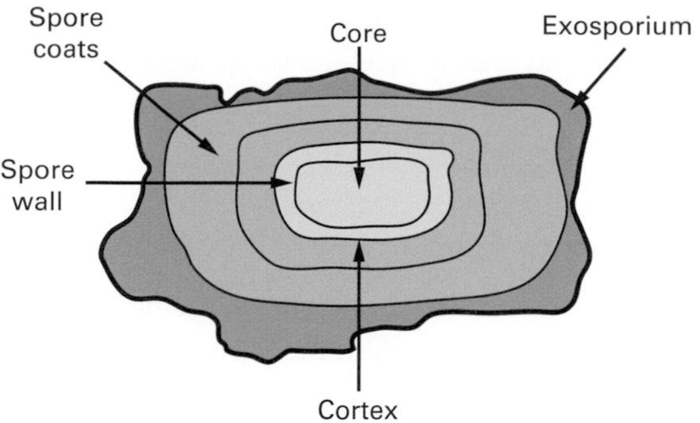

Figure 3.7 Diagram of endospore structure.

with a high cysteine content, the cortex that consists of loosely cross-linked peptidoglycan and the central core that contains the genome. Characteristic of the spore is the presence of dipicolinic acid and high levels of calcium ions which complex together. The core is also partially dehydrated, containing only 10–30% of the water content of the vegetative cells. Dehydration has been shown to increase resistance to both heat and chemicals. In addition, the pH of the core is about 1 unit lower than the cytoplasm of the vegetative cell and contains high levels of core-specific proteins that bind tightly to the DNA and protect it from potential damage. These core-specific proteins also function as an energy source for the outgrowth or germination of a new vegetative cell from the endospore.

3.4.2 Endospore Formation

Under adverse growth conditions, a single cell gives rise to a single spore due to internal and structural reorganisation. During endospore formation, the vegetative cell undergoes a complex series of biochemical events in cellular differentiation, and many genetically directed changes in the cell that underpin the conversion occur in a series of distinct stages. Sporulation requires that the synthesis of some proteins involved in vegetative cell function ceases and that specific spore proteins are made. This is accomplished by activation of a variety of spore-specific genes such as *spo* and *ssp*. The proteins coded by these genes catalyse a series of events leading ultimately to the production of a dry, metabolically inert but extremely resistant endospore. The whole process can take only a matter of hours to complete under optimal conditions.

3.4.3 Endospore Germination

Although endospores can lie dormant for decades, they can revert back to a vegetative cell very rapidly. Activation of the process may occur through removal of the stress inducer that initiated sporulation. During germination, loss of resistance properties occurs along with a loss of calcium dipicolinate and cortex components, and degradation of the core-specific proteins. Outgrowth occurs, involving water uptake and synthesis of new RNA, proteins and DNA until eventually, after a matter of minutes, the vegetative cell emerges from the fractured spore coat and begins to divide again.

3.5 Bacterial Toxins

Although bacteria are associated with disease, only a few species are disease-producing or pathogenic for healthy individuals (see Chapter 7). Of increasing concern are those organisms that, if presented with the correct set of conditions, can cause disease, that is, opportunist pathogens. Examples include *Staphylococcus epidermidis*, a beneficial organism when present on the skin (its normal habitat) yet potentially fatal if attached to a synthetic heart valve, and *P. aeruginosa*, a non-pathogenic environmental organism but again potentially lethal in immunocompromised patients.

Pathogens cause host damage in a number of ways. In most cases, they produce a variety of molecules or factors that promote pathogenesis, among which are the toxins: products of bacteria that produce immediate host-cell damage. Toxins have been classified as either endotoxin, that is, cell-wall-related, or exotoxin, products released extracellularly as the organism grows.

Endotoxin is the lipid A component of LPS (see Section 3.2.2.1). It possesses multiple biological properties including the ability to induce fever, initiate the complement and blood cascades, activate B lymphocytes and stimulate production of tumour necrosis factor. Endotoxin is generally released from lysed or damaged cells. Care must be taken to eliminate or exclude such heat-resistant material from parenteral products and their delivery systems through a process known as depyrogenation (see Chapters 21 and 22).

Most exotoxins fall into one of three categories on the basis of their structure and activities. These are the AB toxins, the cytolytic toxins and the superantigen toxins. The AB toxins consist of a B subunit that binds to a host cell receptor and is also covalently bound to the A subunit that mediates the enzymic activity responsible for toxicity. Most exotoxins (e.g., diphtheria toxin and cholera toxin) are of the AB category. The cytolytic toxins such as haemolysins and phospholipases do not have separable A and B portions but work by enzymatically attacking cell constituents, causing lysis. The superantigens also lack an AB type structure and act by stimulating large numbers of immune response cells to release cytokines, resulting in a massive inflammatory reaction. An example of this type of reaction is *Staphylococcus aureus*-mediated toxic shock syndrome.

3.6 Bacterial Reproduction and Growth Kinetics

3.6.1 Multiplication and Division Cycle

The majority of bacterial cells multiply in number by a process of binary fission. That is, each individual will increase in size until it is large enough to divide into two identical daughter cells. At the point of separation, each daughter cell must be capable of growth and reproduction. While each daughter cell will automatically contain those materials that are dispersed throughout the mother cell (mRNA, rRNA, ribosomes, enzymes, cytochromes, etc.), each must also carry at least one copy of the chromosome. The bacterial chromosome is circular and attached to the cytoplasmic membrane where it is able to uncoil during DNA replication. The process of DNA replication proceeds at a fixed rate dependent on temperature, therefore the time taken to copy an entire chromosome depends on the number of base pairs within it and the growth temperature. For *E. coli* growing at 37 °C, replication of the chromosome will take approximately 45 minutes. These copies of the chromosome must then segregate to opposite sides of the cell before cell division can proceed. Division occurs in different ways for Gram-positive and Gram-negative bacteria. Gram-negative cells do not have a rigid cell wall and divide by a process of constriction followed by membrane fusion. Gram-positive cells, on the other hand, having a rigid cell wall, must develop a cross-wall (see Figure 2.1a in Chapter 2) that divides the cell into two equal halves. Constriction and cross-wall formation take approximately 15 minutes to complete. DNA replication, chromosome segregation (C-phase) and cell division (D-phase) occur sequentially in slow-growing cells with generation times of greater than 1 hour, and are the final events of the bacterial cell cycle. Cells are able to replicate faster than once every hour by initiating several rounds of DNA replication at a time. Thus, partially replicated chromosomes become segregated into the newly formed daughter cells. In this fashion, it is possible for some organisms growing under their optimal conditions to divide every 15–20 minutes. Rod-shaped organisms maintain their diameter during the cell cycle and increase their mass and volume by a process of elongation. When the length of the cell has approximately doubled, then the division/constriction occurs centrally. Coccal forms increase in size by radial expansion, with the division plane going towards the geometric centre. In some genera, the successive division planes are always parallel. Under such circumstances, the cells appear to form chains (i.e., streptococci). In staphylococci, successive division planes are randomised, giving dividing clusters of cells the appearance of a bunch of grapes. Certain genera, for example, *Sarcina*, rotate successive division planes by 90° to form tetrads and cubical octets. The appearance of dividing cells under the microscope can therefore be a useful initial guide to identification.

3.6.2 Population Growth

When placed in favourable conditions, populations of bacteria can increase at remarkable rates, given that each division gives rise to two identical daughter cells, then each has the potential to divide again. Thus, cell numbers will increase exponentially as a function of time. For a microorganism growing with a generation time of 20 minutes, one cell will have divided three times within an hour to give a total of eight cells. After 20 hours of continued division at this rate, the accumulated mass of bacterial cells would be approximately 70 kg (the weight of an average man). Ten hours later, the mass would be equivalent to the combined body weight of the entire population of the UK. Clearly this does not happen in nature; rather, the supply of nutrients becomes exhausted and the organisms grow considerably more slowly, if at all.

The time interval between one cell division and the next is called the *generation time*. When considering a growing culture containing thousands of cells, a mean generation time is usually calculated. As one cell doubles to become two cells, which then multiply to become four cells and so on, the number of bacteria n in any generation can be expressed as:

$$\text{1st generation } n = 1 \times 2 = 2^1$$
$$\text{2nd generation } n = 1 \times 2 \times 2 = 2^2$$
$$\text{3rd generation } n = 1 \times 2 \times 2 \times 2 = 2^3$$
$$x\text{th generation } n = 1 \times 2^x = 2^x$$

For an initial population of N_0 cells, as distinct from one cell, at the xth generation the cell population will be:

$$N = N_0 \times 2^x$$

where N is the final cell number, N_0 the initial cell number and x the number of generations. To express this equation in terms of x, then:

$$\begin{aligned}\log N &= \log N_0 + x \log 2,\\ \log N - \log N_0 &= x \log 2,\\ x &= \left(\log N - \log N_0\right) / \log 2 = \left(\log N - \log N_0\right) / 0.301\\ &= 3.3\left(\log N - \log N_0\right)\end{aligned}$$

The actual generation time is calculated by dividing x into t, where t represents the hours or minutes of exponential growth.

3.6.2.1 Growth on Solid Surfaces

If microorganisms are immobilised on a solid surface from which they can derive nutrients and remain moist, cell division will cause the daughter cells to form a localised colony. In spite of the small size of the individual organisms, colonies are easily visible to the naked eye. Indeed, microbial growth can often be seen on the tonsils of an infected individual or as colonies on discarded or badly stored foods. In the laboratory, solidified growth media are deployed to separate different types of bacteria and also as an aid to enumerating viable cell numbers. These media comprise a nutrient soup (broth) that has been solidified by the addition of agar (see Chapter 2). Agar melts and dissolves in boiling water but will not resolidify until the temperature is below 45 °C. Agar media are used in the laboratory either poured as a thin layer into a covered dish (Petri dish or plate) or contained within a small, capped bottle (slant). If suspensions of different species of bacteria are spread on to the surface of a nutrient agar plate, then each individual cell will produce a single visible colony. These may be counted to obtain an estimate of the original number of cells. Different species will produce colonies of slightly different appearance, enabling judgements to be made as to the population diversity. The colour, size, shape and texture of colonies of different species of bacteria vary considerably and form a useful diagnostic aid to identification. Transfer of single colonies from the plate to a slant enables pure cultures of each organism to be maintained, cultured and identified.

3.6.2.2 Growth in Liquids

When growing on a solid surface, the size of the resultant colony is governed by the local availability of nutrients. These must diffuse through the colony. Eventually growth ceases when the rate of consumption of nutrients exceeds the rate of supply. When grown in liquids, the bacteria, being of colloidal dimensions and sometimes highly motile, are dispersed evenly through the fluid. Nutrients are therefore equally available to all cells. When considering growth of bacterial populations in liquids, it is necessary to consider whether the environment is closed or open with respect to the acquisition of fresh nutrient. Closed systems are typified by batch culture in closed glass flasks. In these, waste products of metabolism are retained and all the available nutrients are present at the beginning of growth. Open systems, on the other hand, have a continual supply of fresh nutrients and removal of waste products.

Liquid Batch Culture (Closed)

Figure 3.8 shows the pattern of population growth obtained when a small sample of bacteria is placed within a suitable liquid growth medium held in a glass vessel. As the increase in cell numbers is exponential (1, 2, 4, 8, 16, *etc.*), then during active growth a logarithmic plot of cell number against time gives a straight line (B). This period is often referred to as the *logarithmic growth phase*, during which the generation or doubling time may be calculated from the slope of the line. However, the exponential phase is preceded by a *lag period* (A), during which time the inoculum adapts its physiology to that required for growth on the available nutrients. As growth proceeds, nutrients are consumed and waste materials accumulate. This has the effect of reducing the rate of growth (*late logarithmic phase*) towards an eventual halt (*stationary phase*, C). Starvation during the stationary phase will eventually lead to the death of some of the cells and adaptation to a dormant state in others (*decline phase*, D). Patterns of growth such as this occur within inadequately preserved pharmaceutical products, in water storage tanks and in industrial fermentations.

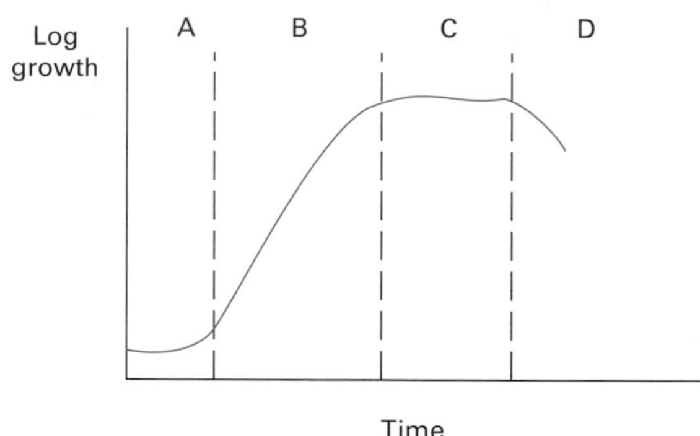

Figure 3.8 Typical bacterial growth curve in closed batch liquid culture: (A) lag or adaptive phase; (B) logarithmic or exponential phase; (C) stationary phase; (D) decline phase.

Growth in Open Culture

Except under circumstances of feast–famine, growth of bacteria in association with humans and in our environment is subject to a gradual but continuous provision of nutrients and a dilution of waste products. Under such circumstances, the rate of growth of bacteria is governed by the rate of supply of nutrients and the population size. Accordingly, bacteria in our gastrointestinal tracts receive a more or less continuous supply of food and excess bacteria are voided with the faeces (indeed, bacteria make up >90% of the dry mass of faeces). In many situations, the bacteria become immobilised, as a biofilm, upon a surface and extract nutrients from the bulk fluid phase.

3.6.3 Growth and Genetic Exchange

For many years, it was thought that bacteria, dividing by binary fission, had no opportunity for the exchange of genetic material and could only adapt and evolve through mutation of genes. This is not only untrue but masks the profound ability of bacteria to exchange and share DNA across diverse genera. This is of particular significance because it enables bacterial populations to adapt rapidly to changes in their environment, whether this is related to the appearance of a novel food or to the deployment of anti-bacterial chemicals and antibiotics. Three major processes of genetic exchange can be identified in bacteria – transformation, transduction and conjugation. Further details of these processes are given in Chapter 13 dealing with the development and spread of antibiotic resistance.

3.6.3.1 Transformation

In 1928, Griffith noticed that a culture of *Streptococcus pneumoniae* that had mutated to become deficient in capsule production could be restored to its normal capsulate form by incubation with a cell-free filtrate taken from a culture of the normal strain. While this discovery preceded the discovery of DNA as the genetic library and was only poorly understood at the time, it demonstrated the ability of certain types of bacteria to absorb small pieces of naked DNA from the environment that may recombine into the recipient chromosome. The process has become known as transformation and is likely to occur naturally in situations such as septic abscesses and in biofilms where high cell densities are associated with death and lysis of significant portions of the population. Transformation is also exploited in molecular biology as a means of transferring genes between different types of bacteria.

3.6.3.2 Transduction

Viruses are discussed more fully elsewhere (see Chapter 5); however, there is a group of viruses, called bacteriophages, which have bacterial cells as their hosts. These bacteriophages inject viral DNA into the host cell. This viral DNA is then replicated and transcribed at the expense of the host and assembled into new viral particles. Under normal circumstances, the host cell becomes lysed in order to release the viral progeny, but in exceptional circumstances, rather than enter a replication cycle, the viral DNA becomes incorporated, by recombination, into the chromosome of the bacterium. This is known as a *temperate phage*. The viral DNA thus forms part of the bacterial chromosome and will be copied to all daughter cells. Temperate phage will become active once again at a low frequency and phasing between temperate and lytic forms ensures the long-term survival of the virus. Occasionally during this transition back to the lytic form, the excision of the viral DNA from the bacterial chromosome is inaccurate. The resultant virus may then either be defective, if viral DNA has been lost, or it may carry additional DNA of bacterial origin. Subsequent temperate infections caused by the latter virions will result in this bacterial DNA having moved between cells: a process of gene movement known as *transduction*. As the host range of some bacteriophages is broad, such processes can move DNA between diverse species.

3.6.3.3 Conjugation

Conjugation is thought to have evolved through transduction, and relates to the generation of defective viral DNA. This can be transcribed to produce singular viral elements, which cannot assemble or lyse the host cell. Such DNA strands are known as *plasmids*. They are circular and can either be integrated into the main chromosome, in which case they are replicated along with the chromosome and passed to daughter cells, or they are separate from it and can replicate independently. The simplest form of plasmid is the F-factor (fertility factor); this can be transcribed at the cell membrane to generate an F-pilus within the cell envelope and cells containing an F-factor are designated F^+. The F-pilus is a hollow appendage that is capable of transferring DNA from one cell to another, through a process that is very similar to the injection of viral DNA into a cell during infection. In its simplest form, an unassociated F-factor will simply transfer a copy to a recipient cell, and such a transfer process is known as conjugation. Integration with, and dissociation of, the F-factor with the chromosome occurs randomly. When it is in the integrated form, designated Hfr (high frequency of recombination), not only can a copy of the plasmid DNA be transferred across the F-pilus but so also can a partial or complete copy of the donor chromosome. Subsequent recombination events incorporate the new DNA into the recipient chromosome.

Just as the excision of temperate viral DNA from the host chromosome could be inaccurate, and lead to additions and deletions from the sequence, so too can the F-factor gather chromosomal DNA as the host cells change from Hfr to F^+. In such instances, the plasmid that is formed will transfer not only itself but also this additional DNA into recipient cells. This is particularly significant because the unassociated plasmid can replicate autonomously from the chromosome to achieve a high copy number. It can also be transferred simultaneously to many recipient bacteria. If the transported DNA encoded a mechanism of antibiotic resistance (see Chapter 13), it would not be difficult to imagine how whole populations could rapidly acquire the resistance characteristics.

3.7 Environmental Factors that Influence Growth and Survival

The rate of growth of a microbial population depends on the nature and availability of water and nutrients, temperature, pH, the partial pressure of oxygen and solute concentrations. In many laboratory experiments, the microorganisms are provided with an excess of complex organic nutrients and are maintained at optimal pH and temperature. This enables growth to be very rapid and the results visualised within a relatively short time period. Such idealised conditions rarely exist in nature, where microorganisms not only compete with one another for nutrients but also grow under suboptimal conditions. Particular groups of organisms are adapted to survive under particular conditions; thus, Gram-negative bacteria tend to be aquatic, whereas Gram-positive bacteria tend to prefer more arid conditions such as the skin. The next two sections of this chapter will consider separately the physicochemical factors that affect growth and survival of bacteria, and the availability and nature of the available nutrients.

3.7.1 Physicochemical Factors that Affect Growth and Survival of Bacteria

3.7.1.1 Temperature

Earlier in this chapter, various classes of bacteria (thermophile, mesophile, etc.) were described according to the range of temperatures under which they could grow. The majority of bacteria that have medical or pharmaceutical significance are mesophiles and have optimal growth temperatures between ambient and body temperature (37 °C). Individual species of bacteria also have a range of temperatures under which they can actively grow and multiply (permissive temperatures). For every organism, there is a minimum temperature below which no growth occurs, an optimum temperature at which growth is most rapid and a maximum temperature above which growth is not possible (Figure 3.9). As temperatures rise, chemical and enzymic reactions within the cell proceed more rapidly, and growth becomes faster until an optimal rate is achieved. Beyond this temperature certain proteins may become irreversibly damaged through thermal lysis, resulting in a rapid loss of cell viability.

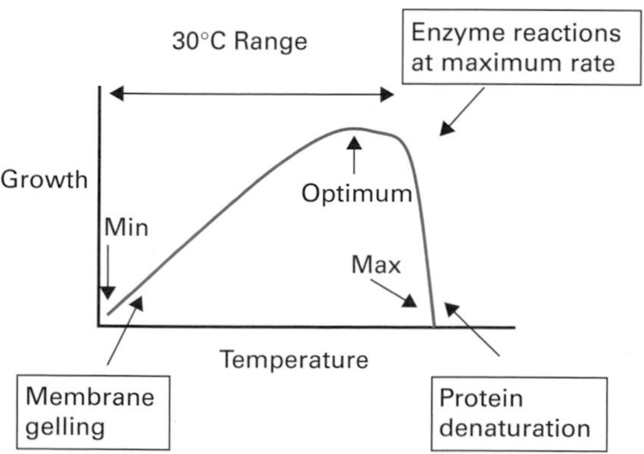

Figure 3.9 The effect of temperature on bacterial growth.

The optimum temperature for growth is much nearer the maximum value than the minimum, and the range of the permissive temperatures can be quite narrow (3–4 °C) for obligate pathogens yet broad (10–20 °C) for environmental isolates, reflecting the range of temperatures that they are likely to encounter in their specialised niches. If the temperature exceeds the permissive range, then provided that lethal temperatures are not achieved (approximately 60 °C for most Gram-negative mesophiles) the organisms will survive but not grow. Temperatures of 105 °C and above are rapidly lethal and can be deployed to sterilise materials and products. Generally, bacteria are able to survive temperatures beneath the permissive range provided that they are gradually acclimatised to them.

3.7.1.2 pH

As for temperature, each individual microorganism has an optimal pH for growth and a range about that optimum where growth can occur albeit at a slower pace. Unlike the response to temperature, pH effects on growth are bell-shaped (Figure 3.10), and extremes of pH can be lethal. Generally, those microorganisms that have medical or pharmaceutical significance have pH growth optima of between 7.4 and 7.6 but may grow suboptimally at pH values of 5–8.5. Thus, growth of lactobacilli within the vaginal vault reduces the pH to approximately 5.5 and prevents the growth of many opportunist pathogens. Accordingly, the pH of a pharmaceutical preparation may dictate the range of microorganisms that could potentially cause its spoilage.

3.7.1.3 Water Activity/Solutes

Water is essential for the growth of all known forms of life. Gram-negative bacteria are particularly adapted to an existence in, and are able to extract trace nutrients from, the most dilute environments. This adaptation has its limitations because the Gram-negative cell envelope cannot withstand the high internal osmotic pressures associated

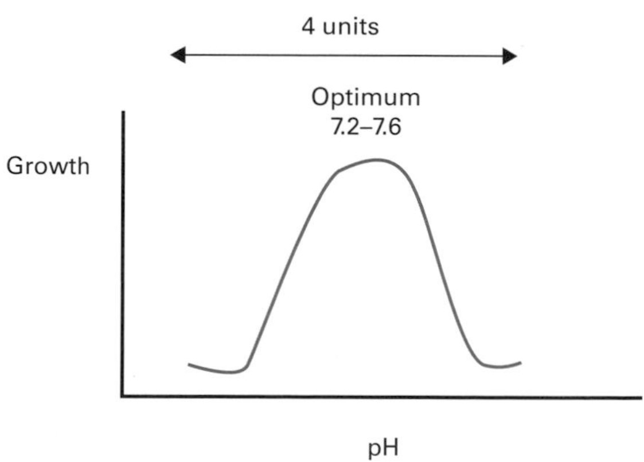

Figure 3.10 The effect of pH on bacterial growth.

with rapid rehydration after desiccation and the organisms are unable to grow in the presence of high concentrations of solute. The availability of water is reflected in the water activity of a material or liquid. Water activity (A_w) is defined as the vapour pressure of water in the space above the material relative to the vapour pressure above pure water at the same temperature and pressure. Pure water by definition has an A_w of 1.00. Pharmaceutical creams might have A_w values of 0.8–0.98, whereas strawberry jam might have an A_w of approximately 0.7. Generally Gram-negative bacteria cannot grow if the A_w is below 0.97, whereas Gram-positive bacteria can grow in materials with A_w of 0.8–0.98 and can survive rehydration after periods of desiccation, hence their dominance in the soil. Yeasts and moulds can grow at low A_w values, hence their appearance on moist bathroom walls and on the surface of jam. The water activity of a pharmaceutical product can markedly affect its vulnerability to spoilage contaminants (see Chapter 17).

3.7.1.4 Availability of Oxygen

For many aerobic microorganisms, oxygen acts as the terminal electron acceptor in respiration and is essential for growth. Alternative terminal electron acceptors are organic molecules whose reduction leads to the generation of organic acids such as lactic acid. They can sometimes be utilised under conditions of low oxygen or where carbon substrate is in excess (fermentation), and highly specialised groups of microorganisms can utilise inorganic materials such as iron as electron acceptors (e.g., iron–sulphur bacteria). Different groups of organisms therefore vary in their dependence on oxygen. Those that require oxygen and would die in the absence are known as obligate (strict) aerobes (e.g., *Bacillus subtilis*). When in the cell, oxygen can be broken down to oxygen radicals (O_2^-) which are poisonous. To be able to survive these, a bacterium must be able to produce the enzyme superoxide dismutase (SoD). This catalyses the reaction which converts the oxygen radical (superoxide: O_2^-) into ordinary molecular oxygen (O_2) and hydrogen peroxide (H_2O_2); the latter can be further broken down to water and molecular oxygen by the enzyme peroxidase, found in abundance in some bacteria.

There are many bacteria for which oxygen is highly toxic (*obligate anaerobes*, e.g., *Clostridium* species); they are killed by oxygen because they do not possess SoD. Hence, the presence or absence of oxygen within a nutrient environment can profoundly affect both the rate and nature of the microbial growth obtained and is an important consideration when attempting to grow clinical and environmental (manufacturing) contaminants. Strongly oxygen-dependent bacteria will tend to grow as a thin pellicle on the surfaces of liquid media where oxygen is most available. Special media and anaerobic chambers are required to grow obligate anaerobes within the laboratory, yet such organisms persist and actively grow within the general environment. This is because the close proximity of strongly aerobic cells and anaerobes will create an anoxic (much reduced or non-existent oxygen availability) microenvironment in which the anaerobe can flourish. This is particularly the case for the mouth and gastrointestinal tract where obligate anaerobes such as *Bacteroides* and *Fusobacter* can be found in association with strongly aerobic streptococci.

Facultative cells have a biochemical preference. A facultative anaerobe (e.g., *Staphylococcus* spp. or *E. coli*) prefers to grow in the presence of oxygen but can survive and grow in its absence, but at much reduced rates. Biochemically it is more favourable for the organism to grow in the presence of oxygen. Microaerophilic bacteria such as *Helicobacter* and *Campylobacter* require oxygen, but at much reduced levels to that normally found in the general environment (about 1–10%, well below the 21% found in the atmosphere). Aerotolerant bacteria are bacteria with an exclusively anaerobic (fermentative) type of metabolism, but they are insensitive to the presence of O_2. They live by fermentation alone whether or not O_2 is present in their environment.

The inability of oxygen to diffuse adequately into a liquid culture is often the factor that causes an onset of stationary phase, so culture density is limited by oxygen demand. The cell density at stationary phase can often be increased, therefore, by shaking the flask or providing baffles. Diffusion of oxygen may also be a factor limiting the size of bacterial colonies formed on an agar surface.

3.7.2 Nutrition and Growth

Bacteria vary considerably in their requirements for nutrients and in their ability to synthesise for themselves various vitamins and growth factors. Clearly the major elemental requirements for growth will match closely the elemental composition of the bacteria themselves. In this fashion, there is a need for the provision of carbon, nitrogen, water, phosphorus, potassium and sulphur with a minor requirement for trace elements such as magnesium, calcium and iron. The most independent classes of bacteria are able to derive much of their nutrition from simple inorganic forms of these elements. These organisms are called *chemolithotrophs* and can even utilise atmospheric carbon dioxide and nitrogen as sources of carbon and nitrogen. Indeed, such bacteria are, in addition to the green plants and algae, a major source of organic molecules and so they are more beneficial than problematic to humans. The majority of bacteria require a fixed carbon source, usually in the form of a sugar, but this may also be obtained from complex organic molecules such as benzene, paraffin waxes and proteins. Nitrogen can generally be obtained from ammonium ions but is also available by deamination of amino acids, which can thus provide both carbon and nitrogen sources simultaneously. Many classes of bacteria are auxotrophic and can grow on simple sugars together with ammonium ions, a source of potassium and trace elements. Such bacteria can synthesise for themselves all the amino acids and ancillary factors required for growth and division. These bacteria, for example, the pseudomonads and *Achromobacter* species, are generally free-living environmental strains, but they can sometimes cause infections in immunocompromised people. In the laboratory, they can be grown in simple salts media with few, if any, complex supplements. The rate of growth of such organisms depends not only on temperature and pH but also on the nature of the carbon and nitrogen sources. Thus, a faster rate of growth is often obtained when glucose or succinate is the carbon source rather than lactose or glycerol, and when amino acids are provided as sources of nitrogen rather than ammonium salts. If faced with a choice of carbon and nitrogen sources, bacteria will adapt their physiology to the preferred substrate and only when this is depleted will they turn their attention to the less preferred substrate. Growth in liquid cultures with dual provision of substrate such as this is often characterised by a second lag phase during the logarithmic growth period while this adaptation takes place. This is called *diauxic growth* (Figure 3.11).

As the association between bacteria and higher life forms becomes closer, then more and more preformed biosynthetic building blocks become available without the need to synthesise them from their basic elements.

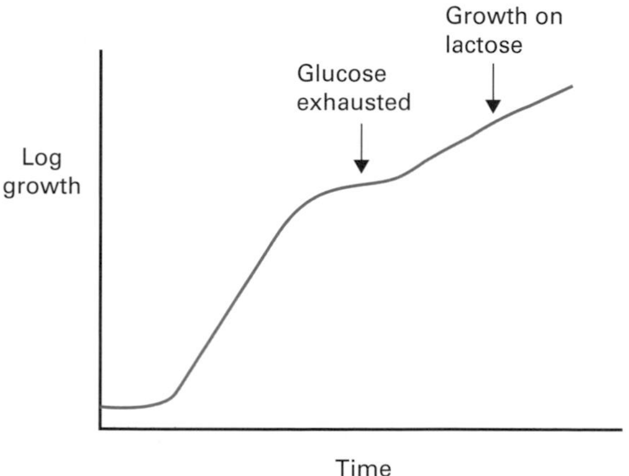

Figure 3.11 Diauxic growth on a mixture of glucose and lactose.

Thus, a pathogenic organism growing in soft tissues will have available to it glucose and metal ions from the blood and a whole plethora of amino acids, bases, vitamins, *etc.*, from lysed tissue cells. While most bacteria will utilise these when they are available, a number of bacteria that have become specialised pathogens have lost their ability to synthesise many of these chemicals themselves and so cannot grow in situations where the chemicals are not provided in the medium. Consequently, many pathogens require complex growth media if they are to be cultured *in vitro*.

The foregoing discussion about the physicochemical and nutritional constraints on bacterial growth has been based on laboratory studies. By definition, the only bacteria that we can describe in this way are those that can be cultured artificially. It cannot be overstated that a majority of bacterial species and genera cannot be cultured in the laboratory. In the past, the presence of such non-culturable bacteria has been attributed to moribund cells. With the advent of modern molecular tools, however, it has now been realised that these organisms are viable. By amplifying their DNA and sequence mapping, the genetic relationship of such bacteria to the culturable ones can be demonstrated and whole new families of hitherto unrecognised bacteria are being identified. It is possible that in the future many disease states currently thought to have no microbiological involvement could be identified as being of bacterial origin. A recent example of this has been the association of *Helicobacter pylori* with gastric ulcers and gastric cancers.

3.8 Detection, Identification and Characterisation of Organisms of Pharmaceutical and Medical Significance

There are many situations in which microorganisms must not only be detected and enumerated but where they must also be identified either to make a specific diagnosis of infection or to ensure the absence of specified bacteria from certain types of product. In such circumstances, various cultural approaches are available that deploy enrichment and selection media. Once a microorganism has been isolated in pure culture, usually from a single colony grown on an agar plate, then further characterisation may be made by the application of microscopy together with some relatively simple biochemical tests. Over the last 30 years, the biochemical characterisation of individual organisms has become simplified by the introduction of rapid identification systems. In recent years, molecular approaches have enabled identification of organisms without the need to culture them.

3.8.1 Culture Techniques

Conventional approaches to microbiological examination of specimens require that they be cultured to assess the total numbers of specific groups of microorganisms or to determine the presence or absence of particular named species. The majority of samples taken for examination contain mixtures of different species, so simple plating on to an agar surface may fail to detect an organism that is present at <2% of the total viable population. Various enrichment culture techniques may therefore be deployed to detect trace numbers of particular pathogens, prior to confirmatory identification.

3.8.1.1 Enumeration

The simplest way in which to enumerate the microorganisms that contaminate an object or liquid sample is to dilute that sample to varying degrees and inoculate the surface of a predried nutrient agar with known volumes of those dilutions (see Chapter 2). Individual viable bacteria that are able to grow on the nutrients provided and under the conditions of incubation will produce visible colonies that can be counted and the numbers related back to the original sample. Such counting procedures are often lengthy and tedious; the number of colonies formed might not relate to the viable number of cells, as clumps of cells will only produce a single colony and they will only detect a particular subset of the viable bacteria present in the sample that can grow under the chosen conditions. Accordingly, a variety of different media and cultural conditions are deployed to enumerate different categories of organism.

A number of techniques are currently being developed in order to speed up the enumeration process, although some of these rapid enumeration techniques indirectly measure the most probable number of viable cells.

Enumeration Media

Enumeration media will only ever culture a subset of cells towards which the medium and incubation conditions are directed. Thus, simple salts media with relatively simple sugars as carbon sources and trace levels of amino acids are often used to enumerate bacteria associated with water (e.g., R2A medium). Such plates may be incubated under aerobic or anaerobic conditions at a range of temperatures. Different temperatures will select for different subsets of cells; therefore, any description of a viable bacterial count must specify the incubation conditions. In medical microbiology, temperatures akin to the human body are often deployed because only those bacteria able to grow at such temperatures are likely to cause infection. However, psychrophilic Gram-negative bacteria (growing in water at 10 °C) can be a major source of bacterial pyrogen, so a variety of incubation temperatures are often used in monitoring pharmaceutical waters and products. Highly nutritious media, for example, blood agar, are also used as enumeration media. This is particularly the case when looking for microorganisms such as staphylococci that are usually found in association with animals and humans. Such agar plates may be deliberately exposed to air (settle plates) and the number of colonies formed related to the bacterial content of a room. In the pharmaceutical industry, microbiological monitoring will generally report the total aerobic count and, less commonly, the total anaerobic counts obtained on a moderately rich medium such as tryptone soya agar. Sometimes inhibitors of bacterial growth (e.g., Rose Bengal) can be added to a medium in order to select for moulds.

Rapid Enumeration Techniques

The detection and quantification of components of bacterial cells are considerably faster than those approaches requiring the growth of colonies, and estimates of total viable cell number can thereby be obtained within minutes rather than hours and days.

Some of the rapid methods that have been used for bacteria and other microorganisms, for example, bioluminescence, epifluorescence and impedance techniques, have been described in Chapter 2, but there are other rapid methods that have found more limited application; these will be considered here. In the examination of pharmaceutical waters and aqueous pharmaceutical products, electronic particle counters, for example, Coulter counters, can be used to determine bacterial concentration, although these instruments do not discriminate between living and dead cells. Similar counters are available that are able to analyse particles found in air. More advanced imaging and counting techniques, such as those employing fluorescence-activated cell sorters combined with specific vitality stains, do offer the potential to differentiate between viable and injured/dead bacteria and are being developed for this purpose. Other rapid techniques aim to detect microbial growth rather than to visualise individual cells and colonies. As bacteria grow in liquid culture, they not only alter the conductivity of the culture (see Chapter 2), but also generate small quantities of heat. The time taken to detect this heat can be directly related to the numbers of viable cells present by means of microcalorimeters. The metabolism of growing cultures can also be followed by manometric techniques to measure oxygen consumption or carbon dioxide production. Once again these are considerable improvements over conventional culture, but unlike particle counting and bioluminescence can only detect those organisms that are able to grow in the chosen medium.

None of the rapid techniques are able to isolate individual organisms. They do not therefore aid in the characterisation or identification of the contaminants, although growth-based techniques can employ liquid selective media (see below) to give presumptive information.

3.8.1.2 Enrichment Culture

Enrichment cultures are intended to increase the dominance of a numerically minor component of a mixed culture such that it can be readily detected on an agar plate. Enrichment media are always liquid and are intended to provide conditions that are favourable for the growth of the desired organism and unfavourable for the growth of other likely isolates. This can be achieved either through manipulation of the pH and tonicity of the medium or by the inclusion of chemicals that inhibit the growth of unwanted species. Thus, MacConkey broth contains bile salts that will inhibit the growth of non-enteric bacteria and may be used to enrich for Enterobacteriaceae. Several serial passages through enrichment broths may be made, and after enrichment it is not possible to relate the numbers of organisms detected back to that in the original sample.

3.8.1.3 Selective Media

Selective media are solidified enrichment broths, so again they are intended to suppress the growth of particular groups of bacteria and to allow the growth of others. The methods of creating this situation are the same as for enrichment broths. Thus, mannitol salt agar will favour the growth of micrococci and staphylococci, and cetrimide agar will favour the growth of pseudomonads. The use of selective media is an adjunct to characterising the nature of contaminants. Counts of colonies obtained on selective solid media are often documented as presumptive counts, so, for example, colonies formed on a MacConkey agar (containing bile salts) might be cited as a presumptive coliform count.

3.8.1.4 Identification Media (Diagnostic)

Identification media contain nutrients and reagents that indicate, usually through some form of colour formation, the presence of particular organisms. This enables them to be easily detected against a background of other species. In this fashion, inclusion of lactose sugar and a pH indicator into MacConkey agar facilitates the identification of colonies of bacteria that can ferment lactose. Fermentation leads to a reduction in pH within these colonies and can be detected by an acid shift in the pH indicator, usually to red. Lactose-fermenting coliforms, for example, *Escherichia* spp. and *Klebsiella* spp., can therefore be easily distinguished from non-fermentative coliforms, such as *Salmonella* spp. and *Shigella* spp. Similarly, the inclusion of egg-yolk lecithin into an agar gives it a cloudy appearance that clears around colonies of organisms that produce lecithinase (a virulence factor in staphylococci). While there are numerous types of selective and diagnostic media available, they can only be used as a guide to identification, but microscopy and biochemical or genetic characterisation are much more definitive.

3.8.2 Microscopy

Observation of stained and wet preparations of clinical specimens (blood, pus or sputum) and isolated pure cultures of bacteria from the manufacturing environment provides rapid and essential information to guide further identification. The application of simple stains such as the Gram stain can divide the various genera of bacteria into two convenient broad groups. The size and shapes of individual cells and their arrangement into clusters, chains and tetrads will also guide identification, as will specific stains for the presence of endospores, capsules, flagella and inclusion bodies. Examination of wet preparations can give an indication as to the motility status of the isolate, and these procedures all represent an important first stage in the identification process.

3.8.3 Biochemical Testing and Rapid Identification

The differing ability of bacteria to ferment sugars, glycosides and polyhydric alcohols is widely used to differentiate the Enterobacteriaceae and in diagnostic bacteriology generally. Fermentation can be indicated by pH changes in the medium with or without gas production visualised by the collection of bubbles in inverted tubes. More specialised media examine the ability of certain strains to oxidise or reduce particular substrates. There are many hundreds of individual biochemical tests available that each separately seek the presence of a particular enzyme or physiological activity. Taxonomic studies have led to the recognition that certain of these tests in combination characterise particular species of bacteria. Various long-established manuals such as *Bergey's Manual* (Holt et al 1994) and *Cowan and Steel's Manual for the Identification of Medically Important Bacteria* (Barrow and Feltham 2004) provide a logical and sequential framework for the conduct of such tests. Identification of particular species and genera by such processes is time-consuming, expensive and may require numerous media and reagents.

This process has become simplified in recent years by the development of rapid identification methods and kits. The latter often use multiwell microtitration plates that can be inoculated in a single operation either with an inoculated wire or with a suspension of a pure culture. Each individual well contains the medium and reagents for the conduct of a single biochemical test. Identification kits vary in their complexity and also in the precision of the identification made. Simple kits may perform only 8–15 tests, while more complex ones are capable of performing 96 simultaneous biochemical evaluations. Scoring of each test and entry into a computer database then allows the pattern of test results to be compared with a large panel of organisms and a probability of identity calculated. As different sets of tests will be required for different classes of bacteria, guidance as to the initial choice of kit is given on the basis of the Gram stain reaction, and the results of oxidase and catalase tests performed directly on isolated colonies. In large diagnostic laboratories and in quality assurance laboratories, automated systems are deployed that can inoculate, incubate and analyse hundreds of individual samples at a time.

3.8.4 Molecular Approaches to Identification

The need to identify microorganisms rapidly has led to the development of a number of molecular identification and characterisation tools. Increasingly, these have become routinely adopted in the analytical or diagnostic laboratory and will continue to be so in the future. The last few years have produced a revolution in the development of very sensitive, rapid, automated and reliable molecular methods used for identifying and differentiating for a variety of various species. A wide range of genome-based methods, particularly those that are polymerase-chain-reaction-based (for example, pulsed field gel electrophoresis, multilocus sequence typing and extragenic palindromic deoxyribonucleic acid sequencing), are useful in identifying bacteria as a complementary or alternative tool to phenotypic methods. One technique (denaturing gradient gel electrophoresis; DGGE) isolates and amplifies 16S ribosomal DNA, and, following sequencing of the bases, compares this with known sequences held in a reference library. This approach enables phylogenetic relationships to be derived even for those bacteria that have not previously been identified. Other systems examine the patterns of key constituents of the cells such as fatty acids and assign identities based on similarity matches to known reference cultures.

Molecular approaches can be especially useful when attempting to detect a particular species. Thus, gene probes carrying fluorescent dyes can be used in hybridisation procedures with the collected clinical material. Examination under the fluorescent microscope will show the targeted organism as fluorescent against a background of non-fluorescent organisms.

3.8.5 Pharmaceutically and Medically Relevant Microorganisms

Microorganisms of medical and pharmaceutical relevance can be broadly classified into those organisms that are harmful or problematic, and those that can be used to our advantage. Some microorganisms, depending on the situation, can fall into both categories. Microorganisms cause some of the most important diseases of humans and animals and they can also be found as major contaminants of pharmaceutical products. On the other hand, many large-scale industrial processes, for example, antibiotic production, are based on microorganisms, and selected species can be used to test disinfectant efficacy and to monitor sterilisation procedures. Tables 3.3 and 3.4, respectively, list examples of some of the more pharmaceutically relevant beneficial and problematic microorganisms. Specific texts should be referred to for more detailed descriptions.

Table 3.3 Examples of some pharmaceutically useful bacteria.

Organism	Characteristics	Pharmaceutical relevance
Actinomyces spp.	Gram-positive, filamentous rods	Antibiotic production
Bacillus atrophaeus (formerly *Bacillus subtilis*)	Gram-positive rod, aerobic, spore-former	Used to validate and monitor dry heat and ethylene oxide sterilisation processes
Bacillus pumilus	Gram-positive rod, aerobic, spore-former	Used to validate and monitor radiation sterilisation processes
Bordetella pertussis	Gram-negative rod, aerobe	Vaccine against whooping cough
Brevundimonas (formerly *Pseudomonas*) *diminuta*	Gram-negative, microaerobic rod	0.22 μm filter challenge test
Clostridium sporogenes	Gram-positive rod, anaerobe, spore-former	Used to confirm anaerobic growth conditions
Clostridium tetani	Gram-positive rod, anaerobe, spore-former	Vaccine against tetanus
Corynebacterium diphtheriae	Gram-positive rod, aerobe	Vaccine against diphtheria

Table 3.3 (Continued)

Organism	Characteristics	Pharmaceutical relevance
Escherichia coli	Gram-negative enteric rod, facultative anaerobe	Kelsey–Sykes disinfectant capacity test
		Preservative limit test
Geobacillus stearothermophilus (formerly *Bacillus stearothermophilus*)	Gram-positive rod, aerobic, spore-former	Used to validate and monitor moist heat sterilisation processes
Haemophilus influenzae type b	Gram-negative rod, aerobe	Vaccine against Hib infections
Leuconostoc mesenteroides	Gram-positive rod	Dextran production
Neisseria meningitidis	Gram-negative cocci, aerobic	Vaccine against meningitis C
Pseudomonas aeruginosa	Gram-negative, microaerobic rod	Alginate production
		Kelsey–Sykes disinfectant capacity test
Proteus vulgaris	Gram-negative, aerobic rod	Kelsey–Sykes disinfectant capacity test
Salmonella enterica serovar Typhi	Gram-negative enteric rod, facultative anaerobe	Chick–Martin/Rideal–Walker disinfectant coefficient test
Staphylococcus aureus	Gram-positive, facultative anaerobe, catalase-positive cocci	Kelsey–Sykes disinfectant capacity test
		Preservative limit test

Table 3.4 Examples of some pharmaceutically problematic bacteria.

Organism	Characteristics	Pharmaceutical relevance
Bacteroides fragilis	Gram-negative enteric rod, anaerobe	Wound infections
Bordetella pertussis	Gram-negative rod, aerobe	Causative agent of whooping cough
Campylobacter jejuni	Gram-negative enteric spiral rod, microaerophilic	Severe enteritis
Clostridium tetani	Gram-positive rod, anaerobe, spore-former	Causative agent of tetanus
Corynebacterium diphtheriae	Gram-positive rod, aerobe	Causative agent of diphtheria
Escherichia coli	Gram-negative enteric rod, facultative anaerobe	Food poisoning, severe enteritis
Haemophilus influenzae	Gram-negative rod, aerobe	Causative agent of infantile meningitis and chronic bronchitis
Legionella pneumophila	Gram-negative rod, aerobic	Causative agent of Legionnaires' disease
Mycobacterium tuberculosis	Gram-positive, acid-fast rod, aerobe	Causative agent of tuberculosis
		Disinfectant resistance
		Intracellular pathogen
Pseudomonas aeruginosa	Gram-negative, microaerobic rod	General environmental contaminant
		Quintessential opportunist pathogen
		High resistance to antibiotics and microbicides
		Biofilm-former
Salmonella spp.	Gram-negative enteric rods, facultative anaerobes	Varying degrees of food poisoning, typhoid fever
Staphylococcus aureus	Gram-positive, facultative anaerobe, catalase-positive cocci	Skin contaminant
		Food poisoning
		Toxic shock syndrome
		Pyogenic infections
Staphylococcus epidermidis	Gram-positive, facultative anaerobe, catalase-positive cocci	Implanted medical device/prosthetic device contaminant
		Biofilm-former
Streptococcus spp.	Gram-positive, catalase-negative cocci; many are facultative anaerobes	Causative agents of tonsillitis and scarlet fever

References

Barrow, G. and Feltham, R.K.A. (ed.) (2004). *Cowan and Steel's Manual for the Identification of Medical Bacteria*, 3e. Cambridge: Cambridge University Press.

Holt, G.H., Krieg, R.N., Sneath, A.H.P., Stanley, T.J., and William, S.T. (1994). Bergey's Manual of Determinative Bacteriology, 9e. Williams and Wilkins, Baltimore, USA.

Further Reading

Bauman, R.W. (2017). *Microbiology with Diseases by Body System*, 5e. San Francisco, CA: Pearson Benjamin Cummings.

Berg, J.M., Tymoczko, J.L., Gatto, G.J., and Stryer, L. (2019). *Biochemistry*, 9e. San Francisco, CA: W. H. Freeman & Co.

Delves, P.J., Martin, S.J., Burton, D.R., and Roitt, I.M. (2017). *Essential Immunology*, 13e. Oxford: Wiley-Blackwell.

Flemming, H.-C., Wingender, J., Szewzyk, U. et al. (2016). Biofilms: an emergent form of bacterial life. *Nat. Rev. Microbiol.* 14: 563–575.

Gould, G.W. (1985). Modification of resistance and dormancy. In: *Fundamental and Applied Aspects of Bacterial Spores* (ed. G.J. Dring, D.J. Ellar and G.W. Gould), 371–382. London: Academic Press.

Madigan, M.T., Bender, K.S., Buckley, D.H. et al. (2020). *Brock Biology of Microorganisms*, 16e. New Jersey: Pearson.

Sutherland, I.W. (2001). Biofilm exopolysaccharides: a strong and sticky framework. *Microbiology* 147: 3–9.

4

Fungi

Kevin Kavanagh

Professor of Microbiology, Department of Biology, Maynooth University, Maynooth, Co. Kildare, Ireland

CONTENTS

4.1 What Are Fungi?

Yeast, such as brewers' yeast, and moulds, such as *Penicillium chrysogenum* which produces the antibiotic penicillin, are classified as fungi. Yeast cells tend to grow as single cells which reproduce asexually in a process known as budding, although a minority of species (e.g., *Schizosaccharomyces pombe*) reproduce by fission. Many yeast species are capable of sexual reproduction and the formation of spores. By contrast, moulds (or filamentous fungi) grow as masses of overlapping and interlinking hyphal filaments (Figure 4.1) and reproduce by producing masses of spores or conidia in a variety of structures. This division between yeast and moulds based on growth morphology is not clear-cut, since some yeast can produce hyphae under specific conditions (e.g., *Candida albicans*), while many normally filamentous fungi possess a yeast-like phase at some point in their life cycle. Fungi are eukaryotic organisms, that is, their cells possess a nuclear membrane surrounding the nucleus; consequently there are many strong similarities between the biochemistry and genetics of fungal cells and vertebrate (human) cells. This partly explains why it can be difficult to kill pathogenic fungi, since agents that are toxic to them can also be toxic

Hugo and Russell's Pharmaceutical Microbiology, Ninth Edition. Edited by Brendan F. Gilmore and Stephen P. Denyer.

Companion website: https://www.wiley.com/go/HugoandRussells9e

to human cells. Fungi are widely distributed in nature, occurring as part of the normal flora on the body of warm-blooded animals, as decomposers of organic matter and as animal and plant pathogens. Medically, fungi are an extremely important group of microbes being responsible for a number of superficial infections of the skin (e.g., athlete's foot) and potentially fatal systemic diseases in humans (Table 4.1). By contrast, however, a significant number of fungi are of great benefit to humanity in terms of the production of alcoholic beverages, bread, enzymes and antibiotics (Table 4.2). Further, they have also been utilised for a range of molecular biological applications such as the production of recombinant proteins (e.g., glucagon and ecallantide).

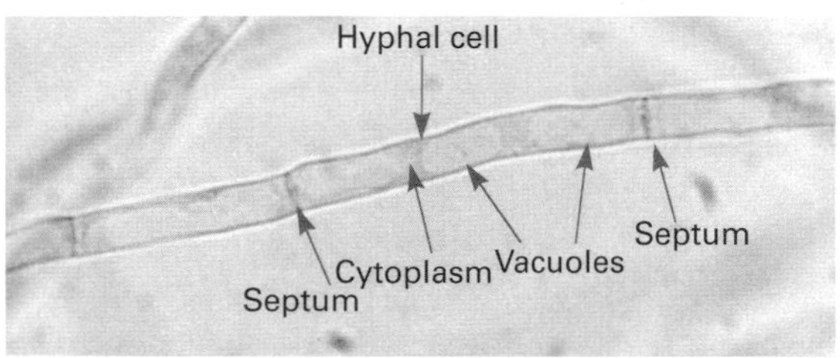

Figure 4.1 Septate hyphae of *Aspergillus fumigatus*.

4.2 Structure of the Fungal Cell

The typical yeast cell is oval in shape and is surrounded by a rigid cell wall which contains a number of structural polysaccharides and may account for up to 25% of the dry weight of the cell wall (Figure 4.2). Glucan accounts for 50–60%, mannan for 15–23% and chitin for 1–9% of the dry weight of the wall, respectively, with protein and lipids also present in smaller amounts. The thickness of the cell wall may vary during the lifetime of the cell; the average thickness in the yeast *C. albicans* varies from 100–300 nm. Glucan, the main structural component of the fungal cell wall, is a branched polymer of glucose which exists in three forms in the cell, that is, β-1,6-glucan, β-1,3-glucan and β-1,3–β-1,6-glucan complexed with chitin. Mannan is a polymer of the sugar mannose and is found in the outer layers of the cell wall. The third principal structural component, chitin, is concentrated in bud scars which are areas of the cell from which a bud has detached. Proteins and lipids are also present in the cell wall and under some conditions may represent up to 30% of the cell wall contents. Mannoproteins form a fibrillar layer that radiates from an internal skeletal layer which is in turn formed from the polysaccharide component of the cell wall. The innermost layer is rich in glucan and chitin, which provides rigidity to the wall and is important in regulating cell division.

Table 4.1 Examples of fungal diseases and selected causative agents.

Type of mycosis	Disease	Species name
Superficial	Pityriasis versicolor	*Malassezia furfur*
	White piedra	*Trichosporon beigelii*
Cutaneous	Tinea pedis (athlete's foot)	*Trichophyton rubrum*
	Onychomycosis (nail infection)	*Trichophyton rubrum*
	Tinea capitis (scalp ringworm)	*Trichophyton tonsurans*
Subcutaneous	Chromoblastomycosis	*Fonsecaea pedrosoi*
	Mycetoma	*Acremonium* spp.
Systemic	Blastomycosis	*Blastomyces dermatitidis*
	Histoplasmosis	*Histoplasma capsulatum*
	Coccidioidomycosis	*Coccidioides immitis*
	Paracoccidioidomycosis	*Paracoccidioides brasiliensis*
Opportunistic	Candidosis (superficial/systemic)	*Candida albicans*
		Candida glabrata
		Candida parapsilosis
	Aspergillosis	*Aspergillus fumigatus*
	Pneumonia	*Pneumocystis carinii*

Table 4.2 Examples of economically important fungi.

Fungal species	Application
Filamentous fungi	
Agaricus bisporus	Edible mushroom
Aspergillus, *Penicillium* spp.	Enzymes (catalase, lipase, amylase, etc.)
Aspergillus spp. + *Saccharomyces* spp.	Sake (rice wine)
Fusarium graminearum	Single-cell protein
Penicillium chrysogenum	Penicillin production
Penicillium notatum	Enzyme (glucose oxidase)
Penicillium roqueforti	Cheese flavouring (Roqueforti 'blue' cheese)
Yeast	
Pichia spp.	Gene expression system
Saccharomyces cerevisiae	Bakers' yeast – bread
	Brewers' yeast – beer, wine, cider, etc.
	Enzyme (invertase)
	Gene expression system
	Dietary supplement

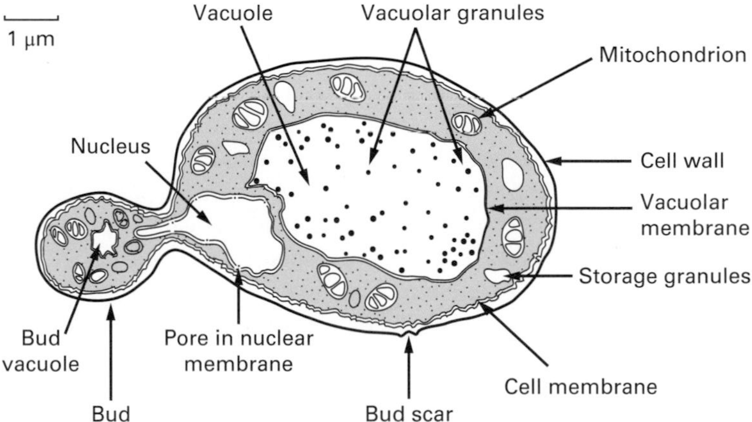

Figure 4.2 Diagrammatic representation of a 'typical' yeast fungal cell.

Enzymatic or mechanical removal of the cell wall leaves an osmotically fragile protoplast which will burst if not maintained in an osmotically stabilised environment. Incubation of such protoplasts in an osmotically stabilised agar growth medium will allow the re-synthesis of the wall and the resumption of normal cellular functions. The ability to generate fungal protoplasts affords the possibility of fusing protoplasts from distantly related fungi to generate strains with novel biotechnological application.

The periplasmic space is a thin region that lies directly below the cell wall. It contains secreted proteins that cannot pass out through the wall and is thus the location for a number of enzymes required for processing nutrients prior to their entry into the cell core. The cell membrane or plasmalemma is located directly underneath the periplasmic space and is a phospholipid bilayer which contains phospholipids, lipids, protein and sterols. The plasmalemma is approximately 10 nm thick and, in addition to being composed of phospholipids, also contains globular proteins. The dominant sterol in fungal cell membranes is ergosterol which is the target of the antifungal agent amphotericin B. Sterols are important components of the plasmalemma and create regions of rigidity within the fluidity provided by the phospholipid bilayer.

Most of the cell genome is concentrated in the nucleus; this is surrounded by a nuclear membrane which contains pores to allow communication with the rest of the cell (shown in Figure 4.2). The nucleus is a discrete organelle and, in addition to being the repository of the DNA, also contains proteins in the form of histones. Yeast chromosomes vary in size from 0.2 to 6 megabases (Mb) and the number per yeast cell is also variable with *Saccharomyces cerevisiae* having as many as 16, while the fission yeast *S. pombe* has as few as 3. In addition to the genetic material in the nucleus, the yeast cell often has extra-chromosomal information in the form of plasmids. For example, a 2 μm plasmid is present in *S. cerevisiae*, although its function is unclear, and there are killer plasmids in the yeast *Kluyveromyces lactis* which encode a toxin.

Actively respiring fungal cells possess distinct mitochondria which serve as the 'power-house' of the cell. The enzymes of the tricarboxylic acid cycle (Krebs cycle) are located within the matrix of the mitochondrion, while electron transport and oxidative phosphorylation occur in the mitochondrial inner membrane. The outer membrane contains enzymes involved in lipid biosynthesis. The mitochondrion is a semi-independent organelle possessing its own DNA and capable also of producing proteins using its own ribosomes which are referred to as mitoribosomes.

The typical fungal cell contains a vast number of ribosomes which are usually present in the form of polysomes – lines of ribosomes strung together by a strand of mRNA. Ribosomes are the site of protein biosynthesis. The system which mediates the export of proteins from the cell involves a number of membranous compartments including the Golgi apparatus, the endoplasmic reticulum and the plasmalemma. In addition, the vacuole is employed as a 'storage space' where nutrients, hydrolytic enzymes or metabolic intermediates are retained until required.

4.3 Medical Significance of Fungi

Fungi represent a significant group of pathogens capable of causing a wide range of diseases in humans under specific conditions (see Table 4.2). While the majority of fungi appear to be harmless, it is worth bearing in mind that a normally non-pathogenic fungus can cause a clinically relevant problem if the immune system is compromised as a result of therapy (e.g., immune suppression for receipt of an organ transplant) or disease (e.g., human immunodeficiency virus [HIV] infection or cancer). In the case of profound immunosuppression, the range of fungi that can present as capable of inducing disease is considerable.

The most frequent fungal pathogens of humans can be divided into three broad groups: yeasts, moulds and dermatophytes. The yeast *C. albicans* is the most frequently encountered human fungal pathogen, being responsible for a wide range of superficial and systemic infections. The superficial infections include oropharyngeal and genital candidosis, the former occurring predominantly in HIV-positive individuals, geriatrics and premature infants, and often arising when a weakened or immature immune system is present. Genital candidosis is very common and approximately 75% of women are affected by vulvovaginal candidosis (VVC) at stages during their life with a further 5–12% suffering from recurring bouts of infection over a prolonged period of time.

The mould *Aspergillus fumigatus* is the dominant fungal pulmonary pathogen of humans and generally presents as a problem in those with pre-existing lung disease or damage. In addition to pulmonary infection, other sites may be affected including the brain, kidneys and sinuses depending upon the level of immunocompromise suffered by the individual. Groups particularly susceptible to colonisation by *Aspergillus* species include those with cavities due to tuberculosis, patients affected with asthma or cystic fibrosis and those with profound immunosuppression due to leukaemia (neutropaenia). Aspergillosis presents as a serious problem in patients immunosuppressed in advance of organ transplantation. Pulmonary infections caused by *Aspergillus* spores released from hay and inhaled by farm workers are recognised and sometimes referred to as 'farmer's lung'.

Dermatophyte is the term applied to a range of fungi capable of colonising the skin, nails or hair. The principal dermatophytic fungi are *Trichophyton*, *Microsporum* and *Epidermophyton* species. The most commonly encountered dermatophytic infections are athlete's foot (infection of the foot) and ringworm (fungal infection of the scalp or skin).

Fungi can produce toxic secondary metabolites known as mycotoxins. These often have greatest health impact as contaminants of fungally spoiled foodstuffs, particularly poorly stored crops. Such toxins include: aflatoxins (*Aspergillus* spp.), ochratoxin (*Aspergillus* and *Penicillium* spp.), citrinin (*Penicillium* spp.) and patulin (*Aspergillus* and *Penicillium* spp.). Although there is a theoretical possibility of such toxins arising from contaminated pharmaceuticals, there is no evidence that this has occurred (see Chapter 17).

4.4 Antifungal Therapy

The choice and dose of an antifungal agent will depend upon the nature of the condition, whether there are any underlying diseases, the health of the patient and whether antifungal resistance has been identified as compromising therapy. Part of the difficulty in designing effective antifungal agents lies in the fact that fungi are eukaryotic organisms, so agents that will kill fungi may also have a deleterious effect on human tissue. The ideal antifungal drug should target a pathway or process specific to the fungal cell (see Chapter 12), thereby reducing the possibility of damaging tissue and inducing unwanted side effects. There are four principal classes of antifungal agents in clinical use today (see also Chapter 11).

4.4.1 Polyene Antifungals

Polyene antifungals are characterised by having a large macrolide ring of carbon atoms closed by the formation of an internal ester or lactone (Figure 4.3). In addition, polyenes have a large number of hydroxyl groups distributed along the macrolide ring on alternate carbon atoms. This combination of highly polar and non-polar regions within the molecule renders the polyenes amphipathic, that is, having hydrophobic and hydrophilic regions in the one molecule, which assists solubility in lipid membranes.

The principal polyenes are amphotericin B and nystatin. Amphotericin B is produced by the bacterium *Streptomyces nodosus* and its activity is due to the ability to bind ergosterol, which is the dominant sterol in fungal cell membranes, and consequently increase membrane permeability by the formation of pores (Figure 4.4). This action leads to fungal cell injury and death by the loss of intracellular contents through the pores. Amphotericin B is active against a broad range of fungal pathogens and is considered the 'gold standard' against which the activity of other antifungal

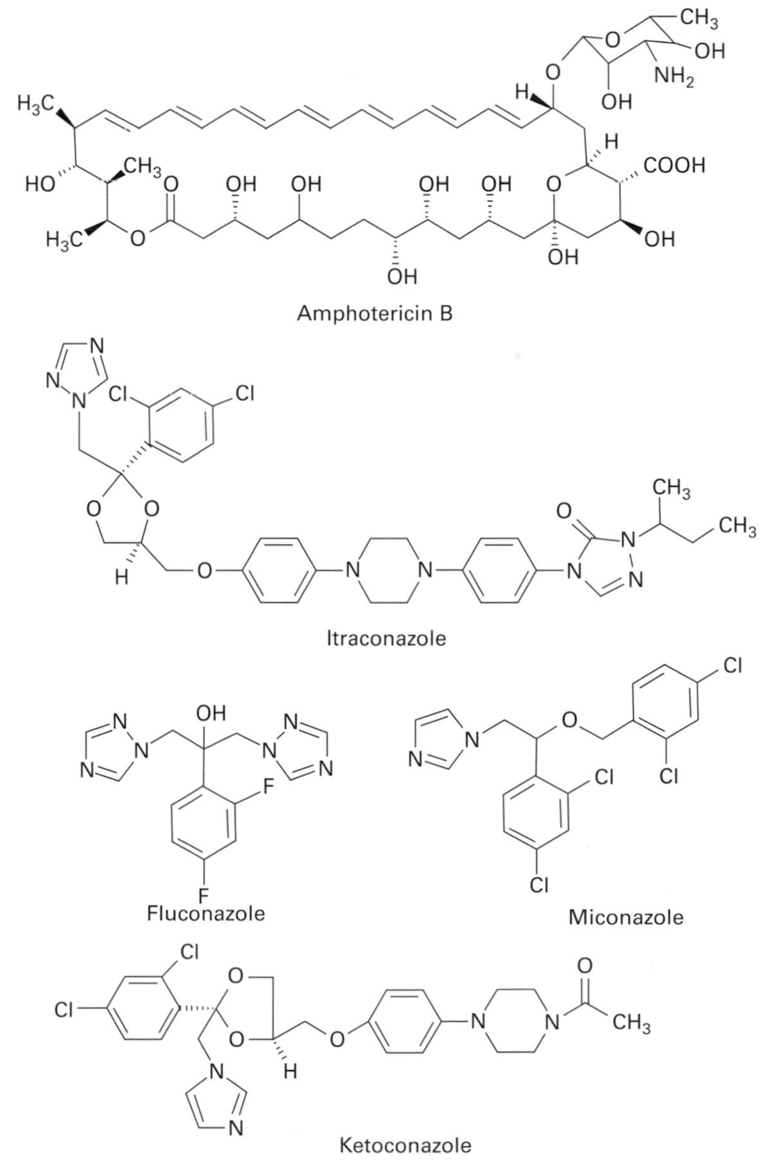

Figure 4.3 Structures of polyene (amphotericin B) and azole (itraconazole, fluconazole, miconazole and ketoconazole) antifungal agents.

Amphotericin B

Itraconazole

Fluconazole

Miconazole

Ketoconazole

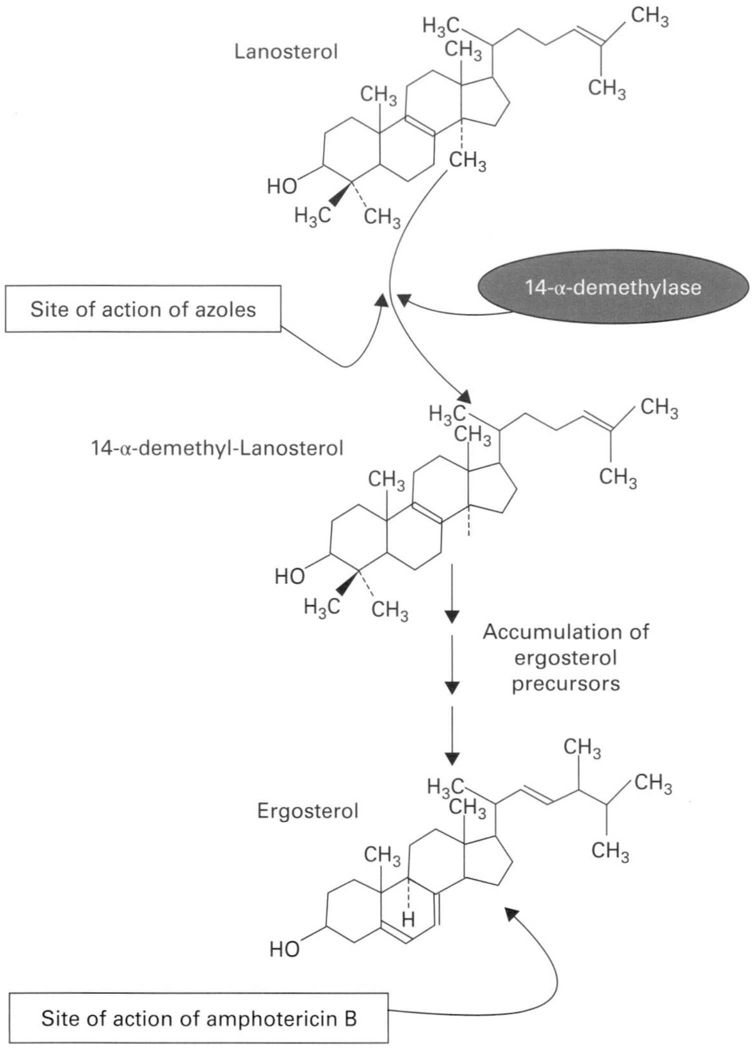

Figure 4.4 Modes of action of polyene (amphotericin B) and azole antifungal agents.

agents is often compared. Amphotericin B can lead to renal damage during prolonged antifungal therapy. Due to this renal toxicity, the drug tends to be reserved for severe cases of systemic fungal disease (e.g., invasive aspergillosis or systemic candidosis); promisingly, recent formulations in which the agent is encapsulated within liposomes have been shown to be of reduced toxicity.

Nystatin was discovered in 1950 and exhibits the same mode of action as amphotericin B, but tends to be of lower solubility, which has restricted its use to the treatment of topical infections. Although nystatin was effective for the treatment of conditions such as oral and vaginal candidosis, its use has been overtaken by the introduction of azole antifungal drugs.

Resistance to polyene antifungals is rare clinically, although it can be induced experimentally in the laboratory by altering the ergosterol content of the fungal cell membrane.

4.4.2 Azole Antifungals

The first generation of azole antifungals revolutionised the treatment of mucosal and invasive fungal infections, and azoles are still the most widely used group of antifungal agents. The azole derivatives are classified as imidazoles and triazoles on the basis of whether they have two or three nitrogen atoms in the five-membered azole ring (Figure 4.3). The azoles in routine clinical use are clotrimazole, miconazole, econazole and ketoconazole, while drugs such as itraconazole, fluconazole and voriconazole are finding important applications in the treatment of systemic infections. Azoles function by interfering with ergosterol biosynthesis by binding to the cytochrome-P450-mediated enzyme known as 14α-demethylase ($P450_{DM}$). This blocks the formation of ergosterol by preventing the demethylation of lanosterol (a precursor of ergosterol) (Figure 4.4). This results in a reduction in the amount of ergosterol in the fungal cell membrane which leads to membrane instability, growth inhibition and cell death. An additional consequence of the block in ergosterol biosynthesis is the build-up of toxic intermediates which can prove fatal to the cell.

Azoles exhibit a broad spectrum of activity *in vitro* being capable of inhibiting the growth of most *Candida*, *Cryptococcus* and *Aspergillus* species, and the dermatophytes. Miconazole was the first azole used to treat systemic fungal infections, but demonstrated a number of toxic side effects. Ketoconazole produced high serum concentrations upon oral administration but had poor activity against aspergillosis. In addition, ketoconazole was associated with a range of side effects which limited its applicability. Newer triazoles such as fluconazole and itraconazole have increased the options for dealing with fungal infections. Fluconazole was introduced for clinical use in 1990, is water soluble and shows good penetration and deposition into the pulmonary tissues, it also reaches high levels in the cerebrospinal fluid and the peritoneal fluids. Fluconazole has proved highly effective in the treatment of infections caused by *C. albicans* but shows limited activity against *Aspergillus*. Itraconazole, available for clinical use in the late 1980s, was the first azole with proven efficacy against *Aspergillus*. Itraconazole is effective in treating severe *Aspergillus* infections and exhibits both fungicidal and fungistatic effects. Upon ingestion, itraconazole undergoes extensive hepatic metabolism which yields up to 30 metabolites, a number of which retain antifungal activity. Itraconazole is currently available as an intravenous formulation and is widely used for the treatment of severe *Aspergillus* infection in this form. Fluconazole and itraconazole demonstrate significantly reduced side effects compared to ketoconazole. Novel azole drugs with increased ability to inhibit the fungal 14α-demethylase are also becoming available. These agents, which include voriconazole, posaconazole and ravuconazole, have a wider spectrum of activity than fluconazole and it has been suggested that some of them show fungicidal effects to some species (e.g., *Aspergillus* spp.). Voriconazole is one of the newest second-generation triazole antifungal drugs and it shows good activity against pulmonary aspergillosis and cerebral aspergillosis.

The use of azoles in therapy is being increasingly compromised by the appearance of resistance, particularly among yeasts of the genus *Candida*. Mutations in the *erg3* gene disrupt the formation of ergosterol and lead to increased accumulation of 14α-methylfecosterol which can substitute for ergosterol in the fungal cell membrane, thus conferring resistance. Mutation of the *erg11* gene results in alterations in the structure of 14α-demethylase and reduced binding by azoles, particularly fluconazole. Overexpression of *erg11* leads to increased levels of 14α-demethylase, meaning that insufficient amounts of azole can accumulate in the cell to bind to all copies of the enzyme. Cells express a number of different efflux pumps (e.g., major facilitator super family [MFS] and the adenosine triphosphate [ATP]-binding cassette super family) which normally expel xenobiotics from the cell and maintain homeostasis. Elevated abundance of efflux pumps in yeast cells can lead to expulsion of the antifungal drug before toxic levels can be achieved. For example, in *Candida dubliniensis*, increased expression of the multidrug resistance mutation 1 (MDR1) efflux family confers fluconazole resistance (Figure 4.5).

Clinical resistance to azole antifungal drugs is still very uncommon in *A. fumigatus*, but recently a number of environmental isolates have developed resistance to azoles, particularly itraconazole. It appears that the widespread use of triazole fungicides in agriculture to control the growth of pathogenic fungi in plants may be selecting for resistance in *A. fumigatus* populations which then have the potential to infect patients.

4.4.3 Echinocandins

The echinocandins are a relatively new group of antifungal agent and are semi-synthetic lipopeptides comprising a cyclic hexapeptide core connected to a lateral fatty acid chain. Three compounds from this group are currently in use: caspofungin, micafungin and anidulafungin (Figure 4.6). Unlike conventional antifungal therapy that targets ergosterol or its synthesis, the echinocandins prevent the synthesis of β-1,3-glucan, the major polymer of the fungal cell wall. This wall is essential to the fungus as it provides physical protection, maintains osmotic stability, regulates cell shape, acts as a scaffold for proteins, mediates cell–cell communication and is the site of a number of enzymatic reactions. Glucan is synthesised by β-1,3-glucan synthase which is composed of two subunits; echinocandins prevent the formation of this enzyme complex and thus β-1,3-glucan synthesis is prevented. Inhibition of β-1,3-glucan synthesis disrupts the structure of the growing cell wall, resulting in osmotic instability and ballooning-out of the intracellular contents as a result of high internal osmotic pressure leading, at high drug concentrations, to cell lysis.

Caspofungin has demonstrated *in vitro* antifungal activity against various filamentous fungi and yeasts. It has activity against different *Aspergillus* species including *A. fumigatus*, *A. flavus*, *A. niger* and *A. terreus*, but is considered to be more fungistatic than fungicidal. Conversely, caspofungin is particularly fungicidal against a range of *Candida* species including species that are resistant (e.g., *C. krusei*) or isolates that are less susceptible

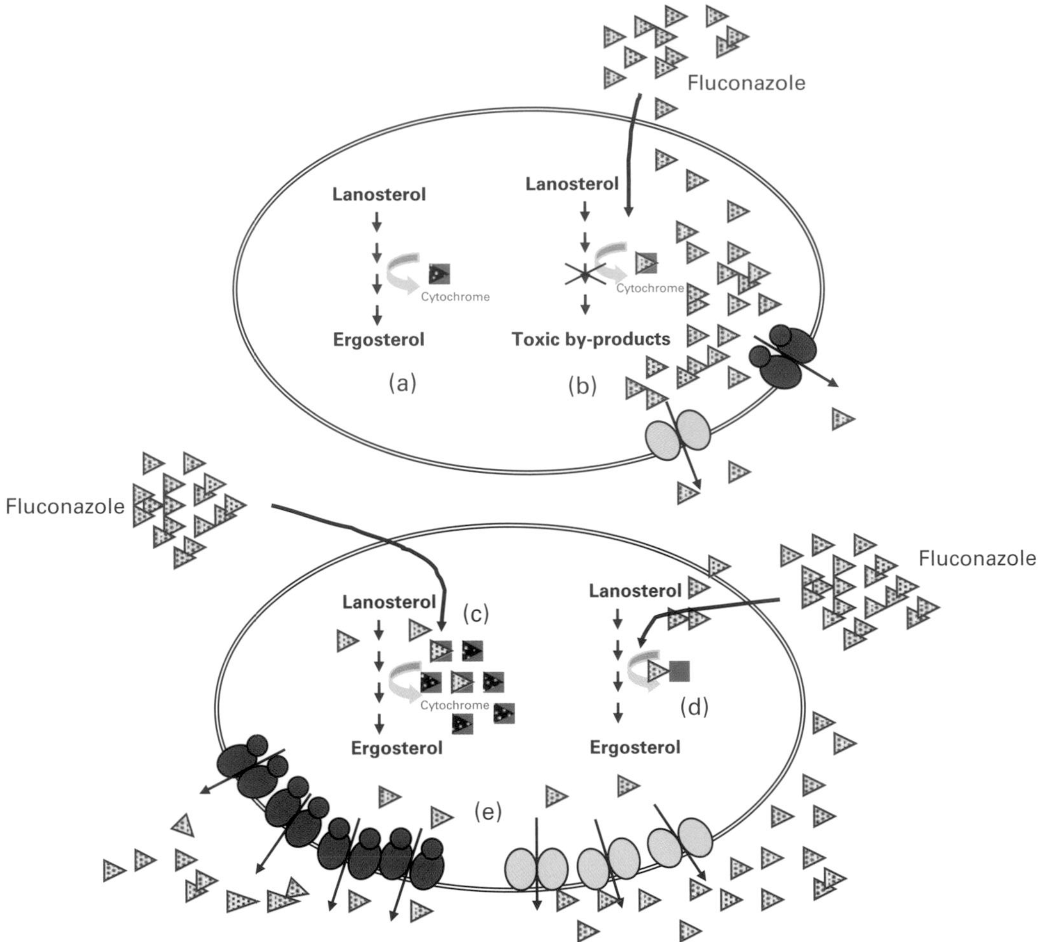

Figure 4.5 Mechanism of resistance to azole drugs commonly exhibited in *Candida albicans*: (a) ergosterol biosynthesis is catalysed by lanosterol 14α-demethylase (cytochrome); (b) azoles (e.g., fluconazole) inhibit the activity of 14α-demethylase leading to a build-up of toxic by-products in the cell and a reduction in the amount of ergosterol in the membrane; (c) overexpression of genes coding for 14α-demethylase leads to an abundance of the enzyme to which fluconazole binds; (d) alterations at the active site of the enzyme prevent the azoles binding; (e) increased abundance of transmembrane efflux pumps prevents toxic concentrations of drug being achieved in the cell.

(e.g., *C. dubliniensis* and *C. glabrata*) to azoles, or resistant to amphotericin B. Caspofungin shows little or no activity against a range of fungi including *Cryptococcus neoformans*, *Fusarium* spp. and *Histoplasma capsulatum*.

The fungal cell wall represents an attractive target and the echinocandins have proven to be a safer alternative to conventional antifungal therapies (i.e., polyenes and azoles). Echinocandins display a unique mode of action which results in defects in cell wall morphology and osmotic instability. As the cell wall is an essential component for stability and ultimately virulence, the targeting of the wall by echinocandins results in the efficient destruction of the fungal cell. Resistance to echinocandins is rarely encountered, but those cases that have been recorded have usually involved strains of *C. glabrata* that also show resistance to azoles. To avoid future problems with resistance, research will need to clarify the precise interactions of the echinocandins with the target enzyme, and fully examine the cell's complex response to this agent.

4.4.4 Synthetic Antifungal Agents

Flucytosine is a synthetic fluorinated pyrimidine which has been used as an oral antifungal agent and demonstrates good activity against a range of yeast species and moderate levels of activity against *Aspergillus* species. Two modes of action have been proposed for flucytosine. One involves the disruption of protein synthesis by the inhibition of DNA synthesis, while the other possible mode of action is the depletion of amino acid pools within the cell as a result of inhibition of protein synthesis. In general, yeast cells increase in size when exposed to levels of flucytosine lower than the minimum inhibitory concentration (MIC) and display alterations in their surface morphology, both of

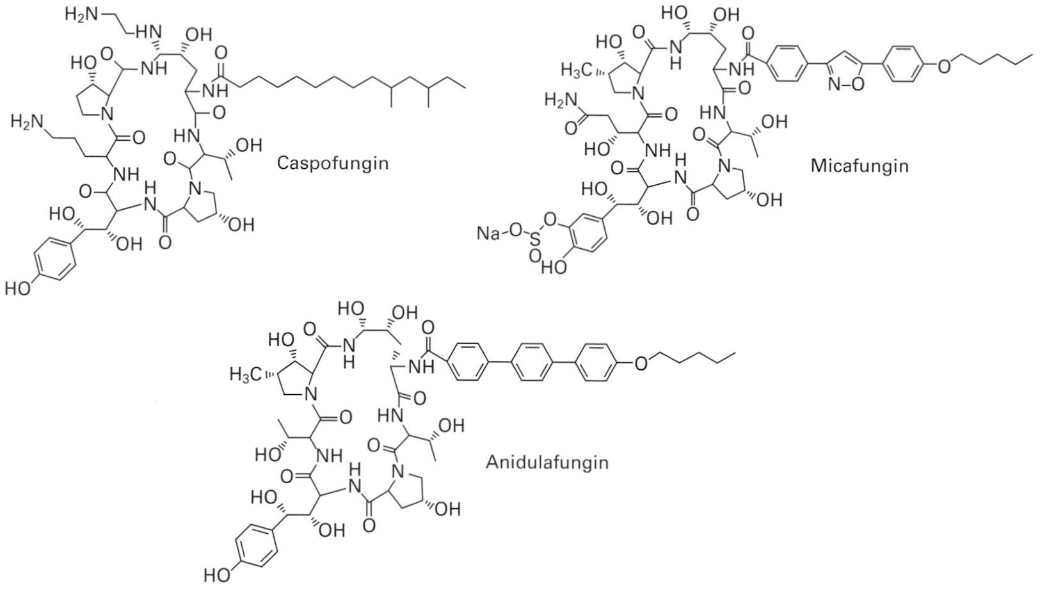

Figure 4.6 Structure of echinocandins.

which can be interpreted as a result of an imbalance in the control of cellular growth. Many fungi are inherently resistant to flucytosine or develop resistance after a relatively short exposure, and resistance has been attributed to alteration in the enzyme (cytosine deaminase) required to process flucytosine once inside the cell or to an elevation in the amount of pyrimidine synthesis. The problem of resistance has limited the use of flucytosine so that now it is generally used in combination with another antifungal agent (e.g., amphotericin B) where it can potentiate the effect of the second agent.

Functionalised allylamines (e.g., terbinafine and naftifine) inhibit the action of squalene epoxidase, an enzyme important for the conversion of squalene to squalene-2,3-epoxide which is an intermediate in the ergosterol synthesis pathway; a build-up of intracellular squalene can prove toxic for the fungal cell. Allylamines bind effectively to the *stratum corneum* because of their lipophilic nature and are therefore useful in the topical treatment of dermatophyte infections. Terbinafine, given orally, is the drug of choice for fungal nail infections.

4.5 Medically Important Fungal Pathogens of Humans

4.5.1 *Candida albicans*

The yeast *C. albicans* is an opportunistic fungal pathogen which can be present as a normal part of the body's microflora. *C. albicans* can induce a variety of superficial infections including oral and genital candidosis (often referred to as 'thrush') (Figure 4.7) and a range of systemic infections which can be difficult to diagnose, hard to treat and are frequently fatal. Systemic infection often leads to colonisation of the kidney, spleen and brain. Infection of the gastrointestinal tract is frequently seen in diabetics, cancer patients and people with acquired immunodeficiency syndrome (AIDS); the oesophagus is a common infection site, rendering swallowing difficult. The urinary tract can also be a site of candidosis which may be due to renal infection, other underlying disease(s) or cystitis. The presence of an indwelling urinary catheter may also predispose to *Candida* infection.

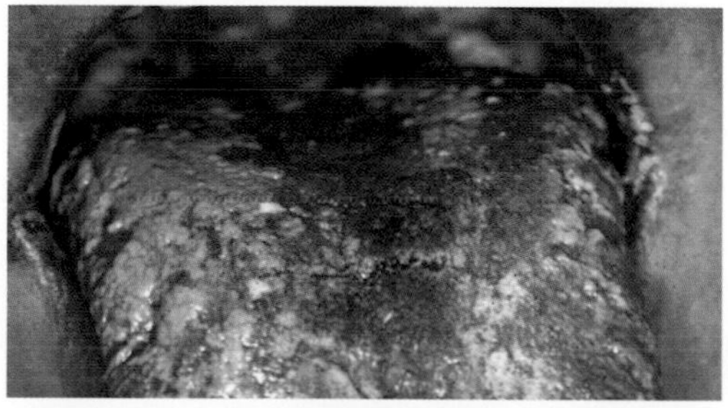

Figure 4.7 Oral candidosis. Note growth of yeast colonies (white plaque) on surface of tongue.

A range of factors are capable of pre-disposing the individual to superficial or systemic *Candida* infections. Factors which impair the host's immune system such as the presence of underlying disease (AIDS, cancer, diabetes, etc.), the use of immunosuppressive therapy during organ transplantation and broad-spectrum antibiotic therapy can leave the individual susceptible to candidosis. Other factors that may predispose to *Candida* infection include the presence of indwelling catheters and skin damage as a result of burns or other trauma.

C. albicans displays a variety of virulence factors which aid colonisation and persistence in the body. One of the most important of these factors is the ability to adhere to host tissue using a variety of mechanisms (Figure 4.8). The importance of adherence may be illustrated by the ability of *C. albicans* to attach to various mucosal surfaces and to withstand forces which might lead to its removal from the body, such as the bathing/washing action of body fluids. A hierarchy exists among *Candida* species indicating that the more common etiological agents of candidosis (*C. albicans* and *Candida tropicalis*) are more adherent to host tissue *in vitro* than relatively non-pathogenic species such as *C. krusei* and *Candida guilliermondii*.

Adherence to host tissue is achieved through a combination of specific and non-specific mechanisms. Specific adherence mechanisms include ligand–receptor interactions, while non-specific mechanisms include electrostatic forces, aggregation and cell surface hydrophobicity.

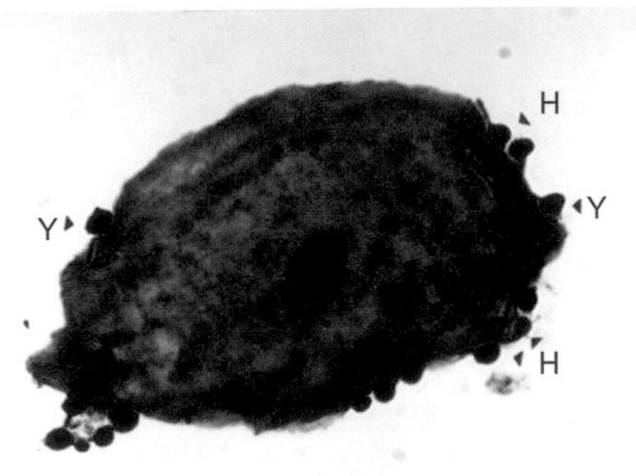

Figure 4.8 Cells of *C. albicans* (arrows) adhering to a human buccal epithelial cell. Y, yeast cells; H, hyphal cells.

Non-specific interactions, which occur over longer distances, are the primary mechanism involved in the initial adherence process and are reversible. Non-specific adherence subsequently becomes irreversible, however, as shorter-range specific interactions come into play that involve the ability of the yeast to recognise a variety of host cell receptors/ligands using cell-surface molecules. Adherence to host tissue gives *C. albicans* the ability to form biofilms (see Chapter 8) which protect the yeast from the host's immune response and form a focal point for dissemination throughout the body.

C. albicans can exist in two morphologically distinct forms: budding blastospores or hyphae (Figure 4.9a,b). The yeast can switch between each form and is usually encountered in tissue samples in both morphological forms (Figure 4.10). The hyphae are capable of thigmotropism (contact sensing) which may assist in finding the line of least resistance between and through layers of cells in tissue. *C. albicans* produces a range of extracellular enzymes which facilitate adherence and/or tissue penetration. Phospholipase A, B, C and lysophospholipase may function to damage host cell membranes and facilitate invasion. *C. albicans* produces a range of acid proteinases which have been shown to aid adherence and invasion but which also play an important role in the degradation of the immunoglobulins IgG and IgA. There are now known to be at least 10 members of the secreted aspartic proteinase (SAP) family and these have a low pH optimum which may assist in the colonisation of the vagina. Haemolysin production by *C. albicans* has also been documented and seems to be important in allowing the yeast to access iron released from ruptured red blood cells. An important immune evasion tactic of *C. albicans* is the ability to bind to platelets via fibrinogen-binding ligands which results in the fungal cell being surrounded by a cluster of platelets.

C. albicans is capable of giving rise to a variety of interconvertible phenotypes which can be considered as

(a)

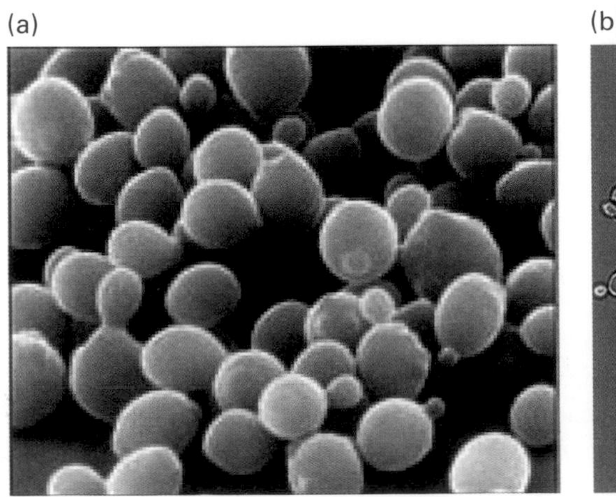

(b)

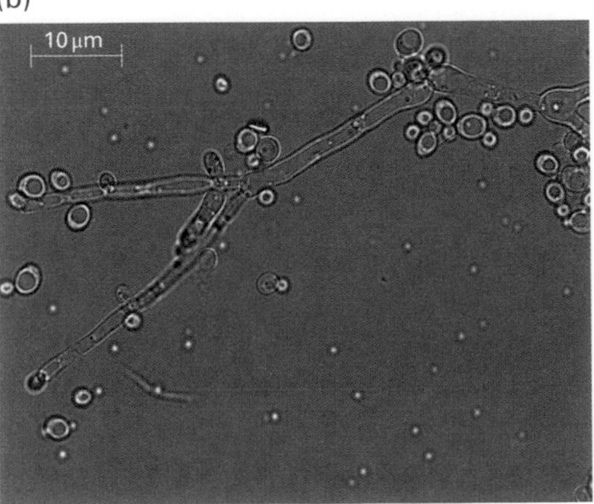

Figure 4.9 (a) Blastospores and (b) hyphae of *Candida albicans*.

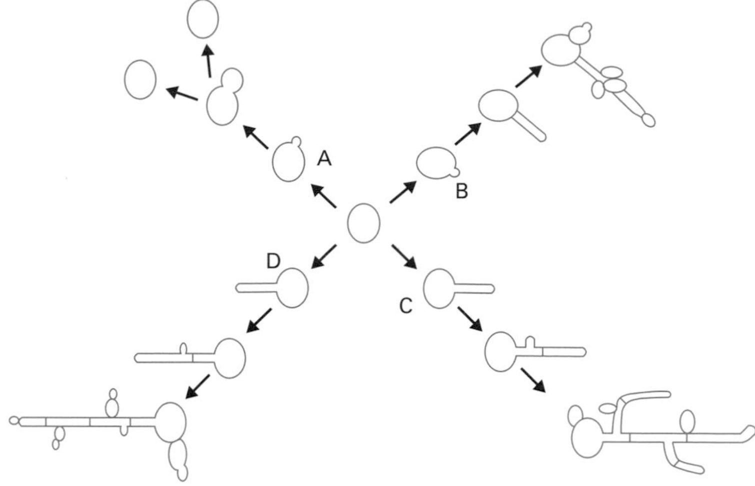

Figure 4.10 Growth morphologies of *Candida albicans*: (A) budding morphology; (B) hyphal formation; (C) germ-tube formation leading to hyphal formation; (D) pseudohyphal formation.

providing an extra dimension to the existing virulence factors associated with this yeast. A number of switching systems have been identified and phenotypic switching may have evolved to compensate for the lack of variation achieved in other organisms that utilise sexual reproduction. Phenotypic switching allows the yeast to exploit micro-niches in the body and alters a variety of factors (e.g., antifungal drug resistance, adherence and extracellular enzyme production) in addition to the actual phenotype and so may be considered as the 'dominant' or 'controlling' virulence factor.

In terms of tissue colonisation and invasion, adherence is the initial step in the process. Once the yeast has adhered, enzymes (phospholipase and proteinase) can facilitate further adherence by damaging or degrading cell membranes and extracellular proteins. Hyphae may be produced and penetrate layers of cells using thigmotropism to find the line of least resistance. The passage through cells is undoubtedly aided by the production of extracellular enzymes. Once endothelial cells are reached, enzymes may assist in the degradation of tissue and allow the yeast to enter the host's blood stream where phenotypic switching or coating with platelets may be used to evade the immune system. While in the blood stream, the haemolysin may function to lyse blood cells and release iron which is essential for growth. Escape from the blood stream involves adherence to the walls of capillaries and passage across the wall.

4.5.2 *Aspergillus fumigatus*

A. fumigatus is a saprophytic fungus which is widely distributed in nature where it is frequently encountered growing on decaying vegetation and damp surfaces (Figure 4.11). *A. fumigatus* can present as an opportunistic pathogen of humans and is the commonest etiological agent of pulmonary aspergillosis, being responsible for 80–90% of cases. While the incidence of disease due to *Aspergillus* species is less than that due to *Candida,* aspergillosis results in a greater mortality.

A. fumigatus produces a number of extracellular enzymes which facilitate growth in the lung and dissemination through the body. Phospholipase production has been shown in clinical isolates of this fungus with optimal production occurring at 37 °C. This enzyme plays a crucial role in tissue degradation and may facilitate exit of the fungus from the lung into the blood stream. Fungal proteases are responsible for tissue degradation and neutralisation of the immune system and probably evolved to allow the fungus to degrade animal and plant material. Elastin constitutes almost 30% of lung tissue and many *A. fumigatus* isolates display elastinolytic activity, while isolates incapable of elastinase production display reduced virulence in mice. *A. fumigatus* produces two elastinases: a serine protease and a metalloproteinase. Apart from their direct role in tissue degradation, *A. fumigatus* proteases (in particular the serine protease) may also function as allergens which may be important in the induction and persistence of allergic aspergillosis. Local inflammation due to the presence of proteases results in airway damage and *in vitro* studies have shown that proteases are capable of inducing epithelial cell detachment from basement membranes. Such desquamation may partly explain the extent of damage seen in the lungs of asthmatic and cystic fibrosis patients affected with allergic aspergillosis. In addition, proteases induce the release of the proinflammatory IL-6 and IL-8 cytokines in cell lines derived from airway epithelial cells which may induce a mucosal inflammatory response and subsequent damage to the surrounding tissue.

The production and secretion of toxins into surrounding tissues by the proliferating fungus is regarded as an

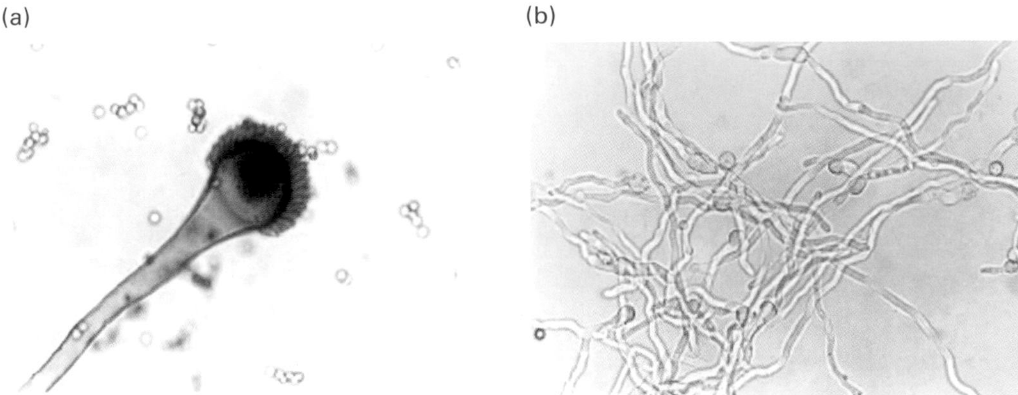

Figure 4.11 (a) Conidiophore and (b) germinating conidia after incubation of *Aspergillus fumigatus* at 37 °C.

important virulence attribute and may facilitate fungal growth in the lung. Gliotoxin is the main toxin produced by *A. fumigatus*, others include helvolic acid, fumigatin and fumagillin. It is believed that toxins play a significant role in facilitating the colonisation of the lung by the fungus, since they can act to retard elements of the local immunity (e.g., gliotoxin inhibits the action of neutrophils). Significantly, *Aspergillus* species that do not produce toxins to the same extent as *A. fumigatus* isolates are rarely seen in clinical cases.

4.5.3 *Histoplasma capsulatum*

H. capsulatum is a dimorphic fungus which is the cause of histoplasmosis, the most prevalent fungal pulmonary infection in the USA. Histoplasmosis is common among AIDS patients but is also found among infants and elderly people living in endemic areas who may be susceptible to infection due to impaired immune function. The mortality rate among infants exposed to a large dose of *H. capsulatum* may be 40–50%. *H. capsulatum* grows in the mycelial form in soil, while in tissue it is encountered as round budding cells. Its natural habitat is soil that has been enriched with the droppings of bats or birds, and disturbance of such soil by natural (e.g., wind) or human (e.g., agriculture) activities releases large numbers of airborne spores that upon inhalation can establish pulmonary infection in individuals or in populations distant from the original source of spores.

Upon inhalation of *H. capsulatum,* pulmonary macrophages engulf the yeast cells and provide a protected environment for that yeast to multiply and disseminate from the lungs to other tissues. The ability to survive within the hostile environment offered by the macrophage is the key to the success of *H. capsulatum* as a pathogen. Normal individuals who inhale a large number of *H. capsulatum* spores can develop a non-specific flu-like illness associated with fever, chills, headache and chest pains after a 3-week incubation period that resolves without treatment. Chronic pulmonary histoplasmosis is seen in men in the 45–55-year age group who may have been exposed to low levels of spores over a long period of time. The condition is progressive, and leads to a loss of lung function and death if untreated.

4.5.4 *Cryptococcus neoformans*

C. neoformans is an encapsulated yeast that is most frequently associated with infection in immunocompromised patients particularly those with AIDS where meningitis is the most common clinical manifestation. *C. neoformans* is a facultative intracellular pathogen that is capable of surviving and replicating within macrophages and withstanding the lytic activity within these cells. In order to survive within macrophages, *C. neoformans* appears to accumulate polysaccharides within a cytoplasmic vesicle. As part of its survival strategy, *C. neoformans* also produces melanin, which has the ability to bind and protect against microbicidal peptides. In addition, melaninisation may allow the cell to withstand the effects of harmful hydroxyl radicals and so survive in hostile environments. The capsule of *C. neoformans* is a virulence factor in that it protects the cell from the immune response, and capsular material (glucuronoxylomannans) induces the shedding of host cell adherence molecules required for the migration of host inflammatory cells to the site of infection, thus explaining the reduced inflammatory response to this yeast.

In immunocompromised patients, pulmonary infection can lead to disseminated forms of the disease where the eyes, skin, and bones become infected. Cryptococcal meningitis is particularly associated with AIDS patients where it is a major cause of death. While cryptococcosis may be controlled by antifungal therapy, in AIDS patients there is a danger of relapse unless that therapy is constantly maintained.

4.5.5 Dermatophytes

The dermatophytes are a group of keratinophilic fungi which can metabolise keratin, the principal protein in skin, nails and hair (Figure 4.12a,b). Tinea capitis is defined as the infection of the hair and scalp with a dermatophyte, usually *Microsporum canis* or *Trichophyton violaceum*. In Europe and North Africa, *T. violaceum* may be responsible for approximately 60% of cases of tinea capitis. This condition is characterised by a mild scaling and loss of hair and, in some cases, it may be contagious. Tinea corporis is characterised by infection of the skin of the trunk, leg and arms with a dermatophyte and is usually caused by *Trichophyton* spp., *Microsporum* spp. or *Epidermophyton floccosum*. Lesions are itchy, dry and show scaling. Typically, lesions retain a circular morphology and the condition is often referred to as 'ringworm'. Tinea cruris is seen where the skin of the groin is infected with a dermatophytic fungus, usually *E. floccosum* or *Trichophyton rubrum*. This condition is highly contagious via fomites (towels, sheets, etc.) and up to 25% of patients show recurrence following antifungal therapy. Tinea pedis presents as a dermatophyte infection of the feet; it is very common and easily contracted. The principal fungi responsible for this condition are *T. rubrum* and *E. floccosum* and the sites of infection may include the webs of the toes, the sides of the feet or the soles of the feet. Tinea manuum is a fungal infection of the hands and can be caused by a range of fungi most notably *Trichophyton mentagrophytes*. Infection is often seen in association with eczema and can result from transmission of fungi from another infected body site. Tinea unguium is defined as infection of the fingernails or toenails and is often described as onychomycosis which includes infections due to a range of other fungi, bacteria and nail damage associated with certain disease states (e.g., psoriasis).

4.6 Emerging Fungal Pathogens

In recent years, a number of fungal species previously regarded as non-pathogenic have emerged as causes of disease in certain groups of patients (e.g., HIV-positive patients, cancer patients and transplant patients). While a number of these fungal species may have been causing disease previously, their emergence as significant pathogens is a cause of great concern. Undoubtedly, the ability to keep immunocompromised patients alive for long periods is providing a set of novel niches for fungi, as is the introduction of novel drugs and therapies. This section will focus on a number of emerging fungal pathogens and demonstrates how the availability of novel opportunities has facilitated the appearance of this group of fungal pathogens.

4.6.1 *Saccharomyces cerevisiae*

The yeast *Saccharomyces cerevisiae* is widely distributed in nature and has been used for millennia in the production of bread and alcoholic beverages, and can be consumed directly as a dietary supplement. Traditionally, it is better known as brewer's or baker's yeast. Due to the ease with which it can be genetically and biochemically manipulated, it is probably the most studied and best characterised organism on the planet. Recently, a considerable number of reports have implicated this yeast as a cause of disease in immunocompromised patients but also in those with no

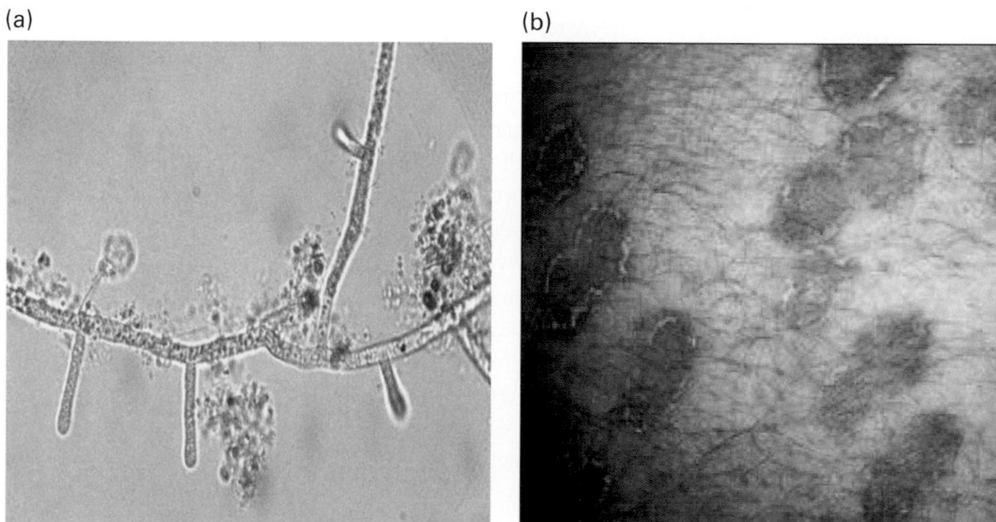

Figure 4.12 Dermatophytic infections. (a) Hyphae of *Microsporum canis* and (b) a dermatophytic infection of the skin.

apparent predisposing conditions. As a result, *S. cerevisiae* is no longer regarded as a GRAS ('generally regarded as safe') organism, but is now classified as a Biosafety Level 1 pathogen indicating that it can cause superficial or mild systemic infections in certain instances. This change of status has serious implications for industries using this yeast and indicates that, in cases of impairment of the immune system, what was once regarded as a harmless yeast is capable of causing life-threatening illness.

S. cerevisiae has been implicated in a number of superficial and systemic cases of disease and often in patients who have no apparent predisposing illness. In the majority of cases, it has been found in association with other microbes, but in a significant number of instances it was identified as the sole pathogen. It has been identified as a cause of vulvovaginitis in women, being responsible for up to 5% of cases, and is responsible for pneumonia and widespread dissemination in AIDS patients. Other conditions attributed to this yeast include septicaemia, postoperative peritonitis and the induction of fever and coughs in transplant patients. In one instance, a bone marrow transplant (BMT) patient taking a self-prescribed course of brewer's yeast tablets developed a fever, cough and chest pains. *S. cerevisiae* was isolated from the lung and identified as the source of the infection. In relation to BMT patients, the contamination of food with *S. cerevisiae* is now regarded as a potential source of infection.

Isolates of *S. cerevisiae* that have been associated with disease display a number of attributes that facilitate their persistence and dissemination in the host. Clinical isolates show the ability to grow at 42 °C, which is significantly greater than the upper temperature range for brewing yeast. This ability is regarded as important, since febrile patients can reach this temperature and it is therefore advantageous for a pathogenic microorganism to survive at this elevated temperature. Pathogenic isolates are capable of producing a number of extracellular enzymes such as acid proteinases and phospholipases which play a role in modulating the immune system's response to infection and allow the degradation of cell membranes, respectively. Isolates also demonstrate the ability to grow in a pseudohyphal form which may assist in the penetration of tissue. Brewing strains of *S. cerevisiae* are known to flocculate at the end of the fermentation process and this phenomenon is also seen in pathogenic isolates where it plays a role in obstructing capillaries, particularly in the brain, with concomitant damage to surrounding tissue. Pathogenic isolates adhere to epithelial tissue via a proteinaceous adhesin which is critical to the survival of the yeast in areas where it could be washed away by the action of swallowing as in the mouth. Potentially, the most important attribute of virulent isolates is their ability to alter their phenotype. In clinical isolates of *S. cerevisiae,* this ability contributes to the yeast's persistence in the body where, in complement factor 5 mice, isolates were capable of persisting in the brain for up to 7 days without being cleared.

Conventional therapy for superficial or systemic *S. cerevisiae* infection relies upon the use of azoles or polyenes. Interestingly, clinical isolates demonstrate a high level of resistance to fluconazole which has been regarded as the first choice for the treatment of *C. albicans*-induced superficial candidosis in HIV-positive individuals. While the mechanism that confers resistance to fluconazole in *S. cerevisiae* is still poorly characterised, it is thought to be mediated via a multidrug efflux pump which would remove the drug from the cell before it can act.

4.6.2 Non-*albicans Candida* Species

The rather cumbersome term 'non-*albicans Candida* species' covers a range of *Candida* species that have emerged as significant human pathogens in recent years. The principal species are *C. dubliniensis*, *C. krusei*, *C. glabrata* and recently *Candida auris,* although it must be emphasised that other *Candida* species may be problematic in specific situations. All the emerging *Candida* species share a number of common characteristics, that is, they were either unknown or regarded as inconsequential pathogens until recently and their emergence as significant causes of disease has occurred by exploiting a series of novel niches produced either as a result of therapy or disease.

C. dubliniensis was first identified in 1995 in samples taken from HIV-positive patients suffering from oropharyngeal candidosis. Upon streaking samples on CHROMagar plates, *C. albicans* appeared green but the newly discovered *C. dubliniensis* produced colonies displaying a different shade of green. The yeast is similar to *C. albicans* in many ways but displays different carbohydrate assimilation and DNA restriction patterns. This yeast has been identified in HIV-positive and -negative populations from many parts of the world and is now the dominant cause of oral candidosis in the former group. The discovery of *C. dubliniensis* demonstrates that the provision of a novel niche allows previously unrecognised pathogens to emerge and outcompete the perceived dominant pathogen.

C. krusei was regarded as a harmless, transient commensal being commonly found in the environment (on fruit) and on the human body, but now it is regarded as a significant cause of disease in HIV-positive patients, diabetics and cancer patients (both solid tumour and leukaemia where it is capable of colonising the gastrointestinal, respiratory and urinary tracts). In terms of virulence attributes, *C. krusei* demonstrates a reduced ability to adhere to epithelial cells compared to *C. albicans,* although it does display a high cell-surface hydrophobicity which allows it stick to and colonise catheters and implants. Its main virulence attribute is the high level of inherent resistance to fluconazole. Upon the introduction of this drug in 1990 to treat oropharyngeal candidosis in AIDS patients and systemic candidosis in transplant patients, there was a reduction in the number of cases of disease caused by *C. albicans*. However, the elimination of this yeast may have facilitated the emergence of *C. krusei* as the dominant fungal pathogen in certain classes of patient

C. glabrata has emerged in recent years as a serious cause of disease in neutropaenic cancer patients and has been responsible for mortality rates of 5–38% in some surveys. It appears to be a particular problem in the late stages of haematological malignancies where mortality rates of 70–100% have been described. The incidence of *C. glabrata* infection has increased in recent years, and it is now the fourth most commonly isolated *Candida* species and this increase may be attributable, in part at least, to an alteration in local epidemiology. Since *C. glabrata* is common among leukaemia patients and bone marrow recipients, a range of other risk factors such as prolonged hospitalisation, use of cytotoxic drugs and catheterisation may also play a role in its prevalence. *C. glabrata* is recognised as being a yeast of relatively low virulence, but its emergence as a serious pathogen has been attributed to it being partially resistant to fluconazole. In addition, other factors that may have contributed to its appearance as a serious pathogen have been identified as azole prophylaxis which eliminates *C. albicans* but not *C. glabrata* or *C. krusei* and local factors such as the use of broad-spectrum antibiotics or vascular catheters or the presence of neutropaenia as part of the disease state.

C. auris was first classified as an emerging pathogen in June 2016, but retrospective studies have suggested infections due to this yeast go back as far as 2009. This yeast is capable of inducing superficial and systemic infection and is a particular problem in intensive care units where person-to-person spread occurs. It can produce a mortality rate of 60% and isolates show a high level of resistance to fluconazole and, in some cases, amphotericin B.

4.6.3 *Penicillium marneffei*

Until recently, *Penicillium marneffei* was regarded as a very rare and inconsequential cause of disease in humans. Now, however, it is considered the most frequent cause of fungal disease in AIDS patients who reside in, or have visited, South-East Asia. The principal areas of infection are Thailand and southern China, although cases have been reported from Malaysia, Taiwan, Japan and Hong Kong. While the nature of the infection in humans is well-characterised, the natural habitat or reservoir of this fungus is still unknown, although it may be soil or decaying vegetation. *P. marneffei* is an asexual, dimorphic fungus growing as a mycelium at 37 °C in tissue and as single cells at 28 °C. It reproduces by a process known as fission. In the yeast form of growth, it can be difficult to distinguish microscopically from *H. capsulatum* and *C. neoformans,* so monoclonal antibody-based assays specific for the detection of mannoproteins associated with *P. marneffei* have been developed. Polymerase chain reaction (PCR) fingerprinting is also used to identify *P. marneffei* and to distinguish between infecting strains.

Infection in humans follows inhalation of fungal material, and in AIDS patients dissemination throughout the body can result. Pulmonary involvement is often seen particularly in AIDS patients, but the conditions most associated with infection are fever, weight loss, anaemia, skin lesions and liver and spleen inflammation. The condition is fatal if untreated with antifungal drugs. While the condition responds well to therapy if it is initiated at an early stage, relapse is common in AIDS patients and continuing antifungal therapy may be required. Due to the immunocompromised nature of AIDS patients, other infections such as tuberculosis and pneumonia are often seen alongside *P. marneffei* infection.

4.7 Antibiotic Production by Fungi

Perhaps one of the most important discoveries regarding the beneficial use of fungi for humans was the identification in 1929 by Sir Alexander Fleming that an isolate of *Penicillium notatum* produced a substance capable of killing Gram-positive bacteria. This compound was subsequently identified as penicillin and was the first member of the β-lactam class of antibiotics to be discovered (Figure 4.13a). Other members of this class include the cephalosporins, the penems and the carbapenems (see Chapter 11). These compounds function by inhibiting peptidoglycan synthesis in bacteria and their use has helped reduce the significance of the Gram-positive bacteria as a cause of infection. Subsequent to the identification of penicillin production by *P. notatum,* a screen revealed that *P. chrysogenum* was a superior producer. Following a series of mutagenic and selection procedures, the strain used in conventional fermentations is now capable of producing penicillin at a rate of 7000 mgl^{-1} compared to the 3 mgl^{-1} of Fleming's *P. notatum* isolate. A typical penicillin fermentation yields three types of penicillin, namely, F, G and V. The latter can be used directly; however, penicillin G is modified by the action of penicillin acylase to give a variety of semi-synthetic penicillins which show resistance to the action of bacterial penicillinases which are implicated in conferring antibacterial drug resistance.

Other clinically useful antimicrobial compounds produced by fungi include fusidic acid (Figure 4.13b), which is produced by *Fusarium coccineum* and is used in the treatment of bacterial infections of the skin and eyes, and griseofulvin

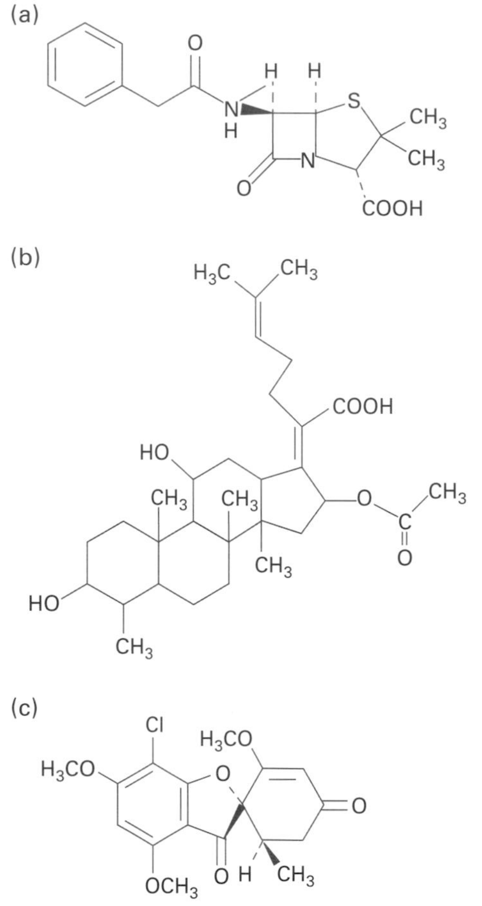

Figure 4.13 Chemical structure of antimicrobial compounds produced by fungi: (a) penicillin; (b) fusidic acid; (c) griseofulvin.

(Figure 4.13c), produced by *Penicillium griseofulvum*, which is used to treat intractable dermatophyte infections.

The majority of antibiotics obtained from fungi are produced by fermentation, and most are secondary metabolites, production of which occurs in the stationary growth phase and is linked to sporulation. Catabolite repression can inhibit antibiotic production and one way to avoid this is to use low levels of glucose in the fermentation medium or to obtain a mutant which is not catabolite-repressed. The chemical content of the medium must be monitored, since high levels of nitrogen or phosphate can retard antibiotic production. One problem that seriously affects the productivity of antibiotic fermentations is feedback inhibition where the antibiotic builds to high intracellular levels and retards further production or kills the cell. One means by which to reverse this is to introduce low levels of the antifungal agent amphotericin B, which increases membrane permeability, leading to a decrease in intracellular antibiotic levels and a concomitant increase in production.

Antibiotic production can be maximised by optimising production as a result of random mutagenesis and selection. Another approach has been to fuse or mate high-producer strains with good secretors. Rational selection is a process whereby a chelating agent is introduced into the fermentation medium to complex all the metal ions present; this has a consequential beneficial effect on antibiotic production. More recently, genetic manipulation has been employed to express the genes for antibiotic production in another species which offers the possibility of producing hybrid antibiotics with novel targets.

Further Reading

Bondaryk, M., Kurzątkowski, W., and Staniszewska, M. (2013). Antifungal agents commonly used in the superficial and mucosal candidiasis treatment: mode of action and resistance development. *Adv. Dermatol. Allergol./Postępy Dermatol. Alergol.* 30: 293–301.

Gupta, V.K., Mach, R.L., and Sreenivasaprasad, S. (ed.) (2015). *Fungal Biomolecules: Sources, Applications and Recent Developments*. New York: Wiley Blackwell.

Hamad, M. (2012). Innate and adaptive antifungal immune responses: partners on an equal footing. *Mycoses* 55: 205.

Kavanagh, K. (ed.) (2018). *Fungi: Biology and Applications*, 3e. Chichester: Wiley Blackwell.

Kullberg, B.J. and Arendrup, M.C. (2015). Invasive candidiasis. *N. Engl. J. Med.* 373: 1445–1456.

Kwon-Chung, K.J. and Sugui, J.A. (2013). *Aspergillus fumigatus* – what makes the species a ubiquitous human fungal pathogen? *PLoS Pathog.* 9: e1003743.

Larkin, E., Hager, C., Chandra, J. et al. (2017). The emerging *Candida auris*: characterization of growth phenotype, virulence factors, antifungal activity, and effect of SCY-078, a novel glucan synthesis inhibitor, on growth morphology and biofilm formation. *Antimicrob. Agents Chemother.* 61: e02396–e02316.

Li, J., Nguyen, C.T., and Garcia-Diaz, J. (2015). Role of new antifungal agents in the treatment of invasive fungal infections in transplant recipients: isavuconazole and new posaconazole formulations. *J. Fungi.* 1: 345–366.

Mayer, F.L., Wilson, D., and Hube, B. (2013). *Candida albicans* pathogenicity mechanisms. *Virulence* 4: 119–128.

Pasqualotto, A.C., Thiele, K.O., and Goldani, L.Z. (2010). Novel triazole antifungal drugs: focus on isavuconazole, ravuconazole and albaconazole. *Curr. Opin. Investig. Drugs.* 11: 165–174.

Pound, M.W., Townsend, M.L., and Drew, R.H. (2010). Echinocandin pharmacodynamics: review and clinical implications. *J. Antimicrob. Chemother.* 65: 1108–1118.

Sanglard, D. (2016). Emerging threats in antifungal-resistant fungal pathogens. *Front. Med.* 3: Article 11.

Tobudic, S., Kratzer, C., and Presterl, E. (2012). Azole-resistant *Candida* spp. – emerging pathogens. *Mycoses* 55: 24–32.

5

Viruses and Other Acellular Infectious Agents: Characteristics and Control

Timofey Skvortsov[1] *and Jean-Yves Maillard*[2]

[1] *Lecturer in Microbial Biotechnology and Bioinformatics, School of Pharmacy, Queen's University Belfast, Belfast, UK*
[2] *Professor of Pharmaceutical Microbiology, School of Pharmacy and Pharmaceutical Sciences, Cardiff University, Cardiff, UK*

CONTENTS

Hugo and Russell's Pharmaceutical Microbiology, Ninth Edition. Edited by Brendan F. Gilmore and Stephen P. Denyer.

Companion website: https://www.wiley.com/go/HugoandRussells9e

5.1 Introduction

Viruses were first discovered at the end of the nineteenth century, although the symptoms they cause were identified much earlier. One of the earliest pieces of evidence is the symptoms of poliomyelitis in an Egyptian priest depicted on a hieroglyph. Virus discovery came about when the cause of an infectious disease (rabies) could not be explained by the presence of bacteria. Unlike bacteria, the 'infectious materials' were not retained by filtration and thus viruses were then referred to as 'filterable agents' or 'filterable viruses' (the term 'virus' was adopted from the Latin word for poison). Until the advent of electron microscopy in the 1940s, only the chemical nature of viruses (i.e., proteins and nucleic acid) could be identified and their infectivity was mainly studied in animal models. The observation of a virus by electron microscopy and the development of cell tissue culture started the golden era of virology. Since then, a large number of viruses have been isolated, their structure identified and their replication understood, leading to the design of potent antiviral drugs and effective vaccines. Progress in virology over the last 50 years has been considerable, leading to the eradication of smallpox following a worldwide vaccination programme, and the likely future eradication of poliovirus, which currently remains in circulation in the wild only in two countries, Afghanistan and Pakistan. For the first time in human history, an infectious disease (smallpox) has been vanquished. Despite such an achievement, much progress is still required to combat other viruses. For example, despite large financial investment and high-profile studies, a cure or vaccine for human immunodeficiency virus (HIV) is still not available, although the use of modern antiretroviral therapy (ART) allows for efficient control of infection, keeping the virus load at undetectable levels and thus significantly increasing the life expectancy of HIV-positive individuals and preventing the transmission of the virus during sexual contacts. The results of latest studies in stem cell therapy and genome editing indicate that complete eradication of HIV from the body of an infected individual is technically possible, but it is difficult to predict when (and if) these approaches will be introduced into clinical practice. The number of commercially available antivirals continues to grow, although it is still limited, especially when compared to the number of antibiotics. Within the last few years, diseases caused by viruses in humans and animals have reminded us that viral infections can easily spread and cause epidemics and pandemics. Recent examples are 'swine flu' and 'avian flu', both caused by influenza viruses, epidemics caused by Ebola and a number of arboviruses, including Zika, West Nile and dengue viruses, and outbreaks of foot and mouth virus affecting cattle, sheep and pigs that had important economic consequences in the UK and mainland Europe. In May 2022, a monkeypox outbreak started from a cluster of infections in the United Kingdom and spread internationally.

One of the most worrying recent developments is the emergence of coronaviruses as a new global public health threat. In the past two decades, three novel coronaviruses have emerged and caused outbreaks in different parts of the world: severe acute respiratory syndrome coronavirus (SARS-CoV) in 2002, Middle East respiratory syndrome-related coronavirus (MERS-CoV) in 2012, and severe acute respiratory syndrome coronavirus 2 (SARS-CoV-2) in 2019. This latter outbreak has resulted in the global pandemic of coronavirus disease 2019 (COVID-19). Recognising that these novel coronaviruses are of zoonotic origin, it is likely that another major outbreak will happen in the foreseeable future. In this regard, global warming alters the distribution ranges of some viral vectors, such as mosquitoes and ticks. Furthermore, the accelerating rates of growth of the world population and associated economic activities (including human encroachment into natural ecosystems and increasing interconnectivity through globalisation) have created the optimal conditions for cross-species transmission. Reducing global biodiversity due to climate change could further exacerbate the problem by increasing the number of competent hosts for a virus. It is now becoming clear that successful prevention and management of such emerging zoonotic viral diseases are only possible through the holistic 'One Health' approach, which takes interconnections between human, animal and environmental health into consideration. This further emphasises the critical importance of better knowledge and understanding of the ecology, biology and epidemiology of different viruses and the available and potential preventive and therapeutic approaches to viral infections.

5.2 General Structure of Viruses

Viruses are extremely diverse in size and in structure (Figure 5.1). The smallest known virus is approximately 17 nm in size (porcine circovirus 1), while the largest is 1500 nm (*Pithovirus sibericum*). In simplistic terms, a virus consists of viral nucleic acid within a protein core, the *capsid* (also referred to as the coat), possibly surrounded by a lipidic *envelope* (Table 5.1). In reality, there are many differences between viruses in terms of nucleic acid, capsid structure, number of coats and envelope composition. Such differences account for the high diversity of viruses and the differences in their properties, notably their resistance to antiviral drugs and viricidal agents. Latest research suggests that viruses are polyphyletic, that is, have no

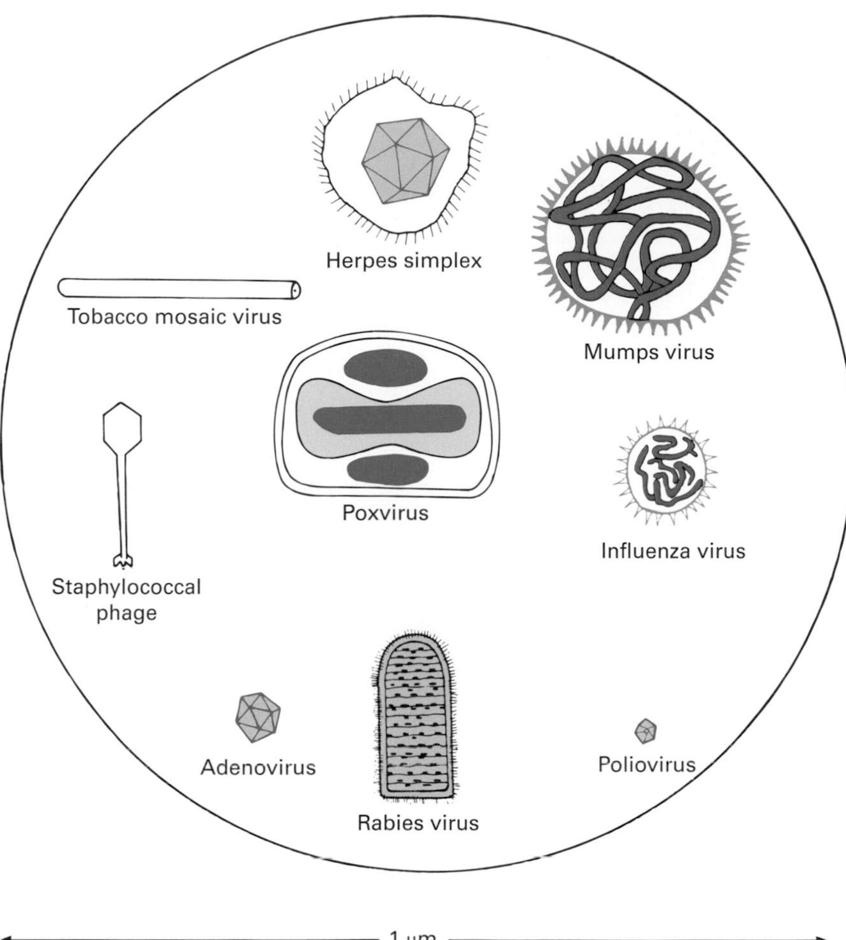

Figure 5.1 The morphology of a variety of virus particles. The large circle indicates the relative size of a *Staphylococcus* bacterial cell.

single evolutionary origin and have developed independently several times during evolutionary history. This makes viral classification (Figure 5.2) extremely complicated and no general methodology for classification of viruses is commonly accepted at the moment. The decision to assign a certain virus to a specific taxon is made by the International Committee on Taxonomy of Viruses (ICTV) mainly based on the information derived from the genomic sequences of viruses, complemented with many additional physical attributes and chemical properties of viral particles, including, for example, their overall structure and morphology. The complete up-to-date taxonomy of viruses can be found in the latest ICTV Report on Virus Classification and Taxon Nomenclature.

5.2.1 Viral Nucleic Acid

The viral genome is composed of either DNA or RNA. It can be double-stranded (ds) or single-stranded (ss), linear (e.g., poliovirus) or circular (e.g., hepatitis B virus), containing several segments (e.g., influenza A virus – eight segments of negative-sense single-stranded RNA) or one molecule (e.g., poliovirus). Seven groups can be distinguished depending on their nucleic acid content (Table 5.2) – this system is known as the Baltimore classification. Viruses that contain positive-sense ssRNA (e.g., poliovirus) can have their genome translated directly by the host ribosomes. The nature of the viral nucleic acid is important for the effectiveness of antiviral treatments (see below). For example, to replicate within the host cell retroviruses such as HIV require a specific virus-encoded enzyme, a reverse transcriptase, to convert their ssRNA into ssDNA. This enzyme is a primary target site of many antiviral drugs.

On some occasions, the viral genome itself has been shown to be infectious, that is, to cause an infection. Such an observation is important when one considers viricidal agents that damage the viral capsid or envelope but not the viral nucleic acid. Furthermore, in laboratory conditions, the phenomenon of *multiplicity reactivation* has been observed with poliovirus whereby random damage to viral capsid and nucleic acid following treatment with

Table 5.1 Structure and clinical importance of mammalian viruses, including emerging ones.

Family	Genus	Virus	Characteristics	Clinical importance
DNA viruses				
Poxviridae	*Orthopoxvirus*	Variola	Large particles 200–250 nm; complex symmetry	Variola is the smallpox virus; it produces a systemic infection with a characteristic vesicular rash affecting the face, arms and legs, and has a high mortality rate
		Monkeypox virus (MPX)	Large complex enveloped virus, similar in size and morphology to other orthopoxviruses	Causes a systemic infection accompanied by enlarged lymph nodes and a characteristic vesicular rash similar in manifestation to smallpox; cases are normally milder, but the infection can be fatal, especially in individuals with weakened immune system. Two major clades (I and II) are in circulation, with clade I causing more severe disease
		Vaccinia	Large complex enveloped virus, approximately 360 nm in length and 250 nm in diameter	Vaccinia has been derived from the cowpox virus and has been used to immunise against smallpox. It also offers protection against viruses related to smallpox (such as monkeypox virus). A vaccine based on a modified vaccinia virus (Ankara strain) was approved for the prevention of monkeypox in 2019
Adenoviridae	*Mastadenovirus*	Various human adenoviruses (HAdV) in seven species (A to G)	Icosahedral particles 80 nm in diameter	Commonly cause upper respiratory tract infections; tend to produce latent infections in tonsils and adenoids; will produce tumours on injection into hamsters, rats or mice. Adenovirus serotype 14 is known to cause severe and potentially fatal respiratory infections
Herpesviridae	*Simplexvirus*	Herpes simplex virus 1 (HSV-1); formally known as human alphaherpesvirus 1 (HHV-1) Herpes simplex virus 2 (HSV-2); formally known as human alphaherpesvirus 2 (HHV-2)	Enveloped, icosahedral particles 150 nm in diameter	HSV-1 infects oral membranes in children; >80% are infected by adolescence. Following the primary infection, the individual retains the HSV-1 DNA in the trigeminal nerve ganglion for life and has a 50% chance of developing 'cold sores'. HSV-2 is responsible for recurrent genital herpes
	Varicellovirus	Varicella zoster virus (VZV); formally known as human alphaherpesvirus 3 (HHV-3)	Enveloped, icosahedral particles 150 nm in diameter	Causes chickenpox in children; virus remains dormant in any dorsal root ganglion of the CNS; release of immune control in elderly people stimulates reactivation resulting in shingles

Table 5.1 (Continued)

Family	Genus	Virus	Characteristics	Clinical importance
	Cytomegalovirus	Human cytomegalovirus (HCMV or simply CMV); formally known as human betaherpesvirus 5 (HHV-5)	Enveloped, icosahedral particles 150 nm in diameter	CMV is generally acquired in childhood as a subclinical infection. About 50% of adults carry the virus in a dormant state in white blood cells. The virus can cause severe disease (pneumonia, hepatitis, and encephalitis) in immunocompromised patients. Primary infections during pregnancy can induce serious congenital abnormalities in the foetus. Latent CMV infection may result in certain forms of cancer
	Rhadinovirus	Kaposi's sarcoma-associated herpesvirus (KSHV); formally known as human gammaherpesvirus 8 (HHV-8)	Enveloped, icosahedral particles 150 nm in diameter	Causes Kaposi's sarcoma, a type of cancer affecting skin and lymph nodes. The skin lesions are of characteristic purple colour. Opportunistic HHV-8 infections are common in people with AIDS
	Lymphocryptovirus	Epstein–Barr virus (EBV); formally known as human gammaherpesvirus 4 (HHV-4)	Enveloped, icosahedral particles 150 nm in diameter	Infections occur by salivary exchange. In young children they are commonly asymptomatic, but the virus persists in a latent form in lymphocytes. Infection delayed until adolescence often results in glandular fever. In tropical Africa, a severe EBV infection early in life predisposes the child to malignant facial tumours (Burkitt's lymphoma)
Hepadnaviridae	*Orthohepadnavirus*	Hepatitis B virus (HBV)	Spherical enveloped particle 42 nm in diameter enclosing an inner icosahedral 27 nm nucleocapsid	The cause of hepatitis B, a dangerous liver infection. In areas such as South-East Asia and Africa, most children are infected by prenatal transmission. In the Western world, the virus is spread through contact with contaminated blood or by sexual intercourse. There is strong evidence that chronic infections with HBV can progress to liver cancer (hepatocarcinoma)
Papillomaviridae	Multiple genera	Human papillomaviruses (HPV)	Naked icosahedral particles 50 nm in diameter	Multiply only in epithelial cells of skin and mucous membranes causing warts. There is strong evidence that some types are associated with cervical cancer and certain other genital cancers. Human papillomavirus 16 and 18 account for 70% of cervical cancer cases. HPV vaccines are available
Polyomaviridae	*Alphapolyomavirus*	Merkel cell polyomavirus (MCV); formally known as human polyomavirus 5	Naked icosahedral particles 50 nm in diameter	Oncogenic virus, causes Merkel cell carcinoma, a rare skin cancer

(Continued)

Table 5.1 (Continued)

Family	Genus	Virus	Characteristics	Clinical importance
	Betapolyomavirus	BK virus (human polyomavirus 1) JC virus (human polyomavirus 2)	Naked icosahedral particles 50 nm in diameter	BK virus causes polyomavirus-associated nephropathy and haemorrhagic cystitis. JC virus is associated with progressive multifocal leukoencephalopathy (PML), a rare but severe disease of the brain; up to 50% of PML cases are fatal
Parvoviridae	*Erythroparvovirus*	Human parvovirus B19	Small (22–24 nm in diameter), non-enveloped particles with icosahedral symmetry	This virus causes 'fifth disease' (erythema infectiosum); the infection is typically contracted during childhood. Although the disease generally manifests as a mild rash and resolves within a few days without complications, in rare cases infections might be more dangerous. In pregnant women, parvovirus B19 infections might infrequently lead to miscarriage
	Dependoparvovirus (also classified as a subviral agent – satellite virus; see Sections 5.8 and 5.10)	Adeno-associated dependoparvovirus A (also known as AAV-1 to AAV-4) Adeno-associated dependoparvovirus B (AAV-5)	Small (20–24 nm in diameter), non-enveloped particles with icosahedral symmetry	Adeno-associated viruses infect humans, but do not cause any diseases and elicit very weak immune response. These properties make AAVs attractive vector platforms for gene therapy
RNA viruses				
Orthomyxoviridae	*Alphainfluenzavirus* *Betainfluenzavirus*	Influenza A virus Influenza B virus	Enveloped particles, 100 nm in diameter with a helically symmetric capsid; haemagglutinin and neuraminidase spikes project from the envelope; genome consists of 8 −ssRNA linear fragments, encapsidated by nucleoprotein	These viruses are capable of extensive antigenic variation, producing new types against which the human population does not have effective immunity. These new antigenic types can cause pandemics of influenza. In natural infections, the virus only multiplies in the cells lining the upper respiratory tract. The constitutional symptoms of influenza are probably brought about by absorption of toxic breakdown products from the dying cells on the respiratory epithelium
Paramyxoviridae	*Orthorubulavirus*	Mumps virus (MuV)	Enveloped particles variable in size, 110–170 nm in diameter, with helical capsids	Infection in children produces characteristic swelling of parotid and submaxillary salivary glands. The disease can have neurological complications, for example, meningitis, especially in adults. In rare cases, MuV infection may lead to reduced male fertility
	Morbillivirus	Measles virus (MeV)	Enveloped particles variable in size, 120–250 nm in diameter, helical capsids	Very common childhood fever; immunity is lifelong and second attacks are very rare. The virus is very infectious
	Henipavirus	Nipah virus	Spherical enveloped particles, around 150 nm in diameter, helical capsids	Infects pigs, bats and humans. Causes fevers, headaches and cough; 40–75% of infected people die. Infections in animals are not normally fatal. Considered an emerging infectious disease of zoonotic origin

Table 5.1 (Continued)

Family	Genus	Virus	Characteristics	Clinical importance
Rhabdoviridae	*Lyssavirus*	Rabies virus (RabV)	Bullet-shaped particles, 75–180 nm, enveloped, helical capsids	The virus has a very wide host range, infecting all mammals so far tested; dogs, cats and cattle are particularly susceptible. The incubation period of rabies is extremely varied, ranging from 6 days up to 1 year. The virus remains localised at the wound site of entry for a while before passing along nerve fibres to the central nervous system, where it invariably produces a fatal encephalitis
Reoviridae	*Rotavirus*	Rotavirus A Rotavirus B Rotavirus C	The virion has a triple capsid structure – the inner core is surrounded by two additional concentric icosahedral shells producing particles 80 nm in diameter; the genome is segmented and consists of 11 linear dsRNA segments	A very common cause of gastroenteritis in infants, with Rotavirus A responsible for more than 90% of cases. It is spread through poor water supplies and when standards of general hygiene are low (faecal-oral transmission). In developing countries, it is responsible for about a million deaths each year
Picornaviridae	*Enterovirus*	Poliovirus (PV) is one of three serotypes of human enterovirus C (PV-1, PV-2 or PV-3)	Naked icosahedral particles 28 nm in diameter	One of a group of enteroviruses common in the gut of humans. The primary site of multiplication is the lymphoid tissue of the alimentary tract. Only rarely do they cause systemic infections or serious neurological conditions such as encephalitis or poliomyelitis
		Various human rhinoviruses	Naked icosahedra 30 nm in diameter	The common cold viruses, causing around 50% of cases; there are over 100 antigenically distinct types, hence the difficulty in preparing effective vaccines. The virus is shed copiously in watery nasal secretions
	Hepatovirus	Hepatitis A virus (HAV)	Naked icosahedra 27 nm in diameter	Responsible for 'infectious hepatitis', an inflammation causing damage to the liver. The virus is spread by the oral–faecal route especially in children. Also associated with sewage contamination of food or water supplies
Matonaviridae	*Rubivirus*	Rubella virus (RuV)	Spherical particles 70 nm in diameter; a tightly adherent envelope surrounds an icosahedral capsid	Causes rubella (German measles) in children, mainly manifesting as a spotty rash. An infection contracted in the early stages of pregnancy can induce severe multiple congenital abnormalities, for example, deafness, blindness, heart disease and mental retardation

(*Continued*)

Table 5.1 (Continued)

Family	Genus	Virus	Characteristics	Clinical importance
Flaviviridae	*Flavivirus*	Yellow fever virus (YFV)	Spherical particles 50 nm in diameter with an inner core surrounded by an adherent lipid envelope	The virus is spread to humans by mosquito bites; the liver is the main target; necrosis of hepatocytes leads to jaundice and fever, with a mortality rate up to 90%
		Zika virus (ZIKV)	Spherical particles 50 nm in diameter with an inner core surrounded by an adherent lipid envelope	The virus is spread to humans by mosquito bites; the initial infection is either asymptomatic or mild and generic (e.g., fever, joint pain, and headache). Mother-to-child transmission during pregnancy can result in microcephaly or other brain development abnormalities in the foetus. Zika virus infections are also found to be implicated in the rare Guillain–Barré syndrome (GBS), a rapidly developing autoimmune disease causing muscle weakness, including the muscles of the respiratory system
		Dengue virus (DENV)	Spherical particles 50 nm in diameter with an inner core surrounded by an adherent lipid envelope	Causes dengue fever. A specific skin rash is a characteristic sign of the disease. DENV is widespread in South America and South Asia, infecting almost 400 million people in the world every year; the fatality rate in severe cases, characterised by haemorrhage and hypotension, can be up to 2.5%
		Japanese encephalitis virus (JEV)	Spherical particles 50 nm in diameter with an inner core surrounded by an adherent lipid envelope	The majority of infections are asymptomatic or mildly symptomatic. In approximately 0.4% of cases it causes Japanese encephalitis, a severe inflammation of the brain, resulting in neurological damage and fatality rates of up to 30%
	Hepacivirus	Hepatitis C virus (HCV)	Spherical particles 60 nm in diameter consisting of an inner core surrounded by an adherent lipid envelope	The virus is spread through blood transfusions and blood products. Induces a hepatitis which is usually milder than that caused by HBV. Infection might result in hepatocarcinoma
Filoviridae	*Ebolavirus*	Ebola virus	Long filamentous rods composed of a lipid envelope surrounding a helical nucleocapsid 1000 nm long, 80 nm in diameter	The virus is widespread among populations of monkeys. It can be spread to humans by contact with body fluids from the primates. The resulting haemorrhagic fever has a 90% case fatality rate

Table 5.1 (Continued)

Family	Genus	Virus	Characteristics	Clinical importance
Retroviridae	*Deltaretrovirus*	Human T-cell leukaemia virus (HTLV-1)	Spherical enveloped virus 100 nm in diameter; icosahedral cores contain two copies of linear RNA molecules and reverse transcriptase	HTLV is spread inside infected lymphocytes in blood, semen or breast milk. Most infections remain asymptomatic but after an incubation period of 10–40 years in about 2% of cases, adult T-cell leukaemia can result
	Lentivirus	Human immunodeficiency virus 1 (HIV-1) Human immunodeficiency virus 2 (HIV-2)	Differs from other retroviruses in that the core is cone-shaped rather than icosahedral	HIV is transmitted from person to person via blood or genital secretions. The principal target for the virus is the $CD4^+$ T-lymphocyte cells. Depletion of these cells induces immunodeficiency
Unassigned (subviral agent – satellite virus; see Section 5.10)	*Deltavirus*	Hepatitis delta virus (HDV)	An RNA-containing virus that can only replicate in cells co-infected with HBV. Nucleocapsid is formed by HDV antigen, but the lipid envelope of HDV is decorated by HBV proteins	The presence of the satellite HDV exacerbates the pathogenic effects of HBV producing severe hepatitis
Coronaviridae	*Betacoronavirus*	Severe acute respiratory syndrome-related coronavirus (SARS-CoV) Middle East respiratory syndrome-related coronavirus (MERS-CoV) Severe acute respiratory syndrome-related coronavirus 2 (SARS-CoV-2)	Large roughly spherical (average diameter 125 nm) enveloped particles with bulbous surface projections	Causes respiratory tract diseases ranging from the common cold (approximately 25% of cases) to a much more serious and potentially fatal severe acute respiratory syndrome (SARS, MERS and COVID-19 pandemic)
Caliciviridae	*Norovirus*	Norovirus (also referred to as the Norwalk virus)	Small (23–40 nm diameter) non-enveloped icosahedral RNA virus	Called the 'winter vomiting bug', norovirus is the most common cause of gastroenteritis characterised by sudden onset of severe vomiting and diarrhoea
Pneumoviridae	*Orthopneumovirus*	Human respiratory syncytial virus (RSV)	Enveloped, spherical particles (average diameter 150 nm); helical capsid	Causes respiratory tract diseases, responsible for about 70% of bronchiolitis cases in infants
Hantaviridae	*Orthohantavirus*	Human hantaviruses	Enveloped, spherical particles (average diameter 100 nm); helical capsid; genome consists of 3 −ssRNA linear segments	Depending on the virus, can cause one of two fatal diseases: hantavirus haemorrhagic fever with renal syndrome (HFRS) or hantavirus pulmonary syndrome (HPS)

(*Continued*)

Table 5.1 (Continued)

Family	Genus	Virus	Characteristics	Clinical importance
Arenaviridae	*Arenavirus*	Lassa mammarenavirus (LASV)	Enveloped, spherical particles (average diameter 150 nm); helical capsid; genome consists of 2 −ssRNA linear segments	Causes Lassa fever. The virus is endemic to rodents of several West African countries. Transmission to humans can occur through contact with household items and food contaminated by rat faeces or urine. The disease is asymptomatic in 80% of cases, but in about 1 in 5 results in severe disease, affecting internal organs (such as the liver, kidneys, and spleen). About 15% of those with severe clinical manifestation of Lassa fever die
Hepeviridae	*Orthohepevirus*	Hepatitis E virus	Quasi-enveloped (the envelope is not always present) icosahedral particles about 33 nm diameter	The virus is spread through contaminated water and food products. Induces a hepatitis which might be fatal in pregnant women and immunocompromised individuals
Togaviridae	*Alphavirus*	Chikungunya virus	Enveloped, spherical viral particles 65–70 nm in diameter; capsid icosahedral	Spread by mosquitoes, the symptoms of the infection include fever and joint pains. Fatality rate is about 0.1%

CNS, central nervous system; SARS, severe acute respiratory syndrome; MERS, Middle East respiratory syndrome; COVID-19, coronavirus disease 2019.

hypochlorite, a microbicide intensively used for surface disinfection, resulted in complementary reconstruction of an infectious particle by hybridisation of the gene pool of the inactivated virus. This again underlines the necessity of rendering the viral nucleic acid non-infectious following a viricidal treatment.

5.2.2 Viral Capsid

The function of the capsid is to protect the viral nucleic acid from detrimental chemical and physical conditions (e.g., disinfection). The capsid is composed of a number of proteinaceous subunits named *capsomeres* genetically encoded by the viral genome. The nature and association of the capsomeres are fundamental for the virus, as they give the shape of the capsid, but also provide the virus with resistance to chemical and physical agents. The assembly of the capsomeres results in two main different architectural styles – icosahedral and helical symmetries (Figure 5.3); in mammalian viruses, a more complex structure can be found, where several proteinaceous structures envelop the viral genome core (e.g., poxviruses and rhabdoviruses). The majority of bacterial viruses (bacteriophages) also show a complex structure consisting of a capsid head, a tail and tail fibres (see Section 5.9.1). The nature of the capsomeres in certain viruses allows for the self-assembly of the capsid within the host cell. The capsomeres are held together by non-covalent intermolecular forces. Such assembly also allows the release of the viral genome following dissociation of the non-covalently bonded subunits. These subunits offer considerable economy of genetic information within the viral genome, since only a small number of different subunits contribute to the formation of the capsid. Viruses with an icosahedral capsid usually have capsomeres in the form of pentons and hexons. The number of these subunits varies considerably between viruses: for example, adenovirus is constructed from 240 hexons and 12 pentons, whereas the poliovirus is composed of 20 hexons and 12 pentons, forming a much smaller structure. Viruses with a helical capsid (e.g., influenza and mumps viruses) have their subunits symmetrically packed in a helical array, appearing like coils of

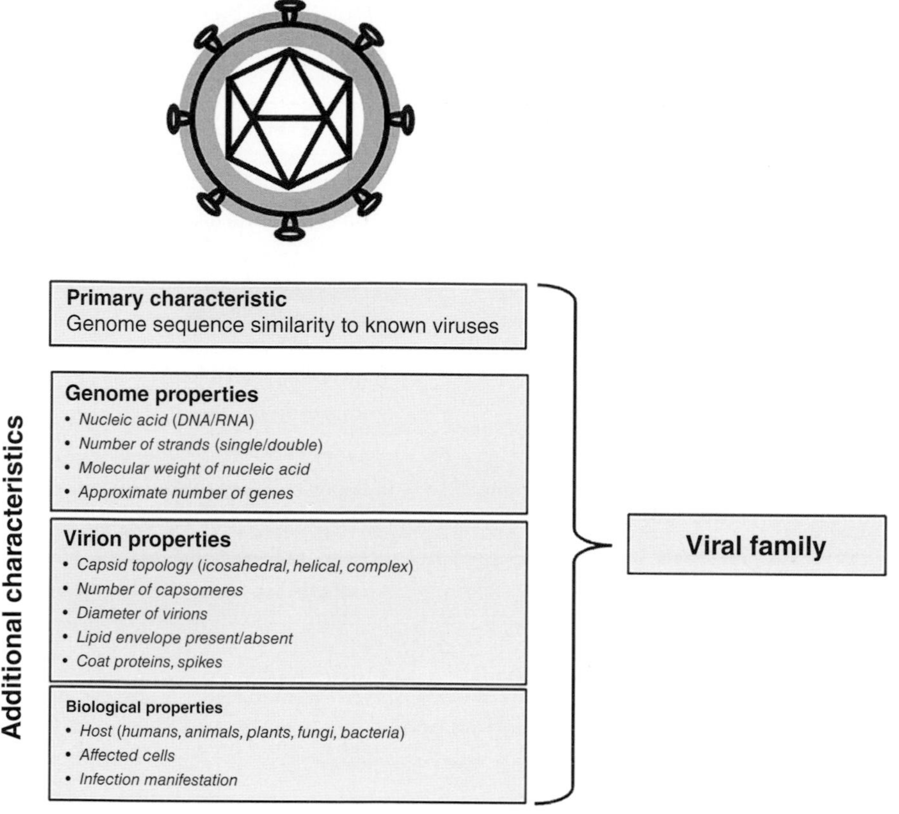

Figure 5.2 Classification of viruses. Some of the main attributes used in classification are listed. Each viral family is defined by a specific combination of these and other traits. Genome sequence similarity of the newly described viruses to the already classified ones serves as the principal classification characteristic.

wound rope under electron microscopy. Although the core of such a virus is hollow, the viral nucleic acid is embedded into ridges on the inside of each subunit and does not fill the hollow core. Such a close association between viral nucleic acid and capsid proteins can explain the damage caused to the nucleic acid following disaggregation of the capsid after chemical or physical treatments.

5.2.3 Viral Envelope

The viral capsid can be surrounded by a lipidic envelope, which originates from the host cell. The envelope is added during the replication process or following excision of the viral progeny from the host cells. The envelope can come from the host cell nuclear membrane (e.g., herpes simplex virus [HSV]), endoplasmic reticulum–Golgi intermediate compartment (e.g., coronaviruses) or the cytoplasmic membrane (e.g., influenza virus). One characteristic of the viral envelope is that host proteins are excluded, but proteins encoded by the viral genome are present. These viral proteins play an important serological role. Enveloped viruses are generally considered to be the most susceptible to chemical and physical conditions and do not survive well on their own outside the host cell (e.g., on surfaces), although they can persist longer in organic matter (e.g., blood, exudates, and faeces). Lipids in viruses are generally phospholipids from the host envelope, although glycolipids, neutral fats, fatty acids, fatty aldehydes and cholesterol can be found. In some cases, lipids can also facilitate the entry of the virus into the host cell.

5.2.4 Viral Envelope-associated Proteins

In addition to these structures, viral proteins and glycoproteins can be found protruding from the viral capsid or embedded in the envelope, either individually or as multimeric units. These structures are known as *peplomers* or spikes and usually serve as viral receptors. They are important for viral infectivity, as they recognise the host cell receptor site conveying viral specificity. Certain peplomers may have enzymatic activity, such as the neuraminidase of influenza viruses. In bacteriophages, these structures can take the shape of tail fibres.

Table 5.2 Examples of types of nucleic acid in human and bacterial viruses.

Group	Nucleic acid	Family	Example
I	dsDNA	*Herpesviridae, Poxviridae, Papillomaviridae, Adenoviridae, Polyomaviridae*	Herpes simplex virus, cytomegalovirus, poxvirus, papilloma virus, adenovirus, JC virus
		Myoviridae, Siphoviridae, Podoviridae	Enterobacteria bacteriophages T4, λ and P22
II	ssDNA	*Parvoviridae, Anelloviridae*	Human parvovirus B19, human torque teno viruses
		Inoviridae, Microviridae	Filamentous bacteriophages, including M13, phiX174
III	dsRNA	*Reoviridae*	Rotaviruses
		Cystoviridae	*Pseudomonas* virus phi6
IV	+ssRNA with mRNA identical in base sequence to virion RNA	*Picornaviridae, Coronaviridae, Flaviviridae*	Poliovirus, hepatitis A virus, rhinovirus, SARS-CoV-2, Zika virus
		Leviviridae	Bacteriophages MS2, Qβ
V	−ssRNA with mRNA complementary in base sequence to virion RNA	*Orthomyxoviridae, Paramyxoviridae, Filoviridae, Pneumoviridae*	Influenza, paramyxovirus, measles, mumps, Ebola virus, RSV
VI	+ssRNA with DNA intermediate in their growth	*Retroviridae*	HIV, HTLV-1
VII	dsDNA with RNA intermediate in their growth	*Hepadnaviridae*[a]	HBV

[a] *Hepadnaviridae* genome contains partially dsDNA and partially ssDNA, with a capped ssRNA oligomer attached to the 5′ end of one of the DNA strands.

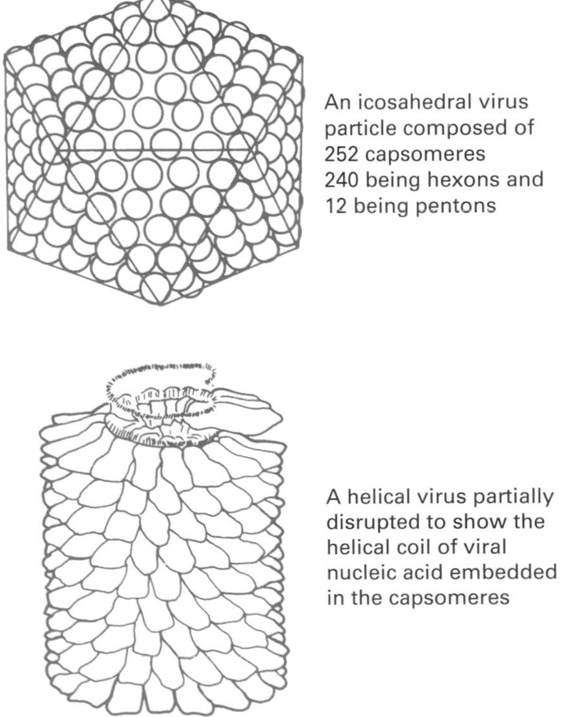

Figure 5.3 Icosahedral and helical symmetry in viruses.

5.3 Virus–Host Cell Interactions

Viruses need to interact with a host cell, as they cannot reproduce on their own. They have no metabolism and cannot synthesise their own proteins, lipids or nucleic acids. Thus, viruses can be considered as true obligate intracellular parasites that grow within living cells and use their energy and synthetic machinery to produce viral components. The production and egress of viruses from the host cell will result in cell death, although this might not be immediate. Following the replication of one virus within the host cell, hundreds of new viruses (virus progeny or *virions*) can be released and infect adjacent cells (within a tissue). The propagation from one infected cell to new cells, and the subsequent destruction of tissue or cells, provides signs of the viral disease. If viruses enter the bloodstream or the lymphatic system, they will be distributed throughout the whole body, causing systemic infection.

On the basis of host specificity, three major viral groups can be distinguished: (i) viruses of bacteria, also known as bacteriophages, (ii) viruses of archaea and (iii) eukaryotic viruses. Eukaryotic viruses are a large and diverse group, which consists of viruses infecting eukaryotic microorganisms, plants, fungi, animals (including invertebrates) and humans. Viruses are usually very specific and rarely cross species barriers, although there are some exceptions, such as rabies, influenza and certain coronaviruses (e.g., SARS-CoV, MERS-CoV) that can cause diseases in both animals and humans. Viruses can also be asymptomatic in certain hosts where they do not cause an infection; the host becomes a reservoir and can transmit the virus to a susceptible recipient (e.g., transmission of yellow fever virus to humans by mosquitoes).

Viruses can interact with the host cell in five different ways: (i) multiplication of the virus and destruction of the host cell upon release of the viral progeny, (ii) multiplication of the virus and release of the virions without the immediate destruction of the host cell, (iii) survival of the virus in a latent stage without noticeable changes to the infected cell, (iv) survival of the infected cell in a dramatically altered or transformed state (e.g., transformation of a normal cell to one having the properties of a cancerous cell) and (v) incorporation of the viral nucleic acid in the host cell genome without noticeable changes to the infected cell. The interaction with the host cell will vary between viruses, but will generally follow one of these five routes.

There is a great diversity in viral infections and viral diseases. Many viral infections are asymptomatic or 'silent' whereby the virus replicates within the host but does not produce symptoms of a disease. Other common infections produce some mild symptoms, such as a low-grade fever and a 'runny nose'. This is the case of the common cold, caused by rhinoviruses, from which patients make a full recovery within a few days. At the other end of the spectrum, some viruses kill their host very quickly following infection, as in the case of haemorrhagic viruses such as the Ebola virus. On other occasions, a range of symptoms can be observed in different hosts. This has been the case recently with 'swine flu' caused by a new strain of H1N1 influenza virus A, which produced a range of symptoms, from a slight fever to full influenza including a high fever, vomiting, and dizziness. Another recent example of such varying interactions are the effects caused by SARS-CoV-2 infection: while the majority of infected persons will develop some symptoms of the disease, about 20–30% of infections will not cause any noticeable illness and will progress and resolve asymptomatically. Other problematic viruses might not cause immediate symptoms, but following the systematic destruction of host cells will lead to an incurable disease, for example, HIV and oncogenic (tumour) viruses.

5.3.1 Coronaviruses

Coronaviruses, including SARS-CoV-2, the agent responsible for the COVID-19 pandemic, are enveloped, spherical +ssRNA viruses about 120 nm in diameter. The surface of the viral particle is decorated by spikes consisting of the spike glycoprotein (S) trimers. Once SARS-CoV-2 enters the alveoli, principally through inhalation, it binds to cellular angiotensin-converting enzyme-2 (ACE-2) receptors present on the surface of type II alveolar cells. This initiates the process of endocytosis. Two other proteins present on the host cell surface, the serine proteases furin and TMPRSS2 (transmembrane serine protease type 2), are essential for initial proteolytic cleavage and processing of the virus' spike protein, making the fusion of the endosomal and viral envelope membranes possible. This releases the genomic positive-stranded viral RNA into the cytoplasm, where it is first directly translated into a number of polyproteins, which undergo proteolytic cleavage and become processed into the RNA-dependent RNA polymerase (RdRp) and a number of other non-structural proteins. The replication process of SARS-CoV-2 occurs in *viral factories*; these are special structures formed in cells upon infection with certain groups of viruses that increase the efficiency of replication and assembly of viral particles and protect the viral nucleic acids from defence mechanisms of the host cell. In the case of coronaviruses, these structures take the form of double membrane vesicles derived from membranes of the Golgi complex and the endoplasmic reticulum. Viral transcription and replication result in the production of structural proteins, from which new virions are then assembled. Finally, the mature virus particles are released from the infected cell via exocytosis following which they can infect adjacent cells.

Direct damage by the virus as well as damage from a hyperinflammatory response will eventually lead to destruction of the infected cells, which is the main cause of pathology associated with COVID-19. The dysfunctional immune response, commonly referred to as a 'cytokine storm', leads to the accumulation of a protein-rich fluid in the alveoli, causing shortness of breath, pneumonia and progressively alveolar collapse resulting in hypoxia, acute respiratory distress syndrome (ARDS) and multiorgan failure. SARS-CoV-2 can cause a number of additional complications, including direct damage to organs that express ACE-2 receptors, such as the heart, gastrointestinal tract, kidneys and liver. In severe disease, blood coagulation might occur, with blood clots forming in the lungs and elsewhere. Severe cases, including the ones resulting in death, are more prevalent in older people and those with a pre-existing long-term condition such as cardiovascular disease, diabetes, respiratory disease, hypertension or cancer. A noticeable proportion of people recovered from COVID-19 appear to experience long-lasting symptoms and disabilities, which include, among others, extreme fatigue, shortness of breath, and loss of the senses of smell and taste. This post-COVID-19 syndrome is known as 'long

COVID', but there is still limited data on how it should be managed and whether its effects are permanent or not.

Treatment of COVID-19 is largely symptomatic. While several antiviral compounds are approved for emergency use in a number of countries and more are in development (discussed in Section 5.7.1.6), supportive care remains the main approach to management of the disease.

5.3.2 Human Immunodeficiency Virus (HIV)

HIV is an enveloped virus with a cone-shaped capsid containing two copies of a +ssRNA molecule and the enzymes reverse transcriptase (RT), protease and integrase. The viral genome contains nine genes, encoding 16 proteins in total. Three major genes are: *gag*, coding for structural proteins (matrix, capsid, nucleocapsid and p6); *pol*, coding for key viral enzymes (RT, protease and integrase); and *env*, encoding the envelope glycoproteins (gp120 and gp41). The genes *tat* and *rev* encode essential proteins regulating host metabolism, while the remaining genes encode accessory proteins. Seventy glycoprotein spikes (gp120) project from the envelope and interact specifically with the CD4 protein receptor on the T helper lymphocyte (see Chapter 9). The HIV core penetrates the cell cytoplasm following membrane fusion and is uncoated, releasing two RNA molecules and the enzymes, including the reverse transcriptase, into the cytoplasm. The RNA is copied by RT into ssDNA, which is then duplicated to form a dsDNA copy of the original viral RNA genome. This DNA moves into the host cell nucleus where it is integrated as a *provirus* into a host cell chromosome.

The provirus can lie dormant in the cell or can be expressed, producing viral mRNA and proteins, thereby resuming the multiplication cycle producing virions. The viral mRNA is *polycistronic*, producing *polyproteins* (Gag and Pol) that need to be processed (cleaved) by a specific virus-encoded protease. Following the assembly of viral proteins and viral RNA, the virions bud off the infected cells.

Some of the latest studies, conducted in mice, demonstrate that HIV-1 proviruses can be eliminated from the infected cells by a combination of currently used antiretroviral chemotherapy and CRISPR/Cas9 gene editing (see Chapter 24). This approach remains highly experimental and will require additional development and validation before it can be used for human treatment, but raises hopes that HIV infections will be curable in the foreseeable future. Current therapy allows HIV-positive individuals to maintain a high count of $CD4^+$ T helper lymphocytes by regulating the viral load produced by infected cells (untreated, up to 10^{10} viral particles can be produced continuously per day). Indeed, the ultimate decrease in $CD4^+$ T helper cells (below 200 ml^{-1} of blood), indicating the progression of HIV infection to the stage of acute immunodeficiency syndrome (AIDS), seriously compromises the host immune system and allows infection by a range of opportunist pathogens including fungi, protozoa, bacteria and other viruses. Currently, antireteroviral therapies (ART) combining two reverse transcriptase inhibitors and another antiviral agent, such as a protease inhibitor, reduce the number of HIV particles to undetectable levels and slow the progression of the disease by restoring and maintaining the number of $CD4^+$ T helper lymphocytes. However, while this prevents the further transmission of the virus, this triple therapy does not eliminate the virus completely. Patients who stop using the drugs experience a rapid rebound in levels of the virus in the blood and progression of the disease. The inability to eliminate the virus completely calls for lifelong therapy that is prohibitively expensive for countries with very limited health budgets.

5.3.3 Oncogenic Viruses

It is estimated that approximately one in eight of human cancers has a viral origin. Virus-infected cells change dramatically, acquiring the characteristics of tumour cells exhibiting uncontrolled growth. For example, the Epstein–Barr virus (EBV) has been associated with the formation of lymphomas and nasopharyngeal carcinomas, the hepatitis B and C viruses with hepatocellular carcinoma, human papilloma viruses with cervical cancer, human T-cell lymphotropic virus type 1 with adult T-cell leukaemia/lymphoma syndrome and Kaposi's sarcoma-associated herpesvirus (KSHV) with skin or mucous membrane cancers.

There are no identified single mechanisms by which viruses induce tumours. One direct mechanism involves the acquisition of viral genes whose products disrupt the metabolic and regulatory pathways of the host cell, resulting in oncogenic transformation. In certain situations, the malignant transformation might be caused by a chronic inflammation resulting from a long-term infection with a virus, such as in case of HCV infections. Other events, such as environmental or dietary exposures to chemical carcinogens, might increase the chances for cancer to occur in the virus-infected host cells. For example, there might be an association between EBV and malaria to trigger Burkitt's lymphoma in young children in Africa. EBV and consumption of smoked fish might trigger nasopharyngeal carcinoma in adults in China. The development of liver cancer following infection with hepatitis B virus (HBV) might be triggered by high alcohol consumption, smoking and exposure to fungal toxin (aflatoxins), events that damage the liver.

It is known that the viral genome of oncogenic viruses (oncoviruses) can integrate with the host DNA. Indeed, viral DNA has been recovered from infected cells. Following integration of the provirus, the regulation of cell growth and division can be affected. There is currently no means of eradicating proviruses. However, progress in the prevention of papillomavirus has been made by designing an effective vaccine linked to a successful vaccination programme that is now responsible for an important decrease in cervical cancer cases.

5.4 Multiplication of Human Viruses

The objective of the replication cycle is to ensure the multiplication of the virus with the formation of identical viral progeny. Viruses differ in their replication cycle and the time to produce and release new virions. The multiplication cycle of human viruses is generally slow, from 4 to more than 40 hours. Bacterial viruses are generally faster and can take as little as 20 minutes to replicate within the bacterial host. The replication cycle can be divided into six distinct phases (attachment, penetration, uncoating, gene expression and replication, assembly and virion release) (Figure 5.4); these are common to all viruses, although the detail within each phase varies greatly between viruses. Understanding the viral multiplication process is crucial for the development of new antiviral drugs as well as repurposing existing ones.

5.4.1 Attachment to the Host Cell

Viral attachment to the cell surface can be divided into three phases: (i) an initial contact mainly dependent on Brownian motion, (ii) a reversible phase during which electrostatic repulsion is reduced and (iii) irreversible changes in virus-receptor–host-receptor configuration that initiates viral penetration through the cell membrane.

All viruses possess *receptors* on their surface, usually in the form of glycoproteins embedded in the viral envelope or protruding as spikes from the viral capsid. These structures recognise and bind receptors on the host cell and provide the virus with its high specificity, although different

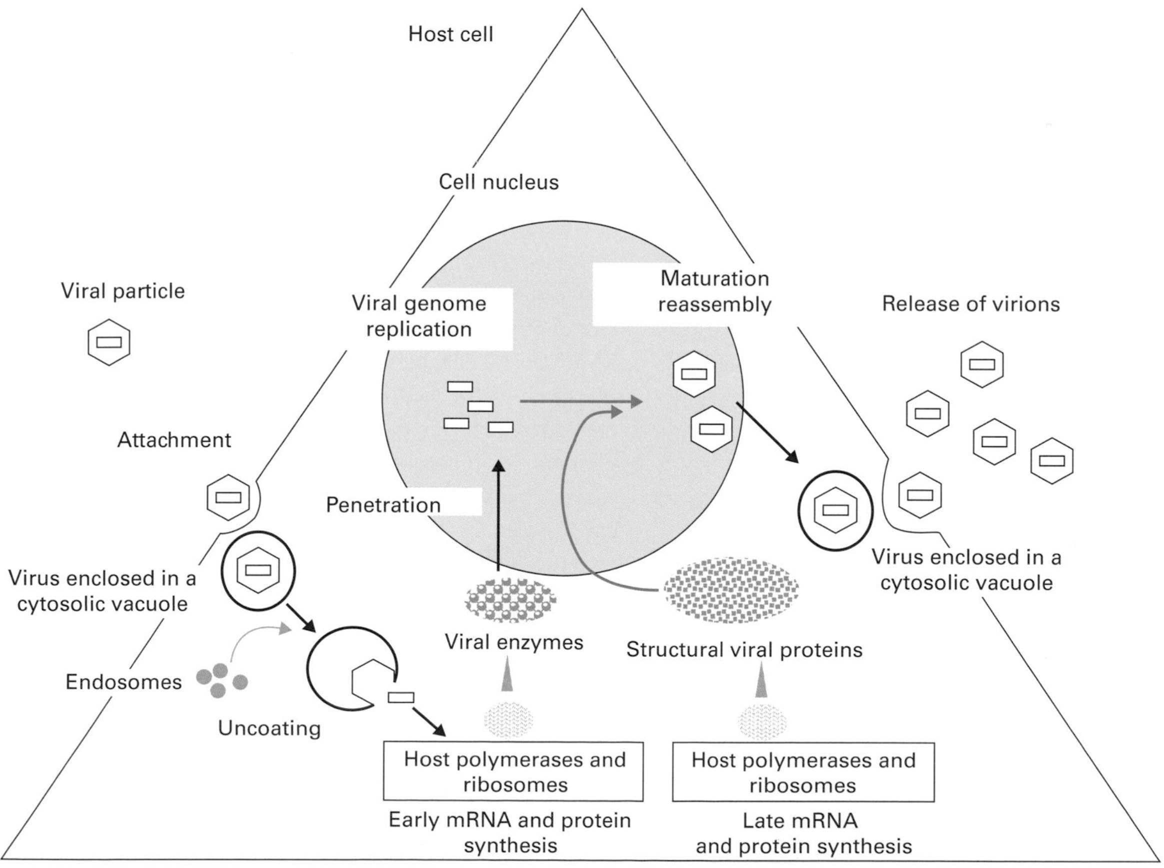

Figure 5.4 General diagrammatic representation of the production and release of viral particles from an infected cell. Specific details may vary depending on the virus.

viruses might share the same receptor. The virus–cell recognition event is similar to any protein–protein interaction in that it occurs through a stereospecific network of hydrogen bonds and hydrophobic forces. For example, the haemagglutinin receptor of influenza virus binds the terminal glycoside residues of gangliosides (cell surface glycolipids) of the target cell leading directly to the virus particle adhering to the cell. Similarly, the interaction between the HIV receptor (i.e., gp120) and the T-lymphocyte receptor (i.e., CD4) has been intensively studied, as well as the interaction between the ACE-2 receptor of lung type II alveolar cells and the S protein of SARS-CoV-2. This is important for antiviral drug development, as it allows the identification of chemical compounds and approaches that could interfere with this process, preventing viral infections of the host cells.

5.4.2 Penetration of the Viral Particle

Following the irreversible attachment of the virus to the host cell, penetration of the virus through the cell membrane is initiated following either of two energy-dependent mechanisms, endocytosis or fusion. A third mechanism has been identified in those bacteriophages that can inject their nucleic acid into the bacterium (see Section 5.9.1). During endocytosis, the association between virus receptor and host receptor triggers a number of mechanisms that cause the cell membrane to engulf the virus particle forming a cytosolic vacuole. This process is widespread among non-enveloped viruses, but is also used with some enveloped viruses such as influenza (orthomyxoviruses) and SARS-CoV-2 (coronaviruses). In case of SARS-CoV-2, it has been shown Delta variants primarily infect cells via the fusion mechanism, while Omicron relies on endocytosis. Certain enveloped viruses (e.g., herpes simplex virus, and HIV) can penetrate following fusion of their envelope with the host cell membrane, liberating the viral capsid within the cell cytoplasm.

5.4.3 Uncoating of the Viral Particle

Following penetration of the virus in a vacuole or directly into the cell cytoplasm, the viral nucleic acid then needs to be released from the capsid/coat(s) to initiate viral replication. This is the *uncoating* process. For viruses that penetrate by endocytosis, the acidification of the cytosolic vacuoles following endosome fusion induces a conformational change in the capsid and the release of viral nucleocapsid (some helper proteins are associated with the viral nucleic acid) into the cytoplasm. For certain viruses, such as rotaviruses, only a partial uncoating is necessary for the expression of the viral genome. The release of the nucleocapsid from vacuoles can occur in the cytoplasm, close to the nucleus or within the cell nucleus.

5.4.4 Replication of Viral Nucleic Acids and Translation of the Genome

This stage of viral replication ensures that (i) the host cell synthetic machinery is taken over by the virus, and (ii) the viral genome is replicated. The structure, size and nature of the viral genome are extremely diverse and thus this stage of the viral multiplication cycle reflects this diversity. Three main mechanisms are, however, common to all viruses: the transcription of viral genes into viral mRNA, the translation of the viral genome into proteins and the replication of the viral genome. Early transcription and translation, usually occurring immediately after the release of the nucleocapsid in the cytoplasm, are also common, and ensure the production of early proteins such as viral polymerases, and the hijacking of the cell synthesis machinery. In addition, some viruses can encode genes, the products of which regulate the host synthetic processes according to the needs of the virus (e.g., *tat* gene in HIV).

The replication and transcription of the viral genome depend on the type of nucleic acid carried by the virus (Table 5.2) and require the activity of a polymerase, which can be either encoded in the viral genome or come from the host. Viruses are known to utilise all four possible types of polymerases: DNA-dependent DNA polymerases, DNA-dependent RNA polymerases, RNA-dependent RNA polymerases and RNA-dependent DNA polymerases (reverse transcriptases), with the latter two types of polymerase being unique to viruses. For example, the positive-strand RNA genome in viruses such as the poliovirus or SARS-CoV-2 can be used directly as mRNA following its release into the host cell. Negative-strand RNA (e.g., in influenza virus) is transcribed into a positive RNA complementary in base sequence to the parent RNA using an RNA-dependent RNA polymerase carried by the virus. In dsDNA viruses (e.g., adenoviruses), the nucleic acid passes into the nucleus where it is usually transcribed by a host DNA-dependent RNA polymerase. In some viruses (e.g., poxvirus), this enzyme is contained within the virus and released during uncoating, allowing the viral genome to be replicated in the cell cytoplasm. In retroviruses (e.g., HIV), a single-stranded proviral DNA is produced from the viral ssRNA by the HIV reverse transcriptase. This unique enzyme acts both as an RNA- and DNA-directed DNA polymerase, and has associated RNAase activity. The proviral DNA can be transported to the cell nucleus where it can be integrated within the cell host genome by a viral integrase.

In comparison to host polymerases, viral polymerases often demonstrate higher processivity, being able to synthesise long chains of nucleic acids without dissociating from the template. At the same time, their fidelity is often lower, resulting in frequent misincorporation of nucelotides during DNA or RNA synthesis and thus a higher mutation rate of viral genomes compared to prokaryotic and eukaryotic organisms. In general, mutation rates of dsDNA viruses are the lowest, while ssDNA viruses usually accumulate mutations at a faster rate. The majority of viruses with RNA genomes mutate even faster due to the activity of their error-prone polymerases, to the extent that some viruses (including such important pathogens as HCV and HIV), instead of having a defined and relatively stable genome sequence, are known to exist as a population consisting of a spectrum of viable mutant variants of approximately equal ecological fitness collectively known as a *viral quasispecies*. Such high mutation rates and the resulting genetic diversity at the population level significantly expedite evolution and allow for high adaptability of viral quasispecies whereby, upon the exposure to a new environmental stress factor, beneficial mutants will be quickly selected from the existing pool of genetic variants and a new quasispecies will form around them. A rapid accumulation of mutations making a viral quasispecies resistant to an antiviral drug or an immune response could be seen as an example of this process. Conversely, with the mutation rates this high, such viruses are dangerously close to the error threshold – the mutation rate after which the level of detrimental and lethal mutations becomes too high, reducing the overall fitness of the quasispecies or even driving it to extinction. Certain antiviral drugs (e.g., ribavirin) exploit this vulnerability, increasing viral mutation rates above the error threshold and thus inducing lethal mutagenesis.

It should be noted that, although error-prone polymerases are frequently found in viral species, some viral polymerases have proofreading activity, which improves the overall accuracy of replication. For example, the DNA-dependent DNA polymerase of the dsDNA bacteriophage phi29 has a proofreading domain and is characterised by both high processivity (it can amplify the 20 kbp genome of the phage in a single event, without dissociating from the template) and accuracy, which is estimated to be 1–2 orders of magnitude higher than that of Taq polymerase, the enzyme frequently used in the polymerase chain reaction (PCR). Among RNA viruses, coronaviruses (including SARS-CoV-2) are unique, as their RNA-dependent RNA polymerase complexes (replicases) also have proofreading activity, resulting in lower mutation rates of coronaviruses compared to other RNA viruses, which makes the development of antivirals against coronaviruses particularly challenging. This additional proofreading functionality of replicases probably can be explained by the size of coronaviral genomes – at approximately 26–32 kbp they are the longest of all RNA viruses and thus their replication requires higher accuracy. Nevertheless, coronaviruses still have relatively high mutation rates and evolve rapidly (see Section 5.6), although slower than comparable RNA viruses (e.g., influenza viruses).

One important difference between the eukaryotic host cell and the virus is in the nature of their mRNA. Host cell mRNA codes directly for functional proteins, whereas some viral mRNAs are *polycistronic*, which means several distinct proteins are encoded within a single piece of mRNA. This implies that the virus needs to use a virus-specific protease to cut at the correct place within the *polyprotein* formed by translation of such an mRNA to produce functional viral proteins.

Late protein synthesis during the replication cycle concerns the production of structural components (e.g., capsomeres) of the new virions and proteins required for the release of viral particles from the infected cell.

5.4.5 Maturation or Assembly of Virions

Towards the end of the multiplication process, large amounts of viral material accumulate within the host. Viral capsid starts to form from individual structural proteins. In certain viruses (e.g., poliovirus), the capsid self-assembles. The replicated viral genome and some viral proteins become packaged within the capsid. Most non-enveloped viruses accumulate within the cytoplasm or nucleus and are only released when the cell lyses. Packaging of viral components can occur within the cytoplasm, in the cell nucleus or, in the case of certain viruses such as SARS-CoV-2, in viral factories. For example, with influenza virus, the capsomeres are transported to the cell nucleus where they combine with the viral RNA and assemble into helical capsids. The envelope of enveloped viruses originates from the host membrane structures. With the influenza virus, viral proteins such as neuraminidase and haemagglutinin migrate to the cell membrane, displacing cell protein. The assembled nucleocapsids pass out from the nucleus to the cytoplasm and as they impinge on the altered cytoplasmic membrane they cause it to bulge and bud off completed enveloped particles from the cell. In the herpesvirus, the envelope originates from the nuclear membrane. The nucleocapsid assembles into the nucleus and it acquires its envelope as it passes through the inner nuclear membrane. The complete virus is then incorporated into a vesicle which migrates to the cell surface.

The maturation of viruses and their assembly is not well understood at present. The presence of chaperone proteins

Table 5.3 Cultivation of viruses to produce vaccines.

Virus	Cultivation
Hepatitis A virus	Human diploid cells
Coronaviruses	Human or mammalian continuous cell lines (e.g., African green monkey kidney cells Vero E6 and Vero CCL-81)
Influenza virus	Fertilised hen's eggs – membrane bounding the amniotic cavity
Smallpox	Fertilised hen's eggs – chorioallantoic membrane
Measles and mumps	Chick embryo cells
Rubella	Human diploid cells
Human herpesvirus 3 (shingles, herpes zoster)	Human diploid cells
Rabies virus	Chick embryo cells or in human diploid cells
Varicella zoster virus	Human diploid cells
Tick-borne encephalitis virus	Chick embryo cells
Yellow fever virus	Chick embryos
Poliovirus	Human diploid cell line, continuous cell line or primary, secondary or tertiary monkey kidney cells
Baculovirus (recombinant vaccine)	Insect vector

may play an important role in the interaction between the viral nucleic acid and the structural proteins.

5.4.6 Release of Virions into the Surrounding Environment

At the end of the multiplication process, the mature virions are released from the host cell. This can occur in a number of different ways. For most non-enveloped viruses, the virus progeny accumulates within the host cell cytoplasm and is released following cell lysis. Some viruses (e.g., bacteriophages) produce lytic enzymes (endolysins) or proteases to lyse the host enabling the release of infectious particles, although the host often self-disintegrates as it cannot maintain normal housekeeping functions during a viral infection. Enveloped viruses are usually released by a budding process over a period of hours. Ultimately the host cell will die following damage to its metabolism and homeostatic functions during viral replication.

5.5 Cultivation of Human Viruses

The study and identification of viruses (for diagnosis) depend on our ability to propagate them, but viruses replicate only within living cells. In the early days of virology, viruses were propagated in a host. To some extent, this is still the case today with the use of the chick embryo (see below). However, progress in cell and tissue culture has revolutionised the cultivation of many viruses, enabling a better understanding of their replication properties, more rapid diagnosis and the easier production of vaccine (Table 5.3).

5.5.1 Cell Culture

Cells to support the growth of human viruses are usually derived from humans or other primates, or from rodents. Cell cultures may be divided into three types according to their history: (i) primary, (ii) secondary and (iii) continuous cell cultures. Primary and secondary cells are usually diploid cell lines. Primary cell lines are derived directly from an intact tissue such as human embryo kidney or monkey kidney. Secondary cell cultures are derived from primary cultures, usually those arising from embryonic tissue. These cells are more homogenous, better characterised, but might not be as susceptible to viral infection as primary cell lines. In addition, a limited number of subcultures can be performed with these cells, generally up to a maximum of about 50 before the cells degenerate. Continuous cell lines are usually derived from malignant tissue (e.g., HeLa cells derived from a cervical carcinoma) and have the capacity to multiply indefinitely *in vitro*.

In principle, cell culture for propagating viruses relies on the growth of cells in a semiconfluent monolayer attached to a surface (e.g., the bottom of a flask). To subculture, the cells are separated from the monolayer or relevant tissue usually with trypsin to form a suspension of single cells. These suspended cells are then used to seed a new flask. Following growth at 37 °C, cells will multiply, attach to the surface and form a new monolayer within a few days. The media used to grow the cells consist of basic nutrients and salts (the composition of the medium varies depending on the type of cell) supplemented with serum (usually bovine albumin) to provide growth factors; antibiotics and antifungals are included to prevent bacterial and fungal contamination in such a rich growth medium.

The established cell monolayer will support viral replication from which viruses can be harvested. Many types of viruses, upon inoculation of a cell culture, will produce a characteristic morphological change in the infected cells. This is called a *cytopathic* effect and usually indicates cell death. The cytopathic effect can take the form of cell shrinkage or ballooning, or the detachment of cells from the surface of the flask; in some instances, cellular effects will be detected using various staining solutions. Cytopathic effects usually spread to adjacent cells and will result in local lysis and the formation of a clear zone (*plaque*) that can easily be identified following staining. These plaques are used for the enumeration of viruses assuming one plaque results from an initial infection by one virus.

To confirm the identity of a viral pathogen (e.g., herpes simplex virus, cytomegalovirus, or influenza), viruses are grown in cell culture and, following the appearance of a cytopathic effect, the identity of the virus is confirmed using an appropriate viral antiserum labelled with a fluorescent dye.

Mammalian cells used for vaccine production are obtained from an approved cell bank. All such cells need to be checked for infectious agents and tumourigenicity (in the case of live vaccines). Such cells are also characterised biochemically (isoenzyme analysis), immunologically (histocompatibility antigens) and by cytogenetic markers, and are shown to be free from contaminating cells (nucleic acid fingerprint analysis). Depending on their origin, cells will be examined for the absence of specific infectious agents, for the absence of bacterial, fungal and mycoplasma contaminants and for retroviruses; techniques used to do this include product-enhanced reverse transcriptase (PERT) assay, transmission electron microscopy and, if necessary, infectivity assays. The same controls apply to insect cells.

5.5.2 The Chick Embryo

Fertile chicken eggs, 9–11 days old, are used as a convenient cell system to grow a number of human pathogenic viruses. Their usefulness derives from the many types of different tissues found in the eggs, tissues that will support the growth of different viruses (Table 5.3). The use of chicken eggs is expensive, and cell culture is preferred wherever possible. The use of chicken eggs for the production of vaccine is necessarily subject to many controls. The eggs have to be free from specific pathogens and originate from healthy flocks. The processing of the fertilised eggs must be conducted under aseptic conditions in an area where no other infectious agents or cells are handled at the same time.

5.5.3 Animal Inoculation

Some animals (e.g., rodents and primates) have to be used to culture certain viruses in order to study antiviral and vaccine effectiveness, and also as a source of cell lines for cell cultures. The use of animals follows strict ethical guidelines and is very costly. A number of controls ensuring that the animals are free from diseases must be observed. Where animals are used to grow viruses or to test an antiviral or vaccine, growth of the virus is indicated by signs of disease or death.

5.6 Viral Epidemics and Pandemics

When a disease affects a large proportion of a population, it is called an *epidemic*. A *pandemic* is an especially dangerous epidemic, occurring over a wide geographic area and affecting a large proportion of the world's population. Epidemics and pandemics happen in circumstances when the population as a whole is susceptible to the disease and the methods of detection, prevention and control are either not available or not effective. The lack of immunity to an infectious agent in a population facilitates its transmission and is most often caused by the absence of prior exposure to that agent, which happens when such a pathogen is either novel or a recently formed mutated strain, or as a consequence of insufficient numbers of individuals immunised against the pathogen in the population.

Under certain favourable circumstances, if the initial outbreak is not detected and contained in time, viral infections capable of human-to-human transmission, especially respiratory and gastrointestinal ones, can rapidly spread through communities and entire populations. Some of the worst of recent epidemics and pandemics have been caused by viral agents, including multiple influenza epidemics, the ongoing HIV pandemic, epidemics of Ebola and measles, and the COVID-19 pandemic.

COVID-19 is a new and highly dangerous illness and as such has become the focus of very intensive research. It is caused by SARS-CoV-2 betacoronavirus, a member of the *Coronaviridae* family, which includes viruses that cause respiratory and intestinal illnesses in humans and animals. Although usually associated with mild respiratory disease (e.g., colds caused by betacoronaviruses OC43 and HKU1), coronaviruses were the cause of SARS in 2002 and MERS in 2012. On 31st December 2019, the first cases of pneumonia of unknown cause were identified in Wuhan, Hubei Province, China. Several of the early cases had visited a live animal market and so the newly discovered virus, named in February 2020 by the ICTV as SARS-CoV-2, is thought to be of zoonotic origin. Although at the time of writing (August 2022) the natural host of SARS-CoV-2 has not yet been identified, it appears to be closely related to the bat coronavirus RaTG13 (96% identical at the whole genome level); several studies also reported high similarity of the virus to pangolin (scaly anteater) coronaviruses, thus both animals have been considered to be possible vectors to the human population. The SARS-CoV-2 human coronavirus spread rapidly beyond national borders and COVID-19 was declared a pandemic by the World Health Organization on 11th March 2020.

The COVID-19 virus appears to spread more easily than influenza and is more contagious than SARS; without control measures the median R_0 (the basic reproduction number, a number of people an infected individual is expected to infect in a community with no pre-existing immunity to a particular pathogen) is in the region of 2.5–3 for early (ancestral) strains and higher for more recently evolved variants such as Delta and Omicron, while for seasonal influenza it is around 1.3. Replication in RNA viruses is error-prone, leading to the rapid accumulation of mutations. However, SARS-CoV-2 appears to have a mutation rate lower than many other RNA viruses such as influenza virus, norovirus and HIV and this may limit strain variation. Nevertheless, as the virus constantly mutates and evolves, new variants have emerged. The majority of mutations are either neutral or detrimental for the virus, but some mutations will result in its increased ecological fitness, such as improving transmissibility of the virus or reducing the efficiency of immune response. For example, the mutation that led to replacement of aspartate (D) in the 614th position of the SARS-CoV-2 spike protein with glycine (G) was first reported in January 2020. The new variant of the virus with D614G mutation had completely replaced the original one globally by July 2020, raising concerns that the virus was becoming more transmissible. To monitor the evolution of the virus and identify and track strains with particularly important mutations (variants of concern), many countries implemented COVID-19 surveillance systems, based on routine sequencing of viral genomes isolated from samples collected from infected individuals. By January 2021, about 44% of all SARS-CoV-2 genomic sequences in international public databases were generated by the national monitoring system of the UK (COVID-19 Genomics UK Consortium). The bioinformatics analysis of the available sequencing data identified that several lineages of SARS-CoV-2 were prevalent globally. One particular lineage, known as the lineage B.1.1.7, or Alpha in WHO classification, was detected in samples from Kent in December 2020. This variant, designated by Public Health England as the Variant of Concern 202012/01 (VOC-202012/01), is characterised by the presence of 17 mutations changing sequences of viral proteins. More recently emerged SARS-CoV-2 variants, Delta (B.1.617.2) and Omicron (B.1.1.529), in particular, accumulated further mutations, which resulted in their increased virulence (Delta) and transmissibility (Omicron). The accumulation of mutations in the viral genome, especially in the spike protein, raises a number of concerns about the future effectiveness of vaccines. Laboratory testing has demonstrated that a number of the vaccines developed by March 2021 indeed had reduced effectiveness against some novel variants of SARS-CoV-2, prompting vaccine manufacturers to initiate research into modifying their vaccines to address this.

A future concerning development would be the acquisition of mutations by the virus that would make it easier to infect animals, similar to what happened during the 2009 influenza pandemic. Here, the human influenza H1N1 virus which originated in pigs, crossed into humans, spread globally and finally jumped back into pigs, causing a disruption to the pork industry in a number of countries. The H1N1 virus continues to circulate in pigs. It is known that SARS-CoV-2 can infect domestic cats and minks. The infection of minks at mink farms in the Netherlands and Denmark resulted in the culling of millions of animals and significant economic losses. There is a risk that the SARS-CoV-2 could develop mutations allowing for better human-to-animal and animal-to-animal transmissions, thus potentially creating a new reservoir of viruses in animals from which the disease could re-emerge. White-tailed deer in the United States are known to be highly susceptible to SARS-CoV-2 infections and animal-to-animal transmissions have been detected. Finally, a case in which a veterinarian from Thailand acquired SARS-CoV-2 from an infected domestic cat was reported in June 2022. While such cases remain rare, this once again highlights the importance of the 'One Health' approach to infectious diseases.

As of August 2022, the global case fatality ratio (CFR) for COVID-19 appears to be around 1.1% with close to 600 million cases worldwide and 6.5 million deaths, a fatality level around 25 times higher than common flu (estimated 4 billion cases each flu season). For comparison, the death rate for the Spanish flu of 1918 is estimated at 1–2% (of 500 million cases), for the 2009 swine flu pandemic 0.01–0.08% (from 1.6 billion cases), for 2002 SARS it was 9.6% (of 8096 cases) and for MERS in 2012, 34.4% (of 2494 cases). Both CFR and R_0 vary significantly between different countries due to differences in population structure, genetics and the standard of care available, usually improving over time as new treatments become available. For example, as of August 2022, the CFR for COVID-19 in Singapore is close to 0.15%, while in two countries with the highest COVID-19 death rates, Yemen and Sudan, it is 18.1% and 7.9%, respectively. It should be noted that estimates for low-income countries might be highly unreliable if cases are underreported. For comparison, the CFR in the

United Kingdom is 0.8%, which is higher than in Ireland (0.5%), but lower than in the United States (1.1%).

SARS-CoV-2 has emerged only recently as a pathogen, and so there is little clarity as to whether the virus will become endemic (circulating permanently in the global human population) and whether its transmission will vary seasonally, although the latest data suggest that this most likely will be the case. However, we do know that it is transmitted through direct and indirect contact with respiratory aerosols and droplets in a manner similar to the other respiratory viruses such as the four human coronaviruses that have circulated in the population for many decades. These coronaviruses, usually associated with mild cold symptoms, tend to spread alongside influenza during the winter in temperate regions.

As with other viruses with similar transmission mechanisms, control measures have been a significant feature for managing the pandemic caused by SARS-CoV-2. Transmission is mainly by close contact between people, most often via aerosols and droplets released by coughing, sneezing and talking, but less commonly by transfer from contaminated surfaces to the face; transmission via air conditioning systems is unlikely. The virus can survive in droplets for up to 3 hours and on surfaces of stainless steel for up to 72 hours.

To control the outbreak, national authorities responded by implementing travel restrictions, screening travellers, local and national lockdowns, workplace hazard controls and facility closures. Personal preventative measures employed included: hand-washing, the wearing of masks and face coverings in public, maintaining distance between people, monitoring and self-isolation; personal protective equipment (PPE) was issued to front-line healthcare workers. Shortages of clinical equipment, particularly ventilators, PPE and testing materials, were experienced on a global scale in the first several months of the pandemic.

One of the most important approaches helping to keep the infection spread under control is timely identification of infected persons. Many countries increased their testing capacity and contact-tracing capabilities in order to do so. Two main techniques were routinely used. The first approach detects the ongoing viral infection and is based on the use of the PCR for detection of viral RNA fragments. The second detects the presence of antibodies against SARS-CoV-2 and thus can be used for confirmation of previous exposure to the virus. Both of these methods require a sample of nasopharyngeal secretions, but other secretions or bodily fluids, such as blood, faeces and urine, can also be used for diagnostic testing.

Recently, an approach called *wastewater surveillance* has become popular in the UK and several other countries. It is based on continuous sampling and monitoring of community wastewater (untreated sewage) for the presence of viral genetic material using PCR, which can be further supplemented with DNA sequencing for a reliable identification of the viral variants. This approach allows for measuring levels of infection within the sampled community (such as city district, town, or a prison), monitoring infection rate trends (increasing or decreasing), timely identification of potential outbreaks and enables identification of novel viral variants in circulation. An interesting finding of such surveillance conducted in New York City (USA) was the detection of cryptic lineages of SARS-CoV-2, which are virus variants that are rarely or never detected in clinical samples. A potential explanation could be that they originate from either unsampled human COVID-19 infections or a non-human animal reservoir. Another example of the utility of wastewater surveillance was the detection of a poliovirus from sewage samples collected in London between February and May 2022, which allowed the UK Health Security Agency (UKHSA) to begin a timely investigation into its community source.

Alongside infection monitoring and control and contact tracing, effective immunisation is a critical measure in the management of a pandemic. As soon as the scale and seriousness of the COVID-19 pandemic had been realised, an unprecedented international initiative to find efficient antiviral drugs, develop vaccines and accelerate clinical testing was implemented. Six main approaches in vaccine development were explored (see also Chapter 10): a viral vector vaccine, a DNA vaccine, an RNA vaccine, a live-attenuated vaccine, a vaccine based on the inactivated virus and a protein-based vaccine (subunit vaccine). Before undergoing clinical trials, candidates had to show that they could induce protective immunity, not immunopathology, as was unfortunately experienced in early attempts to develop a SARS-CoV vaccine after the virus emerged in 2002. By March 2021, 12 different vaccines were authorised for use in at least one country, 85 more were in different stages of clinical testing and 225 in preclinical testing. The rate at which new vaccines were developed, tested, manufactured and deployed was astonishing: the first vaccine in the world (outside clinical trials) was administered in the UK on the 8th December 2020, just 343 days after the disease was reported for the first time. By the end of March 2021, more than 50% of the adult population of the UK had been vaccinated either once or twice and more than 400 million people in the world had received at least one dose of the vaccine.

As noted in Section 5.1, an outbreak of another disease of viral origin, monkeypox, was detected in May 2022. The initial cases were reported from the UK in individuals who had recently travelled to Nigeria where monkeypox is endemic. The disease began to spread internationally and by the end of August 2022 more than 40,000 cases had been reported from over 90 countries in total. On 24th July 2022, monkeypox was declared to be a public health emergency of international concern (PHEIC) by the WHO. Monkeypox clinical manifestations are superficially similar to those of deadly smallpox (fever, rash, formation of characteristic blisters all over the body), but the disease is usually milder and less likely to be fatal; the case fatality rate of the clade II variants that caused the initial outbreak in the UK is normally around 1%. Nevertheless, monkeypox is a dangerous infectious disease; moreover, the ease and speed of the global spread, and the fact that the new variants are genetically more distant from previously studied isolates than would be expected based on the assumed speed of viral evolution, make this a reason for concern. Two antivirals, cidofovir, an inhibitor of viral DNA-dependent DNA polymerases, and tecovirimat, a novel drug inhibiting the egress of newly formed viral particles through binding to an envelope protein, were shown to be effective against monkeypox. While no specific vaccine against monkeypox exists, vaccines developed against smallpox provide adequate protection as smallpox and monkeypox belong to the same *Orthopoxvirus* genus of the *Poxviridae* family of dsDNA viruses. By the end of August 2022, several countries had initiated preventive vaccination against monkeypox among healthcare workers involved in the treatment of monkeypox patients and had begun offering post-exposure vaccines to individuals at risk. Unsurprisingly, since smallpox was eradicated by 1980, the production and supply of vaccines remains limited.

5.7 Control of Viruses

5.7.1 Antiviral Chemotherapy

A number of antivirals are in use in the UK for a range of viral infections, including HIV, herpesvirus infections, viral hepatitis, influenza and respiratory syncytial virus (RSV). Antiviral treatments are particularly important for persons at high risk, notably immunocompromised patients. Most antivirals are prodrugs that need to be activated within the cell, usually by a kinase and other cellular enzymes.

Antivirals can act at different stages of the viral replication cycle, with the most effective treatments targeting unique viral enzymes, such as proteases, polymerases and the reverse transcriptase (Table 5.4 and Chapter 11). A number of targets are being investigated to prevent viral attachment to the host cell: competition for CD4 receptors using a pentapeptide identical in sequence to the terminal amino acids of HIV gp120; inhibition of HSV ribonucleotide reductase; competition for the cell receptor using a hexapeptide fusion sequence at the N-terminus of the influenza haemagglutinin viral receptor. Proteases are particularly important at certain stages of a virus life cycle, including the uncoating process, which is necessary for the release of viral genetic material into the host cell, and for the cleavage of viral polypeptide gene products, thus making protease inhibitors (e.g., saquinavir) particularly disruptive. The replication of viral DNA is also a well-exploited target with the use of nucleoside analogues (e.g., aciclovir which is incorporated into viral and cellular DNA instead of guanine), non-nucleoside analogues (e.g., nevirapine and foscarnet) and oligonucleotides (Table 5.5). These nucleic acid oligomers with base sequence complementarity to conserved regions of proviral DNA have found successful use in the prevention of viral mRNA function. Oligonucleotide-based therapeutic agents are specific, efficient and generally well-tolerated. Although oligonucleotide-based antivirals are not currently used in the UK, several are in phase I or II clinical trials. The inhibition of HIV reverse transcriptase has led to the synthesis of many successful antivirals (Table 5.4). The release of the mature virions after the multiplication process can also be blocked. This is the case for neuraminidase inhibitors (e.g., zanamivir and oseltamivir) which prevent the shedding of virions.

Unfortunately, antiviral chemotherapy is associated with a number of problems. Many viral diseases only become apparent after extensive viral multiplication and tissue damage have occurred, delaying treatment onset. Many antivirals are toxic (e.g., nucleoside analogues), since viral replication often depends on the use of host cell enzymes. There is also scope for improving the pharmacokinetic properties of antivirals, providing a better penetration and retarding drug degradation. The use of prodrugs has improved drug adsorption. Finally, antiviral monotherapy often leads to the development of virus resistance. Emerging HIV resistance has been well documented and current treatments are based on a triple therapy.

5.7.1.1 HIV

There is no cure for HIV infections as yet. The role of antivirals is to slow or halt disease progression. Since their discovery and use, these drugs (Table 5.4), called antiretrovirals, have considerably prolonged the life expectancy of patients, although not without some significant side effects. Antiretroviral treatments aim to reduce HIV plasma levels by as much and for as long as possible. Several antiretroviral drugs are usually given together to avoid emerging viral resistance. Initiation of HIV treatment (ART) is therefore complex and involves two nucleoside reverse transcriptase inhibitors and a third antiretroviral agent, such as a non-nucleoside reverse transcriptase inhibitor, protease inhibitor or integrase inhibitor. Alternative regimens are possible

Table 5.4 Current antiviral drugs in use in the UK (based on BNF 83), classified according to their mechanism of action.

Mechanism of action	Viral infection	Name
Ribonucleotide analogue (RNA polymerase inhibitor)	SARS-CoV-2 (COVID-19)	Remdesivir
Ribonucleoside analogue (increases number of mutations)	SARS-CoV-2 (COVID-19)	Molnupiravir
Nucleoside reverse transcriptase inhibitor (NRTI)	HIV	Zidovudine (AZT)
	HIV	Abacavir
	HIV	Emtricitabine
	HIV	Lamivudine
Nucleotide reverse transcriptase inhibitor (NtRTI)	Chronic hepatitis B, HIV	Tenofovir disoproxil
	Chronic hepatitis B, HIV	Tenofovir alafenamide
	Chronic hepatitis B	Adefovir dipivoxil
HIV protease inhibitor	HIV	Atazanavir*
	HIV	Darunavir*
	HIV	Fosamprenavir (prodrug of amprenavir)
	HIV	Lopinavir (only in combination with ritonavir)
	HIV	Ritonavir
	HIV	Tipranavir
Non-nucleoside reverse transcriptase inhibitor	HIV	Efavirenz
	HIV	Etravirine
	HIV	Nevirapine
	HIV	Doravirine
	HIV	Rilpivirine
Inhibition of HIV–host fusion	HIV	Enfuvirtide
Attachment inhibitor	HIV	Fostemsavir (prodrug of temsavir)
Antagonist of CCR5 chemokine receptor	HIV	Maraviroc
Inhibitor of HIV integrase	HIV	Raltegravir
	HIV	Bictegravir
	HIV	Cabotegavir
	HIV	Dolutegravir
	HIV	Elvitegravir
Inhibitor of viral DNA polymerase	Herpes viruses	Aciclovir
	Herpes zoster and genital herpes	Famciclovir (prodrug of penciclovir)
	Herpes simplex, herpes zoster	Valaciclovir (ester of aciclovir)
	Cytomegalovirus	Ganciclovir
	Cytomegalovirus	Valganciclovir (ester of ganciclovir)
	Cytomegalovirus	Cidofovir
Immunostimulant	Herpes simplex	Inosine pranobex (stimulates cell-mediated immune response – mode of action unknown)
	Chronic hepatitis B	Peginterferon alfa
Cytomegalovirus DNA terminase complex inhibitor	Cytomegalovirus	Letermovir
Inactivation of virus-specific DNA polymerase and reverse transcriptase	Cytomegalovirus, herpes simplex	Foscarnet

(*Continued*)

Table 5.4 (Continued)

Mechanism of action	Viral infection	Name
Nucleoside and nucleotide analogues; interference with viral nucleic acids synthesis	Hepatitis C, RSV, adenovirus, influenza	Ribavirin
	Chronic hepatitis C	Sofosbuvir
	Chronic hepatitis B	Entecavir
NS3/NS4A protease inhibitors (used in different combinations with NS5A inhibitors)	Chronic hepatitis C	Grazoprevir
	Chronic hepatitis C	Glecaprevir
	Chronic hepatitis C	Voxilaprevir
NS5A inhibitors	Chronic hepatitis C	Elbasvir
	Chronic hepatitis C	Pibrentasvir
	Chronic hepatitis C	Ledipasvir
	Chronic hepatitis C	Velpatasvir
Inhibition of viral neuraminidase	Influenza	Oseltamivir
	Influenza	Zanamivir
Monoclonal antibody	RSV	Palivizumab

*, effect can be enhanced by the pharmacokinetic enhancer cobicistat; NS3/NS4A, hepatitis C virus (HCV) protease; NS5A, non-structural protein 5A, required for HCV replication.

Table 5.5 Oligonucleotide therapies.

Methods	Principles	Effect
Antisense nucleotides	Production of an RNA sequence complementary to single-stranded viral RNA	Triggers the formation of double-stranded duplex, inhibiting viral RNA replication
Antigen methods	Formation of triple helix of DNA	Inhibits transcription
Decoy methods	Production of synthetic decoys corresponding to a specific nucleic-acid sequence which binds virally encoded regulatory proteins	Inhibits transcription
Ribozymes	Production of RNA molecules (oligo(ribo)nucleotides)	Cleave other RNA sequences at specific sites

following treatment failure and deterioration of a patient's condition. The use of antiretrovirals for prophylaxis after exposure is also possible, where a patient has been exposed to HIV-contaminated materials (e.g., needle injury). Such use follows guidelines available locally (e.g., hospital) or nationally (e.g., Department of Health and Social Care, British HIV Association [BHIVA] and the British Association for Sexual Health and HIV).

The immune reconstitution syndrome and the lipodystrophy syndrome have been associated with antiretroviral treatments. The latter includes fat redistribution, insulin resistance, hyperglycaemia and dyslipidaemia. In addition, these antivirals can be damaging to liver function and have been associated with osteonecrosis following long-term combination treatments. A number of side effects are commonly associated with the use of antiretrovirals: gastrointestinal disturbance, anorexia, pancreatitis, liver damage, dyspnoea, cough, headache, insomnia, dizziness, fatigue, blood disorders, myalgia, arthralgia, rash, urticaria and fever. Protease inhibitors are metabolised by cytochrome P450 and therefore have a significant potential for drug interactions. Non-nucleoside reverse transcriptase inhibitors have been shown to interact with a number of drugs metabolised in the liver. They have been associated with a number of side effects such as rash, psychiatric and central nervous system disturbances and even fatal hepatitis. Nevertheless, BHIVA guidelines recommend to start antiretroviral therapy immediately after the confirmation of HIV infection and continue it indefinitely, as this minimises the loss of $CD4^+$ lymphocytes, which outweighs the risks from side effects.

5.7.1.2 Herpesvirus Infections

Herpesviridae is a family of viruses that include the herpes simplex virus, chickenpox (varicella), shingles (herpes zoster) and cytomegalovirus. Mild herpes simplex virus infections in healthy individuals are treated with a topical antiviral drug (e.g., treatment of cold sores). However, for primary herpetic gingivostomatitis, a change of diet and analgesics are recommended. For severe infections (e.g., neonatal herpes infection and infection in immunocompromised patients), a systemic antiviral drug is used (Table 5.4). Antiviral treatments for chickenpox are recommended in patients at risk and in neonates to reduce risks of severe disease. In healthy adults, treatment taken within 24 hours of the appearance of a rash may decrease the duration and severity of symptoms. Systemic antivirals are used to decrease the severity and duration of shingles when taken within 72 hours of the onset of rash. Antivirals for herpes are also associated with a number of side effects which vary depending on the drug, but may include nausea, vomiting, stomach pain, headache, fatigue, rash, and an increase in serum and urine uric acid. Antivirals for the treatment of cytomegalovirus are usually given to immunocompromised patients and they tend to be more toxic with notable nephrotoxicity (e.g., cidofovir) and a number of documented side effects (e.g., ganciclovir and foscarnet).

5.7.1.3 Viral Hepatitis

Hepatitis B and C are major causes of viral chronic hepatitis. The initial treatment for acute hepatitis B is with interferons (peginterferon alfa-2a) which may reduce the risk of chronic infection. However, the use of interferon is limited by a poor response rate in patients and frequent relapse. A number of antivirals are licensed for the treatment of chronic hepatitis B (Table 5.4). The choice of antivirals depends upon the initial response to peginterferon alfa, emerging viral resistance and co-infection with HIV. For the treatment of chronic hepatitis C, a combination of ribavirin and peginterferon alfa is recommended, although the choice and duration of treatment depend upon the viral genotypes and viral load. These antivirals are also associated with a number of side effects including nausea, vomiting, abdominal pain and diarrhoea.

5.7.1.4 Influenza

Two antivirals are recommended for the treatment of influenza according to the National Institute for Health and Care Excellence (NICE) guidelines (Table 5.4). Oseltamivir was extensively used for the prevention and control of the swine flu outbreak in the UK in 2009. Following an intensive use, at least two major limitations in the usefulness of the drug have been identified. First, the drug needs to be taken within a few hours of the onset of symptoms, which proved very difficult with a range of mild 'cold-like' to severe 'flu-like' symptoms reported. Second, the side effects, especially in young children and adolescents, have been very severe, prompting many parents to stop the medication, decreasing the willingness to give the antivirals to children who have been possibly exposed to the virus.

5.7.1.5 Respiratory Syncytial Virus

RSV is responsible for severe bronchiolitis notably in infants. A monoclonal antibody (palivizumab) or an antiviral drug (ribavirin) is indicated for the treatment of RSV (Table 5.4). The antiviral is associated with a number of severe side effects.

5.7.1.6 SARS-CoV-2

No curative treatment is currently available, but remdesivir has been approved for management of severe COVID-19 cases in many countries. Remdesivir is a prodrug, which is converted into its active form through the action of a number of cellular enzymes. The resulting active ribonucleotide analogue acts as an inhibitor of viral RNA-dependent RNA polymerase. Remdesivir was originally developed for treatment of hepatitis C and RSV infections, but proved ineffective. It was later used for treatment of Ebola infections. Remdesivir was repurposed for treatment of COVID-19 soon after the start of the pandemic, but the results of later clinical trials were inconclusive. In November 2020, the World Health Organization (WHO) issued a recommendation against the use of remdesivir for COVID-19 treatment. The antiviral is associated with a number of side effects, including nausea, respiratory failure and liver damage.

A massive international effort to discover new and repurpose existing drugs for treatment and prevention of COVID-19 continues. Three main approaches are being investigated: (i) antivirals that interfere with different stages of SARS-CoV-2 life cycle; (ii) antibodies against the virus' components, either derived from convalescent plasma or produced as recombinant proteins (e.g., sotrovimab, a neutralising monolconal antibody) and (iii) immune system modulators that normalise the inflammatory response. The largest clinical trial of several potential COVID-19 treatments, RECOVERY, began in the UK in March 2020. One of the important findings was the discovery of positive effects for the immunosuppressant dexamethasone in patients requiring respiratory support and the monoclonal antibody tocilizumab, targeting interleukin 6 (IL-6). Both dexamethasone and tocilizumab were found to significantly reduce the risk of death in patients with severe COVID-19. The trial also demonstrated the ineffectiveness of a hydroxychloroquine and lopinavir/ritonavir combination in people hospitalised with COVID-19.

Several drugs that inhibit cellular components necessary for replication of the virus are being actively studied, such as camostat mesylate, an inhibitor of the cellular protease transmembrane serine protease 2 (TMPRSS2), essential for viral entry into lung cells. A number of other approaches are being investigated, such as cell-based therapies and RNA-based therapeutic agents, including antisense oligonucleotides. Finally, many pharmaceutical and biotechnology companies and research institutions are conducting computational screening of promising compounds for *in vitro* testing against SARS-CoV-2, powered by artificial intelligence.

By June 2022, several additional options had become available for COVID-19 treatment, including the antiviral molnupiravir, a prodrug whose activated form is incorporated into viral RNA during its synthesis causing increased mutation rate and making the majority of viral progeny defective. Another recent drug is paxlovid, a combination of nirmatrelvir, a 3C-like protease inhibitor which inactivates SARS-CoV-2 protease, thus preventing cleavage of viral polypeptides and interfering with the viral replication process, and ritonavir, an inhibitor of cytochrome CYP3A, which delays nirmatrelvir inactivation by human host enzymes and thus increases the duration of its pharmacological action. It is worth noting that, as the virus continues evolving, some of the currently used drugs will become ineffective, necessitating continued research into new antivirals.

5.7.2 Vaccination

It is always better to prevent a disease than to treat it. Vaccination is undoubtedly the most successful measure against microbial infections, and particularly viral infections. Remarkably, human protection against smallpox was achieved by Jenner in 1796 with the inoculation of cowpox, well before the 'germ theory' of disease was postulated. A worldwide vaccination programme initiated in 1966 led to the eradication of smallpox in 1980. The poliovirus is almost completely eradicated following an intensive worldwide vaccination programme by the World Health Organization.

Vaccines are preparations containing antigens that elicit a specific and active immunity against an infecting agent (see Chapter 10); they can induce the innate and the adaptive (cellular and humoral) parts of the immune system (see Chapter 9). There are currently a number of viral vaccines available against a diverse range of human viruses (Table 5.6). The success of vaccination relies on the prevention of a disease from occurring. Vaccination is particularly indicated to protect persons at risk (e.g., hepatitis B and varicella zoster vaccines for healthcare workers), prior to travelling (hepatitis A virus, Japanese encephalitis, yellow fever, and tick-borne encephalitis virus) or to prevent cancer (human papillomavirus [HPV] vaccine preventing cervical cancer). A vaccine can also be given to protect from a viral outbreak (e.g., measles, mumps and rubella vaccine [MMR]), where success is greatly influenced by the level of uptake within a susceptible population, or following exposure to rabies.

Viral vaccines are prepared using different methods, the most common being the use of live attenuated viruses, inactivated viruses or viral components (subunits). Viruses or their components can be prepared from animals, fertilised hen's eggs, in suitable cell cultures (see Section 5.5) or in suitable tissues, or in cultures of genetically engineered

Table 5.6 Examples of viral vaccines.

Vaccine	Type
Hepatitis A vaccine	Formaldehyde-inactivated hepatitis A virus
Hepatitis B vaccine	Inactivated HBV surface antigen (HBsAg)
HPV vaccine	Virus-like particle composed of the major capsid protein (L1) of HPV types 6, 11, 16 and 18
Influenza vaccine	Formaldehyde-inactivated influenza virus
Japanese encephalitis vaccine	Inactivated Japanese encephalitis virus
MMR vaccine	Live attenuated viruses
Poliomyelitis vaccines	Inactivated poliomyelitis vaccine (injection)
	Live poliomyelitis vaccine (oral)
Rabies vaccine	Inactivated rabies virus
Rotavirus vaccine	Live attenuated rotavirus
SARS-CoV-2 vaccines	Multiple types: RNA, protein subunit, non-replicating vector, inactivated virus; additional types are in development
Tick-borne encephalitis vaccine	Formaldehyde-inactivated tick-borne encephalitis virus
Varicella zoster vaccine	Live attenuated varicella zoster virus
Yellow fever vaccine	Live attenuated yellow fever virus

HBsAg, hepatitis B virus surface antigen; HPV, human papillomavirus; MMR, measles, mumps and rubella.

cells. MMR vaccine and live (oral) poliomyelitis vaccines are based on the use of live attenuated viruses, which are not as virulent as the original virus. The attenuated viruses will cause a strong immune response without causing the disease. Hepatitis A virus and influenza vaccines rely on chemically inactivated (formaldehyde or propiolactone) virus particles or components (surface antigens). Hepatitis B virus vaccine is a recombinant vaccine where the viral DNA encoding for a virus surface antigen (hepatitis B surface antigen [HBsAg]) is expressed in yeast (*Saccharomyces cerevisiae*) or mammalian cells (Chinese hamster ovary cells or other suitable cell lines). The surface antigen is then purified. HPV vaccine contains virus-like particles and recombinant capsid protein expressed in yeast or using a baculovirus as an expression system.

It should be noted that most viral vaccines contain one or more adjuvants, for example, aluminium salts (antigens are absorbed to the aluminium salts) or monophosphoryl lipid A, to increase or modulate the host immune response to the antigens.

A promising alternative approach for vaccine development harnesses the host's own synthetic machinery to prepare isolated viral components, usually surface protein, which upon release to the circulation elicit the necessary protective immune response. Vectors in this instance include genetically engineered non-pathogenic viral carriers, whether non-replicating (e.g., adenoviruses) or replicating (e.g., vesicular stomatitis virus [VSV]), DNA plasmids and messenger RNA coding for the viral surface protein gene. Of the seven different COVID-19 vaccines currently procured for the use in the UK (Table 5.7), five fall into this category. Finally, some more experimental approaches are being explored, including peptide vaccines and dendritic-cell-based vaccines (i.e., live dendritic cells that are challenged with an antigen *ex vivo* and then delivered back into the patient). It should be noted that new vaccines have to be developed when the mutations of the virus lead to changes in antigens that render the original vaccines less effective. In August 2022, the UK became the first country to approve a dual vaccine (Spikevax) developed by the US company Moderna to target both the original SARS-CoV-2 strain and the latest Omicron variant, against which previously developed vaccines had become less efficient.

Immunoglobulin may play a role in the protection of patients with a compromised immunity against viral infections. Human normal immunoglobulin (HNIG) is prepared from a pool of donated human plasma that has been checked to be non-reactive for hepatitis B surface antigen, hepatitis C virus and HIV (types 1 and 2), but contains immunoglobulin G (IgG) and antibodies against viruses that are prevalent in the general population including hepatitis A, measles, mumps, rubella and varicella. Intramuscular normal immunoglobulin is thus used to protect against hepatitis A virus in immunocompromised patients visiting areas where the disease is highly endemic and to protect against or attenuate measles infection in immunocompromised patients. It can also be used for pregnant women against rubella virus, where the risk of termination of pregnancy is unacceptable.

Disease-specific immunoglobulins are prepared from a pool of plasma obtained from specific human donors who have high levels of the specific antibody required, such as the ones who have recently recovered from an infectious disease (convalescent plasma). Disease-specific hepatitis B immunoglobulin is used following accidental inoculation by a risk material (e.g., needlestick injury) or for infants born from mothers infected with the virus. Disease-specific rabies immunoglobulin is available following the bite of an animal suspected of carrying the disease or originating from an area where the disease is endemic. Disease-specific varicella zoster immunoglobulin is indicated for individuals who are at a high risk such as neonates whose mothers develop chickenpox, or for those exposed to the virus while requiring intensive care or prolonged special care, and for immunocompromised individuals. Convalescent plasma

Table 5.7 SARS-CoV-2 vaccines to be used in the UK. All vaccines use the spike protein of SARS-CoV-2 or its fragments as antigens.

Vaccine type	Vaccine manufacturer	No. of doses ordered	Status (as of June 2022)
Non-replicating vector (adenovirus)	Oxford/AstraZeneca (UK/Sweden)	100 million	Approved and in deployment
Non-replicating vector (adenovirus)	Janssen (Netherlands/USA)	20 million	Approved, deployment pending
mRNA	Pfizer/BioNTech (USA/Germany)	189 million	Approved and in deployment
mRNA	Moderna (USA)	77 million	Approved and in deployment
mRNA	CureVac (Germany)	50 million	Phase III clinical trials
Protein subunit	GlaxoSmithKline/Sanofi Pasteur (UK/France)	60 million	Phase III clinical trials
Protein subunit	Novavax (USA)	60 million	Approved, deployment pending

was trialled against COVID-19, but the results of several studies showed that while the treatment is safe, it is ineffective.

5.7.3 Viricidal Effects of Chemical and Physical Agents on Viruses

Viruses are generally transmitted via surfaces and therefore the use of viricidal disinfectants on hard surfaces and viricidal antiseptics on skin is important. In addition, viruses are often associated with organic materials, such as secretions from the host, blood and faeces, which enable them to persist on surfaces for longer periods of time (weeks, months, and rarely years) and to survive better viricidal challenges.

In general, viruses are not particularly resistant to chemical or physical agents, although some exceptions exist. In terms of susceptibility to viricidal agents, small non-enveloped viruses (e.g., poliovirus) are more resistant than large enveloped viruses (e.g., HIV, influenza and SARS-CoV-2), the lipid-rich envelope being damaged easily by chemical and physical agents. Membrane-active agents, such as cationic microbicides, alcohols and biguanides are particularly effective in inactivating enveloped viruses. The susceptibility of large non-enveloped viruses varies, but it is generally considered to be between that of the small naked and large enveloped viruses, however some rotaviruses are proving particularly difficult to destroy.

The viricidal activity of microbicides (antiseptics and disinfectants) varies and not all agents show a strong viricidal activity against non-enveloped viruses (e.g., cationic biocides, phenolics and alcohols). In addition, microbicidal activity depends upon a number of factors, such as concentration, contact time, presence of soiling and formulation (see Chapters 18 and 19). Soiling is particularly an issue with water- and food-borne viruses. Indeed, even enveloped viruses can survive for many days on a soiled surface even when exposed to microbicides. Viricidal formulations often contain several microbicides (e.g., combinations of quaternary ammonium compounds [QACs], QACs and biguanides combined or QACs or biguanides in combination with alcohols) as well as other excipients which might improve the efficacy of a particular microbicide. In addition to the influence of added excipients, formulation pH will also impact on efficacy. The interactions between microbicides and viruses have been poorly studied. In general, viruses present only a few target sites to microbicides, mainly the envelope (when present), glycoproteins, the capsid and viral nucleic acid (see Chapter 20). Some microbicides (e.g., cationic agents) are likely to interact with the envelope and glycoproteins, inhibiting viral infectivity, without altering the viral capsid and genome. The main target site is most probably the capsid which has been shown to be severely damaged in the presence of highly reactive microbicides such as aldehydes (e.g., glutaraldehyde) and oxidising agents (e.g., peracetic acid and hydrogen peroxide). Less reactive microbicides, such as the QACs and biguanides (e.g., chlorhexidine), have been shown to damage viral capsid to a lesser extent, explaining the limited activity of these agents against non-enveloped viruses. The viral genome is the infectious part of the virus and is the ideal target for microbicides. The destruction/alteration of the viral nucleic acid would ensure complete viral inactivation. However, only a limited number of reactive microbicides, mainly oxidising agents (e.g., hydrogen peroxide and chlorine dioxide), have been shown to penetrate within the capsid and damage viral nucleic acid, or to damage viral nucleic acid released from a damaged capsid. The nature of the association of the viral nucleic acid with the capsid also plays a role in the susceptibility of the virus to chemical and physical agents. Viruses with a helical capsid structure might be more susceptible, since the destruction/alteration of capsid is more likely to cause damage to the viral nucleic acid which is closely associated to this type of structure.

Physical agents such as heat and irradiation are viricidal and play an important role in the control of viral contaminants in pharmaceutical products. Most viruses are susceptible to exposure to temperatures above 60 °C for 30 minutes. Such susceptibility is used for the inactivation of viral contaminants, such as HIV, in blood products. However, other viruses such as the hepatitis B virus are less susceptible and appropriate assurance of the absence of such a virus is needed. Viruses survive well at low temperatures and they can be routinely stored at −40 °C to −70 °C. In addition to thermal processes, UV irradiation and ionising radiation (γ-ray and accelerated electrons) are viricidal mainly following the destruction of the viral nucleic acid. Ionising irradiation and thermal processes are used for terminal sterilisation processes applied to medical and pharmaceutical products (see Chapter 21). Finally, a number of novel sterilisation approaches are being actively investigated, such as the use of supercritical carbon dioxide and low-temperature atmospheric-pressure plasma. Preliminary data suggest that both approaches are efficient and can rapidly inactivate viruses, including coronaviruses, on various surfaces.

5.7.4 Control of Viruses in Pharmaceutical Products

The presence of certain viruses needs to be controlled in pharmaceutical products derived from human and animal origin. This includes blood products such as human plasma for fractionation intended for the manufacture of human antithrombin III, human coagulation factors VII, VIII, IX and XI, dried prothrombin complex, dried fibrinogen, normal immunoglobulin, human α-1-proteinase inhibitor and human von Willebrand factor, for which tests for the presence of antibodies against HIV-1 and HIV-2, HBsAg and antibodies against hepatitis C virus are required. For the urine-derived urofollitropin (obtained from post-menopausal women), tests for hepatitis virus antigens and HIV antigen are needed.

The risk of a pharmaceutical product being contaminated by viruses depends mainly on the origin of the product component (e.g., species, organ or tissue), the history of the donor, the amount of material used, the manufacturing process and its capacity to remove/destroy any contaminants. In addition, the infectivity and pathogenicity of possible viral contaminants must be taken into consideration, notably when considering the route of administration of the medicinal product (i.e., transdermal delivery would carry less risk than an injection). A risk assessment is generally carried out for these products containing a component from human or animal origin, which takes into consideration factors affecting the potential level of infectious particles and those related to the use of the product.

Thus, stringent controls are applied to the raw materials, in process samples and to the final product. In addition, one or more validated procedures to remove or destroy viruses can be applied. The type of inactivation measures used must be validated against a range of representative viruses (i.e., enveloped, non-enveloped, DNA and RNA viruses) with different degrees of resistance to that type of treatment. Furthermore, early inactivation limits the extent of contamination. For the preparation of vaccines, the inactivation process must ensure that it does not affect the antigenicity while killing the virus and other potential contaminants such as mycoplasmas; for example, for the preparation of influenza vaccine, the inactivation process chosen must cause minimum alteration of the haemagglutinin and neuraminidase antigens.

5.8 Biotechnological Applications of Viruses

As already mentioned in relation to modern methods of vaccine production, certain viruses or virus components are now used as vectors for the delivery of genes to targeted cells. A number of viruses are being used in gene transfer medicinal products (GTMP) and these include adenoviruses (Ad), poxviruses, retroviruses, lentiviruses, adeno-associated viruses (AAV) and herpesviruses. Viral vectors for human use are freeze-dried or liquid preparations of recombinant viruses, genetically modified to transfer genetic material to human somatic cells *in vivo* (i.e., injected directly into the patient's body) or *ex vivo* (i.e., transferred into host cells before administration).

There are different approaches for the design and construction of viral vectors. The chosen approach depends upon the type of virus used. The procedure aims to minimise the risk of generating replicating viruses or to eliminate *helper viruses* (functional viruses, co-infection with which is required for the replication-defective viruses to produce infectious virions) when used during production. In addition, a number of stringent controls are performed ensuring the complete genetic and phenotypic characterisation of the viral vector is carried out. These include the complete sequence of the genome of the viral vector, verification of genomic integrity of the vector, determination of the concentration of the infectious vector, residual host-cell protein and DNA and residual reagents including antibiotics.

For retrovirus-derived vectors, genetic modification aims to ensure that the recombinant retroviruses are rendered replication-incompetent. Recombinant adeno-associated virus vectors (rAAV) are deficient adeno-associated viruses in which certain genes (i.e., *cap* and *rep*) necessary for viral replication have been replaced. A helper virus is thus needed during production of the rAAV and must be eliminated from the final GTMP. The resulting vector is essentially a proteinaceous nanoparticle containing the required DNA fragment (transgene) and cannot replicate on its own in host cells. As with other viral vectors, the sequence integrity of the viral genes and expression cassette as well as genetic stability need to be controlled, and the absence of wild-type virus (e.g., AAV) verified.

Some viruses, actively infecting and killing cancer cells, can be used to treat specific cancers. Such viruses are called *oncolytic viruses*. In addition to their direct destructive effects, oncolytic viruses elicit a strong immune response against the cancer cells infected with the virus, further improving the therapeutic effect. An example of such an oncolytic-virus-based drug is talimogene laherparepvec, licensed for the use in the UK against unresectable metastatic melanoma and available as a solution for intralesional injections. This biopharmaceutical drug product (biological) is a genetically engineered herpes simplex virus 1, carrying a copy of the granulocyte–macrophage colony-stimulating factor (GM-CSF); this is a cytokine that promotes the production of granulocytes from stem cells, stimulates neutrophil migration and production of pro-inflammatory cytokines and attracts dendritic cells to the site of infection. Clinical trials have demonstrated that the combined lytic effect of the virus and the systemic anti-tumour immune response it induces by post-lysis release of tumour-derived antigens and GM-CSF make talimogene laherparepvec an efficient treatment option.

Among other applications of viruses deserving a mention are their use as biopesticides (e.g., baculoviruses against the codling moth) and as a source of important enzymes for molecular biology, such as the topoisomerase

I of vaccinia virus used for TOPO cloning and Moloney murine leukaemia virus reverse transcriptase (M-MLV RT).

5.9 Bacterial Viruses

5.9.1 Overview

Bacteriophages (phages) are viruses that infect only bacteria. They were first described at the end of the nineteenth century. They are typically 20–200 nm in size and are highly diverse in their structure and host range, and it is likely that all bacterial species can be infected by a phage. Phages are extremely specific in their host range and some will only infect a specific bacterial strain. Such a high specificity is used for bacterial typing as discussed below. The most studied phages are complex ones (e.g., *Escherichia* T4 phage) sometimes referred to as 'tadpole-shaped' consisting of a head (often icosahedral) that contains the viral genome and a tail, whose function is to recognise the host receptor, attach and subsequently serve as a nucleic acid injection device (Figure 5.5). Indeed, one of the main differences between such tailed phages and common mammalian viruses is that these phages inject their viral genome inside the host cell. Tailed phages (*Caudovirales*) are thought to be the oldest known group of viruses and are evolutionarily related to herpesviruses, with which they share certain features, such as a dsDNA genome, icosahedral capsid and sequence similarity of a number of genes.

Phages have proved to be very useful genetic tools over the years, since they are easy to propagate to high concentration and easy to study. Because of their similarity to mammalian viruses, it is not surprising that phages have been used to elucidate the viral multiplication cycle, and their study has led to many discoveries such as mRNA, the understanding of the genetic code and the control of genes, contributing to important advances in molecular biology and biotechnology.

From the study of phage replication cycles, two main scenarios have emerged, one resulting in the lysis of the bacterial host – the *lytic cycle* – and the other resulting in the viral nucleic acid being integrated into the host genome – the *lysogenic cycle* (Figure 5.6). Infection with a lytic phage, also called *virulent* phage, results in the replication of the phage within the susceptible bacteria and the release of infectious phage progeny from the host cell following cell lysis. Such a lytic property is used to enumerate phages. Phages inoculated on to a lawn of a susceptible host bacterium form clear 'holes' (plaques) which result from phage infection and lysis of a bacterial host and the release of phage progeny, subsequently infecting, replicating in and lysing adjacent cells, ultimately forming these *plaques* which are easily identifiable with the naked eye (Figure 5.7). Since each of these plaques is assumed to result from the infection from a single phage, the number of plaques counted is used to represent the number of phages.

In the lysogenic cycle, the viral nucleic acid which has integrated the host genome is called *prophage*, and the host cell that contains the viral genome *lysogenic*. Following infection with lysogenic phages, both lytic and lysogenic responses can be observed. The integration of the prophage ensures that the viral genome is passed on to the daughter cells following bacterial cell replication (vertical gene transfer). Lysogeny is an extremely common phenomenon and through evolution most bacteria will host several prophages. It is now accepted that phages have played an important part in bacterial evolution. Indeed, sequencing of the whole bacterial genome often indicates the presence of prophages (or their remnants) that have become disabled with time. On occasions, a prophage dormant in its host can be reactivated and resume a lytic cycle. Upon excision from the host genome, the prophage can take adjacent bacterial genes that become incorporated in the virion and transmitted to a new susceptible host cell. Genes carried on the prophage can then be expressed in the new host. This

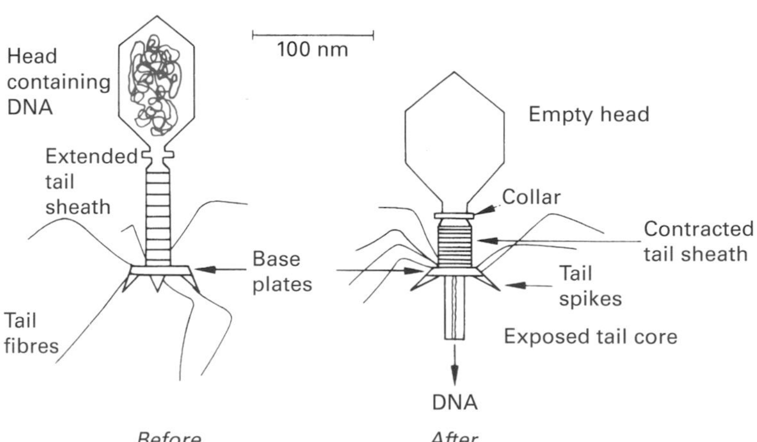

Figure 5.5 *Escherichia* T4 phage (a member of the *Myoviridae*) structure before and after tail contraction. While all tailed phages inject their genetic material into the host cell with the help of the tail structure, only *Myoviridae* have a contractile tail sheath.

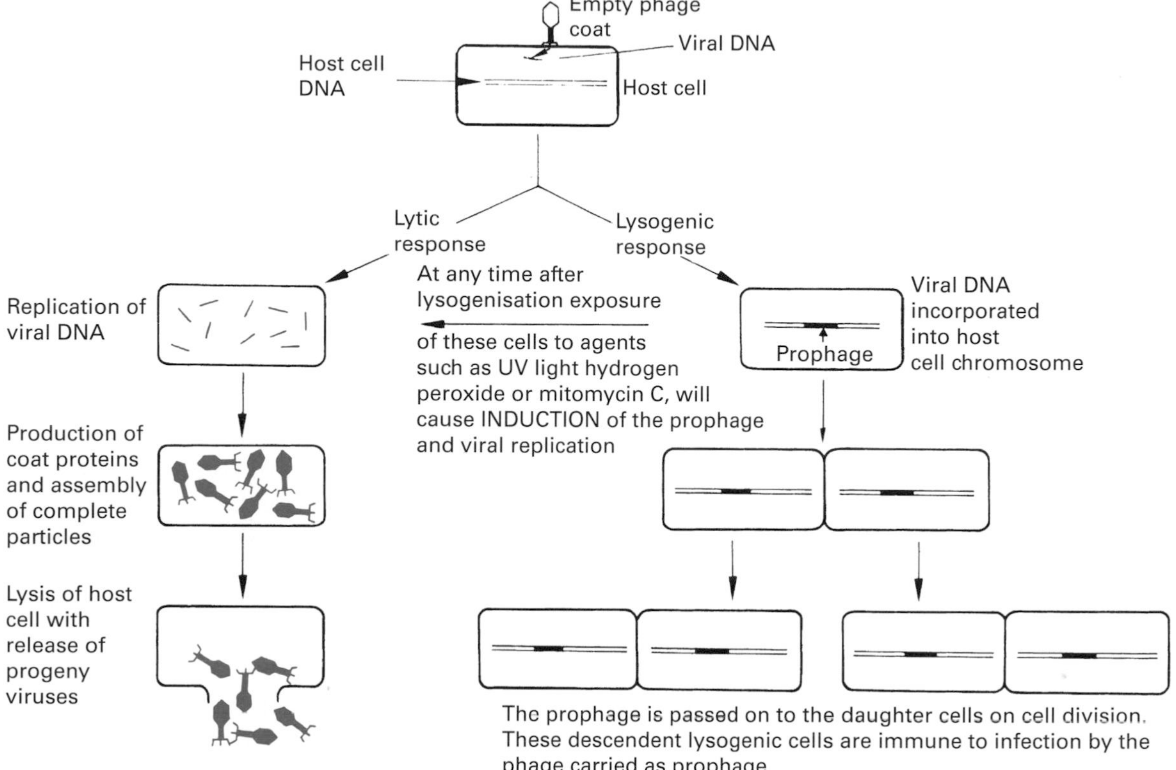

Figure 5.6 Scheme to illustrate the lytic and lysogenic responses of bacteriophages.

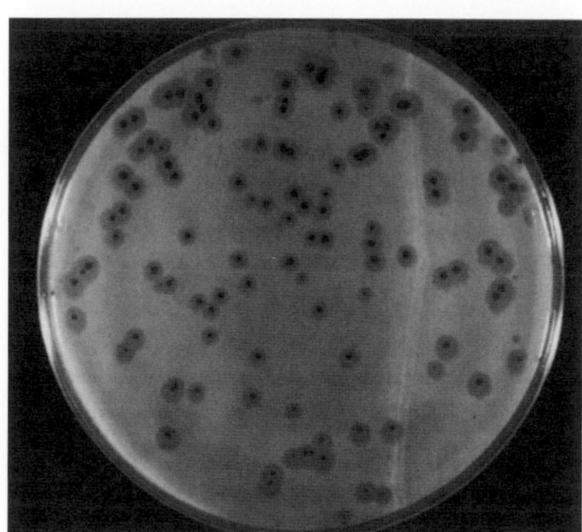

Figure 5.7 Plaques formed by phage on a plate seeded with *Bacillus subtilis*.

process is called *specialised transduction* and is responsible for horizontal gene transfer between bacteria. A related mechanism of horizontal gene transfer, which is characteristic of purely lytic phages, is called *generalised transduction*. In the case of generalised transduction, the phage particle is filled by random fragments of the chromosomal or plasmid DNA present in the host cell instead of the phage DNA and transferred to another bacterial cell in the same way as in specialised transduction. Sometimes, genetic factors transferred by transduction encode for antibiotic-resistant determinants and/or virulence factors such as toxins. The induction of prophages to a lytic cycle can be artificially triggered by exposure to chemical and physical agents such as mitomycin C and ultraviolet light. If the use of lytic phages might be appropriate to kill bacteria, the use of lysogenic phages is best confined to the genetic engineering of bacteria.

5.9.2 Bacteriophages and Their Products as Antibacterial Agents

The discovery of the lytic property of phages quickly resulted in their use as a potential bactericidal agent at the beginning of the twentieth century, to combat bacteria responsible for dysentery outbreaks, first against *Vibrio cholerae* (through the work of Hankin) and then *Shigella shiga* (through the work of d'Herelle). Phages targeting bacteria causing a number of diseases such as anthrax, scarlet fever, cholera and diphtheria were quickly isolated, but with the exception of 'cholera' phages these did not result in useful treatments. The introduction of antibiotics in the early 1940s resulted in the end of phage therapy in the West, although it continues in Poland and in the former Soviet Union, especially in Georgia and Russia, where it was used to treat a variety of bacterial infections in both the First and Second World Wars and is still used nowadays in clinical practice (Chapter 26).

The misuse and overuse of antibiotics have led to the emergence and dissemination of bacterial pathogens resistant to multiple antibiotics. It has been estimated that by 2050 up to 10 million deaths each year and a cumulative $100 trillion economic losses could be caused by drug-resistant bacterial infections. With the ever-increasing risks posed by the worsening global antibiotic-resistance crisis, there has been a renewed interest in the use of phages to control bacterial infection and product contamination, and this has led to the licensing of phage products for a number of applications; the use of phages to combat *Listeria monocytogenes* in ready-to-eat meat and poultry products was authorised by the US Food and Drug Administration (FDA) in 2006 and in cheeses by the EU Commission in 2009. Phage preparations are also successfully employed in agriculture and aquaculture, notably against *Erwinia amylovora*, which causes fire blight, and *Lactococcus garvieae*, the cause of a serious fish disease. Although a number of off-the-shelf phage therapeutics intended for human use are available in several Eastern European countries, none so far have been licensed in the UK, EU or the USA. Despite numerous reports demonstrating efficacy and safety of phage therapy, many problems preventing its wider adoption still remain unsolved, including issues associated with phage stability, resistance development in bacteria and a limited number of available phages against certain pathogens. One of the main hurdles is regulatory, but clinical trials are underway. In the UK, a phase I/II clinical trial of the phage-based product to combat *Pseudomonas aeruginosa* in ear infection (otitis) was successfully conducted in 2009. More recent trials, including the major 'PhagoBurn' phase I/II clinical trial of a bacteriophage cocktail to treat burn wounds infected by *P. aeruginosa*, were less conclusive, but still provided important information about the safety and efficiency of phage preparations and helped to identify issues to be solved for successful commercialisation of phage products.

Personalised phage therapy has been successfully used as a compassionate treatment option against systemic infections caused by multidrug-resistant bacteria. In 2017, a US citizen, who contracted a life-threatening *Acinetobacter baumannii* infection while on holiday in Egypt, was cured with a phage cocktail. More recently, in 2019, a cystic fibrosis patient with a disseminated drug-resistant *Mycobacterium abscessus* infection was treated with a combination of natural and genetically engineered phages at the Great Ormond Street Hospital in London. The patient, who was in critical condition, made a successful recovery. As of March 2021, phage therapy centres operate in Georgia, Poland, Belgium, and the USA.

There are a number of ways to prepare a phage product. 'Natural' phages from the environment can be selected on the basis of their activity and incorporated into a product on the basis that they are lytic and do not contain any detrimental genes encoding, for example, antibiotic resistance or bacterial virulence factors. Often several phages (a cocktail) attacking the same species or strain are added to the product to minimise the risk of emerging bacterial resistance. Non-replicating phages have been used with some degree of success, but in this case the lytic effect is short-lived. Genetically modified phages have also been used, whereby detrimental genes can be removed and phage virulence genes added. Another advantage of using genetically modified phages is commercial where patents might be easier to file. Finally, lysogenic phages can be used following treatment to remove their lysogenic property.

Phage-based products can be developed using phage components, mainly phage lytic enzymes which are employed during phage penetration and during virion release from the host cell. Natural or genetically engineered phage lytic enzymes (e.g., endolysins) can be harvested and used on their own to lyse/kill bacteria (Chapter 26). A number of skincare products containing an endolysin from a *Staphylococcus aureus* phage are produced by a biotechnology company in the Netherlands. Another group of phage enzymes, polysaccharide depolymerases, are being actively investigated as antivirulence therapeutics. Phage depolymerases do not kill bacterial cells, therefore minimising the risk of resistance development, but act instead as biofilm-dispersing agents, degrading capsular polysaccharides and exopolysaccharides produced by bacteria. As biofilms protect bacteria from antibiotics and the host's immune response, polysaccharide depolymerases could become another approach to deal with antibiotic-resistant pathogens.

The use of phages for surface disinfection and antisepsis or for the treatment of a bacterial infection (phage therapy) is at an early stage and further work is needed to develop appropriate phage-based products, notably the effect of the different routes of administration on phage viability and effectiveness. Animal studies have shown that the route of administration is crucial for phage efficacy. Phage therapy is unlikely to supplant antibiotic therapy in the future; however, it is highly probable that commercially available phage products will increase, as the advantages of phage therapy outweigh its disadvantages (Table 5.8 and Chapter 26). In addition, phage therapy can be used in

Table 5.8 Some advantages and disadvantages of phage therapy.

Advantages	Disadvantages
Highly specific	High specificity requires pathogen identification Need for 'custom' treatments based on organisms present
Replicate at site of infection Less frequent dosing required Active against bacterial biofilms	Bacterial resistance can emerge – the use of a cocktail containing several distinct phages is often proposed
No reported side effects	Phage therapy could result in toxic shock from bacterial lysis; that is, release of bacterial components such as lipopolysaccharide wall material Potentially immunogenic
Easy to isolate and propagate Phages can be developed against a wide range of bacterial hosts It is believed that every bacterium will possess at least one phage due to natural selection	The genomes of selected phages need to be sequenced to ensure they do not contain unwanted genes
Can be easily manipulated; for example, incorporated into capsules, for ease of delivery	Quality assurance controls are complex and will need to address biological variation, phage yield, and endotoxin limits
Development and production costs may be less than a new antibiotic	

combination with antibiotic treatment, as it has been shown that the use of such combinations results in a synergistic effect, reducing or preventing the development of resistant variants.

5.9.3 Other Applications of Bacteriophages

The high specificity of phage against their host leads to other applications. *Phage typing* is a method that differentiates distinct strains of the same bacterial species on the basis of their susceptibility to a standardised panel of lytic phages. This has been particularly relevant with bacteria such as *Salmonella enterica* serovar Typhi and to some extent *S. aureus* that can be 'typed' during an outbreak, and thus provides some important epidemiological information. Molecular techniques based on genetic differences are now preferred for *S. aureus*.

A further application for phage is in developing rapid diagnostics, notably against slow-growing bacteria such as *Mycobacterium tuberculosis*. Here such developments as thermosensitive fluoromycobacteriophage, a reporter phage containing a fluorescent reporter gene which does not lyse cells at 37 °C, offer methods for labelling viable mycobacteria for subsequent paraformaldehyde fixing and detection by fluorescence microscopy.

Although tailed phages are the best studied and the most commonly used, another group of phages, called *filamentous phages*, deserves a special mention. Filamentous phages are long, rod-shaped bacteriophages, whose single-stranded genomic DNA is covered with multiple copies of coat proteins. Their replication cycle is unique; the bacterial cells which become chronically infected with filamentous phages will continuously produce and extrude virions, without lysing. Filamentous phages are used for the production of recombinant *phagemids*, cloning vectors combining properties of plasmids and filamentous phages. Phagemids can replicate in bacterial cells as plasmids but can also be packaged into the capsid of a filamentous phage, a property making the phage display technique possible. Phage display is used to study protein–ligand interactions and for improving the affinity of antibodies and other proteins to their binding partners. Phagemids carrying a gene encoding a protein of interest fused with a coat protein of a phage could be transformed into bacterial cells, which then start producing phage particles. The phages displaying the fusion proteins with the highest affinity to a specific ligand on their surface could be selected and the whole process repeated, if necessary, to further improve the binding properties of the protein of interest. One half of the 2018 Nobel Prize in Chemistry was awarded for the development of the phage display method.

The study of interactions of phages and bacteria has led to a very important discovery. A cellular system called CRISPR/Cas9 is one of the restriction/modification systems that some bacteria use to recognise and cut foreign DNA (including phage and plasmid DNA). It is possible to engineer this system to recognise and introduce a double-stranded break into any specific DNA sequence. Such artificial CRISPR/Cas9 systems are very powerful and precise gene-editing tools, allowing the target DNA molecule to be modified by introducing or removing virtually any sequence (see Chapter 24). Emmanuelle Charpentier and Jennifer Doudna were awarded the 2020 Nobel Prize in Chemistry for their discovery of the CRISPR-Cas9 system as a tool for gene editing.

Bacteriophages also serve as a source of enzymes for molecular biology (e.g., phi29 DNA polymerase and T4 DNA ligase). They can be used as probiotics and microbiome modulators, gene vectors and vaccine platforms, biological tracers and as surrogates for dangerous viruses (e.g., SARS-CoV-2) in the testing of sterilisation and filtration equipment. Finally, due to their desirable physical characteristics (their uniform size and ability to self-assemble), phages are studied for nanotechnological applications, such as for production of nanoparticles or surface modification.

5.10 Subviral Infectious Agents and Prions

Although we can think of viruses as some of the most primitive life forms on Earth, this is not entirely true. Some viruses are truly large and complex, such as the amoeba-infecting viruses *Mimivirus* and *Pandoravirus*, comparable in size to some bacteria and with genomes of 1.2 and 2.5 million bp in length, respectively. At the other end of the spectrum are acellular infectious agents that are smaller and simpler than viruses, collectively known as *subviral agents*. Many of these are important pathogens of plants and animals, including humans.

Satellites are encapsidated subviral agents that resemble viruses but require a helper virus to complete the replication cycle. The degree to which satellites depend on helper viruses varies significantly. For example, in the case of AAV, the helper virus is only required to stimulate the cell to enter a stage in which the AAV can replicate. On the other hand, the hepatitis D virus (HDV) is much more significantly dependent on its helper, the HBV. Hepatitis D virus has a circular negative-sense ssRNA genome of 1700 nucleotides (nt) in length encoding a single polypeptide, the hepatitis D antigen, from which the HDV nucleocapsid is assembled. The HDV virion is covered by HBV envelope proteins and requires the activity of a number of other HBV proteins for release from the infected cell. It has been shown that the viral hepatitis resulting from a superinfection with HDV of a person already chronically infected with HBV significantly increases the severity of the disease and leads to serious complications, including liver cirrhosis and liver failure, which often proves fatal.

Even more minimal than satellites are *viroids*, unencapsidated circular ssRNA molecules between 250 and 400 nt, that do not encode any proteins. These naked RNAs are, nevertheless, infectious and replicate autonomously in their host plants (all known viroids are plant parasites). While many viroids are benign, some of them cause economically important diseases, such as coconut cadang-cadang viroid (CCCVd), which infects coconut palms and related plants. The infection is always fatal. It is estimated that in the Philippines about 40 million palms have been lost to CCCVd infections, with associated economic losses of about $100 per tree.

The causative agents of the neurodegenerative diseases bovine spongiform encephalopathy (BSE), scrapie in sheep and Creutzfeldt–Jakob disease (CJD) in humans used to be referred to as slow viruses. However, it is now clear that they are caused by a distinct class of infectious agents termed *prions* that have unique and disturbing properties. They can be recovered from the brains of infected individuals as rod-like structures which are oligomers of a 30-kDa glycoprotein. In contrast to all other currently known infectious agents, they are devoid of nucleic acid. Prions are extremely resistant to heating and ultraviolet irradiation and fail to produce an immune response in the host. Just how such proteins can replicate and be infectious has only recently been understood. It seems that a glycoprotein (designated PrPc) with the same amino acid sequence as the prion (PrPsc) but with a different tertiary structure is present in the membranes of normal neurons of the host. The evidence suggests that the prion form of the protein interacts with the normal form and alters its configuration to that of the prion. The newly formed prion can then in turn modify the folding of other PrPc molecules. In this way, the prion protein is capable of autocatalytic replication. As the prions slowly accumulate in the brain, the neurons progressively vacuolate. Holes eventually appear in the grey matter and the brain takes on a sponge-like appearance. The clinical symptoms take a long time to develop, up to 20 years in humans, but the disease has an inevitable progression to paralysis, dementia and death.

It is now clear that the large-scale outbreak of BSE that began in the UK during the 1980s resulted from feeding cattle with supplements prepared from sheep and cattle offal. The recognition of this fact led to changes in animal feed policies and eventually to the imposition of a ban on the human consumption of bovine brain, spinal cord and lymphoid tissues that were considered to be potentially infectious. Unfortunately, people had been consuming potentially contaminated meat for a number of years. Concerns that the agent had already been disseminated to humans in the food chain were realised in 1996 with the advent of a novel human disease that was called variant or vCJD. This condition was unusual, as it attacked young adults with an average age of 30 rather than the 60-year-olds who typically succumb to classical sporadic CJD. Studies on the experimental transmission of prions to mice provided evidence that vCJD represents infection by the BSE agent. The pathology in the mouse brain induced by the vCJD agent and the incubation time of the disease are different from that of classical CJD and very similar to that of BSE. Gel electrophoresis of the polypeptides from the brains of infected mice revealed that the different transmissible spongiform encephalitis agents have characteristic molecular signatures. These signatures are based on the lengths of protease-resistant fragments and the glycosylation patterns on the prion molecules. The patterns from vCJD agent were very different patterns from those of the classical CJD, but remarkably similar to those formed by BSE.

Since 1996, there has been a slow but gradual increase in the numbers of confirmed cases of vCJD. By October 2022, the number of deaths in the UK from vCJD had reached 178. As the average incubation time for vCJD is not yet known, it is difficult to estimate how many more cases will develop. The results of a study published in October 2013 suggest that approximately 1 in 2000 people in the UK may be infected with vCJD but are currently asymptomatic carriers.

The measures taken to protect the public have extended beyond food safety and now include health practices such as managing the risk of iatrogenic transmission during surgery, hormone therapy and dural grafts. These actions will hopefully have prevented any further human infections, but sadly no effective treatment is available for those who have already contracted the disease.

Further Reading

Altamirano, F.L.G. and Barr, J.J. (2019). Phage therapy in the postantibiotic era. *Clin. Microbiol. Rev.* 32: e00066–e00018.

BHIVA guidelines for the treatment of HIV-1-positive adults with antiretroviral therapy 2015 (2016 interim update). *British HIV Association (BHIVA).* (https://www.bhiva.org/hiv-1-treatment-guidelines)

British National Formulary 83 (2022) BMJ Publishing Group Ltd. and Royal Pharmaceutical Society, London. (The most recent volume should be consulted. New editions of the BNF appear at regular intervals and it is available online at https://bnf.nice.org.uk)

British Pharmacopoeia (2021) The Stationery Office, London. (The most recent volume should be consulted; it is also available online at https://www.pharmacopoeia.com)

Cihlar, T. and Fordyce, M. (2016). Current status and prospects of HIV treatment. *Curr. Opin. Virol.* 18: 50–56.

Connelly, D. and Robinson, J. (2020). The race to stop COVID-19. *Pharm. J.* 304: 168–169.

Connelly, D. (2022). Monkeypox: a visual guide. *Pharm. J.* 309: 7964; 309 (7964) DOI:10.1211/PJ.2022.1.151922

De Clercq, E. and Li, G. (2016). Approved antiviral drugs over the past 50 years. *Clin. Microbiol. Rev.* 29: 695–747.

Deeks, S., Overbaugh, J., Phillips, A., and Buchbinder, S. (2015). HIV infection. *Nat. Rev. Dis. Primers* 1: 15035.

Frank, T.D., Carter, A., Jahagirdar, D. et al. (2019). Global, regional, and national incidence, prevalence, and mortality of HIV, 1980–2017, and forecasts to 2030, for 195 countries and territories: a systematic analysis for the global burden of diseases, injuries, and risk factors study 2017. *Lancet HIV* 6: e831–e859.

Gibbs, E.P.J. (2014). The evolution of one health: a decade of progress and challenges for the future. *Vet. Rec.* 174: 85–91.

House, N.N.C., Palissery, S., and Sebastian, H. (2021). Corona viruses: a review on SARS, MERS and COVID-19. *Microbiology Insights* 14: 1–8.

Hu, B., Guo, H., Zhou, P., and Shi, Z.-L. (2020). Characteristics of SARS-CoV-2 and COVID-19. *Nat. Rev. Microbiol.* 19: 141–154.

ICTV Report on Virus Classification and Taxon Nomenclature. *International Committee on Taxonomy of Viruses (ICTV).* (https://talk.ictvonline.org/ictv-reports/ictv_online_report)

Krammer, F., Smith, G.J.D., Fouchier, R.A.M. et al. (2018). Influenza. *Nat. Rev. Dis. Primers* 4: 3.

Lamers, M.M. and Haagmann, B.L. (2022). SARS-CoV-2 pathogenesis. *Nat. Rev. Microbiol.* 20: 270–284.

Maillard, J.-Y. (2001). Virus susceptibility to biocides: an understanding. *Rev. Med. Microbiol.* 12: 63–74.

Mesri, E.A., Feitelson, M.A., and Munger, K. (2014). Human viral oncogenesis: a cancer hallmarks analysis. *Cell Host Microbe* 15: 266–282.

Parry, C. (2021). Antivirals for COVID-19: five questions that must be answered. *Pharm. J.* 307: 7954; 307 (7954) DOI:10.1211/PJ.2021.1.111364

Scheckel, C. and Aguzzi, A. (2018). Prions, prionoids and protein misfolding disorders. *Nat. Rev. Genet.* 19: 405–418.

Soto, C. (2006). *Prions: The New Biology of Proteins*. London: CRC Press.

Strauss, J.H. and Strauss, E.G. (2008). Subviral agents. In: *Viruses and Human Disease*, 345–368. Amsterdam: Elsevier.

Tao, K., Tzou, P.L., Nouhin, J. et al (2021). SARS-CoV-2 antiviral therapy. *Clin. Microbiol. Rev.* 34(4): DOI:https://doi.org/10.1128/CMR.00109-21

6

Protozoa

Tim Paget

Professor of Medical Microbiology, School of Medicine, University of Sunderland, UK

CONTENTS

Hugo and Russell's Pharmaceutical Microbiology, Ninth Edition. Edited by Brendan F. Gilmore and Stephen P. Denyer.

Companion website: https://www.wiley.com/go/HugoandRussells9e

6.1 Introduction

6.1.1 Protozoa

The classification of protozoa has been surrounded by uncertainty and this term is perhaps best used informally to describe a group of single-celled eukaryotes which include amoebae, flagellates and ciliates. These organisms can range in size from microns (e.g., *Plasmodium falciparum*, 1–14 μm depending on growth phase) to several millimetres in length. Protozoa are either free-living or parasitic, feeding on organic matter such as other microorganisms or organic tissues. Of the parasitic protozoa, *Plasmodium* spp. is the most significant to humans with an estimated 241 million infections worldwide causing annual deaths of between 400,000 and 600,000. In free-living form, protozoa are abundant in aqueous and soil environments and can be found associated with larger multicellular organisms. Interestingly, many free-living protozoa ingest bacteria as a nutrient source and their presence within protozoa can have an unforeseen health impact. A good example is found with amoeba, where several species have become hosts for pathogenic bacteria forming natural reservoirs for organisms such as *Mycobacterium tuberculosis* and *Legionella pneumophila*. This association can lead to the airborne transmission of bacteria protected from external stresses, including disinfection; this has resulted in pulmonary infections such as Legionnaires' disease which is associated with biofilm aerosols released from air-conditioning units and cooling towers.

6.1.2 Parasitism

Parasitism is a specific type of interaction between two organisms that has many features in common with other infectious processes, but host–parasite interactions often operate over a longer timescale than those seen with other pathogens. This extended process results in significant host–parasite interaction at the cellular and organismal levels. It is known that some parasites alter the behaviour of the host, while others, such as *Giardia lamblia*, induce biochemical and physiological changes in the host cells and tissues at the site of infection (the duodenal epithelium) that persist after infection is cleared. Many parasites have a life cycle that often involves several hosts; this means that survival and transmission between different hosts require the parasite to exhibit more than one morphologically and physiologically distinct form.

6.1.3 Habitats

Parasites inhabit a wide range of habitats within their hosts. Some parasites will inhabit only one site throughout their life cycle, but many move to various sites within the body. Such movement may require the formation of different morphological forms, and this will often produce a significant change in the physiology and morphology of the parasite because of environmental differences arising in the new locality. Parasites moving from the gut to other tissues, for example, will encounter higher levels of oxygen, changes in pH and significant exposure to the host immune response. When a life cycle involves more than one host organism, these changes are even greater. The reasons why parasites move to various sites within the host would seem to be driven by evasion of host immune attack and to aid transmission. There is also evidence through the evolutionary record that co-evolution of parasites along with their host species and genera has occurred.

6.1.4 Physiology of Parasitic Protozoa

Parasitic protozoa, like their free-living counterparts, are single-celled eukaryotic organisms that utilise flagella, cilia, or amoeboid movement for motility. The complexity of some parasite life cycles means that some species may exhibit, at different times, more than one form of motility. All pathogenic protozoa are heterotrophs, using carbohydrates or amino acids as their major source of carbon and energy. Some parasitic protozoa utilise oxygen to generate energy through oxidative phosphorylation, but many protozoan parasites lack functional or 'typical' mitochondria or have mitochondria that do not function like those in mammalian cells. As a result of this adaptation, many parasites exhibit a fermentative metabolism that functions even in the presence of oxygen. The reason for the utilisation of less efficient fermentative pathways is not clear, but it is presumably due in part to the fact that such parasites survive in environments where oxygen is only present occasionally or at low levels. For some parasites, oxygen is toxic, and they appear to utilise it possibly to remove it and thus maintain an anaerobic metabolism.

The metabolism of parasites is highly adapted, with many possessing unique organelles such as kinetoplasts and hydrogenosomes. Many synthetic pathways that are found in other eukaryotes are absent in this group because many important metabolic intermediates or precursors such as lipids, amino acids and nucleotides are actively scavenged from their environment. This minimises energy expenditure, which is finely balanced in parasites, and means that the membrane of parasitic protozoa is necessarily rich in transporters. Secretion of haemolysins, cytolysins, proteolytic enzymes, toxins and antigenic and immunomodulatory molecules that reduce host immune response also occurs in pathogenic protozoa. It should be noted by readers that the introduction of genomic, proteomic, metabolomic and transcriptomic technologies into parasitology research over the past 10–15 years has uncovered additional metabolic pathways in many parasites, opening up new avenues for drug research and the potential use of re-purposed drugs (examples of this will be given later in this chapter).

Survival of parasites is partly due to their high rate of reproduction, which may be either sexual or asexual; some organisms such as *Plasmodium* exhibit both forms of reproduction in their life cycle. Simple asexual fission is characteristic of many amoebae, but some species which utilise this form of reproduction also undergo nuclear division in the cystic state (cysts are forms required for survival outside the host) with each nucleus giving rise to new trophozoites (the growing, motile and pathogenic form).

6.2 Blood and Tissue Parasites

This section considers the life cycles, diseases and pathology of some blood and tissue parasites; this is not an exhaustive list but covers some of the most important species. These diseases are commonly associated with travel to tropical and subtropical countries, but diseases such as leishmaniasis are frequently seen in southern Spain and France. It should also be noted that climate change is altering the geographical distribution of many parasitic diseases.

6.2.1 Malaria

Malaria has been a major disease of humankind for thousands of years. Despite the availability of drugs for treatment, it is still one of the most important infectious diseases of humans. Data on malaria incidence, mortality and morbidity have been collated since the 1950s, and in 2019 (the last full data set available) it was estimated that there were 229 million cases of malaria with the number of deaths estimated to be in the range of 400,000–600,000; levels of mortality have decreased but overall infection numbers have remained similar over the past 10 years. The World Health Organization (WHO) has launched several initiatives from the 1970s onwards to control malaria in Africa and Asia; however, these have had varying levels of success due to factors such as increasing levels of drug resistance in the parasite, as well as geopolitical changes in the regions where this parasite is endemic. Protozoa of the genus *Plasmodium* cause malaria with four species being responsible for the majority of disease in humans: *P. falciparum*, *Plasmodium vivax*, *Plasmodium ovale* and *Plasmodium malariae*. *P. falciparum* and *P. vivax* account for the vast majority of cases, although *P. falciparum* causes the most severe disease. Other species of plasmodia infect reptiles, birds and other mammals. Malaria is spread to humans by the bite of female mosquitoes of the genus *Anopheles* but transmission by inoculation of infected blood and through congenital routes is also seen. These mosquitoes feed at night and their breeding sites are primarily in rural areas.

6.2.1.1 Disease

The most common symptom of malaria is fever, although chills, headache, myalgia and nausea are frequently seen and other symptoms such as vomiting, diarrhoea, abdominal pain and cough occasionally appear. In all types of malaria, the periodic febrile response (fever) is caused by rupture of mature schizonts (one of the cell forms arising as part of the life cycle). In *P. vivax* and *P. ovale* malaria, fever occurs every 24–48 hours, whereas in *P. malariae* it is typically every 72 hours. In *P. falciparum* malaria, fever is usually irregular, showing no distinct frequency. Apart from anaemia, most physical findings in malaria are often non-specific and offer little help in diagnosis, although enlargement of some organs may be seen after prolonged infection. If the diagnosis of malaria is missed or delayed, especially with *P. falciparum* infection, potentially fatal complicated malaria may develop. The most frequent and serious complications of malaria are cerebral malaria and severe anaemia.

6.2.1.2 Life Cycle

Plasmodia spp. have a complex life cycle (Figure 6.1) involving a number of stages and two hosts. The human infective stage comprises the sporozoites (approximately 1–7 μm in size), which are produced by sexual reproduction in the midgut of the mosquito (vector) and migrate to

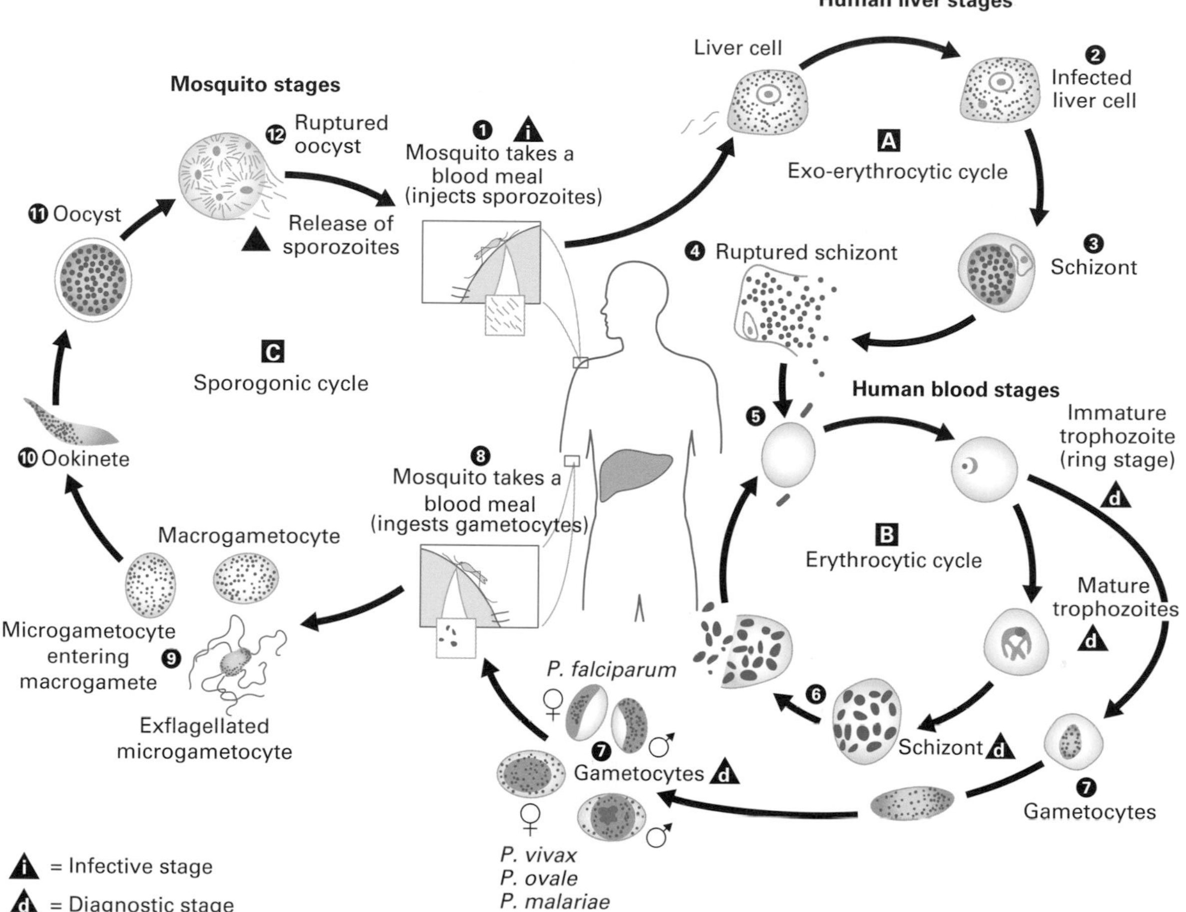

Figure 6.1 The malaria parasite life cycle involves two hosts. During a blood meal, a malaria-infected female *Anopheles* mosquito inoculates sporozoites into the human host (1). Sporozoites infect liver cells (2) and mature into schizonts (3), which rupture and release merozoites (4). (Of note, in *P. vivax* and *P. ovale,* a dormant stage [hypnozoites] can persist in the liver and cause relapses by invading the bloodstream weeks or even years later.) After this initial replication in the liver (exo-erythrocytic schizogony, A), the parasites undergo asexual multiplication in the erythrocytes (erythrocytic schizogony, B). Merozoites infect red blood cells (5). The ring-stage trophozoites mature into schizonts, which rupture releasing merozoites (6). Some parasites differentiate into sexual erythrocytic stages (gametocytes) (7). Blood-stage parasites are responsible for the clinical manifestations of the disease. The gametocytes, male (microgametocytes) and female (macrogametocytes), are ingested by an *Anopheles* mosquito during a blood meal (8). The parasite's multiplication in the mosquito is known as the sporogonic cycle (C). While in the mosquito's stomach, the microgametocytes penetrate the macrogametes, generating zygotes (9). The zygotes in turn become motile and elongated (ookinetes) (10), which invade the midgut wall of the mosquito where they develop into oocysts (11). The oocysts grow, rupture and release sporozoites (12), which make their way to the mosquito's salivary glands. Inoculation of the sporozoites into a new human host perpetuates the malaria life cycle (1).

its salivary gland. When an infected *Anopheles* mosquito bites a human, sporozoites are injected into the bloodstream and enter liver parenchymal cells within approximately 30 minutes of inoculation. In these cells, the parasite differentiates into a spherical, multinucleate schizont which may contain 2000–40,000 uninucleate merozoites. This process of growth and development is termed *exo-erythrocytic schizogony*. This exoerythrocytic phase usually takes between 5 and 21 days, depending on the species of *Plasmodium*; however, in *P. vivax* and *P. ovale,* the maturation of schizonts may be delayed for up to 1–2 years. These 'quiescent' parasites are called *hypnozoites*. Clinical illness is caused by the erythrocytic stage of the parasite life cycle; no disease is associated with sporozoites, the developing liver stage of the parasite, the merozoites released from the liver or gametocytes.

The common symptoms of malaria associated with the erythrocytic stage of the life cycle of the parasites are due to the rupture of erythrocytes when erythrocytic schizonts mature (Figure 6.2a). This release of parasite and host cellular material triggers a host immune response linked to the formation of pro-inflammatory cytokines, reactive

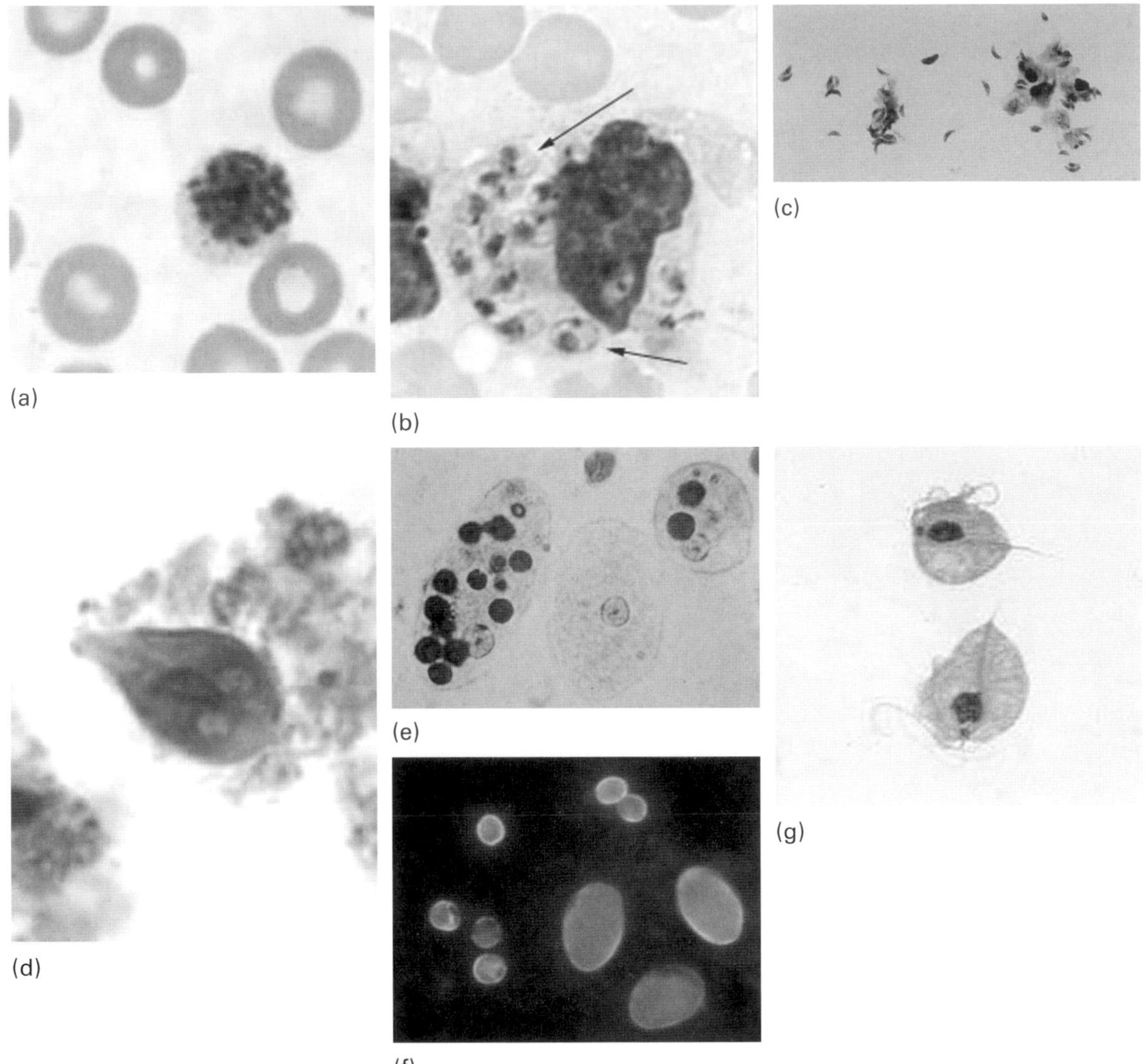

Figure 6.2 (a) Mature schizonts of *Plasmodium vivax*. *P. vivax* schizonts are large, have 12–24 merozoites, and may fill the red blood cells (RBC). RBCs are enlarged 1.5–2 times and may be distorted. Under optimal conditions, Schüffner's dots may be seen. (b) *Leishmania tropica* amastigotes within an intact macrophage. (c) *Toxoplasma gondii* trophozoites in the bronchial secretions from an HIV-infected patient. (d) Trophozoites of *Giardia intestinalis*. Each cell has two nuclei and is 10–20 μm in length. (e) Trophozoites of *Entamoeba histolytica* with ingested erythrocytes, which appear as dark inclusions. (f) Oocysts of *Cryptosporidium parvum* (upper left) and cysts of *Giardia intestinalis* (lower right) labelled with immunofluorescent antibodies. (g) Trophozoites of *Trichomonas vaginalis*.

oxygen intermediates and other cellular mediators. Pro-inflammatory molecules play a prominent role in pathogenesis and are likely responsible for the fever, chills, sweats, weakness and other systemic symptoms associated with malaria. In *P. falciparum* (this species is associated with most deaths due to malaria), infected erythrocytes adhere to the endothelium of capillaries and postcapillary venules, leading to obstruction of the microcirculation and localised anoxia. Anaemia is also seen in malaria infections and directly relates to the percentage of erythrocytes infected (percentage parasitaemia). The cause of this anaemia primarily involves haemolysis or phagocytosis of parasitised erythrocytes and ineffective erythropoiesis, but is also thought to include several other factors.

6.2.2 Trypanosomatids

The family Trypanosomatidae consists of two genera, *Trypanosoma* and *Leishmania*. These are important pathogens of humans and domestic animals and the diseases they cause constitute serious medical and economic problems. Because these protozoans have a requirement for haematin obtained from blood, they are classed as *haemoflagellates*. The life cycles of both genera involve insect and vertebrate hosts, and the parasite exhibits up to eight life-cycle stages. Trypanosomatids have a unique organelle called the kinetoplast, a special part of the mitochondrion which is rich in DNA. Two types of DNA have been found in the kinetoplast: *maxicircles* that encode many mitochondrial enzymes, and *minicircles*, which serve a function in the process of RNA editing. RNA editing is a mechanism that amplifies genetic and proteomic plasticity by allowing the production of alternative protein products from a single gene. Replication of trypanosomatids occurs by single or multiple fission, involving first the kinetoplast, then the nucleus and finally the cytoplasm. There are four major diseases associated with this group: Chagas disease is caused by *Trypanosoma cruzi*; sleeping sickness (African trypanosomiasis) is associated with *Trypanosoma brucei*; cutaneous and mucocutaneous leishmaniasis are caused by a range of species including *Leishmania tropica*, *Leishmania major*, *Leishmania mexicana*, *Leishmania amazonensis* and *Leishmania braziliensis*; and visceral leishmaniasis, which is also known as kala-azar, is typically caused by *Leishmania donovani*.

6.2.2.1 American Trypanosomiasis (Chagas Disease)

Chagas disease begins as a localised infection that is followed by a more disseminated disease (parasitaemia) with ultimate colonisation of internal organs and tissues. The first sign of infection is often the development of a small tumour (chagoma) on the skin at the site of a bite or wound that has become infected by faeces from one of several genera of triatomine bugs (*Triatoma*, *Rhodnius* and *Panstrongylus*). Symptoms of the disease include fever, oedema and myocarditis (inflammation of the heart muscle) with or without heart enlargement, and meningoencephalitis in children. The acute disease is frequently subclinical and patients may become asymptomatic carriers; this chronic phase may result, after 10–20 years, in cardiopathy. Human trypanosomiasis is seen in almost all countries of the Americas, including the southern USA, but the main foci are in poor rural areas of Latin America.

T. cruzi exhibits two cell types in vertebrate hosts, a blood form termed a trypomastigote, and in the tissues (mainly heart, skeletal and smooth muscle, and reticuloendothelial cells) the parasite occurs as an amastigote (Figure 6.3). Trypomastigotes ingested when the insect takes a blood meal from an infected host transform into epimastigotes in the intestine. Active reproduction occurs and in 8–10 days metacyclic trypomastigote forms appear which are flushed out of the gut with the faeces of the insect. These organisms can penetrate the vertebrate host only through the mucosa or abrasions of the skin; hence, transmission does not necessarily occur at every blood meal. Within the vertebrate, the trypomastigotes transform into amastigotes, which, after a period of intracellular multiplication at the portal of entry, are released into the blood as trypanosomes; these invade other cells or tissues, becoming amastigotes again.

The pathology of the infection is associated with inflammatory reactions in infected tissues. Infection with *Trypanosoma*, more specifically its surface proteins and glycoproteins, induces a polyclonal B-cell activation and lytic antibody production in the host (see Chapter 9), consequentially leading to the destruction of the infected tissue which can cause acute myocarditis when heart tissue is involved. An autoimmune pathological process is seen and is initiated by parasite damage to cardiac tissue. This pathology seems to be mediated by T lymphocytes (CD4+) and by the production of cytokines; this also induces a polyclonal activation of B lymphocytes and the secretion of large quantities of autoantibodies. Parasite enzymes may also cause cell and tissue damage.

6.2.2.2 African Trypanosomiasis (Sleeping Sickness)

Sleeping sickness (African trypanosomiasis) is caused by *T. brucei*, of which there are two morphologically indistinguishable subspecies: *T. brucei rhodesiense* and *T. brucei gambiense*. After infection, the parasite undergoes a period of local multiplication, and then enters the general circulation via the lymphatic system. Recurrent fever, headache, lymphadenopathy and splenomegaly may occur. Later, signs of meningoencephalitis appear, followed by somnolence (sleeping sickness), coma and death.

T. brucei, unlike *T. cruzi*, multiplies in the blood or cerebrospinal fluid. Trypanosomes ingested by a feeding fly must reach the salivary glands within a few days, where they reproduce actively as epimastigotes attached to the microvilli of the salivary gland subsequently transforming into metacyclic trypomastigotes, which are found free in the lumen. Around 15–35 days after infection, the fly becomes infective through its bite.

The pathology of infection is due to inflammatory changes associated with an induced autoimmune demyelination of nerve cells. Interestingly, the immunosuppressive action of components of the parasite's membrane is probably responsible for frequent secondary infections such as pneumonia. Liberation of common surface antigens (the mechanism involved in immune evasion) in every trypanolytic crisis (episode of trypanosome lysis) leads to antibody and cell-mediated hypersensitivity reactions. It is believed that some cytotoxic and pathological processes are the result of biochemical and immune mechanisms.

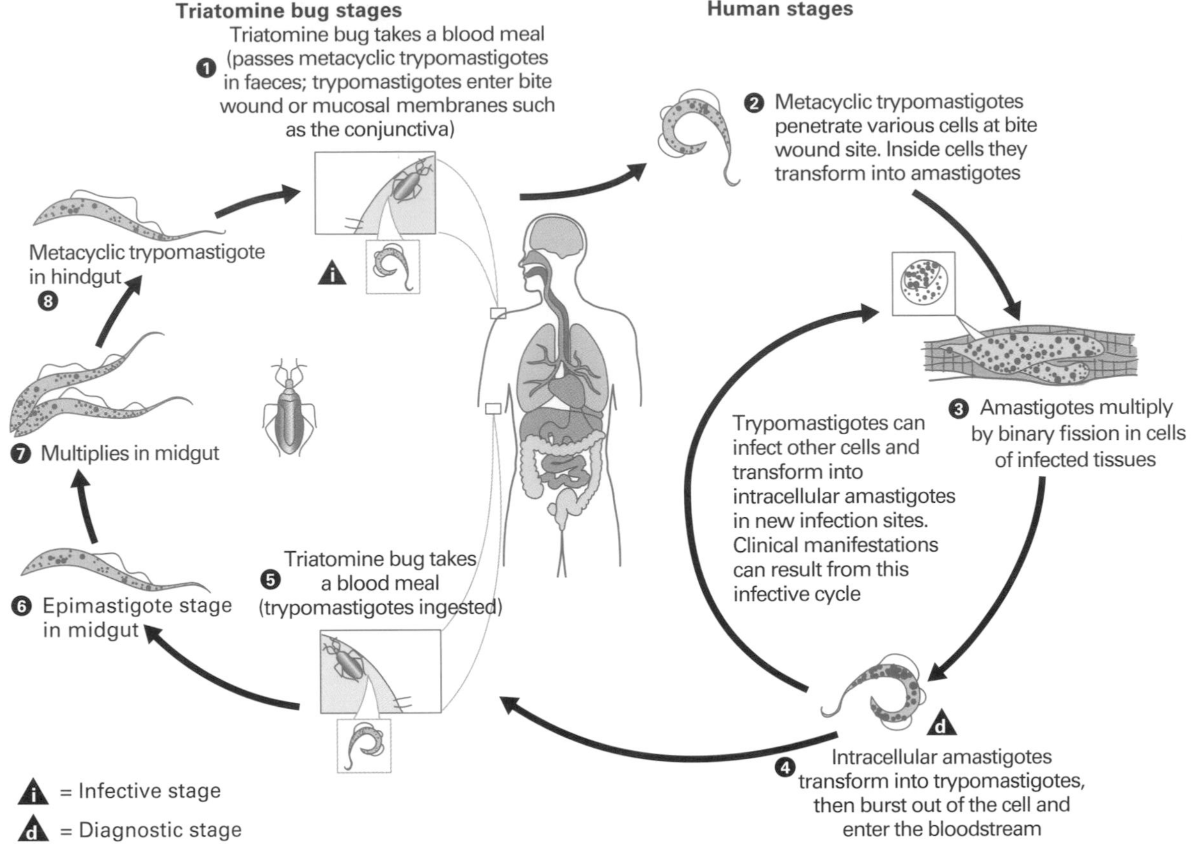

Figure 6.3 An infected triatomine insect vector (or 'kissing' bug) takes a blood meal and releases trypomastigotes in its faeces near the site of the bite wound. Trypomastigotes enter the host through the wound or through intact mucosal membranes, such as the conjunctiva (1). Common triatomine vector species for trypanosomiasis belong to the genera *Triatoma*, *Rhodnius* and *Panstrongylus*. Inside the host, the trypomastigotes invade cells, where they differentiate into intracellular amastigotes (2). The amastigotes multiply by binary fission (3) and differentiate into trypomastigotes, and then are released into the circulation as bloodstream trypomastigotes (4). Trypomastigotes infect cells from a variety of tissues and transform into intracellular amastigotes in new infection sites. Clinical manifestations can result from this infective cycle. The bloodstream trypomastigotes do not replicate (different from the African trypanosomes). Replication resumes only when the parasites enter another cell or are ingested by another vector. The 'kissing' bug becomes infected by feeding on human or animal blood that contains circulating parasites (5). The ingested trypomastigotes transform into epimastigotes in the vector's midgut (6). The parasites multiply and differentiate in the midgut (7) and differentiate into infective metacyclic trypomastigotes in the hindgut (8). *Trypanosoma cruzi* can also be transmitted through blood transfusions, organ transplantation, transplacentally and in laboratory accidents.

6.2.2.3 Cutaneous and Mucocutaneous Leishmaniasis

Leishmaniasis is the term used for diseases caused by species of the genus *Leishmania* that are transmitted by the bite of infected sandflies. The lesions of cutaneous and mucocutaneous leishmaniasis are localised to the skin and mucous membranes. Visceral leishmaniasis is a much more severe disease, which involves the entire reticuloendothelial system, and is discussed in Section 6.2.2.4. Cutaneous leishmaniasis appears 2–3 weeks after the bite of an infected sandfly as a small cutaneous papule; this slowly develops and often becomes ulcerated and subject to secondary infections. Secondary or diffuse lesions may develop. The disease is usually chronic but may occasionally be self-limiting. Leishmaniasis from a primary skin lesion may involve the oral and nasopharyngeal mucosa. *Leishmania* species that infect humans are all morphologically similar and only exhibit one form, the intracellular amastigotes (3–6 μm long and 1.5–3 μm in diameter) (Figure 6.2b). Promastigotes are found in the sandfly.

In mammalian hosts, amastigotes are phagocytosed by macrophages, but resist digestion and divide actively in the phagolysosome (Figure 6.4). The female sandfly ingests parasites in the blood meal from an infected person or animal and these pass into the stomach where they transform into promastigotes, and multiply actively. The parasites attach to the walls of the oesophagus, midgut and hindgut of the fly, and some eventually reach the proboscis and are inoculated into a new host.

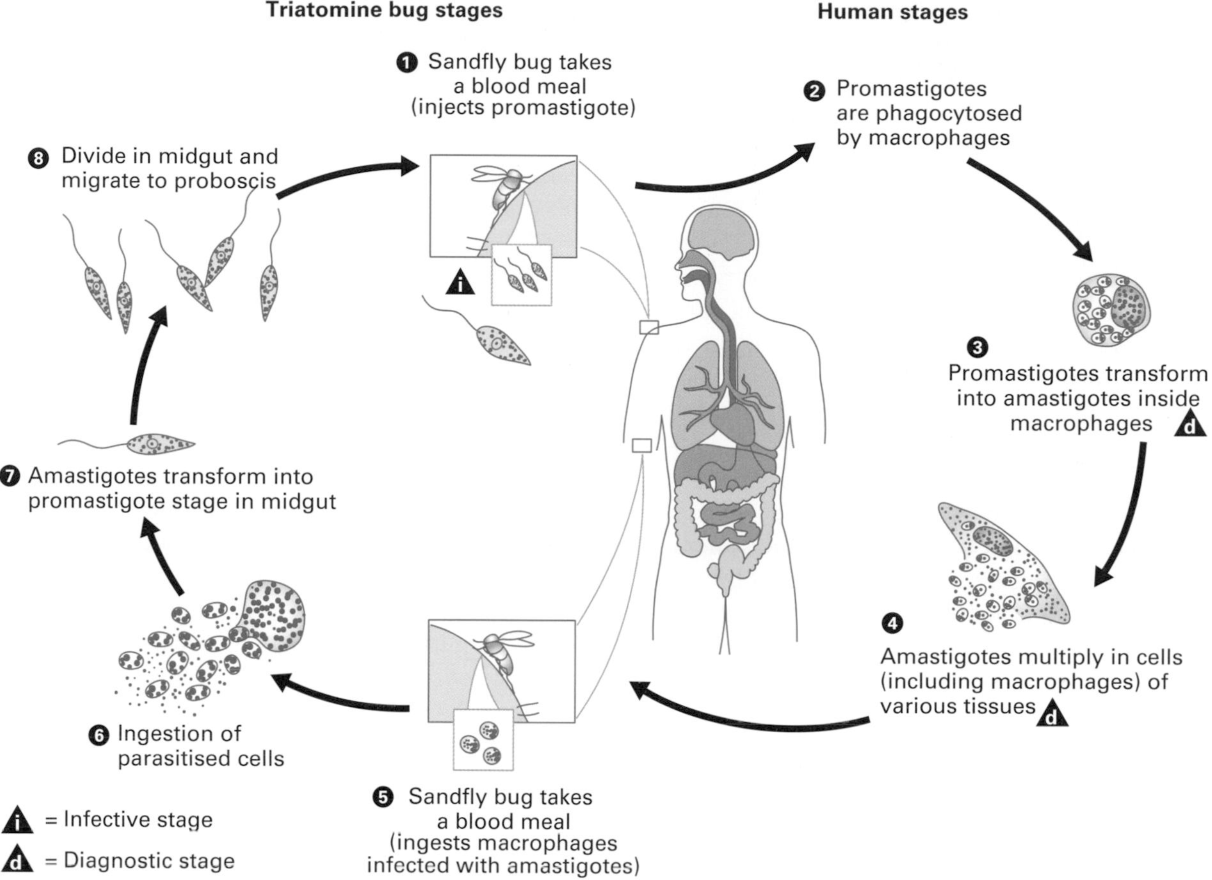

Figure 6.4 Leishmaniasis is transmitted by the bite of female phlebotomine sandfly. The sandfly injects the infective stage, promastigotes, during blood meals (1). Promastigotes that reach the puncture wound are phagocytosed by macrophages (2) and transform into amastigotes (3). Amastigotes multiply in infected cells and affect different tissues, depending in part on the *Leishmania* species (4). This originates the clinical manifestations of leishmaniasis. Sandfly become infected during blood meals on an infected host when they ingest macrophages infected with amastigotes (5) and (6). In the sandfly's midgut, the parasites differentiate into promastigotes (7), which multiply and migrate to the proboscis (8).

The obvious symptoms of this infection are caused by the uptake of parasites by local macrophages. Host response to infection produces tubercle-like structures designed to limit the spread of infected cells. Some lesions may resolve spontaneously after a few months but other types may become chronic, sometimes with lymphatic and bloodstream dissemination. In infections due to *L. braziliensis*, there is a highly destructive spread of infected macrophages to the oral or nasal mucosa. In *L. mexicana*, *L. amazonensis* and *Leishmania aethiopica* infections, the disease becomes more disseminated. The immunological response of the host plays an important factor in determining the precise pathology of the disease and this is apparent from the more severe type of infection seen in individuals with HIV. In Europe and Africa, several rodents may act as reservoirs of the disease, but in countries such as India, transmission can occur in a human–sandfly–human cycle without rodent intervention. In rural semi-arid zones of Latin America, both wild and domestic dogs enter the epidemiological chain and the vector is a common sandfly, *Lutzomyia longipalpis*, abundant in and around houses. The disease is more common in children in both Latin America and the Mediterranean area.

6.2.2.4 Visceral Leishmaniasis (Kala-azar)

Like cutaneous leishmaniasis, visceral leishmaniasis begins with the formation of a nodule at the site of inoculation, but this lesion rarely ulcerates and usually disappears in a few weeks. However, symptoms and signs of systemic disease such as undulating fever, malaise, diarrhoea, organ enlargement and anaemia subsequently develop. In more serious cases of visceral leishmaniasis, the parasites, which can resist the internal body temperature, invade internal organs (liver, spleen, bone marrow and lymph nodes) where they occupy the reticuloendothelial cells. The pathogenic mechanisms of the disease are not fully understood, but enlargement occurs in those organs that exhibit marked cellular alteration such as hyperplasia. Parasitised macrophages replace tissue in the bone marrow. Patients with advanced disease are prone to superinfection with other organisms which are predominantly bacterial.

6.2.3 *Toxoplasma gondii*

The term *coccidia* is applied to a group of protozoa which includes the genus *Cryptosporidium* (see intestinal parasites, Section 6.3), as well as a number of important veterinary parasites. *Toxoplasma gondii* is an intestinal coccidian that exhibits its major pathology in other tissues and organs. *T. gondii* infects members of the cat family as definitive hosts and has a wide range of intermediate hosts. Infection is common in many warm-blooded animals, including humans. In most cases, infection is asymptomatic, but devastating disease can occur congenitally in children as a result of infection during pregnancy. *T. gondii* infection in humans is a global problem; however, the incidence of human infection varies from country to country. The reasons for this variation include environmental factors, cultural habits and the presence of domestic and native animal species. The frequency of postnatal toxoplasmosis acquired by eating raw meat and by ingesting food contaminated by oocysts from cat faeces (oocyst formation is greatest in the domestic cat) is not well established but is thought to be significant. Widespread natural infection is possible because infected animals may excrete millions of resistant oocysts, which can survive in the environment for prolonged periods (months to years). Mature oocysts are approximately 12 μm in diameter and contain eight infective sporozoites.

T. gondii infection in most animals including humans is usually asymptomatic. Severe disease in humans is observed only in congenitally infected children and in immunosuppressed individuals. The most common symptom associated with postnatal infection in humans is lymphadenitis which may be accompanied by fever, malaise, fatigue, muscle pains, sore throat and headache (flu-like symptoms). Typically, infection resolves spontaneously in weeks or months, but in immunosuppressed individuals, a fatal encephalitis may occur producing symptoms such as headache, disorientation, drowsiness, hemiparesis, reflex changes and convulsions. Prenatal *T. gondii* infections often target the brain and retina and can cause a wide spectrum of clinical disease. Mild disease may consist of impaired vision, whereas severely diseased children may exhibit a 'classic tetrad' of signs: retinochoroiditis, hydrocephalus, convulsions and intracerebral calcifications. Hydrocephalus is the least common but most dramatic lesion of congenital toxoplasmosis.

The life cycle of *T. gondii* was only fully described in the early 1970s when felines, including domestic cats, were identified as the definitive host and various warm-blooded animals were recognised as intermediate hosts. *T. gondii* is transmitted by three mechanisms: congenitally, through the consumption of uncooked infected meat and via faecal matter contamination. Figure 6.5 shows the life cycle of *T. gondii*. Cats acquire *Toxoplasma* by ingesting any of the three infectious stages of the organism: (i) the rapidly multiplying forms, tachyzoites; (ii) the dormant bradyzoites (cysts) in infected tissue; and (iii) the oocysts shed in faeces. The probability of infection and the time between infection and the shedding of oocysts vary with the stage of *T. gondii* ingested. Fewer than 50% of cats shed oocysts after ingesting tachyzoites or oocysts, whereas nearly all cats shed oocysts after ingesting bradyzoites. When a cat ingests tissue cysts, the cyst wall is dissolved by intestinal and gut proteolytic enzymes, which causes the release of bradyzoites. These enter the epithelial cells of the small intestine and initiate the formation of numerous asexual generations before the sexual cycle begins. At the same time some of those bradyzoites invade the surface epithelia, while other bradyzoites penetrate the lamina propria and begin to multiply as tachyzoites (trophozoites) (Figure 6.2c). Within a few hours, tachyzoites may disseminate to other tissues through the lymph and blood. Tachyzoites can enter almost any type of host cell and multiply until the cell becomes packed with parasites. The host cell then lyses and releases more tachyzoites to enter new host cells. The host usually controls this phase of infection, and as a result the parasite enters the 'resting' stage in which bradyzoites are isolated in tissue cysts. Tissue cysts are formed most commonly in the brain, liver and muscles. These cysts usually cause no host reaction and may remain dormant for the life of the host. In intermediate hosts, such as humans, the extraintestinal cycle of *T. gondii* is similar to the cycle in cats except that there is no sexual stage.

Most cases of toxoplasmosis in humans are probably acquired by the ingestion of either tissue cysts in infected meat or oocysts in food contaminated with cat faeces. Bradyzoites from the tissue cysts or sporozoites released from oocysts invade intestinal epithelia and multiply. *T. gondii* may spread both locally to mesenteric lymph nodes and to distant organs by invading the lymphatic and blood systems. Focal areas of necrosis (caused by localised cell lysis) may develop in many organs. The extent of the disease is usually determined by the extent of injury to infected organs, especially to vital and vulnerable organs such as the eye, heart and adrenal glands. Opportunist toxoplasmosis in immunosuppressed patients usually represents reactivation of a chronic infection.

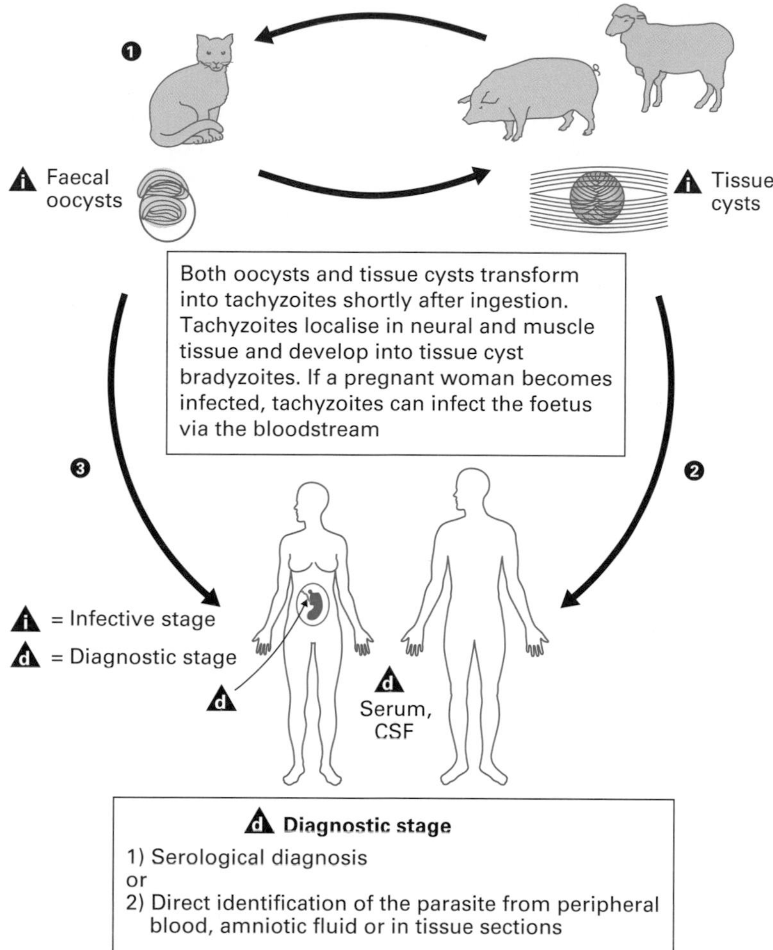

Figure 6.5 Members of the cat family (Felidae) are the only known definitive hosts for the sexual stages of *Toxoplasma gondii* and thus are the main reservoirs of infection. Cats become infected with *T. gondii* by carnivorism (1). After tissue cysts or oocysts are ingested by the cat, viable organisms are released and invade epithelial cells of the small intestine where they undergo an asexual cycle followed by a sexual cycle and then form oocysts, which are then excreted. The unsporulated oocyst takes 1–5 days after excretion to sporulate (become infective). Although cats shed oocysts for only 1–2 weeks, large numbers may be shed. Oocysts can survive in the environment for several months and are remarkably resistant to disinfectants, freezing and drying, but are killed by heating to 70 °C for 10 minutes. Human infection may be acquired in several ways: (i) ingestion of undercooked infected meat containing *Toxoplasma* cysts (2); (ii) ingestion of the oocyst from faecally contaminated hands or food (3); (iii) organ transplantation or blood transfusion; (iv) transplacental transmission; (v) accidental inoculation of tachyzoites. The parasites form tissue cysts, most commonly in skeletal muscle, myocardium and brain; these cysts may remain throughout the life of the host.

6.3 Intestinal Parasites

Gut protozoan parasites include *Entamoeba histolytica*, *G. lamblia*, *Dientamoeba fragilis*, *Balantidium* spp., *Isospora* spp. and *Cryptosporidium parvum*. All these organisms are transmitted by the faecal–oral route and most of them are cosmopolitan in their distribution. A good example of this is *Giardia*, which is found in nearly all countries of the world. In many developed countries, including the UK and USA, it is one of the most commonly identified waterborne infectious organisms. *Cryptosporidium*, like *Toxoplasma*, has a complex life cycle utilising both sexual and asexual reproduction. By contrast, *Giardia* and *Entamoeba* have simple life cycles utilising only asexual reproduction. These latter organisms are members of a small group of eukaryotes that do not have mitochondria. Indeed, it had long been assumed that they had never possessed mitochondria, but recent studies showing the presence of mitochondrial-like enzymes and structural proteins suggest that it is more likely that this organelle was lost through metabolic/physiological adaptation.

6.3.1 *Giardia lamblia* (syn. *intestinalis, duodenalis*)

Giardia duodenalis (syn. *lamblia* and *intestinalis*) is the causative agent of giardiasis, a severe diarrhoeal disease.

The incidence of *Giardia* infection worldwide ranges from 1.5% to 20%, but is probably significantly higher in countries where standards of hygiene are poor. The most common route of spread is via the faecal–oral route, although spread can also occur through ingestion of contaminated water, and these modes of transmission are particularly prevalent in institutions, nurseries and day-care centres. Recent outbreaks and epidemics in the UK, USA and Eastern Europe have been caused by drinking contaminated water from community water supplies or directly from rivers and streams. Many animals harbour *Giardia* species that are indistinguishable from the human infective types. There is now clear evidence from genotyping studies (see Section 6.6.1.2) that the *G. duodenalis* species is made up of several genetically distinct groups which may represent separate species. This has raised the question of the existence of animal reservoirs of *Giardia*. Recent findings of *Giardia*-infected animals in watersheds from which humans acquired giardiasis, and the successful interspecies transfer of these organisms, suggest that human giardiasis can be acquired by zoonotic transfer; however, it is not clear if the major route of transfer is from animal to human or from human to animal.

Giardia exhibits only two life cycle forms: the vegetative binucleate trophozoite (10–20 μm long × 2–3 μm wide) (Figure 6.2d) and the transmissible quadranucleate cyst (10–12 μm long × 1–3 μm wide) (Figure 6.2f). Trophozoites have four pairs of flagella and an adhesive disc, which is thought to help attachment to the intestinal epithelium. Division in trophozoites is by longitudinal fission.

It was long-believed that *Giardia* was a non-pathogenic commensal. However, we now know that *Giardia* can produce disease ranging from a self-limiting diarrhoea to a severe chronic syndrome. Immune-competent individuals with giardiasis may exhibit some or all of the following signs and symptoms: diarrhoea or loose, foul-smelling stools; steatorrhoea (fatty diarrhoea); malaise; abdominal cramps; excessive flatulence; fatigue and weight loss. Infected individuals with an immune deficiency or protein–calorie malnutrition may develop a more severe disease and will exhibit symptoms such as interference with the absorption of fat and fat-soluble vitamins, retarded growth, weight loss, or a coeliac-disease-like syndrome.

Giardia infection is initiated by ingestion of viable cysts (Figure 6.6), the infective dose of which can be as low as one cyst, although infection initiated by 10–100 viable cysts is more likely. As the cysts pass through the stomach, the low pH and elevated CO_2 induce excystation (cyst–trophozoite transformation). From each cyst, two complete trophozoites emerge and these rapidly undergo division, and then attach to the duodenal and jejunal epithelium. Once attached, they will undergo division, and 4–7 days later they will detach and begin to round up and form cysts (encystment). This process is thought to be induced in response to bile. The first cysts are found in faeces after 7–10 days.

The underlying pathology of giardiasis is not fully understood. The trophozoites do not invade the mucosa, and although their presence may have some physical effects on the surface, it is more likely that some of the pathology is caused by inflammation of the mucosal cells of the small intestine causing an increased turnover rate of intestinal mucosal epithelium. The immature replacement cells have less functional surface area and less digestive and absorptive ability. This would account for the microscopic changes seen in infected epithelia. It has been suggested that other mechanisms may exist, for example, toxin production; however, to date no such toxin-like molecule has been identified.

6.3.2 *Entamoeba histolytica*

E. histolytica is the causative agent of amoebic dysentery, another infection transmitted via the faecal–oral route. The severity of this and related pathologies caused by this organism can vary from diarrhoea associated with the intestinal infection to extraintestinal amoebiasis producing hepatic and often lung infection. The prevalence of amoebiasis in developing countries reflects the lack of adequate sanitary systems. It had long been known that most infections associated with *E. histolytica* are asymptomatic or exhibit minimal symptomology, but in the late 1980s, a separate, but morphologically and biochemically similar species, *Entamoeba dispar*, was identified. This organism exhibits limited pathogenicity and, in many cases, produces no symptoms, but is commonly misidentified as *E. histolytica*. This species is the most likely cause of 'asymptomatic *Entamoeba* infection'.

E. histolytica has a relatively simple life cycle and, like *Giardia*, exhibits only two morphological forms: the trophozoite and cyst stages. Trophozoites (Figure 6.2e) vary in size from 10 to 60 μm and are actively motile. The cyst is spherical, 10–20 μm in diameter, with a thin transparent wall. Fully mature cysts contain four nuclei.

Symptoms of amoebic dysentery are associated with mucosal invasion and ulceration. Mucosal erosion causes diarrhoea, the severity of which increases with the level of invasion and colonisation. Symptoms can also reflect the site of the infection. Peritonitis as a result of perforation has been reported in connection with severe amoebic infection. Extraintestinal amoebiasis is usually associated with liver infection, causing abscesses and/or enlargement. The abscess appears as a slowly enlarging liver mass and will cause noticeable pain. Jaundice may also occur due to blockage of the bile ducts. Pleural, pulmonary and pericardial infections result from metastatic spread from the liver, but can also manifest in other parts of the viscera or give

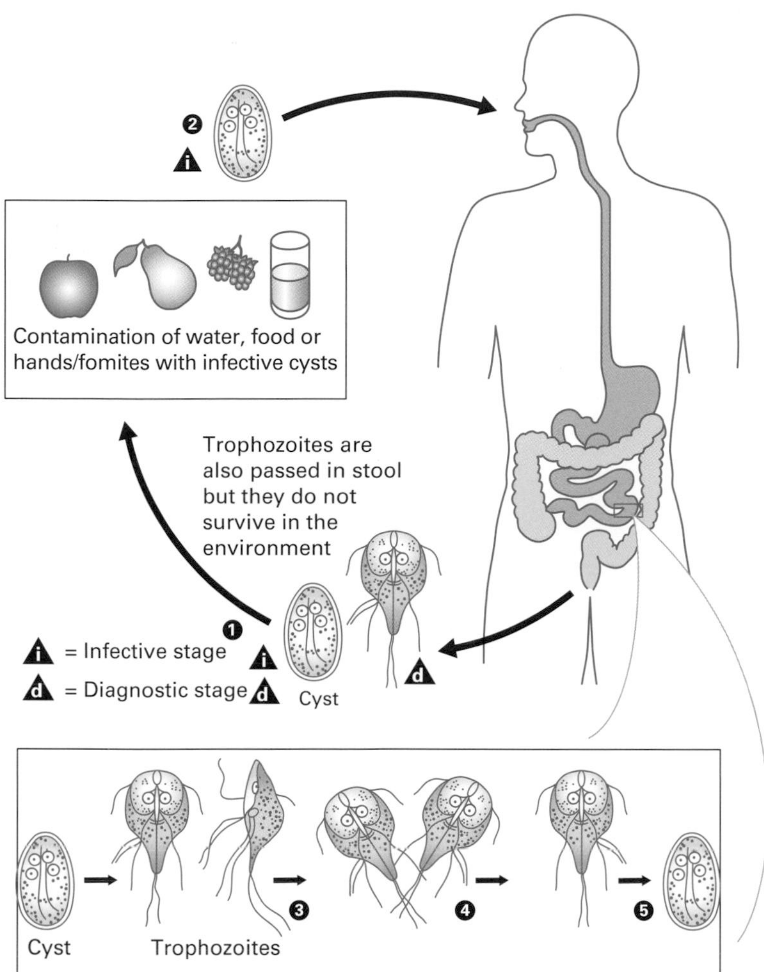

Figure 6.6 Cysts are resistant forms and are responsible for transmission of giardiasis. Both cysts and trophozoites can be found in the faeces (diagnostic stages) (1). The cysts are hardy, and can survive several months in cold water. Infection occurs by the ingestion of cysts in contaminated water, food or by the faecal–oral route (hands or fomites) (2). In the small intestine, excystation releases trophozoites (each cyst produces two trophozoites) (3). Trophozoites multiply by longitudinal binary fission, remaining in the lumen of the proximal small bowel where they can be free or attached to the mucosa by a ventral sucking disc (4). Encystation occurs as the parasites transit towards the colon. The cyst is the stage found most commonly in non-diarrhoeal faeces (5). Because the cysts are infectious when passed in the stool or shortly afterwards, person-to-person transmission is possible. Although animals are infected with *Giardia*, their importance as a reservoir is unclear.

rise to a brain abscess. However, these complications are uncommon.

The life cycle of *E. histolytica* (Figure 6.7) is simple, but the ability of trophozoites to infect sites other than the intestine makes it more complex than that of *Giardia*. Infection is initiated by ingestion of mature cysts, and again, excystation occurs during transit through the gut. After this, trophozoites rapidly divide by simple fission to produce four amoebic cells which undergo a second division; thus, each cyst yields eight trophozoites. Survival outside the host depends on the resistant cyst form.

The pathology of the disease is only partially understood. The process of tissue invasion has been well studied and involves binding and killing of the host cells by specific adhesin molecules and the action of a pore-forming protein, amoebapore. The initial superficial ulcer may deepen into the submucosa and become chronic. Spread may occur by direct extension, by undermining of the surrounding mucosa until it sloughs, or by penetration that can lead to perforation. If the trophozoites gain access to the vascular or lymphatic circulation, metastases may occur first to the liver and then by direct extension or further metastasis to other organs, including the brain.

6.3.3 *Cryptosporidium parvum*

C. parvum is a ubiquitous coccidian parasite that causes cryptosporidiosis in humans; however, other species are known to cause infection in immunocompromised patients and in total this genus comprises 19–20 distinct species

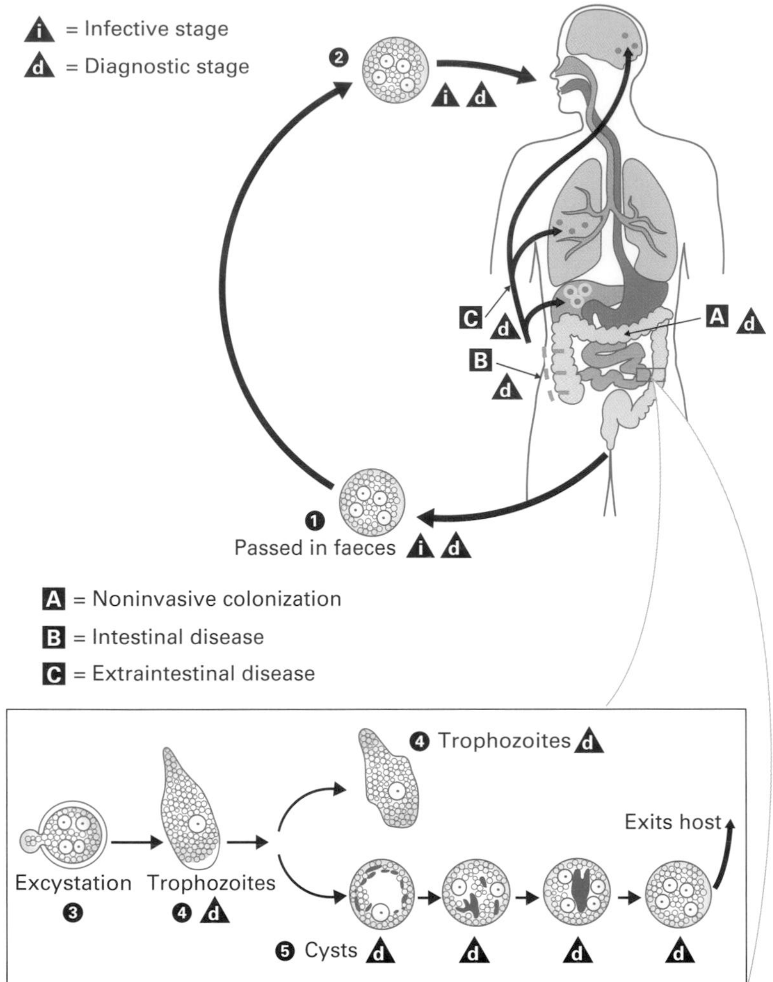

Figure 6.7 Cysts are passed in faeces (1). Infection by *Entamoeba histolytica* occurs by ingestion of mature cysts (2) in faecally contaminated food, water or hands. Excystation (3) occurs in the small intestine and trophozoites (4) are released, which migrate to the large intestine. The trophozoites multiply by binary fission and produce cysts (5), which are passed in the faeces (1). Because of the protection conferred by their walls, the cysts can survive days to weeks in the external environment and are responsible for transmission. (Trophozoites can also be passed in diarrhoeal stools, but are rapidly destroyed once outside the body, and if ingested would not survive exposure to the gastric environment.) In many cases, the trophozoites remain confined to the intestinal lumen (A, non-invasive infection) of individuals who are asymptomatic carriers, passing cysts in their stool. In some patients, the trophozoites invade the intestinal mucosa (B, intestinal disease), or through the bloodstream, extraintestinal sites such as the liver, brain and lungs (C, extraintestinal disease), with resultant pathological manifestations. It has been established that the invasive and non-invasive forms represent two separate species, respectively, *E. histolytica* and *E. dispar*. However, not all persons infected with *E. histolytica* will have invasive disease. These two species are morphologically indistinguishable. Transmission can also occur through faecal exposure during sexual contact (in which case not only cysts but also trophozoites could prove infective).

with species names reflecting the major host specificity of the particular species or genotype. The life cycle of the parasite is complex but is completed in a single host. Infection follows the ingestion of oocysts associated with contaminated water or food. According to the WHO, the health significance of *C. parvum* is high due to the persistence of the organism in the environment. Cattle represent the most important reservoir of *C. parvum* but other mammals, domestic and wild, can be infected and act as carriers of the disease, even if asymptomatic. It is now known that a number of genetically distinct subspecies exist that can be divided into two groups, those organisms that infect humans only, such as *Cryptosporidium hominis*, and those that infect a wider range of hosts such as *C. parvum*. There have been several large outbreaks of this infection in the UK and USA in which water was identified as the initial vehicle for transmission. Members of this genus are intracellular parasites infecting the intestinal mucosal epithelium. The two major life cycle forms are the oval oocyst and the sporozoite.

C. parvum infections are often asymptomatic, but symptoms such as profuse watery diarrhoea, stomach cramps, nausea, vomiting and fever are typical. The symptoms can last from several days to a few weeks in immunocompetent individuals, but in immunocompromised patients infection can become chronic, lasting months or even years. The mean infective dose for immunocompetent people is dependent on the strain of *C. parvum* but is approximately 100 cells, and infants are more vulnerable to infection. Diarrhoea is a major cause of childhood mortality and morbidity as well as malnutrition in developing countries. *Cryptosporidium* is the third most common cause of infective diarrhoea in children in such countries, and consequently it plays a role in the incidence of childhood malnutrition.

Cryptosporidium infection has a higher nutritional impact in boys than girls, because of the need for micronutrients in boys to build up larger muscle mass. Breastfeeding offers some protection against infection. In immunocompromised individuals, *Cryptosporidium* infection causes a severe gastroenteritis, and often the parasites infect other epithelial tissues causing pneumonia; the mortality rate due to *C. parvum* in acquired immunodeficiency syndrome (AIDS) patients is between 50% and 70%. Infection occurs when oocysts (Figure 6.2f) excyst following environmental stimuli (typical intestinal conditions) and parasitise the epithelial cells which line the intestine wall (Figure 6.8). After several further stages of the cycle, two forms of oocyst are produced; soft-walled oocysts reinitiate infection of neighbouring enterocytes, while hard-walled cysts are expelled in the faeces.

Little is known about the mechanism by which these organisms cause disease. They are known to invade cells, but this process is atypical in that the parasites form a vacuole just below the epithelial cell membrane. During infection, a variety of changes are seen such as partial villous atrophy, crypt lengthening and inflammation; these responses are probably due in part to cell damage that occurs during the growth of the intracellular forms. It has also been proposed that parasite enzymes and/or immune-mediated mechanisms may also be involved. It should be remembered, however, that cryptosporidiosis is resolved by the immune system in healthy patients normally within 3 weeks.

6.4 *Trichomonas* and Free-living Amoebae

6.4.1 *Trichomonas* Vaginalis

Trichomonas vaginalis is a common sexually transmitted parasite. Infection rates vary from 10% to 50%, with the highest reported rates found in the USA. Infections are usually asymptomatic or mild, although symptomatic infection is most common in women. Trichomonads are all anaerobes; they contain hydrogenosomes, organelles found in very few other anaerobic eukaryotes and often termed the 'anerobic mitochondria'. A number of functions have been assigned to them, and they have been shown to participate in the generation of adenosine triphosphate (ATP). This organism does not exhibit a life cycle, as only the motile (flagellate/amoeboid) trophozoite (Figure 6.2g) has been seen and division is by binary fission. Trichomonads have a pear-shaped body 7–15-μm long, a single nucleus, three to five forward-directed flagella and a single posterior flagellum that forms the outer border of an undulating membrane.

Trichomoniasis in women is frequently chronic and is characterised by vaginal discharge and dysuria. The inflammation of the vagina is usually diffuse and is characterised by reddening of the vaginal wall and migration of polymorphonuclear leucocytes into the vaginal lumen (these form part of the vaginal discharge).

Because there is no other life cycle form, transmission of trichomonads from host to host must be direct. The inflammatory response in trichomoniasis is the major pathology associated with this organism; however, the mechanisms of induction are not known. It is likely that mechanical irritation resulting from contact between the parasite and vaginal epithelium is a major cause of this response, but the organism produces high concentrations of acidic end products and polyamines, both of which would also irritate local tissues.

6.4.2 Free-living Opportunist Amoebae

The free-living opportunist amoebae are an oft-forgotten group of protozoans. The two major groups, *Naegleria* and *Acanthamoeba*, infect humans and both can cause fatal encephalitis. Both types of infections are rare, with less than 200 cases of *Naegleria fowleri* infection recorded worldwide and approximately 100–200 cases of *Acanthamoeba* ulcerative keratitis occurring in the UK per year. *Acanthamoeba* keratitis is commonly associated with contact lens use and it is thought that infection is caused by a combination of corneal trauma and dirty contact lenses. Both types of amoeba produce resistant cysts and *Naegleria* also exhibits a flagellate form. Both *Acanthamoeba* and *Naegleria* are free-living inhabitants of fresh water and soil, but *N. fowleri* (the human pathogen) reproduces faster in warm waters up to 46 °C. Treatment of water by chlorination or ozonolysis does not entirely eliminate cysts and both amoebae have been isolated from air-conditioning units.

N. fowleri is the causative agent of primary amoebic meningoencephalitis, a rapidly fatal disease that usually affects children and young adults. In all cases, contact with amoebae occurs as a result of swimming in infected fresh

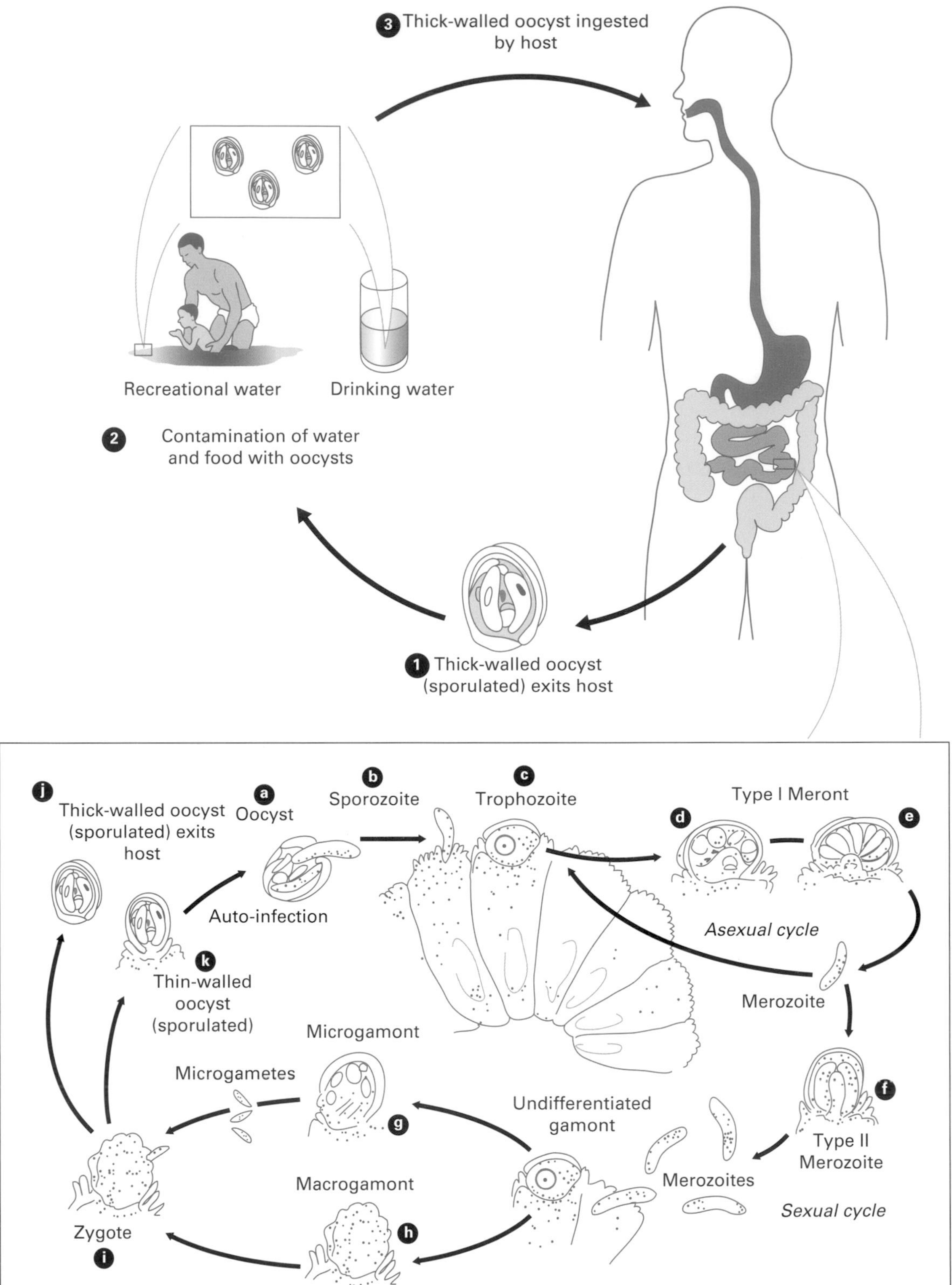

Figure 6.8 Life cycle of *Cryptosporidium*. Sporulated oocysts, containing four sporozoites, are excreted by the infected host through faeces and possibly other routes such as respiratory secretions (1). Transmission of *Cryptosporidium parvum* occurs mainly through contact with contaminated water (e.g., drinking or recreational water). Occasionally, food sources, such as chicken salad, may serve as vehicles for transmission. Many outbreaks in the USA have occurred in water parks, community swimming pools and day-care centres. Zoonotic transmission of *C. parvum* occurs through exposure to infected animals or exposure to water contaminated by faeces of infected animals (2). Following ingestion (and possibly inhalation) by a suitable host (3), excystation (a) occurs. The sporozoites are released and parasitise epithelial cells (b, c) of the gastrointestinal tract or other tissues such as the respiratory tract. In these cells, the parasites undergo asexual multiplication (schizogony or merogony) (d, e, and f) and then sexual multiplication (gametogony) producing microgamonts (male, g) and macrogamonts (female, h). Upon fertilisation of the macrogamonts by the microgametes (i), oocysts (j, k) develop that sporulate in the infected host. Two different types of oocysts are produced, the thick-walled oocyst, which is commonly excreted from the host (j), and the thin-walled oocyst (k), which is primarily involved in autoinfection. Oocysts are infective upon excretion, thus permitting direct and immediate faecal–oral transmission. *Source:* From Juranek (2000). Cryptosporidiosis. In: *Hunter's Tropical Medicine*, 8th edn, ed. G.T. Strickland.

water. The organisms enter the brain via the olfactory tract after amoebae are inhaled or splashed into the olfactory epithelium. The incubation period ranges from 2 to 15 days and depends both on the size of the inoculum and the virulence of the strain. The disease appears with the sudden onset of severe frontal headache, fever, nausea, vomiting and stiff neck. Symptoms develop rapidly to lethargy, confusion and coma and in all cases to date the patient died within 48–72 hours.

Acanthamoeba castellanii, *Acanthamoeba culbertsoni* and other pathogenic *Acanthamoeba* species can cause opportunist lung and skin infections in immunocompromised individuals. Where amoebae spread from such lesions to the brain, they can cause a slowly progressive and usually fatal encephalitis. In addition, *Acanthamoeba* can cause an ulcerating keratitis in healthy individuals, usually in association with improperly sterilised contact lenses. The presence of cysts and trophozoites in alveoli or in multiple nodules or ulcerations of the skin characterises acanthamoebic pneumonitis and dermatitis. Spread of amoebae to the brain produces an encephalitis, characterised by neurological changes, drowsiness, personality changes and seizures in the early stages of infection, which progress to altered mental status, lethargy and cerebellar ataxia. The end point of infection is usually coma followed by death of the patient. *Acanthamoeba* keratitis is characterised by painful corneal ulcerations that fail to respond to the usual anti-infective treatments. The infected and damaged corneal tissue may show a characteristic annular infiltrate and congested conjunctivae. If not successfully treated, the disease progresses to corneal perforation and loss of the eye, or to a vascularised scar over thinned cornea, with impaired vision.

6.5 Host Response to Infection

Mechanisms to control parasitic protozoa are similar to those utilised for other infectious agents; they can be divided into non-specific mechanism(s) and specific mechanism(s) involving the immune system. The best-studied non-specific mechanisms include those that affect the entry of parasites into the red blood cell. The sickle cell haemoglobin trait and lack of the Duffy factor on the erythrocyte surface make the red cell more resistant to invasion by *Plasmodium*. These traits are commonly found in populations from malaria-endemic regions. A second example of a non-specific mechanism is the presence of trypanolytic factors in the serum of humans which confer resistance to *T. brucei*. Although non-specific factors can play a key role in resistance, usually they work in conjunction with the host's immune system.

6.5.1 Immune Response

Unlike most other types of infection, protozoan diseases are often chronic, lasting for months to years. When associated with a strong host immune response, this type of long-term infection is apt to result in a high incidence of immunopathology. Until recently, the importance of the host immune response in controlling many parasite infections was not fully appreciated, but the impact of HIV infection on many parasitic diseases has highlighted this relationship.

Different parasites elicit different humoral and/or cellular immune responses (see Chapter 9). In malaria and trypanosome infections, antibody appears to play a major role in immunity, although for many organisms both humoral and cellular immunities are required for killing of the parasites. Cellular immunity is believed to be the most important mechanism in the killing of *Leishmania* and *Toxoplasma*. Cytokines are involved in the control of both the immune responses and also the pathology of many parasitic diseases. Helper (h) and cytotoxic (c) T cells play major roles in the induction/control of the response. The various subsets of these produce different profiles of cytokines. For example, the Th1 subset produces gamma interferon (IFN-γ) and interleukin-2 (IL-2) and is involved in cell-mediated immunity. By contrast, the Th2 subset produces IL-4 and IL-6 that are responsible for antibody-mediated immunity. The induction of the correct T-cell response is key to recovery. The Th1 subset and increased IFN-γ are important for the control of *Leishmania*, *T. cruzi* and *Toxoplasma* infections, whereas the Th2 response is more important in parasitic infections in which antibody is a major factor. It is important to recognise that the cytokines produced by one T-cell subset can upregulate or downregulate the response of other T-cell subsets; IL-4 will downregulate Th1 cells, for example. The cytokines produced by T and other cell types do not act directly on the parasites but induce changes in the metabolism of glucose, fatty acid and protein in other host cells. Cytokines can also stimulate cell division and, therefore, clonal expansion of T- and B-cell subsets. This can lead to increased antibody production and/or cytotoxic T-cell numbers. The list of cytokines and their functions is growing rapidly, and these chemical messages influence all phases of the immune response. They are also clearly involved in the multitude of physiological responses (fever, decreased food intake, etc.) observed in an animal's response to a pathogen, and in the pathology that results.

6.5.2 Immune Pathology

The protozoa can elicit humoral responses in which antigen–antibody complexes are formed, and these can trigger coagulation and complement systems. Immune complexes have been found circulating in serum and deposited in the kidneys where they may contribute to conditions such as glomerulonephritis. In other tissues, these complexes can also induce localised hypersensitivities. It is thought that this type of immediate hypersensitivity is responsible for various clinical syndromes including blood hyperviscosity, oedema and hypotension.

Another important form of antibody-mediated pathology is autoimmunity. Autoantibodies to a number of different host antigens (e.g., red blood cells, laminin, collagen and DNA) have been demonstrated. These autoantibodies may play a role in the pathology of parasitic diseases by exerting a direct cytotoxic effect on the host cells, for example, autoantibodies that coat red blood cells produce haemolytic anaemia; they may also cause damage through a build-up of antigen–antibody complexes.

Many parasites can elicit the symptoms of disease through the action of their surface molecules such as the pore-forming proteins of *E. histolytica* that induce contact-dependent cell lysis, and trypanosome glycoproteins that can fix and activate complement resulting in the production of biologically active and toxic complement fragments. A range of parasite-derived enzymes such as proteases and phospholipases can cause cell destruction, inflammatory responses and gross tissue pathology.

6.5.3 Immune Evasion

Parasites exhibit several mechanisms that allow them to evade the host immune response. Two such mechanisms are displayed by trypanosomes, which can exhibit both antigenic masking and antigenic variation. Masking means the parasite becomes coated with host components and therefore is not recognised as foreign. In addition, parasites can undergo antigenic variation which results in surface antigens being changed during the course of an infection. The goal of these changes is that the host's immune response is evaded. Parasites can also suppress the host's immune response either to the parasite specifically or to foreign antigens in general. This, however, can cause several problems, as general immune suppression may make the individual more susceptible to secondary infection.

6.6 Detection of Parasites

The detection of parasites in the host and environment (including foods) is vital for proper treatment and for understanding mechanisms of transmission. The use of molecular typing is of major benefit in epidemiology studies and is particularly useful in monitoring the potential for zoonotic transmission in some parasite species such as *Cryptosporidium*.

6.6.1 Methods of Detection

It is not always easy or possible to culture parasites, so detection of these organisms in samples requires the use of methods such as microscopy and DNA amplification. The most commonly used approach is microscopy and this can be applied to clinical as well as environmental samples. For some organisms, this approach remains the 'gold standard' for detection and identification. The advantages of microscopy are speed, cost and availability. In addition, fluorescent-labelled antibodies raised to species-specific antigens can be utilised to help identify organisms to species or subspecies level, and other stains can be used to help determine the viability of cells. Examples of such stains include fluorescein diacetate, which is cleaved by esterases in viable cells releasing fluorescein (gives a green fluorescence), and propidium iodide which is excluded from viable cells but taken up by cells with damaged membranes (gives red fluorescence). However, there are a number of obvious limitations including the requirement for well-trained staff to perform the microscopy, limits of sensitivity of the method and, for some parasites, difficulty in differentiating species based on morphology.

6.6.1.1 Antibody-based Technologies

For the major protozoan parasites, a number of immunology-based methods exist to detect the presence of organisms in clinical samples. These include the use of agglutination, complement fixation and enzyme-linked immunosorbent assay (ELISA). The most commonly used method is the ELISA and this can be employed to detect the presence of antigens in samples (direct assay) or antigen-specific antibodies in patients' serum (indirect). The ELISA method has several advantages in that it can be automated and has good specificity and sensitivity. Although several ELISA-based detection kits are available, their cost can be a limitation to use especially in those developing countries where parasitic infections are endemic. The use of indirect ELISA methods for determining the infection status of the patient can also be difficult because previous exposure to the parasite can cause problems and the immune status of the patients may also impact on antibody production.

6.6.1.2 DNA-based Technologies

The sequences of nucleic acids, either DNA or RNA, can be used to help in the identification of species and individuals. Key gene targets for DNA-based identification of parasites include ribosomal DNA genes, and those encoding for metabolic enzymes and structural proteins. Metabolic enzymes and structural proteins are often used, as their gene sequences exhibit more variability at the DNA sequence level and this allows for greater discrimination at species level particularly when species are genetically very similar. For example, *Cryptosporidium* can be speciated by using a combination of target genes including the *Cryptosporidium* oocyst wall protein (COWP), heat shock protein (hsp70), dihydrofolate reductase (DHFR) and 18S ribosomal DNA. Complete genomes are now available for the major protozoan parasites, and this has helped in the development of improved methods for species identification. These genomes can be accessed at http://eupathdb.org/eupathdb/, and this website links to many other resources including the National Center for Biotechnology Information (http:// http://www.ncbi.nlm.nih.gov).

6.6.1.3 Alternative Methods

Alternative methods are being developed for the detection of parasites; these include mass spectrometry (MS) and biosensors. MS can be used by identifying known surface characteristics of appropriate life cycle forms. This type of MS uses low-energy electrons to generate a fingerprint of the cells. Other mass spectrometry methods can generate fingerprints based on parasite-derived peptides and metabolites. These can be detected easily with a high level of sensitivity and can be used in complex mixtures that would be present in clinical and environmental samples. The development of kits for near-patient testing has driven advances in detection technology and this has generated interest in the use of biosensors. These sensors detect the presence of 'marker molecules' that are specific to a particular pathogen and utilise mechanical, electrochemical or piezoelectric methods to generate a signal that can be detected. Such sensors can be combined onto 'chips' to detect a range of pathogens.

6.6.2 Analysis of Samples

6.6.2.1 Clinical Samples

Diagnosis of parasitic infection is dependent on the demonstration of the parasite in appropriate samples. The type of sample can vary from blood, where preparation can be minimal (e.g., sample of smears for microscopy), to faeces or intestinal aspirates. Faecal samples require more processing: for example, fresh or preserved stools can be concentrated to increase the yield of the parasites by sedimentation using the formol–ether or formol–ethyl acetate techniques or by the faecal parasite flotation method using copper sulphate. These concentrates can be stained for microscopy. For the extraction of DNA from samples, a number of methods exist; however, there are various resin-based kits that will separate DNA from complex biological samples.

6.6.2.2 Environmental Samples

Many parasites have life cycle forms that can survive in the environment. These act to initiate infections in susceptible hosts; for some parasites this only requires ingestion of no more than 10 cells or cysts, thus the ability to detect them in the environment is vital. This section focuses on water and foods, as they are often major routes of transmission for parasites such as *Giardia* and *Cryptosporidium* which are included in the monitoring standards for potable waters (drinking waters) by regulatory bodies in the UK, the European Union and the USA. In addition, food and pharmaceutical companies that utilise water in their processes are required to test for several pathogens, including waterborne parasites. Foods can also be a source of infection, and methods for the detection of pathogens in foods are as important as those for water samples.

As outlined in Section 6.6.1, a number of methods can be used to detect and to identify parasites, but the performance of these techniques will often be impaired when used on real samples. This is due to a number of factors that include:

- the low levels of parasites present;
- the volume of sample required for analysis;
- the presence of other microorganisms;
- the presence of compounds that interfere with detection;
- turbidity of samples (water); and
- high levels of protein, lipids and carbohydrates in samples (foods).

Often these factors combine to make detection difficult. For example, if levels of a parasite in water are low (<1/100 ml), several litres must be collected and analysed. This is possible but would require the sample volume to be reduced for analysis. This can be achieved either by filtration or centrifugation. If the sample contains sediment, both approaches are difficult; however, methods such as tangential flow filtration (fluid passed parallel to the filter) can be used. Waters can also contain organic acids that can inhibit the polymerase chain reaction (PCR) process used to amplify nucleic acid material; thus, these organic acids must be removed from the sample before analysis. DNA-based technology may also fail to detect the presence of a parasite if the DNA present in the sample is degraded, for example, by other organisms. In foods, the process can be even more complex and separation of parasites from the foodstuff is often the factor that impacts most on the limits (sensitivity) of the method.

6.7 Control of Protozoan Parasites

It is now clear that the best approach for the successful control of parasites requires the integration of several methods which draw upon our increasing understanding of their life cycle, epidemiology and host response to infection.

Table 6.1 Common antiprotozoal drugs and their modes of action.

Drug	Mode of action (if known)	Mechanism of selectivity	Target organism(s)
Benzimidazoles	Microtubule function	Differences in the target	*Giardia*, *Trichomonas*
Metronidazole and other nitroimidazoles such as tinidazole and fexinidazole	Nucleic acid synthesis	Activation in the parasite	*Giardia*, *Trichomonas*, *Entamoeba* and *Trypanosoma* spp.
Amphotericin B	Membrane function	Differences in the target	*Leishmania* spp.
Mepacrine (Quinacrine)	Metabolic inhibitor	Differences in the target	*Leishmania* spp. *Giardia* and *Plasmodium* spp.
Pentamidine	Nucleic acid synthesis	Differential uptake	*Leishmania* spp.
Stibogluconate (antimonial drug)	DNA replication and transcription; also impacts on ATP biosynthesis	Differences in the target	*Leishmania* spp.
Artemisinin/artesunate / dihydroartemisinin	Protein alkylation and DNA damage via production of reactive oxygen species	Differences in metabolism	*Plasmodium* spp.
Atovaquone	Energy metabolism	Differences in the target	*Plasmodium* spp.
Chloroquine	Nucleic acid synthesis; inhibition of haem degradation	Differential uptake	*Plasmodium* spp.
Dapsone	Cofactor synthesis	Unique target	*Plasmodium* spp.
Piperaquine	Nucleic acid synthesis; inhibition of haem degradation	Differential uptake	*Plasmodium* spp.
Proguanil	Cofactor synthesis	Differences in the target	*Plasmodium* spp.
Pyrimethamine	Cofactor synthesis	Differences in the target	*Plasmodium* spp.
Mefloquine	Nucleic acid synthesis	Differential uptake	*Plasmodium* spp.
Quinine	Nucleic acid synthesis	Differential uptake	*Plasmodium* spp.
Sulphonamides	Cofactor synthesis	Differences in the target	*Plasmodium* spp.
Tetracycline	Protein synthesis	Differential uptake	*Plasmodium* spp.
Benznidazole	Nucleic acid synthesis	Activation in the parasite	*Trypanosoma* spp.
Eflornithine	Amino acid biosynthesis	Differences in the target	*T. brucei gambiense*
Melarsoprol	Energy metabolism in the parasite	Target pathway more important	*T. brucei gambiense*
Primaquine	Energy metabolism	Differences in the target	*Trypanosoma* spp.

6.7.1 Chemotherapy

The origins of chemotherapy are closely linked to the development of antiparasitic agents, but there has been slow progress in identifying new and novel antiprotozoal agents by comparison to that seen for antibacterial and antiviral drugs. With the support of the WHO, the Drugs for Neglected Diseases *initiative* (DNDi, see Section 6.7.1.4) and government-sponsored research, new antiparasitic drugs are slowly coming into the market. Interestingly, there are still a number of protozoan parasite infections such as cryptosporidiosis for which there is no effective treatment.

6.7.1.1 Mechanisms of Action and Selective Toxicity

For many of the commonly used antiprotozoal drugs the modes of action and mechanisms of selective toxicity are well understood, although for some the precise mechanism remains unclear. The most common antiprotozoal drugs and their modes of action are shown in Table 6.1.

Considering the drugs in relation to modes of action, dapsone and the sulphonamides block the biosynthesis of tetrahydrofolate by inhibiting dihydropteroate synthetase, while the 2,4-diaminopyrimidines (proguanil and pyrimethamine) block the same pathway but at a later step catalysed by dihydrofolate reductase.

The drugs that interfere with nucleic acid synthesis include those that bind to the DNA and intercalate with it such as chloroquine, mefloquine and quinine, and pentamidine, which is unable to intercalate but probably interacts ionically. Other compounds such as benznidazole and metronidazole may alkylate DNA through activation of nitro groups via a one-electron reduction step.

Several of these compounds, however, including chloroquine, mefloquine, quinine and metronidazole, have more than one potential mode of action. Chloroquine, for example, inhibits the enzyme haem polymerase, which functions to detoxify the cytotoxic molecule haem that is generated during the degradation of haemoglobin. Metronidazole is reduced in the parasite cell and forms several cytotoxic intermediates, which can cause damage not only to DNA but also to membranes and proteins.

Tetracycline targets protein synthesis in *Plasmodium* via a similar mechanism to that seen in bacteria: inhibition of chain elongation and peptide bond formation. Eflornithine interferes with the metabolism of the amino acid ornithine in *T. brucei gambiense* by acting as a suicide substrate for the enzyme ornithine decarboxylase.

Albendazole has been shown to have significant antigiardial activity, although its mode of action is unclear. In *Leishmania*, amphotericin B binds to ergosterol in the membrane making it leaky to ions and small molecules (e.g., amino acids), while the anti-protozoal drugs atovaquone and primaquine bind to the cytochrome bc_1 complex and inhibit electron flow. The anti-trypanosomal drug melarsoprol is most likely to act by blocking glycolytic kinases, especially the cytoplasmic pyruvate kinase, although it may also disrupt the reduction of trypanothione.

6.7.1.2 Drug Targets and Life Cycle Stages

A confounding issue with parasites, particularly those that have complex life cycles, is that not all parasite life cycle stages exhibit the same level of sensitivity to drugs (Figure 6.9). This has been well described for many years in *Plasmodium* and has been comprehensively reviewed by Delves *et al.* (2012).

For malaria, the various drug types can be used to target key features of the disease; for example, blood schizonticides (drugs that target blood schizonts) can be used to stop the immediate early symptoms of malaria (Figure 6.9). Tissue schizonticides are employed to prevent the relapse of infections caused by *P. ovale* and *P. vivax* due to hypnozoites in the liver stage of their life cycle.

6.7.1.3 Drug Resistance

As with bacteria, drug resistance in some parasites such as *Plasmodium* is a major problem and tends to appear where chemotherapy has been used extensively. In addition, the rapid development of resistance can also be linked to gene rearrangement and recombination that can occur during sexual reproduction. Parasites utilise the same five basic

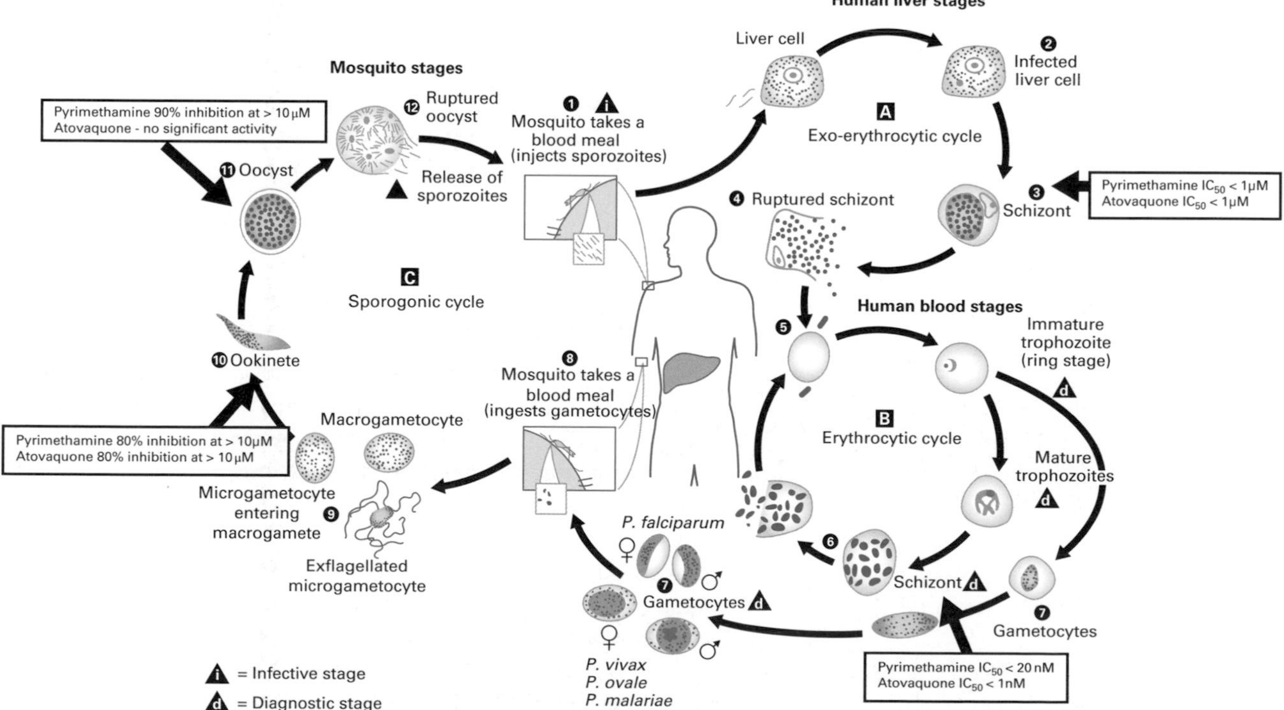

Figure 6.9 Diagram showing the activity of two antimalarial drugs against various life cycle stages of *Plasmodium*. Interestingly, two schizont forms in different environments exhibit different sensitivities. IC_{50}, concentration inhibiting parasite growth by 50%. For a full description of the life cycle stages, see legend to Figure 6.1.

resistance mechanisms that are displayed by bacteria: (i) metabolic inactivation of the drug; (ii) use of efflux pumps; (iii) use of alternative metabolic pathways; (iv) alteration of the target; and (v) elevation of the amount of target enzyme. The problem of resistance is exacerbated by the fact that there are so few drugs available for the control of some parasites.

Drug resistance has led to the introduction of combination therapies for parasites such as malaria with an artemisinin combination therapy (ACTs) becoming the first-line therapy. Artemisinin and its derivatives are highly potent against all asexual blood stream and some gametocyte forms; however, these compounds have short half-lives, and if not used appropriately, this can leave residual parasites that are likely to maintain infection. As a result, ACTs combine artemisinin with a partner drug such as mefloquine that has a longer half-life. In addition, both drugs will have different drug targets and thus ACTs have remained highly effective for over two decades. The effectiveness of ACTs is under threat in some regions such as Southeast Asia where resistance to ACT combination drugs is increasingly prevalent. This has led the WHO to recommend the introduction of a triple ACT combination of dihydroartemisinin with piperaquine and mefloquine. While combination therapies can be adapted to suit the resistance profiles of parasites in particular regions, these changes increase the cost of each medication because of reformulation, additional drug ingredient costs and the reduction in useful lifespan of each new combination.

6.7.1.4 Drug Repurposing

A major problem associated with the development of new drugs for parasitic diseases is the cost of that development; this is significantly compounded by factors already discussed in this section such as the complexity of life cycle stages, the lack of common targets in the various life cycle stages and in addition there are often no good animal models. All of these factors decrease the number of drugs that show activity appropriate for clinical trial and this makes the economics of developing anti-parasitic drugs difficult to justify for most drug companies. Estimates of costs associated with discovering and developing a new anti-parasitic compound may reach $800 million and can take many more than 10 years from inception.

There are many organisations willing to work with drug companies to help drive novel drug developments, significant among these is the DND*i*. This collaborative product development partnership, set up by key research and health institutions most notably from the public sector in neglected disease-endemic countries, has succeeded in bringing forward treatments for malaria, African trypanosomiasis, visceral leishmaniasis and childhood Chagas disease since its inception in 2003. Despite such initiatives, however, approaches other than traditional *de novo* drug discovery must also be used for the development of 'novel' antiparasitic drugs. One such approach is drug repurposing, where a validated molecular target for one disease and well-characterised ligands (drugs) for that target are used as the 'discovery' starting point for another disease; this is often called 'piggybacking'. As well as offering economic benefits, repurposing can also result in reduced time to market if available safety data can be used. Repurposing has become an important approach to target and lead antiparasitic drug development, since proteomic and transcriptomic tools have helped identify previously unknown signalling, regulatory and metabolic pathways in many parasites. One example is glucose-regulated protein (GRP78), a molecular chaperone that is a regulator of the unfolded protein response (UPR) and is found in *P. falciparum*. By screening repurposed chaperone inhibitors previously developed as prospective anti-cancer agents, new drug structures were identified and showed that GRP78 inhibition is lethal to drug-sensitive and -resistant strains of the parasite. Other examples include: histone deacetylase (HDAC) enzyme inhibitors, clinically approved for treating T-cell lymphoma, which can also target a similar enzyme in the parasites causing malaria, leishmaniasis and trypanosomiasis; and kinase inhibitors, again clinically approved for human use, which are under development as potential new drugs for parasitic diseases such as malaria and African trypanosomiasis.

6.7.2 Other Approaches to Control

An early success in malaria control can be attributed to the use of professional spray teams who treated the inside of huts with dichlorodiphenyltrichloroethane (DDT), without any direct involvement of the infected population. However, the problem with pesticides such as DDT is that they lack specificity, and as application is not always well-directed, there is often destruction of a wide range of insects, which may have undesirable side effects. Further problems include the accumulation of pesticide residues in the food chain and pesticide resistance in the target organism. Window screens and bed nets do prevent mosquito bites, however, and there has been a lot of interest in using bed nets impregnated with insecticide. Environmental control was a major strategy used before the development of modern insecticides. A good example of this is mosquito control through the removal of breeding sites by drainage, land reclamation projects, removal of vegetation overhanging water, speeding up water flow in canals and periodic drainage and drying out of canals. Life cycle forms that enter the water system, such as cysts and oocysts of *Giardia* and *Cryptosporidium*, can present a major public health problem. These forms are often resistant to common disinfection methods and require physical removal from waters. Cysts and oocysts can be destroyed by use of proper sewage treatments such as anaerobic digestion, but these systems require regular maintenance in order to remain effective.

6.7.2.1 Biological Control

Biological control is an active but still developing area. Genetic control of insect vectors, particularly the use of irradiated sterile males, has been widely publicised, and the release of chemically sterile males has been attempted to control anopheline mosquitoes. Other similar methods include the release of closely related species within the environment in order to produce sterile hybrids. Genetically modified mosquitoes that are resistant to *Plasmodium* infection have been successfully used in large-scale field trials. Larvivorous fish have also been employed for mosquito control; other organisms considered for the same purpose include bacteria, fungi, nematodes and predatory insects. One of the best-studied agents is the bacterium *Bacillus thuringiensis*; the spore or the isolated toxin from this species can be used as a very effective and specific insecticide.

6.7.2.2 Vaccines and Vaccine Development

Where exposure to infection is likely to occur, killing the parasite as it enters the host is a sensible approach to control. There are two options available, chemoprophylaxis or vaccination. Unfortunately, long-term chemotherapy can have adverse side effects and, in the absence of symptoms, members of the at-risk population may fail to take the treatment. Vaccination would seem to be the ideal method of parasite control, as lifelong resistance may result from just a single treatment. Despite a huge amount of effort, the only successful parasite vaccines are those for the control of veterinary parasites. However, there has been significant success with the development of recombinant vaccines for the control of malaria and it is likely that DNA vaccines may be of use in the control of parasites. In this method, the DNA encoding an important parasite protein is injected into host cells and the foreign 'vaccinating' protein is synthesised in or on the surface of the cell. This intracellular foreign protein enters the cell's major histocompatibility complex (MHC) class 1 pathway resulting in a cell-mediated immune response. By contrast, a protein that is extracellular enters the MHC class 2 pathway, which results primarily in an antibody or humoral response. Innate defence regulator (IDR) peptide-mediated responses to infection have also been identified as important for parasite control and this has also opened up new areas for the development of vaccine candidates. Furthermore, recent advances in messenger RNA vaccines (see Chapter 10) now point towards new opportunities for parasite vaccine development.

Despite such technological advances, however, the complexity of parasitic infections may mean that conventional vaccine platforms, such as live attenuated or killed whole parasite, will still prove for some time to be more effective than subunit vaccines, including recombinant protein strategies. Vaccine development for parasitic infections is often hindered by limitations of production and/or inadequate immune responses. Currently, few commercially available vaccines exist to control parasitic protozoal infections; indeed, in 2020, there were only 10 commercially available vaccines for these types of infections, and these were mostly for use in animals.

A selection of current licensed vaccines is shown in Table 6.2. Several others are being evaluated in clinical trials and most of these are against malaria. Information about the strategic approach can be found at the Malaria Vaccine Initiative website (www.malariavaccine.org). In addition, there are vaccines being evaluated for human use against other parasites, for example *Leishmania* vaccines co-administered with BCG (bacillus of Calmette and Guérin) have been under trial for many years. Recently, DNA and viral-vector-based vaccines have been tested in clinical trials including one utilising an adenovirus human serotype 35-based vector encoding the malarial circumsporozoite protein.

Acknowledgement

The life cycle figures for this chapter originate in the copyright-free DPDx website maintained by the United States Center for Disease Control's Division of Parasitic Diseases; this source is gratefully acknowledged.

Table 6.2 Examples of the type of licensed vaccines available for the control of diseases caused by parasitic protozoa.

Target species	Formulation	Effect	Status
Plasmodium falciparum	Circumsporozoite surface protein fragment fused to hepatitis B surface antigen with lipid-based adjuvant	Inhibits sporozoite motility and invasion of hepatocytes	Licensed for use in humans
Leishmania infantum chagasi	Antigen preparation from *Leishmania* (glycoprotein rich) together with amphoteric surfactant	Prevents infection; blocks transmission; increases CD4+, CD8+ and CD21+ lymphocyte levels	Licensed for veterinary use
Leishmania infantum chagasi	*L. infantum* excreted secreted proteins (ESP) with saponins	Increases Th1 antibody-mediated responses, and increases leishmanicidal activity of macrophages via nitric oxide synthase	Licensed for veterinary use
Leishmania infantum chagasi	Recombinant *L. donovani* amastigote stress response protein A2 with saponins	Targets protein A2 which is expressed in amastigotes and involved in resistance	Licensed for veterinary use
Giardia lamblia	Inactivated trophozoites of *Giardia lamblia*	Prevention and treatment of clinical signs and reduction of cyst shedding	Licensed for veterinary use

References

Delves, M., Plouffe, D., Scheurer, C. et al. (2012). The activities of current antimalarial drugs on the life cycle stages of *Plasmodium*: a comparative study with human and rodent parasites. *PLoS Med.* 9 (2): e1001169.

Juranek, D.D. (2000) Cryptosporidiosis. In *Hunter's Tropical Medicine and Emerging Diseases.* 8e (ed. G.T. Strickland), 594–600. Philadelphia: W.B. Saunders Company.

Further Reading

British National Formulary *83* (2022). *Chapter 5: Infection.* London: BMJ Group and Pharmaceutical Press *(A new volume is published every 6 months and the reader is advised to consult the most recent edition.).*

Malaria Vaccine Initiative website (www.malariavaccine.org). PATH, Washington DC.

National Center for Biotechnology Information (2021). Antiparasitic Drugs, *NCBI Bookshelf* https://www.ncbi.nlm.nih.gov/books/NBK544251

Ryan, E.T., Hill, D.R., Solomon, T. et al. (2020). *Eds. Hunter's Tropical Medicine and Emerging Infections*, 10e. Edinburgh: Elsevier.

Sacks, D.L., Peters, N.C. and Bethony, J.M. (2016). Chapter 17 Vaccines against parasites. In: *The Vaccine Book*, 2e (ed. B.R. Bloom and P.-H. Lambert), 331–360. London: Academic Press.

Versteeg, L., Almutain, M.M., Hotez, P.J. and Pollet, J. (2019). Enlisting the mRNA vaccine platform to combat parasitic infections. *Vaccine* 7 (4): 122.e.

Wiser, M. (2010). *Protozoa and Human Disease.* New York: Garland Science.

Thomas, V., McDonnell, G., Denyer, S.P. and Maillard, J-Y. (2010). Free-living amoebae and their intracellular pathogenic microorganisms: risks for water quality. *FEMS Microbiol. Rev.* 34: 231–259.

Part 3

Pathogens and Host Response

7

Principles of Microbial Pathogenicity and Epidemiology

David Allison[1] *and Andrew J. McBain*[2]

[1] *Reader in Pharmacy Education, Division of Pharmacy and Optometry, School of Health Sciences, The University of Manchester, Manchester, UK*
[2] *Professor of Microbiology, Division of Pharmacy and Optometry, School of Health Sciences, The University of Manchester, Manchester, UK*

CONTENTS

7.1 Introduction

Microorganisms are ubiquitous, and most of them are free-living and derive their nutrition from organic and inorganic substrates. The association of humans with such microorganisms is generally harmonious, as the majority of those encountered are benign and, indeed, are often vital to commerce, health and a balanced microbiota. The ability of bacteria and fungi to establish infections of plants, animals and humans varies considerably. Some are rarely, if ever, isolated from infected tissues, while opportunist pathogens such as *Pseudomonas aeruginosa* and *Staphylococcus epidermidis* can establish themselves most commonly in compromised individuals. Only a few species

Hugo and Russell's Pharmaceutical Microbiology, Ninth Edition. Edited by Brendan F. Gilmore and Stephen P. Denyer.

Companion website: https://www.wiley.com/go/HugoandRussells9e

of bacteria may be regarded as obligate pathogens, for which animals or plants are the only reservoirs for their existence (e.g., *Neisseria gonorrhoeae*, *Mycobacterium tuberculosis* and *Treponema pallidum*). Viruses (see Chapter 5), on the other hand, must parasitise host cells to replicate and are therefore inevitably associated with disease. Even among the viruses and obligate bacterial pathogens, the degree of virulence varies, in that some (particularly the bacteria) can potentially coexist with the host without causing overt disease (e.g., *Staphylococcus aureus*), while others will always cause some detriment to the host (e.g., rabies virus). Organisms such as these invariably produce their effects, directly or indirectly, by actively growing on or in the host tissues.

Other groups of microorganisms may cause disease through ingestion of substances (toxins) produced during microbial growth on foods (e.g., *Clostridium botulinum*, botulism; *Bacillus cereus*, vomiting). In this case, the organisms themselves do not have to proliferate in the host for the effects of the toxin to be manifested.

Animals and plants constantly interact with bacteria present within their environment. For an infection to develop, such microorganisms must remain associated with host tissues and increase their numbers more rapidly than they can be either eliminated or killed. This balance relates to the ability of the bacterium to sequester nutrients and multiply in the face of innate defences and a developing immune response by the now compromised host.

The greater the number of bacterial cells associated with the initial challenge to the host, the greater will be the chance of disease. If the pathogen does not arrive at its 'portal of entry' to the body or directly at its target tissues in sufficient number, then an infection will not ensue. The minimum number of viable microorganisms that is required to cause infection and thereby disease is called the *minimum infective number* (MIN). The MIN varies markedly between the various pathogens and is also affected by the general health and immune status of the individual host. The course of an infection can be considered as a sequence of separate events that includes initial contact with the pathogen, its consolidation and spread between and within organs and its eventual elimination (Figure 7.1). Growth and consolidation of the microorganisms at the portal of entry may involve the formation of a microcolony (biofilm, see Chapters 3 and 8). Biofilms and microcolonies are collections of microorganisms that are attached to surfaces and enveloped within exopolymers (biofilm matrix) composed of polysaccharides, glycoproteins, proteins, and DNA, etc. Growth within the matrix not only protects the pathogens against opsonisation and phagocytosis by the host but also modulates their microenvironment and reduces the effectiveness of many antibiotics. The localised

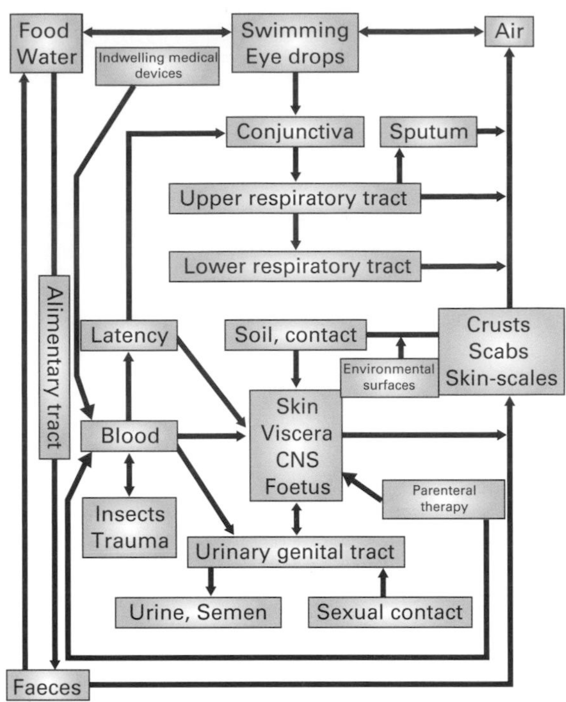

Figure 7.1 Routes of infection, spread and transmission of disease.

high cell densities present within biofilm communities may also initiate production, by the colonising organism, of extracellular virulence factors such as toxins, proteases and siderophores (low-molecular-weight ligands responsible for the solubilisation and transport of iron (III) in microbial cells). These are associated with a phenomenon termed *quorum sensing* (see Section 7.4.2) and help the pathogen to combat the host's innate defences and also promote the acquisition of nutrients. In essence, when a pathogenic microorganism infects the human body, a battle ensues between the host's innate and adaptive immune systems and the pathogen's assorted virulence mechanisms and factors. The outcome of this battle determines whether, and how well, the host survives and recovers.

Viruses are incapable of growing extracellularly and must therefore rapidly gain entry to cells (normally epithelial) at their initial site of entry. Once internalised in the non-immune host, they are to a large extent protected against the non-specific host defences. Following these initial consolidation events, the virus may extend into surrounding tissues and/or disperse, via the blood, plasma, lymph or nerves, to distant tissues to establish secondary sites of infection or to consolidate further. In some instances, viruses can colonise the host indefinitely and remain viable for many years (e.g., the herpesvirus varicella zoster which causes chickenpox, and herpes simplex virus 1 responsible for cold sores), but more generally they succumb to the heightened defences of the host, and to survive must either infect other individuals or survive in the general environment.

7.2 The Human Microbiome

Even though some parts of the human body are free from microorganisms (an *axenic* state), the body harbours millions of mutualistic and commensal symbionts. All of us unwittingly carry populations of bacterial cells on our skin and in our mouth, nasal cavities, vagina and the gastrointestinal tract that outnumber cells carrying our own genome. Internal tissues are normally sterile. *Mutualistic* relationships occur when both organisms (microbial and host cell) benefit from the interactions, whereas *commensalism* is a state in which one member of the relationship benefits without significantly affecting the other. Microorganisms that colonise body surfaces (internal and external) without normally causing disease constitute the *microbiome* (the term microbiome generally refers to a community of microorganisms and their genetic material, e.g., populating a human host, while *microbiota* refers to specific microorganisms living at a particular site). The microbiome thus comprises several distinct microbiotas which are characteristic of the region of the body colonised.

The microbiome is present throughout life and may comprise predominantly bacteria, with some fungi and protozoa, the majority of which are commensal. It is generally believed that the microbiome begins to develop when the amniotic membrane surrounding the unborn child ruptures, allowing contact with vaginal, faecal and skin-associated microorganisms from the mother during childbirth. Microorganisms enter the infant's mouth and nose during passage through the birth canal, colonisation of the upper respiratory tract occurs with the first breath of air and the beginning of the colon microbiota occurs during feeding. The development of the resident microbiota is therefore initiated during the first few months of life. By comparison, transient microbiotas remain in the body for only a few hours, days or months. They are found in the same locations as the resident biota, but cannot persist because of their inability to compete with the established microbiome, to resist elimination by the body's defence mechanisms or to tolerate the chemical and physical changes encountered.

It is now clear that the microbiome is essential for human development. It helps digest our food, regulate our immune system, protect against pathogens and produce vitamins including some B vitamins and vitamin K. Some autoimmune diseases such as diabetes, multiple sclerosis and rheumatoid arthritis are thought to be associated with disruption within the microbiome. This may lead to changes in gene expression and metabolic processes in the microbiome, resulting in an abnormal immune response to host biomolecules and tissue. Obesity and type 1 diabetes both appear to be associated with a less diverse gut microbiota. Microbial metabolites such as short-chain fatty acids can affect gut–brain signaling, affording the gut microbiome with a possible regulatory role in anxiety, mood and cognition.

The substantial metabolic power of the gut microbiota can also influence the pharmacokinetic and pharmacodynamic behaviour of therapeutic agents. At least 150 drugs are now known to be susceptible to biotransformation or bioaccumulation by intestinal bacteria, potentially leading to decreasing bioavailability, or to indirect processes such as enterohepatic recycling which can extend systemic half-lives. This modulation of drug behaviour by the microbiome, which has been termed pharmacomicrobiomics, may well play a part in promoting individual variability in drug-handling.

Changes in the composition of the normal microbiota, for whatever reason (e.g., major changes to diet, antibiotic treatment, hormonal changes, chemotherapy or radiotherapy), may allow one or more members of the microbiome to become opportunistic pathogens. For example, reductions in numbers of protective lactobacilli within the vagina brought about through antibiotic use can allow *Candida albicans*, a minority member of the normal microbiota, to grow more prolifically, resulting in an opportunistic vaginal yeast infection such as vaginal candidiasis. Following appropriate treatment, the normal microbiota is typically re-established in adults. In some areas of the body, such as the gastrointestinal tract, it is claimed that the recolonisation by desired species can be encouraged by administration of probiotics. Probiotics are live cultures of intestinal bacteria that are marketed as conferring a health benefit and preventing digestive problems. Prebiotics (normally fibre-like carbohydrates) that represent preferred or selective growth substrates for beneficial bacteria already present within the digestive tract may also be of benefit. There is also considerable interest currently in the potential therapeutic benefit of faecal transplantation, where faecal material from a healthy individual is administered by enema, colonoscopy or via nasoduodenal tube, in the treatment of *Clostridioides* (formerly *Clostridium*) *difficile* colitis.

7.3 Portals of Entry

7.3.1 Skin

The part of the body that is most widely exposed to microorganisms is the skin. Intact skin is usually impervious to microorganisms, and its surface is of acid pH and contains relatively few nutrients that are favourable for microbial growth. The vast majority of organisms falling on to the skin surface will die, while the survivors must compete with the commensal microbiota for nutrients to grow. These commensals are now known to include a variety of microorganisms (mainly bacteria) with high diversity but relatively low total abundance. These include coryneform bacteria, staphylococci and yeasts, which derive nutrients from compounds such as urea, hormones (e.g., testosterone) and fatty acids found in the apocrine and eccrine secretions. Such organisms are highly adapted to growth in this environment and will normally prevent the establishment of chance contaminants of the skin. Infections of the skin itself, such as ringworm (*Trichophyton mentagrophytes*) and warts (human papillomavirus [HPV]), rarely, involve penetration of the epidermis. Infection can, however, occur through the skin following trauma such as burns, cuts and abrasions, and, in some instances, through insect or animal bites or the injection of contaminated medicines. In recent years, extensive use of intravascular and extravascular medical devices and implants has led to an increase in the occurrence of healthcare-associated infection. Commonly, these infections involve the growth of skin commensals such as *S. epidermidis* when associated with devices that penetrate the skin barrier. The organism grows as an adhesive biofilm on the surfaces of the device, and infection arises either from contamination of the device during its implantation or by growth along it. In such instances, the biofilm may shed bacterial cells to the body and may give rise to a bacteraemia (the presence of bacteria in the blood).

The weak spots, or Achilles heels of the body, occur where the skin ends and mucous epithelial tissues begin (mouth, anus, eyes, ears, nose and urogenital tract). These mucous membranes present a more favourable environment for microbial growth than the skin, in that they are warm, moist and rich in nutrients. Such membranes, nevertheless, possess certain characteristics that allow them to resist infection. Most of them, for example, possess their own highly adapted microbiotas (see Section 7.2) which reduce the chances of infection by any invading organisms through a process termed colonisation resistance. The resident biota varies greatly between different sites of the body. Each site can be additionally protected by physicochemical barriers such as extreme acid pH in the stomach and bile salts in the large bowel, the presence of freely circulating non-specific antibodies and/or opsonins and/or by macrophages and phagocytes (see Chapter 9). Infections may start from contact between thcsc tissues and the potential pathogen. Contact can be direct, from an infected individual to a healthy one, or indirect, and may involve inanimate vectors such as soil, food, drink, air and airborne particles. These may directly contact the body or be ingested or inhaled or enter wounds via infected bed linen and clothing. Indirect contact may also involve animal vector intermediates (carriers).

7.3.2 Respiratory Tract

Air contains a large amount of suspended organic matter and, in enclosed occupied spaces, may hold up to 1000 microorganisms/m^3. Almost all of these airborne organisms are non-pathogenic bacteria and fungi, of which the average person inhales approximately 10,000/day. The respiratory tract is protected against this assault by a mucociliary blanket that envelops the upper respiratory tract and nasal cavity. Both present a tortuous path down which microbial particles travel and impact on these surfaces to become trapped within an enveloping blanket of mucus. Beating cilia move the mucus coating to the back of the throat where it, together with adherent particles, is swallowed. The alveolar regions of the lower respiratory tract have additional protection in the form of alveolar macrophages. To be successful, a pathogen must avoid being trapped in the mucus and swallowed; if deposited in the alveolar sacs it must avoid phagocytosis by macrophages, or if phagocytosed it must resist subsequent digestion by them. The possession of surface adhesins, specific for epithelial receptors, aids attachment of the invading microorganism and avoidance of removal by the mucociliary blanket. Other strategies include the export of ciliostatic toxins (i.e., *Corynebacterium diphtheriae*) that paralyse the cilial bed. As the primary defence of the respiratory tract is the mucociliary blanket, it is easy to envisage how infection with respiratory viruses including coronavirus and influenza virus, which damage respiratory epithelia, or the chronic inhalation of tobacco smoke, which increases mucin production and decreases the proportion of ciliated epithelial cells, increases the susceptibility of individuals to infection.

7.3.3 Intestinal Tract

The intestinal tract must contend with whatever it is given in terms of food and drink. The extreme acidity and presence of digestive enzymes in the stomach will kill many of the bacteria challenging it, and the gastrointestinal tract carries a commensal biota of yeast and bacteria, including lactobacilli, that afford protection by, for example, competing with potential pathogens. Bile salts are mixed with the semi-digested solids exiting from the stomach into the small intestine. These salts not only neutralise the stomach acids but also represent biological detergents or surfactants that can solubilise the outer membrane of many Gram-negative bacteria. Consequently, the small intestine is normally colonised by lower numbers of bacteria than the colon. The lower gut, on the other hand, is highly populated by commensal microorganisms ($10^{12}g^{-1}$ gut tissue) that are often associated with the intestinal wall, either embedded in layers of protective mucus or attached directly to the epithelial cells or attached to particulate food residues. The pathogenicity of incoming bacteria and viruses depends on their ability to survive passage through the stomach and duodenum and their capacity for attachment to, or penetration of, the gut wall, despite competition from the commensal biota and the presence of secretory antibodies (see Chapter 9).

7.3.4 Urogenital Tract

In healthy individuals, the bladder, ureters and urethra are sterile, and sterile urine constantly flushes the urinary tract. Organisms invading the urinary tract must avoid being detached from the epithelial surfaces and washed out during urination. Because the male urethra is long (approximately 20 cm), bacteria must be introduced directly into the bladder, possibly through catheterisation, to initiate an infection. The female urethra is shorter (approximately 5 cm) and is more readily traversed by microorganisms that are normally resident within the vaginal vault. Bladder infections are therefore much more common in the female. Spread of the infection from the bladder to the kidneys can easily occur through reflux of urine into the ureter. As for the implantation of devices across the skin barrier (above), long-term catheterisation of the bladder will promote the occurrence of bacteriuria (the presence of bacteria in the urine) with all of the associated complications.

Lactic acid in the vagina gives it an acidic pH (5.0); this, together with other products of metabolism, inhibits colonisation by most bacteria, except some lactobacilli that constitute the commensal biota. Other types of bacteria are unable to establish themselves in the vagina unless they have become extremely specialised. These species of microorganism tend to be associated with sexually transmitted infections.

7.3.5 Conjunctiva

The conjunctiva is usually free of microorganisms and protected by the continuous flow of secretions from lachrymal and other glands, and by frequent mechanical cleansing of its surface by the eyelid periphery during blinking. Lachrymal fluids contain several inhibitory compounds, together with lysozyme, that can enzymically degrade the peptidoglycan of Gram-positive bacteria such as staphylococci. Damage to the conjunctiva, caused through mechanical abrasion or reductions in tear flow, will increase microbial adhesion and allow colonisation by opportunist pathogens. The likelihood of infection is thus promoted by the use of soft and hard contact lenses, physical damage, exposure to chemicals or damage and infection of the eyelid border (blepharitis).

7.4 Consolidation

To be successful, a pathogen must be able to survive at its initial portal of entry, frequently in competition with the commensal biota and generally while subject to the attention of macrophages and wandering white blood cells. Such survival invariably requires the organism to attach itself firmly to the epithelial surface, eventually forming a biofilm. The initial attachment must be highly specific to displace the commensal microbiota, and subsequently governs the course of an infection. Attachment can be mediated through the provision, on the bacterial surface, of adhesive substances such as mucopeptide and mucopolysaccharide slime layers, fimbriae, pili (see Chapter 3) and agglutinins (see Chapter 9). These are often highly specific in their binding characteristics, differentiating, for example, between the tips and bases of villi in the large bowel and the epithelial cells of the upper, mid and lower gut. Secretory antibodies, which are directed against such adhesions, block the initial attachment of the organism and thereby confer resistance to infection.

The outcome of the encounter between the tissues and potential pathogens is governed by the ability of the microorganism to multiply at a faster rate than it is removed from those tissues. Factors that influence this are the organism's rate of growth, the initial number arriving at the site and their ability to resist the efforts of the host tissues at removing/starving/killing them. The outcome of an encounter between a microorganism and a host can, therefore, be described as a balance between the accumulation of the pathogen and its elimination by the host.

The definition of *virulence* (i.e., the degree of pathogenicity caused by a microorganism) for pathogenic microorganisms must include the MIN. This will vary between individuals, but will invariably be lower in compromised hosts such as those who are catheterised, diabetics, smokers and cystic fibrosis patients, and those suffering trauma such as malnutrition, chronic infection or physical damage. A number of the individual factors that contribute towards virulence are discussed below.

7.4.1 Nutrient Acquisition

Because the initial inoculum of a pathogen is usually too small to cause immediate damage to the host, it must acquire sufficient nutrients to allow it to multiply and increase in number. Not all nutrients, vitamins or growth factors are soluble and present in adequate quantities to allow pathogens to multiply. Moreover, trace elements may also be in short supply and can influence the establishment of the pathogen. One such example is that of iron (Fe^{3+}) which is essential for microbial growth and function. Normally this is complexed with host iron-binding proteins such as lactoferrin or transferrin, resulting in insufficient iron being made available to the pathogen. To survive and multiply, pathogens need to be able to compete with the host (and normal microbiota) for iron. Some bacteria can do this through the production of iron-chelating compounds called *siderophores* which have a greater affinity for iron than the host's iron-binding proteins, while others secrete hydrolytic enzymes that release iron from the host. Some organisms, such as *P. aeruginosa*, possess three or more different mechanisms of iron capture, giving them great versatility. To protect itself from such virulence mechanisms, the host cell can fight bacteria by synthesising siderocalin receptors which competitively bind iron.

7.4.2 Biofilms

Cell attachment (by specific, e.g., pili- or fimbriae-mediated; non-specific, e.g., secretion of exopolymeric substances; or physicochemical interactions), and subsequent biofilm formation, is a means by which pathogens can survive and remain in a favourable environment (i.e., one where there are plenty of nutrients) without getting washed away. As a consequence, bacterial cell numbers and activities can become quite high. Biofilms can form on any surface (e.g., soft tissue, bone, and medical implants) and may contain only one or two species (e.g., *S. aureus*-mediated osteomyelitis) or more commonly several species of bacteria (e.g., dental plaque). Hence, biofilms may be considered as a functional microbial community (see Chapter 8). Within a biofilm, intracellular signalling molecules (e.g., *N*-acyl homoserine lactones) are produced that when sufficient (threshold) concentrations are reached upregulate biofilm-specific genes. This process is known as quorum sensing and is responsible for the formation and maintenance of the biofilm.

Once formed, biofilms can be extremely difficult, if not impossible, to remove. Their size and morphology can help protect the underlying cells, resisting physical forces of removal, phagocytosis and penetration of toxic molecules such as antibiotics. In addition, biofilms allow cells to live in close proximity to each other, thereby facilitating intercellular communication and genetic exchange. Finally, due to their profound resistance, biofilms provide foci of infection which often can only be removed by surgery.

7.4.3 Resistance to Host Defences

Most bacterial infections confine themselves to the surface of epithelial tissue (e.g., *Bordetella pertussis*, *C. diphtheriae* and *Vibrio cholerae*). This is, to a large extent, a reflection of their inability to combat that host's deeper defences. Survival at these sites is largely due to firm attachment to the epithelial cells. Such organisms manifest disease through the production and release of toxins (see below).

Other groups of organisms regularly establish systemic infections after traversing the epithelial surfaces (e.g., *Brucella abortus*, *Salmonella enterica* serovar Typhi, and *Streptococcus pyogenes*). This property is associated with their abilities either to gain entry into susceptible cells and thereby enjoy protection from the body's defences, or to be phagocytosed by macrophages or polymorphs and yet resist their lethal action and multiply within them (e.g., *M. tuberculosis* or *Legionella pneumophila*). Other organisms can multiply and grow freely in the body's extracellular fluids. Microorganisms have evolved several different strategies that allow them to suppress the host's normal defences and thereby survive in the tissues.

7.4.3.1 Modulation of the Inflammatory Response

Growth of microorganisms releases cellular products into their surrounding medium, many of which cause non-specific inflammation associated with dilation of blood vessels. This increases capillary flow and access of phagocytes to the infected site. Increased lymphatic flow from the inflamed tissues carries the organisms to lymph nodes where further antimicrobial and immune forces come into play (see Chapter 9). Many of the substances that are released by microorganisms in this fashion are chemotactic towards polymorphs that tend, therefore, to become concentrated at the site of infection; this is in addition to the inflammation and white blood cell accumulation that are associated with antibody binding and complement fixation. Many organisms have, therefore, adopted mechanisms that allow them to overcome these initial defences. Thus, virulent strains of *S. aureus* produce a mucopeptide (peptidoglycan), which suppresses early inflammatory oedema, and related factors that suppress the chemotaxis of polymorphs.

7.4.3.2 Avoidance of Phagocytosis

Resistance to phagocytosis is sometimes associated with specific components of the bacterial cell wall and/or with the presence of capsules surrounding the cell wall. Classic examples of these are the M-proteins of the streptococci, the polysaccharide capsules of the pneumococci and the alginate-like slime associated with *P. aeruginosa* infections of the cystic-fibrotic lung. The acidic polysaccharide K-antigens of *Escherichia coli* and *S. enterica* serovar Typhi behave similarly, in that (i) they can mediate attachment to the intestinal epithelial cells, and (ii) they render phagocytosis more difficult. Generally, possession of an extracellular capsule and/or slime will reduce the likelihood of phagocytosis.

Microorganisms are more readily phagocytosed when coated with antibody (opsonised). This is due to the presence on the white blood cells of receptors for the Fc fragment of IgM and IgG (discussed in Chapter 9). Avoidance of opsonisation will enhance the chances of survival of a particular pathogen. A substance called protein A is released from actively growing strains of *S. aureus*, which acts by non-specific binding to IgG at the Fc region (see Chapter 9), at sites both close to and remote from the bacterial surface. This blocks the Fc region of bound antibody masking it from phagocytes. Protein A–IgG complexes remote from the infection site will also bind complement, thereby depleting it from the plasma and negating its actions near to the infection site.

7.4.3.3 Survival Following Phagocytosis

Death of microorganisms following phagocytosis can be avoided if the microorganisms are not exposed to the killing and digestion processes within the phagocyte. This is possible if the microorganism can block acidification of the phagosome and its fusion to lysosomes. Such a strategy is employed by virulent *M. tuberculosis*, although the precise mechanism is unknown. Other bacteria seem able to grow within the vacuoles despite lysosomal fusion (*Listeria monocytogenes* and *S. enterica* serovar Typhi). This can be attributed to cell wall components that prevent access of the lysosomal substances to the bacterial membranes (e.g., *B. abortus*, mycobacteria) or to the production of extracellular catalase which neutralises the hydrogen peroxide liberated in the vacuole (e.g., staphylococci).

If microorganisms can survive and grow within phagocytes, they will escape many of the other body defences such as the lymph nodes, and be distributed around the body. As the lifespan of phagocytes is relatively short, such bacteria will eventually be delivered to the liver and gastrointestinal tract where they are 'recycled' and offered a further opportunity to infect.

7.4.3.4 Killing of Phagocytes

An alternative strategy is for the microorganism to kill the phagocyte. This can be achieved by the production of leucocidins (e.g., by staphylococci and streptococci) which promote the discharge of lysosomal substances into the cytoplasm of the phagocyte rather than into the vacuole, thus directing the phagocyte's lethal activity towards itself.

7.5 Manifestation of Disease

Once established, the course of a bacterial infection can proceed in a number of ways. These can be related to the relative ability of the organism to penetrate and invade the surrounding tissues and organs. The vast majority of pathogens, being unable to combat the defences of the deeper tissues, consolidate further on the epithelial surface. Others, including most viruses, penetrate the epithelial layers, but no further, and can be regarded as partially invasive. A small group of pathogens are fully invasive. These permeate the subepithelial tissues and are circulated around the body to initiate secondary sites of infection remote from the initial portal of entry (Figure 7.1).

Other groups of organisms may cause disease through ingestion by the victim of substances produced during microbial growth on foods. Such diseases may be regarded as intoxications rather than as infections and are considered later (Section 7.6.1.1). Treatment in these cases is usually an alleviation of the harmful effects of the toxin rather than elimination of the pathogen from the body.

7.5.1 Non-invasive Pathogens

B. pertussis (the aetiological agent of whooping cough) is probably the best described of these pathogens. This organism is inhaled and rapidly localises on the mucociliary blanket of the lower respiratory tract. This localisation is very selective and is thought to involve agglutinins on the organism's surface. Toxins produced by the organism inhibit ciliary movement of the epithelial surface and thereby prevent removal of the bacterial cells to the gut. A high-molecular-weight exotoxin is also produced during the growth of the organism which, being of limited diffusibility, pervades the subepithelial tissues to produce inflammation and necrosis. *C. diphtheriae* (the causal organism of diphtheria) behaves similarly, attaching itself to the epithelial cells of the respiratory tract. This organism produces a diffusible toxin of low molecular weight, which enters the blood circulation and brings about a generalised toxaemia.

In the gut, many pathogens adhere to the gut wall and produce their effect via toxins that pervade the surrounding gut wall or enter the systemic circulation. *V. cholerae* and some enteropathic *E. coli* strains localise on the gut wall and produce toxins that increase vascular permeability. The result is hypersecretion of isotonic fluids into the gut lumen, acute diarrhoea and, as a consequence, dehydration that may be fatal in young or elderly people. In all these instances, binding to epithelial cells is not essential but increases permeation of the toxin and prolongs the presence of the pathogen.

7.5.2 Partially Invasive Pathogens

Some bacteria, and viruses, can attach to the mucosal epithelia and then penetrate rapidly into the epithelial cells. These organisms multiply within the protective environment of the host cell, eventually killing it and inducing disease through erosion and ulceration of the mucosal epithelium. Typically, members of the genera *Shigella* and *Salmonella* utilise such mechanisms in infections of the gastrointestinal tract. These bacteria attach to the epithelial cells of the large and small intestines, respectively, and, following their entry into these cells by induced pinocytosis, multiply rapidly and penetrate laterally into adjacent epithelial cells. The mechanisms for such attachment and movement are unknown but involve a transition from a non-motile to motile phenotype. Some species of salmonellae produce, also, exotoxins that induce diarrhoea (Section 7.6.1.2). There are innumerable serotypes of *Salmonella* which are primarily parasites of animals but are important to humans in that they colonise farm animals such as pigs and poultry and ultimately infect foods derived from them. *Salmonella* food poisoning (salmonellosis), therefore, is commonly associated with inadequately cooked meats, eggs and also with cold meat products that have been incorrectly stored following contact with the uncooked product. Dependent upon the severity of the lesions induced in the gut wall by enteric pathogens, red blood cells and phagocytes pass into the gut lumen, along with plasma, and cause the classic 'bloody flux' of bacillary dysentery. Similar erosive lesions are produced by some enteropathic strains of *E. coli*.

Viral infections such as influenza and the 'common cold' (in reality several hundred different viruses, including many strains of rhinovirus), and notably coronaviruses including severe acute respiratory syndrome coronavirus 2 (SARS-CoV-2), infect epithelial cells of the respiratory tract and nasopharynx. Release of the virus, after lysis of the host cells, is to the void rather than to subepithelial tissues. The residual uninfected epithelial cells are rapidly infected, resulting in general degeneration of the tracts. Such damage not only predisposes the respiratory tract to infection with opportunist pathogens such as *Neisseria meningitidis* and *Haemophilus influenzae* but also causes the associated fever.

7.5.3 Fully Invasive Pathogens

Invasive pathogens either aggressively invade the tissues surrounding the primary site of infection (active spread) or are passively transported around the body in the blood, lymph and cerebrospinal, axonal or pleural fluids (passive spread). Some especially aggressive organisms move both passively and actively, setting up multiple, expansive secondary sites of infection in various organs. For bacteria and fungi, this will vary depending upon the particular microorganism. Viral pathogens, on the other hand, do need to invade a host cell to complete their replication cycle. For example, the human immunodeficiency virus (HIV) hijacks $CD4^+$ T cells to degrade the host's ability to retaliate with a strong cell-mediated immune (CMI) response. The virus utilises co-receptors (CCR5/CXCr4) to gain access to $CD4^+$ host cells, resulting in a gradual loss of $CD4^+$ cells with attrition of CMI function in the host and an increased susceptibility of the host to other infections (e.g., bacterial pneumonia) or to tumours (e.g., Kaposi's sarcoma).

7.5.3.1 Active Spread

The active spread of microorganisms through normal subepithelial tissues is difficult in that the gel-like nature of the intercellular materials physically inhibits bacterial movement. Induced death and lysis of the tissue cells produce, in addition, a highly viscous fluid, partly due to undenatured DNA. Physical damage, such as wounds, is rapidly sealed with fibrin clots, thereby reducing the effective routes for spread of opportunist pathogens. Organisms such as *S. pyogenes*, *Clostridium perfringens* and, to some extent, the staphylococci can establish themselves in tissues by their ability to produce a wide range of extracellular enzyme toxins. These are associated with killing of tissue cells, degradation of intracellular materials and mobilisation of nutrients. A selection of such toxins will be considered briefly.

- *Haemolysins* are produced by most of the pathogenic staphylococci and streptococci. They have a lytic effect on red blood cells, releasing iron-containing nutrients.
- *Fibrinolysins* are produced by both staphylococci (staphylokinase) and streptococci (streptokinase). These toxins indirectly activate plasminogen and so dissolve fibrin clots that the host forms around wounds and lesions to seal them. The production of fibrinolysins, therefore, increases the likelihood of the infection spreading. Streptokinase may be employed clinically in conjunction with streptodornase in the treatment of thrombosis.
- *Collagenases* and *hyaluronidases* are produced by most of the aggressive invaders of tissues. These can dissolve collagen fibres and the hyaluronic acids that function as intercellular cements; this causes the tissues to break up and produce oedematous lesions.
- *Phospholipases* are produced by organisms such as *C. perfringens* (α-toxin). These toxins kill tissue cells by hydrolysing the phospholipids that are present in cell membranes.
- *Amylases, peptidases* and *deoxyribonucleases* mobilise many nutrients that are released from lysed cells. They also decrease the viscosity of fluids present at the lesion by depolymerisation of their biopolymer substrates.

Organisms possessing the above toxins, particularly those also possessing *leucocidins*, are likely to cause expanding oedematous lesions at the primary site of infection. In the case of *C. perfringens*, a soil microorganism that has become adapted to a saprophytic mode of life, infection arises from accidental contamination of deep wounds when a process similar to that seen during the decomposition of a carcass ensues (gangrene). This organism is most likely to spread through tissues when blood circulation, and therefore oxygen tension, in the affected areas is minimal.

Abscesses formed by streptococci and staphylococci can be deep-seated in soft tissues or associated with infected wounds or skin lesions; they become localised through the deposition of fibrin capsules around the infection site. Fibrin deposition is partly a response of the host tissues but is also partly a function of enzyme toxins such as *coagulase*. Phagocytic white blood cells can migrate into these abscesses in large numbers to produce significant quantities of pus. Such pus, often carrying the infective pathogen, might be digested by other phagocytes in the late stages of the infection or discharged to the exterior or to the capillary and lymphatic network. In the latter case, blocked capillaries might serve as sites for secondary lesions. Toxins liberated from the microorganisms during their growth in such abscesses can freely diffuse to the rest of the body to set up a generalised toxaemia.

S. enterica serovar Typhi, *S. enterica* serovar Paratyphi and *S. enterica* serovar Typhimurium are serotypes of *Salmonella* (Section 7.4.3) that are not only able to penetrate into intestinal epithelial cells and produce exotoxins but are also able to penetrate beyond into subepithelial tissues. These organisms, therefore, produce a characteristic systemic disease (typhoid and enteric fever), in addition to the usual symptoms of salmonellosis. Following recovery from such infection, the organism is commonly found associated with the gallbladder. In this state, the recovered person will excrete the organism and become a reservoir for the infection of others.

7.5.3.2 Passive Spread

When invading microorganisms have crossed the epithelial barriers, they will almost certainly be taken up with lymph in the lymphatic ducts and be delivered to filtration and immune systems at the local lymph nodes. Sometimes this serves to spread infections further around the body. Eventually, spread may occur from local to regional lymph nodes and thence to the bloodstream. Direct entry to the bloodstream from the primary portal of entry is rare and will only occur when the organism damages the blood vessels or if it is injected directly into them. This might be the case following an insect bite or surgery. Bacteraemia such as this will often lead to secondary infections remote from the original portal of entry.

7.6 Damage to Tissues

Damage caused to the host organism through infection can be direct and related to the destructive presence of microorganisms (or to their production of toxins) in particular target organs, or it can be indirect and related to interactions of the antigenic components of the pathogen with the host's immune system. Effects can, therefore, be closely related to, or remote from, the infected organ.

Symptoms of the infection can in some instances be highly specific, relating to a single, precise pharmacological response to a particular toxin, or they might be non-specific and relate to the usual response of the body to particular types of trauma. Damage induced by infection will, therefore, be considered in these categories.

7.6.1 Direct Damage

7.6.1.1 Specific Effects

For the host, the consequences of infection depend to a large extent upon the tissue or organ involved. Soft-tissue infections of skeletal muscle are likely to be less damaging than, for instance, infections of the heart muscle and central nervous system. Infections associated with the epithelial cells that make up small blood vessels can block or rupture them to produce anoxia or necrosis in the tissues that they supply. Cell and tissue damage is generally the result of direct local action by the microorganisms, usually concerning action at the cytoplasmic membranes. The target cells are usually phagocytes and are generally killed (e.g., by *Brucella*, *Listeria* and *Mycobacterium*). Interference with membrane function through the action of enzymes such as phospholipase causes the affected cells to leak. When lysosomal membranes are affected, the lysosomal enzymes disperse into the cells and tissues causing them, in turn, to autolyse. This is mediated through the vast battery of enzyme toxins available to these organisms (Sections 7.4 and 7.5.3.1). If these toxins are produced in sufficient concentration, they may enter the circulatory systems to produce generalised toxaemia. During their growth, other pathogens liberate toxins that possess very precise, singular pharmacological actions. Diseases mediated in this manner include diphtheria, tetanus and scarlet fever.

In diphtheria, the organism *C. diphtheriae* confines itself to epithelial surfaces of the nose and throat and produces a powerful toxin which affects an elongation factor involved in eukaryotic protein biosynthesis. The heart and peripheral nerves are particularly affected, resulting in myocarditis (inflammation of the myocardium) and neuritis (inflammation of a nerve). Little damage is produced at the infection site.

Tetanus occurs when *Clostridium tetani*, ubiquitous in the soil and the faeces of herbivores, contaminates wounds, especially deep puncture-type lesions. These might be the result of minor trauma such as a splinter, or a major one such as a motor vehicle accident. At these sites, tissue necrosis and possibly also microbial growth reduce the oxygen tension to allow this anaerobe to multiply. Its growth is accompanied by the production of a highly potent toxin that passes up peripheral nerves and diffuses locally within the central nervous system. The toxin has a strychnine-like action and affects normal function at the synapses. As the motor nerves of the brainstem are the shortest, the cranial nerves are the first affected, with twitches of the eyes and spasms of the jaw (lockjaw).

A related organism, *C. botulinum*, produces a similar toxin that may contaminate food if the organism has grown in it and if conditions are favourable for anaerobic growth. Meat pastes and pâtés are likely sources. This toxin interferes with acetylcholine release at cholinergic synapses and also acts at neuromuscular junctions. Death from this toxin eventually results from respiratory failure.

Many other organisms are capable of producing intoxication following their growth on foods. Most common among these are the staphylococci and strains of *B. cereus*. Some strains of *S. aureus* produce an enterotoxin which acts on the vomiting centres of the brain. Nausea and vomiting, therefore, may follow ingestion of contaminated foods and the delay between eating and vomiting varies between 1 and 6 hours depending on the amount of toxin ingested. *B. cereus* also produces an emetic toxin but its actions are delayed and vomiting can follow up to 20 hours after ingestion. The latter organism is often associated with rice products and will propagate when the rice is cooked (spore activation) and subsequently reheated after a period of storage.

Scarlet fever is produced following infection with certain strains of *S. pyogenes*. These organisms produce a potent toxin that causes an erythrogenic skin rash that then accompanies the more usual effects of a streptococcal infection.

7.6.1.2 Non-specific Effects

If the infective agent damages an organ and affects its functioning, this can manifest itself as a series of secondary disease features that reflect the loss of that function to the host. Thus, diabetes may result from an infection of the islets of Langerhans, paralysis or coma from infections of the central nervous system, and kidney malfunction from loss of tissue fluids and its associated hyperglycaemia. In this respect, virus infections almost inevitably result in the death and lysis of the host cells. This will result in some loss of function by the target organ. Similarly, exotoxins and endotoxins can also be implicated in non-specific symptoms, even when they have well-defined pharmacological actions. Thus, several intestinal pathogens (e.g., *V. cholerae* and *E. coli*) produce potent exotoxins that affect vascular permeability. These generally act through adenylate cyclase, raising the intracellular levels of cyclic AMP (adenosine monophosphate). As a result of this, the cells lose water and electrolytes to the surrounding medium, the gut lumen. A common consequence of these related, yet distinct, toxins is acute diarrhoea and haemoconcentration. Kidney malfunction might well follow and in severe cases lead to death. Symptomologically, there is little difference between these conditions and the food poisoning induced by ingestion of staphylococcal enterotoxin (above).

7.6.2 Indirect Damage

Inflammatory materials are released not only from necrotic cells but also directly from the infective agent. Endotoxins (e.g., the lipid A component of the lipopolysaccharide) are derived from constituents of the bacterial cell rather than being deliberately exported cellular products. Thus, during the growth and autolysis of Gram-negative bacteria, components of their cell envelopes, such as lipopolysaccharide (see Chapter 3), are shed to the environment. Endotoxins tend to be less toxic than exotoxins and have much less precise pharmacological actions. Indeed, it is not always clear to what extent these can be related to actions by the host or by the pathogen. Reactions include local inflammation, elevations in body temperature, aching joints and head and kidney pain. Inflammation causes swelling, pain and reddening of the tissues, and sometimes loss of function of the organs affected. These reactions may sometimes be the major sign and symptom of the disease.

While various toxic effects have been attributed to these endotoxins, their role in the establishment of the infection, if any, remains unclear. The most notable effect of these materials is their ability to induce a high body temperature (pyrogenicity) (see Chapters 3 and 22). The pyrogenic effect of lipopolysaccharide relates to the action of the lipid A component directly upon the hypothalamus and also to its direct action on macrophages and phagocytes. Elevation of body temperature follows within 1–2 hours. In infections such as meningitis, the administration of antibiotics may cause such a release of pyrogen that the resultant inflammation and fever may be fatal. In such instances, antibiotics are co-administered with steroids to counter this effect. The pyrogenic effects of lipid A are unaffected by moist heat treatment (autoclave). Growth of Gram-negative organisms such as *P. aeruginosa* in stored water destined for use in terminally sterilised products will cause the final product to be pyrogenic. Processes for the destruction of pyrogen associated with glassware, and tests for the absence of pyrogen in water and product, therefore form an important part of parenteral drug manufacture (see Chapter 22).

Many microorganisms minimise the effects of the host's defence system against them by mimicking the antigenic structure of the host tissue. The eventual immunological response of the host to infection then leads to its autoimmune self-destruction. Thus, infections with *Mycoplasma pneumoniae* can lead to the production of antibody against normal group O erythrocytes, with concomitant haemolytic anaemia.

If antigen released from the infective agent is soluble, antigen–antibody complexes are produced. When an antibody is present at a concentration equal to or greater than the antigen, such as in the case of an immune host, these complexes precipitate and are removed by macrophages present in the lymph nodes. When an antigen is present in excess, the complexes, being small, continue to circulate in the blood and are eventually filtered off by the kidneys, becoming lodged in kidney glomeruli and in the joints. Localised inflammatory responses in the kidneys are sometimes then initiated by the complement system (see Chapter 9). Eventually, the filtering function of the kidneys becomes impaired, producing symptoms of chronic glomerulonephritis.

7.7 Recovery from Infection: the Exit of Microorganisms

The primary requirement for recovery is that multiplication of the infective agent is brought under control, so that it ceases to spread around the body and that the damaging consequences of its presence are arrested and repaired. Such control is brought about by the combined functions of the phagocytic, immune and complement systems. A successful pathogen, however, should not seriously debilitate its host; rather, the continued existence of the host must be ensured to maximise the dissemination of the pathogen within the host population. From the microorganism's perspective, the ideal situation is where it can persist permanently within the host and be constantly released to the environment. Although this is the case for a number of virus infections (chickenpox and herpes) and for some bacterial ones, it is not common. Generally, recovery from infection is accompanied by destruction of the organism and restoration of a sterile tissue. Alternatively, the organism might return to a commensal relationship with the host on the epithelial and skin surface.

Where the infective agent is an obligate pathogen, a means must exist for it to infect other individuals before its eradication from the host organism. The route of exit is commonly related to the original portal of entry (Figure 7.1). Thus, pathogens of the intestinal tract are liberated in the faeces and might easily contaminate food and drinking water. Infective agents of the respiratory tract might be exhaled during coughing, sneezing or talking, survive in the associated water droplets and infect nearby individuals through inhalation. Infective agents transmitted by insect and animal vectors may be spread through those same vectors, the insects/animals having been themselves infected by the diseased host. For some 'fragile' organisms (e.g., *N. gonorrhoeae* and *T. pallidum*), direct contact transmission is the only means of spread between individual hosts. In these cases, intimate contact between epithelial membranes, such as occurs during sexual contact, is required for transfer to occur. For opportunist pathogens, such as those associated with wound infections, transfer is less important because the pathogenic role is minor. Rather, the natural habitat of the organism serves as a constant reservoir for infection.

7.8 Epidemiology of Infectious Disease

Spread of a microbial disease through a population of individuals can be considered as *vertical* (transferred from one generation to another) or *horizontal* (transfer occurring within genetically unrelated groups). The latter can be divided into *common source outbreaks*, relating to infection of a number of susceptible individuals from a single reservoir of the infective agent (i.e., infected foods), or *propagated source outbreaks*, where each individual provides a new source for the infection of others.

Common source outbreaks are characterised by a sharp onset of reported cases over the course of a single incubation period (Figure 7.2) and relate to a common experience of the infected individuals (e.g., a contaminated food product). The number of cases will persist until the source of the infection is removed. If the source remains (i.e., a reservoir of insect vectors), the disease becomes endemic to the exposed population, with a constant rate of infection. Propagated source outbreaks, on the other hand, are brought about by person-to-person spread, and show a gradual increase in reported cases over a number of incubation periods and eventually decline when most of the susceptible individuals in the population have been

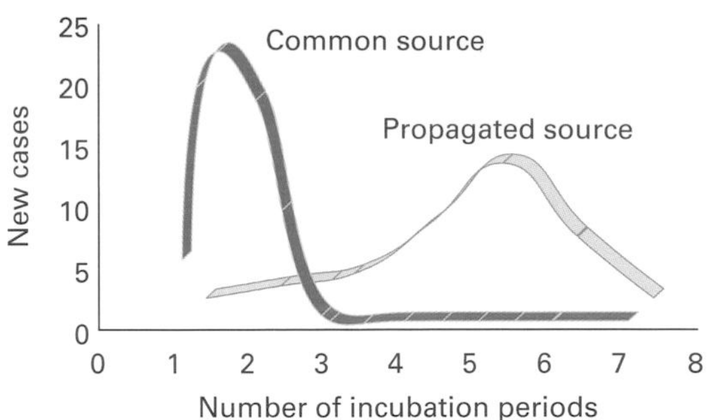

Figure 7.2 Comparison of timescale for common source outbreak and propagated source outbreak infections.

affected (Figure 7.2). Factors that contribute to propagated outbreaks of infectious disease are the infectivity of the agent (I), the population density (P) and the numbers of susceptible individuals in it (F). The likelihood of an epidemic occurring is given by the product of these three factors (i.e., FIP). An increase in any one of them might initiate an outbreak of the disease in epidemic proportions. Thus, reported cases of particular diseases show periodicity, with outbreaks of epidemic proportion occurring only when FIP exceeds certain critical threshold values, related to the infectivity of the agent. Outbreaks of measles and chickenpox, therefore, tend to occur annually in the late summer among children attending school for the first time. This has the effect of concentrating all susceptible individuals in one, often confined, space at the same time. The proportion of susceptible individuals can be reduced through rigorous vaccination programmes (see Chapter 10). Provided that the susceptible population does not exceed the threshold FIP value, then the herd immunity (a form of indirect protection from infectious disease that occurs when a large percentage of the population has become immune to an infection, thereby providing a measure of protection for individuals who are not immune) against epidemic spread of the disease will be maintained.

Certain types of infectious agent (e.g., influenza virus) can combat herd immunity such as this through undergoing major antigenic changes. These render the majority of the population susceptible, and their occurrence is often accompanied by the spread of the disease across the entire globe (pandemics). Emerging viral diseases such as those associated with coronaviruses, i.e., severe acute respiratory syndrome (SARS), Middle East respiratory syndrome (MERS) and coronavirus disease (COVID)-19, are situations where a population may be highly susceptible due to immunological naivety. In such circumstances, a better understanding of the potential for prior exposure to related viruses to confer protection and the development of effective vaccines become research priorities.

Further Reading

Bauman, R.W. (2017). *Microbiology with Diseases by Body System*, 5e. San Francisco, CA: Pearson Benjamin Cummings.

Delves, P.J., Martin, S.J., Burton, D.R. and Roitt, I.M. (2017). *Roitt's Essential Immunology*, 13e. Oxford: Wiley Blackwell.

McCoubrey, L.E. and Basit, A.W. (2022). Addressing drug-microbiome interactions: the role of healthcare professionals. *Pharm. J.* 308, No. 7958.

Mohajeri, M.H., Brummer, R.J.M., Rastall, R.A. et al. (2018). The role of the microbiome for human health: from basic science to clinical applications. *Eur. J. Nutr.* 57 (Suppl.): 1–14.

Ribet, D. and Cossart, P. (2015). How bacterial pathogens colonise their hosts and invade deeper tissues. *Microbes Infect.* 17: 173–183.

Smith, H. (1990). Pathogenicity and the microbe *in vivo*. *J. Gen. Microbiol.* 136: 377–393.

Wilson, M., McNab, R. and Henderson, B. (2007). *Bacterial Disease Mechanisms: an Introduction to Cellular Microbiology*. Cambridge: Cambridge University Press.

8

Microbial Biofilms: Consequences for Health

Brendan F. Gilmore

Professor of Pharmaceutical Microbiology, School of Pharmacy, Queen's University Belfast, Belfast, UK

CONTENTS

8.1 Introduction

Traditionally, microbiologists have grown bacteria as suspension cultures in nutritionally rich media, in order to optimise cell yield. This planktonic mode of growth also became part of the standard assay on which all existing antimicrobials were discovered, developed and selected for clinical use, and continues to be the basis for the selection of antimicrobials for specific patient treatment. It is now recognised however that in most environments, including our own bodies, the predominant mode of growth of bacteria is typically as adherent microcolonies termed *biofilms*; these afford bacteria a number of growth advantages including an inherent lack of susceptibility to antimicrobials. This antimicrobial tolerance differs from classical *genotypic* (genetic) resistance in that this reduced susceptibility

Hugo and Russell's Pharmaceutical Microbiology, Ninth Edition. Edited by Brendan F. Gilmore and Stephen P. Denyer.

Companion website: https://www.wiley.com/go/HugoandRussells9e

disappears when the biofilm is returned to planktonic growth, and is therefore *phenotypic*. Biofilms are characterised by elevated antimicrobial tolerance, and often no correlation exists between planktonic and biofilm antimicrobial susceptibility, posing a significant problem in extrapolating data from standard antibiotic screening approaches to selection of a clinically effective antibiotic for the treatment of infection. Biofilm antimicrobial tolerance is multifactorial, which includes the spatial and structural parameters of the biofilm as well as the increased phenotypic diversity within the biofilm population. Biofilms are believed to be associated with approximately 60% of human bacterial infections including chronic, recurrent and device-related infections; therefore, treatment of biofilm infections has become an important focus in modern clinical medicine. As planktonic susceptibility testing, via the minimum inhibitory concentration (MIC) test (see Chapter 19), provides little guidance in the selection of antimicrobials to treat biofilms, a change in paradigm is required to determine appropriate treatment methods for biofilms and for the discovery of next-generation antimicrobials.

8.2 Biofilms

The ability of microorganisms to grow and form complex communities on submerged surfaces in the marine environment was first described in the 1930s, but the term biofilm was not used until 1975, when it was employed to describe bacterial colonisation of wastewater filters. The importance of biofilm formation in engineered water systems, industrial systems and in the clinical scenario (in chronic as well as indwelling medical-device-associated infections) is now recognised universally. Biofilms are microcolonies of one or more species of bacteria or fungi typically growing adherent to a biotic or abiotic surface, or to each other in aggregates, embedded within a self-produced matrix of polymeric substances (e.g., polysaccharides, extracellular DNA [eDNA] and proteins). Microorganisms within the biofilm exhibit an altered phenotype, compared with the same microorganisms in the planktonic phase, with respect to growth rate and gene transcription.

Biofilms become established in order to allow bacteria to maintain themselves in a niche of their choosing; in this way they can take advantage of nutrient opportunity or other favourable environmental conditions, rather than being mechanically removed by the shear force of, for example, running water in the natural environment or the movement of body fluids and mucins in the body. Biofilms provide a more energy-efficient means of growth, capturing nutrients as they flow past and easily expelling waste. They also provide a more secure environment for sustainability and perseverance, making it difficult for phagocytes, found both in nature and as part of the immune system, to eradicate the biofilm, and protect against protozoan grazing and desiccation. Also, as a biofilm, bacteria and fungi are less susceptible to environmental insults including antimicrobial challenges, allowing them to be more tolerant than their planktonic counterparts to antibiotics found in nature and those used clinically. A schematic of the ‘classical’ biofilm developmental life cycle of bacteria is shown in Figure 8.1. In the centre of the figure, bacteria exist in a mature biofilm that may be formed from many species, as in a consortium formed on the face of a rock in a stream or those found in the mouth as part of our dental plaque. Chemical signals regulate the interactions between members of the biofilm much like hormones regulate the cells of our body. For example, under specific stress conditions, appropriate signalling may lead to an increase in phenotypic diversity within the biofilm to accommodate that stress, or alternatively these signals may cause bacteria to revert to their more motile planktonic phenotype and escape the biofilm to colonise a new surface and establish new microcolonies that will ultimately give rise to a fresh biofilm. Recently, limitations of this five-step biofilm developmental model have been proposed; for example, the model does not describe biofilm formation of non-surface-attached biofilm aggregates, which are increasingly observed in the clinical setting (e.g., in chronic wounds and embedded in viscous mucus within the cystic fibrosis lung) and in the environment. The model was initially based on *P. aeruginosa* biofilm formation *in vitro* and therefore does not reflect the complexity or diversity of biofilms in real-world scenarios, where biofilm formation may not follow the steps described in an orderly, sequential fashion and *P. aeruginosa* may not be a useful ‘model’ organism. Irrespective of the model used to describe this complex process, the overarching hallmark of biofilm formation is the aggregation of bacteria, whether surface attached or not, which creates a unique microbial environment that protects the microorganism within, facilitates cell–cell communication and cooperative activities, and ultimately creates significant challenges for their control in the clinical setting.

8.2.1 Biofilms in Nature and the Consequences for Health

In nature, bacteria often exist as multispecies biofilms; these may allow disseminated pathogens to survive distant from their natural host, thus serving as a nidus for

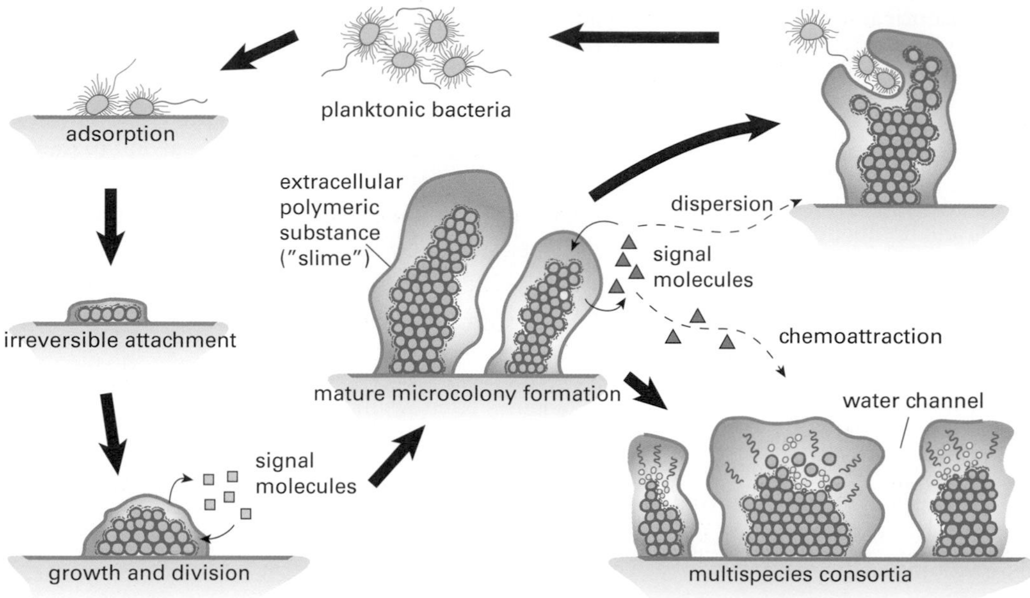

Figure 8.1 The main stages in microbial surface attachment and biofilm formation. *Source:* From Harrison, J.J. et al. (2005) Biofilms. *Am. Sci.*, **93**, 508–515, with permission from *American Scientist*.

reinfection. Examples of this are enteric organisms that form biofilms in drinking-water pipes, engineered water systems in care facilities or in wells. Following an original contamination event, biofilms allow these populations to persevere within the environment, which then serve to shed further organisms into potable water supplies, even after the apparent clearance of the original contamination event. Contamination of our groundwater sources poses particular concerns for the future of our potable water supplies; this threat is accentuated by the long-term stability that biofilms of these contaminants bring into the equation.

8.2.2 Biofilms in the Food Industry

Food-borne outbreaks of infections are often associated with biofilms formed on the hard surfaces of food-processing plants, such as tables, knives, processing equipment and the built environment. The inherent phenotypic resistance of biofilms to many biocides used in the cleaning process in food-processing facilities allows these bacteria to multiply and contaminate food products. Such biofilms act as a reservoir for contaminating microorganisms, including important human pathogens which may be present in multispecies biofilms formed on a range of surface materials commonly employed in the food industry (metals, polymers and glass). The presence of biofilms within the food-processing environment may give rise to a range of challenges, including: microbially induced corrosion of metals and other surfaces; food spoilage and alteration of the organoleptic properties of food due to contamination from microorganisms shed from the biofilm during processing; and, importantly, outbreaks of infections by human pathogens harboured within the biofilm. Outbreaks of food poisoning associated with a range of known biofilm-forming pathogens associated with food-processing environments, including *Listeria monocytogenes*, *Salmonella enterica*, *Bacillus cereus*, *Staphylococcus aureus* and enterohaemorrhagic *Escherichia coli* (including the Shiga toxin [Stx]-producing *E. coli* strain O157:H7), have been reported. In many cases, such strains have been shown to exhibit an enhanced ability to form biofilms and can tolerate harsh conditions associated with specific food-processing environments, including biocide challenges, elevated temperature and pressure. The extended survival times of pathogenic bacteria within 'dry' biofilms which exhibit significantly elevated tolerance to biocides are a major emerging issue in the food industry, with a recent report of *S. enterica* surviving within a desiccated biofilm on stainless steel for more than a year while still retaining the capability to contaminate processed foods. Biofilms in the food-processing environment therefore pose both an economic and a public health threat, and challenges associated with the control of such biofilms have led to the investigation of a range of novel biofilm-control technologies, including ozonation, high-pressure processing, non-thermal (cold) plasma, bacteriophages and antimicrobial peptides.

8.2.3 Biofilms in the Pharmaceutical Industry

The pharmaceutical industry relies heavily on water in its operations. It is widely used as a raw material, ingredient and solvent in the processing, formulation and manufacture of pharmaceutical products and may even be itself a final product. It also finds use for the cleaning and rinsing of such items as mixing vessels and production equipment. Different grades of water are required depending on their use: potable water, purified water and Water for Injection (see Chapter 22).

All aqueous environments are susceptible to biofilm formation which, if not properly controlled, can place product quality and patient health at risk. Water purification, storage and distribution systems are inherent sites for biofilm activity in the pharmaceutical manufacturing environment. A relatively low level of nutrient in pharmaceutical water systems encourages the formation of biofilms at surfaces where nutrients tend to adsorb. This risk is often exacerbated in new water systems as a consequence of poor design. This can be caused by low-quality materials used for pipework, seals and fittings and inappropriate diameter pipes or poorly designed bends, both of which may slow the rate of circulating water. Even in established and properly designed pharmaceutical water systems, biofilms can form during shutdown periods, when low usage of water slows water flow, and following maintenance and repairs. The risk of biofilm formation should be considered at all stages of system design, validation, operation, monitoring and maintenance.

Some system design and operating features can limit risk, such as: smooth internal surfaces; continuous movement of water in tanks and rapid flow in pipework (1–2 m/s); sloping drainage; minimising devices in the water path and the avoidance of 'dead legs' created by overlong pipe branches; installing accessible sampling ports at critical locations; correct heating and sanitisation temperatures, especially for stored water; urgent resolution of water leaks which can allow microbial access; deliberate isolation of maintenance work areas; alarm systems for water failing to meet chemical specification; and established sampling and sanitisation strategies.

Even with good design and management, biofilms can still arise; these are generally detected indirectly through out-of-specification water chemistry and microbial counts. Sometimes compromised water quality is only identifiable from point-of-use samples when microbiological limits are no longer met. The time taken to detect a biofilm from its initial formation is variable, often depending on the shedding of biofilm cell clusters through shear forces and pressure shocks. The management and elimination of biofilms are achieved through elevated temperature (65–80 °C or greater), steaming at 121 °C for 10–15 minutes or treatment with chemicals such as ozone, chlorine, chlorine dioxide, hydrogen peroxide, peracetic acid and sodium hydroxide, depending on system compatibility. Membrane filtration and ultraviolet irradiation can be attempted, but these will not remove the biofilm source. If such treatments fail to work, the only resolution is disassembly of the system and replacement with new fittings.

8.2.4 Biofilms in Healthcare Facilities

Healthcare-associated infections (HCAIs) within healthcare facilities often result from pathogens surviving in the environment as biofilms. Biofilms may facilitate bacterial carriage by patients, healthcare staff or visitors, as for example in the colonisation of nasal passages by methicillin-resistant *Staphylococcus aureus* (MRSA). Biofilms may also become associated with hard surfaces, drains or water pipes within the facility. Infections may be associated with instruments or devices used in hospitals, such as endoscopes contaminated with biofilms, where they have been implicated in the passage of infectious organisms from one patient to another. Whether biofilms form on animate or inanimate surfaces, their recalcitrant nature makes it difficult to remove them from the clinical environment.

8.2.5 Biofilms and Medical Devices

Medical devices have become an essential aspect of patient care, with tens of millions of implantable or indwelling medical devices (such as catheters, endotracheal tubes and artificial joint prostheses) used each year in patients worldwide. However, despite the evolution of such devices and the biomaterials from which they are manufactured, their use *in vivo* is significantly compromised by their seemingly ubiquitous propensity to succumb to microbial colonisation and biofilm formation, leading to *medical-device-associated infection*. Immediately after implantation, the device surface becomes modified by the adsorption of biological materials such as host-derived proteins, extracellular matrix proteins and coagulation products depending on the site. This 'conditioning film' renders the surface of the device favourable for microbial adhesion and is often followed by rapid primary attachment of microorganisms to the material surface and early biofilm formation.

The first report of a biofilm-associated medical-device infection (see Marrie et al., 1982) described the colonisation of an indwelling medical device (an endocardial pacemaker lead) by *S. aureus*. The patient experienced three sequential episodes of *S. aureus* bacteraemia years after the implantation of the device, and despite intensive antimicrobial therapy, the infection was only resolved upon removal of the infected device followed by antibiotic therapy. This case defined the basic characteristics of a biofilm-associated indwelling device infection, namely: inherent tolerance to antibiotic therapy/elevated antibiotic challenge; persistent chronic infection (often latent or asymptomatic) with recurrent exacerbations; blood cultures often culture-negative; and resolution only after removal of the medical device, which acts as a nidus of infection.

The microorganisms responsible for causing medical-device-associated infections may be either from exogenous (e.g., personnel, visitors, healthcare environment and fomites) or endogenous sources (via the migration of microorganisms from normally colonised body sites). Although site-dependent, the main causative organisms of medical-device-associated nosocomial infections are frequently normal skin biota including *S. aureus* and coagulase-negative staphylococci, predominantly *Staphylococcus epidermidis*, which is the most common causative organism of infections related to intravascular catheters and other implanted medical devices. A number of other microorganisms have been shown to be significant causes of medical-device-related nosocomial infections, including *Pseudomonas aeruginosa* (ventilator-associated pneumonia [VAP]), enterococci, *E. coli* (urinary tract infection [UTI] and septicaemia) and *Proteus* species such as *Proteus mirabilis* (UTI, urinary device encrustation and blockage).

At least half of all cases of healthcare-associated infections are estimated to be due to biofilm-mediated, medical-device-associated infections, with medical device use now regarded as the greatest external predictor of healthcare-associated infections. The development of medical-device-associated infections generally necessitates the complete removal and replacement of the device, with the level of clinical intervention depending on the nature and site of the implanted device. Systemic antibiotics (often a combination therapy of two or more antimicrobial agents) represent the conventional approach to the treatment of device-associated infections; however, given the high degree of tolerance to antimicrobial challenge that is a feature of biofilm populations, eradication proves extremely difficult and infection relapses frequently occur. This has led to the development of a range of anti-infective and antimicrobial biomaterials for use in device manufacture, though the long-term efficacy of these devices in the reduction of medical-device-associated infection is an area of considerable debate.

Healthcare-associated infections typically occur at four main body sites (urinary tract, respiratory tract, surgical sites and bloodstream infections), three of which (UTI, pneumonia and bloodstream infections) are commonly associated with the use of indwelling devices. Indeed, around 95% of nosocomial UTIs reported are linked to the use of urological devices (mainly urinary catheters), and more than 85% of nosocomial respiratory infections (mainly VAPs) are device-related. Central venous catheters pose the greatest risk of mortality due to catheter-related bloodstream infections. In the USA, around 250,000 bloodstream infections occur annually, most of which are associated with the use of indwelling intravascular devices, leading to 28,000 deaths each year. Incidences of central-line-associated bloodstream infections (CLABSIs) in the USA declined by 46% over the period 2008–2013, and again between 2015 and 2020 by a further 14% to 21,399 cases annually. Although these represent the most common device-associated infections, it is worth noting that all types of implantable medical devices are susceptible to infection: for example, peritoneal catheter infections in peritoneal dialysis, orthopaedic implant infections and biofilm formation on prosthetic heart valves. In addition to patient morbidity and mortality, device-associated infections impose significant financial burdens on healthcare providers, related primarily to increased hospitalisation time and associated care costs. Despite this, the use of and dependence on implantable, indwelling medical devices increases annually, correlated to an increasing ageing population in industrialised nations.

8.3 Tolerance of Biofilms to Antimicrobials

With the discovery of antibiotics, the world changed. Acute infectious diseases, the leading cause of morbidity and mortality in humans, became treatable, resulting in an increase in life expectancy and quality of life. While infections continue to be a leading contributor to mortality, they are often associated with pre-existing conditions that compromise the patient. However, what became known as the ‘antibiotic era’ is now being compromised itself by the emergence of more and more antibiotic-resistant strains of bacteria that have caused modern medicine to question if we are now entering the ‘post-antibiotic era’ (see Chapter 13).

What is often ignored in these discussions of antimicrobial resistance and our reduced ability to treat infection is the fact that even in the halcyon times of expanding antimicrobial therapy chronic or recurrent infections were poorly resolved with antibiotics. In fact, the designation of these infections as chronic was presumably derived due to their lack of responsiveness to antimicrobial therapy, allowing them to become chronic or to recur in the face of therapy. Diseases such as recurrent ear infections in children, recurrent UTIs in women and medical-device-associated infections were and still remain a challenge to antimicrobial therapy, even when the isolates of these infections have been shown *in vitro* to be susceptible to antibiotics used in their treatment.

It is now recognised that these chronic infections involve bacteria associated within biofilms. Significantly, the US Food and Drug Administration (FDA) and Centers for Disease Control and Prevention (CDC) both state that more than 60% of infections in North America involve biofilms. We also now recognise that the confounding issue in the treatment of chronic infections is the inherent tolerance of biofilms to antibiotics, predicted to have efficacy against the organism on the basis of planktonic susceptibility testing. In fact, Ceri and colleagues demonstrated that for an antibiotic to be effective in biofilms may require a concentration over 1000 times that needed to treat the same planktonic population (Ceri et al. 1999); these are concentrations that cannot be achieved or used safely in the treatment of patients. This altered tolerance to drugs is an adaptation of the biofilm, since bacteria derived from that biofilm show the same susceptibility profile as planktonic bacteria of the same strain when the organisms are returned to planktonic growth.

This reduced susceptibility to antibiotics differs from antibiotic resistance in a number of fundamental ways. First, this tolerance is only demonstrated when the isolate is in the biofilm mode of growth (phenotypic) and is lost when the culture is returned to planktonic growth, hence it is not a permanent genetic change. Secondly, tolerance implies that the biofilm is not killed by the antimicrobial but it may not necessarily be able to grow in the presence of the drug, whereas in resistance the organism can grow in the presence of the antimicrobial. The tolerance of biofilm populations to antimicrobials would imply that, in many chronic infections, microbes are, in fact, exposed to sublethal concentrations of drug, which may have important implications for the development and evolution of classical antimicrobial resistance.

8.4 Mechanisms of Biofilm Tolerance

It is now accepted that the tolerance to antimicrobials characteristic of biofilms is a multifactorial process involving, to some degree or another, a number of different mechanisms contributing to the survival of the population, if not the individual cell. A model for this multifactorial tolerance is shown in Figure 8.2. Contributing to the tolerance of biofilms are factors ranging from the structural components of the biofilm, the physiological potential of cells spread throughout the biofilm and the expression of the genetic phenotypes of disparate populations of cells, all derived from the original clonal population(s) that made up the biofilm.

8.4.1 Biofilm Structure

The hypothesis that the extracellular matrix acts as the gatekeeper for the penetration of antimicrobials into the biofilm, as identified in point 3 in Figure 8.2, has stimulated many studies and engendered a great deal of controversy. When biofilms were first visualised using both transmission and scanning electron microscopy, the dehydrated matrix seen in these original micrographs led to the belief that biofilms were flat and dense structures where the compact and highly charged matrix around the biofilm would prevent penetration of antibiotics into the biofilm; hence, this diffusion barrier would render them resistant to antimicrobial treatment. Stabilisation of the matrix and cross sections through the biofilm revealed a very different picture of the biofilm; however, cells were seen to exist within a highly hydrated matrix containing channels to allow for nutrient transfer into the biofilm and the diffusion of waste out. The matrix is now believed to be composed primarily of bacterially derived carbohydrate, the composition of which is dependent upon the bacterial species, nutrient availability and the growth conditions of the biofilm, and extracellular DNA, with protein and other biomolecules present in lower proportions dependent on the species and nutrient environment. Recently, it has been established that DNA is an important, and ubiquitous, component of the matrix and may be specifically transported into the region; its complete role has yet to be determined. Nevertheless, the matrix DNA is recognised to influence the conformation of the carbohydrate and is hypothesised to serve as a gene pool for the diversity seen within the biofilm, offering a mechanism for horizontal gene transfer between biofilm bacteria potentially contributing to their protection from antimicrobial challenge and host immune cells. The highly anionic charge of this matrix could still play an important role in preventing charged antibiotics from effectively entering the biofilm and thereby still act as a primary inhibitor of antibiotic killing, as was originally proposed. Several studies of antibiotic penetration into biofilms demonstrated that the charge of the antibiotic could affect its penetration. For example, fluoroquinolones (ciprofloxacin, ofloxacin) that are not highly charged easily penetrate the matrix, while the penetration of charged aminoglycosides (tobramycin, gentamicin) is delayed. These studies have not, however, resolved the issue of the importance of the matrix in the resistance of biofilms. The rapid entry of fluoroquinolones, for example, may be only into water channels of the biofilm and not into areas where cells of the biofilm are found, while the delay in entry of aminoglycosides may affect the rate of entry but may not necessarily affect final concentration significantly enough to alter susceptibility of the biofilm. Further, penetration of antimicrobials alone may not be as key an issue as

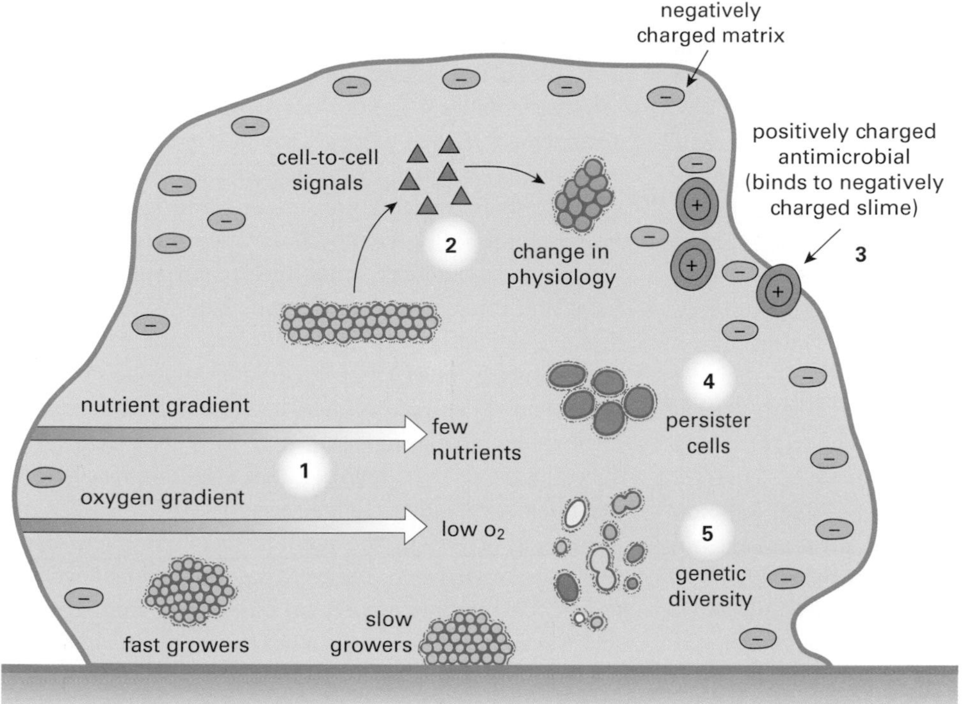

Figure 8.2 Factors contributing to antimicrobial tolerance of biofilms. (1) Low O_2 and decreased nutrient levels near the centre of the microcolony result in slow bacterial growth and hence tolerance to antibiotic drugs which are more effective against fast-growing cells. (2) Intercellular signals can alter biofilm physiology, resulting in expression of molecular efflux pumps which expel antibiotics from the cells allowing the community to grow even in the presence of antimicrobial drug. (3) Negatively charged biofilm matrix may bind positively charged antimicrobials retarding their penetration into the biofilms. (4) Persister cells, a specialised population of cells which do not grow but also do not die in the presence of antibiotic. Persister cells can, upon removal of the antimicrobial challenge, give rise to a normal bacterial colony. (5) Genetic and physiological diversities within the population act as an 'insurance policy', improving the chances that some cells survive any challenge. *Source:* From Harrison, J.J. et al. (2005) Biofilms. *Am. Sci.*, **93**, 508–515, with permission from *American Scientist*.

the physiological state of the cells, which is also affected by the structure and organisation of the biofilm. The diffusion into the biofilm of multiple factors, not limited to just the antibiotics themselves, may impact the biofilm's physiological status, thereby affecting the efficacy of antibiotics against the biofilm.

8.4.2 Biofilm Physiology

The physiological state of the biofilm is also affected by its organisational structure, as diffusion of oxygen, nutrients and waste will ultimately affect all properties associated with growth and sustainability of the biofilm (shown in part 1 of Figure 8.2). Sophisticated experiments based on microelectrode probing of the biofilm and confirmed by dye distribution confocal microscopy assays have established the presence of oxygen and pH gradients within the biofilm. Gradients of nutrients and end products are also implicated in defining the different growth properties throughout the biofilm, which, as described above, have been linked to antibiotic susceptibility. This hypothesis predicts that antibiotics dependent on cell growth for activity will be less effective against biofilms because of the variability of growth within the biofilm. However, biofilms can prove to be as recalcitrant to antibiotics that are not dependent upon cell growth as to those that do. Further, live–dead staining of biofilms does not always correlate with cell death occurring most rapidly at the outer edges of the biofilm, where nutrient and oxygen levels are at their highest and hence where growth should be most rapid. In mixed species biofilms, where each component of the population may exist within its own niche for optimal growth, this model becomes even more complex to understand. The complexity of these interactions will make dissecting the process of antimicrobial tolerance even more challenging. One can, however, argue that targeting one member of a mixed population within the biofilm may alter the susceptibility patterns of other species that are dependent upon symbiotic interactions within the biofilm.

Another focus of study in biofilm resistance related to spatial orientation and physiology has been to look at how biofilms deal with oxidative stress. The mechanism of killing for many antimicrobials, including antibiotics, biocides and metals, is often associated with redox reactions involving various cellular components. These reactions may oxidise sensitive cellular thiol (RSH) groups or result in the production of reactive oxygen species (ROS), such as superoxides, hydroxy radicals or hydrogen peroxide. The regulation of antioxidant pathways within the cell, such as glutathione (GSH) and thioredoxin pathways that manage thiol–disulphide homeostasis, and the *oxyRS*, *soxRS* and *marR* regulons that render cells resistant to ROS, plays an important role in the susceptibility of biofilms to antimicrobials. Indeed, it has been recently proposed that bactericidal antibiotics act via a common ROS-mediated mechanism, but this is the subject of much debate. Despite this, ROS have been shown to contribute and enhance antibiotic-mediated cell death in *Burkholderia cepacia* complex (Bcc) bacteria in the biofilm mode of growth. The difference in oxygen tension in the biofilm and of the cells' response to oxygen stress may prove vital in the survival of biofilms to naturally occurring antibiotics or those used in patient treatment. The role of the redox potential in the response of *E. coli* to metals has demonstrated a very complex picture of these interactions and has shown a difference in mechanisms between planktonic and biofilm populations.

8.4.3 Cellular Signalling and Biofilm Resistance

Our perspective of the microbial lifestyle has changed from one where bacteria exist mainly as solitary independent planktonic populations to one where bacteria form adherent communal populations organised into microcolonies called biofilms. This shift in lifestyle suggests the presence of specific signalling between cells to allow them to organise these complex structures. Many different genes have been identified that can alter biofilm formation or antimicrobial susceptibility, but two global signalling pathways have come to the forefront as biofilm regulators in many different species of bacteria (see point 2 in Figure 8.2). Although models of biofilm formation have been proposed that do not require cell signal molecules, the importance of the following molecules in biofilm formation and antimicrobial resistance is well established and has even led to attempts to develop signal antagonists for the treatment of biofilm-related disease or to enhance the efficacy of existing antimicrobials by returning biofilms to a planktonic-like level of susceptibility.

8.4.3.1 Quorum Sensing

Quorum sensing (QS) has been recognised as a key regulatory process associated with biofilm formation and antibiotic susceptibility. Well studied in *Vibrio fischeri*, QS involves an enzyme LuxI that produces a small signalling molecule, or *autoinducer*, that diffuses out from the cell. Upon reaching a threshold concentration, the autoinducer will then diffuse back into cells, where cellular transcription is altered when the autoinducer binds the transcription regulator LuxR and initiates QS-specific gene expression. In Gram-negative organisms, the autoinducer is typically an acyl-homoserine lactone (AHL), but in some organisms multiple QS systems exist. For example, in *P. aeruginosa*, signalling involves interactions of two distinct AHL compounds, produced by the LuxI homologues Lasl and Rhll, respectively, that interact with their cognate receptors LasR and RhlR. Yet a third signal system, the pseudomonas quinolone signal (PQS), is also active in *P. aeruginosa*. In Gram-positive bacteria, QS is typically carried out by autoinducing peptides. As QS is an integral step in biofilm formation and antibiotic tolerance, it has become a target for new therapeutics. Inhibitors of the QS signal pathway, assayed for their ability to either block biofilm formation, increase biofilm susceptibility to antibiotics or inhibit the expression of QS-dependent genes, without introducing a selective survival pressure (and thus the emergence of resistance) may provide new approaches to the treatment of biofilm-related disease.

8.4.3.2 Cyclic Diguanylate

The universal use of nucleotides as signalling molecules is well recognised in biology. The importance of cyclic diguanylate (c-di-GMP) as a switch to move bacteria from a motile planktonic lifestyle to that of an adherent biofilm is now just being systematically explored. As with other nucleotide regulation systems, two components are involved in the regulatory pathway. The first is responsible for the synthesis of the signal, in this case a diguanylate cyclase (DGC) defined by proteins expressing GGDEF domains. The second component, a phosphodiesterase (PDE), degrades the active signal and is associated with two distinct domains, EAL and HD-GYP. The high level of redundancy of these domains makes understanding the mechanisms by which c-di-GMP regulates biofilm formation and virulence a complex issue, where patterns of temporal and spatial separation remain to be resolved.

8.4.4 Plasticity of Biofilms

The final mechanism by which biofilms become less susceptible to antimicrobials is illustrated in parts 4 and 5 of Figure 8.2. Biofilms are able to give rise to unique subpopulations; in some instances, these may be part of the normal diverse metabolic activity found within the nutrient and oxygen gradients of the biofilm, an example being persister cell populations, or alternatively they may be subpopulations that are derived in response to stress but which are not classically resistant populations according to definitions discussed previously. Being part of a population, as opposed to being a single cell, allows for the adaption of subpopulations within the biofilm through phenotypic expression of unique gene sets, which can ensure the survival of the population as a whole, but often at the expense of individuals within the biofilm. This mechanism can be considered either as altruism in a subset of the population or simply adaptation to the gradients of growth conditions present in the biofilms discussed in Section 8.2 that result in the expression of different phenotypes. There have been many proposed models for phenotypic plasticity of a bacterial population, but we will focus on two prominent hypotheses demonstrated in Figure 8.2. These are persister cell populations and the genetic diversity associated with the 'insurance hypothesis'.

8.4.4.1 Persister Cells

Clonal populations of cells, grown either as a planktonic or biofilm culture, give rise to persistent subpopulations that resist killing by high concentrations of antimicrobials. Persistence is not the same as resistance, as persister populations possess no resistance mechanisms carried on transposable elements. They survive, due to a lack of metabolic activity, but do not grow in the presence of the selective agent; when they are regrown in the absence of the inimical agent, the persister population recapitulates the killing curve of the original population when challenged again with the same antimicrobial. These persister populations typically represent about 0.1% of a logarithmic planktonic culture and up to about 10% of the initial population in a biofilm; they may therefore account for the higher level of antimicrobial tolerance seen in biofilms. While planktonic phase persister cells might be expected to be cleared by the host immune cells, persister cells within a biofilm may be shielded from such clearance mechanisms. Although persister cells were first reported in the 1940s, the molecular mechanisms responsible for their properties are still a subject of debate. Persister cells are not produced in response to a challenge but pre-exist in the population and can be selected from any homogenous population of cells for being a slow-growing, physiologically distinct subpopulation of small cells capable of tolerance to environmental stress. The mechanism by which persistence is manifested remains a focus of many studies. Persistence in *E. coli* has been mapped to the high persistence operon (hip), containing the *hipA* gene that encodes a toxin and the *hipB* gene that encodes an antitoxin that functions as a DNA-binding protein that both binds *hipA* and also autoregulates the expression of the *hip* operon itself. Homologues of the *hip* operon are found across many bacterial genera, suggesting this is a common mechanism of resistance. Interestingly, in *E. coli* and other species, redundant toxin–antitoxin genes have been identified, suggesting the possible specialisation of sets of genes to deal with specific stress factors. Recently, a toxin– antitoxin pair, *yafQ–dinJ*, has been shown to act on biofilm but not planktonic populations to protect them against very specific antimicrobials, which may provide a possible rationale for the redundancy seen in these systems. While antibiotics have proven ineffective against persister cells, the use of mitomycin C and cisplatin (both approved for cancer therapy) has been shown to effectively kill persisters through cross-linking of DNA. Since persister cells are now accepted to be important causative agents in recurrent infections, such approaches may provide an opportunity for the design of combination therapies aimed at eradication of biofilms and their highly antibiotic-tolerant persister subpopulations.

8.4.4.2 Subpopulations of Cells: The 'Insurance Hypothesis'

Biofilms consist of cells that have adapted to a wide range of physiological states associated with the nutritional gradients within the biofilm, and hence even if the biofilm is initiated from a clonal population it will display heterogeneity at both the phenotypic and genotypic levels. This self-generated diversity is enhanced when the biofilm is placed under antimicrobial stress. Persister cell populations, discussed above, represent only one adaptive state that contributes to the increased tolerance of biofilms to antimicrobials. Populations of organisms of any type which comprise diverse subpopulations are expected to perform better in the face of changing environmental conditions, since some subpopulations would be expected to be better placed (or 'fit' in the Darwinian sense of the word) to respond to these changing circumstances. The combination of diverse populations found in the biofilm that contribute to tolerance has been referred to as the insurance hypothesis, where diversity is increased in an attempt to ensure a population will survive the stress of antimicrobial challenge or increased metal or toxin concentrations in nature. This increased survival is a consequence of increased diversity. This is an area of immense interest and a field of study that is just in its infancy. At this point, numerous variants, separated on morphological criteria from challenged populations, have been identified, but the advent of new-generation sequencing has facilitated the screening of these populations for possible mutations that lead to their tolerant phenotype.

8.5 Treatment of Chronic Biofilm Infections

As already stated, chronic, recurrent and device-related infections are now recognised to be associated with biofilm formation. Biofilms, as discussed above, possess multiple mechanisms that render them less susceptible to antibiotic treatment than the same isolate in the planktonic mode of growth. The antibiotics we have today were all selected for efficacy against planktonic cultures and all our diagnostics are based on planktonic assays. Finally, we now recognise that MIC values provide us with little relevant information on how to treat biofilm infections. Clearly, a new paradigm for the treatment of biofilms is needed.

8.5.1 New Biofilm Assays

As part of the development of the next generation of antimicrobials, techniques must be developed and set in place to determine efficacy of these 'new' antimicrobials against cells grown in biofilms. Antimicrobial assays described in Chapter 19 include those targeted at identifying antimicrobials effective against biofilms. It is tempting to speculate that, since screening of all combinatorial libraries of antibiotics was based on efficacy against planktonic targets, potential new antibiotics with efficacy against chronic disease may have been overlooked. The potential for identifying 'next-generation' antibiotics in existing libraries by appropriate biofilm screens is a distinct possibility. The ability to now produce multiple reproducible biofilms of defined target size provides the potential for high-throughput screens for antibiotic efficacy against biofilms. While a range of *in vitro* biofilm assay models now exist, the complexity of treating biofilm infections *in vivo* makes the identification of an appropriate assay/model difficult. To date, guidelines for the diagnosis of biofilm infections have been developed, alongside standardised methods to determine biofilm susceptibility (giving rise to parameters such as minimum biofilm inhibitory concentration [MBIC] and minimum biofilm eradication concentration [MBEC], alongside conventional planktonic susceptibility values of MIC and minimum bactericidal concentration [MBC]). However, insufficient evidence exists currently as to whether or not such *in vitro* tests of biofilm susceptibility should be used to guide clinical choice of antibiotic or to screen for the discovery of new antibiotic compounds.

8.5.2 Better Use of Existing Antimicrobials

Although all existing antimicrobials were selected for their efficacy against planktonic cultures and this efficacy has not always translated to activity against biofilms, it may still be possible to make better use of existing antimicrobials to treat biofilm disease. A marked trend in treating chronic infections of many kinds is the use of antibiotic combinations. The possible existence of synergies between existing antimicrobials represents one area of progress in treating biofilm infections. Rational approaches to the application of combinations of antimicrobials, based on the differences of their targets, have not provided clear use predictions. Most combinations are still empirically derived from past experience. The bioFILM PA™ assay used to select combinations of antibiotics for the treatment of *P. aeruginosa* lung infections in cystic fibrosis patients is one of the first diagnostics to receive regulatory approval (in Canada) and has had a measure of success in the treatment of seriously ill patients. This test has completed clinical trials as a standard diagnostic in cystic fibrosis in Canada and Israel. Based on the Calgary Biofilm Device (see Chapter 19), which is the only high-throughput device for selecting antimicrobials with efficacy against biofilms, this represents one of the first attempts to address the differences in susceptibility of organisms in the biofilm growth mode. In the past decade, the number of standardised tests for determining biofilm susceptibility has increased, but a lack of large-scale clinical trials has left us with insufficient evidence for their widespread acceptance and adoption as standard tests for guiding therapeutic choice of antibiotics.

8.5.3 Next-generation Antimicrobials

It is clear that biofilms represent an important challenge in the treatment of infectious diseases. Biofilms are involved in more than 60% of infections, typically associated with chronic, recurring and device-related infections. Furthermore, we now know that existing antimicrobials have been selected for efficacy against planktonic organisms and are often much less effective against biofilms. What is clearly needed is a paradigm shift for the selection and development of antimicrobials, which will ensure efficacy against biofilms.

8.5.3.1 Conceptual Evaluation of Antibiotics

There is a great deal of discussion about the development of future antibiotics and which is the correct direction to follow. It is noteworthy that every antibiotic on the market has been derived or modified from natural products produced by microbial life forms. It is also interesting to note that these life forms continue to synthesise antibiotics. If they had lost efficacy in nature, one would expect that these organisms would have evolved to stop wasting energy on their synthesis, suggesting that in nature antibiotics continue to have efficacy. The question is then, what disconnect is there between how antibiotics function in nature and how they are used in medicine?

For one thing, in the production of antibiotics, an active compound is purified from the fermentation liquor and tested as an antibiotic against a planktonic target population of bacteria. This approach assumes that the planktonic population is a relevant target for antibiotic selection. It also assumes that other components of the liquor are not important components in the activity of the antibiotic. It is very possible that these discarded components may define activity against the biofilms found in nature. It is more difficult, if not impossible, to bring complex mixtures of active ingredients through regulatory processes; however, this may be the manner by which the active form of antibiotics in nature is able to function against biofilms.

8.5.3.2 Biofilm Assays

It should now be obvious that to find antibiotics capable of treating biofilm infections we require a biofilm assay of antibiotic efficacy. The lack of such an assay and the inability to deal with biofilm infections have in part slowed the acknowledgement of the importance of biofilms in modern medicine. High-throughput screening of antibiotics against biofilms must be achieved for this field to move forward. More diagnostics like the bioFILM PA™ assay must be developed, and standardised tests which better represent the *in vivo* scenario should take priority in the method development process. Our understanding of the composition of natural antibiotic fermentations must be better established for us to recognise the synergies that might exist between existing antibiotics and to formulate suitable compositions of ingredients for future antibiotics yet to be discovered.

Acknowledgements

The contribution of Prof Howard Ceri who established this chapter in the previous edition of this book is gratefully acknowledged.

References

Ceri, H., Olsen, M.E., Stremick, C. et al. (1999). The Calgary Biofilm Device: new technology for rapid determination of antibiotic susceptibilities of bacterial biofilms. *J. Clin. Microbiol.* 37 (6): 1771–1776.

Harrison, J.J., Turner, R.J., Marques, L.L.R. and Ceri, H. (2005). Biofilms: A new understanding of these microbial communities is driving a revolution that may transform the science of microbiology. *Am. Sci.* 93: 508–515.

Marrie, T.J., Nelligan, J. and Costerton, J.W. (1982). A scanning and transmission electron microscopic study of an infected endocardial pacemaker lead. *Circulation* 66: 1339–1341.

Further Reading

Amankwah, S., Abdella, K. and Kassa, T. (2021) Bacterial biofilm destruction: a focused review on the recent use of phage-based strategies with other antibiofilm agents. *Nanotechnol. Sci. Appl.* 14: 161–177.

Borriello, G., Werner, E., Roe, F. et al. (2004). Oxygen limitation contributes to antibiotic tolerance of *Pseudomonas aeruginosa* in biofilms. *Antimicrob. Agents Chemother.* 48: 2659–2664.

Bridier, A., Briandet, R., Thomas, V. and Dubois-Brissonnet, F. (2011) Resistance of bacterial biofilms to disinfectants: a review. *Biofouling* 27(9): 1017–1032.

Ciofu, O., Moser, C., Østrup Jensen, P. and Hoiby, N. (2022). Tolerance resistance of microbial biofilms. *Nat. Rev. Microbiol.* https://doi.org/10.1038/s41579-022-00682-4.

Coenye, T., Goeres, D., Van Bambeke, F. and Bjarnsholt, T. (2018). Should standardized susceptibility testing for microbial biofilms be introduced in clinical practice? *Clin. Microbiol. Infect.* 24 (6): 570–572.

Harrison, J.J., Ceri, H. and Turner, R.J. (2007). Multiple metal resistance and tolerance in microbial biofilms. *Nat. Rev. Microbiol.* 5: 928–938.

Flemming, H.-C., Wingender, J., Szewzyk, U. et al. (2016). Biofilms: an emergent form of bacterial life. *Nat. Rev. Microbiol.* 14 (9): 563–575.

Jonas, K., Melefors, O. and Römling, U. (2009). Regulation of c-di-GMP in biofilms. *Fut. Microbiol.* 4: 341–358.

Keren, I., Wu, Y., Inocencio, J. et al. (2013). Killing by bactericidal antibiotics does not depend on reactive oxygen species. *Science* 339 (6124): 1213–1216.

Kim, J.S. and Wood, T.K. (2016). Persistent Persister misconceptions. *Front. Microbiol.* 7: 2134.

Kohanski, M.A., Dwyer, D.J., Hayete, B. et al. (2007). A common mechanism of cellular death induced by bactericidal antibiotics. *Cell* 130 (5): 797–810.

Koo, H., Allan, R.N., Howlin, R.P. et al. (2017). Targeting microbial biofilms: current and prospective therapeutic strategies. *Nat. Rev. Microbiol.* 15 (12): 740–755.

Lawrence, J.R., Korber, D.R., Hoyle, B.D. et al. (1991). Optical sectioning of microbial biofilms. *J. Bacteriol.* 173: 6558–6567.

Lewis, K. (2007). Persister cells, dormancy and infectious disease. *Nat. Rev. Microbiol.* 5: 48–56.

Nadell, C.D., Xavier, J.O. and Foster, K.R. (2008). The sociobiology of biofilms. *FEMS Microbiol. Rev.* 33: 206–224.

Neethirajan, S., Clond, M.A. and Vogt, A. (2014) Medical biofilms - nanotechnology approaches. *J. Biomed. Nanotechnol.* 10: 1–22.

Römling, U. and Galperin, M.Y. (2017). Discovery of the second messenger cyclic di-GMP. *Methods Mol. Biol.* 1657: 1–8.

Rumbaugh, K.P. and Sauer, K. (2020). Biofilm dispersion. *Nat. Rev. Microbiol.* 18 (10): 571–586.

Sandle, T. (2017). Design and control of pharmaceutical water systems to minimize microbial contamination. *Pharm Engin* **37** (4): 44–48.

Steenackers, H.P., Parijs, I., Foster, K.R. and Vanderleyen, J. (2016). Experimental evolution in biofilm populations. *FEMS Microbiol. Rev.* 40 (6): 373–397.

Van Acker, H., Gielis, J., Acke, M. et al. (2016). The role of reactive oxygen species in antibiotic-induced cell death in *Burkholderia cepacia* complex bacteria. *PLoS One* 11 (7): e0159837.

Walters, M.C. III, Roe, F., Bugnicourt, A. et al. (2003). Contributions of antibiotic penetration, oxygen limitation and low metabolic activity to tolerance in *Pseudomonas aeruginosa* biofilms to ciprofloxacin and tobramycin. *Antimicrob. Agents Chemother.* 47: 317–323.

Whiteley, M., Diggle, S.P. and Greenberg, E.P. (2017). Progress and promise of bacterial quorum sensing research. *Nature* 551 (7680): 313–320.

Williams, P. and Cámara, M. (2009). Quorum sensing and environmental adaptation in *Pseudomonas aeruginosa*: a tale of regulatory networks and multifunctional signal molecules. *Curr. Opin. Microbiol.* 12: 182–191.

Wood, T.K., Knabel, S.J. and Kwan, B.W. (2013). Bacterial persister cell formation and dormancy. *Appl. Environ. Microbiol.* 79 (23): 7116–7121.

Yoon, H.S. and Waters, C.M. (2021). The ever-expanding world of bacterial cyclic oligonucleotide second messengers. *Curr. Opin. Microbiol.* 60: 96–103.

9

Immunology

Mark Gumbleton[1] *and Mathew W. Smith*[2]

[1] *Professor of Experimental Therapeutics, School of Pharmacy and Pharmaceutical Sciences, Cardiff University, Cardiff, UK*
[2] *Reader, School of Pharmacy and Pharmaceutical Sciences, Cardiff University, Cardiff, UK*

CONTENTS

Hugo and Russell's Pharmaceutical Microbiology, Ninth Edition. Edited by Brendan F. Gilmore and Stephen P. Denyer.

Companion website: https://www.wiley.com/go/HugoandRussells9e

9.1 Introduction

9.1.1 Historical Perspective and Scope of Immunology

Progress in immunological science has been driven by the need to understand and exploit the generation of immune states exemplified now by the use of modern vaccines. From almost the first recorded observations, it was recognised that persons who had contracted and recovered from certain infectious diseases were not susceptible (i.e., were immune) to the effects of the same disease when re-exposed to the infection. Thucydides, over 2500 years ago, described in detail an epidemic in Athens (which could have been typhus or plague) and noted that sufferers were 'touched by the pitying care of those who had recovered because they were themselves free of apprehension, for no one was ever attacked a second time or with a fatal result'.

Since that time many attempts have been made to induce this immune state. In ancient times, the process of variolation (the inoculation of live organisms of smallpox obtained from the diseased pustules of patients who were recovering from the disease) was practised extensively in India and China. The success rate was very variable and often depended on the skill of the variolator. In the late eighteenth century, Edward Jenner, an English country doctor, observed the similarity between the pustules of smallpox and those of cowpox, a disease that affected the udders of cows. He also observed that milkmaids who had contracted cowpox by the handling of diseased udders were immune to smallpox. Jenner deliberately inoculated a young boy with cowpox, and after the boy's recovery, inoculated him again with the contents of a pustule taken from a patient suffering from smallpox; the boy did not succumb to infection from this first, or any subsequent challenges, with the smallpox virus. Even though the mechanisms of this protection against smallpox were not understood, Jenner's work had shown proof of principle that the harmless stimulation of our adaptive immune system (see Section 9.1.2) was capable of generating an immune state against a specific disease, and thereby provided the basis for the process we now understand as vaccination. The cowpox virus is otherwise known as the vaccinia virus and the term vaccine was introduced by Pasteur to commemorate Jenner's work.

In 1801, Jenner prophesied the eradication of smallpox by the practice of vaccination. In 1967, smallpox infected 10 million people worldwide. The World Health Organization (WHO) initiated a programme of confinement and vaccination with the aim of eradicating the disease. In Somalia in 1977, the last case of naturally acquired smallpox occurred and, in 1979, WHO announced the total eradication of smallpox, thus fulfilling Jenner's prophecy. Many vaccine products are now available designed to provide protection against a range of infectious diseases. Their value has been proven in national vaccination programmes leading to dramatic reductions in morbidity and mortality from such diseases as diphtheria, pertussis, mumps, measles, rubella, hepatitis A and hepatitis B.

Further progress in the understanding of the complex nature and functioning of the immune system has been gained through the recognition that many varied forms of pathology, beyond that of infectious disease per se, have an underlying immunological basis, including such diseases as asthma, diabetes, rheumatoid arthritis and many forms of cancer. A basic knowledge of how the immune system functions is essential for health professionals involved in understanding the nature of disease and rationalising therapeutic strategies. This chapter aims to provide a sound overview of the structure and functioning of the immune system and impart the reader with knowledge which will serve as a platform for the study of more complex specialised texts if and when required.

9.1.2 Definitions and Outline Structure of the Immune System

The primary function of the immune system is to defend against and eliminate 'foreign' material, and to minimise any damage that may be caused as a result of the presence of such material. The term 'foreign' includes not only potentially pathogenic microorganisms but also cells recognised as 'non-self' and therefore foreign such as the human body's own virally infected or otherwise transformed (e.g., cancerous) host cells. Foreign material would also include *allogeneic* (within species) or *xenogeneic* (between species) transplant tissue and therapeutic proteins administered as medicines if they arose from a different species or were of human origin but had undergone inappropriate post-translational modifications during manufacture or contained impurities. It is also possible that small organic-based drugs may form adducts with endogenous proteins leading to the generation of an immunogen. A good example of such adduct formation is that between the serum protein albumin and the glucuronide metabolite of some non-steroidal anti-inflammatory drugs. This adduct is proposed as the basis of some hypersensitivity reactions.

For clarity, there are a number of terms that should be defined at this point. An organism which has the ability to cause disease is termed a *pathogen*. The term *virulence* is used to indicate the degree of *pathogenicity* of a given strain of microorganism. Reduction in the virulence of a pathogen is termed *attenuation*; this can eventually result in an organism losing its virulence completely and it is then said to be *avirulent*.

An *antigen* is a component of the 'foreign' material that gives rise to the primary interaction with the body's immune system. If the antigen elicits an immune response it may then be termed an *immunogen*. Within a given antigen, for example, a protein, there will be *antigenic determinants* or *epitopes*, which actually represent the antigen recognition sites for our *adaptive immune system* (see below). For example, within a protein antigen, an epitope for an antibody response will consist of 5–20 amino acids that form either part of a linear chain or a cluster of amino acids brought together conformationally by the folding of the protein. Antibodies (otherwise known as immunoglobulins – Ig) are produced and secreted into biological fluids by our adaptive immune system, are widely used in *in vitro* diagnostics and have been investigated in therapeutics as a means of targeting drugs to specific sites in the body. A *monoclonal antibody* is an antibody nominally recognising only a single antigen (e.g., a single protein) and within which only a single common epitope (e.g., clusters comprising a common single specific amino acid sequence or pattern) is recognised. By contrast, a *polyclonal antibody* is an antibody nominally recognising only a single antigen but within which a number of different epitopes (e.g., clusters comprising different amino acid sequences or patterns) are recognised.

The immune system is broadly considered to exhibit two forms of response:

- The *innate immune response*, which is non-specific, displays no time lag in responsiveness, and is not intrinsically affected by prior contact with infectious agent.
- The *adaptive immune response*, which displays a time lag in response, involves highly specific recognition of antigen and affords the generation of immunological memory. An example of immunological memory is that provided by the generation of specific lymphocyte memory cell populations following vaccination with an antigen (e.g., diphtheria toxoid). These memory cells reside over a long term in our lymphoid tissue and permit a more rapid and pronounced protective immunological response on future exposure to the same antigen. The adaptive immune system is further subdivided into:
  - *Humoral immunity*, within which the effector cells are *B-lymphocytes* and where antigen recognition occurs through interactions with antibodies.
  - *Cell-mediated immunity*, within which the effector cells are *T-lymphocytes* and where antigen recognition occurs through interactions of peptide antigen (presented on the surface of other cell types) with *T-cell receptors* (TCR) on the plasma membrane of T-lymphocytes. In cell-mediated immunity, the peptide antigen must be presented to T-lymphocytes by other cell types in association with a class of plasma membrane molecules termed *major histocompatibility complex* (MHC) *proteins*.

9.1.3 Cells of the Immune System

A schematic overview of the cells involved in both the innate and adaptive components of the immune response is shown in Figure 9.1. Most of the cells involved in the immune system arise from progenitor cell populations within the bone marrow. The differentiation of these progenitor cells is under the control of a variety of growth factors, for example, granulocyte colony-stimulating factors (G-CSF) or macrophage colony-stimulating factors (M-CSF) released by monocyte and macrophage cells as well as by fibroblasts and activated endothelial cells. These growth factors promote the growth and maturation of monocyte and granulocyte populations within the bone marrow before their release into the lymphoid and blood circulations.

The principal cells of the innate immune system include the following:

- *Mononuclear phagocytic cells*, which are short-lived (<8 hours) monocytes in the blood circulation that migrate into tissues and undergo further differentiation to give rise to the long-lived and key effector cell – the macrophage.
- The *granulocyte cell* populations which include the neutrophil, basophil and eosinophil.
- The *mast cell* which is a tissue-resident cell that is triggered by tissue damage or infection to release numerous initiating factors leading to an inflammatory response.

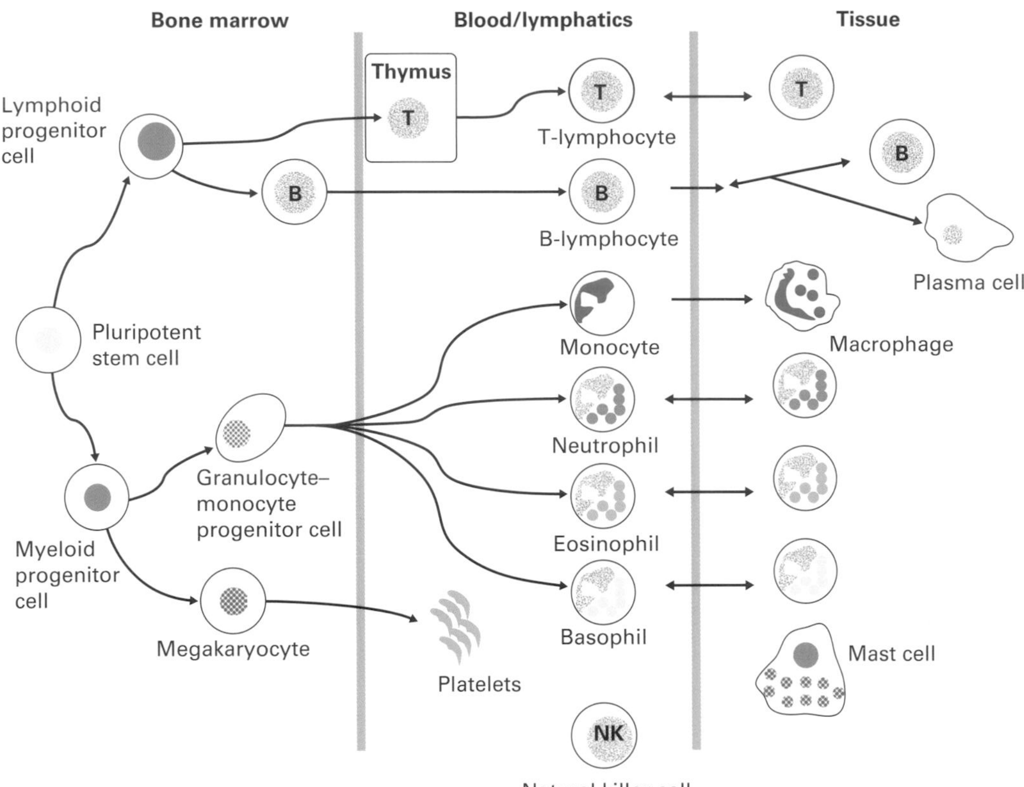

Figure 9.1 An overview of the cells involved in the immune response: both innate and adaptive components. The cells arise from a pluripotent progenitor cell within the bone marrow, with their growth and differentiation controlled by numerous growth factors. The T-lymphocytes differentiate in the thymus gland.

Such initiating factors include histamine, leukotrienes B4, C4 and D4, proinflammatory cytokines (signal proteins released by leucocytes – white blood cells), such as tumour necrosis factor-α (TNF-α), and chemotactic substances such as interleukin-8 (IL-8). The sudden degranulation of the contents of mast cells is also responsible for the acute anaphylactic reactions to bee stings, penicillins, nuts, etc.

- The *natural killer* (NK) cell which has a phenotype similar to that of lymphocytes but lacks their specific recognition receptors. The NK cell exploits non-specific recognition to elicit cytotoxic actions against host cells infected with virus and those host cells that have acquired tumour cell characteristics.

The lymphocyte populations also arise from bone marrow progenitor cells. The B-lymphocytes mature or differentiate in the bone marrow before leaving to circulate in the blood and lymph, while T-lymphocytes undergo maturation in the thymus. Antibodies mediating the effector functions of the humoral immune system are produced and secreted from a differentiated B-lymphocyte cell population termed *plasma cells*.

9.2 The Innate Immune System

9.2.1 Innate Barriers at Epidermal and Mucosal Surfaces

Innate defence against the passage of potentially pathogenic microorganisms across epidermal and mucosal barriers involves a range of non-specific mechanisms. Commensal microorganisms living on mucosal surfaces and on membranes such as skin and conjunctiva constitute one such mechanism (see Chapter 8). These commensals are, under normal circumstances, non-pathogenic, and help prevent colonisation by pathogenic strains. There are also a number of physical and chemical barriers against microbial entry, including the flow of fluid secretions from tear ducts, the urogenital tract and the skin. Many of these secretions possess bacteriostatic or bactericidal activity due to their low pH or the presence of hydrolytic enzymes such as lysozyme (a peptidoglycan hydrolase). Similarly, the mucus barrier covering mucosal surfaces such as the epithelium of the lung serves as a false binding platform for microorganisms, preventing them from interacting with the underlying host cells. In the normal state, the hydrated mucus barrier is efficiently cleared under the driving force of beating cilia. The serious lung infections seen in cystic fibrosis arise because patients are unable to clear the bacteria-laden dehydrated mucus effectively.

9.2.2 Innate Defence Once Epidermal or Mucosal Barriers Have Been Compromised

The function of the innate defence system against microorganisms that have penetrated into interstitial tissues and the vascular compartment relies largely on the processes of phagocytosis (see Section 9.2.2.3) and of activation of the alternative complement pathway (see Section 9.2.2.4). However, the functions of the innate system when exposed to microbial infection are also critical in the recruitment and activation of cells of the adaptive immune response (see later).

The main cells mediating phagocytosis are the mononuclear phagocytic cells and granulocyte cell populations; of the latter, neutrophils are particularly important. For such cells to function, they must possess receptors to sense signals from their environment. In executing their effector functions they need to secrete a range of molecules that will recruit or activate other immune cells to a site of infection.

Before consideration of the process of phagocytosis, an overview of the mononuclear phagocytic cell and granulocyte cell populations is useful.

9.2.2.1 Mononuclear Phagocytic Cells

The mononuclear phagocytic cells include monocytes and macrophages. Monocytes make up approximately 5% of the circulating blood leucocyte population and are short-lived cells (circulating in blood for ≤8 hours), but migrate into tissue to give rise to tissue macrophages. The macrophages constitute a long-lived, widely distributed heterogeneous population of cell types which bear different names within different tissues, such as the migrating Kupffer cell within the liver or the fixed mesangial cell within the kidney glomerulus.

The mononuclear phagocytic cells secrete a wide range of molecules too numerous to list in full here. However, these secretions include:

- Molecules which can break down or permeabilise microbial membranes and thereby mediate extracellular killing of microorganisms, e.g., enzymes (lysozyme or cathepsin G), bactericidal reactive oxygen species and cationic proteins.
- *Cytokines* which can provide innate protective antiviral (e.g., interferon [IFN]-α or -β) and antitumour (e.g., TNF-α) activity against other host cells. A group of cytokines termed *chemokines* can also serve to chemoattract other leucocytes into an area of ongoing infection or inflammation, e.g., IL-8 which attracts neutrophils. Yet another group of cytokines has proinflammatory actions (e.g., IL-1 and TNF-α) which, among other outcomes, leads to activation of endothelial and leucocyte cells promoting increased leucocyte extravasation into tissues and, in the case of IL-1, activation of T-lymphocyte populations.
- *Bioactive lipids* (e.g., thromboxanes, prostaglandins and leukotrienes), which further promote the inflammatory response through actions to increase capillary vasodilation and permeability.

The mononuclear phagocytic cells also possess numerous receptors that interact with their environment. These cells possess, among others:

- Receptors for chemotaxis towards microorganisms, e.g., receptors for secreted bacterial peptides such as formylmethionyl peptide.
- Receptors for complement proteins that serve as leucocyte activators (e.g., C3a and C5a; see Section 9.2.2.4) or complement proteins that serve to coat (opsonise) microorganisms (e.g., C3b). An opsonised microbial surface more readily adheres to a phagocyte membrane, with the opsonin triggering enhanced activity of the phagocyte itself.
- Receptors for promoting adherence, such as lectin receptors interacting with carbohydrate moieties on the surface of the microorganism, or receptors for Fc domains (non-antigen-recognition domains) of antibodies which opsonise microorganisms (e.g., the receptor for the Fc domain of IgG is Fcg), or integrin receptors for cell–cell adhesion (e.g., promoting interaction between a macrophage and T-lymphocyte).
- Receptors for cytokines including those involved in macrophage activation (e.g., IFN-γ) or limiting macrophage mobility (e.g., macrophage inhibitory factor [MIF]) and hence increasing cell retention at a site of infection.

9.2.2.2 Granulocyte Cell Populations

The granulocyte cell populations include the neutrophils, basophils and eosinophils. The short-lived (2–3 days) neutrophil is the most abundant granulocyte (comprising >90% of all circulating blood granulocytes) and is the most important in terms of phagocytosis; indeed, this is the main function of the neutrophil. The receptors and secretions of the neutrophil are similar to those of the macrophage, although notably the neutrophil does not present antigen via MHC class II proteins (see later). The neutrophil is recruited to sites of tissue infection or inflammation by a neutrophil-specific chemotactic factor (IL-8) and is also chemoattracted and activated by some of the same factors described for mononuclear phagocytic cells, including complement protein C3a, bacterial formylmethionyl peptides and leukotrienes. Like macrophages, neutrophils undergo a respiratory burst and are very effective generators of reactive oxygen species.

Eosinophils are poor phagocytic cells and have a specialised role in the extracellular killing of parasites such as helminths, which cannot be physically phagocytosed. Basophils are non-phagocytic cells.

9.2.2.3 Phagocytosis

Macrophages and neutrophils in particular demonstrate a high capacity for the physical engulfment of particles such as microorganisms or microbial fragments from their immediate extracellular environment. This process (Figure 9.2) is made up of a number of steps:

- Chemotaxis of the phagocyte towards the microorganism through signals arising from the microorganism itself (e.g., formylmethionyl peptide), signals arising from complement proteins (e.g., C3a and C5a) generated as part of the activation of the alternative complement pathway (see Section 9.2.2.4) or signals due to release of inflammatory factors (e.g., leukotrienes) secreted by other leucocyte cells situated at the site of an infection.
- Adherence of the microorganism to the surface of the phagocyte (step A in Figure 9.2), involving adhesion through lectin receptors present on the surface of the phagocyte which interact with carbohydrate moieties on the surface of the microorganism; adhesion through complement C3b receptors present on the surface of the phagocyte interacting with C3b molecules that have opsonised the surface of the microorganism; and adhesion through Fc receptors which interact with the Fc domain of antibodies that have opsonised the microbial surface.
- Membrane activation of the phagocyte actin–myosin contractile network to extend pseudopodia around the attached microorganism (step B in Figure 9.2). Membrane activation will also lead to the generation of a 'respiratory burst' by the phagocyte which involves an increase in the activity of the phagocyte membrane NADPH oxidase which converts molecular oxygen into bactericidal reactive oxygen species such as superoxide anion ($\bullet O^-$), hydrogen peroxide (H_2O_2) and, in particular, hydroxyl radicals ($\bullet OH$) and halogenated oxygen metabolites ($HOCl^-$).
- The enclosure of phagocytosed material, initially within a membranous vesicle termed a *phagosome*. Here, cationic proteins such as defensins and reactive oxygen (RO) species begin microbial membrane degradation. This is followed within minutes by fusion of the phagosome with a lysosome to form a phagolysosome, whose contents are at an acidic pH of about 5 which is optimal for the continued active breakdown of microbial structural components (step C in Figure 9.2).

9.2.2.4 Alternative Complement Pathway

The alternative complement pathway fulfils a critical role in innate immune defence. The complement system comprises at least 20 different serum proteins; many are known

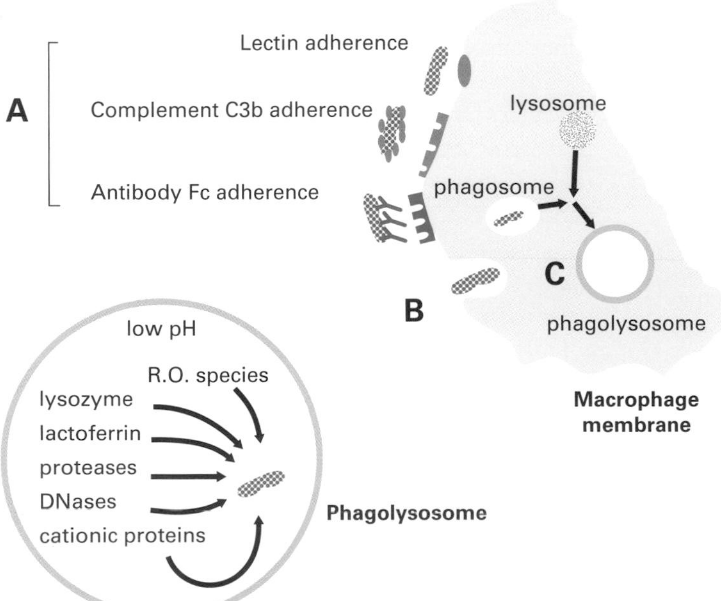

Figure 9.2 Schematic of phagocytosis showing: (step A) adherence of the microorganism to the surface of the phagocyte; (step B) membrane activation of the phagocyte; (step C) enclosure of phagocytosed material within the phagosome and subsequently the phagolysosome. The mediators of the phagolysosome degradation of the microorganism are shown in the enlarged phagolysosome insert. R.O., reactive oxygen.

by the letter C and a number, for example, C3. Many of the complement proteins are *zymogens*, that is, proenzymes requiring proteolytic cleavage to be enzymically active themselves; some are regulatory in function. The cleavage products of complement proteins are distinguished from their precursor by the suffix 'a' or 'b', for example, C3a and C3b, with the suffix 'b' generally denoting the larger fragment that stays associated with a microbial membrane, and the suffix 'a' generally denoting the smaller fragment that diffuses away. The activation of the complement pathway occurs in a cascade sequence, with amplification occurring at each stage, such that each individual enzyme molecule activated at one stage generates multiple activated molecules at the next. In the 'resting' state, in the absence of infection, the complement proteins are inactive or have only a low level of spontaneous activation. The cascade is tightly regulated by both soluble and membrane-bound associated proteins. The regulation of the complement pathway prevents inappropriate activation of the cascade (i.e., when no infection is present) and also minimises damage to host cells during an appropriate complement response to a microbial infection. Complement activation is normally localised to the site(s) of infection.

There are three main biological functions of the alternative complement pathway.

- *Opsonisation of microbial membranes:* this involves the covalent binding of complement proteins to the surface of microbial membranes. This opsonisation or coating by complement proteins promotes adherence of the opsonised microbial component(s) to the cell membranes of phagocytic cells. The complement protein C3b is a potent opsonin.
- *Activation of leucocytes:* this involves complement proteins acting on leucocytes, either at the site of infection or at some distance away, with the result of raising the level of function of the leucocytes in immune defence. For example, C3a is a potent leucocyte chemoattractant and also an activator of the respiratory burst.
- *Lysis of the target cell membrane:* this involves a collection of complement proteins associating on the surface of a microbial membrane to form a membrane attack complex (MAC), which leads to the formation of membrane pores and, ultimately, microbial cell lysis.

Figure 9.3 shows a highly schematised view of the activation cascade for the alternative complement pathway on a

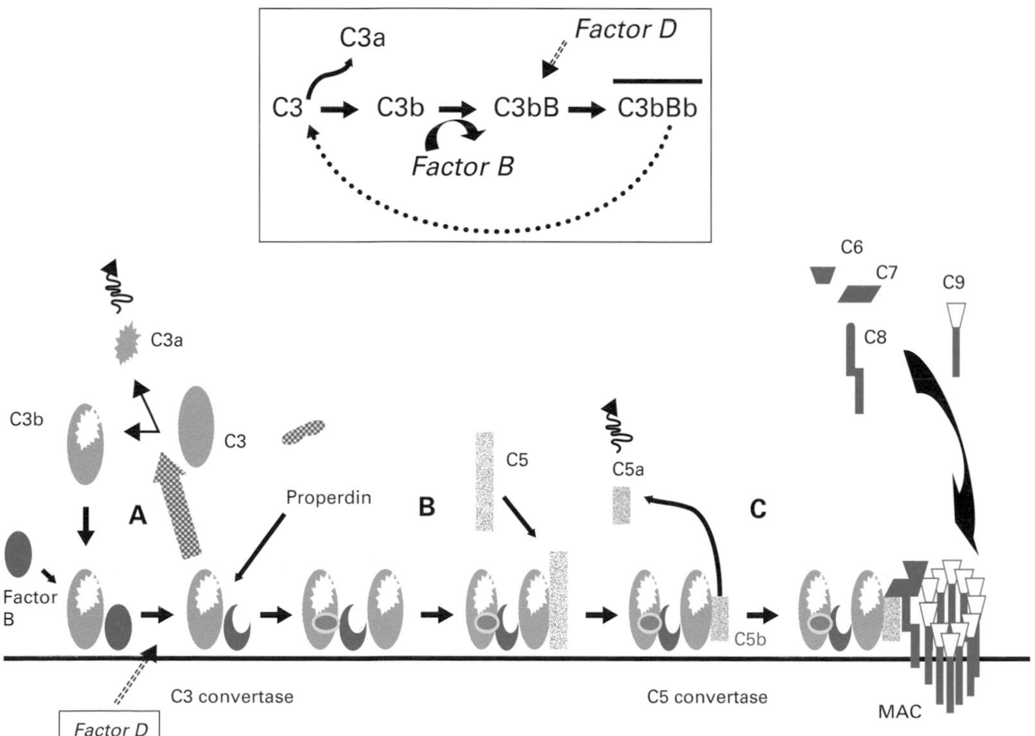

Figure 9.3 A highly schematised overview of the activation cascade for the alternative complement pathway on a microbial membrane surface. In the presence of a microbial membrane, the C3b formed by C3 tickover deposits on the microbial membrane (step A). C3a diffuses away, leading to leucocyte activation. The deposited C3b leads to the generation of a stabilised C3 convertase (step B) which, through a positive feedback loop, leads to the amplified cleavage of more C3. Some C3b associates with the C3 convertase to generate a C5 convertase (step C) which will eventually lead to the generation of a membrane attack complex (MAC).

microbial membrane surface. The activation steps in the alternative pathway are also shown in Figure 9.7, which contrast with the activation steps in the classical complement pathway involving antibody.

The pivotal protein in the alternative pathway is C3 (195 kDa). Under normal circumstances (in the absence of infection), C3 is cleaved very slowly through reaction with water or trace amounts of proteolytic enzyme to give C3b and C3a. The C3b formed is susceptible to nucleophilic attack by water and is rapidly inactivated to give iC3b. The C3a is not generated in sufficient amounts to lead to leucocyte activation and is rapidly inactivated. This normal low-level cleavage of the C3 molecule is termed 'C3 tickover' and it provides low levels of starting material, that is, C3b, which will be required for full activation of the alternative complement pathway in the case of a microbial infection.

In the presence of a microbial membrane, the C3b formed by C3 tickover will be susceptible to nucleophilic attack by hydroxyl or amine groups on the membrane surface, leading to the covalent attachment of C3b to the membrane (step A in Figure 9.3). Once C3b has attached to the membrane, factor B can bind to form a molecule termed C3bB. This complex is stabilised by a soluble protein called properdin. Factor D then enzymically cleaves the bound factor B to generate a molecule termed C3bBb which is the C3 convertase of the alternative pathway (Figure 9.3, inset).

This newly generated stable C3 convertase enzymically cleaves C3 to generate further C3b and C3a molecules, leading to leucocyte activation (by C3a) and greater deposition of C3b on the microbial membrane and hence further generation of C3-convertase molecules. In effect, the microbial membrane has activated a positive feedback loop with cleavage of C3 to generate high amounts of C3b and C3a molecules.

The deposited C3b not only leads to the formation of the C3 convertase but also coats the microbial membrane as an opsonin and so promotes binding to phagocyte cell membranes. Some of the deposited C3b associates with the newly formed C3 convertase to generate a complex termed C3bBb3b, which is the C5 convertase of the alternative pathway (step B in Figure 9.3). This C5 convertase binds the complement protein C5 and cleaves it into C5a (a leucocyte activator) and C5b (an opsonin). The C5b remains associated with the membrane and acts as a platform for the sequential binding of complement proteins C6, C7 and C8 (step C in Figure 9.3). The α-chain of the C8 molecule penetrates into the microbial membrane and mediates conformational changes in the incoming C9 molecules such that C9 becomes *amphipathic* (simultaneously containing hydrophilic and hydrophobic groups). In this form, it is capable of insertion through the microbial membrane where it mediates a polymerisation process that gives the MAC. The MAC generates transmembrane channels within the microbial membrane with the osmotic pressure of the cell leading to an influx of water and eventual microbial cell lysis.

Differences between host cell membranes and microbial cell membranes mean that the cascade is only activated in the presence of microorganisms, so C3 tickover cannot give rise to full activation of the alternative pathway in the absence of microbial membrane. Stable deposition of a functional C3 convertase only occurs on the microbial cell surface. The differences that exist include, for example:

- lipopolysaccharide or peptidoglycan on microbial membranes that promotes the binding of C3b;
- the high sialic acid content of host cell membranes that promotes the dissociation of any C3 convertase formed on host surfaces; and
- the presence of specific host cell membrane proteins that also serve a key regulatory function.

Decay-activating factor (DAF) and complement receptor type 1 (CR1) are host cell membrane proteins that serve to competitively block the binding of factor B with C3b and hence inhibit formation of a C3 convertase; they also promote disassembly of any C3 convertase formed. Membrane cofactor protein (MCP) and CR1 are further host cell membrane proteins that promote the displacement of factor B from its binding with C3b. Host cell membranes also possess a protein, CD59, which prevents the unfolding of C9 – a required step for membrane insertion to form an effective MAC.

9.3 The Humoral Adaptive Immune System

The humoral immune response is mediated through antibody–antigen interactions. B-lymphocytes in their naive state, unstimulated by antigen, possess antibody molecules on their cell membrane, which serve a surveillance function to recognise any invading antigen. A B-lymphocyte that has bound antigen is capable of differentiating into a plasma cell which, under the influence of signals from helper T-cells, produces a fuller repertoire of antibody molecules (i.e., a fuller range of antibody classes), which are then secreted from the plasma cell into the extracellular environment to bring about a range of humoral effector functions.

9.3.1 B-Lymphocyte Antigens

As briefly discussed in Section 9.1.2, a B-cell antigen is a substance or molecule specifically interacting with an antibody, and which may lead to the further production of antibody and an immunological response. Typically, B-lymphocyte antigens are proteins within which all the epitopes consist of clusters of 5–20 amino acid residues. B-lymphocyte epitopes arise most commonly from the three-dimensional folding of proteins (i.e., conformational epitopes), although they may also consist of a sequential linear sequence of amino acids within the polypeptide chain (linear epitopes). As a general rule, there is a gradient of increasing immunogenicity with increasing molecular weight of protein. Further, the higher the structural complexity of the protein or polypeptide antigen, the higher the level of immunogenicity it is likely to exhibit. Thus, a polypeptide comprising a single amino acid such as polylysine will be expected to be a weaker immunogen than a protein of equivalent molecular weight made up of a diverse range of amino acids.

Polysaccharides tend not to be good immunogens for B-lymphocytes. When a polysaccharide serves as the sole immunogen, the humoral response obtained is termed 'T-cell-independent' because the polysaccharide does not elicit helper T-lymphocyte cooperation (see Section 9.4). The consequences of a T-cell-independent humoral response include the lack of production of memory B-cell populations and the lack of synthesis by the plasma cell of the full range of antibody subclasses, that is, T-cell-independent humoral responses mainly involve the production of IgM antibody. For improved immunogenicity, carbohydrate antigens are conjugated to proteins which allow a more effective 'T-cell-dependent' humoral response, that is, one that affords the generation of memory B-cell populations and the synthesis of the full range of antibody subclasses. This strategy is used in a number of current vaccine products; for example, meningococcal group C conjugate vaccine contains the capsular polysaccharide antigen of *Neisseria meningitidis* group C conjugated to *Corynebacterium diphtheriae* protein. Pure nucleic acid and lipid serve as very poor antigens.

9.3.2 Basic Structure of Antibody Molecules

Figure 9.4 shows an antibody monomer with a four-polypeptide subunit structure, where the subunits are linked through disulphide bonding. The basic monomer structure can be considered the same for all the different classes of antibody (see below) even though some may form higher-order structures, for example, IgM is a pentamer made up of five antibody monomer units.

The subunits of the antibody monomer comprise two identical 'heavy' polypeptide chains and two identical 'light' polypeptide chains, with each of these containing a 'constant' region and a 'variable' region. The light-chain variable regions (V_L) and the heavy-chain variable regions (V_H) are the parts of the antibody molecule involved in antigen recognition. Specifically, antibodies produced by different B-lymphocytes or plasma cells will have variable regions possessing different amino acid sequences leading to differences in antibody variable region surface conformation. At the extreme tips of the variable regions are hypervariable domains that serve the specific antigen recognition function discriminating between, for example, diphtheria toxin and tetanus toxin. The structural differences in the variable and hypervariable domains enable different antibodies to recognise different structural epitopes; this meets the needs of the immune system to combat a large and diverse range of antigens.

A horizontal line of symmetry can be drawn through the antibody structure in Figure 9.4, bisecting the molecule into two equivalent halves each containing a single heavy chain and a single light chain and clearly showing the antibody monomer to possess bivalency in its ability to interact with antigen, that is, each antibody monomer can bind two epitopes, although the epitopes bound by a single antibody must be identical. The antigen recognition domain of an antibody monomer is termed the Fab domain. The structure of the constant region of the heavy chain (C_H) does not influence the antigen recognition function of the molecule

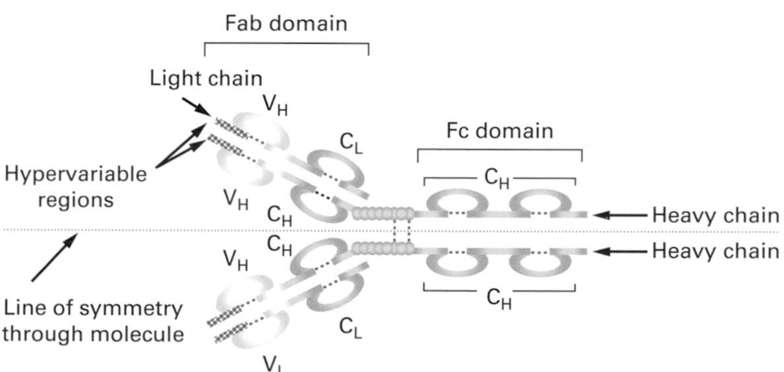

Figure 9.4 An antibody monomer consisting of a four-polypeptide subunit structure, where the subunits are linked through disulphide bonding. The Fab fragment is concerned with antigen recognition, while the Fc region determines the various effector functions of antibodies. A horizontal line of symmetry can be drawn through the antibody structure bisecting the molecule into a single heavy chain and a single light chain and clearly showing the bivalency in antigen recognition. C_H, constant region of heavy chain; C_L, constant region of light chain; V_H, variable region of heavy chain; V_L, variable region of light chain.

but defines the different classes of antibody that are produced and hence the effector functions arising from antigen–antibody interaction; this heavy-chain constant region is termed the Fc domain.

An analogy that may assist visualisation of the function of an antibody molecule is one that views it as a hand (Fab domain) attached to the arm (Fc domain) (Figure 9.4). The palm of the hand (variable region) can take up different shapes to allow the fingertips (hypervariable regions) to gain a very precise interaction with an object (antigen). At the wrist (hinge region), the hand is highly flexible relative to the arm (Fc domain) to allow the hand and fingertips (Fab domain) maximum flexibility to orientate an interaction with objects (antigen). The structure of the arm (Fc domain) does not influence interaction with an object (antigen). Once the object (antigen) has interacted with the fingertips (hypervariable regions) of the hand, the arm (Fc domain) can then mediate a variety of effector functions.

A B-lymphocyte and plasma cell can produce different classes of antibody depending on the stage of immune activation and on the intercellular signals that the B-lymphocyte and plasma cell receive from other effector cells within the immune system. As stated above, the class of antibody is determined by the structure of the Fc domain and the different classes of antibodies possess different effector functions. The basic classes of antibodies are: IgM (heavy-chain constant region defined as μ); IgA (heavy-chain constant region defined as α); IgD (heavy-chain constant region defined as δ); IgG (heavy-chain constant region defined as γ) and IgE (heavy-chain constant region defined as ε). The different classes of antibody can be remembered using the acronym MADGE. In addition to the heavy-chain constant region classes, there are two light-chain constant region classes, κ and λ; however, these do not mediate different antibody effector functions.

Each B-lymphocyte and the plasma cell that derives from it is capable of producing all the different antibody classes. However, all the antibody classes produced by a single B-lymphocyte and its derived plasma cell will recognise only a single epitope, that is, only a single specific set of chemical features within a sequence or pattern of amino acid residues. In other words, all antibodies produced by a single B-lymphocyte, and its derived plasma cell, possess the same Fab domain recognising the same antigenic determinant but clearly may possess different Fc domains capable of mediating different effector functions. Thus, the same epitope can stimulate various different forms mediated via the IgM, IgA, IgD, IgG and IgE classes of humoral immune attack.

Within the antibody pool it is estimated that there are approximately 10^9 different epitope recognition specificities, sufficient to cover the range of pathogens likely to be encountered in life. This enormous diversity in antigen recognition is due to the amino acid sequence diversity in the variable and hypervariable domains of the antibody molecule. However, this large diversity cannot result from the presence of an equivalent number of separate protein-coding genes; the human genome project has estimated there to be only approximately 30,000 protein-coding genes. Rather, the clonal diversity in antigen recognition is due in the main to a process termed *gene rearrangement*, which occurs in each B-lymphocyte during maturation in the bone marrow. For example, the DNA coding for a single heavy-chain molecule will result from the splicing together of genes from four separate regions termed a variable region gene (V), a diversity region gene (D), a joining region gene (J) and a constant region gene (C). There are approximately 100 V genes, 25 D genes and 50 J genes. Gene rearrangement will allow combinatorial freedom for any V, D and J genes to splice together, providing a large number of VDJ combined gene product permutations and hence diversity in antigen recognition. Inaccurate splicing together of the regional genes at the V–D and D–J junctions further increases diversity, as does the process of random nucleotide insertion. The C genes dictate the different classes of antibody and not the antigen recognition specificity. An additional process which occurs in a B-lymphocyte memory cell population while it resides within the lymphoid tissue is that of somatic mutation, in which only very slight changes in antibody Fab domains occur through single base mutations. Sometimes these mutations prove advantageous by increasing the affinity of an antibody to the same original epitope. Under these circumstances, the antibody clone with the highest binding affinity to the original target epitope will proliferate and dominate. The light-chain gene also has V, J and C regions and the V and J genes undergo a similar rearrangement to that described for the heavy chain, and hence further add to diversity. The heavy-chain and light-chain polypeptides are joined together via disulphide bond formation following protein synthesis of the individual heavy and light chains. In summary, all antibodies produced by a single B-lymphocyte and its derived plasma cell are 'programmed' to recognise only a single antigen recognition feature determined by the recombination pattern of the V, D and J genes (heavy chain) and the V and J genes (light chain). The class of antibody is determined by further excisions within the DNA to allow the same VDJ gene combination to lie next to a different C gene, which codes for the structure of the antibody constant region and therefore determines antibody class. The five C gene classes are m, a, d, g and e, although various subclasses also exist. Antibody class switching is not a random process but one that is regulated by helper T-lymphocyte cytokine secretions.

9.3.3 Clonal Selection and Expansion

Within the body there may exist at any one time only a handful of naive B-lymphocytes capable of recognising the same epitope. The meeting of an antigen and a naive B-lymphocyte capable of recognising an epitope within the antigen occurs through the delivery of antigen to lymphoid tissues of the spleen, lymph nodes and local lymphoid tissue within mucosal surfaces (mucosa-associated lymphoid tissue [MALT]) and skin (skin-associated lymphoid tissue [SALT]). This lymphoid tissue is rich in lymphocytes. Further, a proportion of B-lymphocytes will always be recirculating from the lymphoid tissue through the lymph and blood circulations and so is able to encounter circulating antigen.

Antigen will be specifically recognised by IgM molecules present on the surface of the naive B-lymphocyte. Following this antigen-driven selection of a specific B-lymphocyte clone, the clone will undergo repeated cell divisions. Some of the daughter cells will differentiate into short-lived (2–3 days) plasma cells able to secrete antibody of different classes to combat the initial primary antigen exposure. Other clonal daughter cells will become long-lived B-lymphocyte memory cells populating the lymphoid tissue and spreading around the body through the lymph and blood circulations. These cells will provide 'immunological memory' able to generate a more rapid and pronounced secondary response on subsequent exposure to the original antigen (Figure 9.5).

This process of clonal selection and expansion to form memory cell populations is the basis of vaccination. The initial introduction of antigen gives rise to a primary response (Figure 9.6) in which there is a significant latent period before increased serum antibody levels are observed; the main antibody response is IgM production, although some IgG is also synthesised and secreted. On re-exposure to the same antigen a secondary response is elicited. The features of the secondary response include:

- a reduced latent period between antigen challenge and increases in serum antibody (e.g., latent period of 5–7 days for the secondary response against 7–20 days for the primary response); and
- an antibody response dominated by IgG which is more pronounced with higher serum levels achieved.

In the absence of helper T-lymphocyte involvement (T-cell-independent humoral responses, for example, where antigen is carbohydrate alone), B-lymphocyte memory cell populations are not produced, and antibody class switching is restricted. Hence, under these circumstances, the primary and secondary antibody responses to antigen challenge are essentially indistinguishable and exhibit a prolonged latent period, relatively low levels of serum antibody produced and IgM as the main serum antibody.

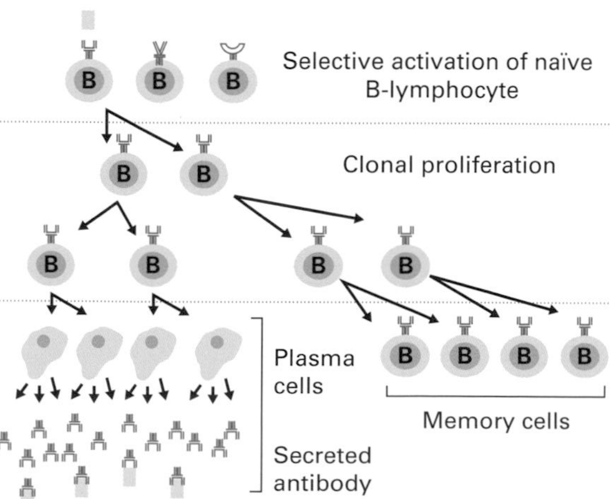

Figure 9.5 Clonal proliferation of B-lymphocytes. Following antigen-driven selection of a specific B-lymphocyte clone, it will undergo repeated cell divisions to give effector cell populations and memory cell populations.

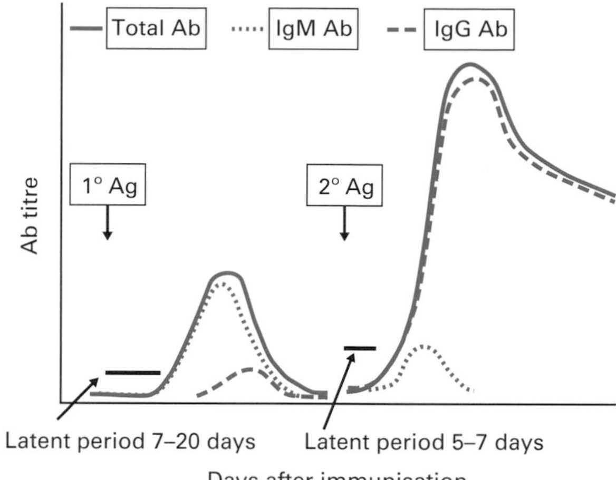

Figure 9.6 Primary and secondary responses to antigen (Ag). A primary response of the humoral system involves a significant latent period before elevated serum antibody (Ab) levels are seen; the major serum antibody generated is IgM. Memory cell populations provide the basis of the secondary response, which displays a significant reduction in the latency period to achieve elevated serum antibody. The antibody serum levels are greater than in the primary response and involve mainly IgG.

9.3.4 Humoral Immune Effector Functions

The humoral immune response is mediated by the initial antibody–antigen interaction, but with the different antibody classes offering a range of effector functions. The effector functions of antibodies include those described below.

9.3.4.1 Cognitive Function on B-Lymphocyte Cell Surface

Antibody on the surface of naive or memory B-lymphocytes serves to recognise and bind specific antigen; IgM serves this main cognitive function. It exists as a pentamer of five monomer units with an antigen valency of 10 and is extremely efficient at binding antigen. IgD appears to function mainly on the surface of B-lymphocytes and may also contribute to cognition in some way.

9.3.4.2 Neutralisation of Antigen by Secreted Antibody

Secreted antibody, in particular IgG, IgA and IgM, can bind antigen and sterically hinder the interaction of such agents as toxins, viruses and bacteria with host cell surfaces. In the circulatory and interstitial fluids, IgG (which exists as a monomer with an antigen valency of 2) is the main antibody that fulfils this role in the secondary response, while IgM is the main antibody produced in the primary response. IgA has specific roles in mucosal immunity.

9.3.4.3 Opsonisation of Antigen

Secreted antibody, in particular IgG, opsonises antigenic material and in so doing promotes association (e.g., through Fcg receptors) of the antigenic material with phagocyte membranes. Occupancy of the Fc receptor by the antibody also serves to activate a phagocyte's killing mechanisms.

9.3.4.4 Mucosal Immunity

Mucosal immunity involves the interaction of antibody with antigen at mucosal surfaces such as those of the gastrointestinal tract, lung or urogenital tract. The major antibody of the mucosal lining fluid is IgA, which exists as a dimer of two monomer units (antigen valency of 4). IgA is actively secreted across mucosal epithelium into the lining fluid; it will neutralise antigen and may also serve as an opsonin. IgA is also present in secretions such as tears and saliva but it has a limited role in systemic immunity.

9.3.4.5 Antibody-dependent Cell Cytotoxicity (ADCC)

Through specific binding to antigen on the surface of membranes perceived as 'foreign', for example, microbial cells or host cells virally infected or otherwise transformed, antibody can direct (through its Fc domains) the close association of 'killing' cells, such as neutrophils, eosinophils, NK cells and even cytotoxic T-lymphocytes, with the 'foreign' membrane. This close association depends on the antibody's Fc domain binding to the respective Fc receptor present on the surface membrane of the 'killing' cell. Such close proximity to the 'foreign' cell enables the efficient and targeted release of cytotoxic molecules into the extracellular environment. IgG is the main antibody of systemic body fluids and is an important mediator of ADCC, although IgE and IgA may undertake this role in certain circumstances, for example, against certain parasites where IgE directs ADCC mediated by eosinophils.

9.3.4.6 Immediate Hypersensitivity

Mast cells express high-affinity receptors (Fce) that bind the Fc domain of IgE antibodies. In the absence of antigen, these receptors are occupied by the IgE monomer (antigen valency of 2) secreted previously from plasma cells. In this circumstance, the IgE molecules are serving a cognitive function which, on appropriate antigen binding, results in aggregation of the membrane-bound IgE and causes immediate mast cell degranulation and release of inflammatory mediators. Mast cells possess in their membranes IgE monomers able to recognise different antigenic epitopes. This contrasts with each single B-lymphocyte, which possesses IgM antibody on its surface membrane that performs a cognitive function but is capable of recognising only a single epitope specificity.

9.3.4.7 Neonatal Immunity

The neonate lacks the ability to mount a full immunological response; accordingly, maternal IgG is transported across the placenta late in pregnancy and is also absorbed across the gastrointestinal tract from breast milk. Maternal IgA secreted into breast milk will also provide mucosal protection for the neonate.

9.3.4.8 Activation of the Classical Complement Pathway

A complement cascade similar to that of the alternative pathway can be activated through specific antibody–antigen interactions. The antibodies that activate the classical complement pathway are IgM and IgG.

Key steps in the activation of the classical pathway are shown in Figure 9.7, where this pathway is also compared to the alternative pathway. In the classical pathway, the initiating step is the specific binding of IgG or IgM to antigen. Once this occurs, a complement protein termed C1 (which comprises a single C1q subunit, two C1r subunits and two C1s subunits) binds to adjacent Fc domains in the antibody–antigen complex. This binding of C1 activates the catalytic activity of the C1r subunits, and in turn the C1s subunits. The activated C1s subunits cleave C4 into C4b and C4a; the latter can diffuse away and serve as a leucocyte activator. The C4b covalently associates with the antibody–antigen complex on the surface of a microbial membrane and can serve as an opsonin. A further complement protein, C2, binds to this membrane complex to give C4b2. The C1s subunit then enzymically cleaves the bound C2a to generate on the membrane a new complex termed C4b2b, which is the C3 convertase of the classical pathway. (In some

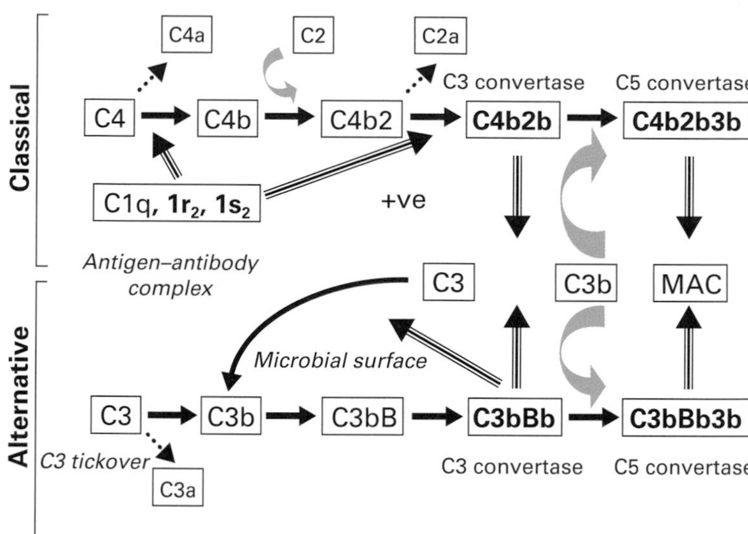

Figure 9.7 The classical and alternative complement pathways.

texts, the C2a is referred to as the larger subunit remaining with the membrane, while C2b is the smaller subunit that diffuses away.) This C3 convertase molecule is distinct from that within the alternative pathway, but it is from this point onwards that parallels can be drawn between the two cascades.

The host proteins that serve key regulatory functions within the alternative pathway (DAF, CR1 factor I and CD59) also serve similar functions within the classical pathway. However, in contrast to the alternative pathway, the activation step in the classical pathway requires specific antibody–antigen interactions. In this context, the C1 protein can only become catalytically active when it is bound to at least two adjacent Fc domains. In the case of the IgG and IgM molecules, the Fc domains will only align adjacent to each other when the corresponding Fab domains bind antigen. Further, when C1 is free in the circulation, it is bound to a protein termed C1 inhibitor (C1-INH) which prevents any possible activation of C1 in the absence of antibody. Once C1 binds to adjacent Fc domains within an antibody–antigen complex, C1-INH is displaced.

The functions of the classical complement pathway are similar to those described for the alternative pathway, that is, opsonisation, leucocyte activation and membrane lysis of target cells. The classical pathway can additionally lead to complement protein deposition on insoluble antibody–antigen immune complexes circulating within blood, and in doing so promote the clearance of such potentially harmful complexes by Kupffer cells of the liver. The presence of two complement pathways provides for rapid (alternative) and specific (classical) activation of a key defence mechanism, and offers greater protection against the development of microbial resistance mechanisms.

9.4 Cell-mediated Adaptive Immune System

Cell-mediated adaptive immune responses are mediated by T-lymphocytes which arise from bone marrow progenitor cells and undergo maturation in the thymus before release into the systemic blood and lymph circulations (Figure 9.1). A number of parallels can be drawn between the B-lymphocyte-mediated immune response and the T-lymphocyte-mediated response. First, membrane-bound antibodies serve the cognitive function for B-lymphocytes, while the cognitive function for T-lymphocytes is served by TCR present on the cell's plasma membrane surface. Second, in response to antigen, T-lymphocytes, like B-lymphocytes, will undergo clonal proliferation and form a population clone of memory T-cells specific for a single epitope. Third, each single B-lymphocyte and plasma cell that derives from it is capable of producing antibodies that will only recognise a single epitope. In the same manner, each single T-cell is programmed to make TCR of only a single specificity able to recognise only a single specific set of chemical features within a T-cell epitope. This is achieved for the TCR in a similar manner to that for antibodies in that different gene segments termed V–D–J are brought together by the process of gene rearrangement into single RNA products. The recombined RNA will code for the polypeptide chains that make up the TCR. When all the possible recombinations are considered, the number of different TCR molecules that an individual can make is in excess of 10^9, a number similar to the primary antigen recognition repertoire of T-cells.

There are two general classes of T-lymphocytes: helper T-lymphocytes and cytotoxic T-lymphocytes. The latter function to kill host cells that have undergone a transformation such as a viral infection or cancer, and they recognise specific antigens on the surface of host cells that have arisen as a result of such cell transformation. Through this specific antigen recognition, the cytotoxic T-cell becomes closely apposed to the target host cell and is activated to synthesise and release cytotoxic secretory products (e.g., pore-forming molecules such as perforins) leading to lysis of the affected host cell. By contrast, the helper T-cell can be viewed as the coordinator of the adaptive immune system, providing appropriate activation signals, in the form of secreted cytokines, to promote the functioning of both the cytotoxic T-cell populations and that of the antibody-producing B-lymphocyte and plasma cell populations. The actions of the helper T-cell populations also promote the function of the innate immune system, for example, IFN-γ released by helper T-cells increases the phagocytic activity of macrophages. The helper T-cells are further divided into T_H1 or T_H2 subpopulations depending on the nature of cytokines they secrete and, as a consequence, the arms of the immune system they predominantly influence. The T_H1 helper T-cells mainly regulate cell-mediated immunity, while T_H2 helper T-cells regulate humoral immunity.

9.4.1 T-Lymphocyte Antigen Recognition and MHC Proteins

Epitopes for T-lymphocytes comprise exclusively linear peptide sequences. T-lymphocytes are unable to respond to carbohydrate, lipid or nucleic acid material and they only respond to a peptide antigen when it is presented to the T-lymphocyte by surface proteins on the plasma membrane of host cells. These surface proteins are termed MHC proteins (see Section 9.1.2) and can be subdivided into two main classes:

- *MHC class I proteins* are expressed on the surface of all nucleated host cell membranes and present peptide antigen to cytotoxic T-lymphocytes.
- *MHC class II* proteins are expressed only on a more specialised group of cells termed antigen-presenting cells (APCs), and present peptide antigen to helper T-lymphocytes.

Such a distinct cellular distribution of MHC proteins and restriction in presentation to discrete T-lymphocyte subpopulations may be remembered by considering the different T-lymphocyte functions. That is, all cells of the body have the potential to become infected with virus and undergo a cancerous change, and hence all cells must have the capacity to be destroyed by the actions of cytotoxic T-cells. As such, all cells of the body must possess MHC I molecules to afford antigen presentation to cytotoxic T-cells. By contrast, as a coordinator cell of the immune system, the helper T-cell must be able to respond to its environment in order to give appropriate signals or 'help' to other immune cells. Specialised APCs with the capacity to phagocytose interstitial proteinaceous material therefore undertake the function of 'environmental sampling'. MHC class II proteins expressed on the surface of APCs will present peptide antigen to helper T-lymphocytes.

APCs include the macrophage tissue cell population, specialised APCs such as dendritic cells within the lymphatic system or Langerhans cells within the skin. B-lymphocytes also serve the function of an APC because they interact with protein antigen through high-affinity surface IgM molecules. Subsequently, they internalise the protein antigen for processing to generate peptides that will be presented by MHC II molecules expressed on the B-lymphocyte cell surface. Another cell type that can serve the function of an APC is the endothelial cell, which can be induced to express MHC II molecules by the action of the cytokine IFN-γ. It should not be overlooked that the APC can itself become infected with virus and undergo cancerous transformation, and therefore the APC, in addition to MHC II molecules, will also express the full complement of MHC I molecules on its surface.

This process of MHC presentation of peptide and interaction with T-lymphocyte receptor is shown in Figure 9.8. A foreign peptide presented by a MHC molecule will be recognised by a TCR expressed on the surface of an appropriate T-lymphocyte. Once a particular TCR recognises a peptide sequence as foreign, intracellular signals to activate the T-cell are sent via the CD3 complex present within the T-cell membrane. The recognition of peptide as foreign will lead to an immune response. Beyond antigen presentation, the interaction between MHC molecule and T-lymphocyte also serves to identify that the T-lymphocyte and host cell membrane arise from the same embryonic tissue. Tremendous inter-individual differences, or more specifically polymorphisms, exist in the MHC proteins within a population. The T-lymphocyte undertakes this MHC surveillance through the possession of accessory molecules. Cytotoxic T-lymphocytes possess $CD8^+$ molecules which interact with MHC I (Figure 9.8a), while helper T-lymphocytes possess $CD4^+$ molecules which interact with MHC II (Figure 9.8b); hence, the use of the terms $CD8^+$ lymphocytes to refer to cytotoxic T-cells and $CD4^+$ lymphocytes to refer to helper T-cells.

9.4.2 Processing of Proteins to Allow Peptide Presentation by MHC Molecules

Peptide epitopes presented by MHC I are derived from the processing of proteins (e.g., a viral protein) synthesised

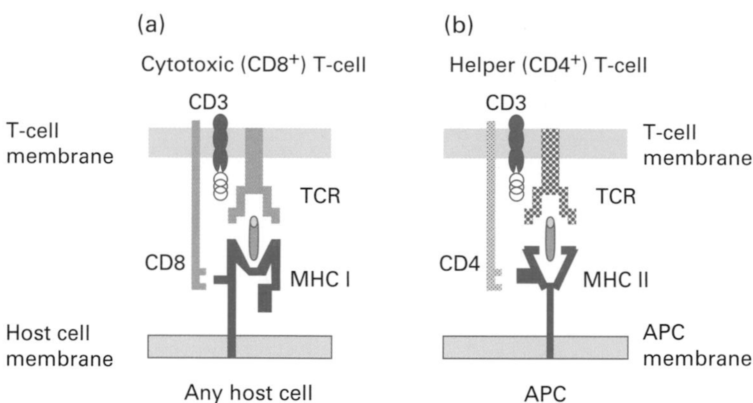

Figure 9.8 The process of MHC presentation of peptide and interaction with T-lymphocyte receptor (TCR). (a) Cytotoxic T-lymphocytes (CD8$^+$) interact with MHC I, while (b) helper T-lymphocytes (CD4$^+$) interact with MHC II. MHC, major histocompatibility complex; APC, antigen-presenting cell.

within the actual cell that eventually will present the peptide to cytotoxic T-lymphocytes. The MHC I molecule is composed of two polypeptide chains, an α-chain which has α1, α2 and α3 domains, and a second polypeptide termed β_2-microglobulin. The α1 and β2 domains form a peptide-binding cleft which can accommodate peptides up to 11 amino acids in length. Figure 9.9a shows the processing of a protein into peptide fragments for presentation by MHC I. The synthesised protein (indicated by an asterisk) is present in the cytoplasm of the cell and is degraded by a subcellular organelle termed a proteasome. The derived peptide fragments are actively transported, via a transporter associated with antigen processing (TAP) peptide transporter, into the lumen of the endoplasmic reticulum (ER) where they fit within the binding clefts of MHC I molecules. From the ER, the MHC I with bound peptide is transported to the trans-Golgi network (TGN), from which it is transported via endosomes to the plasma membrane where the MHC I molecule with bound peptide is accessible to surveillance by cytotoxic CD8$^+$ T-lymphocytes.

Peptide epitopes presented by MHC II are derived from proteins present within the extracellular fluid and are

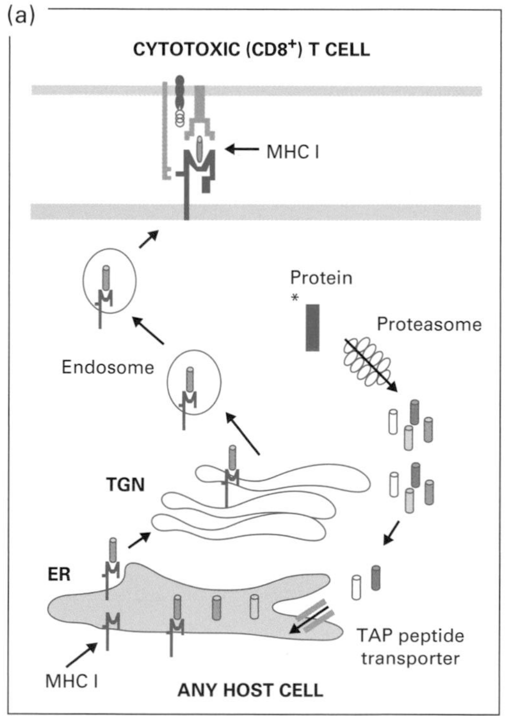

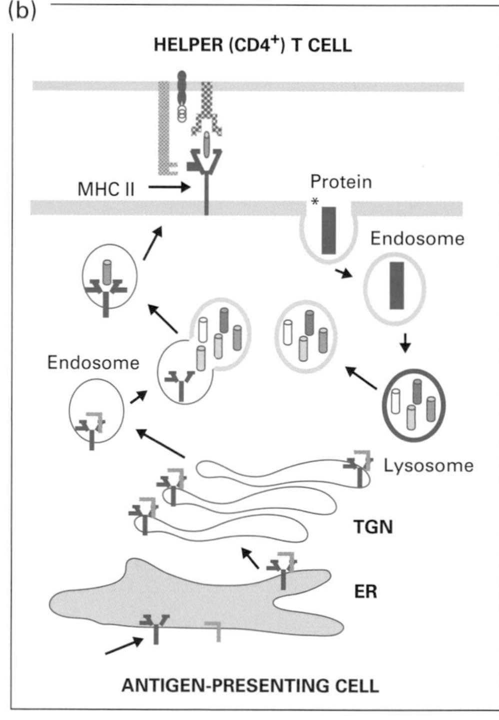

Figure 9.9 Schematic of the processing of a protein into peptide fragments for presentation by MHC. (a) The synthesised protein (*) is present in the cytoplasm of the cell and is degraded into peptide by the proteasome. The derived peptide fragments are presented by MHC I to cytotoxic CD8$^+$ T-lymphocytes. (b) Protein (*) is endocytosed by an antigen-presenting cell and processed into peptide within lysosomes. The derived peptide fragments are presented by MHC II to helper CD4$^+$ T-lymphocytes. MHC, major histocompatibility complex; TGN, trans-Golgi network; ER, endoplasmic reticulum.

presented to helper T-lymphocytes by APCs. The MHC II molecule is composed of two polypeptide chains, an α-chain which has α1 and α2 domains, and a β-chain which has β1 and β2 domains. The α1 and β1 domains form a peptide-binding cleft that can accommodate peptides up to 20 amino acids in length. Figure 9.9b shows the processing of a protein into peptide fragments for presentation by MHC II. In this case, the protein (indicated by an asterisk) is internalised from the extracellular fluid by the APC and restricted to an endosomal compartment without access to the APC's cytoplasm. The endosome delivers the protein to a lysosome compartment which degrades the protein into peptide fragments, after which the peptide fragments are returned to an endosome compartment. In the lumen of the ER, the MHC II molecule becomes associated with another protein termed an invariant chain which blocks access of peptides to the binding cleft of the MHC II molecule; the MHC II–invariant chain complex is transferred to the TGN and then to an endosomal compartment. At this point, the endosomes that contain the processed peptide and the MHC II molecules merge, and the invariant chain disintegrates, allowing peptides access to the MHC-II-binding cleft. The MHC II molecules with bound peptide are transported to the plasma membrane where they are accessible to surveillance by helper $CD4^+$ T-lymphocytes.

9.4.3 More on T-lymphocyte Subpopulations

9.4.3.1 Effector T-helper Cell Subtypes

Following maturation in the thymus, mature but naive $CD4^+$ helper T-cells access the systemic blood and lymphatic circulations. In this naive state, they have yet to be stimulated by antigen. The antigen-driven activation signals involve initially TCR interactions with MHC-presented peptide and subsequent CD3 activation. This is followed by the interaction of a variety of co-stimulatory molecules on the surface of the APC (e.g., CD80 and CD86) with surface receptors (e.g., CD28) on the helper T-cell. Once the helper T-cell is activated, it can proliferate in an autocrine or paracrine fashion driven by secreted IL-2. These proliferating helper T-cells will then differentiate depending on their cytokine environment; for example, IFN-γ and IL-12 drive the differentiation to a T_H1 subpopulation of cells, while IL-4 drives the differentiation to a T_H2 subpopulation of cells.

Apart from IL-2, the main cytokines produced by T_H1 cells are IFN-γ and TNF-β, and the main cell partner for T_H1 cells are the APCs. The T_H1 cells classically promote cell-mediated immune responses maximising the effectiveness of APCs and the proliferation of cytotoxic $CD8^+$ T-cells. Apart from IL-2, the main cytokines produced by T_H2 cells are IL-4, -5, -6, -10 and -13, while the main cell partner for T_H2 cells is the B-cell. The T_H2 cells classically promote the humoral immune responses stimulating B-cells to proliferate, to undergo Ig class switching and increase Ig production and secretion.

The above model of helper T-cell subpopulations and how various cytokines can serve to promote the differentiation pathway to either T_H1 or T_H2 phenotype is recognised to be an oversimplification. However, the basic model serves to emphasise that distinct populations of helper T-cells exist that fulfil many different and varied functions.

9.4.3.2 T-Regulatory Cells

T-regulatory cells (T_{regs}) are a subset of T-lymphocytes that serve an immune suppressor function leading to peripheral tolerance to self-antigens or foreign antigens. T_{regs} are characterised by a $CD4^+/CD8^-$ phenotype, but among a number of other identity markers that these cells display the expression of the Foxp3 transcription factor is the main distinguishing feature. T_{regs} are distinct from those effector T-cells which are induced to switch to secrete immunosuppressive cytokines, as a typical immune response progresses with time from an immunostimulatory to immunoinhibitory character. The T_{regs} represent approximately 10% of all $CD4^+$ T-cells and can acquire the immunosuppressive phenotype in the thymus or via induction in the periphery. In the thymus, this subset of $CD4^+$ T-cells is positively induced by interactions with MHC molecules and the recognition of agonist peptide. This contrasts to the situation for effector T-cells where TCR recognition in the thymus of MHC-presented peptide normally triggers the positive deletion of the affected T-cell. In particular, transforming growth factor (TGF)-β appears particularly important for the expression of the T_{regs} phenotype, while IL-2 as the key T-cell mitogen is also important.

T_{regs} essentially serve to suppress immune responses of effector T-cells, effector B-cells and APCs leading to peripheral immune tolerance. Direct cell–cell contact and cytokine signalling are mechanisms important in mediating their actions. These cells play an important role in self-limiting immune responses. T_{regs} display a number of disease associations, with decreased numbers of T_{regs} or reduced function in a range of autoimmune diseases. T_{regs} also appear to fulfil a role in the active immune evasion of tumours, with the experimental depletion of T_{regs} improving natural anti-tumour immunity and effectiveness of active immunotherapy.

9.4.3.3 γδ T-Cells

The vast majority of T-cells possess a TCR comprising two polypeptide chains, a single α-chain and a single β-chain.

$\gamma\delta$ T-cells possess a TCR made of a single γ-chain and a single δ-chain. The antigenic molecules or ligands that activate $\gamma\delta$ T-cells remain essentially unknown, although they appear not to require antigen processing or MHC presentation. These cells have characteristics of both innate and adaptive immune cells possessing a TCR, but also undergo early activation to become capable of phagocytosis and rapid production of cytokines that regulate inflammation and pathogen removal.

9.5 Some Clinical Perspectives

This section is intended to provide a brief overview of some clinical circumstances that exemplify the basic aspects of immune system function discussed previously.

9.5.1 Transplantation Rejection

Transplantation is the process of transferring cells, tissues or organs – termed a graft – from one location to another. An *autologous* graft is a transplant between two sites within the same individual, for example, skin graft from the thigh to the hand. An *allogeneic* graft is a transplant between two genetically different individuals of the same species, for example, kidney transplant from a donor to a recipient individual. A *xenogeneic* graft is a transplant across different species, for example, pig to human.

The tempo of clinical rejection – in kidney transplantation, for example – is often categorised by the following stages:

- *Hyperacute rejection* occurs within minutes to hours following revascularisation of a graft. The cause is due to the presence of preformed circulating antibody (IgG) that reacts with the blood cell antigens (the ABO blood grouping system), or MHC I molecules or other poorly defined antigens. This should now be a rare event clinically, as recipients are tested (cross-matched) before transplantation for the presence of antibodies reactive with cells of the donor.
- *Acute rejection* occurs within weeks to months following transplantation and involves humoral (antibody) and cell-mediated induced cytotoxicity. Damage may be reversed with early diagnosis and more aggressive immunosuppressive therapy.
- *Chronic rejection* occurs many months or even years following transplantation. The pathology is characterised by fibrosis and may require differential diagnosis to distinguish between a chronic rejection event and the recurrence of the original disease that necessitated transplantation in the first place.

The major alloantigens (i.e., antigens responsible for rejection of allogeneic grafts) are the MHC proteins. Although there are two distinct classes of MHC protein (described in Section 9.4.1), the MHC molecules actually have a number of subclasses which vary further in the general nature of peptides that they will accept within their binding clefts. The MHC I molecules are composed of three subclasses, MHC IA, MHC IB and MHC IC, on each nucleated cell of the body; all three subclasses are simultaneously expressed. The MHC II molecules are also made up of three subclasses, MHC II DR, MHC II DP and MHC II DQ, and again on each APC all three subclasses of MHC II molecule are simultaneously expressed. APCs, like other cells in the body, will also express MHC I molecules on their surface in addition to MHC II.

As indicated previously, the major cause of allogeneic tissue transplantation rejection is the polymorphic nature of the MHC phenotype between individuals. Polymorphism in the MHC arises within the population because the genes for each of the MHC subclasses can exist in multiple different forms or alleles. For example, in humans, there are at least 52 different forms of the MHC IB gene and at least 24 different forms of the MHC IA gene. It follows that individuals in a population can possess any one of the 52 different forms of MHC IB gene and any one of the 24 different forms of MHC IA gene, so the number of different combinations for the six classes of MHC proteins is many millions. The situation is further complicated by the fact that each individual inherits and co-expresses a set of MHC I and II genes from each parent. This means that on each nucleated cell of the body there will be co-expressed paternally derived and maternally derived versions of the MHC IA, MHC IB and MHC IC molecules. The same principle will apply for co-expression on APCs of paternal and maternal MHC II protein subclasses.

This tremendous polymorphism is important in immune defence because it allows the broadest possible scope of peptide antigen presentation, and thus the best chance of survival of a population as a whole, but it also confers the very high probability of MHC mismatch during allogeneic transplantation. As a result of the mode of MHC inheritance, the highest probability of an MHC tissue match between individuals who are not genetically identical twins will be that obtained between siblings, where there is a 1 in 4 chance of a sibling possessing an exact match for all the MHC I and MHC II subclasses. The MHC proteins are also termed human leucocyte antigens (HLA), and HLA tissue typing is undertaken routinely before transplantation to gain improved matches between donor and recipient. In kidney transplantation, it has been found that matching the MHC IA, IB and II DR genes in particular appears to improve short- and long-term graft survival.

The main target for the modern immunosuppressants such as cyclosporin and tacrolimus is inhibition of cytokine gene transcription in a highly selective manner in the helper T-lymphocyte populations. The consequence of this is to inhibit helper T-cell autoactivation and helper T-cell co-activation of cytotoxic T-lymphocytes and of B-lymphocytes, and thus considerably 'damp down' cell-mediated and humoral immune responses to the graft.

9.5.2 Hypersensitivity

Hypersensitivity can be defined as an exaggerated response of the immune system leading to host tissue damage. However, some of the immune responses described in the hypersensitivity classification below are, in some circumstances, appropriate responses to invading antigen. For example, a component in what is an appropriate immune response to tissue transplant rejection can be defined as a type II hypersensitivity reaction.

The highly influential Gell and Coombs classification scheme defines four categories of hypersensitivity.

- *Type I – immediate hypersensitivity:* this is also called anaphylactic or acute hypersensitivity. It involves IgE antibody and is mediated via degranulation of mast cells leading to release of preformed factors which promote an influx of immune cells to the site of mast cell activation and initiation of a rapid inflammatory reaction. In the extreme case, the inflammatory response extends beyond the localised site of initiation and affects systemic tissues leading to life-threatening anaphylactic reactions such as those documented to penicillin, to peanut antigen or to bee-sting antigen. Examples of localised type I hypersensitivity include hay fever. The term 'allergy' has become synonymous with type I hypersensitivity.
- *Type II hypersensitivity – antibody-mediated cytotoxicity:* this is caused by antibodies that are directed against cell surface antigens. IgG and IgM are the key antibodies involved that direct cytotoxic events against the cell surface with which they interact. The cytotoxic events include activation of the classical complement pathway leading to the formation of a MAC, and the attraction and activation of killing cells such as NK cells or phagocytes which can bind to the antigen–antibody complex via receptors for antibody Fc domains or complement C3b. Type II hypersensitivity disorders include blood transfusion reactions arising from mismatch of the blood ABO antigens between donor and recipient, or haemolytic disease of the newborn. Autoimmune disorders such as myasthenia gravis, Goodpasture syndrome and autoimmune haemolytic anaemias are initiated by autoantibodies reacting against 'self' tissue.
- *Type III hypersensitivity – complex-mediated:* this involves the formation of large antigen–antibody complexes that circulate in the blood, are usually coated by complement proteins and are removed by phagocytosis. If this process is compromised for any reason, then the antigen–antibody complexes will be deposited in tissue capillary beds, with kidney deposition being clinically the most important site. This deposition of high-molecular-weight antigen–antibody complexes in the glomerular capillaries of the kidney can lead to a condition termed glomerulonephritis which involves disruption of the glomerular basement membrane, destruction of glomeruli and ultimately renal failure which may necessitate organ transplantation. Systemic lupus erythematosus (SLE) is a condition where autoantibodies are directed against the host's DNA and RNA with subsequent complement-coated immune complexes deposited throughout systemic tissues such as in the kidney, skin, joints and brain.
- *Type IV hypersensitivity – cell-mediated:* this results from inappropriate accumulation of macrophages at a localised site, and may or may not involve the presence of antigen. Under conditions of ongoing localised infection or inflammation, macrophages release proteases, which destroy infected or otherwise damaged tissue. However, with the inappropriate recruitment and/or activation of excessive numbers of macrophages, continuing damage to normal tissue may result, leading to chronic inflammation. The recruitment and activation of macrophages in type IV hypersensitivity is augmented by the activity of helper T-lymphocytes (specifically the T_H1 subpopulation). Examples of type IV hypersensitivity include granuloma formation and contact dermatitis. Granulomas are initiated and maintained by the recruitment of macrophages into the site of a persistent source of antigen or toxic material. A granuloma is a fibrotic core of tissue composed of tissue cells and macrophages surrounded by lymphocytes and then further surrounded by layers of calcified collagenous material. Sarcoidosis is a granulomatous disease of unknown cause but characterised by granuloma nodule formation in the lung and skin, among other sites.

9.5.3 Autoimmunity

Autoimmunity is defined as an immune response against 'self' where the target is an autoantigen. The term 'autoimmune disease' by implication identifies autoimmunity as leading to pathology. Autoimmune disease is considered to be a disorder of adaptive immunity leading to the presence of autoreactive lymphocytes responding to self-antigens. Autoimmune disease ranges from organ-specific (e.g., thyroid, such as Hashimoto's thyroiditis) to non-organ-specific or systemic disease (e.g., SLE), which causes widespread inflammation and tissue damage affecting organs such as the joints, skin, lungs and kidneys. The development of autoimmunity reflects both the presence of susceptibility genes and environmental triggers (usually infections) and may be caused by different types of immune reactions (antibody- and/or T-cell-mediated), but fundamentally there is a loss of tolerance to 'self'.

Within the adaptive immune system, protective mechanisms at several levels prevent 'self-reactivity' responses from occurring, mechanisms which can be viewed as 'central' or 'peripheral' in nature. Here, 'central' refers to the induction of tolerance to self-antigens by the process of clonal elimination lymphocytes in the primary lymphoid organs (bone marrow and thymus). By contrast, peripheral induction of tolerance includes an array of mechanisms involving lymphocyte exposure (or failure of exposure) to self-antigen in non-activating form or the lack of the co-incidence of co-stimulatory signals in the environment of the self-antigen and potentially 'self-reactive' lymphocyte.

Clonal elimination through 'central' induction of tolerance involves thymus immature T-lymphocytes undergoing a process of positive and negative selection as part of their maturation. Positive selection involves the promotion of growth for those T- lymphocytes able to interact with MHC class I and II molecules on thymic epithelial cells, that is, T-lymphocytes that are CD8-/CD4-positive; T-lymphocytes lacking this interaction undergo deletion. The surviving clones are then subject to negative selection, involving the deletion of T- lymphocyte clones that recognise self-antigens expressed in conjunction with MHC class I or II molecules on thymic dendritic cells or macrophages. If a clonal T-lymphocyte interaction during this negative selection stage is of a high affinity, then that lymphocyte clone will be deleted by apoptosis; if the interaction is of low affinity, the T-lymphocyte clone may escape the negative selection and enter the periphery as mature fully functional lymphocytes. In the bone marrow, a comparative process of negative selection occurs for B-lymphocytes, where immature B-lymphocytes expressing surface IgM are exposed to multivalent self-antigens. If immunoglobulin cross-linking occurs at this stage, then apoptosis will be initiated. Autoreactive B-lymphocytes that escape this initial negative selection undergo mutational changes in 'antigen' receptor to further minimise autoreactivity. B-lymphocytes escaping these processes enter the periphery as mature fully functional lymphocytes.

Although the vast majority of autoreactive lymphocyte clones are removed during the establishment of central tolerance, it is peripheral mechanisms regulating the reactivity of potentially 'self-reactive' clones that have escaped to the periphery which are a particular focus in the aetiology and predisposition of autoimmune disease. The peripheral induction of tolerance is termed 'anergy', and when applied to specific lymphocyte clones, 'clonal anergy'. Peripheral anergy can occur by occupation of lymphocyte receptors by 'self-antigen', but in a non-activating form such as the presence of soluble antigen that renders lymphocytes unresponsive or marks them for apoptosis; for example, B-cells responding to self-antigen in the periphery usually undergo Fas-mediated apoptosis or become anergic. Further, self-antigens may occupy lymphocyte receptors but simply fail to be activated due to the presence of T_{regs} or the lack of appropriate co-stimulatory signals such as cytokines, or failure in engagement with activated immune cells or the presence of anergic effector cells. While the processes promoting peripheral anergy will be more complex than described here (see, for instance, Actor, 2019), failure in any one of the multiple regulatory mechanisms may lead to self-destructive immune responses.

Fundamentally, most autoimmune diseases arise from overcoming peripheral anergy, with disease generally considered to arise through one or more of the following:

Infectious-/damage-/stress-induced inflammation: inflammation, whatever the cause, is considered a key contributor in the development of autoimmune disease. Here, the inflammatory environment may allow peripheral anergy to be overcome. For example, inflammation may reverse the functionality of anergic antigen-presenting cells which would otherwise fail to provide the necessary co-stimulation to an autoreactive lymphocyte. Alternatively, the inflammatory environment may change the balance of T_{regs} to $T_{effectors}$, the latter including autoreactive clones or anergic autoreactive lymphocytes. The impact here would be conversion to an autoresponsive state.

Molecular mimicry by microbial antigens: here, an infecting microorganism presents an antigen within which an epitope exists that closely resembles an epitope within the host, this host epitope being part of a 'self-antigen' (i.e., a host protein against which self-reacting lymphocytes exist in the periphery but where anergy against this self-antigen is observed). Significantly, however, the infection presents high amounts of the respective microbial cross-reactive epitope with accompanying inflammation; taken together, this may overcome the peripheral anergy and allow lymphocyte autoreactivity to occur and progress. Once primed by the microbial antigen, a high avidity lymphocyte autoreaction could be chronically stimulated. Such a circumstance might follow infection with certain strains of group A streptococcal bacteria. These bacteria express a cell wall protein resembling an epitope found in the human protein myosin. Autoreactive lymphocytes then attack heart muscle and valves among other tissues with the condition following a relapsing/remitting pattern. 'Epitope spreading' (see below) has a role in persistence, with the inflammation and tissue damage expanding autoimmune epitopes in other proteins such as collagen and laminin.

Defects in immune regulation: here, innate defects in a patient's immune function and regulation exist that undermine the ability to maintain the state of peripheral anergy. Broadly, such defects can extend from cellular deficiencies such as reduced numbers of T_{regs} or antigen-presenting cells, through changes in the expression and responsiveness of immune cell surface molecules (e.g., MHC molecules or receptors necessary to mediate peripheral apoptosis or anergy), to abnormalities in cytokine production and function.

Alterations in the state of 'immunologic silence': this is also referred to as 'epitope spreading' and describes the process whereby new epitopes previously hidden from autoimmune attack (physically sequestered or processed by antigen-presenting cells only in very low amounts insufficient to activate central deletion or peripheral anergy) become accessible at higher levels. This is considered to occur by damage-induced exposure to tissue which then reveals to the immune system the respective 'self-antigen' together with an appropriate inflammatory environment. For example, pemphigus is a disease that causes blisters and sores on the skin or mucous membranes. Autoantibodies in pemphigus are directed against desmogleins, a family of desmosomal cadherins key to cell–cell adhesion. Initially, the target is the autoantigen desmoglein-3 which gives rise to blistering in the mucosal membranes of the mouth. Immune attack on desmoglein-3 primes an immune response against the related skin isoform desmoglein-1 with patients then experiencing blistering of the skin.

Among many other factors, genetics clearly has some role in the predisposition to autoimmune disease, with some conditions showing a much stronger genetic correlation than others. Both HLA and non-HLA genes are associated with autoimmune disease; however, and not surprisingly given their role in antigen presentation to T-lymphocytes, evidence linking predisposition and autoimmunity is much stronger for the HLA genes. For example, HLA-B8 and HLA-DR3 are common in organ-specific autoimmune disease; type 1 diabetes has a greater association with HLA-DR3, -DR4, -DQ2 and -DQ8 alleles; rheumatoid arthritis with HLA-DR4 allele; Graves' disease with HLA-DR3 and Hashimoto's thyroiditis with HLA-DR3 and -DR5 alleles. Quite remarkable is that greater than 90% of Caucasian patients with ankylosing spondylitis (AS) express an HLA-B27 allele. Some of the most studied autoimmune diseases are briefly described below.

Rheumatoid arthritis is caused by an autoimmunity against antigens in the synovial tissue and cartilage of joints and against the patient's own IgG molecules. Indeed, a distinctive feature is the presence of 'rheumatoid factor' within the patient's plasma and synovial spaces. Rheumatoid factor is a collection of autoantibodies directed against the Fc domain of the patient's own IgG molecules. Immune complex formation and activation of the innate immune components, and of macrophages, dendritic cells and $CD4^+$ and $CD8^+$ T-lymphocytes, lead to further immune cell extravasation into the joints with elevated levels of pro-inflammatory cytokines, for example, TNF-α and destructive proteases, all of which perpetuate inflammation. As the condition progresses, cartilage destruction and bone erosion bring deformity to joints and disability.

AS is an autoimmune process with chronic inflammatory disease of bone and joints, particularly the vertebral joints of the spine. The vertebral joints in AS patients contain raised numbers of lymphocytes and antigen-presenting cells. In the autoimmune attack, the collagen of the joints is destroyed and the fibrocartilage then progressively ossifies with the replacement bone causing the vertebrae to fuse, thereby damaging the spinal column and compromising patient mobility.

Type 1 diabetes mellitus occurs where there is an autoimmune driven loss or dysfunction in pancreatic beta cells that produce insulin. As a consequence, the body's processing of glucose is affected and glucose cannot enter into cells effectively, causing blood glucose levels to rise. When diabetes is chronically poorly controlled, vascular damage ensues which can result in vision loss, kidney failure and damage to the heart and nerves and peripheral blood flow which can lead to tissue necrosis. Autoimmune attack on insulin-producing beta cells is caused by autoantibodies and autoreactive T-cells recognising epitopes of the beta cell enzyme, glutamic acid decarboxylase and the protein tyrosine phosphatase IA-2. The functionality of T_{reg} cells is also considered compromised with effector T-lymphocytes more resistant to T_{reg}-cell-mediated suppression.

Multiple sclerosis (MS) is an autoimmune disease primarily affecting the brain and spinal cord. Autoreactive T-lymphocytes target the myelin sheath, for example, myelin basic protein, proteolipid protein and myelin oligodendrocyte glycoprotein, resulting in nerve demyelination, inflammation and axonal injury and loss. MS patients experience chronic, progressive widespread sensory impairment, motor weakness and disability. Molecular mimicry may have a role with the epitope of an Epstein–Barr virus protein resembling an epitope in myelin basic protein.

Myasthenia gravis is an autoimmune disease that leads to progressive severe muscle weakness caused by autoantibodies against acetylcholine (ACH) receptors in motor-end plates of neuromuscular junctions. These autoantibodies can bind to the ACH receptor serving as blocking or antagonist antibodies preventing the binding of ACH to its cognate receptor and hence failure of the muscle to respond to normal neuronal impulses which then leads to progressive muscle weakness.

Autoimmune thyroiditis comprises two major types: Graves' disease which is an autoimmune hyperthyroidism and Hashimoto's disease which is an autoimmune hypothyroidism. The thyroid gland bears receptors (TSH-R) for thyroglobulin stimulating hormone (TSH). The interior surface of the thyroid is filled with thyroid colloid – mainly thyroglobulin and the membrane-bound enzyme, thyroid peroxidase (TPO). TSH interacts with TSH-R to upregulate the activity of TPO which in conjunction with thyroglobulin leads to the synthesis of thyroxine (T4) or triiodothyronine (T3), the thyroid hormones; these are then released into the circulation and contribute to the control of the body's metabolic rate.

In Hashimoto's thyroiditis, thyroglobulin and TPO are the two major antigens. Anti-thyroglobulin antibodies are found in 95% of patients with Hashimoto's disease, a condition with effects ranging from subclinical disease to complete destruction of the thyroid gland. It is characterised by the presence of autoantibodies in the thyroid, and in some cases organ infiltration with NK cells and autoreactive T-lymphocytes that facilitate autodestruction of the thyroid tissue. The clinical picture is that associated with insufficient thyroid hormone production with symptoms of fatigue, depression, goitre (thyroid enlarged in size) and weight gain. Biochemically, the profile is one of raised plasma TSH with low T3 and T4 levels.

In Graves' disease, autoantibodies against the TSH-R act as an agonist, leading to excessive stimulation and overactivation of the thyroid gland and the overproduction of thyroid hormones. Biochemically, the profile is one of suppressed TSH, raised T4 and T3, and antibodies against the TSH-R receptor. Clinically, patients display symptoms of hyperthyroidism, including weight loss, increased metabolism, hand tremors, palpitations, insomnia and fatigue. A classic physical symptom (for 50% of patients) is a change in the eye socket orbit, exophthalmos or 'protruding eyes', believed to be caused by an interaction between the receptor antibodies and epitopes on the orbital fat tissue.

Autoimmune haemolytic anaemia arises where autoantibodies against antigens found on red blood cells (RBCs) result in RBC destruction leading to haemolysis. There are two RBC cell surface antigens that serve as targets, the rhesus antigens (Rh antigens) targeted by IgG autoantibodies and which account for the vast majority of cases, and the surface I antigen targeted by IgM autoantibodies. Primary autoimmune haemolytic anaemia is where there is no link to any other condition, whereas in secondary disease there is a link such as to rheumatoid arthritis, SLE, Hashimoto's thyroiditis or other conditions which affect the immune system. Certain infections and drugs (e.g., penicillins and erythromycin) can also trigger autoimmune haemolytic anaemia which remits once the inciting intervention is removed.

SLE involves autoantibodies against a range of targets including DNA and ribonuclear proteins and histone nucleolar antigens. The high levels of 'antinuclear' autoantibodies are a characteristic of the pathology. Autoantibodies also exist against non-nuclear targets, which is indicative of polyclonal lymphocyte stimulation with abnormalities in B-lymphocyte regulation rather than antigen-specific activation of an abnormal clone(s) of autoreactive lymphocytes. These autoantibodies form immune complexes that eventually deposit or target tissues triggering inflammation and tissue damage. The condition is one of a chronic remitting/relapsing multisystem autoimmune disease with clinical manifestations that include skin rashes (vasculitis), arthritis, glomerulonephritis, possibly also haemolytic anaemia and thrombocytopenia. Multiple elements of the immune system can be disrupted in SLE patients with individuals more vulnerable to opportunistic infections.

9.5.4 Therapeutic Monoclonal Antibodies

Therapeutic antibodies belong to the group of medicinal products termed 'biologics' or biopharmaceuticals which also includes enzymes, hormones, cytokines, clotting factors and vaccines. Year-on-year biological products make up a growing proportion of new medicinal products approved. Development times for biologics are similar to, or possibly shorter than, those for small-molecule drugs and their probability of success (POS) is good, for example, 20–25% of preclinical stage biologics survive to market stage. However, quality control measures are often more challenging and rigorous for therapeutic proteins to avoid errors introduced during manufacturing, for example, unintended glycosylation, methylation or phosphorylation or a structural change that could alter the molecule's activity in the body (see also Chapter 23). Biologics also display potential for immunogenicity with severe adverse effects. Therapeutic antibodies consistently show a significant presence in the yearly top 10 global sales of drugs.

Following their description in Section 9.1.2, a monoclonal antibody preparation is one within which all of the contained antibodies recognise only a single common epitope, that is, a common single specific amino acid sequence or pattern. In other words, they are from the same clonal origin. By contrast, a polyclonal antibody preparation is one where the antibodies are a heterogeneous

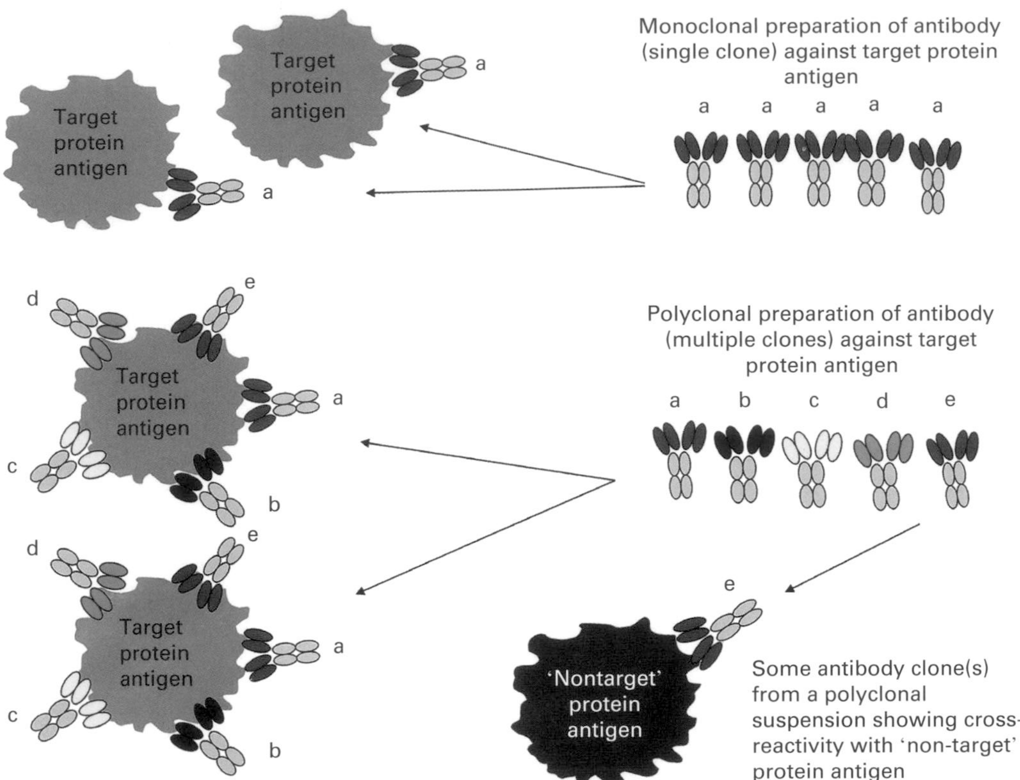

Figure 9.10 Schematic showing the distinction between monoclonal and polyclonal preparations and their epitope-specific binding to target and non-target antigens. Each letter refers to a different antibody clone. Both monoclonal and polyclonal preparations can bind to the desired target protein. However, with a polyclonal mixture, there is a greater probability a clone(s) may also bind to non-target protein with resultant adverse effects.

mix of different antibody clones: here, each clone recognises its own distinct epitope while still nominally recognising the same protein antigen (Figure 9.10).

The advantage of a monoclonal antibody preparation includes greater batch-to-batch reproducibility and high specificity with reduced cross-reactivity to non-target protein antigen. Polyclonal antibodies, however, can have an overall higher affinity of binding to antigen simply due to multiple different putative epitopes in the target protein, although there is also a greater chance of cross-reactivity to non-target proteins, a feature less conducive to their use as therapeutic agents.

The ability to manufacture monoclonal antibodies by means of large-scale tissue culture cell lines (hybridoma technology) was first described by Köhler and Milstein in 1975. Their transformational work derived a number of cell lines secreting anti-sheep red blood cell antibodies. The cell lines were made by the fusion of mouse myeloma and spleen cells harvested from the same immunised mouse donor. Therapeutic monoclonal antibodies now represent the fastest-growing pharmaceutical development sector. From the first therapeutic monoclonal antibody approved in 1986, and indicated for the reversal of kidney transplant rejection (muromonab-CD3, Orthoclone OKT3®), to June 2021, there have been 105 therapeutic monoclonal antibody approvals in the USA and/or Europe with approximately 40% of these approvals targeting malignant disease. A few hundred more monoclonal antibodies are in clinical trial for a range of diseases from cancer to immune/inflammatory conditions. The suffix for all monoclonal antibodies is 'mab', but beyond this there is a uniform naming nomenclature (International Nonproprietary Names – INN) for all therapeutic monoclonal antibodies in a system overseen by the WHO, last updated in 2017.

Beyond the nature of the target and of the constant region of the mAb, for example, the IgG isoform, there are a number of different general types of mAbs determined by their overall mouse to human composition. Specifically:

- *Murine mAbs*: murine (mouse) mAbs represent the first type of mAb approved and exemplified by the approval in 1986 of muromonab-CD3, and later by the anti-CD20 murine mAbs which covalently bind therapeutic radionuclide, e.g., ibritumomab (2002, 2004) which is indicated for non-Hodgkin lymphoma. Of the 105 mAbs approved by June 2021, just six are of the murine type.

The major issue with murine antibodies is their reduced ability to elicit effector functions through engagement of the murine mAb Fc domain with human Fc IgG receptors (FcγR) present on host effector cells. Further, murine mAbs exhibit a significantly greater risk of eliciting a hypersensitivity immune response in the patient, that is, the murine mAb itself serving as an immunogen. These issues bring a high risk of failure in clinical development, with murine mAbs only being progressed for the most serious conditions and where effective treatment represents an unmet medical need. Notwithstanding these constraints, murine mAbs continue to be developed and approved, e.g., inolimomab, whose target is IL-2Rα indicated for graft versus host disease, and omburtamab, a radionuclide conjugated to I^{131} indicated for central nervous system (CNS)/leptomeningeal metastases from neuroblastoma.

Subsequent evolutions in mAb technologies have been directed towards reducing therapeutic antibody immunogenicity through reduced composition of murine sequences while maintaining antibody effectiveness for antigen interaction. These innovations in antibody type include chimeric, humanised and fully human mAbs.

- *Chimeric mAbs:* chimeric (mouse/human) mAbs involve modification to the original hybridoma technology whereby genetic engineering affords substitution of the original murine mAb constant regions with sequences from human immunoglobulin. Abciximab (1994/1995) targeting GPIIb/IIa for the prevention of blood clots in angioplasty was the first chimeric approved, followed by rituximab (anti-CD20; non-Hodgkin lymphoma, 1997/1998), basiliximab (anti-IL-2R; prevention of kidney transplant rejection, 1998) and infliximab (anti-TNF; Crohn's disease, 1998/1999). Of the 105 mAbs approved by June 2021, 11 are of the chimeric type.
- *Humanised mAbs:* humanised (human/mouse) mAbs involve grafting the murine complementarity-determining regions (CDRs) into a human immunoglobulin framework. Humanisation has reduced the immunogenicity associated with murine mAbs. The antigen affinity of this more radical mAb change is maintained by advances in protein engineering involving computational-guided modelling, the selection of human frameworks capable of supporting murine CDRs when bound to antigen and by 'framework shuffling' involving the murine CDRs fused into pools of human framework sequences which are then screened for affinity binding. Examples of these mAbs include some generally well-known agents, such as: trastuzumab (Herceptin®) (1998/2000), targeting human epidermal growth factor receptor 2 (HER2) and used in breast cancer, and bevacizumab (Avastin®) (2004/2005), targeting vascular endothelial growth factor (VEGF) and indicated for colorectal cancer and glioblastoma. Interestingly, as opposed to the almost universal adoption of the IgG antibody class for full length mAbs, this technology has supported the development of the IgE mAb, omalizumab (2003/2005), used in asthma. Of the 105 approved mAbs mentioned earlier, 50 are of the humanised type.
- *Human mAbs:* human mAbs contain exclusively human sequences and can be generated by transgenic animal technologies, that is, animals such as mice containing a human immunoglobulin germ-line locus, and which, following the respective immunisation of antigen, result in a human antibody response and the capacity to generate *in vitro* hybridomas that produce human antibodies. Alternatively, the technology of phage display (see Chapter 24) can be exploited whereby a library of phage virus is created, and within which each member of the library expresses a unique human antibody variable or Fab region; the diversity of such libraries can be very high, e.g., 10^8 and above. Through the process of *in vitro* biopanning of this phage library against the target antigen (multiple rounds are performed), the antigen-interacting antibody(s) can be enriched and sequenced, which then allows for the genetic engineering of the selected sequences into a suitable human immunoglobulin framework. Of the 105 approved mAbs (June 2021), 38 are of the human type. This type includes adalimumab (Humira®; 2002/2003), the third anti-TNF mAb to be approved which is indicated for a range of chronic/immune inflammatory conditions including rheumatoid arthritis, Crohn's disease and plaque psoriasis. Another example is denosumab, targeting the receptor activator of nuclear factor kappa-β ligand (RANK-L) and used in bone loss as therapy to reduce osteoclast bone resorption. In June 2021, the human mAb aducanumab was approved in the USA by the Food and Drug Administration (FDA) for Alzheimer's disease. Aducanumab binds to aggregated forms of beta-amyloid and recognises amyloid plaques in brain tissue. It was originally derived from cognitively normal healthy aged donors under the rationale of 'reverse translational medicine' whereby antibodies from healthy donors will in some way offer protective actions to efficiently reduce amyloid deposition in the brain.

A further innovation in antibody therapeutics is the development of bispecific antibodies that recognise within the single antibody molecule two distinct antigen targets, that is, a distinct antigen for each of the antibody's (IgG) Fab arms (Figure 9.4). An example of this approach is emicizumab which recognises simultaneously coagulation factors IXa and X, and by binding both promotes their spatial approximation and downstream activation of factor X, thereby mimicking the actions of the clotting cascade. Yet a further adaptation is Roche's 'Brain Shuttle' approach to conjugate to a therapeutic human antibody, gantenerumab, a vector that enhances the transfer of the antibody across the blood–brain barrier (BBB). Gantenerumab binds to aggregated forms of beta-amyloid to promote plaque clearance from the brain parenchyma. The 'Brain Shuttle' vector is conjugated to the Fc domain (Figure 9.4) of the therapeutic antibody and has specificity for the transferrin receptor. This receptor is expressed at high levels in the brain microvascular endothelium and naturally traffics iron-laden transferrin protein from the cerebral capillaries to the brain parenchyma via a receptor-mediated endocytosis process; this brain shuttle gantenerumab is in clinical trial. Recently, a mAb cocktail (casirivimab and imdevimab) has been authorised for emergency coronavirus disease (COVID)-19 pandemic use in 20 countries to reduce the risk of death in patients unable to mount an effective immune response. This mAb combination comprises two virus-neutralising antibodies which bind non-competitively to the receptor-binding domain of the severe acute respiratory syndrome-coronavirus disease-2 (SARS-CoV-2) virus spike protein, also reducing the ability of mutant viruses to avoid treatment. Continued authorisation in some countries has now become subject to demonstrable efficacy against new viral variants.

Almost all of the currently approved mAbs are full-length antibodies that retain the Fc antibody domain. The presence of the Fc domain (Figure 9.4) enables full-length antibodies to bind to microvascular FcRn (the neonatal Fc receptor, which contrary to the name is expressed in adult tissues) through which the antibody will undergo non-destructive recycling within the endothelial cell to return back to the plasma. This recycling facilitates the prolonged elimination half-life of full-length antibodies of typically 21 days, and which clearly is critical for the less frequent (e.g., 2–4 weeks) parenteral administration of therapeutic antibodies. Nevertheless, therapeutic engineered antibody fragments are of interest where the removed antibody elements include the entire constant region (leaving the therapeutic variable fragments Fv alone) or the whole of the Fc domain (leaving the therapeutic Fab domain alone), and in some cases antibody fragments are made from engineering completely new structures (e.g., diabodies and minibodies). Approved antibody fragments include: blinatumomab (2014/2015), a bispecific murine single-chain variable fragment (scFv) against CD19 and CD3 and indicated for acute lymphoblastic leukaemia; ranibizumab (2006/2007), a humanised Fab fragment, and brolucizumab (2019/2020), a humanised scFV fragment, both raised against VEGF-A and indicated for some forms of age-related macular degeneration; and caplacizumab (2018/2019), a humanised bivalent single-domain antibody comprising just two linked variable heavy (V_H) chains that target von Willebrand factor (VWF), indicated for acquired thrombotic thrombocytopenic purpura. Engineered therapeutic antibody fragments are beneficial where the mechanism of action does not depend on the Fc-domain, which itself can lead to an inappropriate activation of Fc receptor-bearing cells and to significant unsafe cytokine release. Further, the reduced size of the antibody fragment will facilitate tissue access, and fragments can also be of value in imaging applications where the long elimination half-life of the full-length antibody can lead to poor tissue contrast.

As generic drugs are to the development of low-molecular-weight drugs, then biosimilars are to the development of biologics. A 'biosimilar' is a biological medicine highly similar to another biological medicine already approved – a form of generic medicine. Biosimilars show high similarity in terms of primary, secondary and tertiary structures, in biological activity and efficacy and in the safety and immunogenicity profile. There may be minor differences in components, for example, in the exact glycosylation level, but these cannot be clinically meaningful, that is, there can be no differences in safety and efficacy. Biosimilars are approved according to the same standards of pharmaceutical quality, safety and efficacy as all biological medicines. Biosimilar competition can offer advantages to healthcare organisations by improving patients' access to safe and effective biological medicines with proven quality. Biosimilar mAbs are developed as the patents expire on existing products.

9.5.5 Immunosuppressants

Immunosuppressants are commonly used for managing autoimmune disease and organ/tissue transplantation. Early immunosuppressive agents, such as corticosteroids, azathioprine and cyclophosphamide, demonstrated significant toxicities arising from their lack of molecular target specificity in respect to the adaptive immune response and in particular T-/B-lymphocyte activation and function including interactions with other immune cells. A major advance in the field was realised with the discovery of the calcineurin inhibitor cyclosporin, isolated from the fungal species *Tolypocladium inflatum*, which significantly improved transplantation success rates. During the 1990s, increased understanding of T-/B-lymphocyte function, chemokine and cytokine signalling and complement pathways resulted in the discovery of novel immunosuppressants including humanised/chimeric anti-CD25 monoclonal antibodies targeting interleukin-2 on activated T-lymphocytes, the mechanistic target of rapamycin (mTOR) inhibitors sirolimus and everolimus, as well as purine antimetabolites such as mycophenolate mofetil. The 1990s also saw the implementation of triple therapy approaches to improve transplant graft survival and mitigate rejection, for example, in a combination of corticosteroids, mycophenolate and cyclosporin.

9.5.5.1 Calcineurin Inhibitors

Calcineurin inhibitors remain the mainstay of immunosuppressive therapy. In the UK, there are two licensed agents cyclosporin and tacrolimus. Cyclosporin, licensed in 1983, was the first in class to be discovered and was identified to have immunosuppressive action in a mouse model without effects on tumour growth, that is, not linked with cytostatic activity. Cyclosporin was the first immunosuppressant to modulate defined subpopulations of immunocompetent cells. Tacrolimus, licensed in 1994, is a macrolide antibiotic and has similar immunosuppressive properties to cyclosporin. Both cyclosporin and tacrolimus inhibit T-lymphocyte production of IL-2 together with other factors that promote the immune response. IL-2 in particular is a key target, as it is a primary T-lymphocyte mitogen. Cyclosporin and tacrolimus bring about their effects by inhibition of the cytoplasmic enzyme calcineurin. Calcineurin dephosphorylates the cytoplasmic component of the nuclear factor of activated T-lymphocytes (NFATc) promoting nuclear transport of NFATc where it binds its nuclear component, nuclear factor of activated T-lymphocytes (NFATn). The NFATn complex serves as a transactivator promoting the transcription of, among other factors, IL-2.

While similar in mechanism of action, tacrolimus and cyclosporin are chemically unrelated with some differences in the adverse effect profile. For example, both agents are associated with nephrotoxicity (although this is more marked with cyclosporin), neurotoxicity (more marked with tacrolimus) and hirsutism (more marked with cyclosporin). Further, disturbances of glucose metabolism/tolerance are a feature of tacrolimus. For both agents, therapeutic drug monitoring is essential to maximise outcomes and prevent toxicity given their narrow therapeutic index. Both agents are metabolised by CYP450 3A4 and therefore these agents are potentially exposed to many drug–drug interactions.

9.5.5.2 Corticosteroids

Corticosteroids, produced in the adrenal cortex, are steroid hormones. There are two main classes of corticosteroids, glucocorticoids and mineralocorticoids, and they are involved in a diverse range of physiological functions with the glucocorticoids implicated in stress and immune response. Synthetic analogues showing preferential and increased glucocorticoid activity have been developed for a wide range of anti-inflammatory and immunosuppressive purposes. Methylprednisolone for example is given at induction to all transplant patients followed by prednisolone for maintenance. Corticosteroids exert their action by binding to intracellular glucocorticoid receptors leading to modulation of the immune response primarily associated with inhibition of cytokine transcription. When corticosteroids bind to their cognate cytoplasmic glucocorticoid receptor, they form a complex that translocates to the nucleus and forms a ligand-occupied glucocorticoid receptor dimer. These dimers bind to glucocorticoid response elements present on glucocorticoid-sensitive genes to activate or inhibit transcription of key factors such as the inhibition of nuclear factor kappa-B (NF-κB) and activator protein-1. As a consequence, corticosteroids suppress key inflammatory proteins including IL-1 and IL-2, thereby inhibiting lymphocyte clonal expansion, and TNF-α, which precipitates a decline in macrophage and neutrophil activity. The long-term use of corticosteroids is not without its complications, leading to a diverse range of adverse effects including a Cushingoid state, gastrointestinal (GI) disturbances, hyperlipidaemia, diabetes, mood alterations and reductions in bone density.

9.5.5.3 Janus Kinase Inhibitors

Janus kinases (JAK) are a family of cytoplasmic non-receptor tyrosine kinases transducing cytokine-mediated signals via the JAK–signal transducer and activator of transcription (STAT) pathway. This pathway is associated with a variety of conditions including cancer and disorders of the immune system. Tofacitinib, an inhibitor of JAK1 and JAK3, is licensed in the UK for the treatment of moderate to severe rheumatoid arthritis and in the USA for ulcerative colitis. It inhibits the activation of several cytokines including IL-2, -4, -7, -9, -15 and -21.

9.5.5.4 mTor Inhibitors

mTOR, the mechanistic target of rapamycin, is a signalling node within the phosphatidylinositol 3-kinase-related family of protein kinases and plays an important role in cell growth and proliferation in response to nutrients. mTOR inhibitors are used as immunosuppressive agents in transplantation and as anti-cancer agents. In the UK, sirolimus is the archetype mTOR inhibitor licensed for maintenance immunosuppression. Sirolimus is a macrolide-like compound that inhibits the mTOR pathway blocking the G1–S phase of the cell cycle. From an immunosuppressive perspective, mTOR inhibitors have actions in lymphocytes and monocytes/macrophages, dendritic cells and natural killer cells. Sirolimus binds to the cytosolic protein FK-binding protein 12 and the resultant complex inhibits the mTOR pathway by binding to mTOR complex 1. In renal transplantation, sirolimus is as effective as cyclosporin in preventing acute rejection and prolonging graft survival, and does not display nephrotoxicity except in combination with calcineurin inhibitors. However, it can delay wound healing and is generally initiated 3 months post surgery and only where intolerance to calcineurin is exhibited. In common with cyclosporin, sirolimus is metabolised by CYP450 3A4 and therefore is susceptible to a variety of drug–drug interactions.

9.5.5.5 Antimetabolites

Azathioprine, a prodrug of 6-mercaptopurine, has been used clinically since the 1950s as an antimetabolite. The metabolites of 6-mercaptopurine are thioguanine nucleotides and they act as purine analogues inhibiting the conversion of inosine monophosphate to adenine and guanine nucleotides. Ultimately, this reduces DNA and RNA synthesis blocking the proliferation of lymphocytes. In addition, the metabolites act as immunomodulatory agents blocking S–G2 cell cycling. Elimination of 6-mercaptopurine is via xanthine oxidase and inhibitors of this enzyme such as allopurinol exacerbate toxicities associated with azathioprine such as bone marrow suppression. The use of azathioprine has largely been superseded with the introduction of mycophenolate mofetil, a prodrug of mycophenolic acid. Mycophenolic mofetil is an inhibitor of inosine monophosphate dehydrogenase which catalyses the synthesis of guanine nucleotides. Unlike other rapidly dividing cells, lymphocytes do not have alternative pathways for producing guanosine nucleotides and therefore mycophenolate mofetil selectively inhibits lymphocyte proliferation.

Beyond the low-molecular-weight immunosuppressive agents highlighted above, monoclonal therapeutic antibodies (mAbs) have an increasing role in immunosuppression, targeting surface receptors on immune cells or autocrine, paracrine and endocrine cytokine signalling (see Section 9.5.4).

9.6 Summary

The immune system is a complex body system whose various functions display a high level of inter-regulation. As such, any attempt to describe the functioning of the immune system within a single chapter will inevitably represent an oversimplification. However, the authors consider this chapter to be a comprehensive, but nevertheless basic, overview of the immune system that will serve as a sound foundation for further reading on the clinical immunological basis of disease or for the consultation of more specialised texts on immunological function.

The discussion in this chapter is structured by delineating the immune system into innate and adaptive responses. The innate system, responding immediately but non-specifically to antigen, is complementary to the adaptive immune system which reacts in a highly specific manner to antigen but which displays a delay in its response. It should not be forgotten, however, that the two systems in terms of their respective functioning are intimately related, showing dependency on each other for the optimal maintenance of health.

Dedication

To Dr Jim Furr (1935–2021), a Cardiff University alumnus and retired lecturer in the School of Pharmacy and Pharmaceutical Sciences, whose teaching in immunology inspired many generations of pharmacists.

Reference

Actor, J.K. (2019). *Introductory Immunology: Basic Concepts for Interdisciplinary Applications*, 2e. Cambridge, Massachusetts: Academic Press.

Further Reading

Abbas, A.K., Lichtman, A.H. and Pillai, S. (2017). *Cellular and Molecular Immunology*, 9e. Amsterdam: Elsevier. (Strong on experimental observations that form the basis for the science of immunology at the molecular, cellular, and whole-organism levels, and the resulting conclusions.).

Delves, P.J., Martin, S.J., Burton, D.R. and Roitt, I.M. (2017). *Roitt's Essential Immunology*, 13e. Oxford: Wiley-Blackwell (Classic introductory text).

Deske, M. and Prinz, I. (2020). Ligand recognition by the γδ TCR and discrimination between homeostasis and stress conditions. *Cell. Mol. Immunol.* 17: 914–924.

Hansen, J., Baum, A., Pascal, K.E. et al. (2020). Studies in humanized mice and convalescent humans yield a SARS-CoV-2 antibody cocktail. *Science* 369: 1010–1014.

Köhler, G. and Milstein, C. (1975) Continuous cultures of fused cells secreting antibody of predefined specificity. *Nature* 256: 495–497.

O'Garra, A. and Arai, N. (2000). The molecular basis of T-helper 1 and T-helper 2 cell differentiation. *Trends Cell Biol.* 10: 542–550. (Overview of cytokine regulation of helper T-cell differentiation into T_H1 and T_H2 subpopulations, and the effector functions of the subpopulations.).

Parkin, J. and Cohen, B. (2001). An overview of the immune system. *Lancet.* 357: 1777–1789.

Playfair, J.H.L. and Chain, B.M. (2012). *Immunology at a Glance*, 10e. Oxford: Wiley-Blackwell. (Pictorial based primer for immunological novices.).

Saravia, J., Chapman, N.M. and Chi, H. (2019). Helper T-cell differentiation. *Cell. Mol. Immunol.* 16: 634–643.

The Antibody Society. Antibody therapeutics approved or in regulatory review in the EU or US. https://www.antibodysociety.org/resources/approved-antibodies. (A useful resource documenting and supporting antibody-related research development and listing pending reviews and approvals).

10

Vaccination and Immunisation

Gavin J. Humphreys[1] and Andrew J. McBain[2]

[1] *Lecturer in Medical Microbiology, Division of Pharmacy and Optometry, School of Health Sciences, The University of Manchester, Manchester, UK*
[2] *Professor of Microbiology, Division of Pharmacy and Optometry, School of Health Sciences, The University of Manchester, Manchester, UK*

CONTENTS

Hugo and Russell's Pharmaceutical Microbiology, Ninth Edition. Edited by Brendan F. Gilmore and Stephen P. Denyer.

Companion website: https://www.wiley.com/go/HugoandRussells9e

10.1 Introduction

People rarely suffer from the same infectious disease twice. Reinfections primarily occur when: (i) the infectious agent exhibits antigenic plasticity such as with the common cold and influenza; (ii) the patient is immunocompromised, due for example to immunosuppressive therapy or immunological disorders or (iii) a significant amount of time has passed after the first infection. Alternatively, the patient may have failed to eliminate the primary infection which remained latent and emerged later in a modified or similar form as, for example, with herpes simplex (oral and genital herpes), herpes zoster (chickenpox) and human immunodeficiency virus/acquired immunodeficiency syndrome (HIV/AIDS).

Immunity against reinfection was recognised long before the discovery of the causal agents of infectious disease. Consequently, efforts were made towards developing treatment strategies that could generate immunity to infection without the individual suffering the infection. An early development was the attempted prevention of smallpox (variola major) through the dermal inoculation of healthy individuals with material taken from active smallpox lesions. Such treatments often produced single localised lesions and commonly, but not always, protected the recipient from contracting full-blown smallpox. The process became known as *variolation* and, unknown to its practitioners, protected against the disease by changing the route of infection of the causal organism from respiratory transmission to cutaneous. Unfortunately, occasional cases of smallpox resulted from such practices and variolated individuals could also (rarely) infect others, resulting in disease. Further developments recognised that immunity developed towards one pathogen may be associated with cross-immunity towards related infectious agents. Cowpox is a viral disease of cattle that can be transmitted to humans. The symptoms are similar to those of smallpox, but considerably less severe. Following the observation that individuals exposed to cowpox were conferred protection against smallpox, Edward Jenner substituted material taken from active cowpox (vaccinia) into the variolation procedures. This conferred much of the protection against smallpox that had become associated with variolation but without the associated risks. This discovery, made over two centuries ago, became known as *vaccination* and heralded a new era in disease control. The term vaccination was originally used to refer to prophylactic measures that use living microorganisms or their products to induce immunity, but the term is now used to refer to all immunisation procedures.

Vaccination is used to protect individuals against infection and to protect communities against epidemic disease. Such public health measures have met with spectacular success, and in instances where there is no reservoir of the pathogen other than in infected individuals and survival of the pathogen outside the host is therefore limited, vaccination has the potential to eradicate the disease permanently. This has already been achieved for smallpox where the coordinated deployment of an effective vaccine over many decades led to the elimination of this disease. The global eradication of smallpox was endorsed by the World Health Assembly on 8 May 1980. Another candidate disease for global eradiation by vaccination is poliomyelitis, where effective vaccination programmes have reduced the annual incidence to fewer than 200 cases worldwide. The virus remains endemic, however, in Pakistan and Afghanistan. The Global Polio Eradication Initiative, collaboratively spearheaded by the World Health Organization (WHO), Rotary International, the US Centers for Disease Control and Prevention (CDC), the Bill & Melinda Gates Foundation, Gavi (a global vaccine alliance) and the United Nations International Children's Emergency Fund (UNICEF), is now actively working towards the eradication of this virus. It has been calculated that eradication is a more cost-effective option than containing the disease, as well as reducing morbidity associated with the residual cases. The effectiveness of poliomyelitis vaccines is clearly indicated by the data shown in Figure 10.1.

10.2 Spread of Infection

Infectious diseases may either be spread from a common reservoir (common source) of the infectious agent that is distinct from the diseased individuals, or through a population by serial transfer from diseased to healthy, susceptible individuals (propagated source).

10.2.1 Common-source Infections

In common-source infections, potential reservoirs of infection include infected drinking water, contaminated water droplets from a cooling tower or contaminated food. In the simplest of cases, the source of the infection is transient (i.e., food sourced to a single retail outlet, or to an isolated

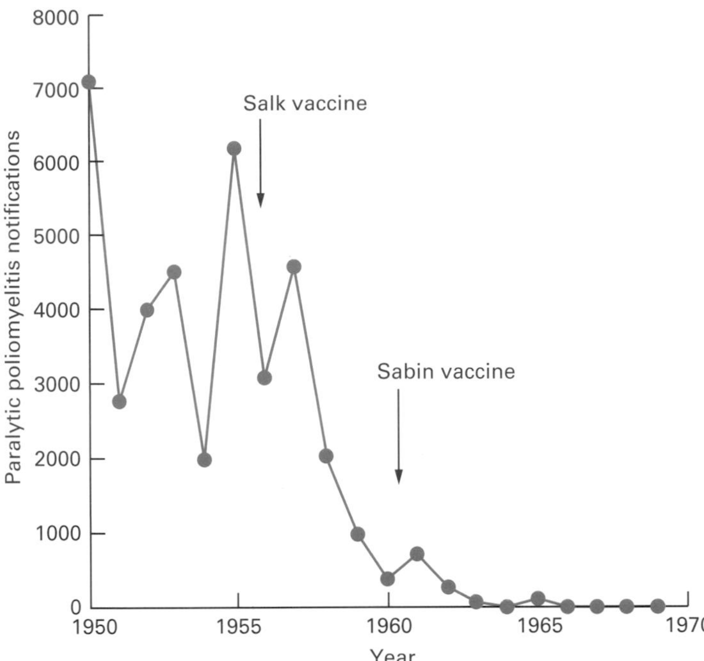

Figure 10.1 Reported incidence of paralytic poliomyelitis in England and Wales during the 1950s and 1960s. After the introduction of vaccination programmes, the incidence of this disease dropped from an endemic incidence of around 5000 cases per year to fewer than 10.

event such as a dinner party). In such instances, the onset of new cases will be phased over a timescale approximately equivalent to one incubation period, and the decline in new cases closely follows the elimination of the source (Figure 10.2). This leads to an acute outbreak of infection, limited to those linked with the source. Such incidents are epitomised by the 1996 outbreak of *Escherichia coli* O157 infections in Lanarkshire, Scotland, that resulted in 5 deaths and left 280 people ill. Similarly, in Clemenstone, South Wales, an outbreak resulted in 157 cases of *E. coli* including the death of a 5-year-old boy in 2005. Both of these outbreaks were linked to a single retail outlet.

If the source of the infection persists beyond the onset, then the incidence of new cases may be maintained at a level that is commensurate with the infectivity of the pathogen and the frequency of exposure of individuals. For those infectious diseases that are transmitted to humans via insect vectors that may act as reservoirs of infection, onset and decline phases of epidemics are rarely observed, other than as reflections of the seasonal variation in the prevalence of the insect. Diseases such as these are generally controlled by public health measures and environmental control of the insect vector with vaccination and immunisation being deployed to protect individuals (e.g., yellow fever vaccination).

10.2.2 Propagated-source Infections

Propagated outbreaks of infection relate to the direct transmission of an infective agent from a diseased individual to a healthy, susceptible one. Mechanisms of such transmission have been described in Chapter 7 and include inhalation of infective aerosols such as with measles, mumps, diphtheria and coronavirus disease (COVID-19); direct physical contact such as may occur with syphilis, herpesvirus and human papillomavirus (HPV); and where sanitation standards are poor, through the introduction of infected faecal material into drinking water (i.e., cholera and typhoid fever) or onto food (e.g., *Salmonella* and *Campylobacter*). The ease of transmission, and hence the rate of onset of an epidemic, relates to the susceptibility status and general state of health of the individuals concerned, the virulence properties of the organism, the route of transmission, the duration of the infective period associated with the disease, behavioural patterns, age of the population group and the population density (e.g., urban versus rural).

In a propagated outbreak, each infectious individual will be capable of transmitting the disease to the susceptible individuals that they encounter during their infectious period. The number of persons to which a single infectious individual might transmit the disease and hence the rate of occurrence of the infection within the population will depend upon the population densities of susceptible and infective individuals, the degree and nature of their interaction and the duration and timing of the infective period. If infectivity precedes the manifestation of the disease, then the spread of the infection may be greater than if these were concurrent. As each infected individual will, in turn, become a source of infection, this may lead to a nearly exponential increase in the incidence of disease. Figure 10.3 shows the incidence of disease within a population group.

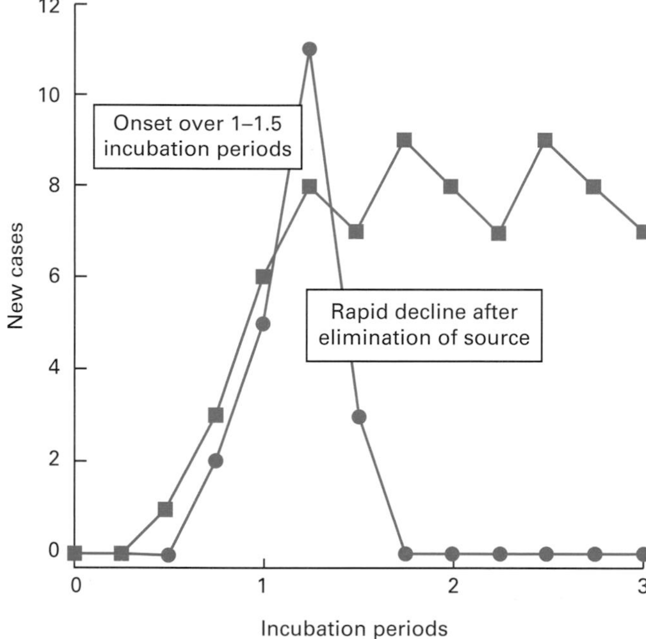

Figure 10.2 Incidence pattern for common-source outbreaks of infection where the source persists (■) and where it is short-lived (●).

This group is perfectly mixed and all individuals are susceptible to the infection. The model infection has an incubation period of 1 day and an infective period of 2 days commencing at the onset of symptoms with recovery occurring 1 day later. For the sake of this illustration, it has been assumed that the reproduction number (R^0) is 2, where each infective individual will infect two others per day until the entire population group has contracted the disease (solid lines). In reality, the rate of transmission can decrease as the epidemic progresses, because recovered individuals may become immune to further infection, reducing the population density of susceptible individuals, and thereby the likelihood of onward transmission. An epidemic is therefore considered to be shrinking when the associated R^0 is less than 1, and may often cease before all members of the community have been infected (Figure 10.3, dotted line). If the proportion of immune individuals within a population group can be maintained above this threshold, then the likelihood of an epidemic arising from a single isolated infection incident is small (this is referred to as *herd immunity*). The threshold level itself is a function of the infectivity of the agent and the population density. Outbreaks of measles and chickenpox, therefore, tend to occur annually in the late summer among children attending school for the first time. This has the effect of concentrating susceptible individuals in one space and thereby reducing the proportion of immune subjects to a value below the threshold for propagated transmission. An effective vaccination programme maintains the proportion of individuals who are immune to a given infectious disease above the critical threshold level for herd immunity. Such a programme will not prevent isolated cases of infection but may prevent these from becoming epidemic.

10.3 Objectives of a Vaccine/Immunisation Programme

There is the potential to develop a protective vaccine/immunisation programme for all infectious diseases, although some pathogens are considerably more challenging candidates than others. Whether or not such vaccines are developed and deployed is related to the severity and economic impact of the disease on the community as well as the effects upon the individual. Various factors governing the likelihood of an immunisation programme being adopted are discussed below, while the principles of immunity and the production and quality control of immunological products are discussed in Chapters 9 and 23, respectively.

10.3.1 Disease Severity

The severity of the disease in terms of its morbidity and mortality, the probability of permanent injury to its survivors and the likelihood of infection must be sufficient to warrant the costly development and use of a vaccine. Thus, although influenza vaccines are constantly reviewed and stocks maintained, the control of influenza epidemics through vaccination is not recommended. Rather, in many influenza vaccination programmes, individuals considered at clinical risk from influenza and eligible paediatric groups, including children aged between 2 and 17 years of age, are protected.

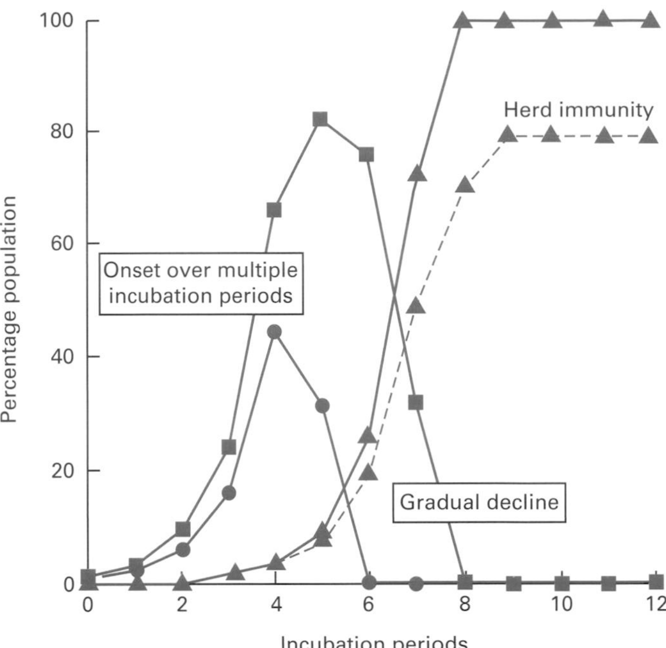

Figure 10.3 Propagated outbreaks of infection showing the incidence of new cases (●), diseased individuals (■) and recovered immune individuals (▲). The dotted line indicates the incidence pattern for an incompletely mixed population group.

Vaccines to be included within national immunisation and vaccination programmes should be chosen to reflect the infection risks within that country. Additional immunisations, appropriate for persons travelling abroad, are intended to protect the at-risk individual, but also to prevent importation of the disease into an unprotected home community.

10.3.2 Vaccine Effectiveness

Vaccination and immunisation programmes seldom confer 100% protection against the target disease. More commonly, the degree of protection is 60–95%. In such instances, although individuals receiving treatment have a high probability of becoming immune, virtually all members of a community must be treated to reduce the actual proportion of susceptible individuals to below the threshold for the epidemic spread of the disease. Anti-diphtheria prophylaxis, which utilises a toxoid, is a highly effective vaccine, whereas the performance of the bacille Calmette–Guérin (BCG) vaccine is variable.

10.3.3 Safety

No medical or therapeutic procedure comes without some risk to the patient, but all possible steps are taken to ensure the safety, quality and efficacy of vaccines and immunological products (see Chapter 23). Common and uncommon adverse events are typically identified through testing in humans (in phase I to III trials). While these vary from vaccine to vaccine, they typically include pain and swelling at the injection site, fatigue and, in some cases, fever. The monitoring of vaccine safety does not stop following regulatory approval and use in the wider community. Very rare and/or long-term adverse events can be monitored through post-marketing surveillance trials (phase IV trials) and reporting by members of the public to the medicines regulator. In the UK, this is achieved through the yellow card scheme, an online platform operated by the Medicine and Healthcare Products Regulatory Agency (MHRA). The risks associated with immunisation procedures are constantly reviewed and balanced against the risks associated with contracting the disease.

10.3.4 Public Perception

Public confidence in the safety of vaccines and immunisation procedures is essential if compliance is to match the needs of the community. The correlation between actual risk and perception of risk is not always reliable, however. Public concern and anxiety in the mid-1970s over the perceived safety of the pertussis vaccine led to a reduction in coverage of the target group from about 80 to 30%. Major epidemics of whooping cough, with over 100,000 notified cases, followed in the late 1970s and early 1980s. By 1992, public confidence had returned and coverage had increased to 92%, with a considerable associated decrease in disease incidence. Similarly, links have been claimed between the incidence of autism in children and the change in the UK from single measles and German measles vaccines to the combined measles, mumps and rubella (MMR) vaccine. Such claims have been proven to be unfounded but have nevertheless decreased the uptake of the MMR vaccine and thereby increased the likelihood and magnitude of measles epidemics. Such issues continue with the current 'anti-vax' movement.

10.3.5 Cost

Low-cost, effective vaccines are an essential component in the global battle against infectious disease. It was estimated that the 1996 costs of the USA childhood vaccination programme, directed against polio, diphtheria, pertussis, tetanus, measles and tuberculosis (TB), was $1 for the vaccines and $14 for the programme costs. Newer vaccines may be considerably more expensive, often putting the costs beyond the budgets of low- and middle-income countries. Issues surrounding vaccine costs and allocation were highlighted during the 2009 H1N1 influenza pandemic, where high-income countries quickly purchased the majority of available vaccine stocks, limiting their global distribution. In 2020, the COVID-19 Vaccine Global Access (COVAX) pillar was created in an attempt to mitigate this problem and provide equitable access to vaccine stocks for participating countries. So far this strategy has not been without problems and has met with shortfalls in funding and vaccine supply, the latter partly as a result of advance-purchase agreements between manufacturers and separate governments.

10.3.6 Longevity of Immunity

The ideal of any vaccine is to provide lifelong protection of the individual against disease. Immunological memory (Chapter 9) depends on the survival of cloned populations of B- and T-lymphocytes (memory cells). Although these lymphocytes can persist in the body for many decades, the duration of protection varies from one individual to another and depends on the vaccine; commonly ranging between 10 and 20 years. Thus, if the immune system is not boosted, either by natural exposure to the organism or by re-immunisation, protective immunity gained in childhood may be lost by the age of 30. Those vaccines that provide only poor protection against disease may have proportionately reduced periods of effectiveness. Equally, vaccines may be less effective and have a shorter duration when administered to neonates. Yellow fever vaccination, which is highly effective, must therefore be repeated at 10-year intervals, while the typhoid vaccine is only effective for up to 3 years. Whether or not immunisation in childhood is subsequently boosted in adolescence or in adulthood depends on the relative risks associated with the infection as a function of age and the longevity of immunity conferred by the vaccine.

10.4 Classes of Immunity

The theoretical background that underlies immunity to infection has been discussed in detail in Chapter 9. Immunity to infection may be passively acquired through the receipt of preformed, protective antibodies or it may be actively acquired through an immune response following deliberate or accidental exposure to microorganisms or their components. Active, acquired immunity might involve either or both of the humoral and cell-mediated responses.

10.4.1 Passive Immunity

Humoral antibodies of the IgG class can cross the placenta from mother to foetus. These antibodies will provide passive protection of the newborn against those diseases which involve humoral immunity and to which the mother is immune. In this manner, most newborn infants in the UK will have passive protection against tetanus, but not against tuberculosis. Protection against the latter relies to a large extent on cell-mediated immunity. Secreted (IgA) antibodies are also passed to the gut of a newborn, together with the first deliveries of breast milk (colostrum). Such antibodies provide some passive protection against infections of the gastrointestinal tract. Maternally acquired antibodies will react with antigens associated with an infection but also with antigens introduced to the body as part of an immunisation programme. Premature immunisation, that is, before degradation of the maternal antibodies, may reduce the potency of an administered vaccine. This aspect of the timing of a course of vaccinations is discussed later.

Administration of preformed antibodies taken from animals, pooled human serum or human cell lines is often used to treat existing infections (e.g., tetanus, diphtheria) or conditions (e.g., venomous snakebite). Pooled serum may also be administered prophylactically, within a slow-release vehicle, for individuals travelling to parts of the world where diseases such as hepatitis A are endemic. Such administrations confer no long-term immunity and may interfere with concurrent vaccination procedures.

10.4.2 Active Immunity

Active immunity (Chapter 9) relates to exposure of the immune system to antigenic materials and the subsequent response. Such exposure might be related to an infection or to the multiplication of an attenuated vaccine strain, or it might be associated with the direct introduction of non-viable antigenic material into the body, for example, a non-living or inactivated vaccine. The route of exposure to antigen will influence the nature of the subsequent immune response. Thus, injection of antigen will lead primarily to humoral (IgG, IgM) production, while exposure of epithelial tissues (gut, respiratory tract) will lead to the production of secretory antibodies (IgA, IgE) and to the stimulation of humoral antibody production.

The magnitude and specificity of an immune response depend upon the duration of the exposure to antigen and on its time–concentration profile. During a naturally occurring infection (or the administration of a live, attenuated vaccine), the concentrations of antigen in the host may be low at the onset and localised to the portal of entry to the host. Since the amounts of antigen are low, they will react only with a highly defined subgroup of lymphocytes. These may transform to produce various antibody classes specific to the antigen and undergo clonal expansion. These immune responses and the progress of the infection may occur simultaneously. With time, microorganisms will produce greater amounts of antigenic materials that will, in turn, react with an increasing number of cloned lymphocytes to produce yet more antibodies. Eventually, the antibody levels may be sufficient to eliminate the infecting organism from the host. Antibody levels will then decline, with the net result of this encounter being the clonal expansion of particular small lymphocytes relating to a highly specific 'immunological memory' of the encounter.

This situation should be contrasted with the administration of a killed or non-living vaccine where the amount of antigen introduced is relatively high when compared with the levels present during the initial stages of an infection. In a non-immune animal, the antigens may react not only with those lymphocytes that are capable of producing an antibody of high specificity but also with those of lower specificity. Antibodies of both higher and lower specificity may react with and remove the residual antigen. The immune response may cease after this initial (primary) challenge. On a subsequent (secondary) challenge (during a course of vaccinations), the antigen will react with residual preformed antibody relating to the first challenge, together with a more specific subgroup of the original cloned lymphocytes. As the number of challenges is increased, the proportion of stimulated lymphocytes that are specific to the antigen rises. After a sufficient number of consecutive challenges, the magnitude and specificity of the immune response match that which would occur during natural infection with an organism bearing the antigen. This pattern of exposure brings with it certain problems. Firstly, as the introduced immunogen will react preferentially with preformed antibody rather than lymphocytes, then sufficient time must elapse between exposures to allow the natural loss of antibody to occur. Secondly, immunity to infection will only be complete after the final challenge with immunogen. Thirdly, low-specificity antibody produced during the early exposures to antigen might be capable of cross-reaction with host tissues to produce an adverse response to the vaccine.

10.5 Types of Vaccine

Vaccines may comprise living, attenuated microorganisms, inactivated or killed microorganisms or purified bacterial and viral components (component vaccines) (see also Chapter 5). Recent innovations include the development of DNA and mRNA vaccines that encode for the antigen when introduced directly into host tissues or vaccines that might be delivered by non-pathogenic bacteria (e.g., *Lactococcus lactis*) or otherwise by viral vectors (e.g., adenovirus). Some aspects of these vaccine classes are discussed below.

10.5.1 Live Vaccines

Live, infective microorganisms, attenuated in their pathogenicity but retaining their ability to infect, can be used to confer protective immunity. Two major advantages stem from the use of live vaccines. First, the immunisation mimics the course of a natural infection such that only a single exposure is required to render an individual immune. Secondly, the exposure may be mediated through the natural route of infection (e.g., oral), thereby stimulating an immune response that is appropriate to a particular disease (e.g., secretory antibody as a primary defence against poliomyelitis virus in the gut with oral polio vaccine [OPV]; see below). Disadvantages associated with the use of live vaccines are also apparent. Live, attenuated vaccines, administered through the natural route of infection, will replicate in the patient and could be transmitted to others. If attenuation is reduced during the replication process, infections might result (see OPV below). A second major disadvantage of live vaccines is that the course of their action, and possible side effects, might be affected by the infection and immunological status of the patient.

10.5.2 Inactivated (Killed) and Component Vaccines

Since these vaccines are unable to evoke a natural infection profile for the release of antigen, they must be administered on several occasions. Immunity may not reach optimal levels until the course of immunisation is complete and, except for toxin-dominated diseases where the immunogen is a toxoid, is unlikely to match the performance of a live vaccine. The specificity of the immune response generated in the patient may initially be low. This is particularly the case when the vaccine is composed of a relatively crude cocktail of killed cells, where the immune response is directed only partially towards antigenic components of the pathogen. This increases the possibility of adverse reactions in the patient. Release profiles of these immunogens can be improved through their formulation with adjuvants (Chapters 9 and 23), and the immunogenicity of certain purified bacterial components, such as polysaccharides, can be improved by their conjugation to a carrier.

10.5.3 DNA Vaccines

A development associated with research into gene therapy has been the use of DNA encoding specific virulence factors of defined pathogens to evoke an immune response. The DNA is introduced directly into tissue cells utilising a transdermal 'gene gun' and is transcribed by the recipient cells. Accordingly, the host responds to the antigenic material produced as though it were an infection. The course of release of the antigen reflects that of a natural infection and, therefore, a highly specific response is invoked. The introduced DNA is eventually lost from the recipient cells and antigen release ceases. Protective immunity has been reported in a trial of a human vaccine for bird flu and a West Nile virus vaccine for horses has been approved. Early phase trials are also underway for COVID-19 DNA vaccines, typically encoding for the viral severe acute respiratory syndrome-coronavirus-2 (SARS-CoV-2) spike protein; these have demonstrated safety and immunogenicity in humans.

10.5.4 mRNA Vaccines

While mRNA vaccines are widely reported as new, the successful use of laboratory-transcribed mRNA in animals was first reported in 1990. Subsequent studies marked this approach as a promising alternative to the traditional routes of vaccine development but were hampered by inefficient delivery systems and issues involving mRNA instability. Decades of research and recent technological advances now permit the production of sufficient yields of stable, synthetic mRNA, and this approach has been employed for the development of vaccines for Zika and influenza virus and more recently in the production and widespread distribution of vaccines for SARS-CoV-2 (see Chapter 5).

mRNA vaccines aim to deliver a genetic code into the host cell which, upon endocytic uptake into the cytoplasm, is instantly translated to produce a protein product. This protein then undergoes post-translational modification before being presented at the cell surface where it can trigger an immune response. This basic concept has some advantages over traditional vaccine design and DNA therapeutics, as: (i) the synthetic mRNA is not able to integrate into the host genome, negating any risk of insertional mutagenesis; (ii) the vaccines are non-infectious because they do not contain an attenuated pathogen and (iii) they can be designed and produced over significantly shorter timescales. Using the COVID-19 pandemic as an example, researchers were able to conceive, test and acquire regulator emergency use approval for the BNT162b2 (now Comirnaty®) mRNA vaccine in less than 1 year. Prior to this, the mumps vaccine had held the record for the shortest timescale at 4 years, with most vaccines taking 10–15 years to develop and approve. While improved delivery systems and nucleoside modification have helped to improve cellular uptake and negate host ribonuclease (RNase)-mediated digestion, respectively, hurdles remain. Some mRNA vaccines require storage through freezing, limiting their use in low-income countries that may lack this form of infrastructure.

10.5.5 Viral Vector Vaccines

Viral vector vaccines use a virus that is unrelated to the causative pathogen to introduce genetic material into a host cell. This subsequently results in endogenous antigen production and the stimulation of an immune response. Antigen production can occur in the presence (replication-competent vector) or absence (replication-defective vector) of further viral replication. Research over the past four decades has identified numerous vectors available for use in humans and typically (although not exclusively) include adenoviruses, poxviruses and rhabdoviruses. Several viral-vector-based vaccines are currently available, including those for Ebola and COVID-19. Vaxzevria utilises a modified chimpanzee virus (ChAdOx1) that encodes for the SARS-CoV-2 spike protein. Trials in humans have shown this vaccine to produce potent humoral and cellular immune responses following two doses.

10.6 Routine Immunisation against Infectious Disease

10.6.1 Poliomyelitis Vaccination

There have been three distinct strains of wild poliovirus (WPV1, WPV2 and WPV3) documented, although coordinated vaccination efforts have resulted in the global eradication of WPV2 and WPV3 in 2015 and 2019, respectively. There are also three phases of the disease. The first is an acute infection of lymphoid tissues associated with the gastrointestinal tract (Peyer's patches), during which time the virus can be found in the throat and in faeces. The second phase is characterised by an invasion of the bloodstream, and in the third phase, the virus migrates from the bloodstream into the meninges. Infections range in severity from asymptomatic (the majority of cases) to paralytic poliomyelitis which may cause permanent neurological damage and muscle paralysis. Paralytic poliomyelitis is a major illness but occurs in only 0.1–2% of cases. It is characterised by the destruction of large nerve cells in the anterior horn of the brain, resulting in varying degrees of paralysis, and unvaccinated adults are at greater risk of paralytic infection than children. The infection is transmitted by the faecal–oral route.

Both live and inactivated/killed vaccines compete in polio prophylaxis. Since the introduction of the inactivated/killed virus (Salk) in 1956 and the live, attenuated virus (Sabin) in 1962, there has been a remarkable decline in the incidence of poliomyelitis (Figure 10.1). The inactivated polio (Salk) vaccine (IPV) contains formalin-killed poliovirus of all three serotypes. On injection, the vaccine stimulates the production of antibodies of the IgM and IgG class that neutralise the virus in the second stage of infection. A course of three injections at monthly intervals produces long-lasting immunity to all three poliovirus types. The live, oral polio (Sabin) vaccine is now less commonly used. Advantages over the IPV vaccine include lower costs and easier administration. OPV contains attenuated poliovirus of each of the three types and is administered, as a liquid, onto the tongue. The vaccine strains infect the gastrointestinal mucosa and oropharynx, promoting the common immune response, and involving both humoral and secretory antibodies. IgA, secreted within the gut epithelium, provides local resistance to the first stages of poliomyelitis infection. OPV, therefore, protects at an earlier stage of the infection than does IPV. Infection of epithelial cells with one strain of enterovirus, however, may inhibit simultaneous infection by related strains. At least three administrations of OPV are therefore given, with each dose conferring immunity to one of the vaccine serotypes. These doses must be separated by a period of at least 1 month to allow the previous infection to lapse. Booster vaccinations are also provided to cover the eventuality that some other enterovirus infection, present at the time of vaccination, had reduced the response to the vaccine strains. Faecal excretion of vaccine virus will occur and may last for up to 6 weeks after administration. Such released virus may spread to close contacts and infect or (re)immunise them. Vaccine-associated poliomyelitis may occur through reversion of the attenuated strains to the virulent wild type, particularly with types II and III and has been estimated to occur once per 4 million doses. Since the introduction of OPV, notifications of paralytic poliomyelitis in the UK have dropped markedly. However, from 1985 to 1995, 19 of the 28 notified cases of paralytic poliomyelitis were associated with reverted vaccine strains (14 recipients and 5 contacts). As the risk of natural infections with poliomyelitis within developed countries has now diminished markedly, the live vaccine strains present the greatest risk. Consequently, OPV has now been replaced with IPV as the polio vaccine of choice in the UK and USA.

10.6.2 Measles, Mumps and Rubella Vaccination

Measles, mumps and rubella (German measles) are infectious diseases with respiratory routes of transmission and infection and each is caused by distinct members of the paramyxovirus group. Each virus only has one serotype. Although the primary multiplication sites of these viruses are within the respiratory tract, the diseases are associated with viral multiplication elsewhere in the host.

10.6.2.1 Measles

Measles is a severe, acute, highly contagious infection that frequently occurs in epidemic form. After multiplication within the respiratory tract, the virus is transported throughout the body, particularly to the skin where a characteristic maculopapular rash develops. Complications of the disease can occur, including measles encephalitis, which can cause permanent neurological injury and death, and subacute sclerosing panencephalitis (SSPE), which is a rare form of progressive encephalitis associated with the persistence of the measles virus that primarily affects children and young adults. It is incurable, although early treatment can slow the progression or improve the remission rate.

A live, attenuated vaccine strain of measles was introduced in the USA in 1962 and to the UK in 1968. A single injection produces high-level immunity in over 95% of recipients. Moreover, as the vaccine induces immunity more rapidly than the natural infection, it may be used to control the impact of measles outbreaks. The measles virus cannot survive outside an infected host. Widespread use of the vaccine, therefore, has the potential, as with smallpox, of eliminating the disease worldwide. Mass immunisation has markedly reduced the incidence of measles, although a 15-fold increase in the incidence was noted in the USA between 1989 and 1991 because of poor compliance with the vaccine. Similar observations can be made in the UK, where vaccine uptake dropped from 95% to approximately 80% between 1995 and 2003. Catch-up campaigns have since helped reverse this trend, with approximately 95% children in 2020 receiving at least a primary dose of MMR vaccine prior to their fifth birthday.

10.6.2.2 Mumps

Mumps virus infects the parotid glands to cause swelling and a general viraemia. Complications include pancreatitis, meningitis and orchitis, the last occasionally leading to male sterility. Infections can also cause permanent unilateral deafness. In the absence of vaccination, infection occurs in more than 90% of individuals by age 15 years. A live, attenuated mumps vaccine has been available since 1967 and has been part of the childhood vaccination programme in the UK since 1988 when it was included as part of the MMR triple vaccine (see below).

10.6.2.3 Rubella

Rubella is a mild, often subclinical infection that is common among children aged between 4 and 9 years. Infection during the first trimester of pregnancy brings with it a major risk of abortion or congenital deformity in the foetus (congenital rubella syndrome [CRS]). Rubella immunisation was introduced to the UK in 1970 for prepubertal females and non-immune women intending to start families. The vaccine utilises a live, cold-adapted strain of the virus. The major disadvantage of the vaccine is that, as with the wild type, the foetus can be infected. While there have been no reports of CRS associated with the use of the vaccine, the possible risk makes it imperative that women do not become pregnant within 1 month of vaccination. Prepubertal females were immunised to extend the period of immunity through the childbearing years. Until 1988, boys were not routinely protected against rubella. Their susceptibility to the virus was thought to maintain the natural prevalence of the disease in the community and thereby reinforce the vaccine-induced immunity in vaccinated, adult females. This proved not to be the case, and, in fact, cases of CRS could be related to the incidence of the disease in younger children within the family. Rubella vaccine is now given to both sexes at the age of about 12 months as part of the MMR programme.

10.6.2.4 MMR Vaccine

The MMR vaccine was introduced to the UK in 1988 for young children of both sexes, replacing the single measles vaccine. It consists of a single dose of a lyophilised preparation of live attenuated strains of the measles, mumps and rubella viruses. The MMR vaccine had previously been deployed in the USA and Scandinavia for a significant number of years without any indication of increased adverse reaction or decreased seroconversion over separate administration of the component parts. Immunisation results in seroconversion to all three viruses in >95% of recipients. For maximum effect, MMR vaccine is recommended for children of both sexes aged 12–15 months but can also be given to non-immune adults. From October 1996, a second dose of MMR was recommended for children aged approximately 4 years to prevent the reaccumulation of sufficient susceptible children to sustain future epidemics.

In 1998, a research paper attempted to associate an increase in autism to the introduction of the triple vaccine. This led to a decreased public confidence in the vaccine. Detailed examination of the data and also the results of several clinical studies have indicated that there is no association between the use of the triple vaccine and autism. This is backed up by over 20 years of successful deployment of the vaccine outside of the UK. Currently, much effort is being made to restore confidence in the vaccine to avoid the lack of compliance leading to the occurrence of measles epidemics.

10.6.3 Tuberculosis

TB is a major cause of death and morbidity worldwide, particularly where poverty, malnutrition and poor housing prevail; almost one quarter of the global population is infected with latent TB. Human infection is acquired by inhalation of *Mycobacterium tuberculosis* or *Mycobacterium bovis*. Tuberculosis is primarily a disease of the lungs, causing chronic infection of the lower respiratory tract, but may spread to other sites or proceed to a generalised infection (miliary tuberculosis). Active disease can result either from a primary infection or from a subsequent reactivation of a quiescent (latent) infection. Following inhalation, the mycobacteria are taken up by alveolar macrophages where they survive and multiply. Circulating macrophages and lymphocytes, attracted to the site, carry the organism to local lymph nodes where a cell-mediated immune response is triggered. The host, unable to eliminate the pathogen, contains the bacteria within small granulomas or tubercles. If high numbers of mycobacteria are present, then the cellular responses can result in tissue necrosis. The tubercles contain viable pathogens that may persist for the remaining life of the host. Reactivation of the healed primary lesions is thought to account for over two-thirds of all newly reported cases of the disease.

The incidence of TB in the UK declined tenfold between 1948 and 1992, to just over 5000 new cases being notified each year. Those most at risk include pubescent children, health service staff and individuals intending to stay for more than 1 month in countries where TB is endemic. However, since 1994, there has been a gradual increase in the number of notified cases in England and Wales to approximately 7000 new cases per year which can be associated with age group (20–45-year-olds more susceptible), sex (males slightly more susceptible), geographical region and ethnicity. The rise in notifications can be attributed to several different factors, including the emergence of multidrug resistance, increased immigration from countries where TB is more prevalent, crowded conditions (e.g., prisons, hostels and wards), a greater number of susceptible individuals now in society (e.g., substance abusers, immunocompromised individuals) and limited training for general practitioners (GPs) in recognising the symptoms of TB. Fortunately, this latter issue has now been addressed, along with the re-emergence of TB research programmes.

A live vaccine is required to elicit protection against TB, and both antibody and cell-mediated immunity are required for protective immunity. Vaccination with BCG, derived from an attenuated *M. bovis* strain, is commonly used in countries where TB is endemic. The vaccine was introduced in the UK in 1953. Efficacy in the UK is over 70%, with protection lasting at least 15 years. In other countries, where the general state of health and well-being of the population may differ adversely, the efficacy of the vaccine is markedly lower than this.

Because of the risks of adverse reaction to the vaccine by individuals who have already been exposed to the disease, a sensitivity test must be carried out before immunisation with BCG. A Mantoux skin test assesses an individual's sensitivity to a purified protein derivative (PPD) prepared from heat-treated antigens (tuberculin) extracted from *M. tuberculosis*. A positive test implies past infection or past, successful immunisation. Those with strongly positive tests may have active disease and should be referred to a chest clinic. However, many people with active TB, especially disseminated TB, seroconvert from a positive to a negative skin test. Results of the skin test must therefore be interpreted with care.

Much debate surrounds the use of the BCG vaccine, a matter of some importance, considering that TB kills around 1.5 million people annually and that drug-resistant strains are increasingly more prevalent. Although the vaccine has demonstrated some efficacy in preventing childhood TB, it has little prophylactic effect against postprimary TB in those already infected. One solution is to bring forward the BCG immunisation to include neonates. Immunisation at 2–4 weeks of age will ensure that immunisation precedes infection, and also negates the requirement for a skin test. Passive acquired maternal antibody to TB is unlikely to interfere with the effectiveness of the immunisation, as immunity relates primarily to a cell-mediated response. Alternative strategies involve improvement of the vaccine, possibly through the introduction into the BCG strain of genes that encode protective antigens of *M. tuberculosis*.

The current UK policy (introduced in September 2005) is to reserve the BCG vaccine for those considered to be at the highest risk based on location or familial links to TB endemic areas. As such, this targeted approach will seek to immunise all infants in areas where the incidence of TB is 40 or more per 100,000; infants with at least one parent or grandparent who was born in a country with a TB incidence of 40 or more per 100,000; previously unvaccinated new immigrants from high-prevalence countries for TB; those who have lived in the same household or had prolonged, close contact with someone with TB; or at-risk workers such as doctors, nurses and social workers.

10.6.4 Diphtheria, Tetanus and Acellular Pertussis (DTaP) Immunisation

Immunisation against these three unrelated diseases is considered together because the vaccines are non-living and are often co-administered as part of the childhood vaccination programme.

10.6.4.1 Diphtheria

This is an acute, non-invasive infectious disease associated with the upper respiratory tract (Chapter 7). The incubation period is 2–5 days, although the disease remains communicable for up to 4 weeks. A low-molecular-weight toxin is produced which affects the myocardium, nervous and adrenal tissues. Death results in 3–5% of infected children. Diphtheria immunisation stimulates the production of an antitoxin that protects against the disease but not against infection/colonisation of the respiratory tract. The immunogen is a toxoid, prepared by formaldehyde treatment of the purified toxin (Chapter 23) and administered while adsorbed to an adjuvant, usually aluminium phosphate or aluminium hydroxide. The primary course of diphtheria prophylaxis consists of three doses starting at 2 months of age and separated by an interval of at least 1 month. The immune status of adults can be determined by the administration of Schick test toxin, which is essentially a diluted form of the vaccine.

10.6.4.2 Tetanus

Tetanus results from the production of a toxin by germinating spores and vegetative cells of *Clostridium tetani* that can potentially infect deep wounds. The organism, which may be introduced into the wound, grows anaerobically at such sites. The toxin is adsorbed into nerve cells and has a profound effect on nerve synapses resulting in spastic paralysis in affected individuals (Chapter 7). Mortality rates are highest in individuals over 60 years of age and the unvaccinated. Tetanus immunisation employs a toxoid and protects by stimulating the production of antitoxin. This antitoxin will neutralise the toxin as the organisms release it and before it can be adsorbed into nerves. As the toxin is produced only slowly after infection, the vaccine, which acts rapidly, may be used prophylactically in non-immunised individuals who have recently suffered a high-risk injury. The toxoid, as with diphtheria toxoid, is formed by reaction with formaldehyde and is adsorbed onto an inorganic adjuvant. The primary course of tetanus vaccination consists of three doses starting at 2 months of age and is separated by an interval of at least 1 month.

10.6.4.3 Pertussis (Whooping Cough)

Whooping cough is caused by the non-invasive respiratory pathogen *Bordetella pertussis* (Chapter 7). This disease may be complicated by bronchopneumonia, or by repeated post-tussive vomiting leading to weight loss and cerebral hypoxia associated with a risk of brain damage. Until the mid-1970s, the mortality from whooping cough was about 1 per 1000 notified cases, with a higher rate for infants under 1 year of age. A full course of vaccine now consists of highly purified selected components of the *B. pertussis* organism (i.e., acellular pertussis) which are treated with formaldehyde or glutaraldehyde and adsorbed onto aluminium phosphate or aluminium hydroxide adjuvants. This vaccine gives considerably lower incidence of local and systemic reactions in comparison to the whole-cell pertussis vaccine that preceded it and gives comparable protection (>80%), although the duration of protection is likely shorter than either natural infection or the whole-cell vaccine. The primary course of pertussis prophylaxis consists of three doses starting at 2 months of age and separated by an interval of at least 1 month. Recently, there has been a global increase in pertussis cases, particularly in young adults. While disease in this age group is generally mild, it serves as a potential reservoir for infection in the very young. In the UK, this has led to the introduction of pertussis vaccination for pregnant women (from 16 weeks gestation) to provide passive immunity in newborns.

10.6.4.4 DTaP Vaccine Combinations and Administration

The primary course of DTaP protection consists of three doses of a combined vaccine to also immunise against polio, *Haemophilus influenzae* type b and hepatitis B (DTaP/IPV/Hib/HepB), each dose separated by at least 1 month and commencing not earlier than 2 months of age. In such combinations, the pertussis component of the vaccine acts as an additional adjuvant for the toxoid elements. Tetanus and diphtheria vaccines are also available both as a combined tetanus/diphtheria/inactivated polio vaccine (Td/IPV) and as a combined diphtheria/tetanus/pertussis/inactivated polio vaccine (DTaP/IPV).

The primary course of pertussis immunisation is followed by an additional vaccine at 3 years and 4 months of age and confers protection for up to 12 years, of note given that the mortality associated with pertussis declines markedly after infancy. The risks associated with tetanus and diphtheria infection, however, persist throughout life and vaccination is therefore repeated at 3 years and 4 months of age and then again at puberty.

10.6.5 Immunisation against Bacteria Associated with Meningitis

10.6.5.1 Meningococcal Immunisation

Meningococcus (*Neisseria meningitidis*) is a bacterium that exclusively colonises and/or infects humans; there is no animal reservoir. It is present as part of the normal microbiota of the pharynx in approximately 10% of individuals but can rarely spread through the bloodstream and to the brain through poorly understood mechanisms, causing meningitis and septicaemia. These are life-threatening, systemic infections; overall mortality from meningococcal disease is approximately 10%, assuming symptoms are recognised and treatment is commenced without delay but rises considerably if there are delays. Diagnosis is therefore considered a medical emergency. At least 13 subtypes or serogroups of meningococcus have been identified, but groups B and C account for the majority of cases in Europe and groups B, C and Y predominating in the Americas. In the UK, group B accounts for approximately 80% of reported cases with groups C, W and Y roughly accounting for the remainder. *N. meningitidis* group A does not normally cause disease in the UK. Historically, this serogroup was an endemic cause of meningitis in other parts of the world, particularly sub-Saharan Africa in an area between Senegal (West Africa) and Ethiopia (East) that has been termed the 'meningitis belt'. However, mass-vaccination programmes from 2010 onwards have meant that epidemics as a result of this serogroup have been largely prevented. It is believed that reasons for the historical hyperendemic incidence of group A meningococcal meningitis in this part of the world include a high incidence of upper respiratory tract infections during the dry (dusty) season, combined with overcrowding, migration and pilgrimages. More recent epidemics in this region have been the result of infection with meningococcal serogroups C and W.

Meningitis accounts for the majority of invasive meningococcal disease; however, in 15–20% of cases, septicaemia predominates and is associated with significantly higher mortality. There are currently vaccines available for capsular groups A, B, C, W and Y of the meningococci. As with the Hib vaccine (see Section 10.6.5.2), the preparations are generally intended to invoke protective immunity towards the polysaccharide component of the bacterium. Early vaccines, composed of purified polysaccharide, worked in adults but had poor efficacy in infants—the most at-risk group. The MenC conjugate vaccine comprises capsular polysaccharide components conjugated to a carrier protein (usually diphtheria or tetanus toxoid). This vaccine is effective in the very young and is therefore suitable for protecting infants. The vaccine is administered along with Hib at 12 months and a single dose is sufficient to immunise individuals over 12 months of age; it has also been used to provide prophylaxis for teenagers, adolescents and young adults. In 2015, a vaccine for capsular group B was approved (Bexsero®) and incorporated into the UK immunisation schedule. It is currently administered as three separate doses between 8 weeks and 1 year of age. Given the ability of this capsular group to mimic host-derived tissue (molecular mimicry), this vaccine is multi-component, comprising recombinant fusion proteins and outer membrane vesicles adsorbed to aluminium hydroxide. A group A vaccine is available for those travelling to areas of the world where the infection is epidemic.

10.6.5.2 *Haemophilus influenzae* Type b Immunisation

H. influenzae can cause infections ranging from bronchitis and otitis media to life-threatening, invasive disease (meningitis and bacteraemia). Invasive infections, which are most common in young children, are normally caused by encapsulated strains of the bacterium that can be serologically differentiated into six typeable capsular serotypes (a–f). Before the introduction of vaccination, Hib was the most prevalent of these in invasive disease. Non-invasive haemophilus disease is most often caused by non-encapsulated strains that are not amenable to typing based on capsular serology. Although the most common form of invasive Hib disease is meningitis, accounting for 60% of cases, Hib can also cause other infections, including pneumonia and pericarditis.

The fatality rate for treated Hib meningitis infections is approximately 5% and complications include deafness and intellectual impairment (in approximately 10% of cases). Hib often forms part of the normal microbiota of the nasopharynx in healthy individuals and the frequency of carriage before the Hib vaccine was introduced was approximately 4 in every 100 for preschool children. Carriage of this bacterium is now rare because of the effectiveness of the Hib vaccination. Hib meningitis is rare in children under 3 months and peaks in its incidence at around 10–11 months of age; infection is uncommon after 4 years of age. Before the introduction of Hib vaccination, the incidence of the disease in the UK was estimated at 34 per 100,000.

The vaccine utilises purified preparations of the polysaccharide capsule of the major serotypes of the bacterium associated with disease. Polysaccharides are poorly immunogenic and must be conjugated onto a protein carrier (diphtheria or tetanus toxoids) to enhance their efficacy. The Hib vaccine is given as part of a combined product of *H. influenzae* type b, diphtheria, tetanus, acellular pertussis, inactivated polio vaccine and hepatitis B surface antigen (DTaP/IPV/Hib/HepB), or as the Hib/MenC conjugate vaccine.

10.6.5.3 Pneumococcal Vaccination

Streptococcus pneumoniae (pneumococcus) is an encapsulated Gram-positive coccus. As with meningococcus and Hib, the capsule is an important virulence factor for this bacterium (non-capsulated strains are normally avirulent). Many different capsular types have been characterised, but approximately 66% of the serious infections in adults and 80% of invasive pneumococcal infections in children are caused by about 10 capsular types. Pneumococci are often part of the normal microbiota of the nasal cavity and associated tissues, but commensal strains are often avirulent. Conversely, invasive infections (i.e., meningitis and septicaemia) are often caused by strains not considered to be normal commensals. *S. pneumoniae* is a versatile pathogen that can cause sinusitis or otitis media (infections of the sinuses or middle ear). The bacterium may also cause deep lung infections (pneumonia), which accounts for its species name, and is also capable of causing systemic infections including bacteraemic pneumonia, bacteraemia and meningitis. The incidence of infection by pneumococci is highest in the winter, and transmission by aerosols or direct contact with respiratory secretions is believed to require either frequent or prolonged close contact. Two distinct vaccines have been developed to protect against this bacterium: the pneumococcal polysaccharide vaccine (PPV) which contains purified capsular polysaccharide from 23 capsular types of bacterium, and the pneumococcal conjugate vaccine (PCV) which comprises capsular polysaccharides from 13 common capsular types. Importantly, PCV is conjugated to protein like the Hib and MenC vaccines. While PPV is an effective vaccine in adults, the effectiveness of pneumococcal prophylaxis is considerably improved in children by protein conjugation; PCV is immunogenic in children and the childhood vaccination schedule recommends that doses be given at 12 weeks of age with a booster at 12 months. The PPV vaccine is recommended for adults over 65 years and at-risk groups aged 2 years or over. It will provide additional prophylaxis to individuals who have already received the PCV vaccine because it protects from additional serotypes.

10.6.6 Human Papillomavirus Vaccination

HPVs are a group of viruses that infect squamous epithelia, including the skin and mucosal surfaces of the upper respiratory and anogenital tracts. Approximately 100 types of HPV have been identified, of which around 40 infect the genital tract. The majority of genital infections are asymptomatic with 90% cases clearing within 2 years of infection, but in some cases may be associated with genital warts and (the reason for the development of the HPV vaccine) cervical cancer. The time between infection and the development of cancers may range from 12 months to over 10 years. It is important to note that HPV is associated with genital and anal cancers in both men and women and also with cancers of the mouth and throat. Importantly, not all types of HPV are carcinogenic; the risk of cancer development associated with different strains is variable and HPV viruses that cause warts (such as HPV types 6 and 11) may be low risk for carcinogenicity and, in some cases, strains are not considered carcinogenic. Genital HPV infections are transmitted primarily through sexual intercourse with infected individuals and the use of condoms reduces the risk of sexual transmission. HPV may also be transmitted vertically from mother to child. Persistent HPV infection with HPV 16 and HPV 18 (high-risk strains) is associated with the majority of cervical and anal cancers. There are, however, strains other than HPV 16 and HPV 18 that are carcinogenic.

The HPV vaccine comprises recombinant subunits expressed in yeast or in cells of insect origin such that the vaccine contains non-infectious, virus-like particles. The current UK vaccine, Gardasil®, affords protection against HPV types 6, 11, 16 and 18 and is used in the prevention of genital warts and premalignant lesions and cancers associated with HPV infection. The vaccine is currently administered to both females and males aged between 12 and 13 as part of a two-dose regime. Two additional vaccines are also licensed for use for HPV and include Cervarix®, a bivalent vaccine (HPV types 16 and 18), and a 9-valent form of Gardasil (Gardasil®9) that covers HPV types 6, 11, 16, 18, 31, 33, 45, 52 and 58. In young females with no prior evidence of HPV infection, these vaccines have been shown in trials to prevent 99% of pre-cancerous lesions caused by HPV types 16 and 18.

10.6.7 COVID-19 Vaccination

COVID-19 is a severe acute respiratory syndrome that was first described in 2019 in Wuhan, China. It is caused by a novel coronavirus, SARS-CoV-2, an enveloped RNA virus that is thought to have transmitted to humans from a zoonotic source, purportedly through direct contact at a wholesale seafood market. The symptoms associated with COVID-19 can vary from person to person, but frequently include onset of a persistent, dry cough, fever and loss of taste and/or smell. Asymptomatic cases of COVID-19 have been reported in up to a third of people. It is estimated that fewer than 5% COVID-19 cases occur in children, with this age group generally experiencing mild disease. Symptoms in this age group may also differ to that in adults, with gastrointestinal involvement more likely. In 2020, a Kawasaki-/toxic shock-like disease was first described in children with COVID-19, later called paediatric inflammatory multisystem syndrome-temporally associated with SARS-CoV-2 (PIMS-TS). While rare (fewer than 0.5% cases), the link between viral infection and this syndrome remains unclear.

Several vaccines are currently available for immunisation against COVID-19 and typically target the SARS-CoV-2 spike (S) protein, a viral component involved in angiotensin-converting enzyme 2 (ACE-2)-binding and viral entry into the host cell. Available vaccines for COVID-19 currently vary geographically and those with WHO emergency-use listing are shown in Table 10.1. In the UK, the COVID-19 vaccines currently utilised include mRNA (Comirnaty and Moderna COVID-19 vaccine) and viral vector (Vaxzevria) platforms (see also Chapter 5). Phase II/III trials of these vaccines demonstrated efficacies of up to 95% and 62.1%, respectively, in preventing symptomatic COVID-19. The analyses of 'real world data' by Public Health England were equally promising, noting up to 90% effectiveness in symptomatic infection prevention regardless of the vaccine type administered. Despite this, the emergence and global spread of novel SARS-CoV-2 variants has led to the prospect of escape mutations. The delta variant raised concerns around reduced vaccine efficacy via a mutation in the viral spike protein (P681R). Initial data for Comirnaty suggested only a modest reduction in efficacy, with two doses providing between 77 and 82% protection against symptomatic disease. Throughout the latter part of 2021, the rise and dissemination of the Omicron variant was similarly marked by a reduction in vaccine effectiveness and importantly, the duration of this effectiveness, prompting a vaccine booster campaign for all eligible adults in the UK. By September 2022, updated bivalent COVID vaccines carrying the mRNA encoding for the spike protein of both the original viral strain and the Omicron BA.1 variant had been approved as a single booster dose by the MHRA, with the aim of eliciting more potent antibody responses to the highly transmissible Omicron sub-variants.

The UK adopted a phased approach to its COVID-19 immunisation strategy with care home residents, the elderly, health care workers and the clinically extremely vulnerable taking initial priority. This, in part, reflects the

Table 10.1 COVID-19 vaccines with WHO emergency-use listing (2022). Data from WHO.

Platform	Vaccine	Country of origin	Dosing
Inactivated virus	BIBP (Sinopharm)	China	×2 injection (3–4 weeks apart)
	CoronaVac (SinoVac Life Sciences)	China	× 2 injection (2–3 weeks apart)
	Covaxin® (Bharat Biotech International)	India	× 2 injection (4 weeks apart)
mRNA	Comirnaty® (Pfizer/BioNTech)	Multinational	×2 injection (3 weeks apart)[a]
	Spikevax (Moderna Biotech)	US	×2 injection (4 weeks apart)
Subunit	Nuvaxovid™/Covovax™ (Novavax/ Serum Institute India)	Czech Republic/India	× 2 injections (3 weeks apart)
Viral vector	Vaxzevria (Oxford University/ AstraZeneca)	UK	×2 injection (4–12 weeks apart)
	Convidecia (CanSino Biologics)	China	× 1 injection
	Covishield™ (Serum Institute of India)	India	× 2 injection (4–12 weeks apart)
	Janssen Vaccine (Johnson & Johnson)	US, Netherlands	×1 injection

[a] Manufacturer recommendations state that Comirnaty® vaccine doses should be separated by a period of 3 weeks. Some countries, including the UK, initially opted to increase this interval to a maximum of 12 weeks to maximise first dose coverage and therefore provide partial protection against hospitalisation within vulnerable populations.

risk of mortality from COVID-19, which increases significantly with age with case fatality rates in excess of 10% reported in individuals aged 75 years and over. In 2021, post-marketing surveillance identified very rare (approximately 10 per million) cases of blood clots with low platelets in individuals up to 16 days post Vaxzevria vaccination. As a result, the MHRA currently recommends the use of this vaccine in individuals aged 40 years and over where the benefits of vaccination significantly outweigh the risk of adverse vaccine events.

10.7 The UK Routine Childhood Immunisation Programme

The timing of the various components of the childhood vaccination programme is subject to continual review. In the 1960s, the primary course of DTaP vaccination consisted of three doses given at 3, 6 and 12 months of age, together with OPV. This separation gave adequate time for the levels of induced antibody to decline between successive doses of the vaccines. Current recommendations (Table 10.2) accelerate the vaccination programme with no reductions in its efficacy. Thus, the MMR vaccination has replaced separate measles and rubella prophylaxis, and BCG vaccination may now be given at birth for infants living in areas of the UK where the annual incidence of TB is 40 per 100,000 or greater and/or those with familial links to high-risk countries. DTaP vaccination occurs at 8, 12 and 16 weeks to coincide with administration of Hib, IPV and HBV as part of the 6-in-1 vaccine. It is imperative that as many individuals as possible benefit from the immunisation programme. Fewer visits to the doctor's surgery translate into improved patient compliance and less likelihood of epidemic spread of the diseases in question. The current recommendations minimise the number of separate visits to the clinic while attempting to maximise the protection generated.

10.8 Immunisation of the Over 65s and Other Risk Groups

In addition to the childhood vaccination schedule, vaccinations are available for individuals over the age of 65 years. These typically cover pneumococcal pneumonia, influenza and shingles, the latter as a result of varicella zoster virus reactivation. Of note, seasonal influenza vaccination in this age category is achieved through the use of an inactivated influenza vaccine given the potential for adverse events associated with the administration of live attenuated viruses in the elderly.

Additional vaccines are available for individuals in special risk categories. Individuals with certain underlying medical conditions may be at increased risk of infectious diseases and as such require vaccinations in addition to those in the UK immunisation schedule to confer protection. Here, vaccinations are considered based upon the specific underlying condition, but

Table 10.2 Schedule for the UK's routine childhood immunisations (2022).

Age	Disease	Vaccine	Administration
8 weeks	Diphtheria, tetanus, pertussis, polio, Hib, hepatitis B	DTaP/IPV/Hib/HepB (6 in 1)	×1 injection
	Meningococcal gp B	MenB	×1 injection
	Rotavirus gastroenteritis	Rotavirus	×1 oral dose
12 weeks	Diphtheria, tetanus, pertussis, polio, Hib, hepatitis B	DTaP/IPV/Hib/HepB (6 in 1)	×1 injection
	Pneumococcal (13 serotypes)	Pneumococcal conjugate vaccine (PCV)	×1 injection
	Rotavirus gastroenteritis	Rotavirus	×1 oral dose
16 weeks	Diphtheria, tetanus, pertussis, polio, Hib, hepatitis B	DTaP/IPV/Hib/HepB (6 in 1)	×1 injection
	Meningococcal gp B	MenB	×1 injection
1 year	Hib and meningococcal gp C	Hib/MenC	×1 injection
	Pneumococcal (13 serotypes)	PCV booster	×1 injection
	Measles, mumps and rubella	MMR	×1 injection
	Meningococcal gp B	MenB	×1 injection
3–17 years	Influenza	Live attenuated influenza vaccine (LAIV)	×1 nasal dose (annually from September)
3 years and 4 months	Diphtheria, tetanus, pertussis and polio	DTaP/IPV	×1 injection
	Measles, mumps and rubella	MMR	×1 injection
12–13 years	HPV (types 16 and 18) associated cancers, genital warts (HPV types 6 and 11)	HPV	×2 injections (6–24 months apart)
14 years	Tetanus, diphtheria and polio	Td/IPV	×1 injection
	Meningococcal gps ACWY	MenACWY	×1 injection

Newborns with HBV-infected mothers will receive a HBV vaccine at birth, 4 weeks and 1 year of age in addition to the 6-in-1 vaccine.
Source: Adapted from the complete immunisation schedule for the UK available from Public Health England. **Policies can and do change. For definitive information, see** https://www.gov.uk/government/publications/the-complete-routine-immunisation-schedule. **Accessed 3rd October 2022.**

broadly aim to protect against pneumococcal, meningococcal, hepatitis and influenza diseases. Separate to underlying medical conditions, categories relating to occupational risks or risks associated with travel abroad should also be considered. Such immunisation protocols include those directed against cholera, typhoid, meningitis (group A), anthrax, hepatitis A and hepatitis B, influenza, Japanese encephalitis, rabies, tick-borne encephalitis and yellow fever.

Acknowledgements

The authors acknowledge the contributions of Peter Gilbert (1951–2008) who was a co-author on previous versions of this chapter. Much of the information in this chapter is developed from the 'Green Book', an authoritative source of information about the composition and schedules for current UK vaccines and immunisation policies.

Further Reading

Amirloo, B. and Jimenez, B.D. (2022). Understanding mRNA vaccine technologies. *Pharm. J.* 308, 7959.

Nash, A., Dalziel, R. and Fitzgerald, J. (2015). *Mims' Pathogenesis of Infectious Disease*, 6e. London: Academic Press.

Public Health England (2013). *Immunisation Against Infectious Disease* (Green Book). London: PHE. https://www.gov.uk/government/collections/immunisation-against-infectious-disease-the-green-book.

Public Health England (2014). *Complete Routine Immunisation Schedule* (regularly updated). London: PHE. https://www.gov.uk/government/publications/the-complete-routine-immunisation-schedule.

Public Health England (2021). *COVID-19 Vaccine Surveillance Report*. London: PHE. https://www.gov.uk/government/publications/covid-19-vaccine-surveillance-report.

Wilson, B.A., Winkler, M.E. and Ho, B.T. (2019). *Bacterial Pathogenesis: A Molecular Approach*, 4e. Washington: ASM Press.

World Health Organization *Status of Covid-19 Vaccines within WHO EUL/PQ Evaluation Process* (regularly updated). Geneva: WHO. https://www.who.int/teams/regulation-prequalification/eul/covid-19.

Part 4

Prescribing Therapeutics and Infection Control

11

Antibiotics and Synthetic Antimicrobial Agents: Their Properties and Uses

Brendan F. Gilmore

Professor of Pharmaceutical Microbiology, School of Pharmacy, Queen's University Belfast, Belfast, UK

CONTENTS

Hugo and Russell's Pharmaceutical Microbiology, Ninth Edition. Edited by Brendan F. Gilmore and Stephen P. Denyer.

Companion website: https://www.wiley.com/go/HugoandRussells9e

11.1 Antibiotic Development, Past and Present

The discovery of penicillin diffusing from cultures of the fungus *Penicillium notatum* by Sir Alexander Fleming in 1928, the subsequent demonstration that extracts from these cultures could be used to successfully treat infections in humans and the isolation of penicillin by Howard Florey, Ernst Chain and Norman Heatley in the early 1940s marked the beginning of what is now considered the 'antibiotic era'. The onset of the Second World War stimulated the development, by American pharmaceutical giant Pfizer, of penicillin into a pharmaceutical agent which could be manufactured on a large scale. Benzylpenicillin was the original antibiotic in this class and the first to be used widely for the treatment of infections. While the study of intermicrobic antagonism (as observed by Fleming between staphylococci and *Penicillium* spp.) had been described previously (by Pasteur and others), and antimicrobial natural and synthetic compounds such as Prontosil (1935, a forebear of the sulphonamides) were already known, it was the discovery and, equally importantly, the painstaking isolation, characterisation and application of penicillin which mark this most decisive moment in mankind's battle against bacterial infection. Since that time, the number of antibiotic agents isolated and identified from natural sources had, until the past few decades, experienced steady growth, though many were unsuitable for widespread and systemic use in humans. From this perspective, penicillin was all the more remarkable, having an antimicrobial, pharmacological and toxicological profile, which rendered it the agent of choice for the treatment of bacterial infections. Indeed, the penicillins are still among the most commonly prescribed antibiotic agents, despite the widespread emergence of antibiotic resistance.

Another antibiotic pioneer, Selman Waksman (discoverer of streptomycin) proposed the original definition of an antibiotic as 'a compound produced by a microbe, which kills or inhibits the growth of another microbe'. This definition was apt for the early discoveries of naturally produced antibiotics such as penicillin, streptomycin, bacitracin, erythromycin, chloramphenicol, vancomycin and numerous others. Advances in medicinal and synthetic chemistry, however, have led to the extensive modification of natural antibiotic molecular scaffolds, and have necessitated a revision of this definition to take into account the fact that many clinically useful agents with antimicrobial activity are either semi-synthetic (i.e., chemical modification of a naturally produced precursor molecule such as 6-aminopenicillanic acid [6-APA] to yield semi-synthetic penicillins) or wholly synthetic (sulphonamides, 4-quinolones and oxazolidinones) in origin. Therefore, a more up-to-date definition of an antibiotic is any substance produced by a microorganism, or a similar substance (produced wholly or partly by chemical synthesis), which in high dilutions (low concentrations) inhibits the growth of other microorganisms. This revised definition therefore encompasses what were traditionally referred to as antimicrobial agents, such as the synthetic sulphonamides and naturally derived antibiotic agents prepared using total synthesis, an approach designed to circumvent isolation and extraction from a natural source (e.g., chloramphenicol) and the semi-synthetic agents (which include the majority of all marketed penicillins). The broader term 'antimicrobial' can be used for any agent which kills or inhibits microorganisms, irrespective of source or concentration used and can therefore include antibiotics, antiseptics, disinfectants and preservative agents.

The 'golden era' of antibiotic discovery began in the 1940s with the introduction of penicillins into clinical use, and the systematic isolation and screening of microorganisms (primarily from soil) for their ability to inhibit or kill pathogenic bacteria. This screening approach, developed by Selman Waksman and which led to the discovery of streptomycin in 1943, became the standard approach to antibiotic research in the pharmaceutical industry, leading to the discovery of the main classes of antibiotics (e.g., tetracyclines, aminoglycosides, macrolides and glycopeptides) in the 1940s through to the 1960s. From the 1960s onwards, these naturally occurring antibiotic scaffolds provided the molecular basis for the development of semi-synthetic versions of, for example, beta-lactams giving rise to first-, second-, and n^{th}-generation compounds in each class, characterised by improved or optimised pharmacological profile and spectrum of activity. By the 1950s and 1960s, wholly synthetic agents (sulphonamides, oxazolidinones and quinolones) were added to the armoury of effective, clinically useful antibiotics. Therefore, despite the recognition of the potential threat posed by the emergence of antibiotic resistance from the very dawn of the antibiotic era, the steady development of new antibiotics by the major pharmaceutical companies throughout the period 1940–1970 meant that the perception that new drugs could replace those to which resistance had developed led to complacency with respect to the widespread and often inappropriate use of antibiotics in clinical, veterinary and agricultural settings. The assumption that the 'antibiotic pipeline' could indefinitely deliver safe and effective antibiotics to stay abreast of, or outpace, the emergence of antimicrobial resistance (AMR) by replacing antibiotics rendered ineffective due to the evolution and emergence of antibiotic-resistance mechanisms in bacteria has proven ill-founded. Despite burgeoning antibiotic resistance from the latter half of the twentieth century onwards, in the past 60 years only one new class of antibiotic, the cyclic lipopeptide daptomycin, has been discovered and approved for clinical use in human infections.

In contrast to the broad-spectrum, safe and pharmacologically acceptable antibiotics discovered and developed during the 'golden era' of antibiotic discovery (1940s–1960s), daptomycin (discovered in 1987, although stalled in development due to concerns over adverse effects, only gaining Food and Drug Administration [FDA] approval in 2003) is narrow-spectrum (active only against Gram-positive bacteria) with a highly restricted profile of clinical indications (complicated skin and soft tissue infections [cSSTI], right-sided infective endocarditis due to *Staphylococcus aureus* and *S. aureus* bacteraemia) and must be administered parenterally due to poor oral bioavailability. In the face of an emerging antibiotic-resistance crisis, the antibiotic pipeline has failed to keep pace with resistance, meaning many previously effective antibiotics are now incapable of treating resistant infections and, with fewer drugs, therapeutic options are dwindling. Clinical reports of infections which are not sensitive to any class of antibiotics are increasing annually.

Since the introduction of antibiotics into clinical practice, deaths from infectious disease have declined by approximately 70%, but antibiotic-resistant infections are rising globally, and are responsible for approximately 1.27 Million deaths annually. The assessment of the current global antibiotic pipeline is particularly bleak, with most of the major pharmaceutical firms having exited the antibiotic research and development space, and with annually declining approvals for new antibiotics coming to the market. The causes for this are primarily economic, as the business model and financial incentives for developing new antibiotics are drastically lacking. The cost–benefit ratio for developing new antibiotics is less favourable than for other types of drugs, for example, those indicated for cancer, hypertension, diabetes and other chronic conditions where the drug is administered daily for long periods of time (in some cases for the lifetime of the patient). The difficulty in identifying compounds with antibiotic activity and acceptable physicochemical and pharmacological characteristics, coupled with high attrition rates in the early stages of development, means that antibiotic development is costly (estimated to be in the region of $1.5 billion), with average annual revenue generated estimated at approximately $46 million, which is insufficient to recover development costs within the short 5–10-year exclusivity period granted to most drugs. Antibiotics are almost invariably taken in short courses and for most patients infrequently; when a new antibiotic is released to the market, physicians (applying the principles of antibiotic stewardship) typically prescribe against strict guidelines to preserve the effective lifetime of the drug by avoiding emergence of resistance through overuse or inappropriate use. Taken together, these factors mean that the economic case for antibiotic research and development is difficult to establish and new business models for antibiotic development are urgently required. A number of new approaches have been proposed and adopted in the past few years, including funding initiatives to cover the costly early developmental/preclinical stages of antibiotic research, encouraging governments to pay pharmaceutical companies for access to new antibiotics (a subscription basis as adopted in the UK in 2020, whereby the UK government will pay pharmaceutical companies in instalments during early stage development in exchange for access to the new agents). Other funding initiatives have been established in the past 5 years aimed at tackling these economic barriers, including CARB-X (with a $500 million budget from governments in the USA, Germany and the UK with charitable organisations including Wellcome) and governmental and privately funded global AMR action funds such as that established by the International Federation of Pharmaceutical Manufacturers & Associations, which aim to bring up to four new antibiotics to the market by 2030. These initiatives aim to de-risk antibiotic research, and improve the economic landscape to encourage major pharmaceutical companies back into the antibiotic research and development arena.

Despite the general stagnation in the antibiotic pipeline, some notable successes provide a much-needed glimmer of hope within this sector. In 2015, researchers in Northeastern University, Boston, USA published the discovery of a new antibiotic, teixobactin, the first report of a new mechanistic class of antibiotic in over 30 years. The compound was discovered from a screen of uncultured soil bacteria, using enhanced culture techniques to overcome the low culture efficiency associated with conventional approaches (approximately 1% of microorganisms can be cultured from most environments, leaving circa 99% uncultured). Teixobactin, isolated from a previously uncultured Gram-negative β-proteobacteria *Eleftheria terrae*, is an unusual 11-amino acid macrocyclic depsipeptide containing 4 D-amino acids, methylphenylalanine and L-*allo*-enduracididine, and a 14-member ring resulting from ring closure between the terminal isoleucine and threonine residues. It has a unique mechanism of action, inhibiting cell wall synthesis via binding to lipid II and lipid III (precursors of peptidoglycan and cell wall teichoic acid, respectively), and is active against several Gram-positive bacteria in both *in vitro* and *in vivo* tests. In 2019, GlaxoSmithKline (GSK) announced the commencement of phase III clinical trials of the first agent in another new chemical class of synthetic antibiotics, gepotidacin, a triazaacenaphthylene bacterial topoisomerase inhibitor, for the treatment of uncomplicated urinary tract infection (uUTIs) and urogenital gonorrhoea. Phase II trials of gepotidacin also showed efficacy in the treatment of acute bacterial skin and skin structure infections. Gepotidacin inhibits two important bacterial enzymes, DNA gyrase and topoisomerase IV, and has activity against antibiotic-resistant bacteria, including fluoroquinolone-resistant strains. Importantly, this antibiotic was developed through a public–private partnership between GSK, the US government Biomedical Advanced Research and Development Authority (BARDA) and the Defense Threat Reduction Agency (DTRA). In a final example, in 2020, researchers at Massachusetts Institute of Technology (MIT) described a deep learning/artificial intelligence (AI) approach to predict antibiotics *in silico* based on structures from chemical libraries. The authors report the discovery of a broad-spectrum bactericidal antibiotic compound, halicin, with an apparently unique mechanism of action based on intracellular iron sequestration leading to the dissipation of the proton motive force. The authors of the study acknowledge that, to date, AI approaches are imperfect and success of the approach in identifying new antibiotic agents will rely on coupling deep learning with appropriate experimentation. These examples of successful discovery and development of new antibiotics demonstrate that it ought to be possible to reverse the trend of low antibiotic approvals, reinvigorate the antibiotic pipeline and avert an impending public health crisis.

11.1.1 Antibiotic Usage

Despite the lack of new antibiotic approvals, there are a large number of antibiotics of diverse mechanistic and chemical classes in widespread use globally. Some of these antibiotics are available only in certain countries, and within countries the list of available antibiotics is subject to regular change, as antimicrobial prescribing/stewardship policies may dictate some compounds are no longer suitable for prescribing, the replacement of old or unsuitable agents in favour of new products and the withdrawal of compounds due to cost or safety concerns. Currently in the UK, there are approximately 80 antibiotics (including antibiotic combinations, for example, lactam–lactamase inhibitor combination products), 20 antifungals and over 50 antiviral agents (greater than 50% of which are antiretrovirals for the treatment of human immunodeficiency virus [HIV]) available for clinical use, with similar numbers in other countries. It cannot be the intention of this chapter, therefore, to describe or mention all of the above drugs, but rather to consider the major antibiotic classes and refer the reader to additional and more detailed sources of information on some of the less frequently prescribed agents.

The various classes of antibiotics will be considered in their order of importance in terms of usage, and frequency of prescribing. Interestingly, this may not coincide with their rank order in terms of annually manufactured quantities by the pharmaceutical industry, given the significant proportion of antibiotic use in animal production, livestock and feed supplements (the O'Neill review estimated that in the USA, 70%, by weight, of medically important antibiotics sold are used in livestock, and over 50% in most countries; see also Chapter 13). However, stringent efforts are being made worldwide to reduce antibiotic consumption in livestock production, with most countries now setting and achieving ambitious targets for antibiotic use reduction.

The World Health Organization (WHO) has developed the Access, Watch, Reserve (AWaRe) classification of antibiotics to assist the development and monitoring of antimicrobial stewardship (see also Chapter 15), and aims to give an indication of appropriateness of antibiotic consumption. Within this classification, antibiotics are classified as Access (first- or second-line antibiotic therapies), Watch (for use only in specific indications due to high resistance potential), or Reserve (last-resort antibiotic therapies). Worryingly, a recent analysis of international antibiotic consumption based on pharmaceutical sales data from 75 countries indicated that in the period 2000–2015, per capita global antibiotic consumption increased by 39%, while consumption of Watch antibiotics increased by 90.9% (increasing from 3.3. to 6.3 defined daily doses [DDDs] per 1000 inhabitants per day), with increases greater in lower-income and middle-income countries (LMICs) than in higher-income countries (HICs). Despite this, per capita antibiotic consumption remains still considerably higher in HICs compared to LMICs. The WHO national level target that 60% of total antibiotic consumption would be from the Access group also decreased, from being met by 76% of countries down to just 55% between 2000 and 2015, indicating a potential decrease in appropriateness of consumption of antibiotics in this time period.

In the UK, antibiotic consumption data are submitted to the European Surveillance of Antimicrobial Consumption Network (ESAC-Net), in addition to publishing data from the English Surveillance Programme for Antimicrobial Utilisation and Resistance (ESPAUR). Between 2014 and 2018, total consumption of antibiotics in England decreased by 9% from 20 DDDs per 1000 inhabitants to 18.2 DDDs per 1000 inhabitants. The UK 5-year national action plan (2019–2024) aims to reduce human antimicrobial use by 15% by 2024, and in food-producing animals by 25% between 2016 and 2020. The majority of antibiotic prescribing (72% in 2018) is in community general medical practice (general practitioner [GP] surgeries). During the coronavirus (COVID-19) pandemic, antibiotic

Table 11.1 Relative frequency of prescribing of antibiotics in the UK, in community and hospital settings, during 2019.

Antibiotic class	Usage
β-Lactams (penicillins)	6.67
β-Lactams (other)	0.36
Tetracyclines	4.74
Macrolides – lincosamides and streptogramins	2.66
Sulphonamides and trimethoprim	0.86
Quinolones	0.49
Aminoglycosides	0.13
Amphenicols (chloramphenicol)	<0.001
Others (including glycopeptides)	1.40

UK antibiotic use in defined daily doses (DDDs) per 1000 inhabitants per day in both community and hospital sectors. Adapted from European Centre for Disease Prevention and Control Antimicrobial Consumption Database.

prescribing trends showed a significant increase in both general practice and the hospital setting, with one study finding that approximately three-quarters of patients hospitalised with COVID-19 were prescribed antibiotics, despite only 8% confirmed to have had a bacterial coinfection.

Table 11.1 shows the distribution of antimicrobial consumption by antimicrobial group, for systemic treatment in the community and hospital sector in the United Kingdom determined from recent (2019) data included in ongoing Europe-wide surveillance of antimicrobial consumption. While variations are likely between relative frequency of antibiotic prescribed between community and hospital sectors, some trends are clear. β-Lactam antibiotics are, by far, the most frequently prescribed class of antibiotic, with penicillins accounting for the majority, far outnumbering the prescribing of other β-lactams including the cephalosporins. Although data are grouped for some antibiotic classes, tetracyclines, macrolides and trimethoprim rank highly. Antibiotics which are administered parenterally (aminoglycosides, glycopeptides) have more restricted prescribing patterns, since they are less likely to be prescribed for outpatient/community use because of issues surrounding administration, which accounts for their lower ranking in this analysis. While the data in this table are part of a Europe-wide consumption surveillance programme, there is variation from country to country according to national trends and prescribing policies.

Detailed discussion of antibiotic mode of action (Chapter 12), antibiotic resistance (Chapter 13) and antibiotic stewardship (Chapter 15) is included elsewhere in this book and the reader is directed to the relevant chapter for further information.

11.2 β-Lactam Antibiotics

For around two decades after their introduction into clinical use, the penicillins were the only category of β-lactam antibiotics available. The 1960s saw the expansion of this family with the introduction of cephalosporins, and later in the twentieth century by carbapenems and monobactams. All β-lactam antibiotics share a common mode of action, disrupting cell wall synthesis through the inhibition of transpeptidases, and all possess the β-lactam nucleus, but they differ widely in other properties including spectrum of activity, pharmacokinetics and activity against antibiotic-resistant bacteria/susceptibility to resistance mechanisms. Structurally, the following major classes of clinically useful β-lactams have been described:

Penams (penicillins): β-lactam nucleus is fused with a five-membered (thiazolidine) ring containing sulphur as the heteroatom (a 4:5 fused ring). Antimicrobial penicillins typically contain an acylamino substituent side chain on the β-lactam ring, the composition of which is important for determining the spectrum of activity and pharmacological properties.

Clavams: β-lactam nucleus is fused with a five-membered heterocyclic ring containing an oxygen atom as the heteroatom. While they possess weak or negligible antimicrobial activity, members of this class are used as inhibitors of β-lactamases (see clavulanic acid in Section 11.2.1).

Carbapenems: contain the 4:5 fused ring lactam of penicillins but with the substitution of carbon for sulphur at position C-1 (no heteroatom) and a double bond between C-2 and C-3 of the five-membered ring.

Cephems (cephalosporins): β-lactam nucleus is fused with a six-membered unsaturated ring containing sulphur as the heteroatom (a 4:6 fused ring).

Oxacephams: analogous to the cephems but containing oxygen instead of sulphur as the heteroatom of the unsaturated six-membered ring.

Monobactams: non-fused β-lactam nucleus with either a methylcarboxylate (nocardicins) or a sulphonate (e.g., aztreonam) functionality providing the acidic moiety required for action against transpeptidases, constructed in the β-lactam nucleus.

11.2.1 Penicillins

The penicillins (general structure shown in Figure 11.1a) are broadly categorised into the following types:

Naturally occurring: for example, those produced by fermentation of moulds such as *P. notatum* and *Penicillium chrysogenum*. Naturally occurring, therapeutically useful

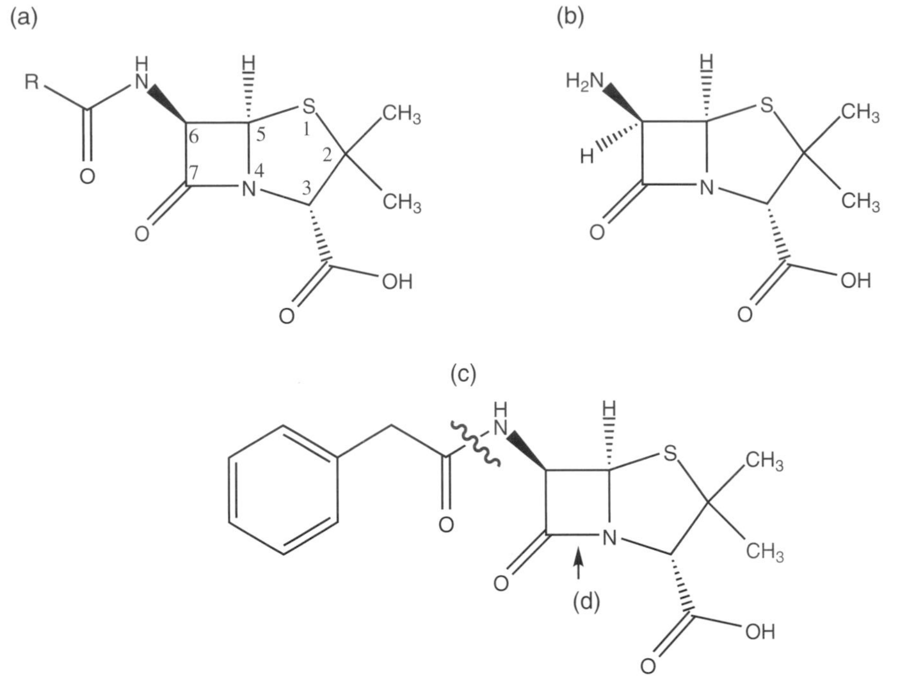

(a) (b) (c) (d)

Figure 11.1 (a) General structure of penicillins with the acyl side chain represented by R. (b) 6-aminopenicillanic acid, 6-APA. (c) Removal of the side chain from benzylpenicillin. (d) Site of action of β-lactamases.

penicillins are few in number, but include the important antibiotics benzylpenicillin (penicillin G) and phenoxymethylpenicillin (penicillin V).

Semi-synthetic: semi-synthetic penicillins were first manufactured in the late 1950s, following the successful isolation of the penicillin nucleus, 6-APA (Figure 11.1b), by scientists at the Beecham Research Laboratories. In order to produce benzylpenicillin, phenylacetic acid ($C_6H_5.CH_2.COOH$), a precursor to the side chain R of benzylpenicillin, is added to the medium in which the *Penicillium* mould is growing. Growth of the penicillin-producing organism in the absence of phenylacetic acid facilitated the identification and isolation of 6-APA, which can be chromatographically resolved from benzylpenicillin.

The discovery of penicillin amidases (acylases) provided a further route to the production of 6-APA from benzylpenicillin, via selective removal of the side chain from benzylpenicillin (Figure 11.1c). Following manufacture of 6-APA using classical fermentation methodologies, differing side chains can be added to the penicillin nucleus which alter the antimicrobial spectrum of activity, pharmacological characteristics and susceptibility to penicillinase enzymes (β-lactamases). The majority of penicillins in widespread use are semi-synthetic agents, such as amoxicillin, methicillin and ampicillin (Figure 11.2).

Sodium and potassium salts of the penicillins exhibit high aqueous solubility, but are susceptible to hydrolysis in solution to the corresponding penicilloic acid, at a temperature-dependent rate. Penicilloic acid lacks antimicrobial activity and is produced at both alkaline and neutral pH. Under acidic conditions, hydrolysis to penillic acid occurs. This susceptibility to hydrolysis, whereby aqueous solutions of penicillins lose approximately 10% or greater of their activity in 24 hours at room temperature, means that penicillins are unsuitable for formulation as aqueous products. Therefore, oral syrups and suspensions are prepared as dry granules for reconstitution in water immediately prior to dispensing, and penicillins for parenteral administration are provided as freeze-dried powders in vials or ampoules. Oral administration of some penicillins, such as benzylpenicillin, is contraindicated, since instability under acidic conditions leads to poor oral bioavailability. For example, benzylpenicillin has a half-life of less than 5 minutes at normal stomach pH (circa pH 1) at 35 °C, whereas ampicillin under the same conditions has a half-life of 600 minutes, making it suitable for oral administration. Both ampicillin and amoxicillin are both sufficiently stable under acid conditions to be taken orally, with amoxicillin having greater bioavailability (being almost completely absorbed from the gut) than ampicillin, which is only 30–60% absorbed. Benzylpenicillin is also rapidly excreted by the kidneys, which may be overcome by formulation of the active drug as sparingly soluble salts

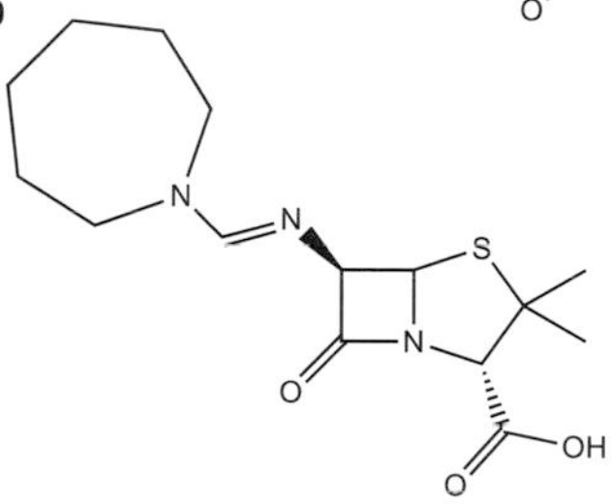

Figure 11.2 Structures of the major semi-synthetic penicillins showing examples of the various side-chain modifications: (1) benzylpenicillin (penicillin G), (2) amoxicillin, (3) phenoxymethylpenicillin (penicillin V), (4) ampicillin, (5) flucloxacillin, (6) ticarcillin, (7) piperacillin, (8) temocillin and (9) pivmecillinam.

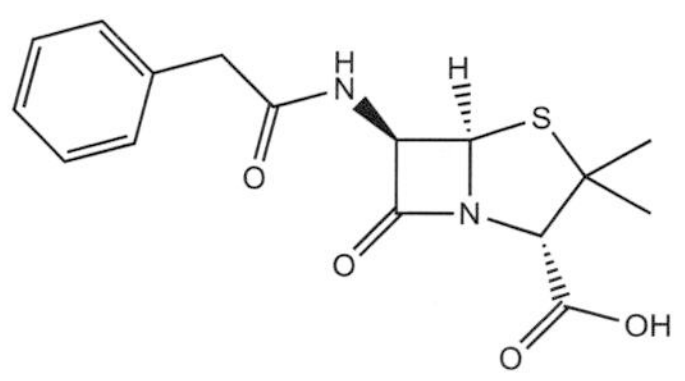

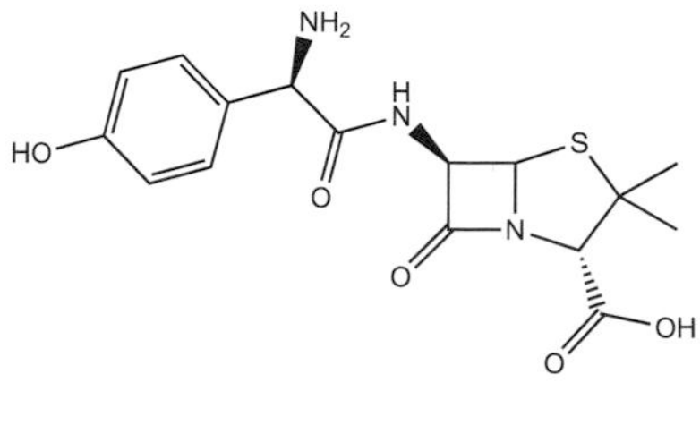

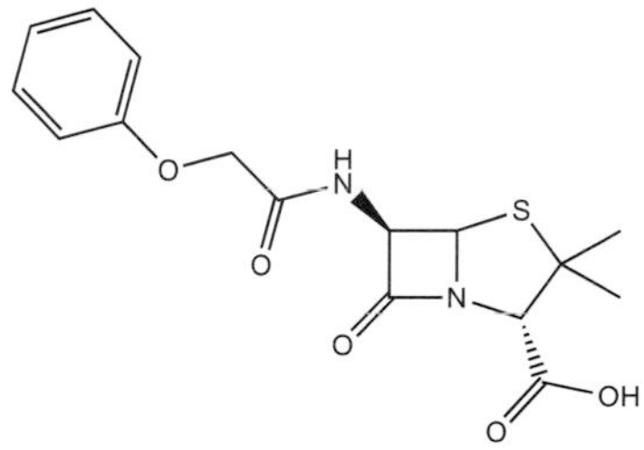

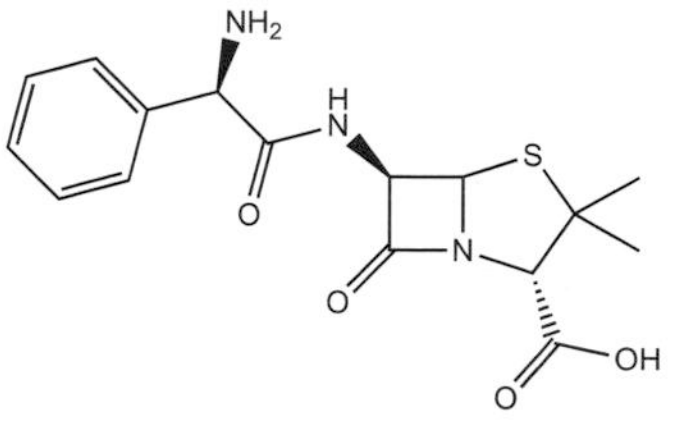

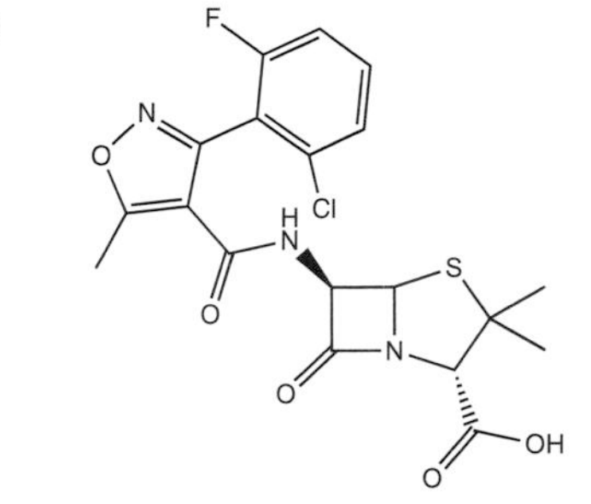

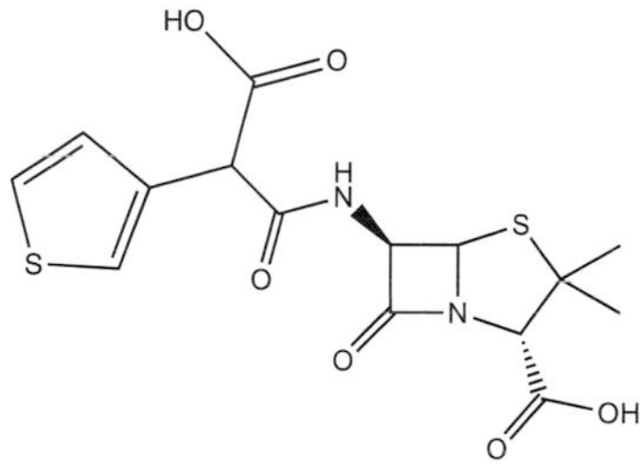

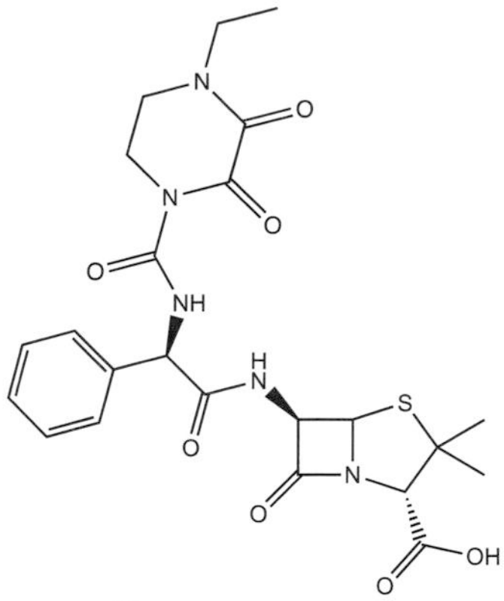

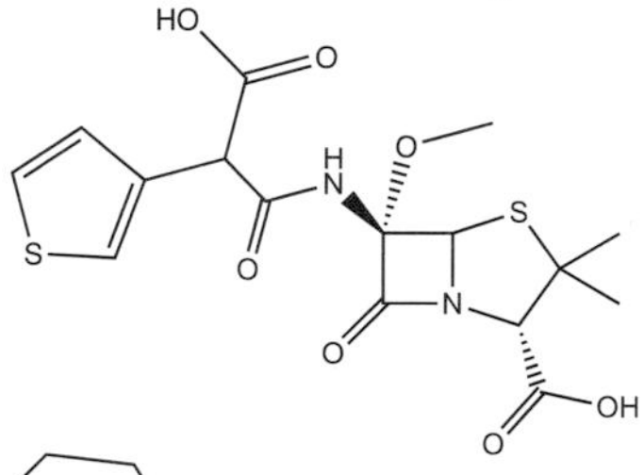

(procaine, benzathine and benethamine) facilitating slow release of benzylpenicillin and maintaining adequately high, continuous plasma concentrations. Probenecid also reduces tubular secretion from the kidney, prolonging the half-life of penicillins.

Many bacteria produce enzymes capable of degrading penicillins and other β-lactam antibiotics, these β-lactamases inactivate penicillins by hydrolysing the amide bond in the β-lactam ring, leading to ring opening and loss of activity; this is a major mechanism of β-lactam resistance. Some semi-synthetic penicillins exhibit insensitivity to β-lactamases (Table 11.2), and are valuable in the treatment of otherwise β-lactam-resistant infections. Clavulanic acid has no significant intrinsic activity but acts as an irreversible inhibitor of β-lactamase enzymes. Clavulanic acid is commonly co-formulated with amoxicillin (UK, Augmentin®) to protect the antibiotic from enzymatic degradation. A full discussion of the classification of β-lactamases and currently available inhibitors and antibiotic inhibitor combinations is provided in Chapter 13.

The development of semi-synthetic penicillins through modification of the 6-APA nucleus has given rise to a large and diverse family of antibiotics. The shortcomings of the natural penicillins (stability, spectrum of activity and susceptibility to hydrolysis by β-lactamase enzymes) were, to varying extents, overcome by medicinal chemistry approaches and semi-synthetic penicillins were approved from the 1960s onwards. Ampicillin, though sensitive to β-lactamases, exhibited an extended spectrum of activity compared to the parent compound, benzylpenicillin, due to the presence of an amino group on the benzyl side chain. The oral absorption of ampicillin was found to be improved by the inclusion of a *p*-hydroxyl group on the benzene ring of the ampicillin side chain to create amoxicillin. Temocillin, a 6α-methoxy derivative of ticarcillin exhibited resistance to Gram-negative β-lactamases. Furthermore, the carboxylic acid substituent on the C3 carbon can be esterified to create lipophilic prodrugs with improved oral bioavailability, which following absorption liberate the active penicillin through the action of hydrolytic tissue esterases. This approach has

Table 11.2 Properties of the common penicillins.

		Activity against			Stability towards β-lactamases from			
Penicillin	**Oral activity**	**Gram-positive**	**Gram-negative**[a]	***Pseudomonas aeruginosa***	***Staphylococcus aureus***	**Gram-negative**	**Doses/day**	**Combined with β-lactamase inhibitor**
1 Benzylpenicillin	−	+	−	−	−	−	4	
2 Phenoxymethylpenicillin	+	+	−	−	−	−	4	
3 Flucloxacillin	+	+	−	−	+	+	4	
4 Ampicillin	+	+	+	−	−	−	4	Sulbactam (not UK)
5 Amoxicillin	+	+	+	−	−	−	3	Clavulanic acid
6 Ticarcillin	−	±	+	+	−	±	3–4	Clavulanic acid
7 Piperacillin	−	+	+	+	−	−	4	Tazobactam
8 Temocillin	−	−	+	−	+	+	2	
9 Pivmecillinam	+	−	+	−	NR	±	3–4	

+, applicable; −, inapplicable; NR, not relevant: pivmecillinam has no effect on Gram-positive bacteria; ±, variable result depending on species and strain.

[a] Except *P. aeruginosa*. All penicillins show some degree of activity against Gram-negative cocci.

Notes:

1) For additional information on β-lactamase-mediated resistance, see Chapter 13.
2) Most penicillins are active against Gram-positive bacteria, although in the case of *S. aureus*, this may depend upon the resistance of the antibiotic to β-lactamase.

been employed to enhance the poor oral absorption of ampicillin, resulting in the development of bacampicillin, pivampicillin and talampicillin. Methicillin, a penicillin synthesised by replacement of one of the amino hydrogens with a 2,6-methoxybenzoyl group exhibits resistance to staphylococcal β-lactamase, whereby the bulky substituent of the side chain hinders enzyme binding; however, due to the emergence of methicillin-resistant *S. aureus* (MRSA), which expresses an additional mutated and β-lactam-insensitive transpeptidase, methicillin has been largely replaced by other β-lactamase-stable penicillins, particularly the orally active flucloxacillin.

Penicillins can also be usefully classified by spectrum of activity:

i) Penicillin G and penicillin V are highly active against Gram-positive cocci, but are highly susceptible to hydrolysis by penicillinases. As a result, both have little or no activity against most strains of *S. aureus*.
ii) The penicillinase-resistant penicillins (methicillin, oxacillin, cloxacillin and dicloxacillin) are less potent against microorganisms which are sensitive to penicillin G (benzylpenicillin), but are effective against penicillinase-producing *S. aureus* and *Staphylococcus epidermidis* that are not methicillin-resistant.
iii) Penicillins which have an extended spectrum of antimicrobial activity to include Gram-negative microorganisms such as *Haemophilus influenzae*, *Escherichia coli* and *Proteus mirabilis* include ampicillin, amoxicillin and bacampicillin. Again, these penicillins are highly sensitive to hydrolysis by broad-spectrum β-lactamases which are now increasingly identified in clinical isolates of Gram-negative pathogens. Extended-spectrum beta-lactamases (ESBLs) are commonly produced by a number of Gram-negative bacteria, especially *E. coli* and *Klebsiella pneumoniae*.
iv) The spectrum of activity of carbenicillin, its indanyl ester (carbenicillin indanyl) and ticarcillin is extended to include *Pseudomonas*, *Proteus* and *Enterobacter* species. However, these penicillins are less effective than ampicillin against Gram-positive cocci and *Listeria monocytogenes*.
v) Mezlocillin, azlocillin and piperacillin have excellent activity against Gram-negative bacteria. In addition, piperacillin retains excellent activity against Gram-positive cocci and *L. monocytogenes*.

11.2.2 Cephalosporins

Cephalosporins are one of the most important and widely prescribed class of antibiotics, which share a similar history of discovery and development, mechanism of action and structure with the penicillins. The initial discovery of cephalosporin was made in 1948, from the fungus *Cephalosporium acremonium*. Crude filtrates from cultures of *C. acremonium* were found to inhibit the *in vitro* growth of *S. aureus*; these filtrates were found to contain three distinct antibiotics, cephalosporin P, N and the penicillinase-stable cephalosporin C. Following the initial discovery, further research was conducted at the Sir William Dunn School of Pathology, Oxford (where the isolation and structural elucidation of penicillin had been performed). The first cephalosporins to be released in the mid-1960s were cephalothin and cephaloridine. Since then, numerous cephalosporins have been synthesised and more than 60 compounds have been marketed in the past 50 years. This section describes the general properties and important characteristics of the cephalosporins by reference to selected examples of these important agents.

As with the penicillins, the isolation of the active nucleus, 7-aminocephalosporanic acid (7-ACA; Figure 11.3a), made it possible to produce multiple modifications, and a battery of useful semi-synthetic cephalosporins were produced. Many of these compounds exhibited improved potency and a superior spectrum of activity compared with the natural parent compound. All cephalosporins possess the six-membered dihydrothiazine ring fused to the four-membered β-lactam ring. The position of the double bond is critical in Δ^3-cephalosporins, since Δ^2-cephalosporins lack antimicrobial activity, irrespective of the side chains present. The presence of two side chains (at carbons 3 and 7; see cephalosporin general structure, Figure 11.4) provides greater scope for structural modification and diversity compared to the penicillins. As is the case with the penicillins, structural

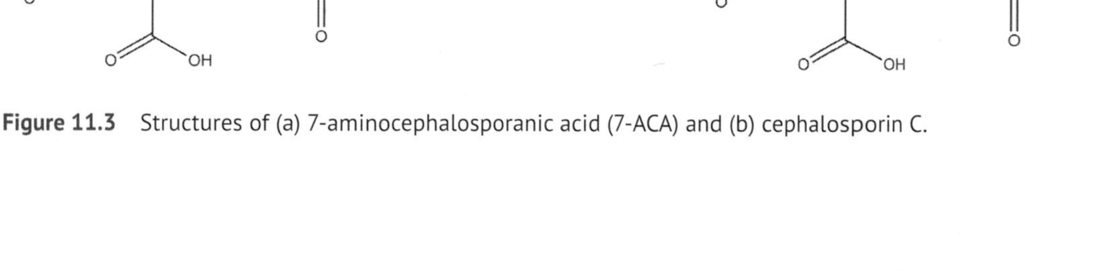

(a) H_2N, H, S, N, O, O, CH_3, O, O, OH

(b) O, HO, NH_2, H N, O, H, S, N, O, O, CH_3, O, O, OH

Figure 11.3 Structures of (a) 7-aminocephalosporanic acid (7-ACA) and (b) cephalosporin C.

modification of these side chains facilitates optimisation of the fundamental properties of the cephalosporins, including acid stability (and therefore oral availability), spectrum of antimicrobial action, pharmacokinetics and stability to β-lactamases. In keeping with several of the penicillins, cephalosporins (especially first-generation compounds) are inducers of β-lactamases.

Cephalosporin C (Figure 11.3b) contains a side chain derived from D-α-aminoadipic acid, condensed with the 7-ACA β-lactam ring system; compounds containing 7-ACA are highly resistant to penicillinases (β-lactamases). Structural modifications at position 7 (R_2; see Figure 11.4) of the β-lactam ring are associated with alterations in antibacterial activity, while modifications at position 3 (R_1; see Figure 11.4) are associated with changes in metabolism and pharmacokinetic properties of the drugs. The cephamycins are similar to the cephalosporins, but have a methoxy group at position 7 of the β-lactam ring of the 7-ACA nucleus. The mode of action of the cephalosporins and the cephamycins is similar to that of the penicillins resulting in an inhibition of bacterial cell wall synthesis.

Cephalosporins are classified into five generations based on antimicrobial activity and temporal discovery; the classification is more clearly defined than with the penicillins, but there is some overlap between generations and some compounds may fall into different classes in different countries. In general, earlier-generation cephalosporins exhibit greater activity towards Gram-positive bacteria, with later generations having increased activity towards Gram-negative microorganisms and an increased resistance to β-lactamase-mediated hydrolysis and inactivation. These are discussed below and summarised in Table 11.3.

First-generation cephalosporins, of which cefalexin and cefazolin are archetypal members, have good activity against Gram-positive bacteria and exhibit moderate activity towards Gram-negative pathogens. Most Gram-positive microorganisms are sensitive to the first-generation cephalosporins, with the exception of enterococci and MRSA. They exhibit good resistance to staphylococcal, but not Gram-negative β-lactamases. In addition, oral cavity anaerobes are generally susceptible with the exception of the *Bacteroides fragilis* group. First-generation cephalosporins are rarely first-choice antibiotics, but may be used as an alternative antibiotic for staphylococcal infections.

Second-generation cephalosporins, including cefaclor, cefoxitin and cefuroxime, generally exhibit an increased activity against Gram-negative microorganisms compared with first- generation agents. Second-generation compounds possess activity against *Enterobacteriaceae* and *H. influenzae*, and exhibit good resistance to both staphylococcal and Gram-negative β-lactamases. However, these agents are much less potent than corresponding third-generation drugs. Cefoxitin, cefotetan and cefmetazole exhibit good activity against the *B. fragilis* group, making them useful agents for dental infections/pre-operative prophylaxis.

Third-generation cephalosporins such as cefotaxime and ceftazidime are generally less potent against Gram-positive cocci than the first-generation agents but are more active against Gram-negatives and the *Enterobacteriaceae*, including ESBL-producing strains. However, widespread evolution and dissemination of ESBLs have somewhat diminished the utility of this generation of compounds. The third-generation agents ceftazidime and cefoperazone are also active against *Pseudomonas aeruginosa*.

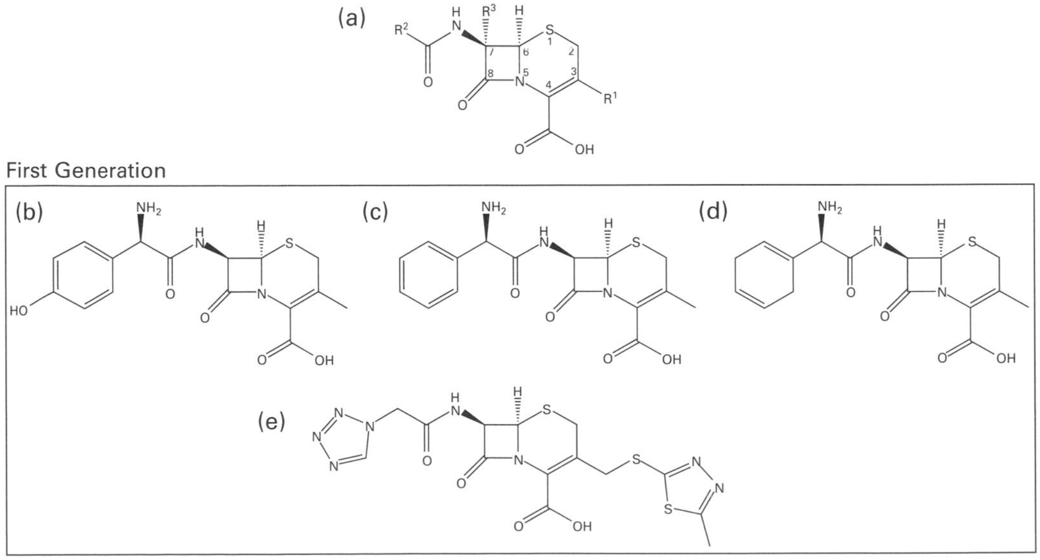

(a)

First Generation

(b) (c) (d) (e)

Figure 11.4 (Continued)

Second Generation

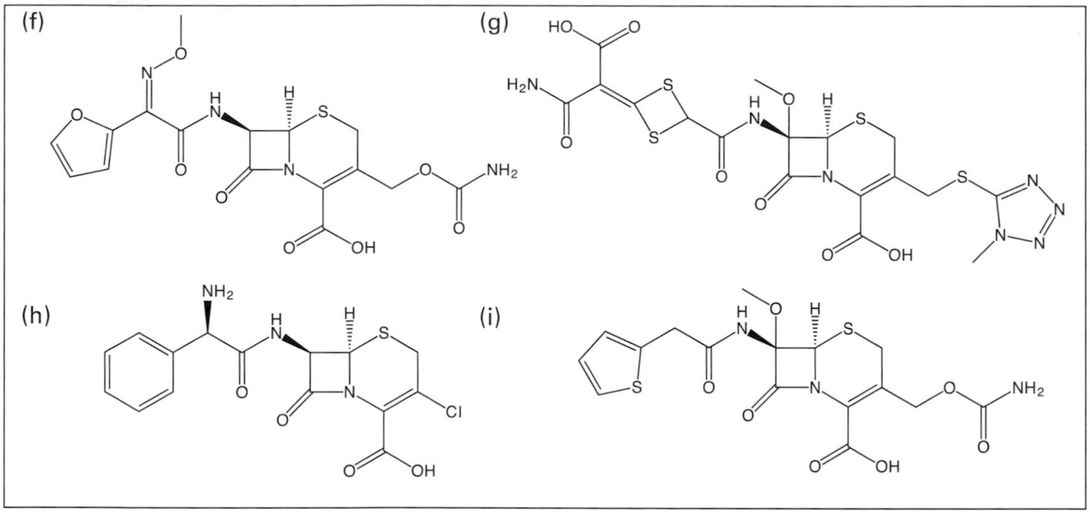

(f) (g) (h) (i)

Third Generation

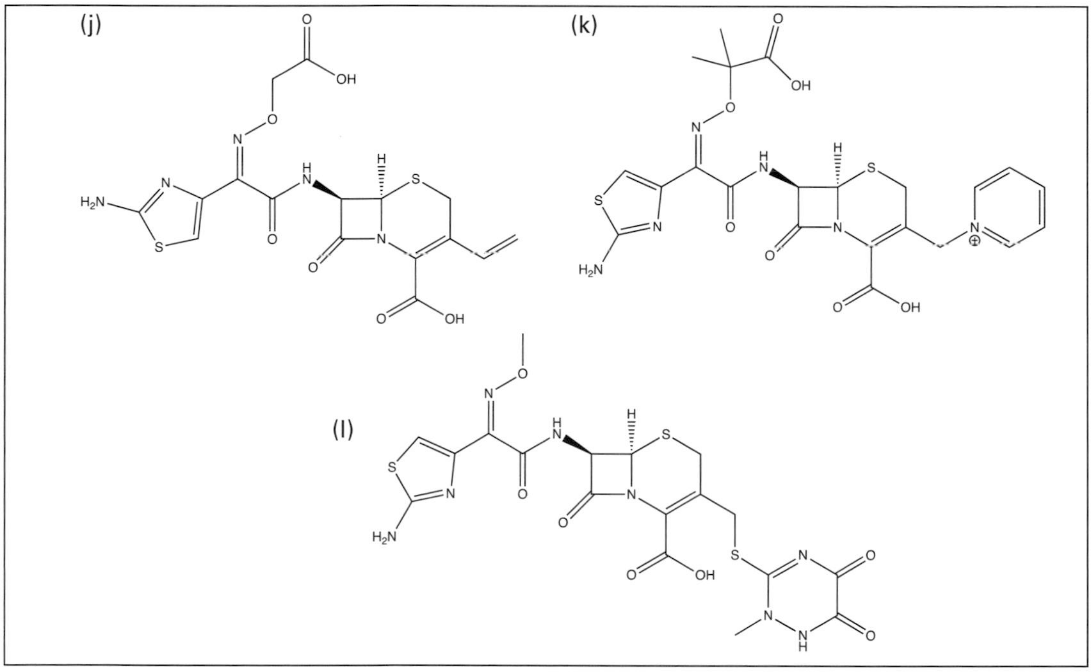

(j) (k) (l)

Fourth Generation

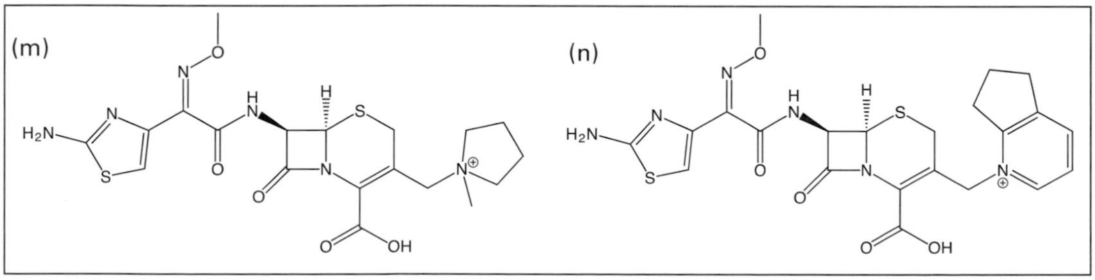

(m) (n)

Figure 11.4 (Continued)

Fifth Generation

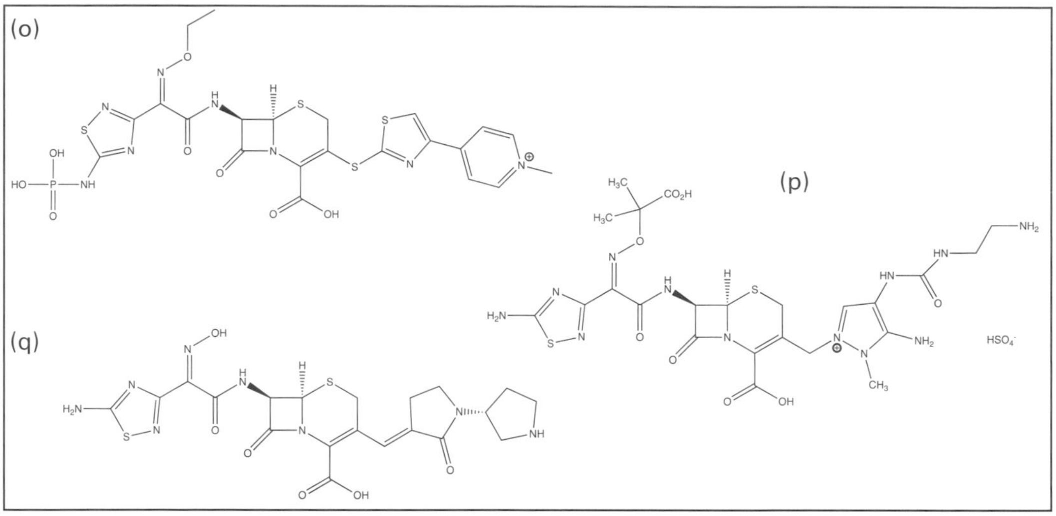

Figure 11.4 Cephalosporin antibiotics: (a) cephalosporin general structure. First generation – (b) cefadroxil; (c) cefalexin; (d) cefradine; (e) cefazolin. Second generation – (f) cefuroxime; (g) cefotetan; (h) cefaclor; (i) cefoxitin. Third generation – (j) cefixime; (k) ceftazidime; (l) ceftriaxone. Fourth generation – (m) cefepime; (n) cefpirome. Fifth generation – (o) ceftaroline fosamil; (p) ceftolozane; (q) ceftobiprole.

Table 11.3 Cephalosporins classified by generation/spectrum of activity.

Generation	Examples	Spectrum of activity
First	Cefazolin Cefalexin Cefadroxil Cefradine	Streptococci[a], *S. aureus*[b]
Second	Cefuroxime Cefaclor Cefoxitin Cefotetan	*E. coli*, *Klebsiella*, *Proteus*, *Haemophilus influenzae*, *Moraxella catarrhalis*. Less active than first-generation agents against Gram-positive bacteria Cefotetan is less active against *S. aureus* than cefuroxime, but with activity against anaerobes including *Bacteroides fragilis* and other *Bacteroides* spp.
Third	Cefotaxime Cefoperazone Cefixime Ceftriaxone Ceftazidime	Activity against *S. aureus*, *Streptococcus pneumoniae* and *Streptococcus pyogenes* comparable to first-generation agents. Less active against *Bacteroides* spp. compared to second-generation agents. Activity against *P. aeruginosa*, *Neisseria gonorrhoeae* and *Enterobacteriaceae*.
Fourth	Cefepime Cefpirome	Comparable activity to third-generation, improved resistance to β-lactamases
Fifth	Ceftaroline Ceftobiprole Ceftolozane	Activity against MRSA, *Enterococcus faecalis* and *L. monocytogenes*

[a] Except penicillin-resistant strains.
[b] Except methicillin-resistant strains. *Source:* Adapted from Nath et al. (2020) and BNF 83 (2022).

Fourth-generation cephalosporins, such as cefepime, exhibit an improved antimicrobial spectrum compared with other agents and have increased stability to hydrolysis by β-lactamases. These are active against methicillin-sensitive *S. aureus* (MSSA), *Streptococcus pneumoniae*, *P. aeruginosa*, *P. mirabilis*, *Citrobacter*, *Enterobacter*, *Providencia*, *Klebsiella* and *Serratia* spp. Cefepime is not active against MRSA, ESBL or Amp-C β-lactamase-producing Gram-negative bacteria.

Fifth-generation cephalosporins include ceftaroline, ceftolozane and ceftobiprole; these have activity against methicillin-resistant staphylococci and penicillin-resistant pneumococci. Ceftaroline is a broad-spectrum antibiotic with excellent activity against MRSA (due to targeted binding to penicillin-binding protein 2a [PBP2a]), *Enterococcus faecalis* and *L. monocytogenes*, and multi-drug resistant *S. pneumoniae*, but lacks activity against *P. aeruginosa* and vancomycin-resistant enterococci (VRE). By contrast, ceftolozane, in combination with the β-lactamase inhibitor tazobactam or avibactam, has activity against *P. aeruginosa*, *Enterobacteriaceae* and other resistant Gram-negative pathogens. Ceftobiprole is active against MRSA and resistant *S. pneumoniae* and Gram-negative bacteria and is indicated for the treatment of hospital-acquired pneumonia.

11.2.2.1 Structure–Activity Relationships

The activity of β-lactam antibiotics relies on their affinity for transpeptidases/PBPs. The primary mechanisms of resistance to β-lactams are through production of β-lactamase enzymes or through expression of altered PBPs (as in MRSA). In order to achieve antimicrobial activity against Gram-negative pathogens, β-lactams must also be able to traverse the outer membrane to gain access to PBPs in the periplasmic space. The outer membrane confers intrinsic resistance to some β-lactams, especially the naturally occurring compounds and the first-generation and some second-generation cephalosporins. Modification of the cephalosporin nucleus (Figure 11.3a) at 7α (R^3; Figure 11.4) by addition of a methoxy group decreases activity against Gram-positive bacteria due to a reduced affinity for PBPs, but increases β-lactamase stability. Cephalosporins with 7α-methoxy groups are termed cephamycins (e.g., cefoxitin). For further information on mechanisms of action and antibiotic resistance, the reader is referred to Chapters 12 and 13.

The general cephalosporin structure and examples of modifications are given in Figure 11.4. Substitution at position R^1, with side chains containing a 2-aminothiazolyl group, for example, in cefotaxime, ceftriaxone and ceftazidime, gives rise to compounds with increased affinity for Gram-negative PBPs and activity against streptococci. An R^1 modification with an iminomethoxy group (—C=N. OCH_3), for example, in cefuroxime, yields compounds with enhanced β-lactamase stability. A propylcarboxyl group at R^1, as in ceftazidime, increases β-lactamase resistance, reduces β-lactamase induction and extends activity to *P. aeruginosa*. The β-lactamase-mediated ring opening in cephalosporins also leads to loss of the substituent at R^2 (unless R^2 is H, e.g., cefalexin) and fragmentation of the molecule. The nature of the R^2 substituent is critical in determining not only the pharmacokinetic properties of the molecule but also activity, since the ability to enter bacterial cells, especially to cross the Gram-negative outer membrane via porins, may be modulated through alterations of the R^2 group. For good oral absorption: (i) the R^2 substituent must be small, non-polar and stable (a methyl group is considered desirable but may decrease antibacterial activity); and (ii) the 7-acyl group, R^1, must be based on phenylglycine and the amino group must remain unsubstituted. As with the penicillins, esterification of the C4 carboxylic acid generates tissue-esterase-activated prodrugs which exhibit enhanced oral absorption (e.g., cefuroxime axetil and cefpodoxime proxetil). The possession of a quaternary nitrogen on the side chain at position 3 reduces the affinity of the cephalosporin for Gram-negative β-lactamases and also makes the molecule zwitterionic, which increases the rate of uptake through porins into the Gram-negative cell.

11.2.3 β-Lactamase Inhibitors

The discovery, from natural product screening, of clavulanic acid, a clavam β-lactam with negligible antimicrobial activity but with broad-spectrum inhibitory activity against staphylococcal penicillinases, resulted in the first combination product, co-amoxiclav (amoxicillin and clavulanic acid), in 1981. Structurally, clavulanic acid is similar to the penicillins but differs in respect of the heteroatom whereby sulphur in the penicillin thiazolidine ring is replaced by oxygen in the clavam oxazolidine ring (Figure 11.5a), and the absence of a side chain at position 6. The general strategy of protecting β-lactamase-labile β-lactams through a

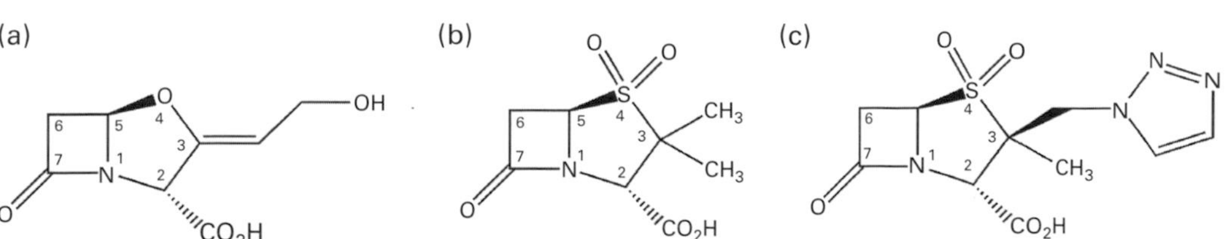

Figure 11.5 Examples of therapeutic β-lactamase inhibitors: (a) clavulanic acid, (b) sulbactam and (c) tazobactam.

combination of antibiotic with β-lactamase inhibitor remains an active and productive avenue in antibiotic research and development, with new combination products approved regularly. Co-amoxiclav remains the most important clinical combination available. Clavulanic acid acts in synergy with both penicillins and cephalosporins, negating the effects of class A β-lactamases and ESBLs and the combination extends the spectrum of activity such that action is against not only *S. aureus* but also *E. coli*, *H. influenzae* and *Klebsiella* spp. against which amoxicillin alone would be ineffective. Clavulanic acid has also been combined with ticarcillin parenterally and shown to be effective against *P. aeruginosa* and other Gram-negative bacteria. Clavulanic acid is primarily active against penicillinases but also shows a modest inhibition of some β-lactamase enzymes active against the cephalosporins.

Following the success of clavulanic acid combinations, a number of penicillanic acid sulphone β-lactamase inhibitors were discovered and two, sulbactam and tazobactam (Figure 11.5b,c) were commercialised. Again, these are β-lactam molecules which resemble penicillin except that the sulphur of the thiazolidine ring is converted to a sulphone and there is no side chain at position 6. Sulbactam exhibits lower inhibitory activity towards the class A β-lactamases than clavulanic acid or tazobactam, but both sulbactam and tazobactam are inhibitors of class C cephalosporinase β-lactamases. Both compounds have been combined with penicillins and cephalosporins; for example, sulbactam is used in combination with ampicillin and cefoperazone, whereas tazobactam may be used in combination with piperacillin, cefoperazone and ceftolozane. Recently, members of a new class of non-β-lactam β-lactamase inhibitors based on diazabicyclooctanones (DBOs) have been successfully brought to market in combination with β-lactams. These compounds exhibit a broad spectrum of inhibitory activity, with class A penicillinases, ESBLs, carbapenemases, class C cephalosporinases and class D oxacillinases effectively inhibited. The first, avibactam, is approved for use with ceftazidime and other combinations are under investigation; relebactam is approved for use in combination with imipenem and cilastatin. In 2017, the cyclic boronate vaborbactam gained regulatory approval for clinical use in combination with meropenem.

Generally speaking, the combination of β-lactamase antibiotics with β-lactamase inhibitors is highly effective and has found application in a range of clinical scenarios where β-lactam antibiotics alone would be ineffective, including in the treatment of hospital-acquired infections, paediatric infections and infections caused by β-lactamase and ESBL-producing Gram-negative pathogens. It would be wise therefore to reserve such combination products for infections confirmed to be due to β-lactamase-producing pathogens (where the β-lactamase is the primary mediator of resistance). Interestingly, nitrocefin, a chromogenic cephalosporin β-lactamase substrate is used for the detection of β-lactamases and ESBLs. A fuller discussion of the current β-lactamase inhibitors in clinical use, and their structures, mechanism of action and the contribution of β-lactamases to β-lactam resistance, is provided in Chapters 12 and 13, respectively.

11.2.4 Carbapenems and Monobactams

Despite the significant volume of penicillin and cephalosporin antibiotics gaining regulatory approval for clinical use in the middle of the last century, the rapid and widespread emergence of resistance (particularly due to β-lactamases) to many of these agents prompted further efforts to discover or design new and diverse antibiotics. Of the many compound classes screened, the most important and useful of these were the carbapenems. The carbapenems comprise a 4:5 fused lactam ring similar to the penicillins but with no heteroatom and a double bond between carbons 2 and 3, as described above in Section 11.2. Thienamycin was the first carbapenem to be described in the late 1970s, and uniquely it possessed both antibacterial and β-lactamase inhibitory activity. The term carbapenem refers to the group of compounds which includes thienamycin and olivanic acid and its derivatives (of which there are no compounds of therapeutic value). Unfortunately, the thienamycins lacked stability and yields from fermentation and purification were low. In addition, thienamycin is unstable in aqueous solution, lacks stability due to reactivity towards nucleophiles (including its own primary amine) and is sensitive to mild base hydrolysis. Given thienamycin's excellent antibacterial spectrum of activity (active against Gram-positive and Gram-negative bacteria, including *P. aeruginosa* and anaerobes) and β-lactamase inhibitory activity, the search for more stable derivatives was undertaken. The *N*-formimidoyl derivative of thienamycin, imipenem (Figure 11.6), exhibited a balance of desirable properties including *in vitro* stability, broad-spectrum activity and resistance to β-lactamases. Imipenem was susceptible to degradation *in vivo* by the renal brush border membrane-bound dipeptidase, dehydropeptidase I (DHP-I), thus necessitating co-administration with the renal dipeptidase inhibitor, cilastatin. Modification of the 1-β position with a methyl group conferred resistance to DHP-I degradation, and therefore meropenem, ertapenem and doripenem may be administered without cilastatin. Ertapenem has similar properties to meropenem but has the advantage of once-daily dosing.

The examination of structure–activity relationships in the early penicillins and cephalosporins led to the

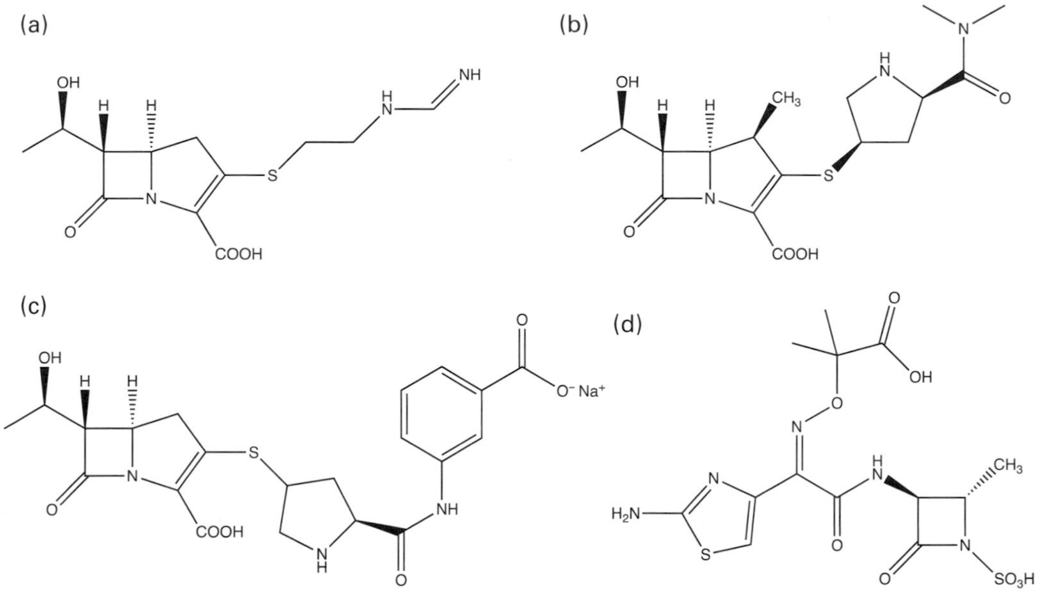

Figure 11.6 Carbapenems and aztreonam: (a) imipenem; (b) meropenem; (c) ertapenem; (d) aztreonam.

expectation that molecules possessing an unfused β-lactam ring would lack antimicrobial activity. However, extended screening and isolation efforts in the 1970s led to the discovery of a wide variety of novel β-lactam antibiotics, not just from fungi but also from bacteria, primarily the actinomycetes. Among these novel bacterially produced β-lactam antibiotics were the monobactams, monocyclic β-lactams bearing a 2-oxoazetidine-1-sulphonic acid moiety and variable side chain groups at the 3 position of the β-lactam ring. Naturally occurring monobactams, such as the nocardicins originally isolated from *Nocardia uniformis* in 1976, exhibit only moderate antimicrobial activity but good stability against β-lactamase-mediated hydrolysis. However, given the success experienced in the development of new penicillin and cephalosporin antibiotics with improved activity, pharmacokinetics and β-lactamase resistance, through structural modification of the β-lactam nucleus, significant research activity was directed towards similar modifications of the monobactam side chain. Thus, while none of the naturally occurring monobactams progressed to clinical use, an analogue produced completely by conventional chemical synthesis, aztreonam, was approved in 1986. The mechanism of action of aztreonam is similar to the other β-lactam antibiotics, but spectrum of activity is somewhat different, essentially lacking activity against Gram-positive bacteria and anaerobes due to low affinity for the PBPs of these organisms; it is, nevertheless, highly active against most Gram-negative bacteria, including *P. aeruginosa*, *Neisseria meningitidis* and *H. influenzae*, since it targets the septum peptidoglycan transpeptidase PBP3 of Gram-negatives with high affinity. Originally, aztreonam was stable to all reported β-lactamase enzymes, but over time with the emergence of ESBLs and serine carbapenemases, the antibiotic was rendered less effective. Aztreonam exhibits synergy with aminoglycoside antibiotics and can be indicated for *P. aeruginosa* infections in cystic fibrosis. Aztreonam remains the only monobactam antibiotic to gain regulatory approval for clinical use, despite several experimental lead compounds being under pre-clinical evaluation.

11.2.5 Hypersensitivity

Penicillins generally exhibit low toxicity, are well-tolerated and are regarded as among the safest antibiotic agents available. Most common side effects are due to hypersensitivity. The most frequent side effect is a rash, occurring in less than 10% of patients, but ampicillin must be used with caution in patients with mononucleosis (glandular fever) where the incidence of rash can be around 90%; ampicillin rash is not regarded as a true penicillin allergy. Penicillin hypersensitivity with anaphylaxis (or penicillin allergy) is a serious but rare side effect of penicillins, occurring in less than 0.004–0.0015% of patients, and most likely to occur with benzylpenicillin and ampicillin. True penicillin allergy is IgE-mediated, and more commonly observed after parenteral administration than oral administration; patients who are sensitive to one penicillin will be sensitive to all other members of the class, as the core penicillin structure is responsible for the hypersensitivity reactions. Benzylpenicillin is the penicillin most likely to result in anaphylaxis. Around 10% of patients allergic to penicillin will also be hypersensitive to cephalosporins. Rashes occur in 1–2.8% of patients, but true anaphylactic reactions to cephalosporins are rare (0.0001–0.1% of patients). There is no increased risk of cephalosporin hypersensitivity with anaphylaxis in patients with penicillin allergy. As a result, oral cephalosporin therapy may be prescribed for patients reporting penicillin allergy. All penicillins have the capacity to cause diarrhoea (and rarely pseudomembranous colitis) due to disruption of the gut microbiota, with orally administered penicillins and ampicillin (since a high proportion remains unabsorbed in the gut and reaches the colon) having a higher incidence. Side effects are also more commonly observed in patients with impaired renal excretion or metabolism. Orally administered cephalosporins (particularly first- and second-generation compounds) may similarly cause diarrhoea and, rarely, pseudomembranous colitis (more common with cefoxitin).

11.3 Tetracyclines

The naturally occurring tetracyclines chlortetracycline and oxytetracycline were originally isolated from *Streptomyces aureofaciens* and *Streptomyces rimosus*, respectively. Tetracycline, demecycline, methacycline, doxycycline and minocycline are all semi-synthetic derivatives. The structure of tetracycline is shown in Figure 11.7b. The tetracyclines are all analogues of polycyclic naphthacene carboxamide.

The tetracyclines (Figure 11.7) are broad-spectrum antibiotics, active against a wide range of Gram-positive and Gram-negative bacteria, both anaerobic and aerobic. In general, however, they are more active against Gram-positive microorganisms. Tetracyclines are also active against some microorganisms which are resistant to cell-wall-active agents, such as *Rickettsia*, *Mycoplasma pneumoniae*, *Chlamydia* spp., *Legionella* spp. as well as *Plasmodium* spp. The availability of superior antimicrobials, coupled with issues of resistance, has limited the use of tetracyclines in the treatment of infections due to Gram-positive microorganisms. Widespread resistance to the tetracyclines is observed in *P. aeruginosa*, *Proteus* spp. and *S. aureus*, but all of the tetracyclines are active against rickettsiae (typhus, Q fever), spirochaetes including *Borrelia burgdorferi* (Lyme disease), *Treponema pallidum* (syphilis) and *Chlamydia* (e.g., trachoma) and *Mycoplasma* spp. Despite the occurrence of widespread resistance, several original tetracyclines are still clinically useful, including tetracycline, oxytetracycline and chlortetracycline, and the semi-synthetic derivatives, doxycycline (1966) and minocycline (1972). A glycylglycine derivative, tigecycline, approved in 2005, exhibits improved potency compared to earlier tetracyclines and is active against some bacteria which have become resistant to these earlier compounds. Tigecycline is useful against MRSA, although most strains of *S. aureus* are resistant to other tetracyclines. The tetracyclines inhibit bacterial

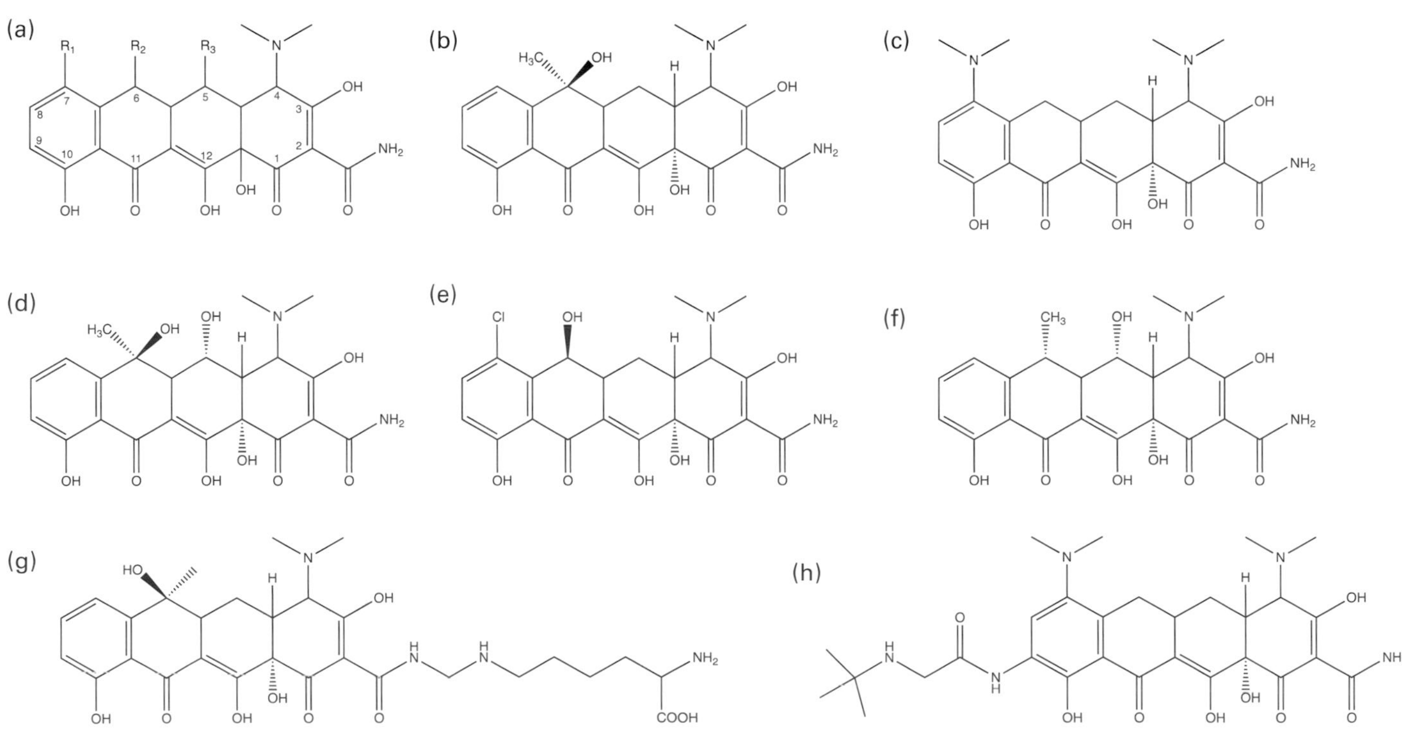

Figure 11.7 Tetracycline antibiotics: (a) tetracycline general structure; (b) tetracycline; (c) minocycline; (d) oxytetracycline; (e) demeclocycline; (f) doxycycline; (g) lymecycline; (h) tigecycline.

protein synthesis by binding to the 30S ribosome, preventing access of aminoacyl-tRNA to the acceptor (a) site on the mRNA–ribosome complex. Tetracyclines enter Gram-negative bacteria via passive diffusion through membrane-spanning porin proteins in the outer membrane and then by active transport across the cytoplasmic membrane. They are bacteriostatic at concentrations achieved in the body, but bactericidal at concentrations used in laboratory tests.

Tetracyclines may be useful alternatives to macrolides and β-lactams for the treatment of common infections including those of the respiratory tract. They may be prescribed for treatment of acne, for eradication of *Helicobacter pylori* (as part of combination therapy) and, in the case of doxycycline, for prophylaxis of *Plasmodium falciparum* malaria. Tetracyclines can achieve high concentrations in the bowel, since they are often poorly absorbed from the gastrointestinal (GI) tract. Absorption (especially of the older agents in the class) may be inhibited by food, milk, divalent and trivalent cations and antacids. Since many of the normal gut bacteria are sensitive to these agents, many aerobic and anaerobic coliforms and Gram-positive spore-forming bacteria may be suppressed. Superinfection (overgrowth) with inherently tetracycline-resistant organisms including *Candida albicans* and other yeasts can occur in the mouth, upper respiratory tract and GI tract as a result. Impaired absorption is less likely with more recent drugs, such as lymecycline, minocycline and tigecycline (twice daily dosing) and also doxycycline which may be administered once daily. The newer tetracyclines are more lipophilic and as a result exhibit good tissue distribution, achieving concentrations in the biliary tract, liver, kidneys and other organs which may exceed those in the blood. Common side effects include nausea and vomiting, and diarrhoea (e.g., a 4–52% incidence with doxycycline has been reported across multiple studies). Tetracyclines may accumulate in teeth (causing staining) and bones, as a result of their calcium-chelating ability and thus tetracycline use is contraindicated in children under 12 years of age and in pregnant women. Tetracyclines may cause hyperpigmentation of the skin, nails and conjunctiva, and doxycycline may cause photosensitivity in up to 20% of patients. Tetracycline use in patients with reduced or impaired kidney function is also contraindicated, as accumulation may lead to tetracycline-associated renal toxicity.

Resistance to tetracyclines develops slowly and is likely to be primarily plasmid-mediated and may come about via three main mechanisms: reduced accumulation, enzymatic inactivation and reduced interaction with the cognate target due to production of ribosome protection proteins. Resistance to one tetracycline usually confers cross-resistance to all other tetracyclines, with the exception of tigecycline; in some cases, tetracycline-resistant *S. aureus* may be sensitive to minocycline. Further information on tetracycline mode of action and resistance is provided in the relevant sections of Chapters 12 and 13, respectively.

11.4 Macrolides

The macrolides (erythromycin, clarithromycin and azithromycin) contain a multi-member lactone ring (14-membered for erythromycin and clarithromycin, and a 15-membered ring in azithromycin), to which are attached one or more deoxy sugars. Erythromycin, the archetypal macrolide, was discovered in the early 1950s from a strain of *Streptomyces erythreus*; both clarithromycin and azithromycin are semi-synthetic derivatives of erythromycin, with the modifications discussed below and shown in Figure 11.8. Erythromycin is bacteriostatic at normal clinically achievable concentrations; however, it can be bactericidal in higher concentrations (a feature of all macrolides) and is most effective against aerobic Gram-positive bacilli. It is not active against most aerobic enteric Gram-negative bacilli, but has modest activity against other Gram-negative organisms, including *Neisseria gonorrhoeae*, *N. meningitidis* and *H. influenzae*. Erythromycin exhibits poor acid stability, resulting in limited absorption and bioavailability. As a result, GI side effects are common and bacteria acquire resistance relatively easily. Mechanisms which produce erythromycin resistance affect all macrolides, meaning that cross-resistance is complete. Because of their similar spectrum of activity to the early penicillins, macrolides may be considered as alternative antibiotics for patients with penicillin allergy.

These shortcomings prompted research into new macrolides, and several semi-synthetic derivatives gained approval; roxithromycin (1987, not approved in USA or UK), clarithromycin and azithromycin (1991) and telithromycin (a 14-membered ketolide, approved 2001, withdrawn 2018). Structural modifications to the original erythromycin structure (methylation of the hydroxyl group at position 6 yields clarithromycin, and azithromycin [strictly an azalide] is characterised by the addition of a methyl-substituted nitrogen atom into the lactone ring) improve both acid stability and tissue penetration and broaden the spectrum of activity. Clarithromycin is slightly more potent than the parent macrolide when used against erythromycin-sensitive strains of streptococci and staphylococci, and has modest potency against *N. gonorrhoeae* and *H. influenzae*. Clarithromycin also exhibits good activity against *Moraxella catarrhalis*, *Chlamydia* spp., *Legionella pneumophila*, *B. burgdorferi* and *M. pneumoniae*. Azithromycin is generally less potent against Gram-positive bacteria (*Streptococcus* spp. and enterococci) than erythromycin, but is more active than either of the other macrolides against *Campylobacter*

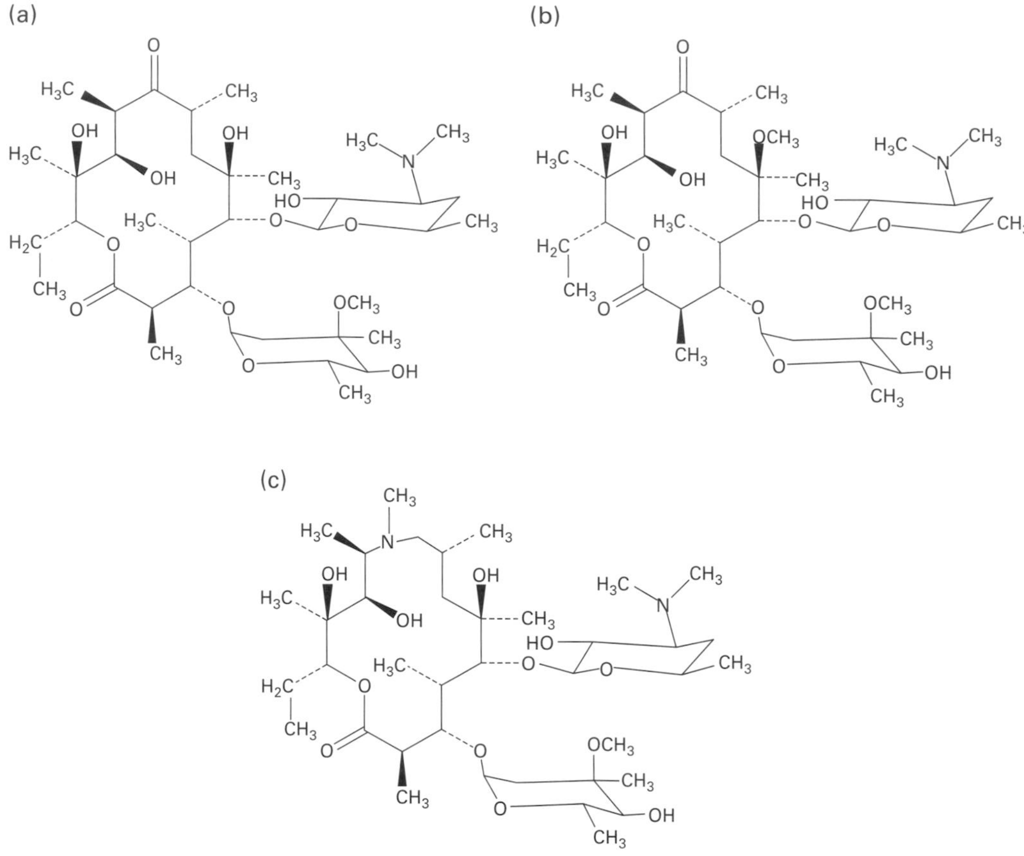

Figure 11.8 Structures of the macrolide antibiotics: (a) erythromycin, (b) clarithromycin and (c) azithromycin.

spp. and *H. influenzae*, and highly active against *Pasteurella multocida*, *M. catarrhalis*, *Chlamydia* spp., *L. pneumophila*, *B. burgdorferi*, *Fusobacterium* spp., *M. pneumoniae* and *N. gonorrhoeae*. The semi-synthetic macrolides afford little additional benefit over erythromycin with respect to activity against staphylococci, streptococci or enterococci but are generally more active against the other organisms discussed above; they also exhibit superior stability and pharmacokinetic profiles and have fewer side effects. The chemical structures of the clinically approved macrolide antibiotics are shown in Figure 11.8.

Macrolides are bacteriostatic agents which inhibit protein synthesis by binding reversibly to 50S ribosomal subunits of sensitive microorganisms. Their activity is pH-dependent, increasing up to pH 8.5. Erythromycin is not thought to interfere with peptide bond formation, but rather to inhibit the translocation of newly synthesised tRNA from the acceptor site on the ribosome to the donor (peptidyl) site. Resistance to macrolides is discussed in the relevant section of Chapter 13; it is usually as a result of efflux from the cell by active membrane efflux pumps, the production of methylase enzymes which modify the ribosomal target, hydrolysis by esterases (produced by *Enterobacteriaceae*) or chromosomal mutations leading to alteration of a 50S ribosomal protein.

Macrolides have a wide range of clinical uses, including *M. pneumoniae* infections, Legionnaire's disease, chlamydia infections, diphtheria, pertussis, infections caused by staphylococci, streptococci and *Campylobacter* spp., *H. pylori* infections (clarithromycin), tetanus, syphilis and mycobacterial infections (*Mycobacterium avium-intracellulare*). Macrolides are exceptionally bitter compounds and oral formulations are often coated for taste-masking and also to protect the antibiotic from acidic conditions encountered in the stomach and small intestine. Given erythromycin's particularly poor acid stability and oral absorption, the drug is generally administered as (most commonly) stearate or ethyl succinate esters. All macrolides are orally active, and are concentrated intracellularly particularly in neutrophils, which increases their transport to sites of infection. Longer elimination half-lives, characteristic of the newer semi-synthetic agents, permit less frequent dosing schedules compared to erythromycin. The macrolides are typically regarded as safe and well-tolerated antibiotics, without serious adverse effects. However, GI disturbances are common with erythromycin

Table 11.4 Properties of clinically available macrolides.

Macrolide	Route	Doses/day	Distinguishing features
Erythromycin	O, IV	2–4	Especially poor acid stability, erratic oral absorption and gastrointestinal side effects
Roxithromycin	O	1–2	Slightly less potent but substantially better oral absorption than erythromycin
Clarithromycin	O, IV	2	Very good acid stability and oral absorption. Tissue concentrations very much higher than those in the plasma
Dirithromycin	O	1	Slightly less active than erythromycin, but long half-life and good tissue concentration
Azithromycin	O	1	More active against Gram-negative bacteria, including *Enterobacteriaceae*, than erythromycin; very high concentration in neutrophils

IV, intravenous; O, oral.

due to poor oral absorption, but much reduced or absent with the other members of this class. The properties of clinically approved macrolides are summarised in Table 11.4.

11.5 Sulphonamides and Trimethoprim

Two classes of antibiotic drugs (the sulphonamides and the diaminopyrimidines /trimethoprim) act at separate stages of the folic acid synthesis pathway, which therefore interferes with downstream DNA synthesis. The active form of the co-enzyme, tetrahydrofolic acid, serves as an intermediate in the transfer of a methyl, formyl or other single carbon fragments in the biosynthesis of purine nucleotides and thymidylic acid. The B vitamin, folic acid, is essential for the biosynthesis of nucleic acids and other important biomolecules, thus inhibition leads to reduction or inhibition of bacterial growth.

Sulphonamides were discovered by Gerhard Domagk in 1935, following his earlier discovery of the curative effect of the red azo dye, prontosil, on mice infected with β-haemolytic streptococci. Prontosil, sulphonamidochrysoidin, the first drug to successfully treat infections and the first of the 'sulpha' drugs, was subsequently found to be converted *in vivo* to sulphanilamide (Figure 11.9a). Sulphonamides are structural analogues of p-aminobenzoic acid (PABA) which competitively inhibit dihydropteroate synthetase, whereas the diaminopyrimidines act later in the pathway to inhibit dihydrofolate reductase. Dihydrofolate reductase generates the active form of the co-enzyme tetrahydrofolic acid. Chemical modification of sulphanilamide (see Figure 11.9a) has led to compounds with improved spectrum of activity or prolonged activity. Once in widespread use, their popularity has declined sharply due to the emergence of widespread cross-resistance and the approval of less toxic, more effective antibiotics. Sulphonamides exhibit broad-spectrum activity against many Gram-positive and Gram-negative pathogens, although this class of antibiotic can be considered to be only moderately potent compared with newer chemotherapeutic agents. They are active against meningococci, *Bordetella pertussis*, *Yersinia pestis*, *Brucella* spp. and *Chlamydia trachomatis*. Mycobacteria are generally resistant, although dapsone is active against *Mycobacterium leprae*. Plasmid-mediated resistance in enterobacteria is common. *P. aeruginosa* is not susceptible to the sulphonamides. A small number of sulphonamides remain in clinical use today, notably topical silver sulphadiazine for burns, and in veterinary medicine. Sulphadiazine itself is indicated for prevention of recurrence of rheumatic fever. Dapsone (Figure 11.9b) was used extensively in the past for the treatment of leprosy and is still indicated (more than 200,000 new cases of leprosy are reported each year) as part of a combination therapy (currently with rifampicin and clofazimine for multibacillary leprosy), although use has declined due to emerging resistance.

In the body, folic acid must be reduced to dihydrofolic acid, then tetrahydrofolic acid in order to become active. It was discovered that a group of synthetic agents, the diaminopyridines, were able to inhibit the dihydrofolic acid reductase enzymes responsible for this reduction. Trimethoprim has a vastly higher affinity for the bacterial enzyme than the mammalian enzyme, facilitating a selectively toxic effect. These dihydrofolate reductase inhibitors were found to act synergistically with sulphonamides, blocking successive steps in the folic acid synthesis pathway. This group comprises mainly 5-substituted 2,4-diaminopyrimidines. Trimethoprim (Figure 11.9c) is the representative antibiotic in this class and is a widely used broad-spectrum antibiotic. When originally introduced in 1969, trimethoprim was included in a combination product with sulphamethoxazole (co-trimoxazole) for treatment of urinary and respiratory

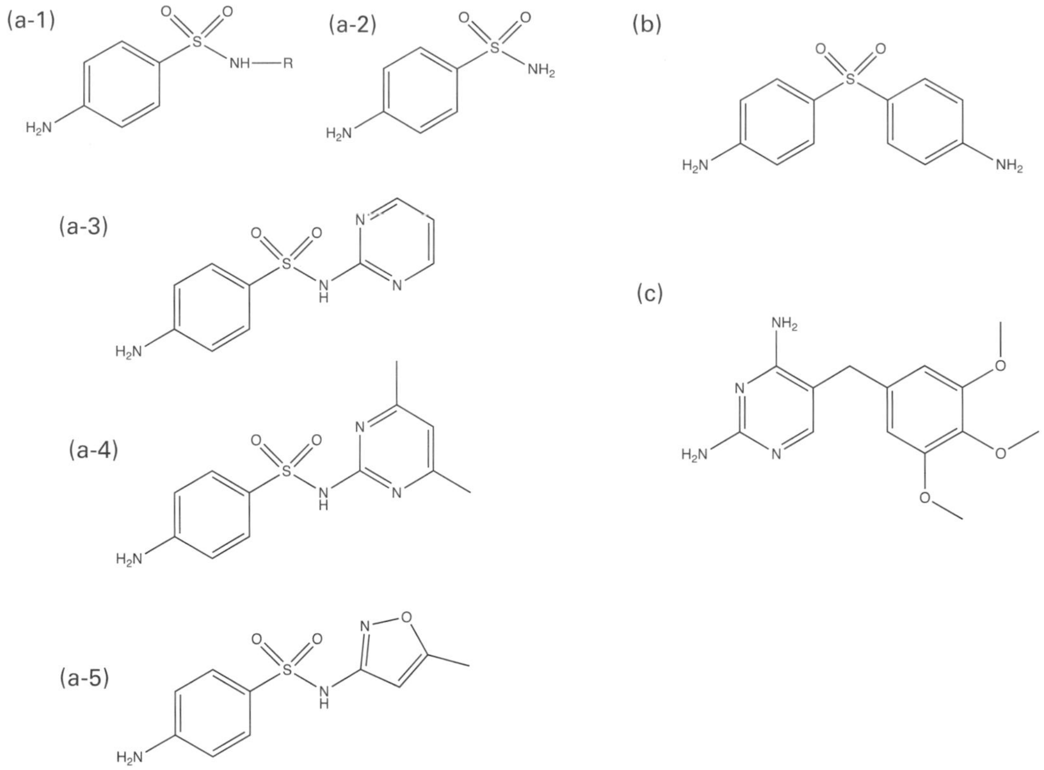

Figure 11.9 (a1–a5) Some sulphonamides: (a-1) sulphonamide general structure; (a-2) sulphanilamide; (a-3) sulphadiazine; (a-4) sulphadimidine; (a-5) sulphamethoxazole; (b) dapsone; (c) trimethoprim.

tract infections. However, pharmacokinetic differences between the two drugs meant that optimal synergistic concentrations were not achieved *in vivo*. It was also noted that the activity of the combination product was primarily due to trimethoprim and that the more toxic sulphamethoxazole contributed little to overall antimicrobial activity. Therefore, trimethoprim was used as a stand-alone antibiotic from the 1970s onwards. The other diaminopyrimidine possessing antimicrobial (anti-protozoal) activity is pyrimethamine, which is used in combination with sulphadoxine for the treatment of malaria (not available in UK or USA) or in combination with sulphadiazine and folinic acid for the treatment of toxoplasmosis in pregnancy.

Trimethoprim–sulphamethoxazole in combination is still indicated for the treatment of susceptible urinary tract infections, *Pneumocystis carinii* pneumonia, hospital-acquired pneumonia, acute exacerbations in chronic obstructive pulmonary disease, diabetic foot ulcer/leg ulcer infections and acute prostatitis. Trimethoprim is active against Gram-positive bacilli and cocci, including *S. aureus* (irrespective of methicillin resistance or lactamase production). It is also active against streptococci, enterococci, *H. influenzae, N. meningitidis, E. coli, K. pneumoniae* and *B. fragilis*. Trimethoprim is widely prescribed for the treatment of urinary tract infections, but increasing resistance means that trimethoprim is frequently replaced by the fluoroquinolones.

11.6 Quinolones

The quinolone antibiotics and the cephalosporins have much in common in terms of their history and development; being first introduced in the early 1960s, and the first members of each class, nalidixic acid and cephalothin, respectively, had limitations in spectrum and pharmacokinetic profiles which limited their applications in therapeutic use. However, both groups were significantly expanded across four generations of compounds in the following decades, with each representing improvements to the spectrum of activity and pharmacological and side effect profiles. The quinolones and cephalosporins, as a result of these improvements and the diversity of approved compounds, currently rank among the most widely used and valuable antibiotics available. To date over 10,000 quinolone antibacterial agents have been synthesised, with nalidixic acid regarded as the progenitor of the new quinolone antibiotics. The general structure of the

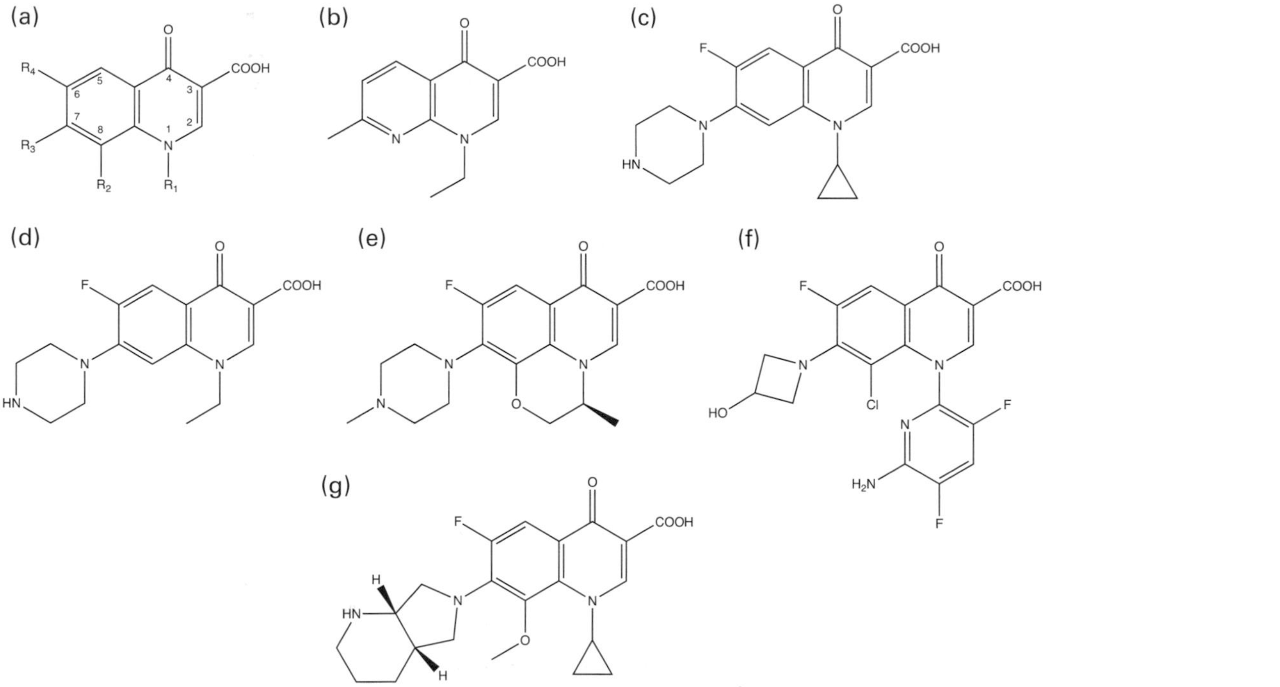

Figure 11.10 Quinolone antibiotics: (a) quinolone general structure; (b) nalidixic acid; (c) ciprofloxacin; (d) norfloxacin; (e) levofloxacin and ofloxacin; (f) delafloxacin; (g) moxifloxacin.

Table 11.5 Properties of the quinolone antibiotics.

Generation	Antimicrobial spectrum
First	Spectrum of activity largely confined to *E. coli* and other enterobacteria e.g., nalidixic acid, cinoxacin, oxolinic acid
Second	Improved activity against enterobacteria, improved spectrum of activity including *P. aeruginosa* and Gram-positive cocci. Compounds characterised by 6-fluoro and 7-piperazinyl groups are known as the fluoroquinolones e.g., ciprofloxacin, norfloxacin
Third	Activity extended against *S. pneumoniae* and other Gram-positive cocci. Some exhibit improved pharmacological properties e.g., levofloxacin, temafloxacin, pazufloxacin
Fourth	Most recent compounds, with improved activity against Gram-positive cocci, including pneumococci and anaerobes e.g., moxifloxacin, gatifloxacin

quinolones, and that of the archetypal member of the first-generation nalidixic acid, are shown below in Figures 11.10a and 11.10b, respectively.

All quinolones are characterised by a dual-ring structure with a nitrogen at position 1, a carbonyl at position 4 and a carboxyl group at position 3. Position 8 may be CH or N (in the case of nalidixic acid) and ring closure may occur between R_1 and R_2 giving a large degree of structural diversity in this group of antibiotics. In general, the following structural modifications give rise to antibiotics with superior properties with respect to antimicrobial efficacy: (i) addition of a fluorine atom at position C-6 (fluoroquinolones) enhances antimicrobial potency and confers anti-staphylococcal activity; (ii) addition of piperazine at group C-7 improves activity against aerobic Gram-negative bacteria and staphylococci; (iii) ring alkylation improves activity against Gram-positives; (iv) addition of a cyclopropyl group at N-1, an amino group at C-5, and a halogen group at C-8 increases activity against *Mycoplasma* and *Chlamydia* spp. and (v) addition of a methoxy group at C-8 targets both topoisomerases I and II, and may reduce the emergence of resistance. A summary of classification and properties of the quinolone antibiotics is provided in Table 11.5.

Nalidixic acid was originally developed as a treatment for urinary tract infections, and, like all first-generation compounds, had a limited spectrum of activity, primarily towards *E. coli* and other *Enterobacteriaceae*. Although there is no universal acceptance of the criteria or definitions for assignment of compounds within the class into generations, the distinguishing feature of first-generation compounds is the absence of a fluorine at position C-6. Thus, these compounds are referred to as 'quinolones', whereas the second, third and fourth generations are termed 'fluoroquinolones' (Figure 11.10a, general structure). First-generation drugs are not widely used, however, while those that followed in the 1980s, for example, ciprofloxacin, norfloxacin, levofloxacin (the L-isomer of ofloxacin) and ofloxacin (Figures 11.10c, 11.10d and 11.10e, respectively), remain in widespread use today; these are first-choice drugs in a range of infections, thanks to their greater activity against Gram-negative bacteria and wider antimicrobial spectrum which includes Gram-positive cocci and *P. aeruginosa*. In addition to sharing the general characteristics of second-generation compounds, the third-generation compounds (e.g., levofloxacin) exhibit greater activity against *S. pneumoniae*, and fourth-generation compounds (delafloxacin and moxifloxacin, Figures 11.10f and 11.10g, respectively) exhibit an extended spectrum of activity against Gram-positives, including *Enterococcus* spp., and activity against anaerobes.

All quinolone antibiotics are bactericidal, and target bacterial DNA gyrase and topoisomerase IV, the latter appears to be the primary target in Gram-positive microorganisms. Bacterial DNA gyrase is the enzyme responsible for the introduction of negative supercoils into DNA to counter the appearance of positive supercoils in the double helix (or over-winding) caused by separation of the two strands, for example, during replication. The α-subunits of DNA gyrase are the primary target of nalidixic acid and the other quinolones. In Gram-positives, topoisomerase IV is not involved in supercoiling but appears to have a role in DNA relaxation and chromosomal segregation. Mammalian topoisomerases are not susceptible to quinolones, permitting selective toxicity against bacteria. The quinolones exhibit good activity against *E. coli* and various species of *Shigella*, *Salmonella*, *Campylobacter* and *Neisseria*. Several intracellular pathogens are also inhibited by the quinolones, including species of *Chlamydia*, *Mycoplasma*, *Legionella*, *Brucella* and *Mycobacterium*. As a result, the quinolones are therapeutically useful in a number of infections including urinary tract infections, prostatitis, sexually transmitted infectious diseases, as well as GI and bone and soft tissue infections.

The quinolones are all orally active and the most common minor side effect is GI disturbance, occurring in 1–7% of patients. Use of fluoroquinolones has been associated with rare cases of tendon damage, tendonitis and rupture, collectively referred to as fluoroquinolone-induced tendinopathy (occurring in 0.14–0.4% of patients). These agents are not generally prescribed in children and are used with caution in athletes as a result. Quinolone resistance, discussed in Chapter 13, occurs primarily through mutations in the quinolone-resistance-determining region of *gyrA* and active efflux from the bacterial cell. Some degree of cross-resistance is observed, which is particularly problematic given their widespread and often inappropriate use in humans and in animals; in the latter instance, they have been overused in the past, especially in Europe, in intensively reared animals for food production.

11.7 Aminoglycosides

The term 'aminoglycosides' is used to represent the group of antimicrobial aminoglycosidic aminocyclitols (amino sugars linked to an aminocyclitol ring via glycosidic bonds). They are bactericidal inhibitors of bacterial protein synthesis. All consist of two or more amino sugars linked via a glycosidic linkage to a hexose (aminocyclitol) nucleus (either streptidine, in streptomycin, or 2-deoxystreptamine, found in all other aminoglycosides). The archetypal aminoglycoside antibiotic is streptomycin, discovered in 1944, but other important family members include gentamicin, tobramycin, amikacin, netilmicin, kanamycin and neomycin. All members of this class of antibiotic exhibit similar pharmacokinetic properties, which are due in part to their polycationic nature. For example, they are poorly bioavailable after oral administration, attain inadequate concentrations in cerebrospinal fluid and all undergo rapid excretion via the kidneys. Significantly, and although these agents represent an important and widely employed class of antibiotic, serious toxicity issues accompany their use and represent a major limitation. Nephrotoxicity (reversible) and ototoxicity (largely irreversible, arising from damage to the eighth cranial nerve) represent the major adverse toxicities associated with the use of aminoglycosides. This toxicological risk is shared by all members of the group. Their susceptibility to emerging resistance, due primarily to enzymatic inactivation (see Chapter 13), and their toxicity profile have limited the use of naturally occurring aminoglycosides, but stimulated the development of several important semi-synthetic aminoglycoside antibiotics that are in widespread use today.

Streptomycin, discovered by Selman Waksman and colleagues in 1943, was the first effective antibiotic for the treatment of tuberculosis (TB) and remains a second-line treatment option for drug-resistant tuberculosis infections. It can also be used as an adjunct to doxycycline in brucellosis but has few other applications. Neomycin, also discovered in the 1940s, is restricted to topical and ophthalmic indications, due to its high toxicity when used systemically. Topically, neomycin is widely available in combination with other antimicrobials and steroids, and is restricted orally (in combination with other antibiotics) to use in bowel sterilisation prior to surgery.

Of the remaining aminoglycosides, the three most important agents in clinical use today are gentamicin, tobramycin and amikacin. Gentamicin and tobramycin are both naturally occurring antibiotics, discovered in the

1960s, while amikacin is a semi-synthetic derivative of kanamycin. The clinical use of both netilmicin and kanamycin has decreased sharply due to their toxicity profile, emerging resistance and the availability of more effective and less toxic aminoglycoside options. Gentamicin is the aminoglycoside of first choice in most circumstances where aminoglycosides are called for, due to long experience of its successful clinical use and its low cost. In common with the other aminoglycosides, gentamicin can be used in the treatment of some urinary tract infections (but not usually as the antibiotic class of first choice), pneumonia (due to Gram-negative bacilli), meningitis (caused by some species of *Pseudomonas* or *Acinetobacter*), sepsis (where the causative organism is *P. aeruginosa*, used often in combination with an antipseudomonal penicillin) and topical infections. Although frequently used therapeutically in synergistic combination, penicillins and aminoglycosides should never be mixed in the same container, since the penicillin inactivates the aminoglycoside to a significant degree.

The aminoglycosides are rapidly bactericidal, with the rate of kill dependent on dose. One characteristic common to all members is a residual post-antibiotic effect where antibacterial activity persists after the plasma concentrations of the drug have fallen below the minimum inhibitory concentration (MIC), with the duration of this effect also being dose-dependent. Aminoglycosides typically have a once-daily dosage regime as a result. Monitoring of aminoglycoside serum levels, to avoid potentially toxic high serum levels or subtherapeutic concentrations, is an integral part of aminoglycoside therapy.

11.8 Glycopeptides

Glycopeptides are natural glycosylated cyclic/polycyclic non-ribosomal peptides of large molecular size produced by several actinomycete soil bacteria. They inhibit bacterial peptidoglycan synthesis by binding to the carboxy-terminus of the D-alanyl-D-alanine dipeptide residue of the muramyl-pentapeptide precursor, thus preventing cell wall cross-linking. Until recently, the only two clinically important members of this family were vancomycin and teicoplanin, but the semi-synthetic lipoglycopeptide derivatives dalbavancin, telavancin and oritavancin have gained regulatory approval in the past decade. Vancomycin was introduced into clinical use in 1958, but its activity against MRSA has made it increasingly valuable and it is now often the agent of choice for these infections. It is a large, amphoteric, complex tricyclic glycopeptide with a molecular mass of 1500 Da. Like other glycopeptide antibiotics, vancomycin primarily exhibits bactericidal activity against aerobic and anaerobic Gram-positive bacteria at or near its MIC, and lacks activity against most Gram-negative bacteria, since it is unable to pass through their outer membrane. Vancomycin is active against some *Clostridioides* species, including *Clostridioides difficile*. Streptococci, such as *Streptococcus pyogenes*, *S. pneumoniae* and the viridans streptococci, are also highly susceptible to vancomycin, as are *Corynebacterium* species (diphtheroids) and most *Actinomyces* species. Gram-negative bacilli and mycobacteria are not susceptible, or are resistant, to vancomycin. Vancomycin is also useful in the treatment of infections where penicillin or cephalosporin patient hypersensitivity exists. It is the drug of choice in the treatment of antibiotic-induced pseudomembranous colitis, most commonly associated with administration of antibiotics such as clindamycin and lincomycin. Vancomycin has no fungicidal/fungistatic activity. Enterococci are broadly susceptible to vancomycin; however, resistant strains of *Enterococcus faecium* and *E. faecalis* are increasingly isolated from clinical samples. For a full discussion of vancomycin-resistance mechanisms, the reader is directed to Chapter 13. Vancomycin is not absorbed significantly from the GI tract when administered orally. It is generally delivered as the hydrochloride via dilute intravenous infusion, and adverse effects include nephrotoxicity; ototoxicity has previously been cited as a side effect, but few cases have been reported and even with long-term vancomycin administration risk of ototoxicity is now regarded as low.

Because of vancomycin's potential toxicity, its poor penetration into bile and cerebrospinal fluid, the necessity for twice-daily dosing and pain on intramuscular administration (which limits delivery to the intravenous route), scope existed for an alternative glycopeptide where these deficiencies were reduced or eliminated; this led to the introduction of teicoplanin in the 1990s. Teicoplanin is a mixture of six distinct antibiotic glycopeptides produced by *Actinoplanes teichomyceticus*, and is similar to vancomycin with respect to spectrum of activity, mechanism of action and chemical structure. However, teicoplanin possesses more fatty acid side chains, making the molecule more acidic, which allows formulation as the sodium salt (which can be given by both the intravenous and intramuscular routes); it is also more lipophilic, which improves teicoplanin tissue penetration and extends half-life. This allows teicoplanin (and the newer semi-synthetic lipoglycopeptides, see below) to be administered once daily, rather than twice. Teicoplanin has slightly higher potency against target bacteria, compared to vancomycin, and a better toxicity profile.

The newer members of the glycopeptide family, the lipoglycopeptides, also inhibit cell wall peptidoglycan synthesis, but may also lead to membrane disruption due to membrane anchoring and, in the case of oritavancin, dimerisation of the molecules at the membrane. Oritavancin and telavancin cause membrane destabilisation and leakage, and exhibit dose-dependent bactericidal activity, and are more potent inhibitors of transglycosidase. Telavancin, derived from vancomycin, exhibits improved potency against Gram-positive bacteria, including those resistant to vancomycin. Dalbavancin does not appear to destabilise bacterial membranes in the same way as oritavancin and telavancin, despite having a lipophilic side-chain moiety. Telavancin has a half-life of 8 hours, whereas both dalbavancin and oritavancin have extended half-lives in humans of over 300 hours, allowing once-weekly dosing. Dalbavancin and oritavancin are both currently indicated for the treatment of acute bacterial skin and skin suture infections, and telavancin for hospital-acquired pneumonia, known or suspected to be caused by MRSA (where other antibiotics cannot be used).

11.9 Antitubercular Drugs

The antibiotics used for the treatment of TB belong to a variety of chemical classes, but they are considered together in this section, since most of them are used exclusively for the treatment of tuberculosis and therapy extends over prolonged periods of time, during which resistance development is a significant possibility. The risk is minimised by using a combination of two or three antibiotics, thus they are considered together, since it represents their normal pattern of use. All current treatment regimens are based on multiple agents, reducing the likelihood of spontaneous acquisition of resistance to all components. The World Health Organization recommends directly observed therapy (DOT) for optimal therapeutic outcomes, with concurrent culture-based phenotypic drug susceptibility testing (DST), to rapidly detect emerging resistance and to allow adjustments to therapy. In resource-limited environments, however, where a significant proportion of the global TB infection burden exists, such infrastructure may not be available, potentially limiting efficacy of treatment and increasing the potential for resistance to emerge and for its dissemination.

Tuberculosis may be caused by bacteria of the *Mycobacterium tuberculosis* complex (*M. tuberculosis*, *Mycobacterium africanum*, *Mycobacterium bovis* or *Mycobacterium microti*). Mycobacteria possess an unusual cell envelope which limits drug penetration, and they exhibit slow growth during established infections, often persisting with low metabolic rates approaching dormancy for long periods of time. As a consequence, therapeutic options are limited. Since therapeutic regimens generally require 4-6 months of treatment, antibiotics which are orally available are preferable. This is also necessary because patients who are unsupervised are more likely to adhere to regimens involving oral medicines, and in many countries it would not be feasible for patients to travel to clinics for daily administration of injectable antibiotics. As a result, the therapeutic options for the management of TB are limited, since a number of conventional antibiotics are deemed inappropriate. The ideal antitubercular drug should be bactericidal, rather than bacteriostatic or inhibitory to growth of the causative organism. Mycobacteria are primarily intracellular pathogens, capable of surviving and reproducing within human cells (including macrophages) despite the host immune response. Therefore, therapy relying on the normal immune system to clear infection following the administration of bacteriostatic antibiotics is unlikely to be effective.

The aminoglycoside, streptomycin (Section 11.7), was the first effective treatment for tuberculosis. Introduced in the 1940s, its use as a monotherapy for TB was short-lived because of the ease and rapidity with which resistance to a single agent emerged. Isoniazid, introduced in the early 1950s, was first used in combination with streptomycin, and then with rifampicin after the latter was introduced in 1967. The combination of isoniazid and rifampicin remains the mainstay of tuberculosis therapy today, although other drugs have been added to the treatment regimen, such as pyrazinamide and ethambutol. Multidrug-resistant tuberculosis has become one of the most significant antibiotic resistance threats to human health globally (see Chapter 13), with *M. tuberculosis* exhibiting several levels of resistance to both first-line and second-line antibiotics.

Isoniazid (isonicotinic acid hydrazide [INH]) is a prodrug which is activated by the enzyme catalase–peroxidase, KatG, endogenously produced by *M. tuberculosis* and other members of the *M. tuberculosis* complex. Activation of isoniazid leads to the inhibition of mycolic acid production, depriving the mycobacterial cell wall of critical components. Specifically, activation of isoniazid leads to the inhibition of InhA, a mycobacterial enoyl reductase involved in the synthetic pathway of mycolic acid, by forming a covalent adduct with the nicotinamide adenine dinucleotide (NAD) cofactor. Rifampicin (and related compounds) inhibits DNA-dependent RNA polymerase, thus preventing the transcription of RNA from the DNA template. Rifampicin is bactericidal and is effective in targeting slow-growing and dormant microorganisms, while isoniazid is bactericidal and targets aerobically growing bacteria. Pyrazinamide, a prodrug converted to pyrazinoic acid by the action of *M. tuberculosis* pyrazinamidase and putatively leading to inhibition of coenzyme A synthesis, is active at low pH; and by virtue of this property, is lethal to bacteria within the necrotic foci characteristic of early infection, but is less useful in later infection where those foci have resolved. Ethambutol is a bacteriostatic antibiotic which targets the arabinosyltransferase enzymes of *M. tuberculosis* encoded

Table 11.6 Properties of selected antitubercular antibiotics.

Antibiotic	Status	Route	Properties
Isoniazid	1	O, IM or IV	Side effect of peripheral neuropathy, preventable with pyridoxine
Rifampicin	1	O or IV	Colours the urine red; induces liver enzymes so oral contraception is less effective
Pyrazinamide	1	O	Used with caution in patients with poor liver function
Ethambutol	1	O	Visual acuity check required before therapy and plasma drug monitoring required during use
Streptomycin	2	IV	Plasma drug monitoring required during use
Capreomycin	2	IM	Hearing and balance function and serum potassium checks recommended before and during treatment
Cycloserine	2	O	Avoided in patients with a history of epilepsy and neurological and psychiatric problems

1, first-choice therapy; 2, second-choice therapy; IM, intramuscular; IV, intravenous; O, oral.

by the genes *embA*, *embB* and *embC*, which are involved in cell wall biosynthesis. The main function of this antibiotic is to prevent resistance emerging to other antibiotics in the regimen, rather than shortening the course of therapy; it may be associated with some severe side effects including visual impairment and (rarely) tubulointerstitial nephritis.

The current standard treatment regime for patients with active tuberculosis is delivered in two phases. In the initial phase of 2 months, a combination of four drugs, rifampicin, ethambutol hydrochloride, pyrazinamide and isoniazid, modified according to drug susceptibility/resistance testing is administered. After this initial phase, treatment is continued with rifampicin and isoniazid (with pyridoxine hydrochloride) for a further 4 months in patients without central nervous system involvement. In the case of tuberculosis caused by bacteria resistant to first-line drugs, second-line agents may be introduced to the regimen and the duration extended. The status of streptomycin in the treatment of TB is equivocal, since it is rarely used in the UK, it is not regarded as first-line by the European Respiratory Society but may be used in treatment in the USA and other countries. The WHO considers streptomycin a second-line antibiotic, to be used only if amikacin is not available or resistance to amikacin is demonstrated (and only if susceptibility to streptomycin has also been established).

Second-line antibiotics are becoming increasingly important in the treatment of TB globally, as the burden of antibiotic resistance increases. Drug-resistant TB is caused by bacteria which are shown to be resistant to at least one first-line antibiotic, while multidrug-resistant TB (MDR-TB) is caused by bacteria resistant to isoniazid and rifampicin. Extensively drug-resistant TB (XDR-TB) is caused by bacteria resistant to isoniazid and rifampicin, fluoroquinolones and at least one of three injectable second-line drugs. Second-line drugs include amikacin, kanamycin or capreomycin; the newer fluoroquinolones moxifloxacin or levofloxacin; and linezolid, delamanid and bedaquiline. Several of the antitubercular drugs have specific contraindications, or require monitoring during use. These features are summarised in Table 11.6.

Rifampicin is the only first-line antitubercular antibiotic which is also employed for treatment of non-mycobacterial infections. It inhibits the growth of most Gram-positive and many Gram-negative bacteria (but not pseudomonads or *Enterobacteriaceae*), such as *E. coli*, *Proteus* spp., *Klebsiella* spp. and *Pseudomonas* spp. Rifampicin is also active against *S. aureus* and coagulase-negative staphylococci at low concentrations. Rifampicin is also highly effective against *N. meningitidis*. Rifampicin resistance occurs rapidly when used alone, both *in vitro* and *in vivo*, so should be used in combination with another antibiotic, such as vancomycin, in the treatment of staphylococcal infections. Rifabutin, a semi-synthetic rifamycin, is indicated for the prophylaxis of *M. avium* complex infections in immunocompromised patients, for *H. pylori* eradication (in combination with other drugs) and in the treatment (as part of a multi-antibiotic regimen) of pulmonary tuberculosis and non-tuberculous mycobacterial infections.

11.10 Newer Antibiotics for MRSA and Other Gram-positive Cocci Infections

In addition to MRSA, vancomycin- and gentamicin-resistant enterococci (VRE and GRE, respectively) and penicillin-resistant *S. pneumoniae* have become increasingly prevalent, with the numbers of antibiotic agents remaining effective continuing to decline. The emergence of vancomycin-intermediate *S. aureus* (VISA) and vancomycin-resistant *S. aureus* (VRSA), or glycopeptide-intermediate strains (GISA) in general, poses particular concerns and has accelerated the introduction of new antibiotics intended for the treatment of Gram-positive cocci infections.

The first of these newer antibiotics, approved in 1999, is a fixed ratio combination of two synergistic streptogramin agents, quinupristin and dalfopristin (70:30), which exhibit dose-dependent bactericidal activity and prolonged post-antibiotic effect. This combination, administered intravenously, is recommended for the treatment of serious infections with vancomycin-resistant *E. faecium* and multidrug-resistant strains of staphylococci and pneumococci. The second, linezolid (Figure 11.11a), is the archetypal member of the oxazolidinone class of antibiotics and gained regulatory approval in 2000. It is an orally active, fully synthetic bacteriostatic agent, which acts at an earlier stage of protein synthesis than do other antibiotics aimed at this target. As a result of this, there is no cross-resistance with other drugs acting to inhibit bacterial protein synthesis. Linezolid is primarily active against Gram-positive organisms including staphylococci, streptococci, enterococci, Gram-positive anaerobic cocci and rods. It has negligible activity against Gram-negative bacteria. Clinically, linezolid is indicated for the treatment of vancomycin-resistant *E. faecium* infections, hospital-acquired pneumonias caused by both methicillin-sensitive and methicillin-resistant *S. aureus*, community-acquired pneumonia caused by penicillin-susceptible strains of *S. pneumoniae* and skin and soft tissue infections caused by Gram-positive bacteria including methicillin-resistant *S. aureus*. Linezolid should be reserved as a drug of last resort for the treatment of infections caused by multidrug-resistant microorganisms. Linezolid resistance has been reported but at very low frequency. Daptomycin (2003), a lipopeptide exhibiting a novel mode of bactericidal action, binds Ca^{2+}, forming micelle-like assemblies which deliver the antibiotic to the bacterial membrane in a detergent-like form, destabilising the membrane and causing leakage of cytoplasmic components; it is considered unlikely that cross-resistance with existing drugs will arise. It is active against Gram-positive bacteria only, and has activity against VRE and staphylococci. It is administered intravenously, and is indicated for the treatment of complicated skin and soft tissue infections caused by Gram-positive bacteria and for right-sided infectious endocarditis caused by *S. aureus*.

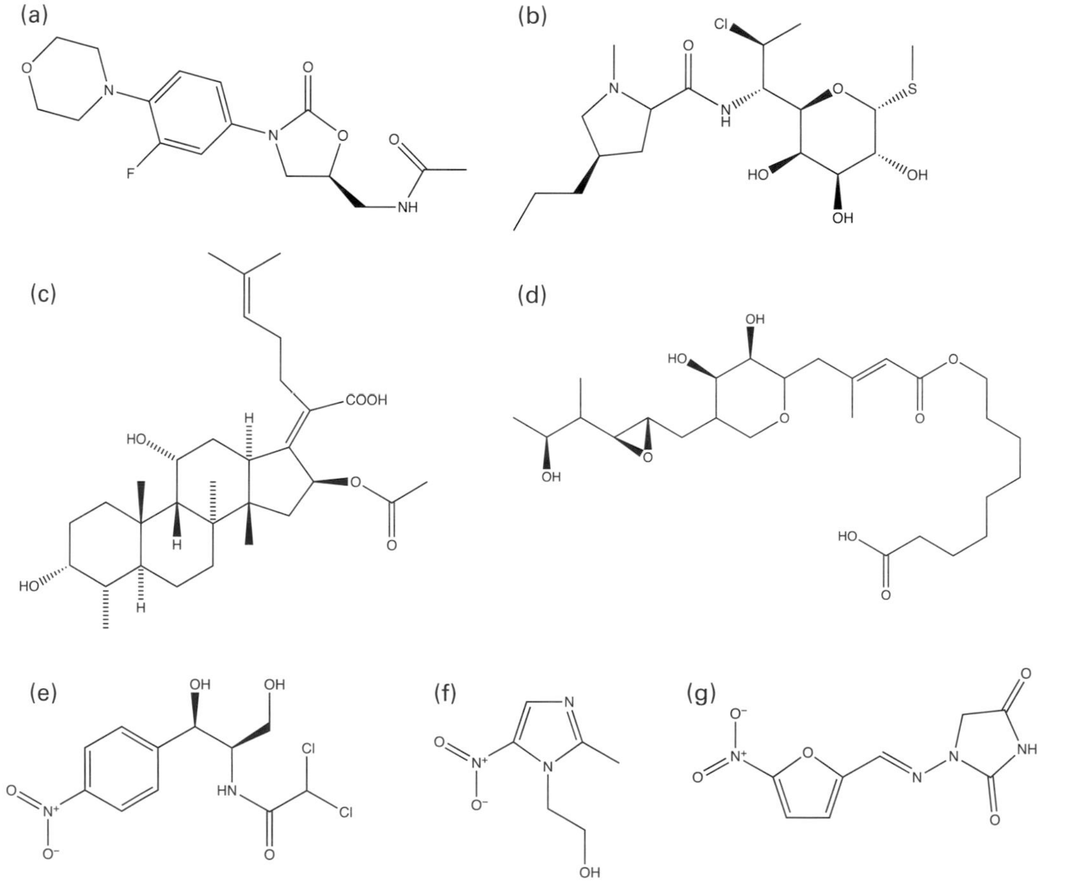

Figure 11.11 Miscellaneous antibiotics: (a) linezolid; (b) clindamycin; (c) fusidic acid; (d) mupirocin; (e) chloramphenicol; (f) metronidazole; (g) nitrofurantoin.

11.11 Miscellaneous Antibacterial Antibiotics

11.11.1 Clindamycin

Clindamycin, a bacteriostatic lincosamide antibiotic, is a synthetic derivative of the amino acid *trans*-L-4-*n*-propylhygrinic acid, attached to a thiolated derivative of an octose. The chemical structure of clindamycin is shown in Figure 11.11b. It is active against Gram-positive cocci (including MRSA, but not *E. faecalis*) and is similar in spectrum of activity to erythromycin against pneumococci, *S. pyogenes* and viridans streptococci (including some strains resistant to macrolides). Clindamycin is more potent than erythromycin against anaerobic bacteria, especially *B. fragilis*. All aerobic Gram-negative bacilli are resistant. Clindamycin has some activity against the protozoa *P. falciparum* and *Plasmodium vivax*.

Clindamycin binds exclusively to the 50S subunit of bacterial ribosomes and inhibits protein synthesis. Erythromycin, clarithromycin and chloramphenicol act at sites on the ribosome which are in close proximity, despite being unrelated structurally. Binding of one of these antibiotics may therefore inhibit the binding, and hence activity, of the others. Macrolide resistance due to methylation of the binding site on the ribosome may produce clindamycin resistance, but activity is not affected by macrolide efflux pumps. Plasmid-mediated resistance to clindamycin has been reported in *B. fragilis*. The streptogramins have a similar mechanism of action but cross-resistance with clindamycin or the macrolides is not observed. Clindamycin is primarily indicated for oral treatment of staphylococcal bone and joint infections, osteomyelitis, peritonitis, cellulitis, intra-abdominal sepsis, diabetic foot infections, falciparum malaria (with or following quinine) and for MRSA in bronchiectasis, bone and joint infections and skin and soft tissue infections. Clindamycin may also be used topically for the treatment of acne vulgaris and bacterial vaginosis. Alongside oral cephalosporins, clindamycin is one of the antibiotics most commonly associated with pseudomembranous colitis caused by *C. difficile*, which has placed significant limitations on its routine use.

11.11.2 Fusidic Acid

Fusidic acid (Figure 11.11c), a steroid-like, bactericidal antibiotic isolated from the fungus *Fusidium coccineum*, forms a stable complex with an elongation factor, EF-G, involved in the translocation process with guanosine triphosphate (GTP), which provides free energy to drive the process. One round of translocation occurs, with hydrolysis of GTP to guanosine diphosphate (GDP); the resulting complex which forms (fusidic acid–EF-G–GDP–ribosome) prevents further peptidyl chain elongation. Fusidic acid is practically restricted to use against staphylococci, primarily in topical infections, but also has activity against other Gram-positive bacteria, although streptococci are relatively resistant and Gram-negative bacteria are completely resistant. It is active against penicillin-resistant strains of *S. aureus*, including MRSA. Resistance arises relatively easily under *in vitro* conditions, but is relatively uncommon in clinical isolates.

11.11.3 Mupirocin

Mupirocin (pseudomonic acid A, Figure 11.11d) is isolated from *Pseudomonas fluorescens* and is active primarily against staphylococci and most streptococci. Mupirocin has an epoxide containing monic acid tail, which is an analogue of isoleucine. This acts as a competitive inhibitor of bacterial isoleucyl-tRNA synthetase specifically. *E. faecalis* and Gram-negative bacilli are inherently resistant, and plasmid-mediated resistance has been described in clinical isolates of *S. aureus*. Its use is largely confined to the topical treatment of *S. aureus* infections, including pre-surgical MRSA nasal decolonisation where it is claimed to be more effective than chlorhexidine or fusidic acid.

11.11.4 Colistin

Colistin, or polymyxin E as it was originally known, is the only member of the polymyxin group of peptidyl antibiotics currently in clinical use. It is a non-ribosomally synthesised polypeptide, consisting of a cyclic heptapeptide, with an N-terminally acylated tripeptide side chain. It is poorly absorbed from the GI tract and is administered parenterally, topically or by inhalation. It is active against many Gram-negative bacteria, but not cocci, *Serratia marcescens* and *Proteus* spp. Colistin, available as either the sodium salt (for oral or topical use) or most commonly the sulphomethate sodium salt, where the primary amines are converted to their corresponding aminomethanesulphonic acid sodium salt (for parenteral administration or inhalation), is primarily indicated for serious infections caused by Gram-negative pathogens in patients with limited treatment options and for chronic *P. aeruginosa* pulmonary infections in patients with cystic fibrosis (CF). It is also active against *Acinetobacter baumannii* where it may be used in the treatment of infected burns and wounds. The first reports of plasmid-mediated resistance to colistin emerged in 2016, in *E. coli* isolated from food animals, and was followed by rapid global dissemination of the dominant *mcr*-1 resistance gene (see Chapter 13). Once widespread, the use of colistin in animal feed and food production is now banned or restricted in several countries in an attempt to preserve the clinical efficacy of the drug.

11.11.5 Chloramphenicol

Although a naturally occurring antibiotic, chloramphenicol (Figure 11.11e) is manufactured by total chemical synthesis. Chloramphenicol targets peptidyl transferase, the enzyme which links amino acids in the growing peptide chain, and thereby halts peptidyl chain elongation, resulting in a reversible, rapidly bacteriostatic effect. It binds with high specificity to the 50S subunit of 70S ribosomes, and may inhibit the interaction of drugs which bind to similar sites on the ribosome (erythromycin and clarithromycin). It has a broad spectrum of activity, but aplastic anaemia, a dose-related side effect, may result from treatment in a proportion of patients and has limited the use of chloramphenicol as a systemic antibiotic. It is now primarily indicated for life-threatening infections particularly those caused by *H. influenzae* and typhoid fever (*Salmonella typhi*), and more commonly, as a topical antibiotic for superficial ophthalmic infections, bacterial infections in otitis externa and in veterinary use. A rare but potentially fatal side effect of chloramphenicol occurs in premature neonates and infants, whereby excessively high serum levels of the drug impair myocardial contractility and result in circulatory collapse, referred to as 'grey baby syndrome': this is characterised by pallid cyanosis (ashen grey skin tone), abdominal distension and circulatory collapse.

11.11.6 Metronidazole and Other Nitroimidazoles

The nitroimidazoles are a group of synthetic antimicrobials with an unusual spectrum of activity quite unlike any other family of drugs. They are useful for bacterial and protozoal infections and some members of the group exhibit anti-helminthic activity also. However, their activity against anaerobic microorganisms and those proliferating in low redox environments has proven their most important and clinically useful attribute. The 5-nitroimidazoles are similar in mode of action, structure, uses and toxicity and can be distinguished primarily on the basis of their pharmacokinetics. The archetypal antibiotic in the class, metronidazole (Figure 11.11f), is the only member of the group still clinically used. Metronidazole, like the other nitroimidazoles, is considered a prodrug, requiring reduction of the nitro group for activity, which occurs in low redox environments. It is this feature which allows them to kill cells growing under anaerobic conditions, and certain anaerobic protozoa. The highly reactive nitro radical anion species formed targets DNA (causing strand beaks) and possibly other critical biomolecules. This mode of action could damage DNA in any cell type regardless of its taxonomic status, but the fact that sufficiently reducing conditions do not arise in mammalian cells explains the lack of toxicity in humans.

Metronidazole was introduced in the 1960s, initially for the treatment of vaginitis caused by the protozoan *Trichomonas vaginalis*, but it was shown much later to exhibit excellent activity against common anaerobic pathogens (such as *B. fragilis*, *B. melaninogenicus*, *Fusobacterium* spp., *Clostridium perfringens*, *Veillonella* spp. and *Propionibacterium* spp.), as well as microaerophilic species including *H. pylori* and *Gardnerella vaginalis*. The trichomonacidal activity of metronidazole remains particularly useful against *T. vaginalis*, alongside other susceptible protozoa including *Entamoeba histolytica* and *Giardia lamblia* (*Giardia intestinalis*). Currently, metronidazole is used alone or in combination with other antibiotics, for the treatment of a wide variety of bacterial infections, summarised in Table 11.7. For treatment of amoebiasis, giardiasis

Table 11.7 Some common bacterial infections for which metronidazole may be used.

Bacterial infection	Examples of causative organism(s)	Drugs with which metronidazole may be combined
Vaginosis	*Gardnerella vaginalis*	Often used alone
Gastroduodenal ulcers	*Helicobacter pylori*	Clarithromycin and amoxicillin
Dental infections (gingivitis)	*Streptococcus* and *Fusobacterium* species	Used alone or with amoxicillin
Gut flora reduction prior to surgery	*Bacteroides* spp. and other colon bacteria	Gentamicin or cefuroxime
Infected bedsores or tumours	Various anaerobes	Quinolones
Pelvic inflammatory disease	*Neisseria gonorrhoeae* and *Chlamydia trachomatis*	Doxycycline + ceftriaxone, or ofloxacin

or trichomonas vaginitis, metronidazole is typically used alone. It is available in more dosage forms (oral, topical, injectable, suppositories) than most other antibiotics, and orally is usually administered two or three times daily. Toxicity or major side effects are relatively uncommon, but alcohol should be avoided during, and for 48 hours after, administration, as it can cause a disulfiram-like reaction in some patients when taken concomitantly.

11.11.7 Nitrofurantoin

Nitrofurantoin (Figure 11.11g) is the only remaining member of the nitrofuran group of antibiotics still in clinical use. Antimicrobial nitrofurans are synthetic agents based on the 5-nitro-2-furaldehyde molecule. The 5-nitro group is a prerequisite for antimicrobial activity and, as with metronidazole, must be reduced in order to exhibit activity. The nitrofurans are activated by enzymatic reduction of the parent molecule, forming highly reactive species resulting in DNA damage. Nitrofurans, and in particular nitrofurantoin, are broad-spectrum bacteriostatic agents, though bactericidal at higher concentrations, they are active against Gram-positive cocci and Gram-negative enteric bacteria. Following oral administration, plasma concentrations achieved are very low, with a significant fraction of the drug rapidly excreted in the urine. It is therefore indicated exclusively for infections of the urinary tract, including lower urinary tract infections, cystitis and catheter-associated urinary tract infections. The size of the drug crystals in tablet formulations is proposed to affect the dissolution of the drug, with macrocrystalline nitrofurantoin exhibiting slower dissolution and steadier release patterns. The activity of nitrofurantoin is substantially greater in acidic urine, which is at odds with common, current symptomatic approaches to treatment of cystitis which rely on elevation of urinary pH to alkaline pH values, using potassium citrate or similar compounds. Interestingly, nitrofurantoin is one of the few antibiotics to which resistance development has not significantly increased since its introduction, prompting a degree of renewed interest in this antibiotic and its related compounds.

11.12 Antifungal antibiotics

Invasive fungal infections, or mycoses, have emerged as significant clinical challenges in the treatment of immunocompromised patients, leading to increased morbidity and mortality. In addition, the emergence of antifungal resistance to clinically important antifungal antibiotics over the past several decades prompted the research and development of newer antifungal drugs (see also Chapter 4). For much of the second half of the twentieth century, nystatin, amphotericin and griseofulvin were the principal therapeutic options available, supplemented with a range of synthetic imidazoles which found application primarily in superficial rather than systemic fungal infections. The clinical development of the triazole antifungals, fluconazole and itraconazole, in the 1980s marked a significant advancement and expansion of the antifungal armamentarium. More recently, a new class of antifungal targeting the fungal cell wall, the echinocandin lipopeptides, further increased the range of clinical options available for severe fungal infections.

Lack of toxicity is, as always, of paramount importance, but differences between bacterial and fungal cells in both structure and biosynthetic processes mean that the low-toxicity antibacterial antibiotics are usually inactive against fungi. Since fungi are eukaryotic, fewer differences exist between human and fungal cells, compared to bacterial and human cells, making selective toxicity harder to achieve. While fungal infections tend to be less virulent than bacterial or viral infections, they nonetheless pose major threats to patients with compromised or depressed immune systems, or the critically ill, particularly in the case of systemic mycoses.

11.12.1 Azoles

The azoles may be considered as two sub-groups; the older imidazole antifungal drugs which were introduced primarily as topical products or pessaries for the treatment of superficial infections caused by dermatophytic fungi (skin pathogens), *Malassezia* (formerly *Pityrosporum*) species (implicated in flaky skin and dandruff) and *C. albicans* (thrush), and the newer, more versatile and in some cases more expensive, triazole drugs.

11.12.1.1 Imidazoles

The imidazoles are a large and diverse group of compounds, which exhibit activity against bacteria and protozoa (metronidazole and tinidazole), helminths (mebendazole) and fungi (clotrimazole, miconazole, ketoconazole, econazole and tioconazole). Table 11.8 lists infections for which the common imidazole antifungals are employed. A number of other imidazole antifungals are available in various countries. As shown in the table, the imidazoles are available in a wide variety of dosage forms, but most have the same uses. As with all azoles, the imidazoles inhibit ergosterol synthesis, by inhibiting the terminal enzymatic conversion of lanosterol to ergosterol, a key component of the fungal cell membrane. Depletion of fungal cell membrane ergosterol leads to either fungistatic or

Table 11.8 Antifungal imidazoles.

Drug	Common formulations	Clinical uses
Clotrimazole	T, P, VC, Pdr, S, Soln	Dermatophytoses, pityriasis or *Candida* in the skin, vagina or ear
Miconazole	T, P, VC, Soln, Pdr	Oral, intestinal, skin or vaginal *Candida* infections, dermatophytoses and pityriasis
Econazole	T, P	Dermatophytoses, pityriasis and skin or vaginal *Candida*
Sulconazole	T	Dermatophytoses, pityriasis and skin or vaginal *Candida*
Ketoconazole	T, Sham, Tab	Oral systemic treatment of dermatophytoses or candidal infections resistant to other drugs or patients intolerant to them
Tioconazole	NS	Fungal infections of finger and toenails

NS, nail solution; P, pessary; Pdr, powder; S, spray; Sham, shampoo; Soln, solution or gel for external or oral use; T, topical cream, oral gel or ointment; Tab, tablets; VC, vaginal cream.

fungicidal activity, although most imidazoles are considered fungistatic when clinically used, unless for prolonged treatment times and at elevated concentrations. Clotrimazole is primarily indicated for topical application for the treatment of cutaneous candidiasis and vaginal yeast infections, and dermatophyte (tinea) infections. Oral clotrimazole, administered as a lozenge, may be employed in the treatment of oropharyngeal candidiasis. However, it is not well absorbed when taken orally. Miconazole has a similar spectrum of activity and is primarily used for cutaneous and mucocutaneous fungal infections, including vaginal and vulval candidiasis. As with clotrimazole, miconazole is poorly absorbed after oral administration but may be used orally for the treatment of intestinal fungal infections. Limited absorption from the GI tract is a benefit in this scenario, but systemic absorption should be considered in terms of potential drug interactions. Ketoconazole is primarily employed for cutaneous tinea infections, cutaneous candidiasis and seborrhoeic dermatitis (including treatment and prophylaxis of dandruff where *Malassezia* spp. is implicated). Ketoconazole also achieves greater oral absorption from the GI tract and has previously been indicated for the treatment of blastomycosis, histoplasmosis, coccidioidomycosis and paracoccidioidomycosis. However, its use has been largely superseded by newer, less toxic and more effective drugs. Ketoconazole participates in numerous drug interactions associated with systemic absorption when taken orally and this has further limited its applications. Therefore, its use as an orally administered antifungal drug is restricted to situations where resistance or patient tolerance to newer drugs is an issue.

11.12.1.2 Triazoles

The triazoles have become the most important class of antifungal drugs for the treatment of systemic fungal infections. The first drugs in this class, fluconazole (Figure 11.12a) and itraconazole, were introduced in the 1980s, followed in the early 2000s by voriconazole, posaconazole and isavuconazole. Fluconazole is absorbed to a greater extent from the GI tract than itraconazole, and is primarily active against dermatophytes, pityriasis and *Candida* infections. Both fluconazole and itraconazole are active against *Cryptococcus neoformans* and are therefore valuable in the treatment of cryptococcosis which, although uncommon, can be life-threatening in immunocompromised patients. Both are active against *Histoplasma capsulatum*, *Paracoccidioides brasiliensis* and *Blastomyces dermatitidis*, but have little activity against *Candida glabrata* and *Candida krusei*. Itraconazole is indicated for similar infections to fluconazole, but it is also active against *Aspergillus* spp. and is therefore commonly selected as an alternative to amphotericin B (see Section 11.12.2 below) in cases of systemic *Aspergillus* infections and other rare systemic mycoses (more common in the immunocompromised). Itraconazole is more frequently associated with hepatic toxicity than fluconazole.

Triazoles have the same mode of action as the imidazoles, targeting ergosterol synthesis. Later generations of triazole antifungals, including itraconazole, posaconazole and voriconazole, inhibit the enzyme lanosterol 14-α-demethylase with higher affinity, which is thought to account for their extended spectrum of activity. While neither fluconazole nor itraconazole exhibits activity towards *Fusarium* spp. or members of the order Mucorales, voriconazole and posaconazole are active against these fungi, and also *Aspergillus* spp., *C. glabrata* and *C. krusei*. These agents are therefore indicated for the treatment of invasive aspergillosis, and as an alternative to amphotericin B in the treatment of mucormycosis (posaconazole and isavuconazole are also active against the Mucorales), serious infections caused by *Scedosporium* spp., *Fusarium* spp. or invasive fluconazole-resistant *Candida* spp. The triazoles

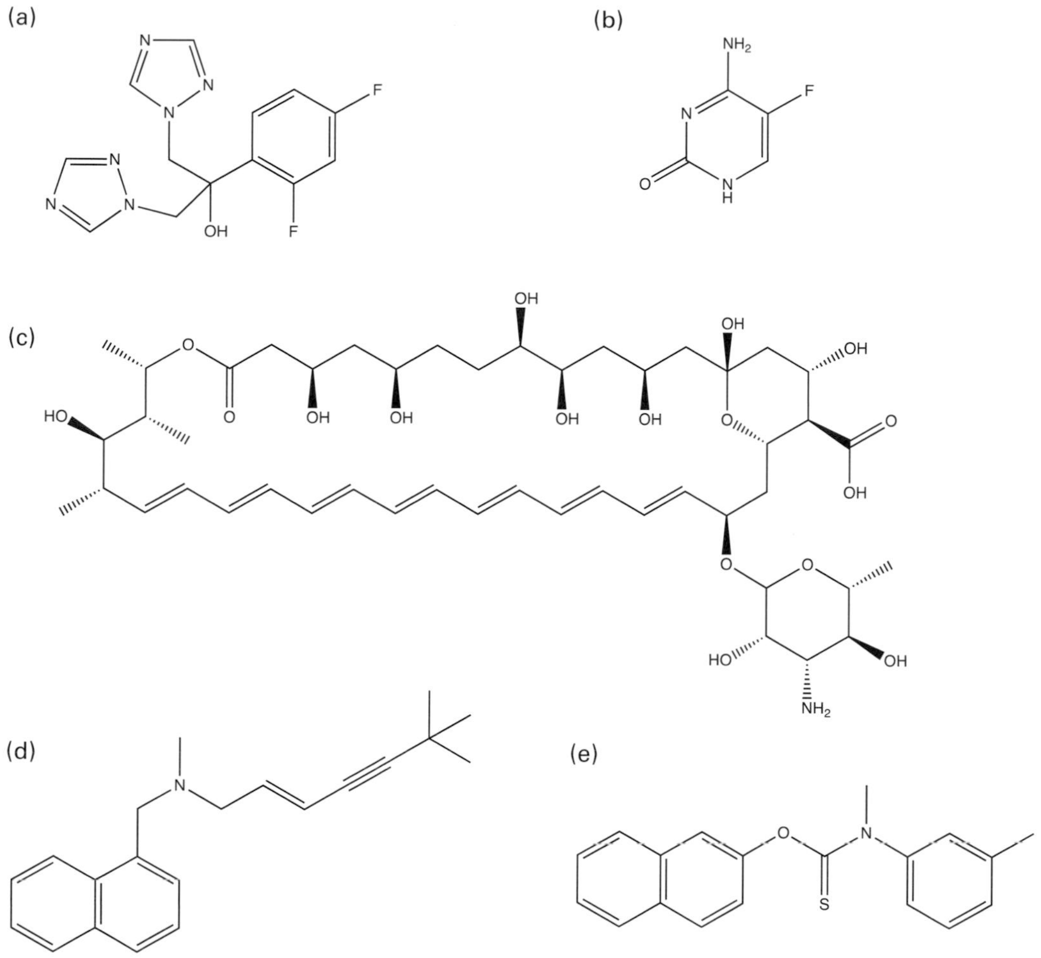

Figure 11.12 Antifungal agents: (a) fluconazole; (b) flucytosine; (c) amphotericin; (d) terbinafine; (e) tolnaftate.

are also used in the treatment and prophylaxis of fungal infections in immunocompromised patients at high risk of systemic fungal infections (e.g., following bone marrow transplantation, HIV-infection or high-dose immunosuppressive therapy). Resistance to triazoles has been described in *Candida* spp., related to efflux pump expression and target modification, and reduced susceptibility in the biofilm mode of growth. The emergence and spread of hospital-acquired triazole-resistant candidal infections are concerning, and triazole resistance has also been described in *C. neoformans* and *Aspergillus fumigatus*.

11.12.2 Polyenes

Polyene antifungals are natural compounds, characterised by the presence of a macrolide ring and a hydrophobic region consisting of a sequence of four to seven conjugated double bonds. The only clinically important polyenes are amphotericin B (Figure 11.12c) and nystatin. Amphotericin B consists of seven conjugated double bonds, a free carboxylic acid group, an internal ester bond in the macrolide ring and a glycoside side chain with a free primary amino group. It acts by binding to membrane ergosterol, which leads to the formation of ion channels in the fungal cell membrane and the leakage of K+ ions and concentration-dependent cell death. Amphotericin B is active against most fungal pathogens and is indicated for life-threatening systemic mycoses, representing a more toxic but potentially more effective alternative to itraconazole. It has been used in the treatment of coccidioidomycosis, cryptococcal meningitis, systemic candidiasis and histoplasmosis in patients living with HIV. It is also licensed for the treatment of oropharyngeal and oesophageal candidiasis, and fungal toenail/fingernail infections (onychomycosis). Amphotericin B is practically insoluble in water, and is either poorly or not absorbed when administered orally or intramuscularly. As a result, it is delivered by intravenous injection under strict medical supervision, where it is formulated in either lipid- or liposomal-based formulations. These formulations exhibit lower toxicity and improved stability when compared to conventional aqueous formulations, permitting higher dose therapies to be employed.

Nystatin is administered orally for the local treatment of oral candidiasis and oral and perioral infections. Since it is not orally bioavailable, it is suitable for treating intestinal candidiasis. Nystatin is formulated either as an oral suspension for treatment of *C. albicans* infections, or as a cream in combination with other agents (including neomycin sulphate, chlorhexidine, benzalkonium chloride, hydrocortisone, clobetasone or oxytetracycline) for a variety of topical infections where a broad-spectrum antifungal antibiotic is deemed beneficial. It is rarely indicated for the treatment of other fungal infections, however, and parenteral nystatin is associated with severe toxicity and is therefore too toxic to be administered by injection.

11.12.3 Echinocandins

The echinocandins are a novel class of semi-synthetic lipopeptide antifungal antibiotics which target the biosynthesis of 1,3-β-D-glucan through non-competitive inhibition of the 1,3-β-D-glucan synthase enzyme complex. Glucan and chitin are key components of the fungal cell wall (see Chapter 4), and so inhibition of glucan synthesis in susceptible fungi leads to loss of integrity of the cell wall and dose-dependent fungicidal activity. The echinocandins have also been shown to enhance neutrophil activity against *Aspergillus* spp. The three clinically useful echinocandins are anidulafungin, caspofungin and micafungin. All three compounds exhibit similar broad-spectrum fungicidal activity against *Candida* spp. and inhibitory activity against *Aspergillus* spp. Caspofungin, the first member of the class, is indicated for the treatment of invasive aspergillosis, invasive candidiasis and empirical therapy of systemic fungal infections in patients with neutropaenia. It is given as an intravenous infusion, and is useful where infections are unresponsive to either amphotericin or itraconazole. Both anidulafungin and micafungin are also intravenously administered for the treatment of invasive candidiasis. Like caspofungin, they tend to be reserve drugs both to minimise the risk of resistance development and also due to cost considerations. Resistance to the echinocandins is uncommon, but has been described in clinical isolates of *C. glabrata* from patients receiving prolonged therapy.

11.12.4 Other Antifungal Agents

Flucytosine (5-fluorocytosine [5-FC], Figure 11.12b) is a narrow-spectrum antifungal agent which causes RNA miscoding and inhibits DNA synthesis. It is water-soluble and orally bioavailable and exhibits activity against yeasts such as *Candida* spp. and *C. neoformans*. It has little or no activity against *Aspergillus* spp. Flucytosine is normally used in combination with fluconazole, or in synergistic combination with amphotericin for severe systemic candidiasis and cryptococcal meningitis. This combination allows amphotericin to be used at lower effective doses, reducing the risk of toxicity. Terbinafine (Figure 11.12d) is an allylamine antifungal agent which acts as an inhibitor of ergosterol biosynthesis. It is fungicidal and orally effective against a broad range of dermatophytes and yeasts. It is the drug of choice for the treatment of fungal nail infections and may be applied topically or administered orally. Griseofulvin was the first orally active therapeutic agent for the treatment of dermatophyte infections and is still indicated for treatment of infections of the skin, scalp, hair and nails, but usually only when topical therapy has failed. Its use has largely been supplanted by newer, more effective agents and its current main indication is for the treatment of tinea capitis (a highly contagious infection of the scalp) caused by *Trichophyton tonsurans*. Tolnaftate (Figure 11.12e) is a synthetic thiocarbamate which is used topically in the treatment or prophylaxis of tinea infections (commonly referred to as ringworm, despite being a fungal infection). Amorolfine is similarly used for tinea infections, though its primary indication is treatment of fungal nail infections (onychomycosis or tinea unguium) by transungual application as a nail lacquer.

11.13 Antiviral Drugs

The vast majority of the antibacterial and antifungal agents described in this chapter exhibit little or no activity against viruses, because they target structures or metabolic enzyme systems found only in bacterial and fungal cells. In contrast to other microorganisms, viruses do not possess the metabolic enzymes necessary for their own replication. Viruses are obligate intracellular parasites, and after entry to the host cell the virus uses either enzymes already present or induces the biosynthesis of new ones in the host cell, in order to synthesise and express the individual components of the viral particle or virion. These components are then assembled and the virion released from the host cell, either by lytic release (rupture of the host cell) or membrane budding (acquiring an external lipid envelope in the process). In a number of cases, the virion contains a small number of key enzymes necessary to initiate or complete replication. Such enzymes are expressed in the host cell prior to packaging within the capsid and release of the mature virion which then goes on to infect another host cell. Viruses effectively hijack the metabolic machinery of the infected host cell to replicate and, as a result, offer very few unique targets in the viral replication pathway which may be exploited for the development of selectively toxic antiviral

Table 11.9 Antiviral drugs used in the treatment of selected viral infections.

Herpes	Cytomegalovirus	Viral hepatitis B	Influenza	Respiratory syncytial virus
Aciclovir	Cidofovir	Adefovir	Oseltamivir	Palivizumab
Famciclovir	Foscarnet	Entecavir	Zanamivir	Ribavirin
Foscarnet	Ganciclovir	Lamivudine		
Penciclovir	Letermovir	Telbivudine		
Valaciclovir	Valaciclovir	Tenofovir		
Inosine pranobex	Valganciclovir	Interferon-α		

drugs, that is, antivirals which inhibit or inactivate the virus without harming the human host. In addition, antiviral agents must cross the host cell membrane in order to be effective, unless targeting the initial binding and entry or release of the virus from the host cell. A complete discussion of viral life cycles and their control is provided in Chapter 5.

The first reported cases of acquired immune deficiency syndrome (AIDS) in the USA in 1981 were quickly followed in 1983 by the discovery of a retrovirus which was the likely causative agent of AIDS, subsequently identified as the HIV. Prior to the identification of HIV, the number of clinically effective, synthetic antiviral drugs was extremely limited. The HIV/AIDS pandemic provided a major stimulus for fundamental research into the structure and reproduction of viruses generally, and in particular retroviruses. This, together with a better understanding of the role certain viruses play in the development of specific cancers (oncogenic viruses), more sophisticated rapid diagnostic methods and the availability of technology for the rapid and inexpensive whole genomic sequencing of viral genomes of important pathogenic viruses, has led to a wealth of new antiviral drugs. Table 11.9 lists a selection of agents currently indicated for a range of viral infections, while Table 11.10 lists the range of drugs, by mechanistic class, that are used exclusively for the treatment of HIV infection. Although these antiviral drugs may be usefully classified on the basis of shared chemical structure (Figure 11.14) or by mode of action, most are indicated or approved for use against only a limited number of viruses, and, more commonly, against just a single virus. Therefore, the most convenient and useful way of considering antiviral drugs is often on the basis of the viral infections they are intended to treat.

Table 11.10 Mechanisms of action of common antiretroviral drugs.

Mechanism of action	Examples
Nucleoside reverse transcriptase inhibitors (nucleoside analogues)	Abacavir, didanosine, emtricitabine, lamivudine, tenofovir, zidovudine
Protease inhibitors	Atazanavir, darunavir, fosamprenavir, lopinavir, nelfinavir, ritonavir, saquinavir, tipranavir
Non-nucleoside reverse transcriptase inhibitors	Doravirine, efavirenz, etravirine, nevirapine, rilpivirine
Integrase inhibitors	Bictegravir, dolutegravir, elvitegravir, raltegravir
Fusion inhibitor	Enfuvirtide
CCR5 antagonist	Maraviroc
Pharmacokinetic enhancers (activity boosters with no intrinsic antiviral action)	Cobicistat, low-dose ritonavir

11.13.1 Human Immunodeficiency Virus

The HIV is a retrovirus (an RNA virus that uses the enzyme reverse transcriptase to reverse-transcribe its RNA genome into DNA, which is subsequently inserted into the host genome by the enzyme integrase) which is the causative agent of AIDS. HIV causes immunodeficiency by infecting and killing host immune cells, particularly T-helper cells also known as CD4 cells. Depletion of CD4 cells to below 200 cells μl^{-1} of plasma, accompanied by opportunistic infections and any of a range of AIDS-defining illnesses/malignancies, confirms the diagnosis of AIDS. The prognosis of patients with HIV and AIDS has improved significantly, thanks to the introduction of highly active antiretroviral therapy (HAART), characterised by the use of agents in combination. There exists a large and increasingly diverse range of antiretroviral agents available to treat HIV, which are used under specialist direction. A detailed account of the characteristics of each individual antiretroviral drug is beyond the scope of this chapter; however, it is possible to gain an understanding of the principles of HIV chemotherapy by considering the unique life cycle of the virus (Figure 11.13), paying particular attention to unique

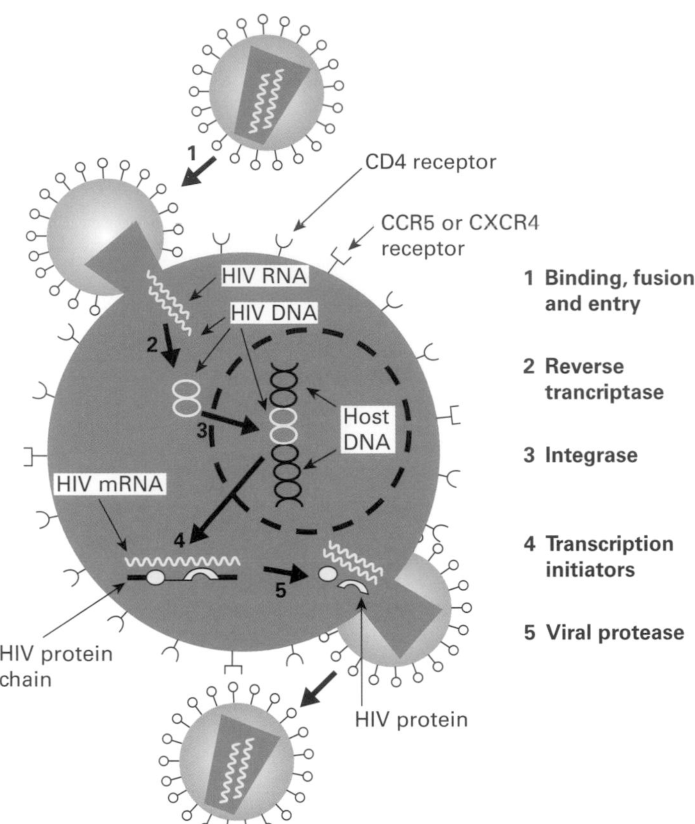

Figure 11.13 HIV life cycle showing stages vulnerable to antiretroviral drugs.

targets in its replication cycle and the mode of action of drugs in current use.

Initiation of HIV infection of CD4/T-helper cells occurs when the envelope glycoprotein gp120, which decorates the surface of the HIV envelope, binds receptors exclusive to T-helper cells, namely, the surface receptor CD4. Upon binding, a conformational change takes place in the CD4 receptor, allowing two other cell surface proteins, chemokine co-receptor (CCR5 or CXCR4), to bind gp120, mediating the fusion of the viral envelope and the host cell membrane with the introduction of the viral capsid into the cytoplasm of the host cell. The CCR5 chemokine receptor antagonist, maraviroc, which inhibits the interaction of gp120 with the CCR5 receptor, is approved for the treatment of patients infected with CCR5-tropic HIV, in combination with other antiretroviral drugs. Following binding, fusion of the viral envelope with the host cell membrane, and subsequent release of the HIV RNA into the host cell, may be inhibited by the HIV-fusion inhibitor, enfuvirtide, which binds the gp41 subunit of the viral envelope glycoprotein, inhibiting conformational changes necessary for fusion to occur. Enfuvirtide is licensed for treatment of HIV in combination with other antiretrovirals for resistant infections, or for patients intolerant to other antiretroviral drug regimens. Once fused, the viral matrix and capsid proteins undergo dissolution in the cytoplasm and viral enzymes and RNA are released. The single-stranded viral RNA is used as a template from which a complementary strand of DNA is synthesised by viral reverse transcriptase, using host nucleotides. Reverse transcriptase is a unique target for HIV chemotherapy and several nucleoside analogue inhibitors of reverse transcriptase, and non-nucleoside reverse transcriptase inhibitors (see Table 11.10) have been approved for the treatment of HIV infection. The first drug approved (in 1987) for treatment of HIV, zidovudine (or azidothymidine [AZT], Figure 11.14d), is a nucleoside reverse transcriptase inhibitor initially developed to treat cancer; it still remains a key component of HIV chemotherapy. Nucleoside and non-nucleoside reverse transcriptase inhibitors make up the backbone of first-line HAART regimens.

As viral replication progresses, the single strand of complementary DNA is duplicated into linear double-stranded DNA which combines with viral enzyme HIV-integrase (packaged in the original viral particle and released at the stage of fusion and entry) and passes into the host nucleus. Integrase cuts the host cell chromosome and inserts the double-stranded proviral DNA into the chromosome, establishing a lifelong infection. This step may be inhibited by integrase inhibitors such as raltegravir (newer drugs include dolutegravir and elvitegravir). Integrase inhibitors are now considered first-line drugs, but were originally

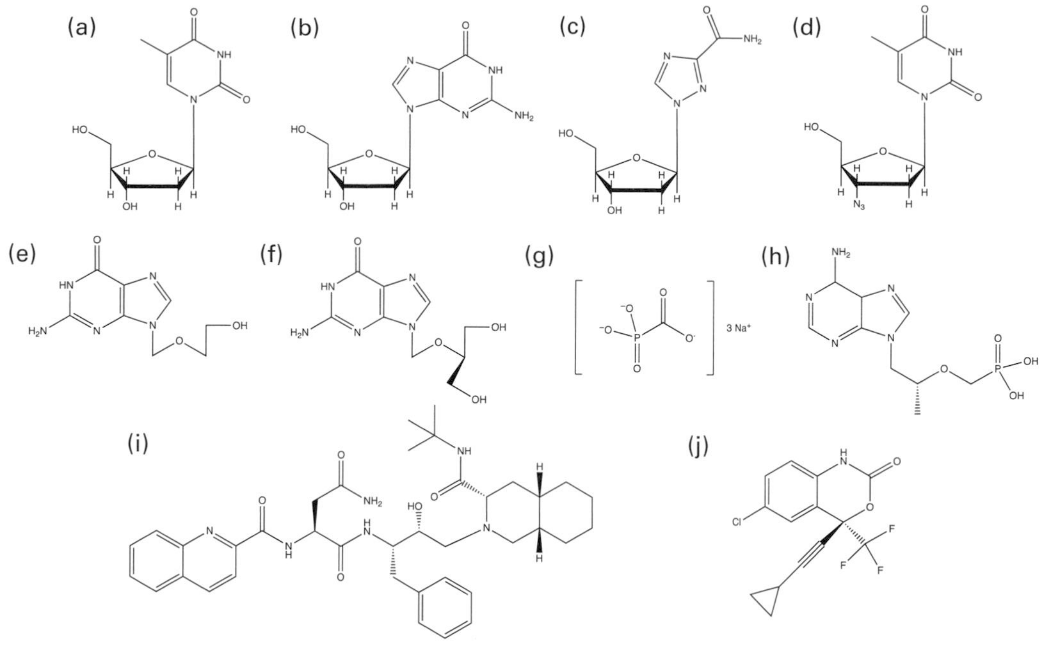

Figure 11.14 Structures of nucleosides and selected antiviral agents: (a) thymidine; (b) guanosine; (c) ribavirin; (d) zidovudine; (e) aciclovir; (f) ganciclovir; (g) foscarnet; (h) tenofovir; (i) saquinavir; (j) efavirenz.

reserved for the treatment of HIV infections resistant to other antiretrovirals. The provirus may remain latent within the host chromosome until activated by regulatory proteins which cause the viral DNA to be transcribed into viral mRNA by RNA polymerase. These viral mRNAs encode several viral proteins, which are ribosomally synthesised as Gag-Pol polyproteins which must be cleaved into individual proteins by the action of the HIV aspartyl protease to become functional. HIV protease cleaves the Gag-Pol polyprotein at nine distinct cleavage sites, yielding functional viral enzymes and structural proteins. Inhibitors of HIV aspartyl protease, known as protease inhibitors (atazanavir, for example), are also important first-line antiretroviral drugs, and are used in combination with other antiretrovirals to avoid development of resistance and to reduce toxicity.

HIV infection is incurable, but strict adherence over many years to a HAART regimen, using a combination of drugs, can achieve undetectable viral loads in infected patients, thus preserving immune function, reducing mortality and morbidity associated with chronic HIV infection and reducing or completely preventing onward HIV transmission; this has been shown to substantially extend survival in patients living with HIV infection. The combination of antiretrovirals in HAART regimens also minimises toxicity associated with individual classes of drugs and reduces or delays the emergence of resistance to individual agents. In general, HAART regimens comprise three or more drugs in combination. Treatment is typically initiated (in patients who are treatment-naïve) with two nucleoside reverse transcriptase inhibitors as a backbone with one other antiretroviral drug, either a non-nucleoside reverse transcriptase inhibitor, a boosted protease inhibitor or an integrase inhibitor. In the UK, currently recommended regimens comprise a backbone of emtricitabine and tenofovir, abacavir and lamivudine with the third drug either ritonavir-boosted atazanavir, darunavir or dolutegravir. The concept of a *boosted protease inhibitor* comes about through the observation that low-dose ritonavir (which has no intrinsic antiviral activity) reduces the clearance, and thus increases the duration of effective plasma concentrations, of almost all other protease inhibitors. Synergy is often observed between antiretroviral drugs, both with agents having the same, and different, modes of action. A number of co-formulated HAART drugs are currently available, which aim to reduce pill burden and improve adherence to the regimen.

Adherence to HAART regimens is key to long-term success, and therefore issues of drug toxicity, side effects and adverse effects are often linked to patient non-adherence, therapeutic failure or development of antiviral drug resistance. Antiretroviral drugs exhibit a number of class-specific side effects, many of which are of sufficient severity to make it difficult for patients to maintain the adherence necessary for long-term therapeutic success. In particular, lipodystrophy syndrome, associated with a number of drugs including older antiretrovirals such as zidovudine, stavudine and protease inhibitors, leads to redistribution of body fat, and accompanying metabolic complications including insulin resistance, dyslipidaemia and increased cardiovascular risk and visceral fat accumulation in the liver. Although lipodystrophy may be associated with HIV infection generally, most newer drugs are less commonly associated with this complication. Most antiretroviral drugs are orally active, since any agent which required lifelong daily injections would predispose to non-adherence.

11.13.2 Herpes and Cytomegalovirus Infections

There are eight herpesviruses capable of causing human infection, but of these the most important are:

- the two *herpes simplex viruses*, HSV-1 and HSV-2, which cause cold sores of the face and lips and genital herpes, respectively;
- the *varicella zoster virus*, which causes chickenpox and shingles (herpes zoster);
- the *Epstein–Barr virus* responsible for infectious mononucleosis (glandular fever);
- the *cytomegalovirus* (CMV) which may cause retinitis (inflammation of the retina) and, infrequently, symptoms similar to infectious mononucleosis.

The first three drugs listed for the treatment of herpes simplex infections in Table 11.9, aciclovir (Figure 11.14e), famciclovir and penciclovir, are the most important. Inosine pranobex is an orally active immunomodulator whose efficacy has not been proven; it is indicated for the treatment of mucocutaneous herpes simplex infections, although it has been almost completely superseded by aciclovir. It is also indicated as an adjunctive treatment for genital warts and for subacute sclerosing panencephalitis. The pyrimidine analogue, idoxuridine, is no longer used widely, again having been replaced by aciclovir.

Many antiviral drugs are nucleoside analogues; aciclovir and its prodrug valaciclovir are acyclic analogues of guanosine, and penciclovir and its prodrug famciclovir are guanine analogues. Aciclovir and penciclovir are structurally very similar and both share a common mode of action, inhibiting viral depolymerase causing premature termination of DNA synthesis in virally infected cells. In both cases, for each drug to become active it must be converted to its monophosphate by the action of viral thymidine kinase, which then allows host cellular kinases to di- and tri-phosphorylate the molecule, which then competes with deoxyguanosine triphosphate as a substrate for viral DNA polymerase. Conversion of aciclovir or penciclovir to the corresponding monophosphate does not proceed to any significant degree in uninfected host cells, since the viral thymidine kinase enzyme is several orders of magnitude more efficient at phosphorylating aciclovir and penciclovir than the corresponding mammalian enzyme. Furthermore, selective toxicity is further achieved, as the triphosphate of aciclovir is a much more potent inhibitor of viral DNA polymerase than host cell DNA polymerases. All four drugs (inosine pranobex, aciclovir, famciclovir and valaciclovir) are used primarily in the treatment of herpes simplex and varicella zoster infections; CMV is normally resistant (since it does not produce thymidine kinase) and Epstein–Barr virus shows intermediate sensitivity. Aciclovir is available as oral tablets, topical cream and intravenous infusion. Five times daily dosing is required for aciclovir when administered topically or orally in order to achieve therapeutically effective doses, since aciclovir is only partially absorbed from the GI tract (15–30% bioavailability) and the plasma half-life is 2–3 hours in adults, or 3–4 hours in neonates. The prodrug valaciclovir, which undergoes first-pass metabolism to yield aciclovir, has a much longer half-life and, as a result, the typical dosing frequency is three times daily. Penciclovir is poorly absorbed and has little oral activity and is therefore indicated for topical use in the treatment of cold sores, applied every 2 hours. The orally active famciclovir, indicated for treatment of herpes zoster (shingles), HSV infection and genital herpes, is taken between once and three times daily.

Because CMV does not produce thymidine kinase, it is not normally susceptible to aciclovir, penciclovir or their corresponding prodrugs. Therefore, a different group of agents is used to treat CMV infections. Ganciclovir (Figure 11.14f) is structurally similar to aciclovir but is phosphorylated more efficiently in CMV-infected cells, albeit by a protein kinase, which only poorly converts aciclovir into its monophosphate. It is administered by intravenous infusion for the prevention and treatment of life- or sight-threatening CMV infections in immunocompromised patients or prevention of CMV infection following organ transplantation. Valganciclovir, an orally available valine ester prodrug of ganciclovir, is similarly indicated for CMV retinitis and the prevention of cytomegalovirus disease following organ transplantation from CMV-positive donors. Cidofovir, a nucleoside analogue of cytosine monophosphate, is a selective inhibitor of human cytomegalovirus DNA polymerase which is active against most herpes viruses, but whose primary indication is the treatment of cytomegalovirus retinitis in AIDS patients. Foscarnet, phosphonomethanoic acid (Figure 11.14g), is capable of chelating metal ions and blocks the pyrophosphate binding site in herpes virus DNA polymerase, inhibiting the enzyme. It is indicated for cytomegalovirus disease (where ganciclovir cannot be used) and mucocutaneous herpes simplex virus infections unresponsive to aciclovir in immunocompromised patients.

11.13.3 Viral Hepatitis

Hepatitis, inflammation of the liver, can be caused by various drugs and toxins, but hepatitis due to a viral infection is more common. The viruses most commonly implicated are the hepatitis viruses A–E, which are not related, and in about 5% of cases viral hepatitis is caused by other viruses including herpes viruses, CMV, and Epstein–Barr virus. Hepatitis A virus or Hepatovirus A (formerly known as infectious hepatitis) is a picornavirus containing a single strand of RNA; it causes self-limiting and rarely fatal, food-borne infection that does not result in permanent liver damage. As a result, it is not normally treated with antiviral drugs and no specific treatment exists. It is common in countries where sanitation is poor and vaccination is recommended if an individual is deemed at high risk of infection or travelling to an area where the virus is endemic. Similarly, hepatitis E is generally mild and self-limiting and relatively uncommon and no treatment or vaccine is currently available. The hepatitis E virus is spread via the faecal–oral route, and is an RNA virus belonging to the family *Hepeviridae*. Hepatitis D only affects individuals already infected with hepatitis B virus, which is required for hepatitis D virus to replicate in the body. There is no current treatment for hepatitis D, but vaccination against hepatitis B protects against infection. Therefore, chronic hepatitis B and hepatitis C (HBV and HCV, respectively) pose the greatest threat to public health and require antiviral therapy in their management.

It has been estimated that more than one third of the world's population is infected with HBV and just over a tenth of that number with HCV. The World Health Organization estimates that in 2019, over 296 million people were living with chronic HBV, and 58 million people with HCV. The two infections have several features in common, although the viruses belong to different families. In both cases, the disease can present as either acute or chronic infections, and, in the latter, there may be progression to liver damage and an associated higher risk of contracting hepatocellular carcinoma (primary liver cancer). Acute HBV cases are not normally treated with antiviral drugs, and while that was also formerly the case for HCV, clinical evidence suggests that early treatment of HCV has a higher success rate and shorter treatment time than that required for chronic disease, so this practice is now more common. Early treatment with interferon alpha may reduce the risk of chronic HCV infection.

HBV is unusual in that it is not a retrovirus (it is a partially double-stranded DNA virus of the genus *Orthohepadnavirus*), yet it uses a reverse transcriptase in its replication, one of the few known non-retroviral viruses to do so. For this reason, antiretroviral drugs used to treat HIV infection, lamivudine and tenofovir (Figure 11.14h), are also effective for HBV. In addition, adefovir dipivoxil (a nucleotide analogue), entecavir (a guanosine nucleoside analogue) and telbivudine (a thymidine nucleoside analogue) are also used, typically for 6 months or more for all five drugs. Emtricitabine, a nucleoside (cytosine) reverse transcriptase inhibitor approved for treatment of HIV, has been shown to be effective against HBV. In patients with decompensated liver disease (liver cirrhosis with fluid accumulation in the abdomen), lamivudine or adefovir is recommended (in combination with another antiviral for chronic hepatitis B). Adefovir is effective in lamivudine-resistant HBV infection, but telbivudine should not be used due to the risk of cross-resistance arising. Entecavir is effective in patients not previously treated with nucleoside analogues, but resistance can occur in patients who have received lamivudine. However, it is still indicated for use in HBV patients with compensated liver disease and lamivudine resistance.

There are several genotypes of HCV which exhibit variable drug sensitivities, so the genotype of the infecting virus should be determined, along with viral load before commencing treatment. A combination of ribavirin (a guanosine analogue, Figure 11.14c) and interferon alpha is used for the treatment of acute and chronic HBV and HCV. Interferons are low-molecular-weight proteins produced by virus-infected cells, which themselves induce formation of a second protein inhibiting the transcription of mRNA. Two pegylated variations of interferon alpha are available (peginterferon alpha-2a and -2b) and are indicated in combination with ribavirin for chronic HCV or as monotherapy for chronic HBV or HCV where ribavirin is not tolerated. These pegylated interferons have largely replaced the routine use of standard interferon alpha. Recently, a number of direct-acting antivirals (DAAs) which target stages in the HCV life cycle have been approved. It is now well-established that addition of a direct-acting antiviral to pegylated interferon plus ribavirin results in an improved sustained virologic response (SVR), and so where peginterferon alpha and ribavirin are used in combination, a direct acting antiviral should also be used as standard therapy. These DAAs include inhibitors of the serine protease NS3/4A which cleaves the HCV polyprotein at four sites. Cleavage of the HCV polyprotein is essential for viral replication, and a range of HCV protease inhibitors with variable selectivity for the HCV major genotypes are now available including grazoprevir (most HCV genotypes), telaprevir (HCV genotype 1), boceprevir (HCV genotype 1), simeprevir (HCV genotypes 1 and 4) and paritaprevir (HCV genotypes 1 and 4). In addition, nucleos(t)ide analogue polymerase inhibitors (nucleos(t)ide analogue drugs [NUCs]) are DAAs which bind to the active site of the HCV NS5B RNA polymerase and inhibit replication. Sofosbuvir has been approved for use in interferon-free regimens for treating chronic HCV infections. It is typically used in combination with NS5A inhibitors, discussed below, for genotypes 1 and 4. The non-NUC, dasabuvir (approved in 2014), causes allosteric inhibition of the HCV NS5B RNA polymerase, and is approved for HCV genotype 1 infections. It is administered in a fixed-dose combination of paritaprevir/ritonavir/ombitasvir (a NS5A inhibitor) with or without ribavirin. The final group of direct-acting antivirals for HCV infection are the NS5A inhibitors. These compounds target the non-structural 5A or NS5A protein, which is involved in modulation of host cell interferon response. It is essential for viral replication and assembly, and lacks enzymatic activity. NS5A inhibitors, including ledipasvir, daclatasvir, ombitasvir and elbasvir, target the NS5A protein and are effective for HCV genotype 1; they are licensed for use in combination with other DAAs in the treatment of HCV.

11.13.4 Influenza and Respiratory Syncytial Virus

There are four related influenza viruses, A, B, C and D. Influenza C is relatively rare and causes only mild infections, and influenza D is not known to cause infections in humans, affecting cattle only. Influenza A and B are responsible for seasonal flu epidemics, whilse influenza A viruses are the only ones that cause pandemic flu. Influenza viruses are further divided into subtypes based on two viral surface proteins, hemagglutinin and neuraminidase, of which there are 18 (H1-18) and 11 (N1-11) subtypes, respectively. All influenza viruses replicate in the same way, using the enzyme neuraminidase, a glycoside hydrolase which cleaves terminal sialic acid residues from glycan receptors near the budding site on the surface of infected cells, to liberate the virions from the dying cell. A number of neuraminidase inhibitors have been developed and approved. Of these, oseltamivir (formulated as an ethyl ester prodrug of the active carboxylate to permit oral administration) and zanamivir (administered by inhalation) are available worldwide, while the newer agents laninamivir and peramivir are available only in Japan, China, South Korea and the USA. All drugs are active against influenza A and B, and exhibit no activity against other viruses.

Both oseltamivir (Figure 11.15a) and zanamivir (Figure 11.15b) are most effective if given within 48 hours of the onset of symptoms; in these circumstances they may reduce the duration of symptoms by between 1 and 1.5 days. They may also reduce the risk of complications in elderly patients, those who are hospitalised, patients with chronic disease and children. These agents are also useful for post-exposure prophylaxis of influenza, but should be given as soon as possible after exposure to be effective, certainly within 36 hours (zanamivir) or 48 hours (oseltamivir). There is evidence of viral strains exhibiting reduced susceptibility to oseltamivir, while still retaining sensitivity to zanamivir. Resistance to oseltamivir may be observed in severely immunocompromised patients and, as a result, zanamivir is typically reserved for patients who are severely compromised or where oseltamivir is not suitable. Zanamivir is available as a dry powder for inhalation, or a solution which may be nebulised or administered by intravenous infusion. Neuraminidase inhibitors are not a substitute for vaccination, which remains the most effective approach for preventing illness associated with influenza infections.

Amantadine and rimantadine are drugs which inhibit the M2 protein, an ion channel found in the influenza A but not in the influenza B virus. Both drugs inhibit viral replication at low concentrations. Again, they are effective if given soon after the onset of infection, but widespread resistance has been reported in circulating strains. As a result, M2 inhibitors are no longer recommended for influenza A prevention or treatment.

Respiratory syncytial virus (RSV) is a common seasonal respiratory virus which belongs to the genus *Paramyxovirus*, which includes the viruses which cause measles and mumps. It primarily affects infants under the age of 2 years, where it can cause pneumonia or bronchiolitis

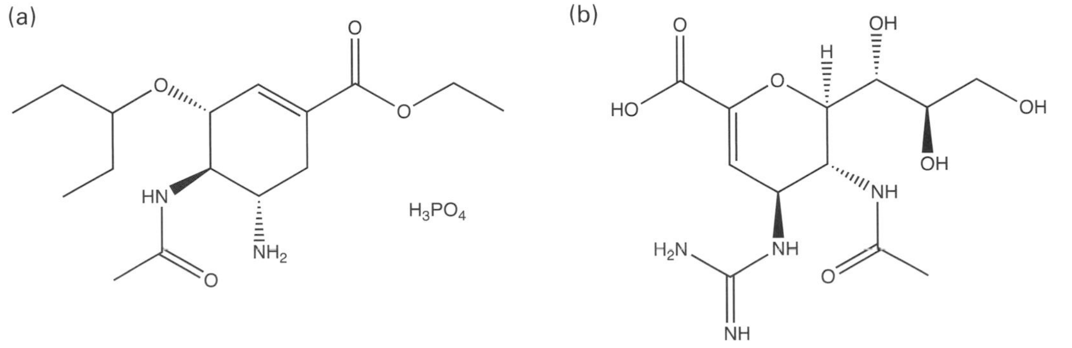

(a) (b)

H_3PO_4

Figure 11.15 Structures of (a) oseltamivir and (b) zanamivir.

which may lead to severe coughing, wheezing, increased respiratory effort and life-threatening respiratory distress. No lasting immunity develops following infection, meaning infants may be subject to repeated infections, and there is currently no available vaccine. Ribavirin (see Section 11.13.1) remains the only licensed antiviral agent for treatment of severe RSV, but its value is doubtful, with trials showing no consistent effect on pulmonary function, hospitalisation times or mortality. Palivizumab, a monoclonal antibody, is used for the prevention of serious lower respiratory tract disease caused by RSV in children at high risk of the disease.

Recently, outbreaks of new respiratory viruses such as the coronaviruses, Middle East respiratory syndrome-coronavirus (MERS-CoV) and severe acute respiratory syndrome-coronavirus-2 (SARS-CoV-2) (the causative agent of COVID-19) have accelerated the efforts to identify new therapeutic candidates, with several agents in early-stage clinical development (see also Chapter 5). Remdesivir (Gilead Sciences), an adenosine analogue prodrug (developed during the Ebola epidemic in 2013) is an RNA polymerase inhibitor licensed for intravenous administration to patients with COVID-19 with pneumonia requiring supplemental oxygen. The experimental drug, molnupiravir (MSD/Ridgeback Biotherapeutics), a ribonucleoside analogue (N4-hydroxycytidine) prodrug which increases the rate of mutations in viral RNA leading to inhibition of replication, received FDA authorisation in December 2021 as an oral antiviral for the emergency treatment of mild to moderate SARS-CoV-2 infection (with at least one risk factor for developing severe illness). The protease inhibitor PF-07321332 (nirmatrelvir, Pfizer) in combination with ritonavir, targeting the 3C-like protease of SARS-CoV-2, also received FDA authorisation for the emergency treatment of COVID-19 in December 2021. Others in clinical trial include another nucleoside analogue with a secondary action on the polymerase enzyme (AT-257, Roche/Atea).

Acknowledgements

The contribution of Dr Norman Hodges who authored this chapter in previous editions of this book is gratefully acknowledged.

References

BNF British National Formulary 83 (March 2022 – September 2022). London: BMJ Group and Pharmaceutical Press *(A new volume is published every 6 months and the reader is advised to consult the most recent edition.).*

Nath, A.P., Balasubramanian, A. and Ramalingam, K.D. (2020). Cephalosporins: an imperative antibiotic over the generations. *Int. J. Res. Pharm. Sci.* 11 (1): 623–629.

Further Reading

Bush, K. and Bradford, P.A. (2016). β-Lactams and β-lactam inhibitors: an overview. *Cold Spring Harb. Perspect. Med.* 6: a025247.

Butler, M.S., Hansford, K.A., Blaskovich, M.A.T. et al. (2014). Glycopeptide antibiotics: back to the future. *J. Antibiot. (Tokyo)* 67: 631–644.

Cohen, J., Powderly, W.G. and Opal, S.M. (ed.) (2017). *Infectious Diseases*, 4e. UK: Elsevier.

Davey, P., Wilcox, M.H., Irving, W. and Thwaites, G. (2015). *Antimicrobial Chemotherapy*, 7e. Oxford: Oxford University Press.

Harrison, C.J. and Bratcher, D. (2008). Cephalosporins: a review. *Pediatr. Rev.* 29 (8): 264–273.

Kruase, K.M., Serio, A.W., Kane, T.R. and Connolly, L.E. (2016). Aminoglycosides: an overview. *Cold Spring Harb. Perspect. Med.* 6: a027029.

Nguyen, F., Starosta, A.L., Arenz, S. et al. (2014). Tetracycline antibiotics and resistance mechanisms. *Biol. Chem.* 395 (5): 559–575.

Papp-Wallace, K.M., Endimiani, A., Taracila, M.A. and Bonomo, R.A. (2011). Carbapenems: past, present and future. *Antimicrob. Agents Chemother.* 55 (11): 4943–4960.

Pham, T.D.M., Ziora, Z.M. and Blaskovich, M.A.T. (2019). Quinolone antibiotics. *Med. Chem. Commun.* 19: 1719–1739.

Redgrave, L.S., Sutton, S.B., Webber, M.A. and Piddock, L.V.J. (2014). Fluoroquinolone resistance: mechanisms, impact on bacteria, and role in evolutionary success. *Trends Microbiol.* 22 (8): 438–445.

Spížek, J. and Rezanka, T. (2017). Lincosamides: chemical structure, biosynthesis, mechanisms of action, resistance, and applications. *Biochem. Pharmacol.* 133: 20–28.

Tooke, C.L., Hinchcliffe, P., Braggington, E.C. et al. (2019). β-Lactamases and β-lactamase inhibitors in the 21st Century. *J. Mol. Biol.* 431: 3472–3500.

Zeng, D., Debabov, D., Hartswell, T.L. et al. (2016). Approved glycopeptide antibacterial drugs: mechanism of action and resistance. *Cold Spring Harb. Perspect. Med.* 6: a026989.

12

Mechanisms of Action of Antibiotics and Synthetic Anti-infective Agents

Peter Lambert

Emeritus Professor of Microbial Chemistry, Aston University, Birmingham, UK

CONTENTS

Hugo and Russell's Pharmaceutical Microbiology, Ninth Edition. Edited by Brendan F. Gilmore and Stephen P. Denyer.

Companion website: https://www.wiley.com/go/HugoandRussells9e

12.1 Introduction

The antibiotics and synthetic anti-infective agents described in Chapter 11 are used to treat infections caused by bacteria, fungi and protozoa. Most exert a highly selective toxic action on their target microbial cells but have little or no toxicity towards mammalian cells. They can therefore be administered at concentrations sufficient to kill or inhibit the growth of infecting organisms without damaging mammalian cells. By comparison, the disinfectants, antiseptics and preservatives described in Chapter 19 are too toxic for systemic treatment of infections. Figure 12.1 illustrates the five broad target areas of the major groups of antibiotics and synthetic agents used to treat microbial infections. Note that most of the agents are selective antibacterials; relatively few agents are available for treatment of fungal or protozoal infections. Study of the mechanism of action reveals the basis for the selective toxicity.

12.2 The Microbial Cell Wall

12.2.1 Peptidoglycan Biosynthesis in Bacteria and Its Inhibition

Peptidoglycan is a vital component of the cell wall of virtually all bacteria. About 50% of the weight of the wall of Gram-positive bacteria is peptidoglycan; smaller amounts occur in mycobacterial walls (30%) and Gram-negative bacterial cell walls (10–20%). It is a macromolecule composed of sugar (glycan) chains cross-linked by short peptide chains (Figure 12.2). The glycan chains contain alternating units of *N*-acetylmuramic acid and *N*-acetylglucosamine. Each *N*-acetylmuramic acid contains a short peptide substituent made up of four amino acids (the stem peptides). A key feature of peptidoglycan is the occurrence of the D-isomers of some amino acids in the stem peptides (particularly D-alanine and D-glutamic acid) and unusual amino acids such as meso-diaminopimelic acid which are

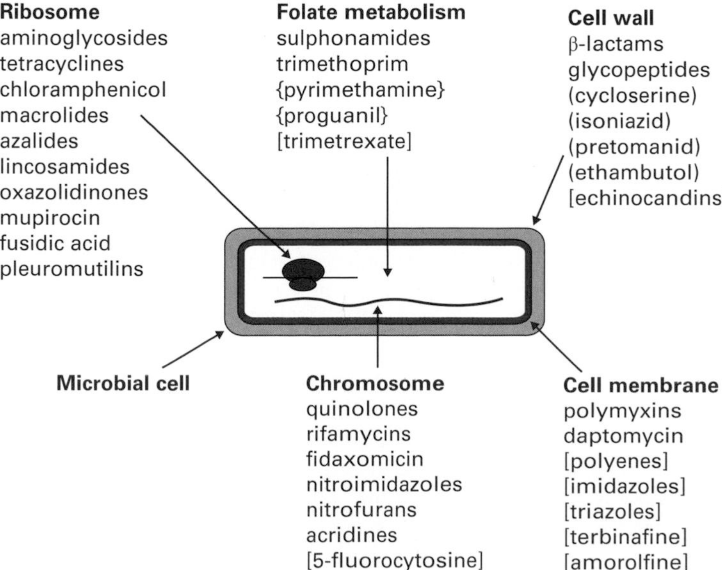

Figure 12.1 Schematic diagram of a typical microbial cell showing the sites of action of the major classes of antibiotics and antimicrobial agents used to treat infections. Agents listed without brackets are used to treat bacterial infections. Agents used against mycobacterial, fungal or protozoal infections are indicated by the use of (), [] and {} brackets, respectively.

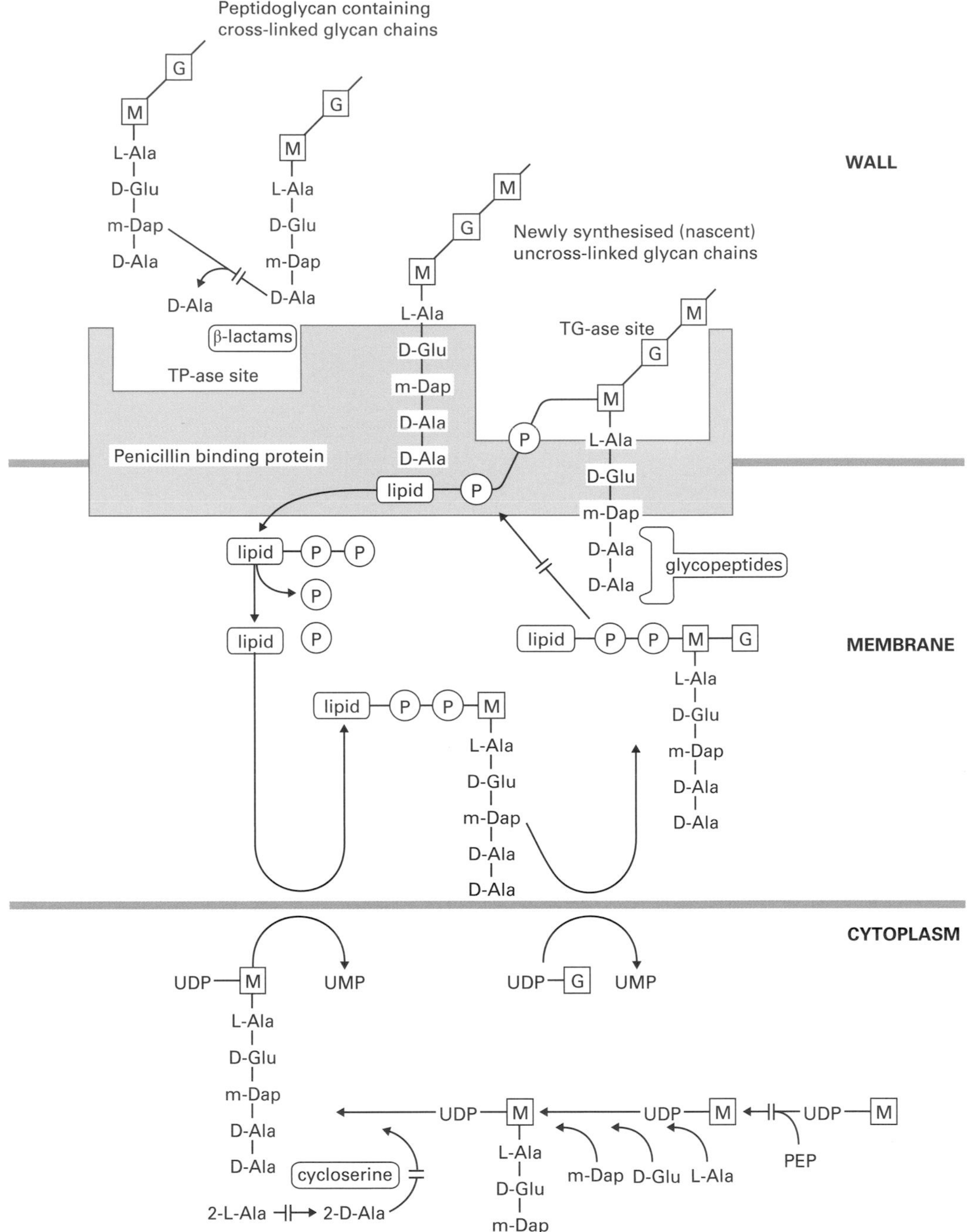

Figure 12.2 Pathway for the biosynthesis of peptidoglycan in bacterial cells showing the sites of action of cycloserine, glycopeptide and β-lactam antibiotics. M, *N*-acetylmuramic acid; G, *N*-acetylglucosamine; UDP, uridine diphosphate; UMP, uridine monophosphate; P, phosphate; PEP, phosphoenolpyruvate; lipid, undecaprenol; TP-ase, transpeptidase; TG-ase, transglycosylase; L-Ala, L-alanine; D-Ala, D-alanine; D-Glu, D-glutamic acid; m-DAP, meso-diaminopimelic acid.

not found in proteins. In some organisms (e.g., *Escherichia coli*), cross-linking of the stem peptides involves a direct peptide bond between the fourth amino acid of the stem peptide on one chain and the third amino acid in the stem peptide on an adjacent chain. In other organisms (e.g., *Staphylococcus aureus*), the linkage is made by a short peptide bridge (e.g., five glycines) between the stem peptides. The precise composition of peptidoglycan varies between different organisms but the overall structure is the same.

In all cases, the peptidoglycan plays a vital role: it is responsible for maintaining the shape and mechanical strength of the bacterial cell. If it is damaged in any way, and particularly if its synthesis is inhibited, then the shape of the cells becomes distorted, they swell and will eventually burst (lyse) as a result of the high internal osmotic pressure. Mammalian cells do not possess a cell wall and contain no other macromolecules resembling peptidoglycan. Consequently, antibiotics which interfere with the synthesis and assembly of peptidoglycan show excellent selective toxicity.

12.2.1.1 D-Cycloserine

D-Cycloserine interferes with the early stage of synthesis of peptidoglycan involving the assembly of the dipeptide D-alanyl-D-alanine. This occurs inside the cytoplasm and involves a racemase enzyme which converts L-alanine to D-alanine and a ligase which couples two D-alanines together (Figure 12.2). Both of these enzymes are inhibited by D-cycloserine, which bears some structural similarities to D-alanine. The antibiotic binds to the pyridoxal phosphate cofactor of the enzymes, effectively preventing them from forming D-alanyl-D-alanine. Subsequent stages of peptidoglycan synthesis, involving coupling of the dipeptide to three other amino acids forming the stem peptide on the uridine diphosphate (UDP)-linked peptidoglycan precursor, UDP-*N*-acetylmuramic acid, are blocked. Note that initially the peptide contains five amino acids, terminating in D-alanyl-D-alanine. The terminal D-alanine is removed on insertion into the cell wall during the final step in which the cross-links are formed between stem peptides on adjacent glycan strands.

12.2.1.2 Glycopeptides – Vancomycin, Teicoplanin, Telavancin, Dalbavancin and Oritavancin

The peptidoglycan macromolecule is assembled in the cell wall by the sequential action of two enzymes (transglycosylases and transpeptidases) which are located on the outer face of the cytoplasmic membrane. To reach the assembly site (i.e., a region of cell wall growth), the precursors, which are assembled in the cytoplasm, must cross the cell membrane. They do this linked to a lipid, undecaprenyl phosphate, which acts as a carrier molecule, cycling between the inner and outer faces of the membrane. The biochemical details of this process are outlined in Figure 12.2. Antibiotics interfering with this stage of peptidoglycan synthesis have been identified, for example, bacitracin, but they have not found major applications in the treatment of infections.

The glycopeptides act at the stage where the peptidoglycan precursors are inserted into the cell wall by the transglycosylase enzyme on the outer face of the cell membrane. This enzyme assembles linear glycan chains that are not initially cross-linked to the existing peptidoglycan in the cell wall. The linear glycan chains are assembled by the transglycosylase by transfer of the growing glycan chain to the disaccharide peptidoglycan precursor on the lipid carrier as it crosses the cell membrane. Glycopeptides block this process by binding, not to the enzyme itself, but to the disaccharide peptidoglycan precursor, specifically to the D-alanyl-D-alanine portion on the stem peptide. The presence of the bulky glycopeptides tightly bound to each D-alanyl-D-alanine residue prevents the transglycosylase from carrying out the transfer reaction. Binding involves formation of a network of five hydrogen bonds between amino acid residues on the glycopeptide antibiotics and D-alanyl-D-alanine. Resistance to this unusual mechanism of enzyme inhibition can result from alteration in the D-alanyl-D-alanine substrate to D-alanyl-D-lactate (Chapter 13), which occurs in glycopeptide-resistant enterococci (e.g., vancomycin-resistant enterococci [VRE]). Vancomycin does not penetrate the cell membrane of bacteria and is thought to bind to the disaccharide-pentapeptides on the outer face of the cytoplasmic membrane. It has been suggested that two vancomycin molecules form a back-to-back dimer which bridges between pentapeptides on separate glycan chains, thus preventing further peptidoglycan assembly. Teicoplanin also binds tightly to the D-alanyl-D-alanine region of the peptidoglycan precursor. However, as a lipoglycopeptide, it may act slightly differently from vancomycin, by locating itself in the outer face of the cytoplasmic membrane and binding the pentapeptide as the precursors are transferred through the membrane. In addition to inhibition of transglycosylase, the modified hydrophobic glycopeptides, telavancin, dalbavancin and oritavancin, also disrupt membrane potential by binding to the lipid carrier.

12.2.1.3 β-Lactams – Penicillins, Cephalosporins, Carbapenems and Monobactams

The final stage of peptidoglycan assembly is the cross-linking of the linear glycan strands assembled by transglycosylation to the existing peptidoglycan in the cell wall. This reaction is catalysed by transpeptidase enzymes, which are also located on the outer face of the cell membrane. They first remove the terminal D-alanine residue from each stem peptide on the newly synthesised glycan chain. The energy released from breaking the peptide bond between the two alanines is used in the formation of a new peptide bond between the remaining D-alanine on the stem peptide and a free amino group present on the third amino acid of the stem peptides in the existing cross-linked peptidoglycan. In many organisms, including *E. coli*, this acceptor amino group is supplied by the amino acid meso-diaminopimelic acid. In other organisms, for example, *S. aureus*, the acceptor amino group is supplied by the amino acid L-lysine. Although there is considerable variation in the composition of the peptide cross-link among different species of bacteria, the essential transpeptidation mechanism is the same. Therefore, virtually all bacteria can be inhibited by interference with this group of enzymes.

The β-lactam antibiotics inhibit transpeptidases by acting as alternative substrates. They mimic the D-alanyl-D-alanine residues and react covalently with the transpeptidases (Figure 12.3). The β-lactam bond (common to all members of the β-lactam antibiotics) is broken but the remaining portion of the antibiotic is not released immediately. The half-life for the transpeptidase–antibiotic complex is of the order of 10 minutes; during this time the enzyme cannot participate in further rounds of peptidoglycan assembly by reaction with its true substrate. The vital cross-linking of the peptidoglycan is therefore blocked while other aspects of cell growth continue. The cells become deformed in shape and eventually burst through the combined action of a weakened cell wall, high internal osmotic pressure and the uncontrolled activity of autolytic enzymes in the cell wall. Penicillins, cephalosporins, carbapenems and monobactams all inhibit peptidoglycan cross-linking through interaction of the common β-lactam ring with the transpeptidase enzymes. However, there is considerable variation in the morphological effects of different β-lactams owing to the existence of several types of transpeptidase. The transpeptidase enzymes are usually referred to as penicillin-binding proteins (PBPs) because they can be separated and studied after reaction with ^{14}C-labelled penicillin. This step is necessary because there

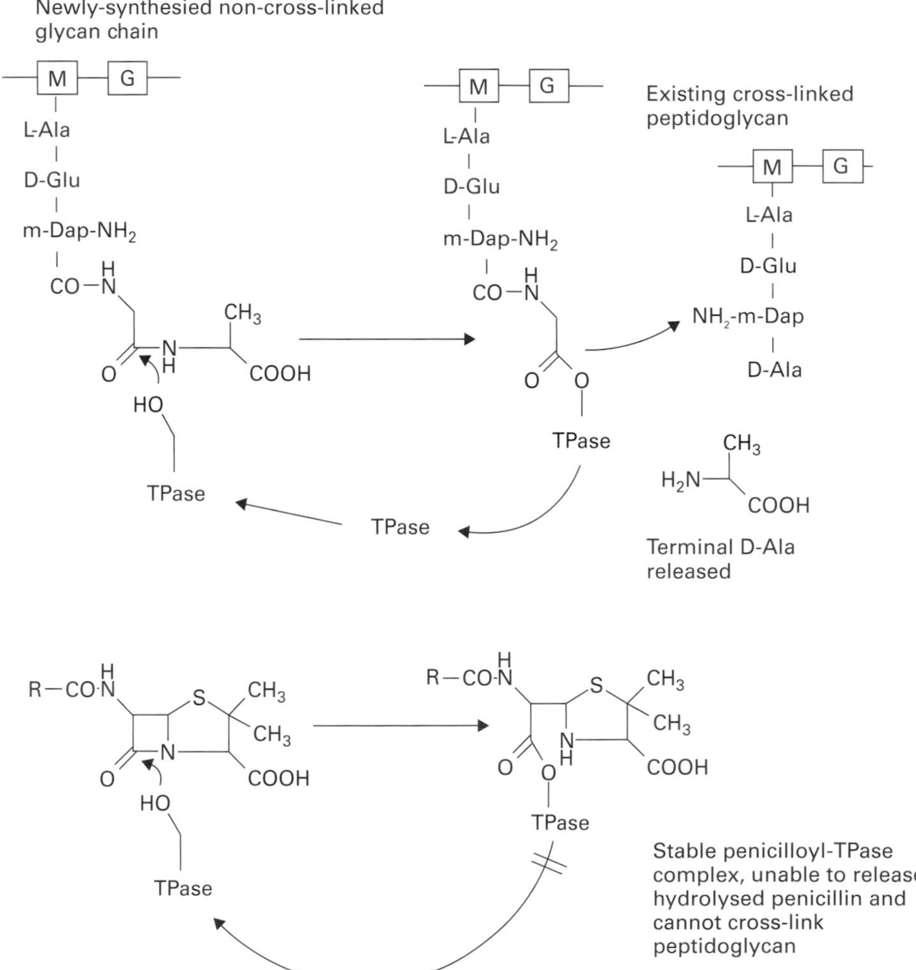

Figure 12.3 The action of transpeptidase (TPase) with its natural substrate (upper) and penicillin G (lower). The —OH group on a serine residue at the active site of the TPase attacks the peptide bond between the terminal D-alanyl-D-alanine residues of the stem peptide in the non-cross-linked glycan chain. The terminal D-alanine is released and a new peptide cross-link is formed with existing peptidoglycan in the cell wall. Penicillin G blocks this process by forming a stable penicilloyl–TPase complex which cannot release the penicillin and therefore cannot form the peptide cross-link in the peptidoglycan. M, *N*-acetylmuramic acid; G, *N*-acetylglucosamine; L-Ala, L-alanine; D-Ala, D-alanine; D-Glu, D-glutamic acid; m-DAP, meso-diaminopimelic acid.

are very few copies of each enzyme present in a cell. They are usually separated according to their size by electrophoresis and are numbered PBP1, PBP2, etc., starting from the highest-molecular-weight species. In Gram-negative bacteria, most of the high-molecular-weight transpeptidases also possess transglycosylase activity, that is, they have a dual function in the final stages of peptidoglycan synthesis with the transglycosylase and transpeptidase activities located in separate regions of the protein structures. Furthermore, the different transpeptidases have specialised functions in the cell; all cross-link peptidoglycan but some are involved with maintenance of cell integrity, some regulate cell shape and others produce new cross wall between elongating cells, securing chromosome segregation prior to cell division. The varying sensitivity of the PBPs towards different β-lactams helps to explain the range of morphological effects observed in treated bacteria. For example, penicillin G (benzylpenicillin), ampicillin and cephaloridine are particularly effective in causing rapid lysis of Gram-negative bacteria such as *E. coli*. These antibiotics act primarily upon PBP1B, the major transpeptidase of the organism. Other β-lactams have little activity against this PBP, for example, mecillinam binds preferentially to PBP2 and it produces a pronounced change in the cells from a rod shape to an oval form. Many of the cephalosporins, for example, cephalexin, cefotaxime and ceftazidime, bind to PBP3 resulting in the formation of elongated, filamentous cells. The lower-molecular-weight PBPs, 4, 5 and 6, do not possess transpeptidase activity. These are carboxypeptidases, which remove the terminal D-alanine from the pentapeptides on the linear glycans in the cell wall but do not catalyse the cross-linkage. Their role in the cells is to regulate the degree of cross-linking by denying the D-alanyl-D-alanine substrate to the transpeptidases but they are not essential for cell growth. Up to 90% of the amount of antibiotic reacting with the cells may be consumed in inhibiting the carboxypeptidases, with no lethal consequences to the cells.

Gram-positive bacteria also have multiple transpeptidases, but fewer than Gram-negatives. Shape changes are less evident than with Gram-negative rod-shaped organisms. Cell death follows lysis of the cells mediated by the action of endogenous autolytic enzymes (autolysins) present in the cell wall which are activated following β-lactam action. Autolytic enzymes able to hydrolyse peptidoglycan are present in most bacterial walls; they are needed to re-shape the wall during growth and to aid cell separation during division. Their activity is regulated by binding to wall components such as the wall and membrane teichoic acids. When peptidoglycan assembly is disrupted through β-lactam action, some of the teichoic acids are released from the cells, which are then susceptible to attack by their own autolysins.

12.2.1.4 β-Lactamase Inhibitors – Clavulanic Acid, Sulbactam, Tazobactam, Avibactam, Relebactam and Vaborbactam

Expression of β-lactamase enzymes is the most important mechanism through which organisms become resistant to β-lactams. Several thousand different β-lactamase enzymes have been described and can be classified according to their amino acid sequences, resulting in classes A, B, C and D enzymes. An alternative nomenclature combines the molecular and biochemical properties into 17 functional groups that describe most β-lactamases. The majority of the enzymes have a serine residue at their active site; other categories of β-lactamase enzymes have zinc atoms at their active sites. A number of successful inhibitors of serine-based enzymes have been developed, including clavulanic acid, sulbactam and tazobactam for use in combination with susceptible β-lactams (amoxicillin, ampicillin and piperacillin, respectively), protecting them from inactivation by the β-lactamases. These inhibitors are hydrolysed by the β-lactamases in the same manner as susceptible β-lactam antibiotics, the β-lactam ring being broken by attack by a serine residue in the active site of the enzyme. Instead of undergoing rapid release from the active site serine, the inhibitors remain bound and undergo one of several different fates. The hydrolysed inhibitors can interact with a second enzyme residue in the active site of the β-lactamase, forming a covalently cross-linked, irreversibly inhibited complex. Newer, non-beta-lactam inhibitors, avibactam, relebactam and vaborbactam (see Chapters 11 and 13), are used in combination with ceftazidime, imipenem/cilastatin and meropenem, respectively. These inhibitors form reversible covalent bonds with the active site serine residues of β-lactamases, including extended-spectrum beta-lactamases (ESBLs) and some carbapenemases. Metallo-β-lactamases pose an increasing clinical problem because they hydrolyse and inactivate nearly all β-lactam-containing antibiotics, including carbapenems. Their control will require the development of specific metallo-enzyme inhibitors.

12.2.2 Mycolic acid and Arabinogalactan Biosynthesis in Mycobacteria

The cell walls of mycobacteria contain an arabinogalactan polysaccharide in addition to the peptidoglycan, plus a variety of high-molecular-weight lipids, including the mycolic acids, glycolipids, phospholipids and waxes. The lipid-rich nature of the mycobacterial wall is responsible for the characteristic acid-fastness on staining and serves as a penetration barrier to many antibiotics. Isoniazid and ethambutol have long been known as specific antimycobacterial agents, exerting no activity towards other bacteria, but their mechanisms of action have only recently been established.

12.2.2.1 Isoniazid

Isoniazid interferes with mycolic acid synthesis by inhibiting an enoyl reductase (InhA) which forms part of the fatty acid synthase system in mycobacteria. Mycolic acids are produced by a diversion of the normal fatty acid synthetic pathway in which short-chain (16-carbon) and long-chain (24-carbon) fatty acids are produced by addition of 7 or 11 malonate extension units from malonyl coenzyme A to acetyl coenzyme A. InhA inserts a double bond into the extending fatty acid chain at the 24-carbon stage. The long-chain fatty acids are further extended and condensed to produce the 60–90-carbon β-hydroxymycolic acids which are important components of the mycobacterial cell wall. Isoniazid is converted inside the mycobacteria to a free radical species by a catalase peroxidase enzyme, KatG. The active free radicals then attack and inhibit the enoyl reductase, InhA, by covalent attachment to the active site.

12.2.2.2 Pretomanid

Pretomanid is active against metabolically active (replicating) and non-replicating (latent) *Mycobacterium tuberculosis*. It is activated by a nitroreductase, generating a number of metabolites and reactive nitrogen species, including nitric oxide (NO). The des-nitroimidazole metabolites kill actively growing *M. tuberculosis* through inhibition of mycolic acid synthesis. Inhibition of non-replicating (latent) *M. tuberculosis* results from respiratory poisoning by the reactive nitrogen species.

12.2.2.3 Ethambutol

Ethambutol blocks assembly of the arabinogalactan polysaccharide by inhibition of an arabinosyl transferase enzyme. Cells treated with ethambutol accumulate the isoprenoid intermediate decaprenylarabinose, which supplies arabinose units for assembly in the arabinogalactan polymer.

12.2.3 Echinocandins – Caspofungin, Anidulafungin and Micafungin

These members of the echinocandin group of antifungal agents have been developed for treatment of serious fungal infections (see Chapter 4). They interfere with the synthesis of the β-1,3-D-glucan polymer in the fungal cell wall. Without the glucan polymer, the integrity of the fungal cell wall is compromised, yeast cells lose their rigidity and become like protoplasts; the effect is especially pronounced in *Candida* and *Aspergillus* species.

12.3 Protein Synthesis

12.3.1 Protein Synthesis and Its Selective Inhibition

Figure 12.4 outlines the process of protein synthesis involving the ribosome, messenger RNA (mRNA), a series of aminoacyl-transfer RNA (tRNA) molecules (at least one for each amino acid) and accessory protein factors involved in initiation, elongation and termination. As the process is essentially the same in prokaryotic (bacterial) and eukaryotic cells (i.e., higher organisms and mammalian cells), it is surprising that there are so many selective agents which act in this area (see Figure 12.1).

Bacterial ribosomes are smaller than their mammalian counterparts. They consist of one 30S and one 50S subunit (the S suffix denotes the size, which is derived from the rate of sedimentation in an ultracentrifuge). The 30S subunit comprises a single strand of 16S ribosomal RNA (rRNA) and over 20 different proteins that are bound to it. The larger 50S subunit contains two single strands of rRNA (23S and 5S) together with over 30 different proteins. The subunits pack together to form an intact 70S ribosome. The equivalent subunits for mammalian ribosomes are 40S and 60S, making an 80S ribosome. Some agents exploit subtle differences in structure between the bacterial and mammalian ribosomes. The macrolides, azalides and chloramphenicol act on the 50S subunits in bacteria but not the 60S subunits of mammalian cells. By contrast, the tetracyclines derive their selective action through active uptake and concentration within microbial cells but only limited penetration of mammalian cells.

12.3.2 Aminoglycoside–Aminocyclitol Antibiotics

Most of the information on the mechanisms of action of aminoglycoside–aminocyclitol (AGAC) antibiotics comes from studies with streptomycin. One effect of AGACs is to interfere with the initiation and assembly of the bacterial ribosome (Figure 12.4). During assembly of the initiation complex, *N*-formylmethionyl-tRNA (fmet-tRNA) binds initially to the ribosome-binding site on the untranslated 5′ end of the mRNA together with the 30S ribosomal subunit. Three protein initiation factors (designated IF-1, -2 and -3) and a molecule of guanosine triphosphate (GTP) are involved in positioning the fmet-tRNA on the AUG start codon of mRNA. IF-1 and IF-3 are then released from the complex, GTP is hydrolysed to guanosine diphosphate (GDP) and released with IF-2 as the 50S subunit joins the 30S subunit and mRNA to form a functional ribosome. The fmet-tRNA occupies the peptidyl site (P-site) leaving a vacant acceptor site (A-site) to receive

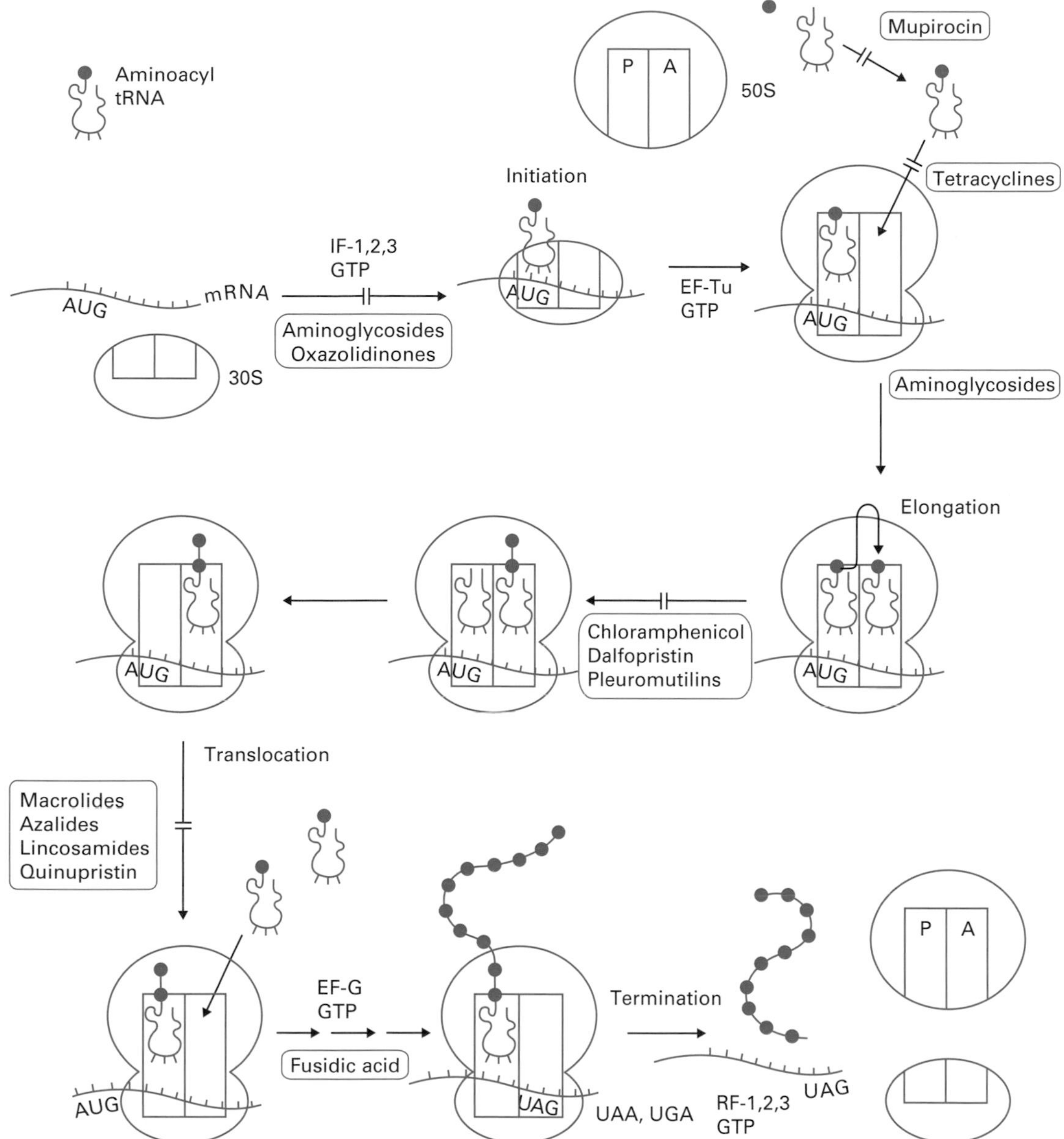

Figure 12.4 Outline of the process of protein synthesis (translation of messenger RNA) in bacterial cells. The four stages of synthesis are shown: initiation, elongation, translocation and termination with the sites of action of antibiotics. AUG is the start codon on messenger RNA (mRNA) specifying the first amino acid in bacterial proteins, *N*-formylmethionine. UAG, UAA and UGA are termination codons specifying no amino acid. 30S and 50S are the subunits of the ribosome. Other protein factors involved in protein synthesis are initiation factors (IF-1, -2 and -3), elongation factors (EF-Tu and EF-G) and release factors (RF-1, -2 and -3). t-RNA, transfer RNA; GTP, guanosine triphosphate; P, peptidyl site; A, acceptor site.

the next aminoacyl-tRNA specified by the next codon on the mRNA. Streptomycin binds tightly to one of the protein components of the 30S subunit. Binding of the antibiotic to the protein, which is the receptor for IF-3, prevents initiation and assembly of the ribosome.

Streptomycin binding to the 30S subunit also distorts the shape of the A site on the ribosome and interferes with the positioning of the aminoacyl-tRNA molecules during peptide chain elongation. Streptomycin therefore exerts two effects: inhibition of protein synthesis by freezing the initiation complex, and misreading of the codons through distortion of the 30S subunit. Simple blockage of protein synthesis would be bacteriostatic rather than bactericidal. As streptomycin and the other AGACs exert a potent lethal action, it seems that the formation of toxic, non-functional proteins through misreading of the codons on mRNA is a more likely mechanism of action. This can be demonstrated with cell-free translation systems in which isolated bacterial ribosomes are supplied with artificial mRNA template such as poly(U) or poly(C) and all the other factors, including aminoacyl-tRNAs needed for protein synthesis.

In the absence of an AGAC, the ribosomes will produce artificial polypeptides, polyphenylalanine (as specified by the codon UUU) or polyproline (as specified by the codon CCC). However, when streptomycin is added, the ribosomes produce a mixture of polythreonine (codon ACU) and polyserine (codon UCU). The misreading of the codons does not appear to be random: U is read as A or C, and C is read as A or U. If such misreading occurs in whole cells, the accumulation of non-functional or toxic proteins would eventually prove fatal to the cells. There is some evidence that the bacterial cell membrane is damaged when the cells attempt to excrete the faulty proteins.

The effectiveness of the AGACs is enhanced by their active uptake by bacteria, which proceeds in three phases. First, a rapid uptake occurs within a few seconds of contact, which represents binding of the positively charged AGAC molecules to the negatively charged surface of the bacteria. This phase is referred to as the energy-independent phase (EIP) of uptake. In the case of Gram-negative bacteria, the AGACs damage the outer membrane causing release of some lipopolysaccharide (LPS), phospholipid and proteins, but this is not directly lethal to the cells. Second, there follows an energy-dependent phase of uptake (EDP I) lasting about 10 minutes, in which the AGAC is actively transported across the cytoplasmic membrane. A second energy-dependent phase (EDP II) which leads to further intracellular accumulation follows after some AGAC has bound to the ribosomes in the cytoplasm. Although the precise details of uptake by EDP I and EDP II are not clear, both require organisms to be growing aerobically. Anaerobes do not take up AGACs by EDP I or EDP II and are consequently resistant to their action.

12.3.3 Tetracyclines

This group of antibiotics is actively transported into bacterial cells, possibly as the magnesium complex, achieving a 50-fold concentration inside the cells. Mammalian cells do not actively take up the tetracyclines (small amounts enter by diffusion alone) and it is this difference in uptake that determines the selective toxicity. Resistance to the tetracyclines occurs through failure of the active uptake system or the action of active efflux pumps, which remove the drug from the cells before it can interfere with ribosome function. Other resistance mechanisms involve ribosomal protection and modification. Protein synthesis by both bacterial and mammalian ribosomes is inhibited by the tetracyclines in cell-free systems. The action is on the smaller subunit. Binding of just one molecule of tetracycline to the bacterial 30S subunit occurs at a site involving the 3′ end of the 16S rRNA, a number of associated ribosomal proteins and magnesium ions. The effect is to block the binding of aminoacyl-tRNA to the A site of the ribosome and halt protein synthesis. Tetracyclines are bacteriostatic rather than bactericidal, consequently they should not be used in combination with β-lactams, which require cells to be growing and dividing to exert their lethal action.

12.3.4 Chloramphenicol

Of the four possible optical isomers of chloramphenicol, only the D-*threo* form is active. This antibiotic selectively inhibits protein synthesis in bacterial ribosomes by binding to the 50S subunit in the region of the A site involving the 23S rRNA. The normal binding of the aminoacyl-tRNA in the A site is affected by chloramphenicol in such a way that the peptidyl transferase cannot form a new peptide bond with the growing peptide chain on the tRNA in the P site. Studies with aminoacyl-tRNA fragments containing truncated tRNA chains suggest that the shape of the region of tRNA closest to the amino acid is distorted by chloramphenicol. The altered orientation of this region of the aminoacyl-tRNA in the A site is sufficient to prevent peptide bond formation. Chloramphenicol has a broad spectrum of activity, which covers Gram-positive and Gram-negative bacteria, mycoplasmas, rickettsia and chlamydia. It has the valuable property of penetrating into mammalian cells and is therefore the drug of choice for treatment of intracellular pathogens, including *Salmonella enterica* serovar Typhi, the causative organism of typhoid. Although it does not inhibit 80S ribosomes, the 70S ribosomes of mammalian mitochondria are sensitive and therefore some inhibition occurs in rapidly growing mammalian cells with high mitochondrial activity.

12.3.5 Macrolides and Azalides

Erythromycin is a member of the macrolide group of antibiotics; it selectively inhibits protein synthesis in a broad range of bacteria by binding to the 50S subunit. The site at which it binds is close to that of chloramphenicol and involves the 23S rRNA. Resistance to chloramphenicol and erythromycin can occur by methylation of different bases within the same region of the 23S rRNA. The sites are therefore not identical, but binding of one antibiotic prevents binding of the other. Unlike chloramphenicol, erythromycin blocks translocation. This is the process by which the ribosome moves along the mRNA by one codon after the peptidyl transferase reaction has joined the peptide chain to the aminoacyl-tRNA in the A site. The peptidyl-tRNA is moved (translocated) to the P site, vacating the A site for the next aminoacyl-tRNA. Energy is derived by hydrolysis of GTP to GDP by an associated protein elongation factor, EF-G. By blocking the translocation process, erythromycin causes release of incomplete polypeptides from the ribosome. It is assumed that the azalides, such as azithromycin, have a similar action to the macrolides. The azalides have improved intracellular penetration over the macrolides and are resistant to the metabolic conversion which reduces the serum half-life of erythromycin.

12.3.6 Clindamycin

This agent binds selectively to a region of the 50S ribosomal subunit close to that of chloramphenicol and erythromycin. It blocks elongation of the peptide chain by inhibition of peptidyl transferase.

12.3.7 Streptogramins – Quinupristin and Dalfopristin

The two unrelated streptogramins, quinupristin and dalfopristin, have been used in combination (in a 30:70 ratio) to treat infections caused by staphylococci and enterococci, particularly methicillin-resistant *S. aureus* (MRSA) and VRE. Their action is synergistic, and is generally bactericidal compared with either agent used alone or compared with antibiotics in the macrolide group. The main target is the bacterial 50S ribosome, with the formulation acting to inhibit protein synthesis. The agents bind sequentially to the 50S subunit; dalfopristin alters the shape of the subunit so that more quinupristin can bind. Dalfopristin blocks an early step in protein synthesis by forming a bond with the ribosome, preventing elongation of the peptide chain by the peptidyl transferase. Quinupristin blocks a later step by preventing the extension of peptide chains and causing incomplete chains to be released. The overall effect is to block elongation. Use of streptogramins is limited by vasculitis, causing pain on intravenous administration.

12.3.8 Oxazolidinones – Linezolid and Tedizolid Phosphate

Oxazolidinones act at the early stage of protein synthesis. By binding to the 50S ribosome subunit near the interface with the 30S subunit, they prevent the formation of the initiation complex between the 30S subunit, mRNA and fmet-tRNA required for bacterial translation. Tedizolid phosphate is an oxazolidinone prodrug; it is converted to the active form, tedizolid, by phosphatases *in vivo*.

12.3.9 Mupirocin

The target of mupirocin is one of a group of enzymes which couple amino acids to their respective tRNAs for delivery to the ribosome and incorporation into protein. The particular enzyme inhibited by mupirocin is involved in producing isoleucyl-tRNA. The basis for the inhibition is a structural similarity between one end of the mupirocin molecule and isoleucine. Protein synthesis is halted when the ribosome encounters the isoleucine codon through depletion of the pool of isoleucyl-tRNA.

12.3.10 Fusidic Acid

This steroidal antibiotic does not act on the ribosome itself, but on one of the associated elongation factors, EF-G. This factor supplies energy for translocation by hydrolysis of GTP and GDP. Another elongation factor, EF-Tu, promotes binding of aminoacyl-tRNA molecules to the A site through binding and hydrolysis of GTP. Both EF-G and EF-Tu have overlapping binding sites on the ribosome. Fusidic acid binds the EF-G–GDP complex to the ribosome after one round of translocation has taken place. This prevents further incorporation of aminoacyl-tRNA by blocking the binding of EF-Tu–GTP. Fusidic acid owes its selective antimicrobial action to active uptake by bacteria and exclusion from mammalian cells. The equivalent elongation factor in mammalian cells, EF-2, is susceptible to fusidic acid in cell-free systems.

12.3.11 Pleuromutilins – Retapamulin and Lefamulin

Pleuromutilins bind to the peptidyl transferase centre of the 50S ribosomal subunit, preventing the correct positioning of tRNAs for peptide transfer in the A- and P-sites, thereby inhibiting peptide bond formation. This mechanism is different to that of other peptidyl transferase inhibitors (chloramphenicol and clindamycin), so cross-resistance to these agents does not occur.

12.4 Chromosome Function and Replication

12.4.1 Basis for the Selective Inhibition of Chromosome Replication and Function

As with protein synthesis, the mechanisms of chromosome replication and function are essentially the same in prokaryotes and eukaryotes. There are, however, important differences in the detailed functioning and properties of the enzymes involved and these differences are exploited by a number of agents as the basis of selective inhibition. The microbial chromosome is large in comparison with the cell that contains it (approximately 500 times the length of *E. coli*). It is therefore wound into a compact, supercoiled form inside the cell. During replication the circular double helix must be unwound to allow the DNA polymerase enzymes to synthesise new complementary strands. The shape of the chromosome is manipulated by the cell by the formation of regions of supercoiling. Positive supercoiling (coiling in the same sense as the turns of the double helix) makes the chromosome more compact. Negative supercoiling (generated by twisting the chromosome in the opposite sense to the helix) produces localised strand separation which is required both for replication and transcription. In a bacterium such as *E. coli,* four different topoisomerase enzymes are responsible for maintaining the shape of DNA during cell division. They act by cutting one or both of the DNA strands; they remove and generate supercoiling, then reseal the strands. Their activity is essential for the microbial cell to relieve the complex tangling of the chromosome (both knotting and chain-link formation) which results from progression of the replication fork around the circular chromosome. Type I topoisomerases cut one strand of DNA and pass the other strand through the gap before resealing. Type II enzymes cut both strands and pass another double helical section of the DNA through the gap before resealing. In *E. coli,* topoisomerases I and III are both type I enzymes, while topoisomerases II and IV are type II enzymes. Topoisomerase II (also known as DNA gyrase) and topoisomerase IV are essential enzymes which are selectively inhibited by the fluoroquinolone group of antimicrobials. Topoisomerase II is responsible for introducing negative supercoils into DNA and for relieving torsional stress, which accumulates ahead of sites of transcription and replication. Topoisomerase IV provides a potent decatenating (unlinking) activity that removes links and knots generated behind the replication fork.

The basic sequence of events for microbial chromosome replication is described below.

12.4.1.1 Synthesis of Precursors

Purines, pyrimidines and their nucleosides and nucleoside triphosphates are synthesised in the cytoplasm. At this stage, the antifolate drugs (sulphonamides and dihydrofolate reductase inhibitors) act by interfering with the synthesis and recycling of the cofactor dihydrofolic acid (DHF). Thymidylic acid (2-deoxythymidine monophosphate [dTMP]) is an essential nucleotide precursor of DNA synthesis. It is produced by the enzyme thymidylate synthetase by transfer of a methyl group from tetrahydrofolic acid (THF) to the uracil base on uridylic acid (2-deoxyuridine monophosphate dUMP) (Figure 12.5). THF is converted to DHF in this process and must be reverted to THF by the enzyme dihydrofolate reductase (DHFR) before the cycle can be repeated. By inhibiting DHFR, the antifolates effectively block the production of dTMP and hence DNA synthesis.

The antifungal agent 5-fluorocytosine also interferes with these early stages of DNA synthesis. Through conversion to the nucleoside triphosphate, it subsequently blocks thymidylic acid production through inhibition of the enzyme thymidylate synthetase (Figure 12.6).

12.4.1.2 Unwinding of the Chromosome

As described in Section 12.4.1, the DNA double helix must unwind to allow access of the polymerase enzymes to produce two new strands of DNA. This is facilitated by topoisomerase II (DNA gyrase) which is a target of the fluoroquinolones. Some agents interfere with the unwinding of the chromosome by physical obstruction. These include the acridine dyes, of which the topical antiseptic proflavine is the most familiar, and the antimalarial acridine mepacrine. They prevent strand separation by insertion (intercalation) between base pairs from each strand, but exhibit very poor selective toxicity.

12.4.1.3 Replication of DNA Strands

The unwound DNA strands are kept unfolded during replication by binding a protein called Albert's protein. A series of enzymes produce new strands of DNA using each of the separated strands as templates. One strand is produced

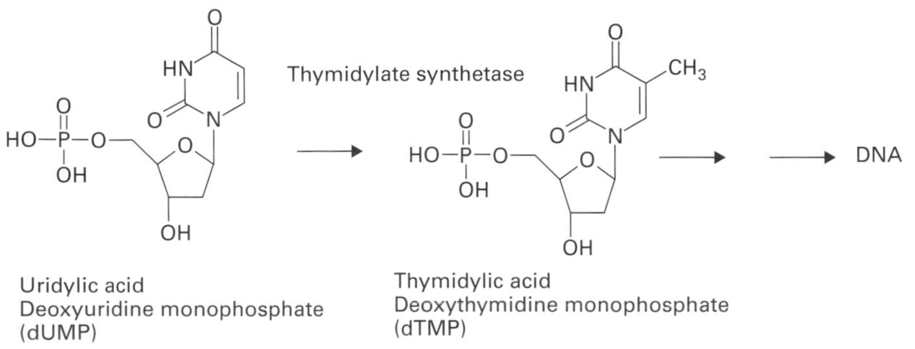

Figure 12.5 Conversion of uridylic acid to thymidylic acid by the enzyme thymidylate synthetase, a vital early stage in the synthesis of DNA.

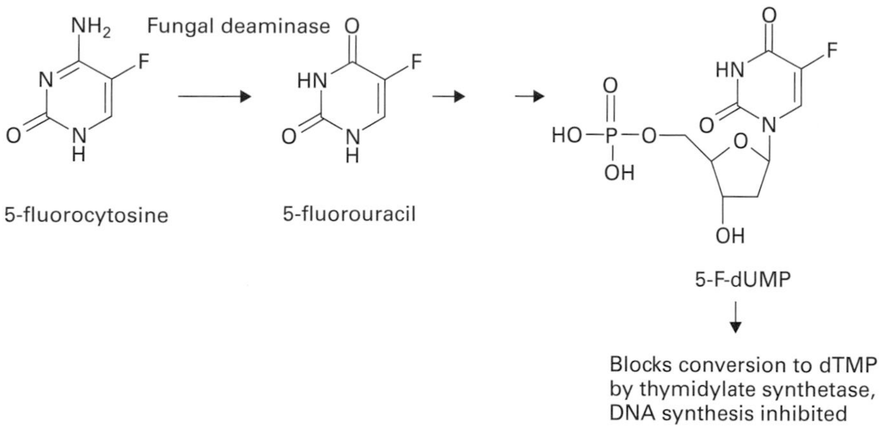

Figure 12.6 Conversion of the antifungal agent 5-fluorocytosine to 5-fluorouracil by a deaminase enzyme inside fungal cells and subsequent inhibition of fungal DNA synthesis through inhibition of thymidylate synthetase. d-UMP, deoxyuridine monophosphate; d-TMP, deoxythymidine monophosphate.

continuously. The other is produced in a series of short strands called Okazaki fragments that are joined by a DNA ligase. The entire process is carefully regulated, with proof-reading stages to check that each nucleotide is correctly incorporated as specified by the template sequence. There are no therapeutic agents yet known which interfere directly with the DNA polymerases.

12.4.1.4 Transcription

The process of transcription, the copying of a single strand of mRNA sequence using one strand of the chromosome as a template, is carried out by RNA polymerase. This is a complex of four proteins (2 α, 1 β and 1 β' subunits) which make up the core enzyme. Another small protein, the σ factor, joins the core enzyme, which binds to the promoter region of the DNA preceding the gene that is to be transcribed. The correct positioning and orientation of the polymerase are obtained by recognition of specific marker sites on the DNA at positions −10 and −35 nucleotide bases before the initiation site for transcription. The σ factor is responsible for recognition of the initiation signal for transcription and the core enzyme possesses the activity to join the nucleotides in the sequence specified by the gene. Mammalian genes possess an analogous RNA polymerase but there are sufficient differences in structure to permit selective inhibition of the microbial enzyme by the semi-synthetic rifamycin antibiotics (rifampicin, rifabutin, rifaximin, rifapentine) and fidaxomicin, a macrocyclic antibiotic used to treat *Clostridium difficile* infection.

12.4.2 Fluoroquinolones

The fluoroquinolones selectively inhibit topoisomerases II and IV, which are not found in mammalian cells. The enzymes, both tetramers comprising two A and two B subunits, are capable of catalysing a variety of changes in DNA topology. The topoisomerases bind to the chromosome at points where two separate double-stranded regions cross. This can be at a supercoiled region, a knotted or a linked (catenane) region. The A subunits (gyrA for topoisomerase II and parC for topoisomerase IV) cut both DNA strands on one chain with a 4 base pair stagger; the other chain is passed through the break which is then resealed. The B subunits (gyrB for topoisomerase II and parE for topoisomerase IV) derive energy for the reaction by hydrolysis of adenosine triphosphate (ATP). The precise details of the interaction are not clear but it appears that the fluoroquinolones do not simply eliminate enzyme function; they actively poison the cells by trapping the topoisomerases as drug–enzyme–DNA complexes in which double-stranded DNA breaks are held together by the enzyme protein alone. The enzymes are unable to reseal the DNA, with the result that the chromosome in treated cells becomes fragmented. The number of fragments (approximately 100 per cell) is comparable to the number of supercoils in the chromosome. The action of the fluoroquinolones probably triggers secondary responses in the cells which are responsible for death. One notable morphological effect of fluoroquinolone treatment of Gram-negative rod-shaped organisms is the formation of filaments. In Gram-positive cocci, topoisomerase IV may be the more important target for fluoroquinolone action.

12.4.3 Nitroimidazoles (Metronidazole, Tinidazole) and Nitrofurans (Nitrofurantoin)

These agents also cause DNA strand breakage, but by a direct chemical action rather than by inhibition of a topoisomerase. Metronidazole is active only against anaerobic organisms. The nitro group of metronidazole is converted to a nitronate radical by the low redox potential within cells. The pyruvate:ferredoxin oxidoreductase (POR) is a major metabolic pathway in anaerobic bacteria and protozoa used for generation of ATP. This system converts metronidazole to its active form which then attacks the DNA, producing strand breakage. Another nitroimidazole (tinidazole) and the nitrofuran (nitrofurantoin) are thought to act in a similar manner.

12.4.4 Semi-synthetic Rifamycins (Rifampicin, Rifabutin, Rifaximin, Rifapentine) and Fidaxomicin

The semi-synthetic rifamycins act upon the β subunit of microbial RNA polymerase by blocking the initiation process, and each molecule of antibiotic neutralises one RNA polymerase molecule. After initiation has commenced, the antibiotic is released from the enzyme which must become dissociated from the DNA in order for it to be affected. The action of these agents is, therefore, to prevent the initiation of new rounds of RNA transcription. They bind in a pocket of the RNA polymerase β subunit deep within the DNA/RNA channel, but at a distance from the active site. Fidaxomicin acts at a site on RNA polymerase that is distinct from the semi-synthetic rifamycin targets. It makes five critical hydrogen bonds with RNA polymerase, involving the elements that mediate conformational changes in the polymerase complex. The fidaxomicin–RNA–polymerase complexes recognise the −35 element but not the −10 element in the promoter region on the DNA upstream of the transcription start site and fail to initiate gene transcription.

12.4.5 5-Fluorocytosine

This antifungal agent inhibits DNA synthesis at the early stages involving production of the nucleotide thymidylic acid (TMP). 5-Fluorocytosine (5-FC) is converted by a deaminase inside fungi to 5-fluorouracil, then to the corresponding nucleoside triphosphate, 5-fluorodeoxyuridine monophosphate (5-F-dUMP) which then acts as an inhibitor of thymidylate synthetase (Figure 12.6). This enzyme normally produces TMP from dUMP by addition of a methyl group (supplied by a folate cofactor, Section 12.4.1.1) to the 5 position of the uracil ring. As this position is blocked by the fluoro group in 5-FC, 5-F-dUMP acts as an inhibitor of the enzyme. 5-FC can be considered as a prodrug; it has the value of being taken up by fungi as the nucleoside, whereas the active triphosphate produced inside the cells would not be taken up because of its negative charge. Although 5-FC is an important antifungal agent in the treatment of life-threatening infections, resistance can occur due to active efflux of the drug from the cells before it can inhibit DNA synthesis.

12.5 Folate Antagonists

12.5.1 Folate Metabolism in Microbial and Mammalian Cells

Folic acid is an important cofactor in all living cells. In the reduced form, tetrahydrofolate (THF), it functions as a carrier of single-carbon fragments, which are used in the synthesis of adenine, guanine, thymine and methionine (Figure 12.7). One important folate-dependent enzyme is thymidylate synthetase, which produces TMP by transfer of the methyl group from THF to UMP. In this and other folate-dependent reactions, THF is converted to DHF, which must be reduced back to THF before it can participate again as a carbon fragment carrier. The enzyme responsible for the reduction of DHF to THF is DHFR which uses the nucleotide $NADPH_2$ as a cofactor. Bacteria, protozoa and mammalian cells all possess DHFR, but there are sufficient differences in the enzyme structure for inhibitors such as trimethoprim and pyrimethamine to inhibit the bacterial and protozoal enzymes selectively without damaging the mammalian form. In the case of protozoa such as the *Plasmodium* species responsible for malaria, the DHFR is a double enzyme which also contains the thymidylate synthetase activity.

There is another fundamental difference between folate utilisation in microbial and mammalian cells (Figure 12.7). Bacteria and protozoa are unable to take up exogenous folate and must synthesise it themselves. This is carried out in a series of reactions involving first the synthesis of dihydropteroic acid from one molecule each of pteridine and *p*-aminobenzoic acid (PABA). Glutamic acid is then added to form DHF, which is reduced by DHFR to THF. Mammalian cells do not make their own DHF, instead they take it up from dietary nutrients and convert it to THF using DHFR.

12.5.2 Sulphonamides

Sulphonamides (e.g., sulphamethoxazole and dapsone) are structural analogues of PABA (Figure 12.8). They competitively inhibit the incorporation of PABA into dihydropteroic acid and there is some evidence for their incorporation into false folate analogues, which inhibit subsequent metabolism. The presence of excess PABA will reverse the inhibitory action of sulphonamides, as will thymine, adenine, guanine and methionine. However, these nutrients are not normally available at the site of infections for which the sulphonamides are used.

12.5.3 DHFR Inhibitors – Trimethoprim, Pyrimethamine, Proguanil and Trimetrexate

Trimethoprim is a selective inhibitor of bacterial DHFR. The bacterial enzyme is several thousand times more sensitive

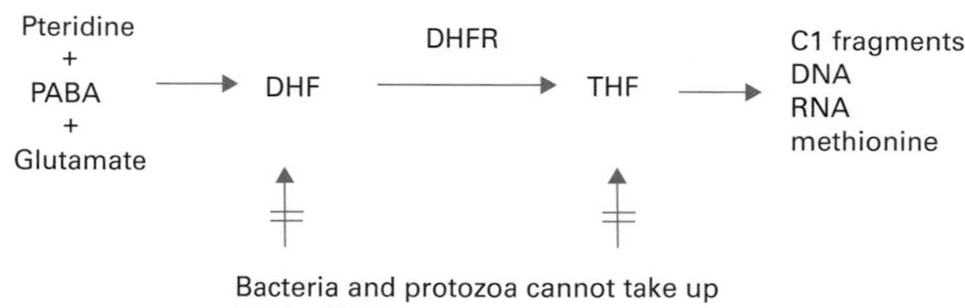

Mammalian cells

DHF —DHFR→ THF → C1 fragments: DNA RNA methionine

Mammalian cells cannot make DHF or THF, DHF is supplied in diet

Figure 12.7 Pathways of folate metabolism and use in microbial cells (upper) and mammalian cells (lower). Bacterial and protozoal cells must synthesise dihydrofolic acid (DHF) from pteridine, *p*-aminobenzoic acid (PABA) and glutamate. DHF is converted to tetrahydrofolic acid (THF) by the enzyme dihydrofolate reductase (DHFR). THF supplies single carbon units for various pathways including DNA, RNA and methionine synthesis. Mammalian cells do not make DHF, it is supplied from the diet; conversion to THF occurs via a DHFR enzyme as in microbial cells.

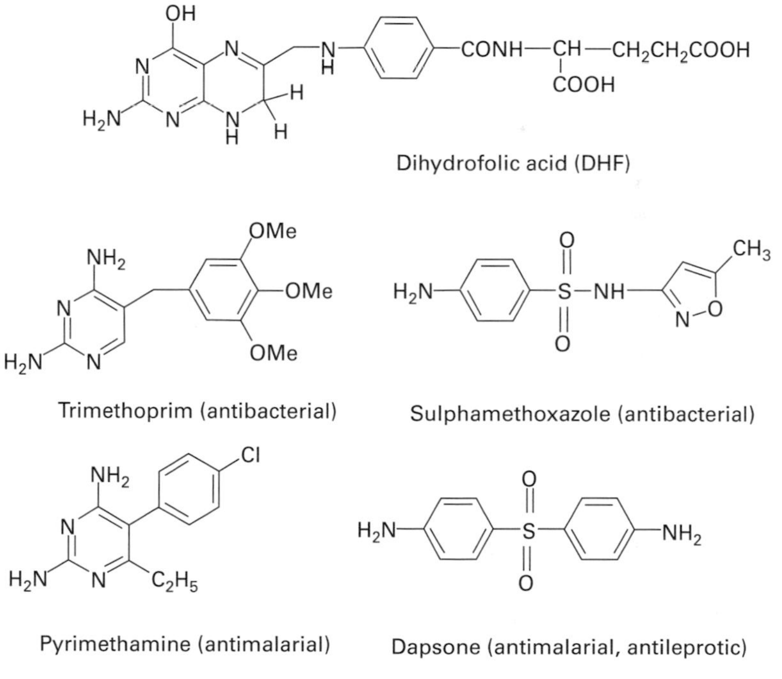

Dihydrofolic acid (DHF)

Trimethoprim (antibacterial)

Sulphamethoxazole (antibacterial)

Pyrimethamine (antimalarial)

Dapsone (antimalarial, antileprotic)

Figure 12.8 Structural relationships between dihydrofolate reductase inhibitors (trimethoprim and pyrimethamine), sulphonamides (e.g., sulphamethoxazole and dapsone) and dihydrofolic acid.

than the mammalian enzyme. Pyrimethamine, likewise, is a selective inhibitor of plasmodial DHFR. Both are structural analogues of the dihydropteroic acid portion of the DHF substrate (Figure 12.8). Crystal structures of the bacterial, plasmodial and mammalian DHFRs, each containing either bound substrate or the inhibitors, have been determined by X-ray diffraction studies. These show how inhibitors fit tightly into the active site normally occupied by the DHF substrate, forming a pattern of strong hydrogen bonds with amino acid residues and water molecules lining the site. Another DHFR is proguanil, a guanidine-containing prodrug which is metabolised in the liver to cycloguanil, an active selective inhibitor of plasmodial DHFR. Methotrexate is a potent DHFR inhibitor that has an analogous structure to the whole DHF molecule, including the glutamate residue. It has no selectivity towards microbial DHFR and therefore cannot be used to treat infections; however, it is widely used as an anticancer agent. A derivative of methotrexate that is used for treatment of *Pneumocystis jirovecii* infections in AIDS patients is trimetrexate. Although it is very toxic to mammalian cells, simultaneous administration of leucovorin (formyl-THF or folinic acid) as an alternative source of folate which cannot be taken up by the organism protects host tissues. DHFR inhibitors can be used in combination with a sulphonamide to achieve a double interference with folate metabolism. Suitable combinations with matching pharmacokinetic properties are sulphamethoxazole with trimethoprim (the antibacterial co-trimoxazole) and dapsone with pyrimethamine (the antimalarial Maloprim).

12.6 The Cytoplasmic Membrane

12.6.1 Composition and Susceptibility of Membranes to Selective Disruption

The integrity of the cytoplasmic membrane is vital for the normal functioning of all cells. Bacterial membranes do not contain sterols and in this respect differ from membranes of fungi and mammalian cells. Fungal membranes contain predominantly ergosterol as the sterol component, whereas mammalian cells contain cholesterol. Gram-negative bacteria contain an additional outer-membrane structure that provides a protective penetration barrier to potentially harmful substances, including many antibiotics. The outer membrane has an unusual asymmetric structure in which phospholipids occupy the inner face and the LPS occupies the outer face. The outer membrane is attached to the peptidoglycan by proteins and lipoproteins. The stability of all membranes is maintained by a combination of non-covalent interactions between the constituents involving ionic, hydrophobic and hydrogen bonding. The balance of these interactions can be disturbed by the intrusion of molecules (membrane-active agents) which destroy the integrity of the membrane, thereby causing leakage of cytoplasmic contents or impairment of metabolic functions associated with the membrane. Most membrane-active agents that function in this way, for example, the alcohols, quaternary ammonium compounds and bis-biguanides (considered in Chapters 18 and 20), have very poor selectivity. They cannot be used systemically because of their damaging effects upon mammalian cells; instead they are used as skin antiseptics, disinfectants and preservatives. A few agents can be used therapeutically: the polymyxins (colistin), which act principally upon the outer membrane of Gram-negative bacteria, and the antifungal polyenes, which act upon fungal membranes. Other antifungal agents, the imidazoles, triazoles and terbinafine act by blocking the synthesis of ergosterol, the major sterol present in fungal membranes (see also Chapter 4).

12.6.2 Polymyxins

Polymyxin E (colistin) is used in the treatment of serious Gram-negative bacterial infections, particularly those caused by *Pseudomonas aeruginosa*. Delivered as the prodrug, colistimethate sodium, it is hydrolysed in the body to release the active form, colistin. Colistin binds tightly to the lipid A component of LPS in the outer membrane of Gram-negative bacteria. The outer leaflet of the membrane structure is distorted, segments of which are released and the permeability barrier is destroyed. The polymyxin molecules can then penetrate to the cytoplasmic membrane where they bind to phospholipids, disrupt membrane integrity and cause irreversible leakage of cytoplasmic components. Their detergent-like properties are a key feature of this membrane-damaging action, which is similar to that of quaternary ammonium compounds. With increasing resistance to the major groups of antibiotics, some multiresistant organisms (e.g., *Acinetobacter* species) remain sensitive only to membrane-active agents such as colistin. However, some Gram-negative bacteria produce LPS that does not bind polymyxins (e.g., *Bacteroides* species and *Burkholderia cenocepacia*) while resistance can occur in some normally sensitive organisms such as *E. coli* and *P. aeruginosa* through modification of their LPS structure (e.g., by addition of aminoarabinose or aminoethanol substituents to the lipid A regions of their LPS).

12.6.3 Daptomycin

This negatively charged bactericidal cyclic lipopeptide binds to the surface of the Gram-positive bacterial cell membrane. The binding is dependent on calcium ions. The acyl tail portion of the compound inserts itself into the cytoplasmic membrane and drug molecules aggregate together forming channels. The leakage of potassium ions from the cells results in inhibition of macromolecular synthesis and cell death.

12.6.4 Polyenes

Amphotericin B and nystatin are the most commonly used members of this group of antifungal agents. They derive their action from their strong affinity towards sterols, particularly ergosterol. The hydrophobic polyene

Figure 12.9 Pathway for synthesis of the essential fungal sterol ergosterol and the sites of inhibition by the antifungal agents terbinafine, imidazoles and triazoles.

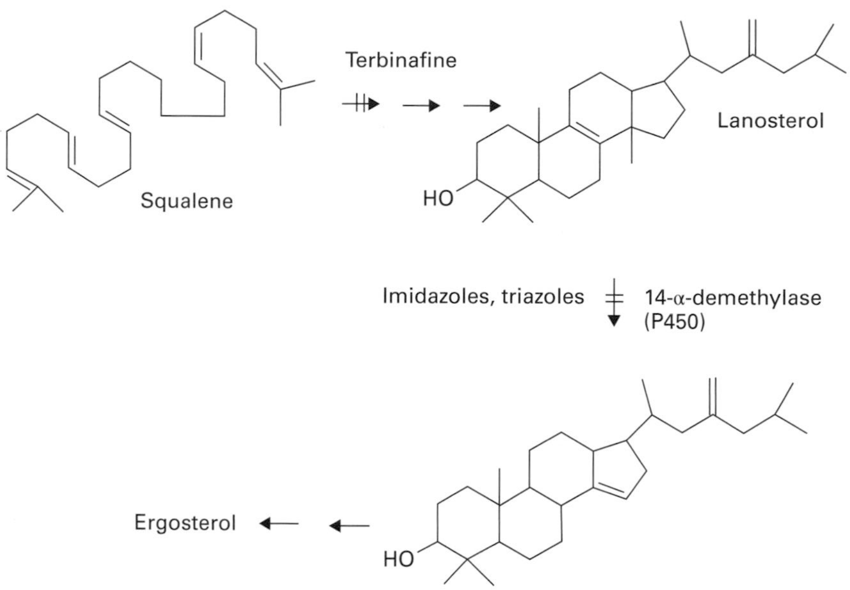

region binds to the hydrophobic sterol ring system within fungal membranes. In so doing, the hydroxylated portion of the polyene is pulled into the membrane interior, destabilising the structure and causing leakage of cytoplasmic constituents. It is possible that polyene molecules associate together in the membrane to form aqueous channels. The pattern of leakage is progressive, with small metal ions such as K^+ leaking first, followed by larger amino acids and nucleotides. The internal pH of the cells falls as K^+ ions are released, macromolecules are degraded and the cells are killed. The selective antifungal activity of the polyenes is poor, depending on the higher affinity for ergosterol than cholesterol. Kidney damage is a major problem when polyenes are used systemically to treat severe fungal infections. The problem can be reduced, but not eliminated by administration of amphotericin as a lipid complex or liposome.

12.6.5 Imidazoles and Triazoles

The azole antifungal drugs act by inhibiting the synthesis of the sterol components of the fungal membrane (see also Chapter 4). They are inhibitors of one step in the complex pathway of ergosterol synthesis involving the removal of a methyl group from lanosterol (Figure 12.9). The 14-α-demethylase enzyme responsible is dependent on cytochrome P-450. The imidazoles and triazoles cause rapid defects in fungal membrane integrity due to reduced levels of ergosterol, with loss of cytoplasmic constituents leading to similar effects to the polyenes. The azoles are not entirely specific for fungal ergosterol synthesis and have some action on mammalian sterol metabolism; for example, they reduce testosterone synthesis.

12.6.6 Terbinafine and Amorolfine

The synthetic allylamine, terbinafine, inhibits the enzyme squalene epoxidase at an early stage in fungal sterol biosynthesis. Acting as a structural analogue of squalene, terbinafine causes the accumulation of this unsaturated hydrocarbon, and a decrease in ergosterol in the fungal cell membrane (Figure 12.9). The synthetic morpholine, amorolfine, inhibits enzymes in the pathway after the 14-α-demethylase. This inhibition depletes ergosterol and causes ignosterol (ergosta-8,14-dienol) to accumulate in the fungal cell membranes.

Further Reading

Baptista, R., Fazakerley, D.M., Beckmann, M. et al. (2018). Untargeted metabolomics reveals a new mode of action of pretomanid (PA-824). *Sci. Rep.* 8 (1): 5084.

Bush, K. and Bradford, P.A. (2019). Interplay between β-lactamases and new β-lactamase inhibitors. *Nat. Rev. Microbiol.* 17 (5): 295–306.

Fernandes, P. (2016). Fusidic acid: a bacterial elongation factor inhibitor for the oral treatment of acute and chronic staphylococcal infections. *Cold Spring Harb. Perspect. Med.* 6 (1): a025437.

Hooper, D.C. and Jacoby, G.A. (2016). Topoisomerase inhibitors: fluoroquinolone mechanisms of action and resistance. *Cold Spring Harb. Perspect. Med.* 6 (9): a025320.

Khoshnood, S., Heidary, M., Asadi, A. et al. (2019). A review on mechanism of action, resistance, synergism, and clinical implications of mupirocin against *Staphylococcus aureus*. *Biomed. Pharmacother.* 109: 1809–1818.

Lin, J., Zhou, D., Steitz, T.A. et al. (2018). Ribosome-targeting antibiotics: modes of action, mechanisms of resistance, and implications for drug design. *Annu. Rev. Biochem.* 87: 451–478.

Lovering, A., Safadi, S.S. and Strynadka, N.C. (2012). Structural perspective of peptidoglycan biosynthesis and assembly. *Annu. Rev. Biochem.* 81: 451–478.

Mosaei, H. and Harbottle, J. (2019). Mechanisms of antibiotics inhibiting bacterial RNA polymerase. *Biochem. Soc. Trans.* 47 (1): 339–350.

Olsufyeva, E.N. and Tevyashova, A.N. (2017). Synthesis, properties, and mechanism of action of new generation of polycyclic glycopeptide antibiotics. *Curr. Top. Med. Chem.* 17 (19): 2166–2198.

Paukner, S. and Riedl, R. (2017). Pleuromutilins: potent drugs for resistant bugs - mode of action and resistance. *Cold Spring Harb. Perspect. Med.* 7 (1): a027110.

Taylor, S.D. and Palmer, M. (2016). The action mechanism of daptomycin. *Bioorg. Med. Chem.* 24 (24): 6253–6268.

Vázquez-Laslop, N. and Mankin, A.S. (2018). How macrolide antibiotics work. *Trends Biochem. Sci.* 43 (9): 668–684.

13

Bacterial Resistance to Antibiotics

Brendan F. Gilmore[1] *and Stephen P. Denyer*[2]

[1] *Professor of Pharmaceutical Microbiology, School of Pharmacy, Queen's University Belfast, Belfast, UK*
[2] *Emeritus Professor of Pharmacy, Universities of Brighton and Sussex, Brighton, UK*

CONTENTS

13.1 Introduction

Antibiotic resistance, or more broadly antimicrobial resistance (AMR), in bacteria is defined as resistance to an antibiotic or antimicrobial agent that was once capable of treating an infection caused by that bacterium. Antibiotic resistance arises when microorganisms survive exposure to an antibiotic through a range of mechanisms. It is both a complex natural and ancient phenomenon, which reflects the constant evolutionary pressures of living within complex microbiota and competition for resources. This competition is characterised by the microbial production of antimicrobial chemicals to control and restrict the growth of competing microorganisms, leading to a Darwinian

Hugo and Russell's Pharmaceutical Microbiology, Ninth Edition. Edited by Brendan F. Gilmore and Stephen P. Denyer.

Companion website: https://www.wiley.com/go/HugoandRussells9e

selection of those microorganisms which are capable of resisting these inimical agents, through intrinsic or acquired mechanisms. Generally, strains capable of resisting antibiotic exposure therefore survive and proliferate, while antibiotic-sensitive strains perish. In the relatively short period of time since the introduction of penicillin into clinical practice in the early 1940s, the discovery and introduction of every new antibiotic has been accompanied by the rapid emergence of resistance, such that resistance to all major classes of antibiotics (see Chapter 11) has now been described. The discovery of antibiotics was accompanied by historical warnings of the potential for bacteria to develop resistance to these new drugs, recognising the risk of an arms race developing between new antibiotic discovery and the evolution of antibiotic-resistant pathogens accelerated by the anthropogenic use of antibiotics to treat infection. For many years, these warnings were largely ignored, since early treatment failure with antibiotic drugs did not represent a significant clinical problem, as other agents with different cellular targets were available. We now realise, however, that the expanding indications for antibiotic agents, which underpin advances in clinical medicine such as cancer chemotherapy, organ transplantation and the widespread use of indwelling medical devices and prostheses, and the introduction of agents with broad-spectrum activity, have led to the emergence of multiple antibiotic-resistance mechanisms. This, along with diminishing therapeutic options as new antibiotic discovery fails to keep pace with the emergence of resistant bacterial pathogens, threatens to bring society to a 'post-antibiotic era' where even simple infections may become impossible to treat.

According to the World Health Organization (WHO), antibiotic resistance now ranks among the greatest threats to global health, food security and development. The O'Neill Review on Antimicrobial Resistance, commissioned by the UK Government to analyse the global problem of rising antibiotic resistance, delivered its final report and recommendations in 2016. Uniquely, the O'Neill Review identified both clinical and economic drivers for antibiotic resistance, and proposed specific actions to address the global problem of antibiotic resistance. Further, O'Neill conservatively estimated deaths associated with AMR at an additional 10 million per year by 2050 (more than cancer and diabetes combined), with a cumulative cost of $100 trillion (equivalent to the entire UK economy from global output each year). A systematic analysis of the global burden of bacterial antimicrobial resistance has estimated the number of deaths attributable to bacterial AMR in 2019 to be 1.27 million.

The US Centers for Disease Control and Prevention (CDC) similarly reported in 2019 that annually in the USA over 2.8 million serious infections are caused by antibiotic-resistant bacteria, with at least 35,000 deaths. The CDC also estimates the healthcare costs associated with multidrug-resistant (MDR) healthcare-associated bacterial infections (caused by six resistant pathogens: methicillin-resistant *Staphylococcus aureus* [MRSA], extended-spectrum cephalosporin resistance in *Enterobacteriaceae*, vancomycin-resistant *Enterococcus* [VRE], carbapenem-resistant *Acinetobacter* species, carbapenem-resistant *Enterobacteriaceae* [CRE] and MDR *Pseudomonas aeruginosa*) at more than $4.6 billion every year. As the number of emerging multidrug-resistant bacterial pathogens increases, the global financial burden of antibiotic resistance, alongside increased patient morbidity and mortality associated with these infections, will continue to rise.

The appearance of resistance to all classes of therapeutically useful antibiotics has led to the identification of antibiotic-resistant bacterial pathogens of particular concern, reflecting the difficulty in treating the infections they cause and recognising the paucity of effective drugs currently available or in the antibiotic pipeline specifically targeted against them. In 2009, the Infectious Diseases Society of America (IDSA) recognised a group of microorganisms (*Enterococcus faecium*, *S. aureus*, *Klebsiella pneumoniae*, *Acinetobacter baumannii*, *P. aeruginosa* and *Enterobacter* species), termed 'the ESKAPE pathogens' from their initial letters, which were responsible for the majority of healthcare-associated infections (HAIs) and which are capable of 'escaping' the inhibitory or bactericidal action of antibiotic agents. The ESKAPE pathogens remain significant multidrug-resistant pathogens in the USA and globally, including MRSA, VRE, *Acinetobacter* species, fluoroquinolone-resistant and MDR *P. aeruginosa*, carbapenem-resistant *Klebsiella* species and *Escherichia coli*. More recently (2017), the WHO have published a list of antibiotic-resistant 'priority pathogens', bacteria which pose the greatest threat to human health and for which few if any new antibiotics are in development (Table 13.1). The list, divided by urgency of need for new antibiotics, catalogues critical, high and medium priority pathogens and is intended to prioritise and encourage research and development of new antibiotic agents. In addition to the IDSA ESKAPE pathogen group, the WHO priority pathogen list highlights the significance of Gram-negative bacteria, which are resistant to multiple antibiotics, as a threat to human health.

13.2 The Origins of Resistance

The discovery of penicillin in 1928, and its subsequent isolation and development as a clinical therapeutic agent in the 1940s, gave rise to a golden era of antibiotic discovery, a period up to the mid-1960s when more than half of all

Table 13.1 Antibiotic-resistant pathogens included in the WHO priority list.

Priority level	Pathogen groups
Priority 1: critical	Carbapenem-resistant *A. baumannii*, carbapenem-resistant *P. aeruginosa*, carbapenem-resistant, extended-spectrum β-lactamase (ESBL)-producing *Enterobacteriaceae* (including *E. coli, Klebsiella, Serratia* and *Proteus* species)
Priority 2: high	Vancomycin-resistant *E. faecium* (VRE), *S. aureus* (methicillin-resistant [MRSA] and vancomycin-intermediate (VISA) and -resistant (VRSA) strains), clarithromycin-resistant *Helicobacter pylori*, fluoroquinolone-resistant *Campylobacter* spp., fluoroquinolone-resistant *Salmonellae* and cephalosporin- and fluoroquinolone-resistant *Neisseria gonorrhoeae*
Priority 3: medium	Penicillin-non-susceptible *Streptococcus pneumoniae*, ampicillin-resistant *Haemophilus influenzae* and fluoroquinolone-resistant *Shigella* spp.

antibiotics in contemporary clinical use (representing almost all of the major classes of clinically useful antibiotics) were discovered. The introduction of antibiotics into clinical use was accompanied by the emergence of antibiotic resistance to those agents, sometimes with worrying rapidity. While this could be interpreted as meaning antibiotic resistance is a modern phenomenon, exclusively linked to the widespread anthropogenic use of antibiotic drugs, modern metagenomic analysis of 30,000-year-old DNA from permafrost sediment cores has demonstrated that antibiotic resistance, represented by a diverse range of genes coding for resistance to β-lactams, glycopeptide and tetracycline antibiotics within this microbiome, was actually an ancient phenomenon predating the widespread use of antibiotics. Similarly, widespread antibiotic resistance has been reported in cultured microorganisms from a cave microbiome estimated to have been cut off from external influences for the last 4 million years. Notwithstanding, it is clear from numerous studies that the anthropogenic use of antibiotics has accelerated the emergence of multidrug resistance over the past 80 years, threatening the very future of the 'antibiotic era'. A multitude of factors, including unregulated and widespread overuse of antibiotics and a lack of investment in the discovery of new antibiotic agents, have contributed to a situation where new clinical agents are being outpaced by the evolution of resistant pathogens. While alternatives to antibiotics are being explored (see Chapter 26), there is still much work to be done before they might realistically find widespread use in clinical medicine. In the meantime, therefore, it is essential that we understand the determinants of resistance and exercise proper controls in the use of our antibiotics.

Bacteria may have *innate*, sometimes called *intrinsic*, resistance to some antibiotic agents, either through variations to the structure of the cell envelope or as a consequence of other structural or functional changes (for details of the cellular and sub-cellular structures of bacteria, see Chapter 3). Intrinsic mechanisms of resistance are summarised in Figure 13.1.

While the origins of antibiotic-resistance genes are unclear, studies have demonstrated that clinical isolates archived before the clinical introduction of antibiotics exhibit antibiotic susceptibility, despite the presence of conjugative plasmids (see Section 13.17.1). This reinforces the idea that the appearance of resistance is related to the clinical and widespread use of antibiotics over the past 80 years; the relatively short period of time that has elapsed since their clinical introduction, however, suggests that mutation of common ancestral genes is unlikely to be the only mechanism by which antibiotic resistance arises. This conclusion is further supported by the discovery of resistance mechanisms in ancient and isolated microbiomes (described above) and indicates that many resistance genes will have derived from the diverse pangenome of environmental microorganisms. Resistance can be disseminated by the horizontal acquisition of genes, mobilised by insertion sequences, transposons and conjugative plasmids, by the recombination of foreign DNA into the chromosome or by mutations in different chromosomal loci. The role of the environment as a reservoir for antimicrobial resistance genes (ARGs) and in the global spread of resistance is recognised. Overuse of antibiotics clearly introduces significant selective pressure leading to the rapid emergence and selection of resistant bacteria which may then lead to genetic exchange of resistance genes within the complex microbiota of the soil, general environment and the gut of animals and humans. The use of antimicrobials in agriculture, where antibiotics were once widely employed as feed additives for growth promotion in food animals, has been, and in some areas of the world still is, a significant driver of antibiotic resistance. It is estimated that some 70% of medically important antibiotic consumption (by weight) in the USA is by animals. Therefore, reduction of antimicrobial use in the agricultural and veterinary sectors is a key target for curbing antibiotic resistance. However, in reducing antibiotic use within the agricultural setting, care must be taken to ensure that this is achieved within the wider confines and principles of good antimicrobial

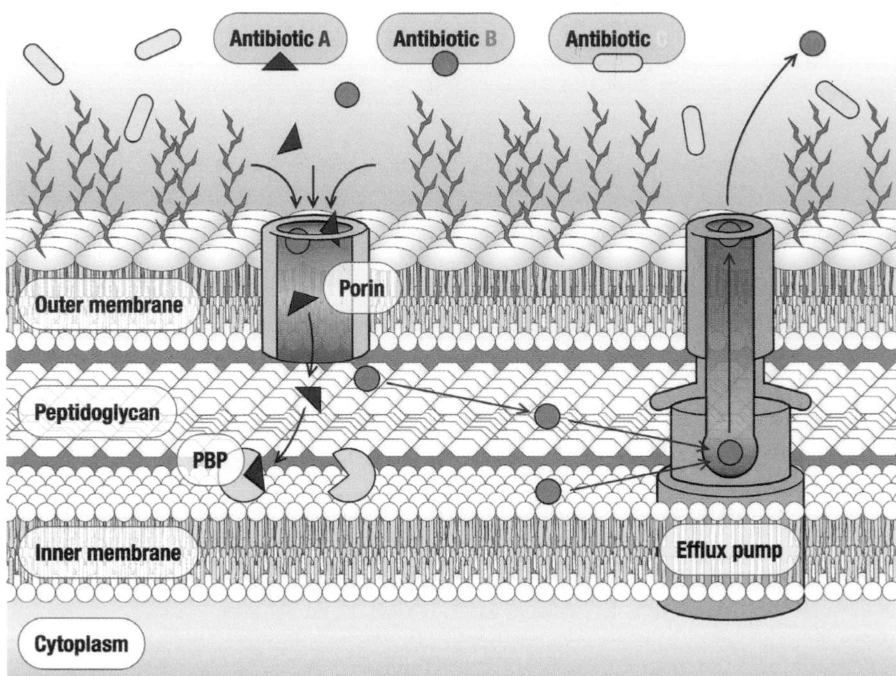

Figure 13.1 Mechanisms of intrinsic resistance: antibiotic A, a penicillin, successfully enters the periplasm and binds to its target, a penicillin-binding protein (PBP), thereby inhibiting peptidoglycan cross-linking. Antibiotic B enters the cell via a porin but is removed by efflux, preventing inhibitory or bactericidal concentrations accumulating in the cell. Antibiotic C is unable to cross the outer membrane and cannot reach its target. *Source:* Adapted from Blair et al. (2015).

stewardship, to avoid (for example) inappropriate shortening of antibiotic treatment courses which may have a negative effect both on animal welfare and the development of resistance.

The mutation process is not a static event and a complex network of factors influences the rate of any mutation and type of mutants that can be selected under antibiotic pressure. Antibiotic concentration, physiological conditions such as nutrient availability and stress can each regulate mutation rates. The structure of a gene is relevant to mutability. Size is not the main factor, as not every mutation in a gene that encodes an antibiotic target leads to resistance. Resistance only occurs by mutations which are both permissive (i.e., not lethal or leading to an unacceptable reduction in 'fitness' or ability to cause infection) and able to produce a resistance phenotype. The probability that such a mutation arises will be proportional to the number of target sites within the gene. In *E. coli*, mutations in the *gyrA* gene, encoding the GyrA subunit of topoisomerase II and leading to fluoroquinolone resistance (Section 13.8), have been identified in at least seven locations, whereas mutational changes in only three positions in the *parC* gene, encoding a subunit of topoisomerase IV, have been observed. As a consequence, the prediction that the mutation rate would be higher in *gyrA* than *parC* is correct. Such observations and predictions cannot be extrapolated to other organisms. Indeed, the opposite is true for fluoroquinolone resistance in *Streptococcus pneumoniae*.

13.3 Mechanisms of Resistance

Resistance to antimicrobial agents typically arises by one or more of the following mechanisms:

- Inactivation (usually enzymatic) of the antibiotic agent by hydrolysis or modification (Figure 13.2a).
- Alteration (or loss) of the antibiotic target through either genetic mutation or post-translational modification (Figure 13.2b).
- Reduced intracellular accumulation of antibiotic either by restricted uptake or increased efflux (Figures 13.1 and 13.9).

In this chapter, in addition to specific examples provided to illustrate each general resistance mechanism above, antibiotic resistance will be examined by agent, with attention drawn to those mechanisms which facilitate resistance to multiple, chemically diverse agents.

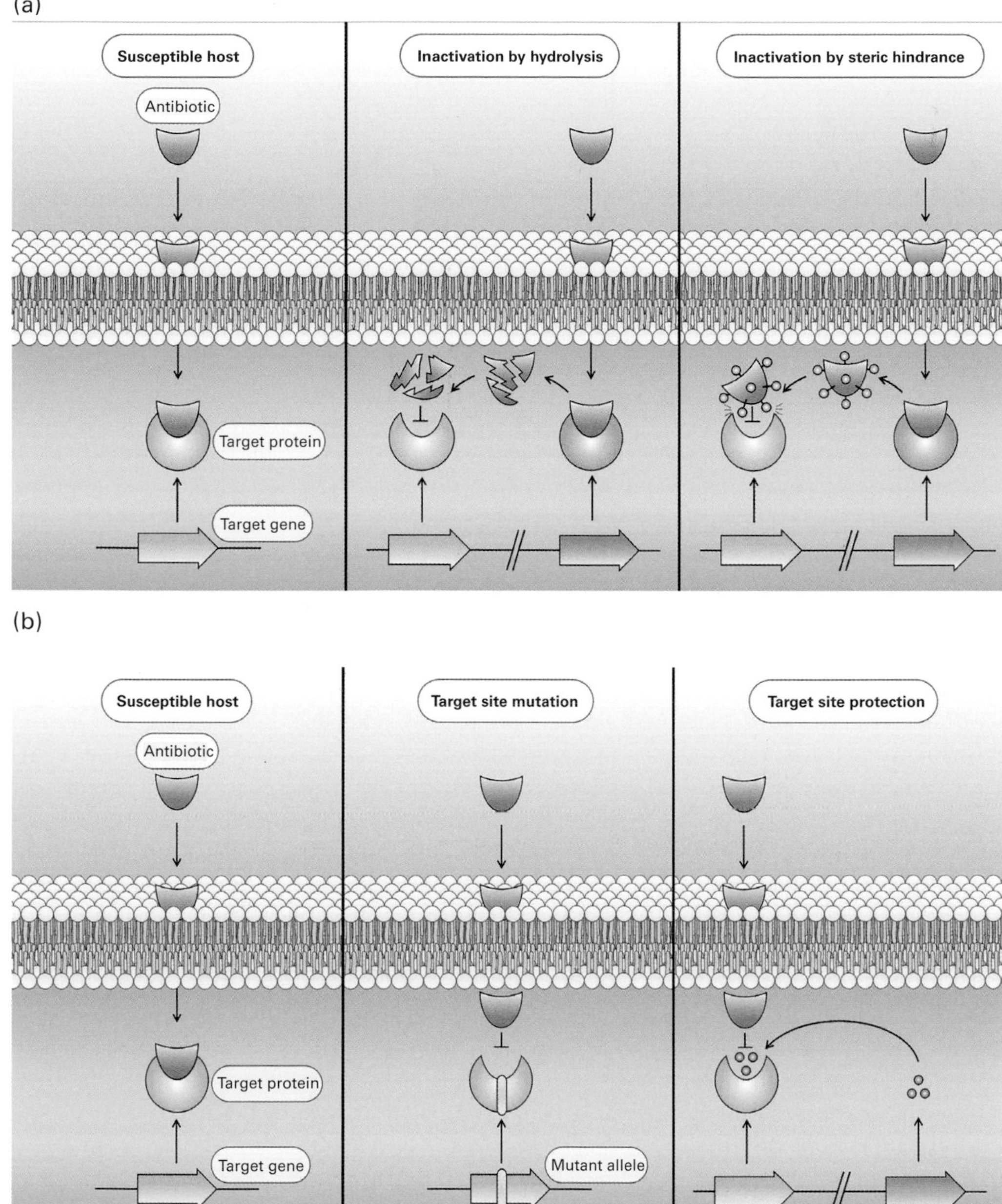

Figure 13.2 (a) Mechanisms of acquired resistance: inactivation of antibiotic. Left – susceptible host, antibiotic reaches and interacts with target; middle – antibiotic inactivated by acquired and expressed antibiotic-degrading enzymes; right – antibiotic structure modified by acquired and expressed enzymes which transfer additional chemical groups to the molecule, preventing antibiotic binding to target. (b) Mechanisms of acquired resistance: target modification. Left – susceptible host, antibiotic reaches and interacts with target; middle – alteration of the target site (arising from mutations to the gene encoding the target protein) leading to the expression of the functional target with reduced or no affinity for the antibiotic; right – target site is modified by addition of chemical groups to the target without loss of functionality, thereby preventing antibiotic binding but without alteration of target gene sequence. *Source:* Adapted from Blair et al. (2015).

13.4 Resistance to β-Lactam Antibiotics

The β-lactam antibiotics were the first antibiotics to be used clinically, and remain the most widely prescribed class of antibiotics globally. Unsurprisingly, the first reports and warnings of emerging antibiotic resistance related to the β-lactams. The β-lactams all bear a 4-member β-lactam ring in their molecular core structure and are represented clinically by the penicillins, cephalosporins, monobactams and carbapenems, as well as in combination with β-lactamase inhibitors; they share a common mode of action. These antibiotics act by inhibiting the late-stage cross-linking of bacterial cell wall peptidoglycan through the inhibition of transpeptidases (otherwise known as penicillin binding proteins [PBPs]). The β-lactam ring is structurally analogous to the natural substrate of the transpeptidase enzyme, the D-Ala-D-Ala terminus of the uncross-linked peptidoglycan precursor N-acetyl-muramyl-pentapeptide. The antibiotic acts as a competitive, irreversible inhibitor of the enzyme which normally catalyses the peptide cross-linking of adjacent peptidoglycan polymers in the synthesis of a functional cell wall, capable of resisting osmotic lysis. Resistance to β-lactam antibiotics is both common and widespread and is most frequently caused by the action of β-lactamases or through mutations in the transpeptidase/PBP target, thereby reducing antibiotic affinity. While reduced uptake and efflux of β-lactams have been reported, they are less significant as a mechanism of resistance to this class of antibiotic.

13.4.1 β-Lactamases

The first report of an enzyme from *E. coli* capable of degrading penicillin was by Ernst Chain in 1940, even before the introduction of penicillin for clinical use. Resistance to penicillin in isolates of *S. aureus* was reported in 1944, and subsequently found to be due to production of the β-lactamase PC1 encoded by *blaZ*. Concerns that β-lactamase enzymes could ultimately compromise the future use of β-lactams led to the search for β-lactamase-stable penicillins, and ultimately the introduction of methicillin in 1960. Since then β-lactamases have been widely reported and represent the major mechanism of resistance to all classes of the β-lactam antibiotics. While belonging to a large and diverse family of enzymes, β-lactamases share the ability to catalyse the hydrolysis of the β-lactam ring, leading to ring opening and loss of structural homology with the D-Ala-D-Ala terminus of the peptidoglycan pentapeptide and consequently loss of affinity for transpeptidases/PBPs.

β-lactamase genes may be chromosomal or plasmid-borne, and can be constitutively or inductively expressed. From protein and nucleotide sequencing data, the number of β-lactamases identified to date (according to the Beta-Lactamase DataBase [BLDB]; Naas et al. 2017) now exceeds 4300. From this data, it is clear that β-lactamases do not constitute a single group of enzymes but belong to multiple classes. Classification systems based on catalytic activity against β-lactam substrates (Bush–Jacoby–Medeiros system) or based on sequence identity (Ambler system) have been proposed. The most commonly adopted system of classification, the Ambler system, proposes that β-lactamases may be subdivided into four distinct classes, A, B, C and D, based on specific conserved sequence motifs and the catalytic mechanism. As with other hydrolytic enzymes, a further division arises based on the nature of the active-site nucleophile. Classes A, C and D have an active-site catalytic serine residue and are thus referred to as the serine-β-lactamases (SBLs), while class B enzymes (in common with other metalloenzymes) utilise metal ion(s) at the active site to coordinate a water molecule which then functions as the nucleophile, and these are referred to as zinc-dependent metallo-β-lactamases (MBLs). As with other druggable enzyme targets, the catalytic mechanism has implications for the design of potent and selective inhibitors of these enzymes; in this context, druggability refers to a biological target, such as a protein, predicted or observed to bind with high affinity to small molecule drugs. Generally, class A enzymes are highly active against benzylpenicillin and include the well-characterised and widely disseminated TEM, SHV, CTX-M and KPC β-lactamases (see below); class B β-lactamases are effective against penicillins and cephalosporins, and include the Verona integron-borne metallo-β-lactamase (VIM) and the NDM β-lactamase (see below). Class C enzymes are usually inducible, but mutation can lead to overexpression. Class D consists of the oxacillinase (OXA) enzymes, which can hydrolyse oxacillin but are also of increasing concern due to their ability to cause carbapenem resistance in the *Enterobacteriaceae* and *A. baumannii*. The general mechanism of hydrolytic ring-opening in β-lactams by the serine β-lactamases is given in Figure 13.3.

As resistance mediated by β-lactamase enzymes increased, agents with greater β-lactam stability were introduced, including cephalosporins, carbapenems and monobactams. Resistance first appeared to clinically relevant β-lactams in organisms such as *Enterobacter cloacae* and *P. aeruginosa*, as a result of mutations to the *ampC* gene and overproduction of the AmpC β-lactamase, a class C enzyme. The *ampC* gene is carried on the chromosome of many Gram-negative pathogens but is not normally expressed. The appearance of β-lactamase-mediated resistance in organisms such as *K. pneumoniae* which lack an inducible AmpC enzyme led to the discovery of plasmid-borne β-lactamases. The first description of a plasmid-borne β-lactamase was the enzyme TEM (named after the patient Temoniera from which the *E. coli* strain was isolated), encoded by the *bla* gene. The SHV (sulphydryl variant) enzyme, a class A limited-spectrum β-lactamase similar to TEM, was discovered initially on the chromosome of *K. pneumoniae* but subsequently mobilised to plasmids; CTX-M (active against cefotaxime, first observed in Munich) and KPC (*K. pneumoniae* carbapenemase) and their variants are now widely disseminated. Extended-spectrum β-lactamases (ESBLs), arising from mutations to TEM and SHV, have altered active-site binding

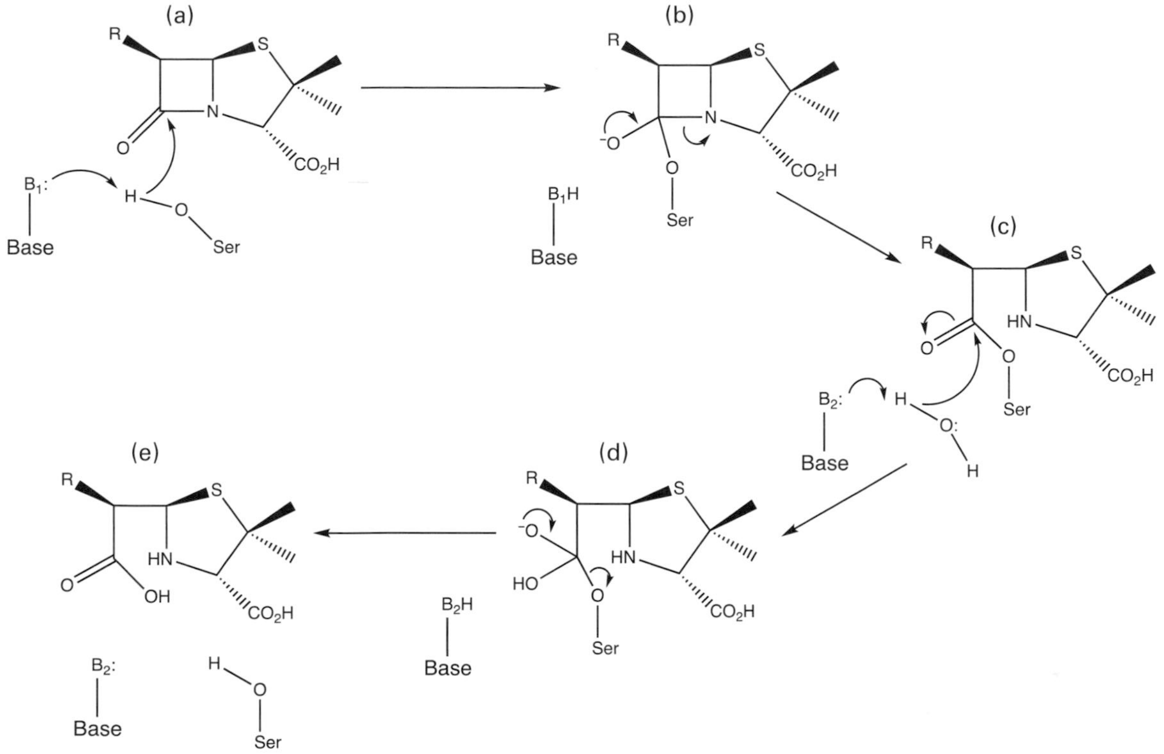

Figure 13.3 General mechanism of hydrolysis of a β-lactam antibiotic by serine β-lactamases. (a) General base B1 activation of active-site serine (Ser), and nucleophilic attack on the amide carbonyl carbon of the β-lactam ring, generating a covalent acyl–enzyme (c) via the tetrahedral oxyanionic acylation transition state (b) (stabilised by positively charged arginine/lysine residues at the active site – not shown). Activation of an incoming water molecule leads to nucleophilic attack on the acyl–enzyme carbonyl of (c) to liberate the penicillinoate (e) β-lactamase reaction product, via a tetrahedral diacylation transition state (d). Complete β-lactam ring opening in (e) is indicated in red. *Source:* Adapted from Tooke et al. (2019).

pockets which can accommodate a wider range of β-lactams, including the larger cephalosporins. The mobilisation of ESBLs on plasmids has led to widespread and globally distributed β-lactam resistance which threatens the clinical effectiveness of several key β-lactams including the cephalosporins. Fortunately, such mutations also increase the binding of clavulanic acid, rendering ESBLs susceptible to β-lactamase inhibitors.

Continued use of the third-generation cephalosporins and the introduction of β-lactamase inhibitor combinations (clavulanate with amoxicillin or ticarcillin, sulbactam with ampicillin, and tazobactam with piperacillin; see Section 13.4.2) have resulted in the appearance of plasmids encoding class C β-lactamases. The first report of a class C β-lactamase carried on a plasmid appeared in 1990 when transmissible resistance to α-methoxy-β-lactam and oxyimino-β-lactam was shown to be mediated by an enzyme whose gene sequence was 90% identical to the *ampC* gene of *E. cloacae*. These enzymes have subsequently been found worldwide. Strains with plasmid-mediated AmpC enzymes are typically resistant to aminopenicillins (ampicillin or amoxicillin), carboxypenicillins (carbenicillin or ticarcillin) and ureidopenicillins (piperacillin). The enzymes also provide resistance to the oxyimino cephalosporins (ceftazidime, cefotaxime, ceftriaxone) and the 7-α-methoxy group (cefoxitin, cefmetazole and moxalactam) as well as the monobactam aztreonam.

The widespread use of β-lactam antibiotics has led to an increasing frequency of infections caused by ESBL-producing pathogens. This has subsequently led to the introduction of carbapenem antibiotics into clinical use, first with imipenem in 1985. Carbapenems are attractive antibiotic agents, since they uniquely exhibit both potent antimicrobial activity and the ability to inhibit the majority of SBLs through the formation of stable acyl–enzyme intermediates. Since their introduction, the use of carbapenems has significantly increased and has been accompanied, predictably, by the emergence of bacteria which carry β-lactamase enzymes capable of hydrolysing carbapenems (carbapenemases). The class A enzyme KPC (encoded by plasmid-borne bla_{KPC}) and its variants are able to avoid inhibition by carbapenem antibiotics and can successfully hydrolyse the lactam ring; bacteria harbouring this enzyme have been responsible for infection outbreaks globally. In 2009, the first report of a specific carbapenemase β-lactamase, referred to as New Delhi metallo-β-lactamase

(NDM-1), was recorded. While the carbapenem-resistant strain *K. pneumoniae* 05-506 harboured the plasmid-borne class B metallo-β-lactamase gene bla_{NDM-1}, NDM-expressing strains are now known to have the gene present on both the chromosome and plasmid, with a high frequency of mobilisation between the two. The NDM metallo-β-lactamase has become one of the most widespread carbapenemases and is responsible for global outbreaks of Gram-negative carbapenem-resistant infections, particularly in *P. aeruginosa*, *E. coli* and *K. pneumoniae*. The bla_{NDM} gene itself is highly mobile and located on conjugative plasmids which often encode additional resistance genes. Both KPC and NDM-1 represent a significant threat to the continued clinical efficacy of the carbapenem family of antibiotics. Indeed, the emergence of isolates of Gram-negative pathogens carrying both ESBLs and carbapenemases has been reported and heralds a worrying clinical scenario of bacteria which are resistant to all current β-lactam antibiotics.

13.4.2 β-Lactamase Inhibitors

In addition to the introduction of semi-synthetic β-lactams with increased stability to β-lactamase-mediated ring opening (see Chapter 11), the discovery of clavulanic acid, a naturally occurring inhibitor of β-lactamase from *Streptomyces clavuligerus*, has led to the development of the semi-synthetic agents sulbactam and tazobactam, facilitating the further extension of spectrum and clinical lifetime of a number of β-lactam antibiotics. These compounds are inhibitors of the class A β-lactamase enzymes (TEM, SHV and CTX-M classes) and have found clinical utility in β-lactam–β-lactamase inhibitor combinations, including the most common combination amoxicillin–clavulanate, as well as ampicillin–sulbactam and piperacillin–tazobactam or ceftolozane–tazobactam. The first-generation β-lactamase inhibitors have found widespread application in the management of infections caused by β-lactamase-producing bacteria, but they are not active against increasingly prevalent β-lactamases, including KPCs.

The search for further β-lactamase inhibitors to extend activity beyond the class A enzymes and against important clinical β-lactamases continues and has led to the successful clinical introduction of two new inhibitor classes, with several other inhibitors or combination products under development. The diazabicyclooctanones (DBOs) are a new class of non-β-lactam β-lactamase inhibitors active against the serine β-lactamases, with avibactam a potent inhibitor of class A (including KPCs which effectively hydrolyse clavulanic acid) and class C enzymes; avibactam in combination with ceftazidime received US Food and Drug Administration (FDA) approval in 2015. The cyclic boronate, vaborbactam, a broad-spectrum inhibitor of class A serine β-lactamases, gained regulatory approval in combination with meropenem in 2017. Vaborbactam exhibits only weak activity against MBLs. While the discovery of agents with pan β-lactamase inhibitory activity, against both serine- and metallo-β-lactamase enzymes, remains the goal, several novel combinations exploiting inhibitors from the two novel classes above are at late stages of development. The structures of clinically approved β-lactamase inhibitors are given in Figure 13.4.

13.4.3 Altered Penicillin-binding Proteins and Methicillin-resistant *Staphylococcus aureus*

Acquisition or mutation of genes leading to an alteration in the structure of penicillin-binding proteins (target alteration) is responsible for resistance to β-lactam antibiotics in *S. pneumoniae* (PBP1a, PBP2b), *Haemophilus influenzae* (PBP3a and PBP3b) and by far the most clinically significant example MRSA. The acquisition of the mobile staphylococcal cassette chromosome *mec* (SCC*mec*) element, carrying the gene *mecA*, confers resistance to the β-lactamase-stable agent methicillin. The *mecA* gene encodes an additional, altered and β-lactam-insensitive penicillin-binding protein, PBP2a. Expression of *mecA* occurs alongside that of the native PBP which is inhibited by methicillin, but cell wall biosynthesis occurs in the presence of the antibiotic due to the uninhibited transpeptidase activity of PBP2a. Although first described in *S. aureus*, many SCC*mec* elements have been found in other *Staphylococcus* species including methicillin-resistant coagulase-negative staphylococci (MR-CoNS) from a wide range of ecological niches other than the hospital environment.

Interestingly, the formation of mosaic genes following transformation can lead to altered PBPs and resistance to penicillins. In *S. pneumoniae*, mosaic *pbp* genes have arisen by recombination with *Streptococcus mitis* and have led to the expression of a β-lactam-insensitive PBP. The mosaic gene, *penA*, in *Neisseria gonorrhoeae* encodes an additional PBP which confers high-level resistance to extended-spectrum cephalosporins, further restricting the therapeutic options for treatment of infections caused by this organism.

13.5 Resistance to Glycopeptide Antibiotics

The glycopeptide antibiotics vancomycin and teicoplanin are used clinically for the treatment of Gram-positive bacterial infections, often as 'last-resort' agents for severe infection. In addition to these actinomycete-derived glycopeptide agents, the second-generation semi-synthetic

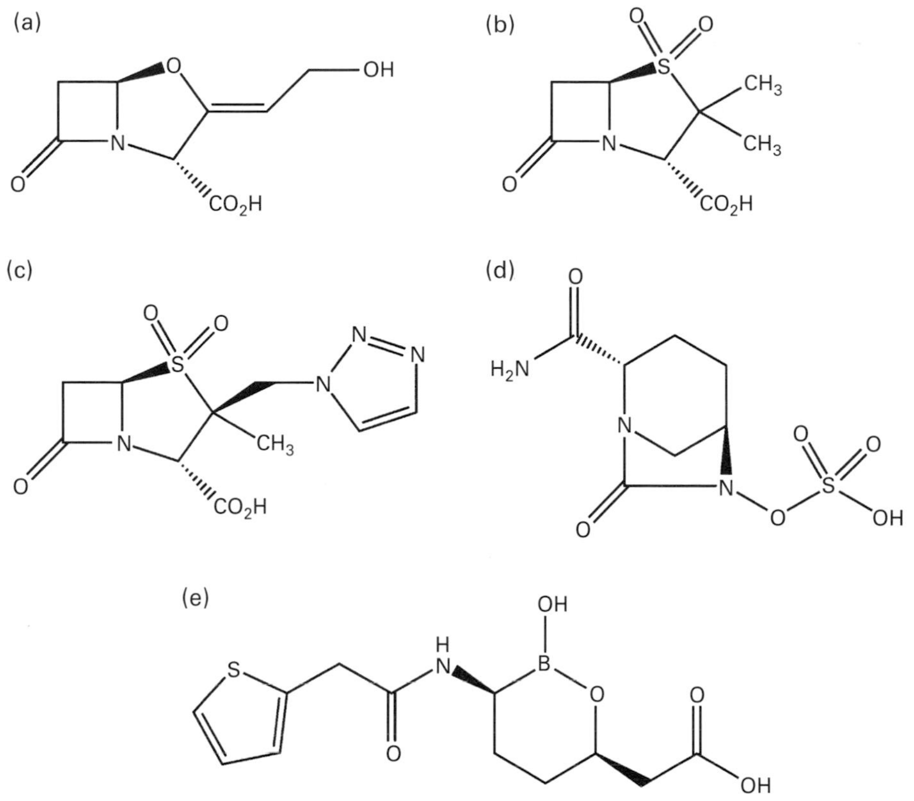

(a) (b) (c) (d) (e)

Figure 13.4 Structures of β-lactamase inhibitors: (a) clavulanic acid, (b) sulbactam, (c) tazobactam, (d) avibactam and (e) vaborbactam.

lipoglycopeptides telavancin, dalbavancin and oritavancin have been developed and approved for the treatment of Gram-positive infections. Glycopeptides are unable to cross the outer membrane of Gram-negative bacteria, which are therefore intrinsically resistant. In Gram-positive bacteria, these agents target late-stage peptidoglycan cross-linking by specifically binding the C-terminal D-alanyl-D-alanine (D-Ala-D-Ala) of the peptidoglycan precursor N-acetyl-muramyl-pentapeptide, forming a complex stabilised by five hydrogen bonds. In so doing, the transglycosylation (polysaccharide backbone polymerisation) and transpeptidation (peptide cross-linking of the polysaccharide backbone) are inhibited. Thus, cell wall synthesis is inhibited, and the accumulation of cell wall cytoplasmic precursors leads to inhibition of nucleic acid and protein synthesis. The lipoglycopeptides, bearing a lipophilic side chain, also interact with the bacterial cell membrane leading to its disruption, the leakage of cytoplasmic components and rapid depolarisation.

Resistance to the glycopeptide antibiotics arises primarily through target modification due to operons encoding enzymes for the synthesis of alternative peptidoglycan precursors which have low affinity for glycopeptide complexation. These enzymes lead to replacement of the C-terminal D-Ala-D-Ala of the peptidoglycan pentapeptide with either D-alanyl-D-lactate (D-Ala-D-Lac) or D-alanyl-D-serine (D-Ala-D-Ser). Nine operons conferring glycopeptide resistance have been reported (vanA-E, vanG and vanL-N), with nomenclature based on the sequence of genes present in the operon showing ligase activity, either D-Ala-D-Lac ligase (*van A*, *vanB*, *vanD* and *vanM*) or D-Ala-D-Ser ligase (*vanC*, *vanE*, *vanG*, *vanL* and *vanN*). The expression of the resistance operon is regulated by a two-component system comprising a sensor histidine kinase (VanS) and a response regulator (VanR). Glycopeptide resistance mediated via a D-Ala-D-Lac phenotype (VanA being the archetypal example of this phenotype, but also VanB, VanD and VanM) requires expression of a ligase (VanA, VanB, VanD and VanM), a dehydrogenase (VanH) and a D,D-dipeptidase (VanX). VanH encodes a D-lactate dehydrogenase/α-keto acid reductase and generates D-lactate, which is the substrate for VanA and the other D-Ala-D-Lac ligases. The organisation of the archetypal *vanA* and *vanC* operons are shown in Figure 13.5. This results in cell wall precursors terminating in D-Ala-D-Lac to which vancomycin binds with very low affinity, with this change in affinity resulting from the loss of one hydrogen bond. The complex formed between vancomycin and D-Ala-D-Ala is stabilised by five

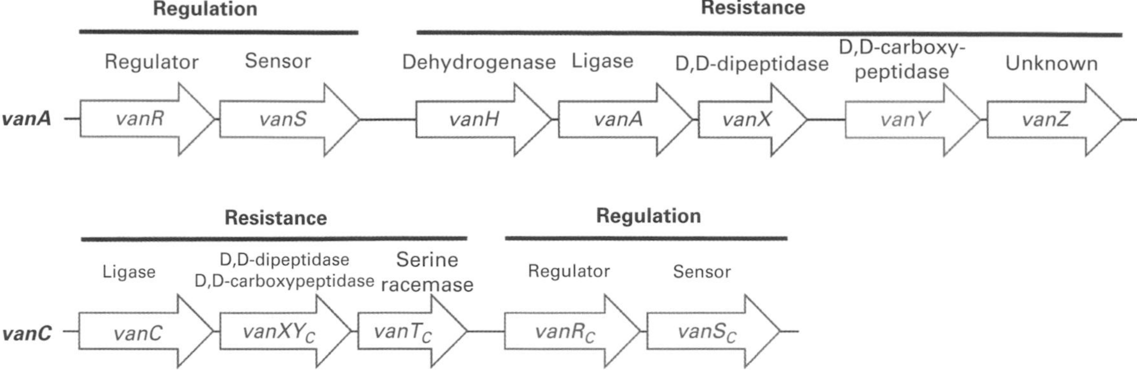

Figure 13.5 Organisation of archetypal vancomycin resistance (*van*) gene clusters, D-alanyl-D-lactate (D-Ala-D-Lac) resistance operon (*vanA*) and D-alanyl-D-serine (D-Ala-D-Ser) resistance operon (*vanC*). Coding sequences are represented by open arrows (with the direction of transcription), green arrows indicate genes necessary for resistance, blue arrows are regulatory genes, orange arrow denotes accessory genes and grey arrows represent genes of unknown function. *Source:* Adapted from Lebreton and Cattoir (2020).

hydrogen bonds, whereas only four bonds can form between vancomycin and D-Ala-D-Lac and the complex is therefore unstable, suffering a 1000-fold decrease in antibiotic activity as a result (Figure 13.6). VanX encodes a D-Ala-D-Ala dipeptidase which can modify endogenous D-Ala-D-Ala precursors. With respect to the D-Ala-D-Ser phenotype, the proteins required for resistance are a D-Ala-D-Ser ligase (VanC, VanE, VanG, VanL and VanN), a D,D-dipeptidase/carboxypeptidase (VanXY, which synthesises the dipeptide D-Ala-D-Ser) and a serine racemase (VanT, which converts L-Ser to D-Ser).

Vancomycin resistance in clinical strains of enterococci (VRE) was first reported in 1988 in Europe, and in the early 1990s in the USA, and found to be VanA-type resistance. The emergence of vancomycin resistance at this time correlates with the increasing use of vancomycin due to increasing incidence of MRSA infections. Phenotypic VanA-type resistance is now the most common and widespread, and confers high-level resistance to vancomycin and teicoplanin. VREs now account for more than 20% of all enterococcal infections and constitute important hospital- and healthcare-acquired pathogens. Genetic analysis of the *vanA* operon indicates a close homology with genes present in the vancomycin-producing strain *Amycolatopsis orientalis*, which suggests that genes originally intended to protect glycopeptide-producing bacteria have, under selective pressure, jumped to other bacteria and are potentially the primary source of glycopeptide resistance genes. VanC resistance is intrinsic and chromosomally encoded in both *Enterococcus gallinarum* and *Enterococcus casseliflavus*, whereas the other eight operons are associated with mobile genetic elements and confer acquired resistance. VanA and VanB resistance are usually acquired via Tn3-type transposons, *Tn1546* and *Tn1547*, which are transposed into plasmids and transferred via conjugation. Transferable VanG and VanN (D-Ala-D-Ser) resistance phenotypes have also been reported. VanA and VanB remain the most common and clinically relevant resistance phenotypes in enterococci, with vanD occasionally detected. By contrast, others have only been detected in the chromosome of some isolated strains of enterococci (e.g., VanE, VanG and VanL in *Enterococcus faecalis* and VanN in *E. faecium*).

13.5.1 MRSA and Reduced Glycopeptide Susceptibility

With an increasing incidence of MRSA infections in the 1980s and 1990s, empirical therapy for these infections, particularly hospital-acquired sepsis, changed to vancomycin. The inevitable consequence of this increased selection pressure was the isolation, in 1997, of the first clinical isolate of *S. aureus* exhibiting reduced vancomycin susceptibility (intermediate resistance). Concomitantly, reports of vancomycin-sensitive *S. aureus* clinical isolates with reduced teicoplanin susceptibility began to emerge. The Clinical and Laboratory Standards Institute (CLSI) now defines three non-susceptible *S. aureus* groups distinct from vancomycin-susceptible *S. aureus* (VSSA): vancomycin-resistant *S. aureus* (VRSA), vancomycin-intermediate *S. aureus* (VISA) and heterogenous vancomycin-intermediate *S. aureus* (hVISA), denoting vancomycin heteroresistance as a result of subpopulations of cells with varying levels of resistance to vancomycin. hVISA has typical minimum inhibitory concentration (MIC) values of $\leq 2\,\mu g\ ml^{-1}$ but has subpopulations with MICs in the intermediate range. The interpretative criteria for susceptibility testing for vancomycin are as follows: strains with MICs $<4\,\mu g\ ml^{-1}$ are considered sensitive, $4–8\,\mu g\ ml^{-1}$ intermediate and $\geq 16\,\mu g\ ml^{-1}$ resistant. The term glycopeptide-intermediate *S. aureus* has also been

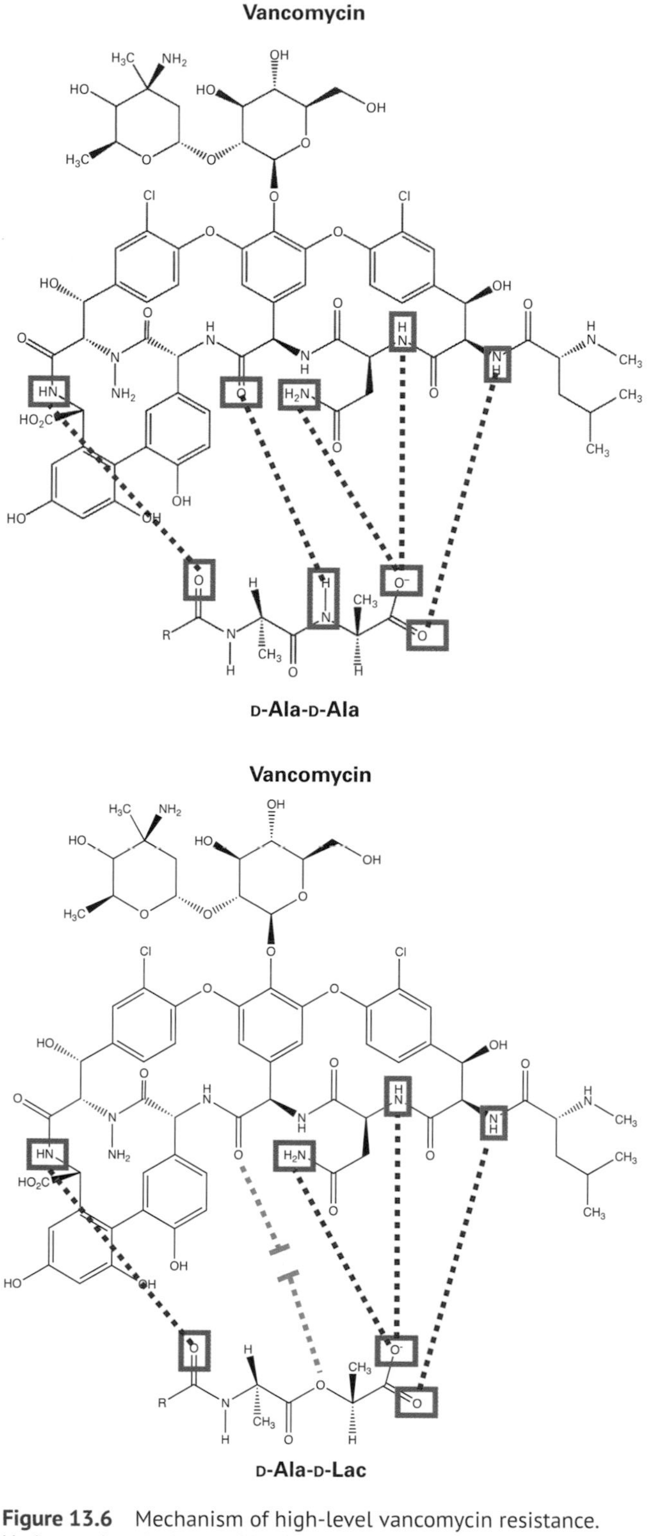

Vancomycin

D-Ala-D-Ala

Vancomycin

D-Ala-D-Lac

Figure 13.6 Mechanism of high-level vancomycin resistance. Hydrogen bonds denoted by dashed red lines. The interaction of vancomycin with D-Ala-D-Ala is stabilised by five hydrogen bonds, while in the case of D-Ala-D-Lac, the substitution of -NH by oxygen in the peptide backbone disrupts formation of a major hydrogen bond with vancomycin, resulting in reduced antibiotic affinity. *Source:* Adapted from Lebreton and Cattoir (2020).

used to denote strains with vancomycin or teicoplanin MICs of 8 μg ml^{-1}.

The transfer of *van* resistance genes from enterococci leading to high-level vancomycin resistance in *S. aureus* was first shown experimentally *in vitro* and in animal models, before the first VRSA clinical isolates appeared in 2002; this firmly established the potential for acquisition of the *vanA* gene from VRE in clinical practice. In a high number of cases, the isolation of VRSA strains alongside VRE from the same patient has been reported, but genetic analysis currently supports the hypothesis that these strains independently acquire the *Tn1546* plasmid carrying a *vanA* operon. Unlike the VRSA isolates, VISA and hVISA do not harbour *vanA*, *vanB* or *vanC* and the mechanism(s) of resistance remain poorly characterised. However, these strains show longer doubling times, decreased susceptibility to lysostaphin, increased cell wall thickness, alteration in cell wall teichoic acid content, reduced autolysis and repression of the staphylococcal global regulator Agr. In addition, increased expression of PBP2 and PBP2a and cell wall precursors are expected to 'trap' vancomycin, alongside reduced expression of PBP4 and reduced levels of peptidoglycan cross-linking (through amidation of glutamine in cell wall muropeptides); these effects are observed in most isolates and all are expected to contribute to intermediate susceptibility to vancomycin.

13.6 Resistance to Aminoglycoside Antibiotics

Aminoglycosides are potent, broad-spectrum antibiotics that are active against both Gram-positive and Gram-negative bacteria exerting their effect by an inhibition of protein synthesis. These agents are hydrophilic aminoglycosidic aminocyclitols (amino sugars linked to a dibasic aminocyclitol ring via glycosidic bonds) possessing a number of amino and hydroxy substituents. At physiological pH, the amine groups are protonated rendering the aminoglycosides polycationic. It is this polycationic nature that affords these agents their affinity for nucleic acids, particularly the acceptor (A) site of 16S ribosomal RNA. The high-affinity binding of aminoglycosides to the A site perturbs its conformation which causes codon misreading by interfering with the accurate recognition of cognate tRNA by rRNA; it may also inhibit translocation of the tRNA from the A to the peptidyl-tRNA (P) site. The aminoglycosides thus promote error-prone protein synthesis, the products of which are released and damage cellular components, primarily the cell membrane. While high-level aminoglycoside resistance as a self-protective strategy in aminoglycoside-producing microorganisms is achieved by methylation of the rRNA, this is *not* a major mechanism of acquired resistance in previously susceptible strains. Clinical aminoglycoside resistance most commonly arises from enzyme-mediated structural modification which compromises the ability of the antibiotic to interact with rRNA leading to a loss of antibacterial activity. Target site modification and efflux mechanisms (intrinsic resistance in *P. aeruginosa* is due to resistance–nodulation–division (RND) efflux pumps and the multiple efflux (Mex)XY-OprM pump) may also have a role to play, with multiple resistance mechanisms often observed in a resistant isolate.

Three major families of aminoglycoside-modifying enzymes (AMEs) have been categorised: the aminoglycoside *O*-phosphotransferases (APHs), the aminoglycoside *O*-nucleotidyltransferases (ANTs) and the aminoglycoside *N*-acetyltransferases (AACs). Respectively, these enzymes have the ability to phosphorylate, adenylate or acetylate susceptible amino or hydroxyl groups at various positions on the aminoglycoside molecule. The largest group of these AMEs is the AACs, which acetylate amino groups on the aminoglycoside scaffold. There are four principal subclasses within the AAC group, classified according to the specific amino group that is acetylated. AAC(1) and AAC(3) acetylate the amino groups at positions 1 and 3 on the 2-deoxystreptamine ring, while AAC(2′) and AAC(6′) modify those amino groups at the 2′ and 6′ positions on the 2,6-di-deoxy-2,6-diaminoglucose ring, respectively (for numbering, see Figure 13.7). In Gram-negative bacteria, the enzyme AAC(6′) confers resistance to tobramycin, amikacin and netilmicin, AAC(3)-IIa to tobramycin, netilmicin and gentamicin and AAC(3)-I to gentamicin. A hybrid enzyme, combining both acetyltransferase and phosphatase activities, AAC(6′)–APH(2″), has been described in *E. faecalis* which confers high-level resistance to most aminoglycosides, including tobramycin. The aminoglycoside phosphotransferases catalyse the adenosine triphosphate (ATP)-dependent phosphorylation of hydroxyl groups on aminoglycosides, resulting in modifications which reduce the ability of the antibiotic to participate in hydrogen bonding with rRNA. Most APHs target the hydroxyl group in the 3′ position, although variants which phosphorylate the 2″ hydroxyl have been reported. The activity of all members of the APHs leads to kanamycin and neomycin resistance, but APH-mediated amikacin and gentamicin resistance has also been described. Finally, the ANTs catalyse the addition of adenosine monophosphate (AMP) to hydroxyl groups at the 2″, 3″, 4′, 6 and 9 positions, with ANT(2″) and ANT(4′) the most clinically relevant. Recently, a novel genomic island encoding six AMEs representing all three AME classes was reported in *Campylobacter coli*. Attempts to circumvent these AMEs have focused on the rational design of structurally modified aminoglycosides, including tobramycin which lacks the 3′ hydroxyl group and is thus not a substrate for APH(3′) and amikacin which has an acylated N-1 group and is therefore not a substrate for several AMEs. Currently, a number of these modified aminoglycoside antibiotics are in preclinical development for the treatment of Gram-negative and non-tuberculous mycobacterial (NTM) infections.

13.7 Resistance to Tetracycline Antibiotics

The tetracycline antibiotics chlortetracycline and oxytetracycline were discovered in the 1940s, and studies of representative populations before their widespread clinical use indicate that emergence of resistance is a relatively modern

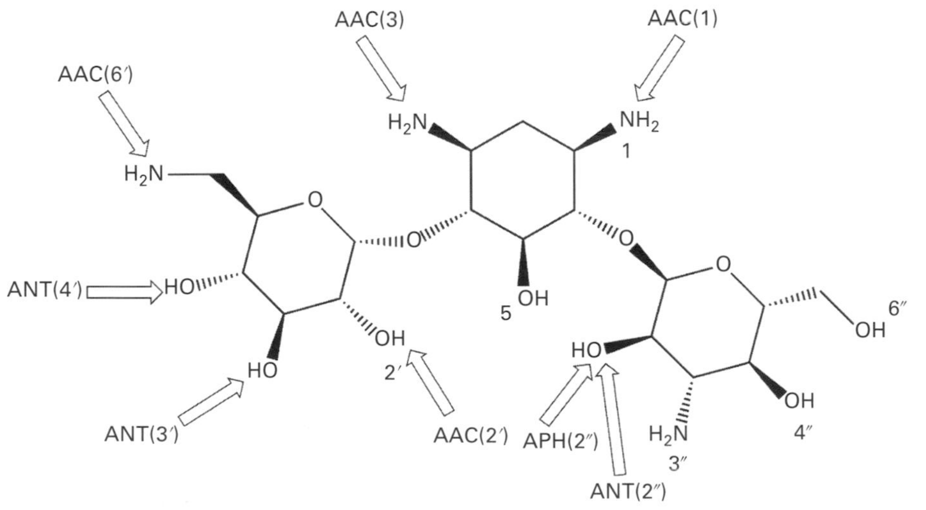

Figure 13.7 Structure of kanamycin A showing the system of ring numbering and sites of action of some aminoglycoside-modifying enzymes. AAC, aminoglycoside *N*-acetyltransferases; ANT, aminoglycoside *O*-nucleotidyltransferases; APH, aminoglycoside *O*-phosphotransferases.

event, following their expanded use in human, animal and agricultural applications. Resistance to tetracyclines is now widespread in both commensal and pathogenic bacteria, due to the acquisition of *tet* genes. The primary mechanisms of tetracycline resistance are efflux and ribosomal (target) protection; tetracycline-inactivating enzymes have been described, although their contribution to clinical resistance remains unclear.

Antibiotic efflux is the main mechanism of acquired resistance to the tetracyclines with more than 28 distinct classes of efflux pump having been described to date. The Tet efflux pumps, such as TetA, belong to the major facilitator superfamily (MFS) of efflux pumps (see also Chapter 20), which exchange a proton (H^+) for a tetracycline-cation (usually Mg^{2+}) complex against a concentration gradient. The intracellular concentration of tetracycline is thus reduced below inhibitory concentrations. Most tetracycline resistance pumps confer resistance to tetracycline but not to second-generation (minocycline, doxycycline) or third-generation glycylcycline (tigecycline) agents. In Gram-negative bacteria, the efflux determinants comprise divergently oriented efflux and repressor proteins that share overlapping promoter and operator regions. The *tet* resistance gene is negatively regulated by a Tet repressor protein, TetR. In the absence of tetracycline, TetR binds to *tet* operators to block transcription of the efflux pump. However, tetracycline binds to TetR leading to its dissociation from the *tet* operator which induces expression of the TetA efflux pump. This mechanism of regulation most likely applies to all of the Gram-negative efflux systems including *tet*(A), *tet*(C), *tet*(D), *tet*(E), *tet*(G) and *tet*(H). The efflux genes, *tet*(K), *tet*(L), *tet*(M) and *tet*(O), are typically associated with Gram-positive bacteria, but may also be found in Gram-negatives. No repressor proteins have been identified for *tet*(K) or *tet*(L) genes, and regulation of plasmid-borne resistance appears to be by translational attenuation, involving stem-loop mRNA structures and tetracycline-induced unmasking of the ribosome-binding site permitting translation of the efflux protein. Regulation of chromosomal *tet*(L) expression involves tetracycline-promoted stalling of ribosome action during translation of early codons of the leader peptide, which normally allows re-initiation of translation at the ribosome-binding site for the structural gene.

Ribosomal protection is mediated by proteins which inhibit the action of tetracycline in stabilising the post-translocational state of the ribosome which prevents delivery of aa-tRNA to the ribosomal A-site. To date, 12 distinct classes of ribosomal protection proteins (RPPs) have been described, with TetO and TetM the most extensively characterised. RPPs are thought to have evolved from *otr*A, which confers protection to the natural oxytetracycline producer, *Streptomyces rimosus*. TetO is commonly found on plasmids, while TetM is usually present on conjugative transposons. Sequence analysis of RPPs indicates that they are GTPases with significant homology to a conserved GTPase, elongation factor EF-G, and are considered paralogues of EF-G which exhibit a specialised function of rescuing translation in the presence of tetracycline agents. Both TetO and TetM exhibit guanosine triphosphate/guanosine diphosphate (GTP/GDP) binding. TetO and TetM bind to the post-translocational state ribosome, and occupy a similar binding site to EF-G. While RPPs confer resistance to first- and second-generation tetracyclines, they have no effect on third-generation agents such as tigecycline.

Tetracycline-inactivating enzymes have been reported in a wide range of environmental, commensal and pathogenic bacteria and confer resistance through alteration of the tetracycline molecule. Tetracycline-resistance determinants, *tet*X and *tet*37, encode oxygen- and reduced nicotinamide adenine dinucleotide phosphate (NADPH)-dependent monooxygenases which hydroxylate a carbon at position C11a between rings B and C in the tetracycline scaffold. This hydroxylation reduces the ability of tetracyclines to coordinate Mg^{2+}, reducing the affinity of the tetracycline–cation complex for the ribosome and rendering the hydroxylated derivative susceptible to decomposition. The clinical importance of tetracycline-inactivating enzymes is unclear and unlikely to be important in resistance to third-generation agents. The widespread emergence of resistance to first- and second-generation tetracyclines has prompted the development of the 9-glycyltetracyclines (9-glycylcyclines) (Figure 13.8). The 9-amino-acylamido derivatives of minocycline exhibited comparable activity to earlier tetracyclines, but modification of the acyl group to include *N,N*-dialkylamine or 9-*tert*-butyl-glycylamido moieties retained the antimicrobial activity of the compounds while allowing activity against strains containing *tet* genes responsible for conferring both efflux and ribosomal protection mechanisms of resistance. Of these compounds, the 9-*tert*-butyl-glycylamido derivative (GAR-936 or tigecycline) gained FDA regulatory approval in 2005 and is indicated for both complicated skin and soft tissue infections and complex intra-abdominal infections.

13.8 Resistance to Fluoroquinolone Antibiotics

The fluoroquinolone antibiotics are synthetic derivates of the quinolones (themselves modifications of 1-alkyl-1,8-naphthyridin-4-one-3-carboxylic acid) whereby the carbon in position 8 of the scaffold is replaced by nitrogen and an addition of a fluorine atom at the sixth position

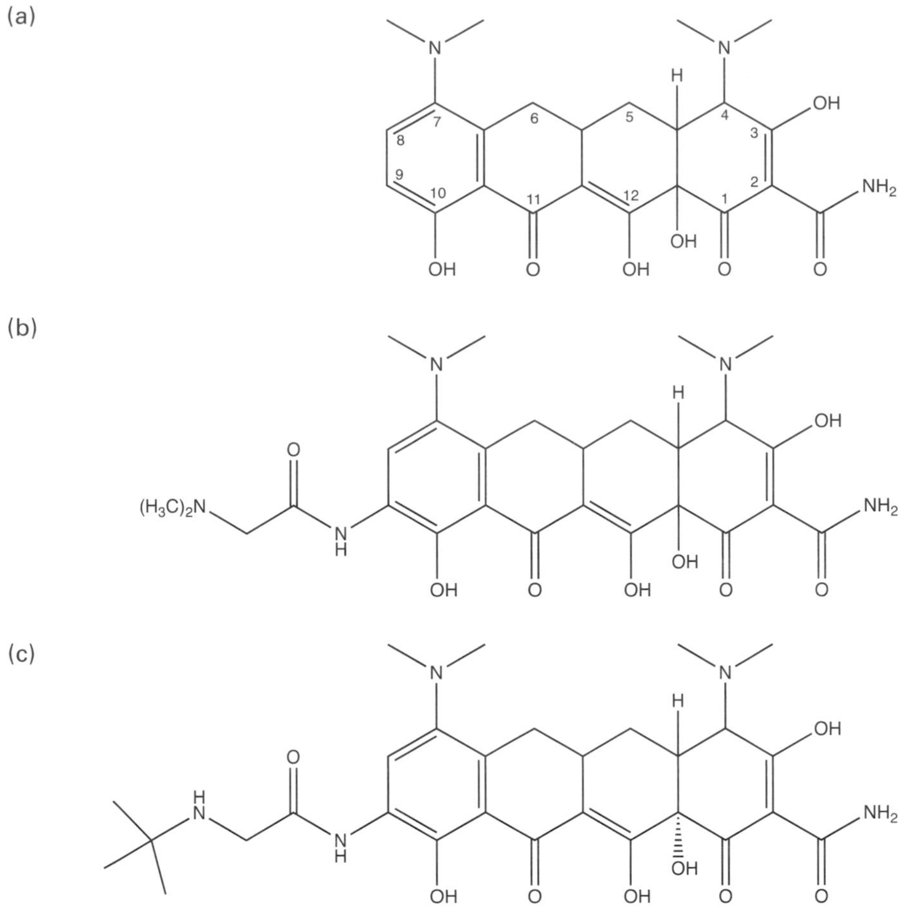

(a)

(b)

(c)

Figure 13.8 Structural modifications at the 9 position of the tetracycline antibiotic minocycline (a) confer compounds (b) 9-(*N,N*-dimethylglycylamido)-minocycline and (c) 9-(*tert*-butyl-glycylamido)-minocycline (GAR-936 or tigecycline) with activity against strains possessing efflux and ribosomal protection resistance mechanisms.

(see Chapter 11). The fluoroquinolones are broad-spectrum, potent antibiotic agents active against both Gram-positive and Gram-negative bacteria, which has led to their widespread use globally in the treatment of both human and veterinary infections. There are now four generations of quinolone/fluoroquinolone antibiotics in clinical use, and resistance has been shown predictably to correlate with consumption of these agents. In the UK, more than 17% of *E. coli* isolates exhibit fluoroquinolone resistance, whereas in Italy over 50% of *K. pneumonia* clinical isolates are resistant. Resistance to fluoroquinolones is now widespread and occurs via a range of mechanisms, primarily target-site mutation and efflux.

Fluoroquinolones bind to and inhibit two bacterial type II topoisomerase enzymes: DNA gyrase and topoisomerase IV, key enzymes in bacterial DNA replication. DNA gyrase introduces negative supercoils into bacterial DNA in order to unwind over-coiled DNA into a relaxed conformation; it can also add further negative supercoils into relaxed DNA giving rise to an under-coiled conformation. Topoisomerase IV facilitates segregation of catenated (linked) chromosomes during cell division. In Gram-negative bacteria, DNA gyrase is the primary target for fluoroquinolones, whereas in Gram-positive bacteria both topoisomerases are inhibited. DNA gyrase and topoisomerase IV are both heterotetrameric proteins, and consist of two copies of two different subunits, either a GyrA and GyrB subunit in DNA gyrase or a ParC and ParE subunit in topoisomerase IV (GrlA and GrlB in *S. aureus*). High-level fluoroquinolone resistance most commonly comes about via mutation in one or more of the genes encoding the topoisomerase subunits (*gyrA*, *gyrB*, *parC* and *parE*). Mutations arise within a short DNA sequence of these genes referred to as the quinolone-resistance-determining region (QRDR), leading to amino acid substitutions for example at Ser83 (*E. coli* numbering) in GyrA whereby the serine (with a side chain hydroxyl group) is replaced by an amino acid bearing a bulky hydrophobic side chain. This substitution leads to a conformational change and a reduction or loss of affinity for fluoroquinolone binding. Mutations in *gyrB* have also been detected but are likely to be less important; similarly, mutations in *parE* leading to resistance are not commonly observed. Interestingly, the fourth-generation fluoroquinolone, moxifloxacin, which targets GyrA and ParC with equal affinity in *S. pneumoniae*, has replaced older second-generation agents such as ciprofloxacin and levofloxacin which primarily target ParC and to which resistance has developed. This has led to an increase in isolates with mutations to both *gyrA* and *parC*. A number of transmissible resistance elements carrying genes encoding quinolone/fluoroquinolone resistance have been reported, frequently occurring on plasmids. These plasmid-mediated quinolone resistance (PMQR) genes were first described in 1998 in a clinical isolate of *K. pneumoniae*. The archetypal gene, *qnr* (now *qnrA*), encodes a protein with homology to immunity proteins such as McbG. The proposed mechanism of resistance is binding of the QnR protein to topoisomerase, preventing the antibiotic interacting with the target enzyme. To date, several families of *qnr* genes have been described. In addition to PMQR efflux genes, a PMQR variant of an aminoglycoside acetyltransferase gene *aac(6′)-lb-cr*, encoding an enzyme capable of modifying some fluoroquinolones, has also been reported.

Topoisomerases are located in the cytoplasm, so fluoroquinolones must cross the cell envelope to access their target. Therefore, changes in outer membrane permeability and mutations leading to downregulation of outer membrane porins are commonly observed in fluoroquinolone-resistant bacteria. In addition, efflux contributes to fluoroquinolone resistance, and has been shown to be essential for high-level fluoroquinolone resistance. The MFS pump NorA in *S. aureus* is expressed weakly in wild-type strains and resistance is thought to occur via mutations leading to increased expression of *norA*. NorA homologues are also present in *S. pneumoniae* and *Bacillus* spp. RND tripartite efflux pumps are also important in Gram-negative bacteria (e.g., *AcrAB-TolC* in *E. coli* and *Salmonella enterica*) which are regulated in part by the multiple-antibiotic resistance (mar) operon (Section 13.17.3). Fluoroquinolones, specifically levofloxacin and moxifloxacin, have become important second-line agents in treating multidrug-resistant *Mycobacterium tuberculosis,* and efflux-mediated resistance has been identified.

13.9 Resistance to Macrolide, Lincosamide and Streptogramin Antibiotics

The macrolide, lincosamide and streptogramin (MLS) group of antibiotics are chemically and structurally distinct but share a common mode of action, inhibiting protein synthesis by binding to target sites on the ribosome. The MLS antibiotic group is primarily active against Gram-positive bacteria, Gram-negative cocci and some intracellular pathogens; typically, Gram-negative bacilli are intrinsically resistant due to the permeability barrier of the outer membrane. In general, resistance to the MLS group arises from target site modification, efflux and drug inactivation mechanisms. Target mutation is also emerging as a mechanism of resistance, with clinical importance in a range of pathogens including *Mycobacterium avium* and *Helicobacter pylori*. Target modification, involving the methylation of adenine in domain V of the 23S rRNA is the most common mechanism of resistance, and leads to cross-resistance between the macrolides, lincosamides and streptogramin B (streptogramin A antibiotics are unaffected and streptogramin A/B combinations remain effective), and is referred to as the MLS_B phenotype. The adenine-N^6-methyltransferase is encoded by a group of *erm* (erythromycin ribosome methylase) genes, and demethylates a single adenosine residue within the domain V region of 23S ribosomal RNA necessary for MLS_B antibiotic binding. Approximately 40 *erm* genes have been described and are most commonly plasmid- or transposon-associated. Expression of *erm* genes may be constitutive or inducible, with four major classes of Erm proteins reported: *erm*(A), *erm*(B), *erm*(C) and *erm*(F), with each class largely confined to a specific bacterial genus. Generally, *erm*(A)/*erm*(C) are considered staphylococcal genes, *erm*(B) streptococcal and enterococcal genes and *erm*(F) *Bacteroides* spp. genes. Inducible expression of *erm* genes leads to resistance in 14- (e.g., clarithromycin, erythromycin) and 15-membered (e.g., azithromycin) ring macrolides only, with sensitivity to lincosamide and streptogramin antibiotics unaffected. An emerging mechanism of resistance to the macrolides, target mutation of domain V of rRNA through mutations at residues A2058 and A2059, has been shown to confer resistance and give rise to an MLS_B or macrolide-lincosamide resistance (ML) phenotype, respectively. Mutations occur in ribosomal RNA (*rrn*) operons in bacteria carrying one or two *rrn* copies, and are responsible for clarithromycin resistance in *M. avium* and *H. pylori*.

Efflux mechanisms contribute to intrinsic resistance in the MLS_B group antibiotics in Gram-negative bacteria, whereas acquisition of genes for efflux-mediated resistance in Gram-positive bacteria constitutes the second major mechanism of macrolide resistance. Expression of *msr*(A) genes (found in *Staphylococcus* spp.) encoding an efflux pump of the ATP-binding-cassette (ABC) transporter superfamily, alongside a contribution from chromosomal genes, leads to a functional efflux pump with specificity for

14- and 15-membered macrolides and streptogramin B (MS_B phenotype). Lincosamides such as clindamycin are unaffected by this efflux mechanism. In a fashion similar to *erm* gene induction, erythromycin and other 14- and 15-membered macrolides induce expression of *msr*(A), whereas streptogramins do not, so streptogramin resistance comes about only after induction by these compounds. Expression of the *mef*(A) gene, encoding an efflux pump of the MFS and found in *Streptococcus* spp. (including *Streptococcus pyogenes*, *S. pneumoniae* and *Streptococcus agalactiae*), leads to macrolide resistance, affecting 14- and 15-membered macrolides. No resistance to 16-membered ring macrolides (e.g., rokitamycin), lincosamides or streptogramins is observed. Acquisition and expression of *vga*(A) and *vga*(B) genes encoding ABC transporter superfamily efflux proteins confer streptogramin resistance in *S. aureus*.

The clinical relevance of drug modification as a resistance mechanism is still unclear, since it appears to confer only low-level resistance to macrolides and lincosamides. The gene *mph*(C) encoding a phosphotransferase capable of inactivating macrolides has been reported in *S. aureus*. In the staphylococci and *E. faecium*, lincosamide nucleotidyltransferase genes *lnu*(A) and *lnu*(B) capable of lincosamide modification and inactivation have been reported.

13.10 Resistance to Chloramphenicol

Chloramphenicol inhibits protein synthesis by binding the 50S ribosomal subunit, preventing the peptidyltransfer step. Decreased outer membrane permeability and active efflux have been identified as factors contributing to chloramphenicol resistance in Gram-negative bacteria. For example, the *cmlA* gene first identified in chloramphenicol-resistant *P. aeruginosa* in 1979 has homology to proteins of the MFS transmembrane transporters, and genes homologous or identical to *cmlA* have been reported in a wide range of Gram-negative bacteria. However, the major resistance mechanism is enzymatic drug inactivation by chloramphenicol acetyltransferase (CAT). CATs have been found in a wide variety of both Gram-positive and Gram-negative bacteria, and while the CAT enzymes share some common attributes, the *cat* genes, typically plasmid-borne, share little homology. CAT enzymes are classified, on the basis of amino acid sequence, into type A and type B. Both families of CAT enzymes, though diverse, inactivate chloramphenicol through *O*- acetylation of the 3-hydroxyl group, which prevents the drug from binding to its target site.

13.11 Resistance to Oxazolidinone Antibiotics

Linezolid, the first of a new class of oxazolidinone antibiotics with a novel target in protein synthesis, gained regulatory approval in the year 2000. Linezolid and tedizolid exhibit a unique affinity for the 50S rRNA of Gram-positive bacteria (twice that of the corresponding molecule in Gram-negatives) and are approved for the treatment of Gram-positive infections, including those caused by MRSA and vancomycin-resistant bacteria (including VRE), pneumonia and complicated skin and soft-tissue infections. Resistance has been reported, though at low frequency, particularly after prolonged clinical administration. The main mechanism of resistance is through ribosomal mutations to oxazolidinone-binding sites, especially mutations in the central loop in the V domain of 23S rRNA genes. Mutation in G257T in the domain V region of 23S rRNA has been reported in linezolid-resistant *S. aureus*, *Staphylococcus haemolyticus*, *Staphylococcus epidermidis* and *E. faecium*. Mutations in L3, L4 and L23 ribosomal proteins are also implicated in oxazolidinone resistance. Acquisition of a plasmid-encoded linezolid resistance gene, *cfr* (chloramphenicol–florfenicol resistance), was shown, in 2007, to render a clinical isolate of MRSA linezolid-resistant and has since been detected in human isolates of *E. faecium* and *S. epidermidis*. The *cfr* gene encodes a methyltransferase of the *S*-adenosylmethionine (SAM) enzyme family, which catalyses the methylation of the 23S rRNA gene at the functionally critical adenosine residue A2503 of the large ribosomal subunit. A novel resistance gene, *optrA*, encoding an ABC-F protein, capable of conferring transferable resistance to both linezolid and tedizolid, was detected in clinical isolates *E. faecium* and *E. faecalis* in 2015. More recently, another ABC-F protein, encoded by *potX*, has been associated with linezolid resistance. The precise role of ABC-F proteins in mediating oxazolidinone resistance is not fully elucidated but they have been shown *in vitro* to bring about ribosomal protection and dose-dependent ribosomal rescue by displacing antibiotics from the ribosome.

13.12 Resistance to Trimethoprim

Trimethoprim competitively inhibits dihydrofolate reductase (DHFR), an enzyme of the folate synthesis pathway, and is primarily indicated for the prophylaxis and treatment of urinary tract infections. In the UK in 2017, surveillance data from the 'English Surveillance Programme for Antimicrobial Utilisation and Resistance' reported that over a third of isolates from patients suffering urinary tract infections were resistant to trimethoprim, with resistance rising especially among the *Enterobacteriaceae*. Trimethoprim resistance in *E. coli* clinical isolates is variable but prevalent, ranging from 10 to 70% of isolates in various parts of the globe. Resistance to trimethoprim can come about through the over-production of host DHFR, alterations in membrane permeability, spontaneous mutation in the structural gene for intrinsic DHFR, expression of a naturally insensitive DHFR enzyme or horizontal acquisition of *dfr* genes encoding resistant DHFR enzymes. To date, more than 30 *dfr* genes have been reported, typically associated with integrons which facilitate horizontal resistance gene transfer; both class 1 and class 2 integrons have been shown to harbour *dfr* gene cassettes. Two major types of *dfr* genes are described, *dfrA* and *dfrB*, based on the size of the gene product, with type A DHFR proteins of between 157 and 187 amino acid residues and the shorter type B DHFR proteins of 78 amino acid residues.

13.13 Resistance to Mupirocin

Nasal carriage of MRSA strains has been identified as a major risk factor in developing surgical site infections (SSIs) post surgery and therefore is an important target for infection control protocols aimed at reducing spread and acquisition. Mupirocin (pseudomonic acid A) is an effective topical antimicrobial and is the most commonly used agent for nasal decolonisation of MRSA/*S. aureus* prior to surgery; high-level resistance has been associated with decolonisation failure. Mupirocin is an analogue of isoleucine and it exerts its antimicrobial activity through the inhibition of protein synthesis via a competitive reversible inhibition of isoleucyl–tRNA synthetase (IRS), the enzyme which conjugates tRNA and isoleucine to form isoleucyl–tRNA. Mupirocin susceptibility for *S. aureus* is characterised, based on MICs, as follows: susceptible (MIC $\leq 4\,\mu g\ ml^{-1}$), low-level mupirocin resistance (MIC $8\text{–}64\,\mu g\ ml^{-1}$), high-level mupirocin resistance $\geq 512\,\mu g\ ml^{-1}$. High-level resistance in *S. aureus* and coagulase-negative staphylococci is usually due to the acquisition of plasmid-mediated *mupA*, which encodes a novel IRS with only 30% homology to the mupirocin-sensitive form. Interestingly, *mupA*-positive strains of *S. aureus* (as determined by polymerase chain reaction [PCR]) which exhibit only low-level mupirocin resistance have been described; however, the *mupA* gene is located on the chromosome and not a plasmid in these strains.

13.14 Resistance to the Polymyxin Antibiotic Colistin (Polymyxin E)

The emergence and rapid increase in cases of serious carbapenemase-producing *Enterobacteriaceae* infections with restricted therapeutic options have led to reliance on tigecycline and colistin (either alone or in combination). Colistin, one of just two polymyxins in clinical use, is a drug of last resort in the management of serious Gram-negative infections. The emergence of these antibiotic-resistant infections has led to an increase in colistin use globally, with the accompanying increased risk of resistance development; this is compounded by the widespread use of colistin as a feed additive in animal production in low- and middle-income countries (LMICs). Polymyxin resistance is caused by the structural alteration of lipopolysaccharide (LPS), specifically the negatively charged lipid A component (see Chapter 3) through chemical substitution of negatively charged phosphate groups, subsequently leading to reduction in polymyxin-binding affinity.

Resistance mechanisms, although regulated differently between species, require expression of genes for the biosynthesis and transfer of the chemical moiety (e.g., 4-amino-L-arabinose, phosphoethanolamine and/or galactosamine) to lipid A, and involve modulation of two-component signal transduction systems (*pmrAB*, *phoPQ*). In some cases, loss of LPS or lipid A production may also lead to high-level polymyxin resistance. For example, in *A. baumannii,* mutations to lipid A biosynthesis genes *lpxA*, *lpxC* or *lpxD* lead to complete loss of LPS. A number of Gram-negative pathogens exhibit intrinsic resistance to polymyxin antibiotics, for example, through production of anionic capsular polysaccharide (*K. pneumoniae*), efflux mechanisms (*Neisseria meningitidis*) or LPS naturally substituted with 4-amino-L-arabinose (*Proteus mirabilis*, *Burkholderia* spp.).

Polymyxin resistance was thought to be exclusively mediated by chromosomal mutations, until 2016, when Liu and colleagues reported for the first-time plasmid-mediated resistance to colistin in commensal *E. coli* from food animals in China. The isolated strain, *E. coli* SHP45, possessed colistin resistance which could be transferred to another strain and was found to be due to a plasmid-mediated gene *mcr-1* (mobile colistin resistance-1). The plasmid could be mobilised to other *E. coli* recipients via conjugation, as well as *P. aeruginosa* and *K. pneumonia*. The gene product, MCR-1, was found to be a member of the phosphoethanolamine transferase enzyme family, which was found to be homologous to the phosphoethanolamine transferase of *Paenibacillus* spp., known producers of polymyxin. It was hypothesised that transfer of this gene to a plasmid occurred from the chromosome of an unknown polymyxin-producing bacteria to *E. coli*. Liu and colleagues stated that 'the emergence of MCR-1 heralds the breach of the last group of antibiotics, polymyxins, by plasmid mediated resistance'. Concerns regarding the transmissibility of *mcr-1* led the Chinese government to ban the use of colistin as a feed additive in 2016. The global dissemination of *mcr*-1 has been rapid, and, since its original description, several plasmid-borne alleles (*mcr*-1 to -9) have been described, although *mcr-1* remains the predominant resistance gene.

13.15 Resistance to the Lipopeptide Antibiotic Daptomycin

Daptomycin, a cyclic lipopeptide antibiotic produced by *Streptomyces roseosporus*, was first discovered by Eli Lilley and Company in the early 1980s. Although targeted for development, toxicity concerns during phase II trials ultimately led to daptomycin being abandoned as a lead compound. Despite this, daptomycin (by now acquired by Cubist Pharmaceuticals) was granted US FDA approval in 2003, for the treatment of infections caused by Gram-positive bacteria. Daptomycin targets the Gram-positive cell membrane in a number of distinct ways: disrupting membrane potential and membrane integrity and targeting lipoteichoic acid synthesis. Despite having restricted clinical indications (complicated skin and soft-tissue infections [cSSIs] and infective endocarditis caused by *S. aureus*) and relatively recent clinical introduction, reports of daptomycin resistance have emerged.

Daptomycin resistance has been reported in *Staphylococcus* spp., *Streptococcus* spp., *Bacillus subtilis* and enterococci. In *Staphylococcus* spp., the mechanisms of daptomycin resistance are not fully understood but they appear to be mediated by an alteration in bacterial cell surface charge (a greater positive charge density at the cell membrane), leading to repulsion of the cationic daptomycin from the cell surface. Daptomycin-resistant *S. aureus* is classically associated with mutations to, or overexpression of, the gene *mprF*, which codes for the bifunctional enzyme MPRF (multiple peptide resistance factor). MPRF catalyses the lysinylation (i.e., addition of a lysine residue, positively charged at physiological pH) of the anionic phospholipid phosphatidylglycerol (PG), then acts as a 'flippase', translocating the lysyl-phosphatidylglycerol (L-PG) from the inner to the outer portion of the membrane. One other mechanism is to interfere with daptomycin oligomerisation within the membrane, following calcium-dependent binding and insertion. In *Staphylococcus* spp. and *Streptococcus* spp., mutations in genes associated with the phospholipid cardiolipin (CL) are associated with resistance, presumably due to changes in the PG to CL ratio in the cell membrane, and an alteration of membrane rigidity. In *S. aureus*, mutations in *pgsA* (phosphatidylglycerol synthase) and *cdsA* (cardiolipin synthase) genes correlated with observed daptomycin resistance, while in *S. mitis* and *Streptococcus oralis*, mutations in the genes *pgsA* and *cdsA* (phosphatidate cytidylyltransferase, a key enzyme in cardiolipin biosynthesis) were associated with daptomycin resistance. The cell envelope stress response, and regulatory changes to genes modulating that stress response, appears important in the emergence of resistance among Gram-positive bacteria, with two-component regulatory systems (TCS), such as the VraSR TCS of *Staphylococcus* spp. and the orthologous LiaSR TCS of *B. subtilis* and enterococci, having been shown to be involved in daptomycin resistance, through regulation of membrane homeostasis.

13.16 Resistance to Antimycobacterial Therapy

Despite remaining one of the top three fatal infectious diseases alongside human immunodeficiency virus/acquired immunodeficiency syndrome (HIV/AIDS) and malaria, tuberculosis (TB) caused by *M. tuberculosis* is not included in the WHO priority pathogen list, since TB is the focus of other WHO programmes (such as the END TB Strategy) having been declared a WHO global health emergency in 1993. Antibiotic resistance in *M. tuberculosis* remains one of the most significant antibiotic resistance threats to human health globally, with *M. tuberculosis* exhibiting several levels of resistance including: rifampicin resistance (RR-TB); multidrug resistance (MDR-TB) defined as resistance to at least two of the most effective anti-TB antibiotics, isoniazid and rifampicin; and extensive drug resistance (XDR-TB), defined as MDR-TB which is also resistant to at least one agent from the two major second-line antibiotics used in MDR treatment regimens (fluoroquinolones [levofloxacin or moxifloxacin] and injectable drugs such as amikacin, kanamycin and capreomycin). The increasing levels of resistance are characterised by longer treatment times, with reduced global success rates. According to the WHO, treatment success rates for resistant TB infections are low. When compared to drug-susceptible *M. tuberculosis* infections where first-line treatment (with proper adherence) results in a cure rate of 83%, infections caused by MDR and XDR variants of *M. tuberculosis* have cure rates of 54 and 28%, respectively.

Significantly, *M. tuberculosis* is intrinsically resistant to a number of antibiotic agents, possessing an unusual cell envelope which limits drug penetration, drug inactivation enzymes and efflux mechanisms. In addition, mycobacterial infections, especially TB, are characterised by slow-growing bacteria, with low metabolic rates approaching dormancy, which results in an inherently low susceptibility to antibiotic challenge. As a result, therapeutic options are limited, since a number of conventional antibiotic agents are not suitable. Rifampicin is effective in targeting slow-growing microorganisms, while isoniazid is bactericidal and targets aerobically growing bacteria. Pyrazinamide, a prodrug converted to pyrazinoic acid by the action of *M. tuberculosis* pyrazinamidase putatively leading to inhibition of coenzyme A synthesis, is active at low pH and is thus well-suited to killing bacteria within necrotic foci characteristic of early infection, but is less useful in later infection where foci have resolved. Current treatment regimens are based on multiple agents, reducing the likelihood of spontaneous acquisition of resistance to all components. However, resistance may occur in patient populations which receive inadequate therapy, due to a lack of access to the complete treatment regimen, the use of individual drugs or as a result of poor adherence. The WHO recommends both directly observed therapy (DOT) for optimal therapeutic outcomes and culture-based phenotypic drug susceptibility testing (DST) for rapid diagnosis of resistance. However, in resource-limited scenarios, such sophisticated infrastructure for observed therapy and drug susceptibility testing may not be available. Resistance can occur to single agents and subsequently lead to multiply drug resistant variants.

Clinically relevant acquired resistance in *M. tuberculosis* typically occurs through chromosomal mutations, via a range of mechanisms with resistance to a given antibiotic class often through multiple mechanisms within one strain. The most common mechanism of acquired resistance is drug target alteration, which can give rise to resistance to antibiotics including, but not limited to, rifamycins, isoniazid, ethambutol, fluoroquinolones, aminoglycosides and linezolid. Resistance to rifamycins (particularly rifampicin) arises from mutations to the active β-subunit site of RNA polymerase, encoded by *rpoB*, which reduces the affinity of rifampicin for its target. A number of antimycobacterial agents are prodrugs, requiring activation at the target cell for antimicrobial activity. As a result, mechanisms which abrogate prodrug activation constitute a major route to resistance in mycobacteria. Mutation of the catalase-peroxidase gene *katG* reduces or abolishes cellular catalase activity, leading to isoniazid resistance, since the catalase-peroxidase activity of KatG is absolutely required for the conversion of isoniazid (isonicotinic acid hydrazide [INH]) to the active hydrazine derivative. In clinical isolates of *M. tuberculosis*, a point mutation in *katG* S315T is observed which retains most of the catalase-peroxidase activity but confers high-level resistance to isoniazid. Low-level rifampicin resistance can also occur through point mutations to *inhA* encoding an enoyl–acyl reductase, leading to its overexpression. Resistance to pyrazinamide, converted by pyrazinamidase encoded by *pncA*, most commonly occurs through mutations to this gene, although gene inactivation by the insertion sequence IS*6110* has been reported. Resistance to streptomycin, amikacin, kanamycin and capreomycin can arise through mutations in the 16S rRNA gene *rrs* (and *rpsL* in the case of streptomycin) leading to drug target alteration. Ethambutol resistance has been reported in a number of mycobacteria, including *M. tuberculosis*. Ethambutol, a first-line antibiotic for the treatment of TB, inhibits the polymerisation of arabinan in the arabinogalactan and lipoarabinomannan of the mycobacterial cell wall, through the inhibition of arabinosyltransferases encoded by the *embB* locus. Resistance occurs through mutations in the embCAB operon (encoding the arabinosyltransferases *embC*, *embA* and *embB*).

13.17 Multiple Drug Resistance

13.17.1 R-Plasmids

A range of mechanisms and examples of multiple antibiotic resistance have been discussed in this chapter. These include significant pathogens such as MRSA which can harbour both small cryptic plasmids and larger plasmids encoding resistance to microbicidal compounds, β-lactams, aminoglycosides and trimethoprim, and multidrug-resistant *M. tuberculosis*. Equally concerning are instances where bacteria exhibit resistance to chemically distinct families of antibiotics in a single biological event. Perhaps the earliest example of this is from 1959, whereby a previously susceptible strain of *E. coli* acquired resistance to several antibiotics through acquisition of a conjugative plasmid (R-factor) from resistant *Salmonella* and *Shigella* isolates. An R-factor, or now more commonly referred to as an R-plasmid, is a plasmid which in addition to genes conferring resistance (r-determinants) to one or several antibiotics, also harbours genes encoding for a resistance transfer factor (RTF) such as conjugative or sex pili, thus facilitating rapid plasmid transfer of resistance through the cell population by conjugation. R-plasmids are now widespread, and those carrying transposons and integrons (see below) are increasingly common, indicating a process of plasmid evolution that has resulted in highly transmissible resistance between strains and mobility between plasmids and chromosomes.

13.17.2 Mobile Gene Cassettes and Integrons

A large number of Gram-negative resistance genes are located in gene cassettes, small mobile elements usually containing a single gene or open reading frame (ORF) and a 59-base element (now referred to as *attC*) forming a specific recombination site (*attl*); this facilitates their recognition by recombinases (integron integrases [Intl]). One or more of these cassettes can be integrated into a specific location on the chromosome termed an *integron*. The cassette cannot move itself, but the recombination site confers mobility because it is recognised by specific recombinases (Intl integrases) encoded by integrons that catalyse integration of the cassette into a specific site within the integron. Thus, integrons can be considered as genetic elements that recognise and capture multiple gene cassettes (gene acquisition systems). As the gene within the cassette typically lacks a promoter, expression depends on correct integration into the integron in order to supply the upstream promoter. To date, five classes of 'mobile' integrons have been identified, all of which are associated with antibiotic resistance. Classes 1, 2 and 3 integrons have been described in clinical isolates, class 4 integrons are limited to *Vibrio cholerae* and a class 5 integron was originally described in *Aliivibrio salmonicida* (formerly *Vibrio salmonicida*) on a tetracycline resistance carrying plasmid pRVS1. Mobile integrons have played a significant role in the spread of antibiotic resistance in Gram-negative bacteria, and continue to evolve under anthropogenic-driven antibiotic selective pressures. Integrons appear capable of acquiring and expressing resistance genes from the pangenome of the microbial biosphere and have global implications for the emergence and evolution of antibiotic resistance.

13.17.3 Chromosomal Multiple Antibiotic Resistance *(mar)* Locus

The multiple antibiotic resistance (*mar*) locus was first described in *E. coli* in 1983, and implicated in cross-resistance to β-lactams, tetracyclines and quinolones. In addition to resistance to structurally unrelated antibiotics, the *mar* locus is implicated in resistance to oxidative stress, chemical disinfectants and organic solvents. The *mar* locus has been subsequently identified as being widely distributed in other enteric bacteria. The locus consists of two divergently transcribed units, *marC* and *marRAB*. Within the locus, *marA* encodes a transcriptional activator which affects expression of more than 60 genes, and controls multidrug efflux pump and porin expression. The Mar phenotype comes about through induction of the *marRAB* operon, leading to expression of MarA. The *marR* gene encodes a repressor of the operon. Mutations in *marO* or *marR* which prevent auto-repression of the operon, or inactivation of MarR following exposure to inducing agents such as salicylate, lead to the Mar phenotype. Recently, the *mar* locus has also been shown to reduce quinolone-induced DNA damage and reduce tetracycline penetration through the outer membrane. A number of effector mechanisms have been identified, including increased expression of the *AcrAB-TolC* multidrug efflux system (see Section 13.17.4) and the *soxRS* regulon. It has also been demonstrated that the *marC* gene is not involved in multiple antibiotic resistance in *E. coli*; however, the cognate function of MarC remains unknown.

13.17.4 Multidrug Efflux Pumps

Bacterial efflux pumps transport molecules, including antibiotics, out of the cell, across the cell and outer membranes, in an energy-dependent manner. Bacterial efflux pumps can have a narrow substrate specificity, leading to the efflux of a single antibiotic or class of antibiotic, or in the case of multidrug efflux pumps, recognise a broad spectrum of substrates leading to excretion of a wide range of compounds, often where little or no structural similarity exists between these substrates. Such pumps are known as MDR pumps, and belong to several families of protein transporters. A feature common to multidrug efflux pumps is a preference for agents with a significant hydrophobic domain or character. Thus, hydrophilic antibiotics such as the aminoglycosides are not typically transported by these pumps. A distinction between Gram-positive efflux systems (which traverse the cell membrane to efflux compounds from the cytoplasm) and Gram-negative efflux systems (which efflux compounds across the cell membrane, peptidoglycan wall and outer membrane) should also be made. A number of well-characterised multidrug resistance pumps in both Gram-positive and Gram-negative bacteria are reported in the literature, with new antibiotic efflux pumps continuing to be discovered in clinical and environmental isolates. While a majority of genes encoding multidrug efflux pumps are found on the chromosome, recent reports have described efflux pump genes mobilised onto plasmids, indicating multidrug efflux could be a transmissible resistance determinant in some situations. In Gram-negative bacteria, the majority of clinically relevant efflux pumps span both cytoplasmic and outer membranes, and of these the RND family of multidrug efflux pumps is the most extensively characterised. These include the *AcrAB-TolC* system in *E. coli* and the MexAB-OprM system in *P. aeruginosa*. The RND family of efflux pumps includes tripartite efflux systems, for example, MexB or AcrB, forming homotrimers in the cell membrane which then associate with a periplasmic adaptor (or linker) protein, such as MexA or AcrA, and finally an outer membrane channel protein such as OprM or TolC, respectively. In *P. aeruginosa*, MexB is predicted to be a proton antiporter with 12 membrane-spanning α-helices, while OprM shows homology with outer membrane channels of systems involved in the efflux of diverse molecules including nodulation signals and alkaline proteases. The structure of the MexAB-OprM efflux pump from *P. aeruginosa* is shown

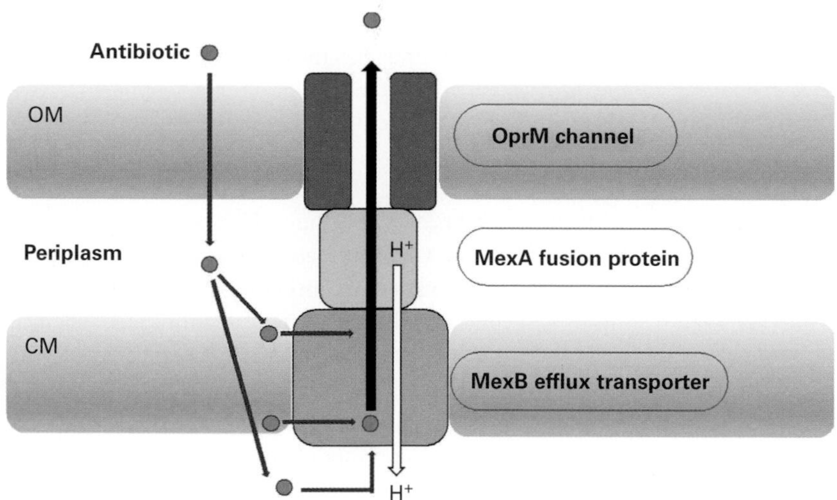

Figure 13.9 Schematic diagram for the MexAB-OprM efflux pump from *Pseudomonas aeruginosa*. Efflux of antibiotic back across the cytoplasmic (CM) and outer (OM) membranes is linked to proton influx, a process known as a proton antiport.

diagrammatically in Figure 13.9. Mutations in regulatory genes, such as *nalB*, cause over-expression of MexAB-OprM and antibiotic resistance. MexB is a proton antiporter, and efflux of this and other RND efflux pumps is proton motive force-dependent.

13.18 Clinical Resistance, MICs, Breakpoints, Phenotypic Resistance and Outcome

The mechanisms of resistance described in this chapter typically result in (and are often discovered as a result of) increases in MIC values. However, this does not always equate to clinical failure. Equally, the MIC value for a particular organism has also often been shown to have no correlation with the concentration required to inhibit or kill the same bacteria when grown as biofilms, which exhibit phenotypic resistance which is reversible upon transition back to the planktonic state. Clinically, MIC values are useful but breakpoint values are more commonly used. Breakpoints are chosen concentrations of an antibiotic which determine whether a pathogen is 'susceptible, standard dose' (S), of intermediate sensitivity now referred to as 'susceptible, increased exposure' (I), or resistant (R) to an antibiotic, and helps predict likelihood of clinical success. If the MIC remains below the breakpoint value, then the antibiotic remains clinically effective. The use of MIC values to guide the clinical selection of antibiotics assumes that MIC values, typically determined in planktonic cultures grown under optimal conditions in complex, sensitivity-test media, correlate to the sensitivity of the same microorganism growing *in vivo*. The antibiotic literature contains numerous examples of treatment failures despite apparent sensitivity in *in vitro* tests. This type of resistance is referred to as phenotypic resistance which relates to the adaptation of the microorganism to growth *in vivo*, which often involves metabolic heterogeny and biofilm formation. Subculture of these organisms onto conventional growth media in the laboratory rarely shows the existence of resistant mutants. Such a lack of sensitivity to antibiotics is usually multifactorial but nutrient depletion, leading to reduced growth rate or dormancy, the formation of persister cells and mode of growth may all contribute to reduced susceptibility/tolerance to antibiotic challenge.

The contribution of microbial biofilms (see Chapter 8) to infection has become increasingly recognised since their first description in medical-device-associated infections in the 1980s. Biofilms are now estimated to be implicated in 60–80% of all human chronic bacterial infections, particularly those associated with indwelling medical devices ranging from urinary catheters and central venous catheters to artificial joints and prosthetic heart valves. A number of chronic, recurrent infections such as chronic and exacerbating pulmonary infections in cystic fibrosis patients are known to involve biofilms composed of microorganisms which are highly tolerant to antibiotic therapy, resist normal clearance mechanisms and adhere to mucosal surfaces. Biofilms, comprising populations of cells attached to a substratum and enclosed within a self-produced extracellular polymeric matrix, typically exhibit altered growth rate and transcription compared to their planktonic counterparts. This metabolic and physiological heterogeneity, in part driven by the microenvironment (including nutrient and oxygen concentrations, redox potential and pH gradients) created within the biofilm matrix, typically results in an overall increase in tolerance or phenotypic resistance to antibiotic and microbicidal agents. Numerous studies in the literature report the lack of correlation between biofilm and planktonic susceptibility, with biofilms often requiring concentrations of antibiotics or microbicides several orders of magnitude higher to achieve eradication than for the same bacteria in the planktonic state. Thus, general biofilm resistance to antibiotic challenge appears to be largely phenotypic. The factors which contribute to the elevated tolerance or phenotypic resistance of biofilms are discussed in Chapter 8.

13.19 Conclusion

Antibiotics have been one of the most transformational discoveries in medicine; however, due to the rapid development of resistance and reduced effort directed towards the discovery of new classes of agents, the antibiotic pipeline is becoming critically depleted. The challenges associated with antibiotic discovery are significant and include: limitations in successfully culturing representative microbiomes from their environment, and a wasteful replication of discovery effort arising from limitations in differentiating similar species in screening programmes. Shortcomings such as these render the discovery process technically challenging, expensive and time-consuming. Since the 'golden era' of antibiotic discovery, few new classes of antibiotics have been described and the lack of effective platforms to deliver lead compounds has meant that the antibiotic pipeline is in a state of stagnation, with many 'big pharma' players having exited the field entirely in the past two decades. The rate at which new antibiotic compounds have been discovered (especially in the last 40 years) has not kept pace with the emergence of resistance. This scenario threatens to undermine the very foundations of our antibiotic security. However, as one era in antibiotic discovery draws to a close, a second era driven by new technologies such as machine learning and artificial intelligence coupled with genomics and proteomics could lead to the discovery of novel targets and compounds, reinvigorating the antibiotic pipeline. New business models built around incentivisation of antibiotic discovery are also necessary to attract the major pharmaceutical players back into the antibiotic discovery arena. In the interim, investment in new technologies and stringent controls aimed at reducing antibiotic use generally are necessary to preserve our current antibiotic armamentarium and to stave off an antimicrobial resistance pandemic.

Acknowledgement

The authors gratefully acknowledge the contribution of Prof Anthony W. Smith, who prepared the earlier versions of this chapter in previous editions of this book.

References

Blair, J.M.A., Webber, M.A., Baylay, A.J. et al. (2015). Molecular mechanisms of antibiotic resistance. *Nat. Rev. Microbiol.* 13 (1): 42–51.

Lebreton, F. and Cattoir, V. (2020). Resistance to glycopeptide antibiotics. In: *Bacterial Resistance to Antibiotics – From Molecules to Man* (ed. B.B. Bonev and N.M. Brown), 51–80. Chichester, UK: Wiley.

Naas, T., Oueslati, S., Bonnin, R.A. et al. (2017). Beta-lactamase database (BLDB) – structure and function. *J. Enzyme Inhib. Med. Chem.* 32: 917–191. (BLDB database website: http://bldb.eu).

O'Neill, J. (2016). Tackling drug-resistant infections globally: final report and recommendations. In: *The Review on Antimicrobial Resistance*, 1–80. London: Wellcome Trust and HM Government.

Tooke, C.L., Hinchcliffe, P., Braggington, E.C. et al. (2019). β-Lactamases and β-lactamase inhibitors in the 21st century. *J. Mol. Biol.* 431: 3472–3500.

Further Reading

Alekshun, M.N. and Levy, S.B. (1999). The mar regulon: multiple resistance to antibiotics and other toxic chemicals. *Trends Microbiol.* 7: 410–413.

Antimicrobial Resistance Collaborators (2022). Global burden of bacterial antimicrobial resistance in 2019: a systematic analysis. *Lancet* 399 (10325): 629–655.

Beyer, P. and Paulin, S. (2020). Priority pathogens and the antibiotic pipeline: an update. *Bull. World Health Organ.* 98 (3): 151.

Boucher, H.W., Talbot, G.H., Bradley, J.S. et al. (2009). Bad bugs, no drugs: no ESKAPE! An update from the Infectious Diseases Society of America. *Clin. Infect. Dis.* 48 (1): 1–12.

Centers for Disease Control and Prevention (CDC) (2019). Antibiotic resistance threats in the United States, 2019. U.S. Department of Health and Human Services, Atlanta, GA. http://www.cdc.gov/DrugResistance/Biggest-Threats.html

Du, D., Wang-Kan, X., Neuberger, A. et al. (2018). Multidrug efflux pumps: structure, function and regulation. *Nat. Rev. Microbiol.* 16: 523–539.

Gygli, S.M., Borrell, S., Trauner, A. and Gagneux, S. (2017). Antimicrobial resistance in *Mycobacterium tuberculosis*: mechanistic and evolutionary perspectives. *FEMS Microbiol. Rev.* 41: 354–373.

Krause, K.M., Serio, A.W., Kane, T.R. and Connolly, L.E. (2016). Aminoglycosides: an overview. *Cold Spring Harb. Perspect. Med.* 6: A027029.

Liu, Y.-Y., Wang, Y., Walsh, T.R. et al. (2016). Emergence of plasmid-mediated colistin resistance mechanism in animals and human beings in China: a microbiological and molecular biological study. *Lancet Infect. Dis.* 16: 161–168.

Mardon, A., Almagen, H., MacDonald, C. et al. (ed.) (2021). *Antibiotic Resistance: An Emerging Pandemic*. Edmonton: GM Press.

Nguyen, F., Starosta, A.L., Arenz, S. et al. (2014). Tetracycline antibiotics and resistance mechanisms. *Biol. Chem.* 395 (5): 559–575.

Piddock, L.J.V. (2006). Multidrug resistance efflux pumps—not just for resistance. *Nat. Rev. Microbiol.* 4: 629–636.

Redgrave, L.S., Sutton, S.B., Webber, M.A. and Piddock, L.V.J. (2014). Fluoroquinolone resistance: mechanisms, impact on bacteria, and role in evolutionary success. *Trends Microbiol.* 22 (8): 438–445.

Singer, A.C., Shaw, H., Rhodes, V. and Hart, A. (2016). Review of antimicrobial resistance in the environment and its relevance to environmental regulators. *Front. Microbiol.* 7: 1728.

Wilson, D.N., Hauryliuk, V., Atkinson, G.C. and O'Neill, A.J. (2020). Target protection as a key antibiotic resistance mechanism. *Nat. Rev. Microbiol.* 18: 637–648.

Word Health Organisation (2017) Global priority list of antibiotic-resistant bacteria to guide research, discovery and development of new antibiotics. https://www.who.int/news/item/27-02-2017-who-publishes-list-of-bacteria-for-which-new-antibiotics-are-urgently-needed

Yong, D., Toleman, M.A., Giske, C.G. et al. (2009). Characterisation of a new metallo-beta-lactamase gene, *bla* (NDM-1), and a novel erythromycin esterase gene carried on a unique genetic structure in *Klebsiella pneumoniae* sequence type 14 from India. *Antimicrob. Agents Chemother.* 53: 5046–5054.

14

Clinical Uses of Antimicrobial Drugs

Hayley Wickens[1] *and Conor Jamieson*[2]

[1] *Consultant Pharmacist Genomic Medicine, NHS Central and South Genomic Medicine Service Alliance, Southampton, UK*
[2] *Regional Antimicrobial Stewardship Lead (Midlands Region), NHS England, Birmingham, UK*

CONTENTS

Hugo and Russell's Pharmaceutical Microbiology, Ninth Edition. Edited by Brendan F. Gilmore and Stephen P. Denyer.

Companion website: https://www.wiley.com/go/HugoandRussells9e

14.1 Introduction

The worldwide use of antimicrobial drugs continues to rise; in 2016, worldwide expenditure on antibiotics was estimated at approximately $40 billion per annum. In the UK, prescribing in general practice accounts for approximately 70% of all antibiotics and largely involves oral and topical agents. Hospital use accounts for just over 20% of antibiotic prescribing, with a much heavier use of injectable agents. Dental practice and other care settings account for the remainder. Although this chapter is concerned with the clinical use of antimicrobial drugs, it should be remembered that these agents are also extensively used in veterinary practice and, to a diminishing extent, in animal husbandry as growth promoters. There is increasing recognition of the importance of a One Health approach to the use of antimicrobials (see also Chapter 5), and how the use of antimicrobials in farming, agriculture and animal health is fundamentally interlinked with the impact of antimicrobial resistance in human health. In humans, the therapeutic use of anti-infectives has revolutionised the management of most bacterial infections, as well as many parasitic and fungal diseases. The availability of highly active antiretroviral agents means that HIV infection is now managed as a long-term condition, and hepatitis C infection can now be cured with direct-acting antivirals (see Chapters 5 and 11). Although originally used for the treatment of established bacterial infections, antibiotics have proved useful in the prevention of infection in various high-risk circumstances; this applies especially to patients undergoing various surgical procedures where perioperative antibiotics have significantly reduced postoperative infectious complications.

The advantages of effective antimicrobial chemotherapy are self-evident, but this has led to a significant problem in ensuring that they are always appropriately used. Prescribers face a dilemma: initial antimicrobial therapy must be effective against all likely infective organisms for the individual presentation, but excessive use of broad-spectrum agents contributes to the development and selection of drug-resistant organisms. Hence, anti-infectives are the only class of drugs where inappropriate use in one patient can jeopardise the efficacy of treatment in other individuals.

Examples of inappropriate antimicrobial use include prescribing in situations where antibiotics are either ineffective, such as viral infections, or where the selected agent, its dose, route of administration or duration of use are inappropriate. Of particular concern is the unnecessarily prolonged use of antibiotics for surgical prophylaxis. Apart from encouraging superinfection by drug-resistant organisms, prolonged use is wasteful of health resources and unnecessarily increases the risk of adverse drug reactions. Thus, it is essential that the clinical use of these agents be based on a clear understanding of the principles that have evolved to ensure safe, yet effective, prescribing. Further information about the properties of antimicrobial agents described in this chapter can be found in Chapter 11.

14.2 Principles of Use of Antimicrobial Drugs

14.2.1 Susceptibility of Infecting Organisms

Drug selection should be based on knowledge of its activity against infecting microorganisms. Selected organisms may be predictably susceptible to a particular agent, and laboratory testing is therefore rarely performed. For example, *Streptococcus pyogenes* is uniformly sensitive to penicillin. By contrast, the susceptibility of many Gram-negative enteric bacteria is less predictable and susceptibility results should be checked for empiric prescriptions. The susceptibility of common bacterial pathogens and widely prescribed antibiotics is summarised in Table 14.1. It can be seen that, although certain bacteria are susceptible *in vitro* to a particular agent, use of that drug may be inappropriate, either on pharmacological grounds or because other less toxic agents are preferred.

14.2.2 Host Factors

In vitro susceptibility testing does not always predict clinical outcome. Host factors play an important part in determining outcome and this applies particularly to circulating and tissue phagocytic activity. Infections can progress rapidly in patients suffering from either an absolute or functional deficiency of phagocytic cells. This applies particularly to those suffering from various haematological malignancies, such as the acute leukaemias, where phagocyte function is impaired both by the disease and also by the use of potent cytotoxic drugs which destroy healthy, as well as malignant, white cells. Under these circumstances, it is essential to select agents that are bactericidal, as bacteriostatic drugs, such as the tetracyclines or sulphonamides, rely on host phagocytic activity to clear bacteria. Widely used bactericidal agents include the aminoglycosides, broad-spectrum penicillins, the cephalosporins and quinolones (see Chapter 11).

In some infections, the pathogenic organisms are located intracellularly within phagocytic cells and therefore remain relatively protected from drugs that penetrate cells poorly, such as the penicillins and cephalosporins. By contrast, erythromycin, rifampicin and the fluoroquinolones readily penetrate phagocytic cells. Legionnaires' disease is an example of an intracellular infection and is treated with macrolides or quinolones.

Table 14.1 Sensitivity of selected bacteria to common antibacterial agents. Note: This summary is not suitable for therapeutic decision-making; in these circumstances local microbiology guidelines should be consulted.

	Staphylococcus aureus (penicillin sensitive)	*Staphylococcus aureus* (penicillin resistant)	*Streptococcus pyogenes* and *Streptococcus pneumoniae*	*Enterococcus*	*Clostridium perfringens*	*Neisseria gonorrhoeae*	*Neisseria meningitidis*
Penicillin V/G	(+)	R	+*	R	+	+*	+
Methicillin, flucloxacillin	+	+*	+	R	R	R	R
Ampicillin, amoxicillin	+	R	+*	+	+	+*	+
Ticarcillin	(+)	R	(+)	R	+	(+)	(+)
Cefazolin	+	+*	+	R	(±)	(+)	(+)
Cefamandole, cefuroxime	+	+	+	R	R	(+)	+
Cefoxitin	+	+	+	R	+	(+)	(+)
Cefotaxime, ceftriaxone	+	+	+	R	+	+	+
Ceftazidime	R	R	R	R	R	R	R
Erythromycin	+	+	+	R	±	±	±
Clindamycin	+*	+*	+*	R	+*	R	R
Tetracyclines	+*	+*	±	±	(+)	+	(+)
Chloramphenicol	+	+	+	±	+	+	+
Ciprofloxacin	±	±	±	±	R	+	+
Gentamicin, tobramycin, amikacin, netilmicin	+	+	R	R	R	R	R
Sulphonamides	+	+	±	R	(±)	±	±
Trimethoprim–sulphamethoxazole	+	+	+	+	R	(+)	(+)

	Haemophilus influenzae	*Escherichia coli*	*Klebsiella* spp.	*Proteus* spp. (indole-negative)	*Proteus* spp. (indole-positive)	*Serratia* spp.	*Salmonella* spp.
Penicillin V/G	R	R	R	R	R	R	R
Methicillin, flucloxacillin	R	R	R	R	R	R	R
Ampicillin, amoxicillin	±	±	R	+	±	R	±
Ticarcillin	(+)	±	±	+	±	±	(+)
Cefazolin	±	+	±	+	R	R	(±)
Cefamandole, cefuroxime	+	+	+	+	+	R	(+)
Cefoxitin	+	+	+	+	+	±	(+)

Cefotaxime, ceftriaxone	+	+	+	+	+	+	(+)
Ceftazidime	R	+	+	+	+	+	(+)
Erythromycin	(±)	R	R	R	R	R	R
Clindamycin	R	R	R	R	R	R	R
Tetracyclines	+	+	±	±	R	R	(+)
Chloramphenicol	+*	+	±	+	±	+	+*
Ciprofloxacin	+	+	+	+	+	+	+
Gentamicin, tobramycin, amikacin, netilmicin	+	+	+*	+	+	+*	(+)
Sulphonamides	±	±	±	±	±	R	±
Trimethoprim–sulphamethoxazole	+	+	+	+	+	R	+

	Shigella spp.	*Pseudomonas* spp.	*Bacteroides fragilis*	Other *Bacteroides* spp.	*Chlamydia* spp.	*Mycoplasma pneumoniae*	*Rickettsia* spp.
Penicillin V/G	R	R	R	+	R	R	R
Methicillin, flucloxacillin	R	R	R	R	R	R	R
Ampicillin, amoxicillin	±	R	R	+	R	R	R
Ticarcillin	(+)	+*	±	±	R	R	R
Cefazolin	(±)	R	R	±	R	R	R
Cefamandole, cefuroxime	(±)	R	R	R	R	R	R
Cefoxitin	(+)	R	+	+	R	R	R
Cefotaxime, ceftriaxone	+	(±)	R	R	R	R	R
Ceftazidime	(+)	+	R	±	R	R	R
Erythromycin	R	R	±	±	+	+	R
Clindamycin	R	R	±	±	R	R	R
Tetracyclines	(±)	R	±	±	+	+	+
Chloramphenicol	±	R	+	+	+	(+)	+
Ciprofloxacin	+	±	R	R	R	+	±
Gentamicin, tobramycin, amikacin, netilmicin	+	±	R	R	R	R	R
Sulphonamides	±	R	R	R	+	R	R
Trimethoprim–sulphamethoxazole	±	R	R	R	±	R	R

+, Sensitive; R, resistant; ±, some strains resistant; ( ), not appropriate therapy; *, rare strains resistant.

14.2.3 Pharmacological Factors

Clinical efficacy is also dependent on achieving satisfactory drug concentrations at the site of the infection; this is influenced by the standard pharmacokinetic factors of absorption, distribution, metabolism and excretion. If an oral agent is selected, gastrointestinal absorption should be satisfactory. However, it may be impaired by factors such as the presence of food, drug interactions (including chelation) or impaired gastrointestinal function either as a result of surgical resection or malabsorptive states. Although effective, oral absorption may be inappropriate in patients who are vomiting or have undergone recent surgery; under these circumstances, a parenteral agent will be required and has the advantage of providing rapidly effective drug concentrations.

Antibiotic selection also varies according to the anatomical site of infection. Lipid solubility is of importance in relation to drug distribution. For example, the aminoglycosides are poorly lipid-soluble and, although achieving therapeutic concentrations within the extracellular fluid compartment, they penetrate the cerebrospinal fluid (CSF) poorly. Likewise, the presence of inflammation may affect drug penetration into the tissues. In the presence of meningeal inflammation, β-lactam agents achieve satisfactory concentrations within the CSF, but as the inflammatory response subsides, drug concentrations fall. Hence, it is essential to administer high doses throughout the treatment of bacterial meningitis, which requires the intravenous route. Other agents such as chloramphenicol are little affected by the presence or absence of meningeal inflammation.

Therapeutic drug concentrations within the bile duct and gallbladder are dependent on biliary excretion. In the presence of biliary disease, such as gallstones or chronic inflammation, the drug concentration may fail to reach therapeutic levels. By contrast, drugs that are excreted primarily via the liver or kidneys may require reduced doses in the presence of impaired renal or hepatic function. The malfunction of excretory organs may not only risk toxicity from drug accumulation, but will also reduce urinary concentration of drugs excreted primarily by glomerular filtration. This applies to the aminoglycosides and nitrofurantoin, where therapeutic failure in urinary tract infections may complicate severe renal failure and increase the risk of side effects, such as peripheral neuropathy with nitrofurantoin.

14.2.4 Drug Resistance

Drug resistance may be an innate or acquired characteristic of a microorganism. This may result from impaired cell wall or cell envelope penetration, enzymatic inactivation, altered binding sites or active extrusion from the cell as a result of efflux mechanisms (Chapter 13). Acquired drug resistance may result from mutation, adaptation or gene transfer. Spontaneous mutations occur at low frequency, as in the case of *Mycobacterium tuberculosis* where a minority population of organisms is resistant to isoniazid. In this situation, the use of isoniazid alone will eventually result in overgrowth by this sub-population of resistant organisms.

Genetic resistance may be chromosomal or transferable on transposons or plasmids. Plasmid-mediated resistance is common among Gram-negative enteric pathogens. By the process of conjugation (Chapter 3), resistance plasmids may be transferred between bacteria of the same and different species and also different genera. Such resistance can code for multiple antibiotic resistance. For example, the penicillins, cephalosporins, chloramphenicol and the aminoglycosides are all subject to enzymatic inactivation, which may be plasmid-mediated. Knowledge of the local epidemiology of resistant pathogens within a hospital, and especially within high-dependency areas such as intensive care and haemodialysis units, is invaluable in guiding appropriate drug selection.

14.2.4.1 Multidrug Resistance

In recent years, multidrug resistance has increased among many pathogens. Resistant Gram-positive pathogens include methicillin-resistant *Staphylococcus aureus* (MRSA), enterococci and *M. tuberculosis*. MRSA strains are resistant to many antibiotics and have been responsible for major epidemics worldwide, usually in hospitals where they affect patients in high-dependency units such as intensive care units, burns units and cardiothoracic units. MRSA have the ability to colonise staff and patients and to spread readily among them. The sensitivity profile of MRSA strains varies and there is now a wide variety of agents to choose from, depending on the antibiogram. Vancomycin remains a common empirical choice when MRSA is suspected or confirmed.

Another serious resistance problem is that of drug-resistant enterococci. These include *Enterococcus faecalis* and, in particular, *Enterococcus faecium*. Resistance to the glycopeptides has again been a problem among patients in high-dependency units.

Extended-spectrum β-lactamase (ESBL)-producing Gram-negative organisms are a problem in hospitals, and are increasingly seen as a cause of urinary tract infection in primary care; ESBLs can hydrolyse most cephalosporins and penicillins, limiting therapeutic options to carbapenems or aminoglycosides. ESBLs can be chromosomally mediated (e.g., *Pseudomonas* spp., *Citrobacter* spp.) or plasmid-mediated (e.g., *Klebsiella* spp.), the latter often being implicated in hospital outbreaks. There have been a number of new agents licensed recently to treat multiresistant Gram-negative organisms. These include both single and combination products such as ceftazidime/avibactam, ceftolozane/tazobactam, cefiderocol, meropenem/vaborbactam and imipenem/cilastatin/relebactam.

Increasing consumption of carbapenems to treat ESBL infections has led to the emergence of carbapenem-resistant organisms (CRO), principally in the *Enterobacterales* spp. but also in other Gram-negative organisms including *Pseudomonas aeruginosa* and *Acinetobacter baumannii*. These organisms can exhibit resistance by either one or a combination of mechanisms such as the production of carbapenemases, porin loss from the outer membrane or expression of efflux pumps. In practice, infections caused by these organisms can be challenging to treat, requiring cocktails of antibiotics including potentially toxic agents such as colistin.

Tuberculosis continues to present a challenge after decades in which the incidence had been steadily falling. Drug-resistant strains have emerged largely among inadequately treated or non-compliant patients. These include the homeless, alcoholic, intravenous drug misusing, HIV-positive and immigrant populations. Resistance patterns vary but usually include rifampicin and isoniazid. Multidrug-resistant, extensively drug-resistant (XDR) and pan-resistant strains of *M. tuberculosis* are now seen. There are new agents available to treat these strains, including delamanid and bedaquiline. The underlying mechanisms of resistance are considered in Chapter 13.

14.2.5 Drug Combinations

Antibiotics are generally used alone, but may on occasion be prescribed in combination. Combining two antibiotics may result in synergism, indifference or antagonism. In the case of synergism, microbial inhibition is achieved at concentrations below that for each agent alone and may prove advantageous in treating relatively insusceptible infections such as enterococcal endocarditis, where a combination of penicillin and gentamicin is synergistically active. Another advantage of synergistic combinations is that it may enable the use of toxic agents where dose reductions are possible. For example, meningitis caused by the fungus *Cryptococcus neoformans* responds to an abbreviated course of amphotericin B when it is combined with 5-flucytosine, thereby reducing the risk of toxicity from amphotericin B.

Combined drug use is occasionally recommended to prevent resistance emerging during treatment. For example, tuberculosis is initially treated with a minimum of three agents, such as rifampicin, isoniazid and pyrazinamide; drug resistance is prevented, which may result if either agent is used alone.

The most common reason for using combined therapy is in the treatment of confirmed or suspected mixed infections where a single agent alone will fail to cover all pathogenic organisms. This is the case in serious abdominal sepsis where mixed aerobic and anaerobic infections are common and metronidazole is added to broad-spectrum agents such as third-generation cephalosporins or piperacillin/tazobactam. Finally, drugs are used in combination in patients who are seriously ill and about whom uncertainty exists concerning the microbiological nature of their infection. This initial 'blind therapy' frequently includes a broad-spectrum penicillin or cephalosporin in combination with an aminoglycoside. If microbiology culture and susceptibility results are available, treatment should be tailored to the most clinically appropriate narrow-spectrum agent, as prolonged use of broad-spectrum agents can drive antimicrobial resistance.

14.2.6 Adverse Reactions

Regrettably, all chemotherapeutic agents have the potential to produce adverse reactions with varying degrees of frequency and severity, and these include hypersensitivity reactions and toxic effects. These may be dose-related and predictable in a patient with a history of hypersensitivity or a previous toxic reaction to a drug or its chemical analogues. However, many adverse events are idiosyncratic and therefore unpredictable.

Hypersensitivity reactions range in severity from fatal anaphylaxis, in which there is widespread tissue oedema, airway obstruction and cardiovascular collapse, to minor and reversible hypersensitivity reactions such as skin eruptions and drug fever. Such reactions are more likely in those with a history of hypersensitivity to the drug, and are more frequent in patients with previous allergic diseases such as childhood eczema or asthma. It is important to question patients closely concerning hypersensitivity reactions before prescribing, as it precludes the use of all compounds within a class, such as the sulphonamides or tetracyclines, while cephalosporins and carbapenems should be used only with caution in patients who are allergic to penicillin, because these agents are structurally related. They should be avoided entirely in those who have had a previous severe hypersensitivity reaction to penicillin.

The incidence of penicillin allergy is overestimated, and approximately 1 in 10 patients will claim a history of allergy, while the true incidence is closer to 1%. Patients with a penicillin allergy label who are treated with antibiotics have longer hospital stays and worse outcomes than non-penicillin-allergic patients, due to the use of less effective or more toxic antibiotic alternatives. For this reason, it is important to differentiate between true allergy and the side effects of penicillin antibiotics, which include nausea and diarrhoea, which many patients assume to be allergy (Shenoy et al. 2019).

Drug toxicity is often dose-related and may affect a variety of organs or tissues. For example, the aminoglycosides are both nephrotoxic and ototoxic to varying degrees; therefore, dosing should be individualised to take account of renal function and body weight. Once-daily dosing has been shown to be less toxic than multiple daily doses. Blood concentrations should be monitored, especially where renal function is abnormal, to avoid toxic effects and ensure efficacy. An example of dose-related toxicity is chloramphenicol-induced bone marrow suppression. Chloramphenicol interferes with the normal maturation of bone marrow stem cells and high concentrations may result in a steady fall in circulating red and white cells and also platelets. This effect is generally reversible with dose reduction or drug withdrawal. This dose-related toxic reaction of chloramphenicol should be contrasted with idiosyncratic bone marrow toxicity which is unrelated to dose and occurs at a much lower frequency of approximately 1:40,000, and is frequently irreversible, ending fatally. Toxic effects may also be genetically determined. For example, peripheral neuropathy may occur in those who are slow acetylators of isoniazid, while haemolysis occurs in those deficient in the red cell enzyme glucose-6-phosphate dehydrogenase (G6PD), when treated with sulphonamides, primaquine, quinolones or nitrofurantoin. G6PD levels should be checked before starting these agents.

14.2.7 Superinfection

Anti-infective drugs not only affect the invading organism undergoing treatment but also have an impact on the normal bacterial flora, especially of the skin and mucous membranes. This may result in microbial overgrowth of resistant organisms with subsequent superinfection. One example is the common occurrence of oral or vaginal candidiasis in patients treated with broad-spectrum agents such as co-amoxiclav. A more serious example is the development of pseudomembranous colitis from the overgrowth of toxin-producing strains of *Clostridioides difficile* present in the bowel flora following the use of clindamycin or broad-spectrum antibiotics, though any antimicrobial can precipitate this condition. *C. difficile*-associated diarrhoea is managed by stopping the offending antibiotic where possible and treatment with oral vancomycin or fidaxomicin. Severe disease is treated with a combination of antibiotics including intravenous metronidazole and oral/colonic vancomycin. Faecal microbiota transplant using stools from health donors is also an effective option. Intravenous immunoglobulin is occasionally used in severe cases, and, rarely, colectomy (excision of part or whole of the colon) may be necessary. Once established, *C. difficile* infection is transmissible, particularly in the hospital setting; isolation of symptomatic patients and strict observation of hygiene practices (e.g., handwashing) are therefore key in preventing outbreaks.

14.2.8 Chemoprophylaxis

An important use of antimicrobial agents is in infection prevention, especially in relationship to surgery. Infection remains one of the most important complications of many surgical procedures, and while perioperative antibiotics are effective and safe in preventing this complication, evidence demonstrates that a single preoperative dose is adequate for many types of surgery, and that withholding prophylaxis altogether for clean procedures is safe. The principles that underlie the chemoprophylactic use of antibacterials relate to the predictability of infection for a particular surgical procedure, in terms of its occurrence, microbial aetiology and susceptibility to antibiotics. Therapeutic drug concentrations present at the operative site at the time of surgery rapidly reduce the number of potentially infectious organisms and prevent wound sepsis. If prophylaxis is delayed to the postoperative period, then efficacy is markedly impaired. It is important that chemoprophylaxis be limited to the perioperative period, the first dose being administered approximately 1 hour before surgery for injectable agents; for many procedures and operative sites, a single dose is now considered sufficient. Prolonging chemoprophylaxis beyond this period is not cost-effective and increases the risk of adverse drug reactions and superinfection. One of the best examples of the efficacy of surgical prophylaxis is in the area of large-bowel surgery. Before the widespread use of chemoprophylaxis, postoperative infection rates for colectomy were often 30% or higher; these have now been reduced to around 5%. For surgery lasting more than 4 hours or with significant blood loss and haemodilution, a second intra-operative dose of antibiotic is recommended, to ensure therapeutic levels are maintained.

Chemoprophylaxis has been extended to other surgical procedures where the risk of infection may be low, but its occurrence has serious consequences. This is especially true for the implantation of prosthetic joints or heart valves. These are major surgical procedures, and although infection may be infrequent, its consequences are serious and on balance the use of chemoprophylaxis is cost-effective.

Examples of chemoprophylaxis in the non-surgical arena include the prevention of pneumococcal infection with penicillin V in asplenia or patients with sickle-cell disease, and the prevention of secondary cases of meningococcal meningitis with rifampicin or ciprofloxacin among household contacts of an index case.

14.3 Clinical Use

The choice of antimicrobial chemotherapy is initially dependent on the clinical diagnosis. In some circumstances, the clinical diagnosis implies a microbiological diagnosis which may dictate specific therapy. For example, typhoid fever is caused by *Salmonella enterica* serovar Typhi, which is generally sensitive to azithromycin, ceftriaxone and ciprofloxacin. However, for many infections, establishing a clinical diagnosis implies a range of possible microbiological causes and requires laboratory confirmation from samples collected, preferably before antibiotic therapy is begun. Laboratory isolation and susceptibility testing of the causative agent establish the diagnosis with certainty and make drug selection more rational. However, in many circumstances, especially in general practice, microbiological documentation of an infection is not possible. Hence, knowledge of the usual microbiological cause of a particular infection and its susceptibility to antimicrobial agents is essential for effective drug prescribing. The following section explores a selection of the problems associated with antimicrobial drug prescribing for a range of clinical conditions.

14.3.1 Respiratory Tract Infections

Infections of the respiratory tract are among the commonest of infections, and account for much consultation in general practice and a high percentage of acute hospital admissions. They are divided into infections of the upper respiratory tract, involving the ears, throat, nasal sinuses and the trachea, and the lower respiratory tract (LRT), where they affect the airways, lungs and pleura.

14.3.1.1 Upper Respiratory Tract Infections

Acute pharyngitis presents a diagnostic and therapeutic dilemma. The majority of sore throats are caused by a variety of viruses; fewer than 20% are bacterial and hence potentially responsive to antibiotic therapy. However, antibiotics have historically been widely prescribed and this reflects the difficulty in discriminating streptococcal from non-streptococcal infections clinically in the absence of microbiological documentation. Clinical prediction scores, such as FeverPAIN, can be used to confirm the likelihood of streptococcal infection, and should be used.

S. pyogenes is the most important bacterial pathogen and this responds to oral penicillin. However, up to 10 days' treatment is required for its eradication from the throat. This requirement causes problems with compliance, as symptomatic improvement generally occurs within 2–3 days.

Although viral infections are important causes of both otitis media and sinusitis, they are generally self-limiting. Bacterial infections may complicate viral illnesses, and are also primary causes of ear and sinus infections. *Streptococcus pneumoniae* and *Haemophilus influenzae* are the commonest bacterial pathogens. Amoxicillin is widely prescribed for these infections, as it is microbiologically active, penetrates the middle ear, is well tolerated and has proved effective; macrolides are an alternative in penicillin allergy. Penicillin V and doxycycline are first-line choices for sinusitis.

14.3.1.2 Lower Respiratory Tract Infections

Infections of the LRT include pneumonia, lung abscess, bronchitis, bronchiectasis and infective complications of cystic fibrosis. Each presents a specific diagnostic and therapeutic challenge, which reflects the variety of pathogens involved and the frequent difficulties in establishing an accurate microbial diagnosis. The laboratory diagnosis of LRT infections is largely dependent upon culturing sputum. Unfortunately, this may be contaminated with the normal bacterial flora of the upper respiratory tract during expectoration. In hospitalised patients, the empirical use of antibiotics before admission substantially diminishes the value of sputum culture and may result in overgrowth by non-pathogenic microbes, thus causing difficulty with the interpretation of sputum culture results. Alternative diagnostic samples include needle aspiration of sputum directly from the trachea or of fluid within the pleural cavity. Blood may also be cultured and serum examined for antibody responses or microbial antigens. In the community, few patients will have their LRT infection diagnosed microbiologically and the choice of antibiotic is based on local or national guidelines, according to severity of infection. The increasing use of point-of-care tests such as C-reactive protein in primary care may help to reduce the prescribing of antimicrobials.

Pneumonia

The range of pathogens causing acute pneumonia includes viruses, bacteria and, in the immunocompromised host, parasites and fungi. Table 14.2 summarises these pathogens and indicates drugs appropriate for their treatment. Clinical assessment includes details of the evolution of the

Table 14.2 Microorganisms responsible for pneumonia and the therapeutic agents of choice.

Pathogen	Drug(s) of choice
Streptococcus pneumoniae	Amoxicillin or clarithromycin or doxycycline
Staphylococcus aureus (methicillin-sensitive *S. aureus*, MSSA)	Flucloxacillin or clindamycin (note: need to investigate for toxin-producing *S. aureus* which will influence drug choice – may require addition of intravenous linezolid plus clindamycin plus rifampicin)
Staphylococcus aureus (MRSA)	Vancomycin or linezolid
Haemophilus influenzae	Co-amoxiclav or clarithromycin or levofloxacin
Klebsiella pneumoniae	Cefotaxime ± gentamicin Note: risk of ESBL production – may require carbapenem
Pseudomonas aeruginosa	Ceftazidime ± gentamicin or piperacillin–tazobactam ± gentamicin Note: risk of ESBL production – may require carbapenem
Mycoplasma pneumoniae	Clarithromycin or doxycycline or levofloxacin
Legionella pneumophila	Clarithromycin or levofloxacin; both if severe
Chlamydia psittaci	Doxycycline or macrolide or quinolone
Mycobacterium tuberculosis	Rifampicin + isoniazid + ethambutol + pyrazinamide[a]
Herpes simplex, varicella/zoster	Aciclovir
Candida spp.	Fluconazole or echinocandins (caspofungin, anidulafungin, micafungin)
Aspergillus spp.	Broad-spectrum triazoles (voriconazole, isavuconazole) or echinocandins (caspofungin, micafungin), or liposomal amphotericin B
Anaerobic bacteria	Benzylpenicillin or metronidazole

[a] Reduce to rifampicin + isoniazid after 2 months, continue for a further 4 months. Different regimens apply for central nervous system involvement, and all regimens should be reviewed in the light of sensitivity testing; ESBL, extended spectrum β-lactamase.

infection, any evidence of a recent viral infection, the age of the patient and risk factors such as corticosteroid therapy or pre-existing lung disease. The extent of the pneumonia, as assessed clinically or by X-ray, is also important.

S. pneumoniae remains the commonest cause of pneumonia and still responds well to penicillin despite a global increase in isolates showing reduced susceptibility to this agent. So-called 'respiratory quinolones' such as levofloxacin and moxifloxacin, which exhibit increased activity against Gram-positive organisms compared to ciprofloxacin, are an alternative. However, quinolones are subject to precautions in use due to rare reports of musculoskeletal, cardiovascular and nervous system adverse events. A number of atypical infections may cause pneumonia and include *Mycoplasma pneumoniae*, *Legionella pneumophila*, psittacosis and occasionally Q fever. With psittacosis, there may be a history of contact with parrots or budgerigars; while legionnaires' disease has often been acquired during hotel holidays in the Mediterranean area. The atypical pneumonias, unlike pneumococcal pneumonia, do not respond to penicillin. Legionnaires' disease is treated with oral fluoroquinolones in moderate disease, or macrolides; in severe disease, a fluoroquinolone, with the addition of a macrolide for the first few days, may be given intravenously. Mycoplasma infections are best treated with either erythromycin or tetracycline, while the latter drug is indicated for both psittacosis and Q fever.

Lung Abscess

Destruction of lung tissue may lead to abscess formation and is a feature of aerobic Gram-negative bacillary and *S. aureus* infections. In addition, aspiration of oropharyngeal secretion can lead to chronic low-grade sepsis with abscess formation and the expectoration of foul-smelling sputum that characterises anaerobic sepsis. The latter condition responds to high-dose penicillin, which is active against most of the normal oropharyngeal flora, while metronidazole may be appropriate for strictly anaerobic infections. In the case of lung abscess, the likelihood of Gram-negative pathogens will guide choice of therapy; if Gram-negative infection is suspected, the agents of choice will be piperacillin–tazobactam or a combination of a quinolone and clindamycin; if the risk of Gram-negative infection is low, then a cephalosporin plus clindamycin, or benzylpenicillin plus metronidazole, should provide adequate cover. Acute staphylococcal pneumonia is an extremely serious infection and requires treatment with high-dose flucloxacillin alone or with other agents.

Cystic Fibrosis

Cystic fibrosis is a multisystem congenital abnormality that often affects the lungs and results in recurrent infections, initially with *S. aureus*, subsequently with *H. influenzae* and eventually leads on to recurrent *P. aeruginosa* infection. The last organism is associated with copious quantities of purulent sputum that are extremely difficult to expectorate. *P. aeruginosa* is a co-factor in the progressive lung damage that is eventually fatal in these patients. Repeated courses of antibiotics are prescribed, and although they have improved the quality and longevity of life, infections caused by *P. aeruginosa* are difficult to treat and require repeated hospitalisation and administration of parenteral antibiotics such as an aminoglycoside, either alone or in combination with an antipseudomonal penicillin or cephalosporin. The dose of aminoglycosides tolerated by these patients is often higher than in normal individuals and is associated with larger volumes of distribution for these and other agents. Some benefit may also be obtained from inhaled aerosolised antibiotics. Unfortunately, drug resistance may emerge and makes drug selection more dependent upon laboratory guidance.

14.3.2 Urinary Tract Infections

Urinary tract infection is a common problem in both community and hospital practice. Although occurring throughout life, infections are more common in pre-school girls and women during their childbearing years than in men, although in the elderly the sex distribution is similar. Infection is predisposed by factors that impair urine flow. These include congenital abnormalities, reflux of urine from the bladder into the ureters, kidney stones and tumours and, in males, enlargement of the prostate gland. Bladder catheterisation is an important cause of urinary tract infection in hospitalised patients.

14.3.2.1 Pathogenesis

In those with structural or drainage problems the risk exists of ascending infection to involve the kidney and occasionally the bloodstream. Although structural abnormalities may be absent in women of childbearing years, infection can become recurrent, symptomatic and extremely distressing. Of greater concern is the occurrence of infection in the pre-school child, as normal maturation of the kidney may be impaired and may result in progressive damage which presents as renal failure in later life.

From a therapeutic point of view, it is essential to confirm the presence of bacteriuria (a condition in which there are bacteria in the urine), as symptoms alone are not a reliable method of documenting infection. This applies particularly to bladder infection, where the symptoms of burning micturition (dysuria) and frequency can be associated with a variety of non-bacteriuric conditions. Patients with symptomatic bacteriuria should always be treated. However, the necessity to treat asymptomatic bacteriuric patients varies with age and the presence or absence of underlying urinary tract abnormalities. In pregnancy, there is a risk of infection ascending from the bladder to involve the kidney. This is a serious complication and may result in premature labour. Other indications for treating asymptomatic bacteriuria include the presence of underlying renal abnormalities such as stones, which may be associated with repeated infections caused by *Proteus* spp. However, asymptomatic bacteriuria in the elderly, particularly women in residential care, does not always represent infection and does not generally require antibiotics.

14.3.2.2 Drug Therapy

The antimicrobial treatment of urinary tract infection presents a number of interesting challenges. Drugs must be selected for their ability to achieve high urinary concentrations and, if the kidney is involved, adequate tissue concentrations. Safety in childhood or pregnancy is important, as repeated or prolonged medication may be necessary. The choice of agent will be dictated by the microbial aetiology and susceptibility findings, because the latter can vary widely among Gram-negative enteric bacilli, especially in patients who are hospitalised. Table 14.3 shows the distribution of bacteria causing urinary tract infection in the community and in hospitalised patients. The greater tendency towards infections caused by *Klebsiella* spp. and *P. aeruginosa* should be noted, as antibiotic sensitivity is more variable for these pathogens. Drug resistance has increased substantially in recent years and has reduced the value of formerly widely prescribed agents such as trimethoprim.

Uncomplicated community-acquired urinary tract infection presents few problems with management. Drugs such as nitrofurantoin, pivmecillinam and fosfomycin are widely used. In non-pregnant women with uncomplicated infection, treatment for 3 days is generally satisfactory and is usually accompanied by prompt control of symptoms; 7 days is usually used in men. Single-dose oral therapy with fosfomycin 3 g has also been shown to be effective in selected individuals. Alternative agents include amoxicillin, cephalexin and trimethoprim (though only if the risk of resistance is known to be low).

It is not necessary to submit follow-up urine samples unless advised to do so by the laboratory; however, recurrent urinary tract infection is an indication for further investigation of the urinary tract to detect underlying pathology that may be surgically correctable. Under such circumstances, and with specialist advice, repeated courses of antibiotics, guided by laboratory sensitivity

Table 14.3 Urinary tract infection: distribution of pathogenic bacteria in the community and hospitalised patients.

Organism	Prevalence (uncomplicated community isolates)	Prevalence (hospital isolates)
Escherichia coli	75%	40%
Klebsiella spp.	6%	11%
Staphylococcus saprophyticus	6%	3%
Enterococci	5%	12%
Group B streptococcus	3%	–
Proteus mirabilis	2%	6%
Pseudomonas aeruginosa	1%	11%
Staphylococcus aureus	1%	3%

Data taken from Cek et al. (2014) and Flores-Mireles et al. (2015).

data, or long-term chemoprophylaxis for up to 6 months may be used. If nitrofurantoin is prescribed long-term, it is important to be aware of the risk of pulmonary toxicity.

Infection of the kidney demands the use of agents that achieve adequate tissue as well as urinary concentrations. As bacteraemia (a condition in which there are bacteria circulating in the blood) may complicate infection of the kidney, it is generally recommended that antibiotics be chosen that achieve high blood concentrations when administered orally, or intravenous agents may be used initially. Agents such as cephalexin, ciprofloxacin and co-amoxiclav, if known to be effective against the target strain, are preferred, because the aminoglycosides, although highly effective and preferentially concentrated within the renal cortex, carry the risk of nephrotoxicity.

Infections of the prostate tend to be persistent, recurrent and difficult to treat. This is in part due to the more acid environment of the prostate gland, which inhibits drug penetration by many of the antibiotics used to treat urinary tract infection. Agents that are basic in nature, such as erythromycin, achieve therapeutic concentrations within the gland, but unfortunately are not active against the pathogens responsible for bacterial prostatitis. Quinolones, however, and trimethoprim/sulphamethoxazole combinations, are useful agents, as they are preferentially concentrated within the prostate and active against many of the causative pathogens. It is important that treatment be prolonged for several weeks, as relapse is common.

14.3.3 Gastrointestinal Infections

The gut is vulnerable to infection by viruses, bacteria, parasites and occasionally fungi. Virus infections are the most prevalent but are not susceptible to chemotherapeutic intervention. Bacterial infections are more readily recognised and raise questions concerning the role of antibiotic management. Parasitic infections of the gut are covered in Chapter 6.

Bacteria cause disease of the gut as a result of either mucosal invasion or toxin production or a combination of the two mechanisms, as summarised in Table 14.4. Treatment is largely directed at replacing and maintaining an adequate intake of fluid and electrolytes. Antibiotics are generally not recommended for infective gastroenteritis, but deserve consideration where they have been demonstrated to abbreviate the acute disease or to prevent complications including prolonged gastrointestinal excretion of the pathogen where this poses a public health hazard.

It should be emphasised that most gut infections are self-limiting. However, attacks can be severe and may result in hospitalisation, and patients who are severely ill or immunocompromised should receive antibiotics. Antibiotics are used to treat severe *Campylobacter* and *Shigella* infections; clarithromycin and ciprofloxacin, respectively, are the preferred agents. Such treatment abbreviates the disease and eliminates gut excretion in *Shigella* infection. The role of antibiotics for *Campylobacter* and *Shigella* infections should be contrasted with gastrointestinal salmonellosis, for which antibiotics are contraindicated as they do not abbreviate symptoms, are associated with more prolonged gut excretion and introduce the risk of adverse drug reactions. However, in severe non-typhoid salmonellosis, especially at extremes of age or in immunocompromised patients or those with a haemoglobinopathy, systemic toxaemia and bloodstream infection can occur and under these circumstances treatment with either ciprofloxacin or cefotaxime is appropriate.

Typhoid and paratyphoid fevers (known as enteric fevers), although acquired by ingestion of the salmonellae

Table 14.4 Bacterial gut infections: pathogenic mechanisms.

Origin	Site of infection	Mechanism
Campylobacter jejuni	Small and large bowel	Invasion
Salmonella spp.	Small and large bowel	Invasion
Shigella spp.	Large bowel	Invasion ± toxin
Escherichia coli		
enteroinvasive	Large bowel	Invasion
enterotoxigenic	Small bowel	Toxin
Clostridioides difficile	Large bowel	Toxin
Staphylococcus aureus	Small bowel	Toxin
Vibrio cholerae	Small bowel	Toxin
Clostridium perfringens	Small bowel	Toxin
Yersinia spp.	Small and large bowel	Invasion
Bacillus cereus	Small bowel	Invasion ± toxin
Vibrio parahaemolyticus	Small bowel	Invasion + toxin

S. enterica serovar Typhi and *S. enterica* serovar Paratyphi, respectively, are largely systemic infections and antibiotic therapy is mandatory; cefotaxime or ceftriaxone is the drug of choice, although azithromycin may be used in mild to moderate disease where drug-resistant organisms are involved. Ciprofloxacin can be used if sensitivity is confirmed; infections from the Middle-East, South and South-East Asia may be resistant. Prolonged gut excretion of *S. enterica* serovar Typhi is a well-known complication of typhoid fever and is a major public health hazard in developing countries. Treatment with ciprofloxacin can eliminate the gallbladder excretion which is the major site of persistent infection in carriers. However, the presence of gallstones reduces the chance of cure.

Cholera is a serious infection, causing epidemics throughout Asia. Although a toxin-mediated disease, largely controlled with replacement of fluid and electrolyte losses, doxycycline, ciprofloxacin or azithromycin have been used to eliminate the causative vibrio from the bowel, thereby abbreviating the course of the illness and reducing the total fluid and electrolyte losses; local outbreak sensitivity testing is useful to guide choice of agent.

Traveller's diarrhoea may be caused by one of many gastrointestinal pathogens (Table 14.4). However, enterotoxigenic *E. coli* is the most common pathogen. While it is generally short-lived, traveller's diarrhoea can seriously mar a brief period abroad, be it for holiday or business purposes. Although not generally recommended, ciprofloxacin is occasionally used as prophylaxis, or rifaximin can be used in patients without complications (e.g., fever or blood in stool).

14.3.4 Skin and Soft Tissue Infections

Infections of the skin and soft tissue commonly follow traumatic injury to the epithelium but occasionally may be blood-borne. Interruption of the integrity of the skin allows ingress of microorganisms to produce superficial, localised infections which on occasion may become more deep-seated and spread rapidly through tissues. Skin trauma complicates surgical incisions and accidents, including burns. Similarly, prolonged immobilisation can result in pressure damage to skin from impaired blood flow. It is most commonly seen in patients who are unconscious.

Microbes responsible for skin infection often arise from the normal skin flora, which includes *S. aureus*. In addition, *S. pyogenes*, *P. aeruginosa* and anaerobic bacteria are other recognised pathogens. Viruses also affect the skin and mucosal surfaces, either as a result of generalised infection or localised disease as in the case of herpes simplex. The latter is amenable to antiviral therapy in selected patients, although for the majority of patients, virus infections of the skin are self-limiting.

S. pyogenes is responsible for a range of skin infections: impetigo is a superficial infection of the epidermis which is common in childhood and is highly contagious; cellulitis is a more deep-seated infection which spreads rapidly through the tissues to involve the lymphatics and occasionally the bloodstream; erysipelas is a rapidly spreading cellulitis commonly involving the face, which characteristically has a raised leading edge due to lymphatic involvement. Necrotising fasciitis is a more serious, rapidly progressive infection of the skin and subcutaneous structures including the fascia and musculature. Despite early diagnosis and high-dose intravenous antibiotics, this condition is often life-threatening and may require extensive surgical debridement of devitalised tissue and even limb amputation to ensure survival. A fatal outcome is usually the result of profound toxaemia and bloodstream spread. Penicillin is the drug of choice for all these infections, usually in combination with other agents such as an aminoglycoside and metronidazole in the case of necrotising fasciitis; in severe instances, parenteral administration is appropriate. Due to increases in drug resistance, topical hydrogen peroxide 1% cream is the first-choice treatment for impetigo; where infection is widespread, or peroxide fails, a topical preparation of fusidic acid or mupirocin, or a short oral course of flucloxacillin or clarithromycin, may be used.

S. aureus is responsible for a variety of skin infections which require therapeutic approaches different from those of streptococcal infections. Staphylococcal cellulitis is indistinguishable clinically from streptococcal cellulitis and responds to flucloxacillin, but generally fails to respond to penicillin owing to β-lactamase production. In hospital-acquired infection, and occasionally in community practice, MRSA must be considered as a possibility, particularly where the patient is known to be colonised. *S. aureus* is an important cause of superficial, localised skin sepsis which varies from small pustules to boils and occasionally to a more deeply invasive, suppurative skin abscess known as a carbuncle. Antibiotics are generally not indicated for these conditions. Pustules and boils settle with antiseptic soaps or creams and often discharge spontaneously, whereas carbuncles frequently require surgical drainage. *S. aureus* may also cause postoperative wound infections, sometimes associated with retained suture material, which may resolve once the stitch is removed. Antibiotics are only appropriate in this situation if there is extensive accompanying soft tissue invasion. Rarely, strains of *S. aureus* may express a toxin complex known as Panton–Valentine Leukocidin (PVL); these strains can cause severe sepsis and an often-fatal necrotising pneumonia in young, otherwise fit, patients. The treatment for such infections usually aims to minimise toxin production using protein synthesis inhibitors such as clindamycin plus rifampicin, in combination with linezolid.

Anaerobic bacteria are characteristically associated with foul-smelling wounds. They are found in association with surgical incisions following intra-abdominal procedures and pressure sores, which are usually located over the buttocks and hips where they become infected with faecal flora. These infections are frequently mixed and include Gram-negative enteric bacilli, which may mask the presence of underlying anaerobic bacteria. The principles of treating anaerobic soft tissue infection again emphasise the need for removal of all foreign and devitalised material. Antibiotics such as metronidazole or clindamycin should be considered where tissue invasion has occurred.

The treatment of infected burn wounds presents a number of peculiar facets. Burns are initially sterile, especially when they involve all layers of the skin. However, they rapidly become colonised with bacteria whose growth is supported by the protein-rich exudate. Staphylococci, *S. pyogenes* and, particularly, *P. aeruginosa* frequently colonise burns and may jeopardise survival of skin grafts, and occasionally, and more seriously, result in bloodstream invasion. Treatment of invasive *P. aeruginosa* infections requires combined therapy with an aminoglycoside, such as gentamicin, and an antipseudomonal agent, such as ceftazidime or piperacillin/tazobactam. This produces high therapeutic concentrations which generally act in a synergistic manner. The use of aminoglycosides in patients with serious burns requires careful monitoring of serum concentrations to ensure that they are therapeutic yet non-toxic, as renal function is often impaired in the days immediately following a serious burn.

14.3.5 Central Nervous System Infections

The brain, its surrounding covering of meninges and the spinal cord are subject to infection, which is generally blood-borne but may also complicate neurosurgery, penetrating injuries or direct spread from infection in the middle ear or nasal sinuses. Viral meningitis is the most common infection but is generally self-limiting. Occasionally destructive forms of encephalitis occur; an example is herpes simplex encephalitis. Bacterial infections include meningitis and brain abscesses, and carry a high risk of mortality, while in those who recover, residual neurological damage or impairment of intellectual function may follow. This occurs despite the availability of antibiotics active against the responsible bacterial pathogens. Fungal infections of the brain, although rare, are increasing in frequency, particularly among immunocompromised patients who either have underlying malignant conditions or are on potent cytotoxic drugs.

The treatment of bacterial infections of the central nervous system highlights a number of important therapeutic considerations. Bacterial meningitis is caused by a variety of bacteria, although their incidence varies with age. In the neonate, *E. coli* and group B streptococci account for the majority of infections, while in the pre-school child *H. influenzae* was the commonest pathogen before the introduction of a highly effective vaccine. *Neisseria meningitidis* has a peak incidence between 5 and 15 years of age, while pneumococcal meningitis is predominantly a disease of adults.

Ceftriaxone is the drug of choice for the treatment of group B streptococcal, meningococcal and pneumococcal infections, but, as discussed earlier, CSF concentrations of penicillin are significantly influenced by the intensity of the inflammatory response. To achieve therapeutic concentrations within the CSF, high doses are required, and in the case of pneumococcal meningitis should be continued for 10–14 days. Resistance among *S. pneumoniae* to penicillin has increased worldwide; in travellers returning from endemic areas, vancomycin may be indicated. Alternative agents include meropenem.

Resistance of *H. influenzae* to ampicillin has increased in the past three decades and varies geographically. Thus, it can no longer be prescribed with confidence as initial therapy, and cefotaxime and ceftriaxone are now the preferred alternatives.

E. coli meningitis carries a mortality of greater than 40% and reflects both the virulence of this organism and the pharmacokinetic problems of achieving adequate CSF antibiotic levels. The broad-spectrum cephalosporins such as cefotaxime, ceftriaxone and ceftazidime have been shown to achieve satisfactory therapeutic levels and are the agents of choice to treat Gram-negative bacillary meningitis. Treatment again must be prolonged for periods ranging from 2–4 weeks.

Brain abscess presents a different therapeutic challenge. An abscess is locally destructive to the brain and causes further damage by increasing intracranial pressure. The infecting organisms are varied, but those arising from middle ear or nasal sinus infection are often polymicrobial and include anaerobic bacteria, microaerophilic species and Gram-negative enteric bacilli. Less commonly, a pure *S. aureus* abscess may complicate blood-borne spread. Brain abscess is a neurosurgical emergency and requires drainage. However, antibiotics are an important adjunct to treatment. The polymicrobial nature of many infections demands prompt and careful laboratory examination to determine optimum therapy. Drugs are selected not only on their ability to penetrate the blood–brain barrier and enter the CSF but also on their ability to penetrate the brain substance. Metronidazole has proved a valuable alternative agent in such infections, although it is not active against microaerophilic streptococci, which must be treated with high-dose benzylpenicillin. The two are often used in combination. Chloramphenicol is an alternative agent.

14.3.6 Fungal Infections

Fungal infections are divided into superficial or deep-seated infections (see also Chapter 4). Superficial infections affect the skin, nails or mucosal surfaces of the mouth or genital tract. By contrast, deep-seated fungal diseases may target the lung or disseminate via the bloodstream to organs such as the brain, spleen, liver or skeletal system.

The fungal infections of the skin and nails include tinea pedis (athlete's foot), tinea capitis and tinea corporis (ringworm), candidal intertrigo (usually groin and submammary regions) and pityriasis (*Malassezia*). A variety of topical and systemic antifungal agents are available. The imidazole class of drugs includes clotrimazole and miconazole, which are highly effective topically. Systemic antifungals used to treat superficial fungal infections include griseofulvin and terbinafine, which is an allylamine. Both agents are ineffective in the treatment of deep-seated fungal infections that may be caused by yeasts (*C. neoformans*), yeast-like fungi (*Candida* spp.) or the filamentous fungi (*Aspergillus* spp.). These produce a variety of syndromes for which different antifungal agents are indicated (Table 14.5). The polyenes include amphotericin B, which after many years remains the agent of choice for the treatment of a wide variety of life-threatening fungal diseases which often complicate cancer chemotherapy, organ transplantation and immunodeficiency diseases, such as AIDS. Nephrotoxicity is common but can be avoided by careful dosing or the use of liposomal formulations. The second major class of systemic antifungals is the triazoles, which include fluconazole and newer, broader-spectrum agents such as itraconazole, voriconazole, posaconazole and isavuconazole. These are extremely well tolerated but may interact with a number of drugs and drug classes such as the sulphonylureas, antihistamines and lipid-lowering agents among others. The echinocandins (caspofungin, anidulafungin, micafungin) are the newest class of antifungal agents, and are increasingly used to treat invasive fungal infections; they have a fungicidal action against *Candida* spp., and are fungistatic against many other organisms, including *Aspergillus* spp.

Table 14.5 Treatment recommendations for selected deep-seated fungal infections.

Infection	Preferred treatment	Alternative treatment
Candida spp.	Echinocandin	Amphotericin B, fluconazole
Cryptococcus neoformans	Amphotericin B ± flucytosine	Fluconazole
Aspergillus spp.	Voriconazole	Amphotericin B, itraconazole, caspofungin
Mucormycosis	Amphotericin B	Isavuconazole

14.3.7 Medical device-associated Infections

A wide variety of medical devices are increasingly used in clinical practice. These range from vasculature and urinary catheters, prosthetic joints and heart valves, shunts and stents for improving the flow of CSF, blood or bile according to their site of use, to intracardiac patches and vascular pumps. Unfortunately, infection is the most frequent complication of their use and may result in the need to replace or remove the device, sometimes with potentially life-threatening and fatal consequences.

Infections are often caused by organisms arising from the normal skin flora, which gain access at the time of insertion of the device. *Staphylococcus epidermidis* is among the most frequent of isolates. Following attachment to the surface of the device, the organisms undergo multiplication with the formation of extracellular polysaccharide material (glycocalyx) which contains slowly replicating cells to form a biofilm (see Chapter 8). Microorganisms within a biofilm are less vulnerable to attack by host defences (phagocytes, complement and antibodies) and are relatively insusceptible to antibiotic therapy despite the variable ability of drugs to penetrate the biofilm.

Management approaches have therefore emphasised the need for prevention through the addition of good sterile technique at the time of insertion. Manufacturers have also responded by using materials and creating surface characteristics of implanted materials inclement to microbial attachment. Likewise, the use of prophylactic antibiotics at the time of insertion of deep-seated devices such as joint and heart valve prostheses has further reduced the risk of infection. Once a medical device becomes infected, management is difficult. Treatment with agents such as flucloxacillin, vancomycin and most recently linezolid is often unsuccessful and the only course of action is to remove the device.

14.4 Antibiotic Policies

14.4.1 Rationale

The plethora of available antimicrobial agents presents both an increasing problem of selection to the prescriber and difficulties for the diagnostic laboratory as to which agents should be tested for susceptibility. Differences in antimicrobial activity among related compounds are often of minor importance but can occasionally be of greater significance and may be a source of confusion to the non-specialist. This applies particularly to large classes of drugs, such as the penicillins and cephalosporins, where there has been an explosion in the availability of new agents over recent years. Guidance, in the form of an antibiotic policy, has a major role to play in providing the prescriber with a range of agents appropriate to his/her needs and should be supported by laboratory evidence of susceptibility to these agents.

In recent years, increased awareness of the cost of medical care has led to a major review of various aspects of health costs. The pharmacy budget has often attracted attention as, unlike many other hospital expenses, it is readily identifiable in terms of cost and prescriber. Thus, an antibiotic policy is also seen as a means whereby the economic burden of drug-prescribing can be reduced or contained. There can be little argument with the recommendation that the cheaper of two compounds should be selected where agents are similar in terms of efficacy and adverse reactions. Likewise, generic substitution is also desirable provided that there is bio-equivalence. It has become increasingly impractical for pharmacists to stock all the formulations of every antibiotic currently available, and here again an antibiotic policy can produce significant savings by limiting the amount and variety of stock held. A policy based on a restricted number of agents also enables price reduction on purchasing costs through competitive tendering. The above activities have had a major influence on containing or reducing drug costs, although these savings have often been lost as new and often expensive preparations become available, particularly in the field of biological and anticancer therapy.

Another increasingly important argument in favour of an antibiotic policy is the occurrence of drug-resistant bacteria within an institution. The presence of sick patients and the opportunities for the spread of microorganisms can produce outbreaks of hospital infection. The excessive use of selected agents has been associated with the emergence of drug-resistant bacteria which have often caused serious problems within high-dependency areas, such as intensive care units or burns units where antibiotic use is often high. One oft-quoted example is the occurrence of a multiple antibiotic-resistant *Klebsiella aerogenes* within a neurosurgical intensive care unit in which the organism became resistant to all currently available antibiotics and was associated with the widespread use of ampicillin. By prohibiting the use of all antibiotics, and in particular ampicillin, the resistant organism rapidly disappeared and the problem was resolved.

One of the most important hospital-acquired pathogens in the early twenty-first century was methicillin-resistant *S. aureus*, which is responsible for a range of serious infections such as pneumonia, postoperative wound infection and skin infections which may in turn be complicated by bloodstream spread. The use of vancomycin and teicoplanin has escalated as a consequence, and in turn has been linked to the emergence of vancomycin-resistant enterococci.

More recently, the increased prevalence of ESBL-producing Gram-negative pathogens in intensive care settings, and further afield, has led to increased usage of carbapenems, and a corresponding rise in carbapenem-resistant *Klebsiella* and *Pseudomonas* species; carbapenem-resistant Gram-negative outbreaks are among the most challenging infection control issues of today.

In formulating an antibiotic policy, it is important that the susceptibility of microorganisms be monitored and reviewed at regular intervals. This applies not only to the hospital as a whole, but to specific high-dependency units in particular. Likewise, general practitioner samples should also be monitored. This will provide accurate information on drug susceptibility to guide the prescriber as to the most effective agent.

14.4.2 Types of Antibiotic Policies

There are a number of different approaches to the organisation of an antibiotic policy. These range from a deliberate absence of any restriction on prescribing to a strict policy whereby all anti-infective agents must have expert approval before they are administered. Restrictive policies vary according to whether they are mainly laboratory-controlled, by employing restrictive reporting, or whether they are mainly pharmacy-controlled, by restrictive dispensing. In many institutions, it is common practice to combine the two approaches.

14.4.2.1 Free Prescribing

The advocates of a free prescribing policy argue that strict antibiotic policies are both impractical and limit clinical freedom to prescribe. It is also argued that the greater the number of agents in use, the less likely it is that drug resistance will emerge to any one agent or class of agents. However, few would support such an approach, which may encourage indiscriminate prescribing and overuse.

14.4.2.2 Selective Reporting

Another approach that is widely practised in the UK is that of selective reporting. The laboratory, largely for practical reasons, tests only a limited range of agents against bacterial isolates. The agents may be selected primarily by microbiology staff or following consultation with their clinical colleagues. The antibiotics tested will vary according to the site of infection, as drugs used to treat urinary tract infections often differ from those used to treat systemic disease.

There are specific problems regarding the testing of certain agents such as the cephalosporins, where the many different preparations have varying activity against bacteria. The practice of testing a single agent to represent first-generation, second-generation or third-generation compounds is questionable, and with the newer compounds susceptibility should be tested specifically to that agent. By selecting a limited range of compounds for use, sensitivity testing becomes a practical consideration and allows the clinician to use such agents with greater confidence.

14.4.2.3 Restricted Dispensing

As mentioned above, the most draconian of all antibiotic policies is the absolute restriction of drug dispensing pending expert approval. The expert opinion may be provided by either a microbiologist or infectious disease specialist. Such a system can only be effective in large institutions where staff are available 24 hours a day. This approach is often cumbersome, may generate hostility and does not necessarily create the best educational forum for learning effective antibiotic prescribing.

A more widely used approach is to divide agents into those approved for unrestricted use and those for restricted use. Agents on the unrestricted list are appropriate for the majority of common clinical situations. The restricted list may include agents where microbiological sensitivity information is essential, such as for vancomycin and certain aminoglycosides. In addition, agents that are used infrequently but for specific indications, such as parenteral amphotericin B, are also restricted in use. Other compounds that may be expensive and used for specific indications, such as broad-spectrum β-lactams in the treatment of *P. aeruginosa* infections, may also be justifiably included on the restricted list. Items omitted from the restricted or unrestricted list are generally not stocked, although they can be obtained at short notice as necessary.

Such a policy should have a mechanism whereby desirable new agents are added as they become available and is most appropriately decided at a therapeutics committee. Policing such a policy is best effected as a joint arrangement between senior pharmacists and microbiologists. This combined approach of both restricted reporting and restricted prescribing is extremely effective and provides a powerful educational tool for medical staff and students faced with learning the complexities of modern antibiotic prescribing.

14.4.2.4 The Antimicrobial Stewardship Team

In an attempt to ensure antimicrobials are prescribed appropriately in hospitals, antimicrobial stewardship teams have emerged to advise and educate staff while monitoring compliance with prescribing policies as well as ensuring good standards of patient management. Typically, these teams comprise, at their core, a consultant in infectious diseases and/or clinical microbiology, and a senior pharmacist specialising in infectious diseases, and may also include infection control practitioners. The team takes a lead in reviewing the therapy of individual patients and setting treatment plans, and, often as part of a wider team, will coordinate the writing and review of antibiotic treatment policies. Other responsibilities may include the education and training of clinical staff, the audit of how well prescribers are adhering to the carefully written policies and the provision of feedback to prescribers. Evidence suggests that this multidisciplinary approach, aligned with targeted and timely feedback, can improve adherence to prescribing policy, reduce drug expenditure and improve patient outcomes. Antibiotic stewardship is discussed further in Chapter 15.

Acknowledgements

The contribution of Prof Roger Finch, who prepared the chapter on Clinical Uses of Antimicrobial Drugs in previous editions of this book, is gratefully acknowledged.

References

Cek, M., Tandoğdu, Z., Wagenlehner, F. et al. (2014). Healthcare-associated urinary tract infections in hospitalized urological patients--a global perspective: results from the GPIU studies 2003-2010. *World J. Urol.* 32 (6): 1587–1594.

Flores-Mireless, A.L., Walker, J.N., Caparon, M., and Hultgren, S.J. (2015). Urinary tract infections: epidemiology, mechanisms of infection and treatment options. *Nature Reviews Microbiology* 13: 269–284.

Shenoy, E.S., Macy, E., Rowe, T., and Blumenthal, K.G. (2019). Evaluation and management of penicillin allergy: a review. *JAMA* 321 (2): 188–199.

Further Reading

Brown, N.M., Goodman, A.L., Horner, C. et al. (2021). Treatment of methicillin-resistant *Staphylococcus aureus* (MRSA): updated guidelines from the UK. *JAC Antimicrob. Resist.* 3 (1): dlaa114s.

Marchello, C.S., Carr, S.D., and Crump, J.A. (2020). A systematic review on antimicrobial resistance among salmonella Typhi worldwide. *Am. J. Trop. Med. Hyg.* 103 (6): 2518–2527.

National Institute for Health and Care Excellence (2021). Clinical knowledge summaries - sore throat, acute https://cks.nice.org.uk/topics/sore-throat-acute (accessed September 2022)

National Institute for Health and Care Excellence (2019). Pneumonia (community-acquired): antimicrobial prescribing, NICE guideline [NG138] www.nice.org.uk/guidance/ng138/chapter/Summary-of-the-evidence#choice-of-antibiotics (accessed September 2022)

National Institute for Health and Care Excellence (2022). Antimicrobial Stewardship https://www.nice.org.uk/guidance/health-protection/communicable-diseases/antimicrobial-stewardship (accessed September 2022)

Public Health England (2020). *English Surveillance Programme for Antimicrobial Utilisation and Resistance Report 2019–2020*. London: Public Health England.

Watts, V., Brown, B., Ahmed, M. et al. (2020). Routine laboratory surveillance of antimicrobial resistance in community-acquired urinary tract infections adequately informs prescribing policy in England. *JAC Antimicrob. Resist.* 2 (2): dlaa022.

15

Antibiotic Prescribing and Antimicrobial Stewardship

Rebecca Craig

Senior Lecturer (Education), School of Pharmacy, Queen's University Belfast, Belfast, UK

CONTENTS

15.1 The Need for Antimicrobial Stewardship

> Antibiotics are one of the most powerful tools we have against infection. Resistance to these drugs therefore places much of modern medicine in jeopardy. A key component of our response to this problem is to ensure people use antibiotics appropriately.
>
> *(Chief Medical Officer for England, Professor Chris Whitty, 2019)*

15.1.1 The Problem of Antibiotic Resistance

Since their discovery in the 1940s, antibiotics have revolutionised medicine, and many of the procedures that are now considered routine – transplantation, cancer treatment, the care of premature babies and several forms of surgery – would be impossible without them. Yet, unfortunately, and largely because they have been taken for granted, antibiotics are becoming less effective as a result of bacterial resistance, and the pace of development of new

Hugo and Russell's Pharmaceutical Microbiology, Ninth Edition. Edited by Brendan F. Gilmore and Stephen P. Denyer.

Companion website: https://www.wiley.com/go/HugoandRussells9e

antibiotics is currently insufficient to address this problem. It was recognised from the start of the antibiotic era that bacteria had the potential to develop resistance to antimicrobial drugs, but it took considerable time before the perception of antibiotic resistance changed from one in which it was regarded as unusual to one where it was expected; in other words, a recognition that long-term efficacy was the exception, and resistance was the rule.

The emergence towards the end of the twentieth century of the antibiotic-resistant pathogens described in Chapter 13 brought with it both the prospect of untreatable infections, where the organisms responsible were resistant to all available agents, and a growing sense of urgency to take steps to preserve the usefulness of the antibiotics currently available. Antibiotic-resistant organisms are an increasing problem, accounting for at least 33,000 deaths in Europe, and an excess of 2.8 million infections and 35,000 deaths annually in the USA, with indications that the true mortality may be 4–5 times greater. Global mortality from antimicrobial-resistant infection, currently estimated to be at least 1.27 million per annum, is on a trajectory, unless curbed, towards an annual mortality of 10 million by 2050. Additionally, the damage to the economy, due to healthcare costs and the effect on sustainable food production, could place 24 million people in extreme poverty by 2030. Healthcare costs arising from antibiotic-resistant infections are already significant, costing at least \$20 billion per annum in direct costs alone in the USA, and £180 million per annum for the National Health Service (NHS) in the UK. Regardless of the economic harm, the cost of antibiotic resistance should, of course, be measured primarily in terms of the suffering that results from the failure of antibiotics to cure infections against which they were formerly effective; from this perspective, the cost is immeasurable.

The pathogens responsible for antibiotic-resistant infections can arise both in the home and the hospital environment, but it is in the latter that they are considerably more prevalent and problematic. Hospital-acquired infections account for a substantial number of deaths each year and the treatment of such infections is time-consuming, difficult and costly. There are also less obvious consequences of resistance: when first-line drugs cease to be effective, it may be necessary to revert to more toxic alternatives. *Acinetobacter* infections are an example of this circumstance because the organism is naturally multidrug-resistant and the incidence of isolates resistant to all first-line antibiotics has risen from 5 to 60% within 20 years in the USA, with carbapenem resistance now above 90% in some countries. Therefore, colistin, a drug that became virtually obsolete in the 1960s because of the significant risk of kidney damage is now, for many patients, the most likely antibiotic choice. Similarly, β-lactam-resistant *Enterobacteriaceae*, which can cause a range of severe infections including bloodstream infections and ventilator-associated pneumonia, could once be treated with carbapenems, but the emergence and rapid rise of carbapenem-resistant *Enterobacteriaceae* has resulted in colistin now also being one of the last-resort therapies for these infections. A further cause of concern for these infections is that colistin resistance has recently been detected in several countries.

15.1.2 The Challenge of New Antibiotic Development

Unfortunately, antibiotics have, to a certain extent, become victims of their own success: the more effective an antibiotic is, the shorter the likely duration of treatment, so the more difficult the cost recovery for the company which developed it. Many courses of antibiotic treatment last for a week or less, so the sales accruing from them are significantly inferior to those from therapies for chronic conditions such as diabetes or hypertension. Additionally, due to global efforts to ensure affordable and much needed access, the price that can be charged for new antibiotics is often much lower than may be charged for other new therapeutics.

These economic constraints, together with (i) increasing pressure to use antibiotics sparingly, and reserving most new antibiotics as last-resort treatments, (ii) the expectation that the drug will ultimately become less effective due to resistance and (iii) difficulties in establishing clinical trials for antibiotics that satisfy the US Food and Drug Administration (FDA) criteria, particularly for the small patient cohorts involved, all combined to create a climate in which antibiotics became an unattractive commercial proposition. Antibiotic development is undoubtedly the only area of pharmaceutical development where the aim is for the final product to be used as sparingly as possible. Larger pharmaceutical companies are therefore continuing to exit the antibiotic research and development arena, leaving small- and medium-sized enterprises, including biotechnology companies, to assume the task. This is not an ideal prospect, and has resulted in a sometimes insurmountable financial burden, and even bankruptcy, for such companies, highlighting the need for new sustainable investment approaches if the resistance problem is to be tackled seriously.

The divestment policies of large pharmaceutical companies, and accompanying reduction in the number of new antibiotics coming into use, has therefore exacerbated the problem of antibiotic resistance. The resultant decreasing trend in the number of FDA antibiotic approvals between the late 1980s and the early to mid-2010s is demonstrating some signs of reversal, albeit limited. One positive step for the antibiotic development process has been the Limited Population Pathway for Antibacterial and Antifungal Drugs mechanism enacted by US Congress in 2016, which allows new antibiotics that treat serious or life-threatening infections to be studied in smaller clinical trials.

To encourage and guide antibiotic research and development, the World Health Organization (WHO) produced the Global Priority Pathogens List in 2017, which categorises organisms as critical, high or medium priority based on the urgency of the need for development of new antibiotics (Table 15.1). Four of the eight antibiotics approved since 2017 are active against the critical priority carbapenem-resistant *Enterobacteriaceae*. However, the majority of new antibiotics are modifications of existing classes of antibiotics (e.g., β-lactams), rather than entirely new chemical entities. Furthermore, most antibiotics that have been recently approved, or which are currently in development, only offer marginal benefits over existing antibiotics in terms of spectrum of activity and ability to overcome resistance.

At the time of writing, of the 43 antibiotics in the pipeline (i.e., in clinical development), over 60% have activity against the pathogens on the Global Priority Pathogens List, but only 13 have activity against at least one of the three critical priority organisms, and only 2 target all three. An additional concern is that only 3 remain active in the presence of New Delhi metallo-β-lactamase 1 (NDM-1), which can render bacteria resistant to most β-lactams, including carbapenems. A further 27 non-traditional antibacterial agents (e.g., biologicals) are also in clinical development, but these do not alter the narrative, and the higher cost of therapies such as monoclonal antibodies may be prohibitive to their use in low- and middle-income countries. Nevertheless, despite the limitations to these new and in-development antibiotics, they are still a valuable addition to the ever-narrowing range of treatment options.

15.1.3 The Need for Alternative Approaches to Antibiotic Use

The increasing frequency in the new millennium of infections due to the so-called 'ESKAPE' pathogens (*Enterococcus faecium*, *Staphylococcus aureus*, *Klebsiella* species, *Acinetobacter baumannii*, *Pseudomonas aeruginosa* and extended-spectrum β-lactamase-producing strains of *Escherichia coli* and *Enterobacter* species) (see Chapter 13), together with the depleted pipeline of new antibiotics from the pharmaceutical industry, has increased the momentum of measures to preserve what is increasingly being seen as an invaluable, and perhaps irreplaceable, resource that society has a duty to pass on to future generations.

This was highlighted at a United Nations (UN) General Assembly high-level meeting on antimicrobial resistance in 2016, which discussed the urgent necessity for countries to enact policies to tackle antimicrobial resistance. The gravity of the situation is indicated by this being only the fourth occasion in UN history for the General Assembly to discuss a health topic. In this meeting, and in a later UN interagency coordination group report entitled 'No Time

Table 15.1 World Health Organization Global Priority Pathogens List for research and development of new antibiotics (WHO 2019).

Critical Priority	
Acinetobacter baumannii	Carbapenem-resistant
Pseudomonas aeruginosa	Carbapenem-resistant
Enterobacteriaceae	Carbapenem-resistant, third-generation cephalosporin-resistant
High Priority	
Enterococcus faecium	Vancomycin-resistant
Staphylococcus aureus	Methicillin-resistant, vancomycin-resistant
Helicobacter pylori	Clarithromycin-resistant
Campylobacter spp.	Fluoroquinolone-resistant
Salmonellae	Fluoroquinolone-resistant
Neisseria gonorrhoeae	Third-generation cephalosporin-resistant, fluoroquinolone-resistant
Medium Priority	
Streptococcus pneumoniae	Penicillin-non-susceptible
Haemophilus influenzae	Ampicillin-resistant
Shigella spp.	Fluoroquinolone-resistant

to Wait: Securing the Future from Drug-Resistant Infections' (2019), the need for a One Health approach was emphasised. One Health is an approach to implementing programmes, policies/legislation and research that recognises the interconnection between human, animal and environmental health, therefore necessitating communication and collaboration across these areas to achieve improved patient health outcomes. This means that efforts cannot be constrained to any one of these sectors, but will require partnership, co-operation and sharing of resources to address the problem of antibiotic resistance. The European Union (EU) One Health Action Plan against Antimicrobial Resistance (AMR), which was adopted by the European Commission (EC) in 2017, therefore provides a framework for action to reduce the prevalence and spread of resistance in human and animal sectors, and increase development of new antimicrobials. The EU AMR One-Health Network meets bi-annually to work towards this end. Following on from the One Health Action Plan, the EC adopted the Pharmaceutical Strategy for Europe in 2020, addressing the poor investment in antimicrobials and inappropriate use of antibiotics, in addition to increasing awareness of antimicrobial resistance both amongst healthcare professionals and the public in the EU. In response to the COVID-19 pandemic, the EU4Health programme 2021–2027 was adopted to provide funding to EU countries to tackle a number of health issues, including reducing the number of antimicrobial-resistant infections.

15.2 Antibiotic Consumption

15.2.1 Relationship between Antibiotic Consumption and Bacterial Resistance

There is widespread agreement, informed by compelling evidence, that greater use of antibiotics predisposes to the development of resistance. The strength of the link between use and resistance varies from one antibiotic to another, but for many antibiotics the connection is irrefutable. However, the situation is complex: there is substantial evidence, for example, that heavy use of one antibiotic may be a risk factor for the acquisition of infections by organisms resistant to other, unrelated antibiotics – heavy cephalosporin use has been shown to increase the risk of vancomycin-resistant enterococci, and fluoroquinolone use has been associated with the prevalence of methicillin-resistant *S. aureus* (MRSA). The selective pressure created by the use of one antibiotic will often select for resistance in others because plasmids within the bacterial cell may carry resistance genes for multiple antibiotics from different chemical groups. If, for example, an organism possessed a plasmid with genes for both rifampicin and gentamicin resistance, constant exposure to gentamicin would represent a selective pressure that afforded an advantage to that organism, so not only would the incidence of isolates with gentamicin resistance be expected to rise, but so too would the incidence of rifampicin-resistant isolates.

Arguments for curtailing antibiotic use in order to restrict resistance development have been supported by both audits and surveys of antibiotic prescribing and costs, and studies that demonstrate the link between reduced use of a particular antibiotic and increased detection of susceptible clinical isolates in that area.

15.2.2 Global Antibiotic Consumption

Antibiotic consumption can be measured in different ways, including by cost and number of prescriptions, but the predominant unit of measurement is the defined daily dose (DDD). This is defined by the WHO as 'the assumed average maintenance dose per day for a drug used for its main indication in adults', and it enables standardised comparison of antibiotic use globally and evaluation of the effects of interventions.

It has been estimated that up to 50% of antibiotic prescribing is either inappropriate (wrong drug, duration, dose, route of administration, etc.) or unnecessary (not required at all). In addition to its association with development of antibiotic resistance, inappropriate antibiotic prescribing contributes to increased morbidity and cost. Global human antibiotic consumption, measured by DDDs, has risen over the past two decades, as has the use of broad-spectrum antibiotics and those antibiotics considered to be last resort. A further trebling in global antibiotic consumption is predicted by 2030. The WHO has classified antibiotics into three groups: 'access', 'watch' and 'reserve', also known as the AWaRe classification, based on the caution required in their use to prevent resistance (Table 15.2). Its aim is to optimise antibiotic monitoring and use, and reduce resistance, without reducing access. The AWaRe classification can be used as a tool for antibiotic stewardship programmes (ASPs) locally, nationally and globally, and has been adopted by many countries worldwide, including the UK, Germany and Bangladesh, in addition to gaining the approval of the G20 nations.

Globally, marked differences in antibiotic use exist, which may reflect overuse in some countries and inadequate access in others. Encouragingly, 50% of antibiotic use worldwide is from those in the 'access' category, with the most frequently used antibiotics being amoxicillin and co-amoxiclav, both of which are also recommended by WHO as first-line treatments for frequently occurring infections.

Table 15.2 World Health Organization (WHO) AWaRe classification of antibiotics.

	Access	Watch	Reserve	Not recommended
Summary	Lower resistance risk than antibiotics in the watch or reserve group Should account for at least 60% of antibiotic consumption in each country by 2023	Broad spectrum Use with caution due to potential to cause resistance and/or side effects Prioritise as targets of antibiotic stewardship programmes	Last resort For treatment of infections caused by multi-drug resistant bacteria Prioritise as targets of national and international antibiotic stewardship programmes	Fixed-dose combinations of multiple broad-spectrum antibiotics
Examples	Amoxicillin, amoxicillin/clavulanic acid (co-amoxiclav)	Second- and third-generation cephalosporins, carbapenems	Colistin, aztreonam, linezolid	Amoxicillin/flucloxacillin combination

Fewer antibiotics are prescribed from the 'watch' category (20–50%), and less than 2% of global antibiotic use is from the 'reserve' group; however, the lack of 'reserve' antibiotics reported from low- and middle-income countries may suggest inadequate access to drugs needed for treatment of multidrug-resistant infections. Indeed, those without access to antimicrobials may number as many as 2 billion, mostly in low- and middle-income countries, and this inaccessibility may be responsible for a mortality of 6 million. Within Europe, antibiotic consumption varies substantially (Figure 15.1), but the higher use in some countries, such as in France, is not necessarily justified by greater infection rates or better cure rates than countries with lower use, such as the Netherlands, therefore suggesting inappropriate prescribing. Similarly, within each country, the differences in antibiotic prescribing rates between regions are rarely attributable to differences in disease incidence alone. For example, in England, one study demonstrated that higher rates of antibiotic prescribing in general practitioner (GP) surgeries (primary care) could be linked with higher GP workload or shorter consultations, rather than higher infection rates alone.

Differences in antibiotic consumption between primary and secondary care are evident globally, with the majority of antibiotic prescribing generally occurring in primary care. In England, approximately 81% of antibiotic prescribing occurs in primary care, yet up to 23% of these prescriptions have been reported as inappropriate – mainly for upper respiratory tract infections, or ear infections. Globally, however, up to 50% of prescribing for these indications in community settings may be inappropriate. In England, the total use of antibiotics decreased between 2013 and 2020, but this was due to decreased use in primary care. Hospital antibiotic use increased; however, the reasons for this are difficult to discern and are likely to be multifactorial. As may be expected, the use of antibiotics in the 'reserve' and 'watch' categories in acute hospital environments in the UK is higher than in primary and community care.

15.2.3 Non-prescription Access to Antibiotics

Throughout the world, there is variation in the ease of availability of antibiotics to the general public. In many countries, antibiotics are supplied without prescription – either because the practice is not illegal, or because the law is not enforced. Supply of antibiotics from community pharmacies without prescription, commonly broad-spectrum antibiotics for acute and self-limiting conditions, is a global concern. Self-medication with antibiotics (obtained via the internet or simply by patients using leftover antibiotics prescribed at an earlier date for unrelated infections) is another practice that leads to uncontrolled and often inappropriate antibiotic use, and so contributes to the resistance problem. Within the UK, only one systemic antibiotic – azithromycin – has been deregulated from a prescription-only medicine (POM) to pharmacy-only (P) status, allowing it to be dispensed within pharmacies without prescription for the defined purpose of treating chlamydial infection. Similar reclassification of other antibiotics, for example, trimethoprim and nitrofurantoin, was abandoned in 2010 – a welcome outcome in light of resistance concerns – and no further antibiotic reclassifications have since been proposed.

Apart from the likely increase in use leading to increased resistance, one of the strongest arguments against the availability of antibiotics without prescription is that it would remove the means by which the consumption of a particular antibiotic could be monitored and correlated with any resistance trends – prescriptions can be counted, but sales in pharmacies and shops are generally not. The ability to operate surveillance systems is an integral component of antibiotic stewardship, so any change in the legal

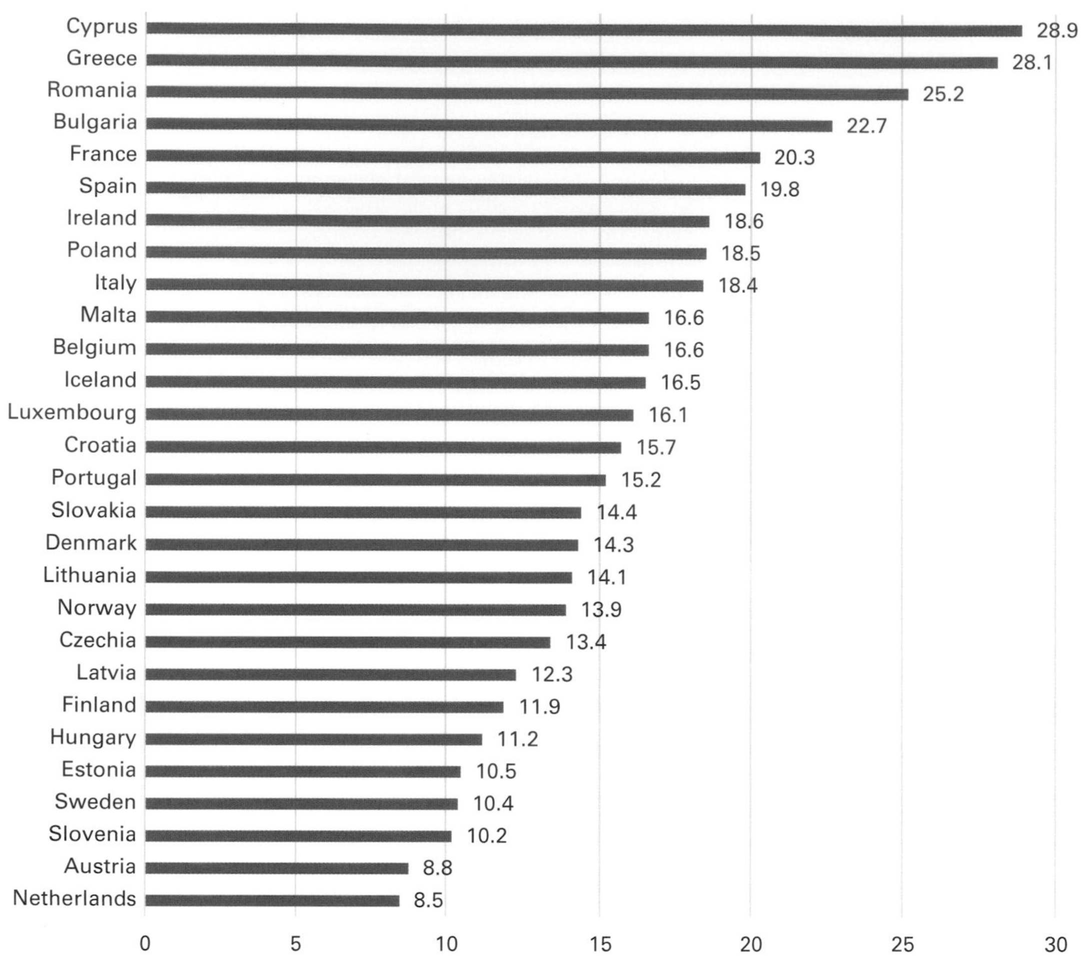

Figure 15.1 Total consumption of systemic antibiotics in Europe in 2020. No data available for Liechtenstein or Germany. *Source:* Data obtained from the European Centre for Disease Prevention and Control (ECDC). UK data not available for 2020, however the figure in 2019 was 18.8.

status of systemic antibiotics to make them available without prescription would undermine the support for prudent antibiotic use.

15.2.4 Non-human Antibiotic Use

The majority of the annual global production of antibiotics is not used in the treatment of human or animal infection. Rather, most of the antibiotic output of the pharmaceutical industry is used as a food additive to increase weight gain in cattle, pigs and poultry, or for routine mass disease prevention in intensive farming environments – some estimates put this proportion above 70% – and yet more is used in plant production, but this fraction is poorly defined. Although antibiotics that are used to treat human infections have been banned as growth promoters in Europe for many years, it is still a common practice in many countries. Even the legitimate use of antibiotics is considerable: the total volume of veterinary antibiotics sold for use in food-producing animals in Europe in 2017 was 6703 tonnes, with the majority being tetracyclines and penicillins. By 2030, global consumption of antibiotics in food animal production is predicted to increase to over 100,000 tonnes. This, therefore, necessitates a global effort to curtail the use of antibiotics for growth promotion – which many see as inappropriate and a likely contributor to resistance development – and to promote prudent prescribing for legitimate use. A recent study demonstrated that reducing antibiotic use in farm animals resulted in up to 32% reduction in multidrug-resistant bacteria in those animals, and an up to 24% reduction in antibiotic-resistant bacteria in humans, although the latter data were less robust. Nonetheless, this demonstrates the potential impact of interventions to reduce antibiotic use in animals.

The EU has taken significant steps towards reducing antibiotic consumption in animals, including introducing new legislation which took effect in 2022 – the Veterinary Medicinal Products Regulation – based on a One Health approach. This will prevent the use in animals of certain antibiotics reserved for human use, and ensure that animal antimicrobials are only available on veterinary prescription. Additionally, an FDA 5-year plan to support veterinary antimicrobial stewardship was released in 2018, and veterinary associations in the UK have produced guidance to support responsible prescribing. The results of efforts can already be seen, with a downward trend in the use of antibiotics in animals in the UK and Europe in recent years, including a 66% decrease in the sales of polymyxins (e.g., colistin) in Europe since 2011.

15.3 Antimicrobial Stewardship Programmes

15.3.1 Definition and Aims of Antimicrobial Stewardship

Resistance to both old and new antibiotics is inevitable, but if the risk and rate of resistance development can be reduced by prudent prescribing and judicious use of the antibiotics currently available, this will ensure their continuing value in infection treatment. Antimicrobial stewardship can be variously defined, but the definition provided by the Infectious Diseases Society of America (IDSA), Society for Healthcare Epidemiology of America (SHEA) and Pediatric Infectious Diseases Society (PIDS) is of benefit:

> Co-ordinated interventions designed to improve and measure the appropriate use of antimicrobial agents by promoting the selection of the optimal antimicrobial drug regimen including dosing, duration of therapy and route of administration.

An ASP, then, can be defined as a strategy to promote appropriate antimicrobial use through implementing evidence-based interventions (WHO). The main aims of an ASP are to:

- improve antimicrobial prescribing;
- improve clinical outcomes for patients;
- minimise the toxicity and adverse events that may be experienced, including secondary infection;
- reduce the costs associated with inappropriate prescribing;
- reduce the selective pressure on bacterial populations;
- reduce resistance levels, or, at the very least, decelerate the development of antibiotic-resistant bacterial strains.

ASPs have consistently demonstrated progress in meeting these aims, therefore warranting their presence as key components of many antimicrobial resistance strategies. The healthcare savings from ASPs routinely outweigh the costs involved in implementing interventions, thus providing further incentive. Additionally, it is estimated that scaling up hospital ASPs could reduce total deaths due to antimicrobial resistance by 54% (in Organisation for Economic Co-operation and Development [OECD] countries).

15.3.2 Components of an ASP

There are no nationally or internationally accepted guidelines on the structure of an ASP, so they vary from country to country and even from one site to another within a geographical region, as they will be influenced by the needs of the area, local resistance patterns and resources, and therefore each must be tailored based on evidence, as required for the particular site of use. However, although there is no harmonised ASP structure, evidence-based guidelines are available regarding the core elements and interventions that should be considered in the design and implementation of an ASP.

15.3.2.1 Core Elements of ASPs

In 2019, the Centers for Disease Control and Prevention (CDC) published a description of the core elements of hospital ASPs in light of growing evidence of antibiotic stewardship and data gathered since the implementation of the first iteration in 2014. Hospitals and long-term care facilities in the USA are now required to implement ASPs that align with these core elements. While US stewardship guidelines have been available since 2007 (then from the IDSA and SHEA) and widely adopted in the USA and elsewhere, the situation in Europe was less uniform until recent years. A technical report produced by the European Centre for Disease Prevention and Control (ECDC) in 2017 formed the basis of EU guidelines for the prudent use of antimicrobials in human health (published by the EC in 2017). The similarities between the EC and the CDC guidelines are evident (Table 15.3).

A multidisciplinary team should be involved, and must include leadership from physicians and pharmacists, ideally as joint leaders. Generally, the team consists of:

- an infectious diseases physician;
- a clinical pharmacist with infectious diseases training;

Table 15.3 Core elements of hospital ASPs as recommended by the CDC (USA) and the EC (Europe). The elements from each have been aligned where possible.

Core elements of hospital ASPs, as recommended by the CDC	Elements of hospital ASPs, as recommended by the EC
Hospital leadership commitment • Dedication of the required resources, including staffing, financial and information technology • Support from groups including clinicians, pharmacy committee, department heads, infection preventionists and microbiology	• Antimicrobial committee with senior management support • Salary support and time for AMS activities, microbiology lab service availability, availability of facility-specific pathogen susceptibility reports
Accountability • Leader(s) who are responsible for the programme management and outcome Pharmacy expertise • Either as leader or co-leader	AMS team • Including clinician, hospital pharmacist and microbiologist
Action • Implement interventions including prospective audit and feedback and preauthorisation, treatment guidelines and pharmacy interventions such as documentation of antibiotic indications and dose optimisation	• Treatment guidelines • Documentation of indication, drug, dose, route and treatment duration in patient records • Policy for preauthorisation or post-prescription review of selected antimicrobial prescriptions
Tracking • Antibiotic prescribing • Impact of interventions • Other outcomes (e.g., patient outcomes)	• Audit of perioperative antimicrobial prophylaxis • Monitoring of quality indicators and quantity metrics of antimicrobial use
Reporting of information on antibiotic use and resistance	Annual report on AMS activities
Education of healthcare professionals and patients	

CDC, Centers for Disease Control and Prevention; AMS, antimicrobial stewardship.

- a medical microbiologist;
- an infection control professional;
- a hospital epidemiologist;
- an information technology specialist.

At least one team member must have training in antimicrobial stewardship. The importance of commitment and involvement from hospital management cannot be overstated. It is easier to gain approval for the necessary budget allocation if there is a publicly stated management goal of improving prescribing. Where preauthorisation for selected antibiotics is a part of the programme, the greater the authority bestowed on the person(s) making the recommendations, the greater the effectiveness of the policy has been shown to be.

While the guidelines do include good clinical practice for stewardship, it is still the responsibility of national/regional/local governments to establish the required measures to ensure prudent antibiotic use. In the UK, the National Institute for Health and Care Excellence (NICE) has published guidance on antimicrobial stewardship in secondary care, alongside a quality standard on antimicrobial stewardship.

15.3.3 ASP Interventions and their Evidence

The IDSA and the SHEA have described evidence-based guidelines for implementing an ASP for inpatient care (emergency, acute or long-term care). These focus on interventions, rather than on the core elements of an ASP, which are already described in detail in the CDC core elements. Twenty-eight interventions are discussed, and five of these are strongly recommended based on the quality of the evidence, among other factors. These are shown in Table 15.4.

Many of these interventions are also addressed in the practical guide to antimicrobial stewardship published by the WHO Regional Office for Europe in 2021 (WHO 2021).

15.3.3.1 Strongly Recommended Interventions

The evidence for preauthorisation and prospective audit and feedback points to these being the most effective stewardship strategies in hospitals. Unsurprisingly, they are also listed as priority interventions in the CDC core elements.

- *Preauthorisation*
  Preauthorisation requires the prescriber to gain approval, usually from a member of the stewardship programme,

Table 15.4 Antimicrobial stewardship recommendations from the IDSA and SHEA, listed according to strength of recommendation. 'Other' recommendations are based on lower-quality evidence, or on good practice; only a selection of other recommendations is presented in the table.

Strongly recommended interventions	Other suggested interventions
1) Preauthorisation and/or prospective audit and feedback 2) Interventions to reduce use of antibiotics associated with a high risk of *Clostridioides difficile* infection 3) Implementation of pharmacokinetic monitoring and adjustment programmes for aminoglycoside in hospitals 4) Greater use of oral antibiotics 5) Implementation of guidelines to reduce therapy to the shortest effective duration	• Didactic education • Facility-specific clinical practice guidelines • Interventions to improve antibiotic use and outcomes in patients with specific infectious diseases • Allergy assessments in patients with a reported β-lactam allergy • Rapid diagnostic testing, culture and routine reporting • Measure antibiotic expenditure based on prescriptions • ASPs in neonatal intensive care units, nursing homes and for terminally-ill patients

before administering the first dose of certain antibiotics. This helps to rationalise the choice of empiric therapy, and prevent unnecessary antibiotic prescribing. It can also provide an opportunity for education of the prescriber, therefore contributing to improved choices on future occasions. Of course, authorisations must be completed in a timely manner to prevent unnecessary delay in therapy, therefore requiring appropriate resources to facilitate this.

- *Prospective audit and feedback*
  In this context, a prospective audit means a review of the future delivery of healthcare to ensure that best practice is being carried out, so a prospective audit with intervention and feedback is a process in which the use of antibiotics is monitored and suggestions made for improvement, where necessary, *while the course of treatment is still in progress*. The feedback element is the provision of information to the prescriber about the drug in question, e.g., local resistance patterns and dose information based upon pharmacokinetic data. Prospective audit and feedback therefore allow the prescriber to prescribe empiric therapy, but this will be reviewed by a member of the ASP, e.g., pharmacist (commonly within 48–72 hours), who will then provide recommendations to optimise or adjust the therapy.

Both approaches have been demonstrated to reduce inappropriate use of antibiotics, achieve cost savings and are associated with no adverse effects. Prospective audit and feedback can significantly reduce antibiotic consumption, but its long-term impact on restricting resistance development is not yet proven. Preauthorisation, however, is associated with a demonstrable increase in susceptible clinical isolates.

- *Interventions to reduce antibiotic use associated with a high risk of Clostridioides difficile infection*
  Evidence demonstrates the utility of hospital ASPs in achieving and sustaining reduced *C. difficile* infection rates. Antibiotic-resistant *C. difficile* infections are rare, although should not be discounted, but it is the relationship between *C. difficile* infections and antibiotic use – most commonly second-, third- and fourth-generation cephalosporins, quinolones, clindamycin and carbapenems – that warrants the inclusion of this intervention in ASPs. *C. difficile* causes at least 125,000 infections at a cost of €3 billion per annum in Europe, with a mortality rate of up to 25%. The general decline in *C. difficile* incidence in England since 2007 is presumedly a testament to decreased use of these high-risk antibiotics, in addition to infection prevention and control measures. However, it should be noted that, likely due to a change in prescribing patterns to avoid using cephalosporins and to use alternative broad-spectrum agents, an increase in the rate of piperacillin–tazobactam and co-amoxiclav-associated *C. difficile* infection has been observed. This reinforces the need for judicial prescribing of all broad-spectrum antibiotics – not just those classified as high risk – to reduce the risk of *C. difficile* infection.
- *Pharmacokinetic monitoring and adjustment (therapeutic drug monitoring)*
  This involves measuring serum antibiotic levels at specific intervals, interpreting the data and then adjusting the dosage to maintain blood levels within the required therapeutic range, therefore optimising efficacy and minimising the risk of side effects. It appears to be of particular benefit in maintaining serum aminoglycoside concentrations within the therapeutic range for intravenous aminoglycoside therapy, resulting in reduced nephrotoxicity (one of the side effects of aminoglycoside overdose) and reduced length of stay, reduced hospital costs and lower mortality.

- *Greater use of oral antibiotics*
  Both increasing the use of initial oral antibiotic therapy and encouraging a timely conversion from intravenous to oral therapy have been shown to reduce the length of hospital stay and drug costs, without adverse effect on efficacy or patient safety. In addition to cost savings, this strategy may also permit earlier removal of intravenous lines which, if in place for too long, facilitate the establishment of infections by skin pathogens such as *Staphylococcus epidermidis*.
- *Reducing therapy to the shortest effective duration*
  This is well supported by evidence, although it is problematic for disease conditions for which a specific effective duration has not been determined. Overall, research indicates similar clinical outcomes with shorter courses when compared to longer courses, including for bacteraemia treatment – even when shortening the duration of therapy by almost half (e.g., reducing from 15 days to 8 days) – with no difference in relapse rate. Reducing the duration of therapy can be supported by evidence-based guidelines (e.g., NICE guidelines), and by the preauthorisation or prospective audit and feedback process.

15.3.3.2 Additional Interventions

- *Education*
  Education of patients to dissuade them from pressurising prescribers for antibiotics – particularly for cold and flu or other viral infections in primary care settings – has established merit. However, passive didactic education of prescribers (using lectures, bulletins, e-mail alerts and teaching sessions) should never be relied upon as a stand-alone strategy for antimicrobial stewardship, particularly in light of the demonstrated lack of sustainability in resultant prescribing changes. Rather, education should be integrated into an ASP, alongside other strategies, and must be included as part of the training of medical, pharmacy, nursing and other healthcare students. Case-based education, as would be provided to the prescriber during preauthorisation or prospective audit and feedback, is noted by the CDC to have more impact, particularly when the education is provided in person.
- *Diagnostic testing*
  The ability to correctly identify the causative organism in a timely manner is necessary for effective stewardship, as the incorrect diagnosis (e.g., misdiagnosing fungal sepsis as bacterial sepsis) can lead to misuse of antibiotics and poor patient outcomes. Diagnostic tests vary in their capabilities and so must be chosen carefully to ensure both their suitability for the clinical situation and their reliability to avoid acquiring misleading results. Traditional diagnostic tests, which often employ genotypic or phenotypic methods, may require more than 72 hours to identify the causative organism, which can therefore delay the start of appropriate therapy. Rapid diagnostic testing, which involves the use of different assays that can provide results in hours or even minutes, rather than days (e.g., peptic nucleic acid fluorescent in situ hybridisation, or polymerase chain reaction [PCR]), is becoming a tangible reality. These diagnostics enable rapid selection or optimisation of treatment and such tests are advocated particularly for bloodstream and acute respiratory tract infections, where early identification of the causative organism is vital. For these infections, rapid diagnostic testing can reduce the time to appropriate treatment, and enable therapy such as vancomycin to be stopped where the test indicates that it is not required for the causative organism. Such tests should be used as part of, rather than separately from, an ASP.
- *Improving antibiotic use in specific diseases*
  There is convincing evidence that practice guidelines and clinical pathways incorporating local resistance patterns can generally improve antimicrobial use. Evidence-based disease state-specific clinical practice guidelines, such as those produced by NICE in the UK, are beneficial when integrated as part of an ASP; if used alone, they may be insufficient to have an impact on prescribing. Such guidelines, or clinical pathways, are intended to reduce the variability both in the quality of care and patient outcomes by the adoption of defined, standardised and sequenced procedures for patients with specific conditions – in this context, infections.
- *Allergy assessment*
  Penicillin allergy is frequently recorded on patient records, but it has been estimated that fewer than 1% of these patients possess a true allergy, yet the resultant avoidance of β-lactam antibiotics in these patients can result in treatment with broader-spectrum alternatives (e.g., carbapenems) that can lead to significant antibiotic resistance and *C. difficile* infection. β-lactam allergy may be assessed with a penicillin skin test, if performed by appropriately trained and resourced staff, who are competent in identification and treatment of anaphylaxis, which can enable optimisation of treatment and circumvent the risks described.

15.3.4 Antimicrobial Stewardship in Primary and Community Care

While guidelines abound for ASPs in secondary care, similarly detailed guidelines around stewardship programmes are not as readily available for community or primary care settings. Certainly, aspects of the CDC and ECDC elements for hospital ASPs (e.g., education, tracking/audit, treatment guidelines, leadership and multidisciplinary input) have

Table 15.5 OECD intervention packages, with associated predicted impact on antibiotic-resistant infection and costs.

	Intervention	Reduction in burden of infection from antibiotic resistance	Cost savings (USD PPP per capita per year)
For hospitals	ASP Increased hand hygiene Improved environmental hygiene	85%	4.1
Community actions	Delayed prescriptions Mass media campaigns Rapid diagnostic tests	23%	0.9
Mixed intervention package	ASP Improved environmental hygiene Mass media campaigns Rapid diagnostic tests	73%	3

ASP, Antimicrobial stewardship programme; PPP, purchasing power parity (allows comparison of cost between countries); USD, US dollars.

utility in primary care. In the UK, resources such as the NICE antimicrobial resistance quality standard and antimicrobial stewardship prescribing pathway cover some aspects of primary care, while the TARGET (Treat Antibiotics Responsibly: Guidance, Education and Tools) antibiotic toolkit provides clear guidance for GPs around antimicrobial prescribing and antibiotic resistance in primary care, and antimicrobial stewardship tools including audit templates and patient self-care information. Therefore, rather than existing as detailed wholistic ASP guidelines such as those provided for hospital, the community and primary care resources provide a series of guidelines to improve prescribing, supplemented by educational strategies (for both prescribers and patients), and promote the use of approaches such as delayed prescriptions. The approaches advocated have demonstrable efficacy in reducing unnecessary antibiotic prescriptions, but what the guidelines often lack in comparison to hospital guidelines is the emphasis of a clearly defined team effort with leadership accountability.

For antimicrobial stewardship to be truly effective across healthcare services, an integrated approach will be required: bacteria know no boundaries between hospital and community, and neither should our stewardship efforts be constrained or halted by these boundaries. It is expected, as healthcare becomes increasingly integrated across different settings, that stewardship approaches also will, and that such integration will in turn, better facilitate the One Health approach promoted by the UN, WHO, EU and others.

15.3.5 ASPs and Infection Prevention and Control Strategies

Curtailment of the use of antibiotics for growth promotion, together with better-targeted and promoted use of vaccines (that would reduce the need for antibiotics), better diagnostic agents which would more rapidly and accurately identify the infecting organism and so inform the selection of the best antibiotic, better epidemiological data and computer analysis to provide early warnings of resistance trends, and changes in other medical practices such as the early removal of catheters and cannulas which are, themselves, a means by which pathogens can enter the body, could all be seen as part of a concerted stewardship programme. But from the perspective of controlling the incidence and spread of antibiotic-resistant organisms, it cannot be over-emphasised that a comprehensive infection control programme (including improving sanitation and hygiene) is of paramount importance (see Chapter 16).

In recognition of the need for a multifaceted approach to tackle the problem of antibiotic resistance, the OECD has proposed three multi-component intervention strategies for this purpose (Table 15.5). In these strategies, ASPs form just one aspect of an overall intervention package, and it is clear that they should always be implemented alongside infection prevention and control programmes. The proposed consequences for antibiotic-resistant infections and cost savings are tremendous, and a strong incentive to ensure inclusion of ASPs as part of a multifaceted approach, rather than in isolation.

15.3.6 The Experience of ASPs during a Pandemic

In March 2020, coronavirus disease 2019 (COVID-19) was declared a pandemic by the WHO (see Chapter 5). From the beginning of the pandemic, there was an increase in the use of broad-spectrum antibiotics, particularly in hospital settings. The uncertainty that surrounded COVID-19 pathology, and the time required to wait for a diagnostic test result, may have increased the likelihood of prescribing antibiotics due to a desire to give patients the best possible chance of survival. Reports from various countries demonstrated that between 71% and 96% of hospitalised COVID-19 patients received antibiotics on admission; however, it is likely that only up to 15% of those patients had bacterial infections, and therefore actually required antibiotics. A proportion of COVID-19 patients have indeed acquired bacterial infections, although more likely secondary to intubation during their hospital stay, rather than having been present at admission. Therefore, recognising the widespread potentially inappropriate use of antibiotics, the WHO recommended the use of antibiotics only for cases of severe COVID-19, where there is an increased risk of secondary bacterial infections and death. Likewise, in the UK, NICE guidelines regarding COVID-19 management only recommended antibiotics if there was a strong clinical suspicion of additional bacterial infection. Neither guidelines recommend the use of antibiotics in patients with mild or moderate COVID-19, in the absence of signs or symptoms of bacterial infection.

The circumstances surrounding the COVID-19 pandemic – particularly at its height - quite understandably put pressure on various elements of ASPs, in part due to social distancing, and in part due to the overwhelming effort to use every resource possible to save lives. In many cases, this led to less stringent adherence to existing ASPs. Studies in the USA, Germany and Italy during the pandemic demonstrated a steady increase in multidrug-resistant Gram-negative bacteria within hospital settings, which could have secondary implications of fatal bacterial co-infection in COVID-19 patients. Not all countries noted the same increase, however, possibly due to differences in antibiotic prescribing. Research in Ireland indicated a reduced adherence to antimicrobial prescribing policies, increased use of broad-spectrum and restricted antibiotics and a reduction in antibiotic educational meetings, and in the screening for multidrug-resistant organisms during the pandemic. The risk with non-adherence to ASPs, however, is the further development of antimicrobial resistance. This therefore led to calls worldwide to redouble stewardship efforts – particularly once antibiotic prescribing guidance for COVID-19 patients was issued – and to ensure the implementation and enhancement of ASPs where necessary.

The WHO recommended five measures to ensure the continuation of ASPs as an integral part of the pandemic response:

- targeted training of healthcare professionals, including identifying signs and symptoms of severe COVID-19 and bacterial co-infection and eliminating unnecessary antibiotic use;
- ensure continuity of essential health services and the regular supply of quality-assured and affordable antimicrobials;
- reduce COVID-19 testing turnaround time to reduce the urge to initiate antibiotics on admission;
- use utmost caution in the use of microbicides for disinfection, prioritising those with no/minimal selection pressure for antibiotic resistance;
- address gaps in research, e.g., rapid and affordable diagnostic tests that differentiate between bacterial and viral respiratory tract infections.

COVID-19 has provided a stark reminder of the difficulties and devastating consequences of the absence of appropriate treatment for an infection. Maintaining ASPs during a pandemic, and modifying as necessary to target recommended areas, will help to prevent a secondary public health emergency in the form of untreatable antibiotic-resistant infections, the consequences of which can perhaps now be more tangibly envisaged.

15.4 Monitoring Antimicrobial Stewardship Programmes

Monitoring and evaluation of the outcomes of both newly implemented ASPs and changes to existing ASPs are imperative to demonstrate continued evidence for the interventions involved, and to facilitate evidence-based decisions regarding further interventions – whether continuation, modification or cessation of an intervention. Processes should also be monitored, for example, to assess if guidelines are being followed. Monitoring is therefore an inherent key element of ASPs. Evaluating the efficacy of a programme, or even of a specific intervention within a programme, is, however, complex due to the paucity of easily measurable outcomes, and due to the interrelationship between the many interventions that may form an ASP, therefore making it difficult to ascribe benefit to any of the interventions individually. In many of the cases reported in medical literature, multiple changes to an established programme have been introduced together, or they have overlapped in time, so that evaluating the contribution of each change becomes complicated. Deciding in advance when a new policy or practice will be implemented and when its effect will be assessed is therefore worthwhile.

The parameters to be measured and the baseline data against which the changes will be judged must be planned in advance. Some outcome measures for ASPs include, but are not restricted to:

- antibiotic consumption and costs, both in total and by specific drug class;

- specific costs associated with prescribing potentially toxic antibiotics, e.g., gentamicin blood level monitoring;
- rates of resistance to specific antibiotics by problem pathogens;
- pharmacy interventions to advise on inappropriate antibiotic use;
- the incidence of hospital-acquired infections.

The input of information technology specialists and hospital epidemiologists to a stewardship management team is important, since they, together, can decide how the data will be recorded and analysed to best effect. Combined with suitable information systems, these aspects are essential to ensure the success of an ASP. There is also the potential to improve antibiotic prescribing by minimising the risk of adverse effects when information systems provide patient-specific warnings on allergies and immune and renal functions and the potential for interaction with the patient's other drugs.

15.4.1 Electronic Surveillance of Antibiotic Use and Resistance

Surveillance and monitoring of antimicrobial resistance are recommended as a priority to support ASPs in all care settings. Surveillance data can help to identify factors that may be linked to the development of resistant strains, and contribute to measuring the efficacy of ASPs, therefore strengthening the evidence base for interventions and antibiotic use. This in turn can inform clinical decisions and policy recommendations. For example, surveillance of antibiotic use and resistance in a hospital or hospital ward over a period of time allows empiric treatment to be modified based on local resistance patterns. It can also help to identify areas which are not compliant with guidelines or local policies and enable interventions to be made as required.

15.4.1.1 Local and National Surveillance

Computer-assisted surveillance is generally preferable to manual monitoring and reporting due to the greater speed and accuracy afforded. The more sophisticated information systems do not simply record data on antibiotic consumption, cost and resistance, but are capable of relating infection control data to antibiotic use, and would be expected to draw attention to situations where a change in use of a particular antibiotic was associated with increasing isolation of a particular pathogen. Such an association does not, of course, mean that one caused the other, but it does raise staff awareness of that potential.

Surveillance can take place at patient level and population level. Patient-level surveillance collects data regarding the specific therapy given to individual patients, while population-level surveillance generally reports aggregated antibiotic use for the particular hospital or unit or, on a larger scale, for a region or country. At patient level, in order to continuously monitor the appropriateness of antibiotic prescribing, knowledge – in real time – is required regarding patient diagnosis, comorbidities, the antibiotic prescribed (including dose, duration, etc.) and the treatment outcome, and it is preferable that these data are collected electronically. Electronic prescribing is increasingly becoming commonplace in secondary care, enabling tracking of prescribing rates and compliance with guidance. Further advances in patient-level diagnostic information will enhance the ability to evaluate the use of diagnostic tools (e.g., rapid diagnostics) and guidelines. As part of its 5-year antimicrobial resistance plan, by 2024, the UK aims for an appropriate diagnostic code to be recorded at each infection consultation (which would remove any ambiguity around the clinical diagnosis when assessing antibiotic use data), alongside ensuring that all NHS hospitals have electronic prescribing systems which can code, audit and provide feedback for surveillance.

Data on local resistance patterns are of paramount importance, and well-structured monitoring programmes should be capable of identifying unforeseen consequences of changes in antibiotic use, such as that arising when one study which, in an attempt to reduce the use of the third-generation cephalosporin ceftazidime, noted a 32% increase in penicillinase-producing *Klebsiella pneumoniae* due to a prescribing shift to piperacillin–tazobactam. Local surveillance data, and updates regarding ASP processes and outcomes, must regularly be fed back to prescribers in a timely manner to enable these data to inform clinical decisions.

15.4.1.2 Multi-country Surveillance

Local AMR surveillance systems provide data pertinent to particular ASPs, but to fully exert their benefit, they should have the capacity to provide data that are easily compared and used not only at a local but also on a national and global level. To effectively compare data across sectors, it must also be harmonised both across different sectors within one country and on a global scale, and many countries now report their data to multi-country systems. In Europe, a degree of harmonisation has been achieved through the European Antimicrobial Resistance Surveillance Network (EARS-Net), which gathers and analyses surveillance data, ensuring standardised reporting and allowing comparability of data across the EU. As can be seen in Figure 15.2, however, more work is required to improve the capacity of resistance monitoring across Europe. The Central Asian and Eastern European Surveillance of Antimicrobial Resistance (CAESAR)

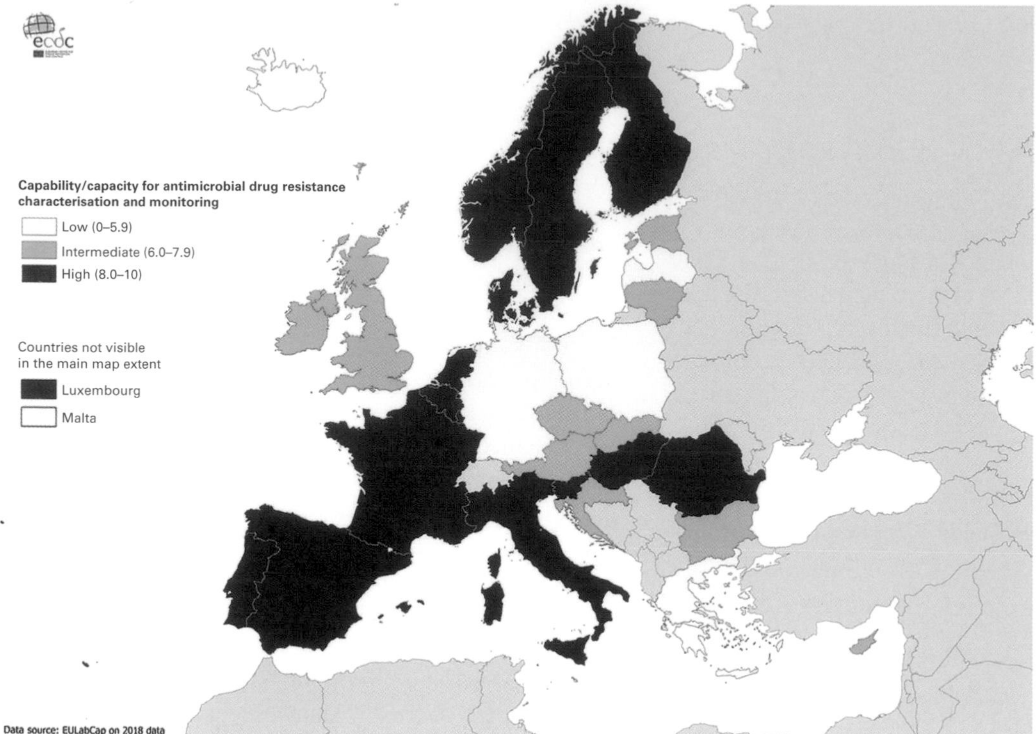

Figure 15.2 Capacity for characterisation and monitoring of antimicrobial drug resistance in Europe. *Source:* Figure obtained from European Centre for Disease Prevention and Control (2019).

similarly harmonises data from countries in that region. The WHO developed the Global Antimicrobial Resistance Surveillance System (GLASS) in 2015, standardising antimicrobial surveillance and harmonising standards globally – the first global system to collect national data in this way. Data from such surveillance systems enable visualisation of the differences in antibiotic resistance patterns from one country to another, and between different regions within the same country.

To be useful, surveillance data must, of course, be available, and should be in an accessible format, as is the case for EARS-Net and GLASS data, and is increasingly true for national data. This enables improved awareness of resistance trends, and accountability for stewardship programmes. As the One Health approach to antimicrobial stewardship is adopted, surveillance is expected to become integrated not only across primary and secondary care, but also across human, animal and plant sectors.

References

European Centre for Disease Prevention and Control (2019). *Surveillance of Antimicrobial Resistance in Europe 2018, in Annual report of the European Antimicrobial Resistance Surveillance Network*. Stockholm: ECDC.

UN Interagency Coordination Group on Antimicrobial Resistance (2019) *No time to wait: Securing the future from drug-resistant infections*. Report to the Secretary-General of the United Nations, IACG. https://www.who.int/docs/default-source/documents/no-time-to-wait-securing-the-future-from-drug-resistant-infections-en.pdf (Accessed 12 September 2022).

World Health Organization (2019). *Antibacterial Agents in Clinical Development – an analysis of the antibacterial clinical development pipeline*. Geneva: WHO.

World Health Organization (2021). *Antimicrobial stewardship interventions: a practical guide*. Copenhagen: WHO Regional Office for Europe.

Further Reading

Barlam, T.F., Cosgrove, S.E., Abbo, L.M. et al. (2016). Implementing an antibiotic stewardship program: guidelines by the Infectious Diseases Society of America and the Society for Healthcare Epidemiology of America. *Clin. Infect. Dis.* 62: e51–e77. https://doi.org/10.1093/cid/ciw118.

Centers for Disease Control and Prevention (2019). *Core Elements of Hospital Antibiotic Stewardship Programmes*. Atlanta: US Department of Health and Human Services (CDC).

Dyar, O.J., Huttner, B., Schouten, J. and Pulcini, C. (2017). What is antimicrobial stewardship? *Clin. Microbiol. Infect.* 23: 793–798.

European Centre for Disease Prevention and Control (2020). *Consumption of antibacterials for systemic use in community and hospital sector in Europe, reporting year 2018*. Stockholm: ECDC.

European Commission (2017). *EU Guidelines on the Prudent Use of Antimicrobials in Human Health (2017/C212/01)*. Stockholm: ECDC.

National Institute for Health and Care Excellence (2015). *Antimicrobial stewardship: systems and processes for effective antimicrobial medicine use NG15*. London: NICE https://www.nice.org.uk/guidance/ng15 (Accessed 12 September 2022).

Organisation for Economic Co-operation and Development (2018). *Stemming the Superbug Tide: Just a Few Dollars More*. OECD Health Policy Studies: OECD Publishing, Paris.

Tang, K.L., Caffrey, N.P., Nóbrega, D.B. et al. (2017). Restricting the use of antibiotics in food-producing animals and its associations with antibiotic resistance in food-producing animals and human beings: a systematic review and meta-analysis. *Lancet Planet. Health* 1: e316–e327. https://doi.org/10.1016/S2542-5196(17)30141-9.

Virdi, P., Steen, J., Martin, A. et al. (2021). The Proliferation of Antimicrobial Resistance Due to COVID-19 Sterilization Practices. *Academia Letters, Article* 3890: https://doi.org/10.20935/AL3890.

16

Infection Prevention and Control: Healthcare-associated Infection

Elaine Cloutman-Green

Consultant Clinical Scientist, Great Ormond Street Hospital, London, UK

CONTENTS

Hugo and Russell's Pharmaceutical Microbiology, Ninth Edition. Edited by Brendan F. Gilmore and Stephen P. Denyer.

Companion website: https://www.wiley.com/go/HugoandRussells9e

16.1 Introduction

At a global level, infectious diseases are currently the leading cause of human death. Among the broad range of infections encountered, those that develop as a complication of treatment provided in a hospital or healthcare environment are a particular concern to health services throughout the world. These may arise from cross-infection or from the patient's own flora, potentially in any healthcare and social care setting, and as a consequence are known as healthcare-associated infections (HCAIs); they remain the most frequent complication of hospitalisation. HCAIs present a major challenge to patient safety and it is estimated that in European healthcare centres one in every eighteen patients will develop at least one HCAI during an acute care hospital stay. HCAIs have an impact not only on individual patients by increasing mortality and morbidity, but they also strain healthcare systems financially and contribute to an increase in antimicrobial resistance (AMR).

An HCAI is defined by the World Health Organization (WHO) as an 'infection occurring in a patient during the process of care in a hospital or other healthcare facility, which was not present or incubating at the time of admission' (WHO 2016). The United Kingdom Department of Health and Social Care defines an HCAI as 'any infection by any infectious agent acquired as a consequence of a person's treatment by the UK National Health Service (NHS), or which is acquired by a healthcare worker (HCW) in the course of their NHS duties'. This definition has significant impact for clinicians and infection prevention and control (IPC) teams in requiring control of transmission routes not just between patients, but across the entire healthcare system.

Therefore, the aims of IPC are to apply microbiological knowledge to the clinical setting and to utilise practical and evidence-based approaches to prevent harm to patients and HCWs. The principal components of IPC interventions are:

- early identification of carriage/infection;
- patient isolation;
- source control, including eradication of carriage if appropriate;
- improved hand hygiene;
- environmental control;
- good antimicrobial stewardship.

16.2 Defining Healthcare-associated Infections

HCAIs encompass a considerable variety of infections across different body sites and systems, caused by a wide range of bacteria, as well as some viruses and fungi. HCAIs may be caused by infectious agents from endogenous or exogenous sources. Exogenous sources are those external to the patient, whereas endogenous sources are from the patient's own body sites.

Identifying colonised and or infected patients is a key factor in limiting HCAI. Colonisation is considered to be the presence of bacteria without induction of any clinical symptoms. This includes the presence of commensals, such as the normal bacteria present in the colon or oral cavity, but importantly also includes asymptomatic colonisation with HCAI-causing organisms, such as methicillin-resistant *Staphylococcus aureus* (MRSA). For many organisms, carriage and colonisation precede infection. It is important therefore to prevent not only infection with a microorganism but also carriage and colonisation.

The National Institute for Health and Care Excellence (NICE 2014) states that HCAIs include any infection contracted:

- as a direct result of treatment in, or contact with, a health or social care setting;
- as a result of healthcare delivered in the community;
- outside a healthcare setting (for example, in the community) and brought in by patients, staff or visitors and transmitted to others (for example, norovirus).

In general, infection or colonisation with any bacteria or fungi detected in the first 48 hours of a healthcare admission is deemed to have been present on admission, and is commonly referred to as community-acquired infection or CAI. This term may be misleading, however, as it can sometimes include patients transferred in from other healthcare facilities and so more accurately indicates acquisition outside of the current healthcare centre.

Viral cross-transmission is suspected when multiple inpatients develop symptoms after being in the hospital environment for over 48 hours and test positive for the same virus; however, it must be noted that for many viruses the incubation period is greater than 48 hours. This results in viral acquisition frequently being counted as HCAI when the virus may have been present but incubating on admission. Different healthcare systems therefore deal with the allocation of viral infections to CAI or HCAI variably, as standardisation is difficult.

Patients particularly susceptible to HCAI include those with severe underlying disease, those admitted for long hospital stays, those of old age and those admitted to intensive care units. It is estimated that of the HCAIs that develop within intensive care units, 40–60% are due to endogenous flora, 20–40% are due to the contaminated hands of HCWs, 20–25% are due to antibiotic-driven change and up to 20% potentially due to environmental contamination.

Patients that have a breach in their natural protective barriers (i.e., skin integrity, mucosal layer conditions) are at particular risk of infection, including risk from their own flora. Breaches may be due to the presence of indwelling devices, such as catheters, or from breaches due to surgical interventions. The Centers for Disease Control and Prevention (CDC; Horan et al. 2008) specify the 'big four' infection types (surgical site infection [SSI], pneumonia [PNEU], bloodstream infection [BSI] and urinary tract infection [UTI]) linked to barrier breaches (Table 16.1). The infection definitions are based on not just time to onset and organism detection, but also other physiological signs, such as increased oxygen requirements, and imaging.

16.2.1 Surgical Site Infections

SSIs can present in a number of different ways depending on where the infecting organism is located. They may be superficial, where the infection affects the wound site itself. More serious infection can be either deep, where the fascial and/or muscle layers are affected, or organ–space where infection occurs within the organ or space where the surgery was undertaken. These SSIs may come from the patient's own normal body flora (e.g., from the intestinal bacteria after abdominal surgery), from nose or skin carriage of wound pathogens such as *S. aureus* by the patient or by cross-infection from other patients or staff as a result of a breakdown in aseptic procedures and proper clinical care. For surgical incisions, every effort must therefore be made to minimise the risk of postoperative wound/surgical site infection, and this may include prophylactic antibiosis to reduce the risk from endogenous flora.

Table 16.1 CDC definitions of HCAI by infection type and time to onset.

Type of infection	CDC timescale
Superficial surgical site infection	Infection occurs within 30 days after the operative procedure
Deep incisional surgical site infection and organ/space surgical site infection	Infection occurs within 30 days after the operative procedure if no implant is left in place, or within 1 year if an implant is in place and the infection appears to be related to the operative procedure
UTI (catheter-associated)	Patient has a urinary catheter or had one removed in the previous 48 hours
BSI (catheter-associated)	Patient has had a cardiovascular access device inserted in place for more than 48 hours
VAP (ventilator-associated pneumonia)	Patient diagnosed with pneumonia where the patient has been on a ventilator for more than 48 hours

Peripheral and decubitus ulcers, commonly known as pressure sores, are a frequent complication following surgical interventions; they can also be linked to any long stay within the healthcare setting. Although not directly related to the surgical site, they are monitored as part of routine clinical observations.

A healthcare professional should assess each patient's pressure ulcer risk. Risk is determined by whether surgery or an invasive intervention has been undertaken and how this has impacted on levels of mobility. Regular assessment should determine if these risk factors alter during the patient's stay. Measures to prevent development of ulcers mainly rely on encouragement of mobility if possible, the use of specially cushioned mattresses and supports and repositioning of patients every 4–6 hours for those who are immobile.

16.2.2 Bloodstream Infections

Potentially the most severe types of HCAI in terms of patient outcomes are BSIs, also known as bacteraemias. The blood and the cardiovascular system should be sterile, and the presence of bacteria in the blood indicates significant clinical risk. Many BSIs are part of infectious diseases themselves and are not linked directly to healthcare risks (e.g., bacterial meningitis, community-acquired pneumonia, acute pyelonephritis), but others are important complications of healthcare.

Almost all hospital treatment in modern medical practice requires invasive procedures with the insertion of various synthetic tubes/catheters and prosthetic devices. Vascular access devices include any device that is left *in situ* within the vascular (blood) system. These can either be short-term peripheral devices, such as cannulae, or frequently longer-term central venous access devices, such as peripherally inserted central catheter (PICC) lines. These devices can present an infection risk from opportunistic pathogens as they breach the natural barrier of the skin, are situated within the circulatory system and are left in place for a prolonged period of time. While the infection may start as a biofilm on the artificial surface of the catheter (see Chapter 8), the organism is readily disseminated throughout the bloodstream and clinical consequences can include infection of cardiovascular structures such as heart valves (endocarditis) or other metastatic sites.

16.2.3 Urinary Tract Infections

The most common form of HCAI is the UTI, often arising from indwelling urinary catheters which become contaminated and colonised with bacteria leading to infection of the bladder and the lower urinary tract, then progressively the ureters and potentially the kidneys (pyelonephritis). These can also be an important source of BSI, as bacteria can then pass from the urinary tract into the blood stream.

16.2.4 Ventilator-associated Pneumonia

During the postoperative period, surgical patients are particularly vulnerable to pneumonia; they will have undergone endotracheal intubation during general anaesthesia, and postoperative discomfort and inactivity may lead to inadequate ventilation of their lungs, as well as an inability (or disinclination) to cough, resulting in postoperative pneumonia. This risk is greatly magnified in patients needing intensive care, and those undergoing prolonged intubation and artificial ventilation; it can also be a significant cause of bacteraemia. Ventilator-associated pneumonia (VAP) is therefore one of the major challenges to successful intensive care.

16.3 Microorganisms Implicated in Healthcare-associated Infection

Traditionally, it has been the view that infections were either caused by specific HCAI pathogens or more rarely by opportunistic pathogens in patients considered at particularly high risk, such as the immunocompromised.

Opportunistic infections are those caused by organisms that are not normally considered to be true pathogens. These opportunistic pathogens include microorganisms found in water, soil and other environmental reservoirs. Infection is caused when these organisms bypass normally protective barriers due to breaches of protective layers, i.e., damaged skin in burns patients, or in individuals with impaired defence mechanisms, such as those with compromised immune systems.

It is now accepted, however, that any organism can be clinically significant if detected in a patient alongside the presence of clinical symptoms. Thus, it is the combination of microorganism alongside exposure and susceptibility that needs to be assessed to determine the likelihood of an HCAI, rather than the organism alone.

For those organisms that are considered to be more frequently associated with HCAI, several countries have made surveillance of these microorganisms mandatory. Mandatory surveillance supports IPC by permitting comparison between centres, benchmarking outcomes and allowing trend analysis on a national scale. These organisms have included MRSA infections (particularly BSI), *Clostridioides difficile*-related infection, Gram-negative BSIs (such as *Escherichia coli*) and some types of surgical site infections. Although national data collection is focused on whole hospitals or hospital groups, effective action within a hospital depends upon the data being assessed and acted upon at individual ward level or within clinical units.

16.3.1 Gram-positive Bacteria

16.3.1.1 Staphylococcal Species

Staphylococcal species are Gram-positive cocci belonging to the Staphylococcaceae family, and were first described in 1882 by Sir Alexander Ogston.

Coagulase-negative Staphylococci

There are over 50 species that fulfil the categorisation of coagulase-negative staphylococcal species; however, coagulase-negative staphylococci (CoNS) are frequently clinically rather than phenotypically defined, and are commonly referred to as the *Staphylococcus epidermidis* group. This group comprises *S. epidermidis* and *Staphylococcus haemolyticus* as the most prevalent species with others included such as *Staphylococcus capitis*, *Staphylococcus hominis*, *Staphylococcus simulans* and *Staphylococcus warneri*.

CoNS are a normal constituent of skin flora with *S. epidermidis* being the most frequently detected, representing more than 65% of CoNS cultured. Infections due to CoNS often involve the presence of prosthetic devices, such as catheters or implanted devices, making these organisms responsible for a wide range of HCAIs, including catheter-related BSI, UTI and SSI. Interpreting microbiological results can be challenging, as detection can represent both sample contamination and true causes of infection.

Staphylococcus aureus

S. aureus, which was named for its golden pigment by Friedrich J. Rosenbach, is a common human pathogen for all age groups that causes skin and soft tissue infections and pneumonia, as well as infections linked to invasive devices. It is a leading human pathogen associated with HCAI worldwide, and can cause both colonisation and infection. In addition to infection, it can also cause toxin-related illness, such as toxic shock and food intoxications, incidents of which can have wider public health implications.

S. aureus is isolated from the anterior nares in about 30% of the population and nasal carriage often precedes infection. It can also colonise other sites such as the throat, perineum and axillae. In England in 2017/2018, there were 12,784 reported incidents of *S. aureus* BSI (including MRSA and methicillin-sensitive *S. aureus* [MSSA]). These BSIs have an estimated mortality rate of 50% in patients with a complicated infection, and 30% in other groups. The main source of transmission within the healthcare setting is believed to be person to person via the hands of HCWs, although it is thought the environment may also play a role, as the organism can survive for long periods on surfaces.

Methicillin-resistant *S. aureus*

The main form of clinically significant resistance in *S. aureus* is resistance to β-lactam agents, including methicillin. β-lactam agents, which include penicillin, are frequently utilised as first-line therapies in both acute and community healthcare settings. The resistance mechanism was first identified in 1981. Resistance is due to the expression of a transpeptidase (penicillin-binding protein 2a [PBP2a]) encoded for by the chromosomal *mecA* gene, which is located on a mobile genetic element known as the staphylococcal cassette chromosome (SCC, see also Chapter 13). When this resistance mechanism is present, the organism is then referred to as MRSA. MRSA strains now account for 20–40% of *S. aureus* detected in hospitals where strains are endemic, such as those within the UK.

Transmission of MRSA is likely to be predominantly via the hands of HCWs. Some 5% of HCWs caring for MRSA-positive patients become long-term colonised with MRSA themselves, from which 5% go on to develop clinical infection. Short-term colonisation is thought to be much more frequent, however, and HCWs carrying MRSA have rarely been demonstrated to be the source of outbreaks; the exact mode of acquisition in these circumstances is therefore unknown.

In recent years, there has been an increase in community infections of both sensitive and resistant *S. aureus* leading to skin and soft tissue infections in otherwise healthy young adults.

16.3.1.2 Vancomycin-resistant Enterococci

Enterococcal spp. are Gram-positive organisms, two of which are common commensals of the human digestive tract, *Enterococcus faecalis* and *Enterococcus faecium*. Vancomycin-resistant enterococci (VRE) were first described in 1988 and have gone on to become important nosocomial pathogens worldwide (see Chapter 13). In 2017, VRE caused an estimated 54,500 infections among hospitalised patients and 5400 estimated deaths in the United States (CDC 2019). Asymptomatic colonisation exceeds infection tenfold, but VRE infections are linked to increased morbidity, mortality and healthcare costs.

Risk factors for VRE acquisition include: disease severity, length of hospital stay and prior antibiotic exposure. Vancomycin resistance does not arise *de novo* in vancomycin-susceptible *Enterococcal* species isolates via spontaneous mutation; instead susceptible patients acquire VRE exogenously, in the context of antibiotic selective pressure. It was previously thought that VRE acquisition was via the hands of HCWs; however, in recent years, the environment is thought to play a greater role in the transmission of VRE.

16.3.1.3 *Clostridioides difficile* (formerly *Clostridium difficile*)

C. difficile is a Gram-positive anaerobe that was first isolated from stools in 1935. *C. difficile* causes disease through the production of enterotoxin A and cytotoxin B which represent the major virulence factors for the organism; however, not all strains carry the toxin genes. *C. difficile* infection (CDI) is due to the presence of a toxin-competent strain in faeces. CDI may be associated with no disease symptoms (colonisation) or with a spectrum of *C. difficile*-associated disease outcomes, ranging from mild diarrhoea to pseudomembranous colitis and toxic megacolon.

Within the USA, a substantial increase in rates of CDI has been observed since 1993, with levels reaching 223,900 cases and approximately 12,800 deaths in 2017 (CDC 2019); CDI has been found to be 21% more common than MRSA infections (not including colonisation). In 2019/2020, the number of hospital-acquired cases of CDI was 13,177 in England. Mortality rates depend on whether the infecting *C. difficile* strain is a toxin hyperproducer or not, but can be as high as 30%; rates are highest among elderly patients who have underlying medical conditions. Risk factors for developing CDI include prior antibiotic use, especially clindamycin, cephalosporins and/or fluoroquinolones.

Patients with CDI excrete between 10^4 and 10^7 *C. difficile* colony-forming units per gram of faeces. Contamination of the environment is common due to aerosolisation of spores during diarrhoeal episodes. This can lead to high levels of environmental contamination, especially in areas such as toilets and side rooms, as well as on the surfaces of equipment. *C. difficile* spores are resistant to disinfectants and can survive for months or even years on surfaces and environmental contamination may lead to outbreaks.

16.3.2 Gram-negative Bacteria

16.3.2.1 *Escherichia coli*

E. coli is the major constituent of the resident facultative anaerobic microbiota in the healthy human digestive tract. It is a Gram-negative bacillus and a member of the Enterobacterales family (previously the Enterobacteriaceae). Up until the 1940s it was generally considered that *E. coli* was non-pathogenic; however, phenotypic and genotypic studies have now demonstrated that pathogenic *E. coli* strains exist and belong to a few subgroups or clonal groups of specific pathotypes.

E. coli is the most common aetiological agent causing UTI infection and is believed to be responsible for 90% of community UTIs and 50% of nosocomial UTIs with infection especially common within elderly patients. It has been estimated that 150 million cases of *E. coli* UTI occur globally per year, and cost about $6 billion for national health resources.

E. coli is also the leading cause of Gram-negative BSIs and is a serious threat in immunocompromised patients, with a case fatality of 5–30%. In the UK, BSIs caused by *E. coli* have increased from 688 in 2002 to 43,294 cases in the year 2019/2020; mandatory reporting of such cases is now required in England. In addition, *E. coli* is a frequent cause of other infections including intra-abdominal infection, meningitis and sepsis. Person-to-person transmission of *E. coli* is believed to be the most likely route of spread within healthcare settings.

The most appropriate therapeutic options for *E. coli* are usually β-lactams or fluoroquinolones; however, increased resistance has been reported in both invasive and non-invasive isolates. Multidrug-resistant strains, such as CTX-M-15 extended-spectrum β-lactamase producers (see also Chapter 13), have emerged worldwide as an important community and hospital pathogen, constituting a serious public health concern as they inactivate first-line therapeutic choices.

16.3.2.2 *Klebsiella* Species

Klebsiella spp. are Gram-negative non-motile organisms first described in 1882 and belonging to the Enterobacterales family. Two features that are associated with virulence are the hyper-production of a thick polysaccharide coat and the presence of the *magA* mucoviscosity gene, which if detected together can lead to more severe clinical outcomes. The genus occupies a diverse range of ecological niches including: soil, water and warm-blooded mammals.

Klebsiella pneumoniae is the most important of the Klebsiella species and accounts for 95% of all *Klebsiella* spp. isolated from clinical samples. *K. pneumoniae* is an important nosocomial pathogen, causing 15% of Gram-negative infections within intensive therapy units (ITUs), and is the second most frequent cause of Gram-negative sepsis. It is also associated with pneumonia, UTIs and wound infections. *K. pneumoniae* infections primarily affect immunocompromised patients and have an associated mortality rate of greater than 50%. This is in part due to the capsule, which is considered to be a significant virulence factor, with certain capsular types being linked to invasive disease, for example, K1, K2, K45 and K57.

Klebsiella isolates associated with HCAI are often linked with antibiotic resistance, including resistance to the carbapenem class of antibiotics, which are used for the most seriously ill patients within ITUs. Resistance to the carbapenem class of antibiotics is due to the production of carbapenemases, enzymes that break down the carbapenem antibiotics. Examples of these resistance mechanisms include: *K. pneumoniae* carbapenemase (KPC) and oxacillinase-type (OXA) β-lactamase, as well as New Delhi metallo-β-lactamase (see also Chapter 13).

It is believed that *Klebsiella* spp. are most frequently acquired from environmental sources in healthcare environments, such as sinks, in addition to direct transmission from other patients. Capacity to survive within the healthcare environment, combined with carriage of antibiotic resistance mechanisms, means that *K. pneumoniae* is capable of causing outbreaks in hospital settings, impacting both paediatric and adult units.

16.3.2.3 *Enterobacter* Species

Enterobacter spp. are Gram-negative proteobacteria belonging to the Enterobacterales family. The main pathogenic species within this genus are *Enterobacter cloacae* and *Enterobacter aerogenes*, the former actually comprising a large complex derived from 12 related genetic clusters. *E. cloacae* rarely causes primary disease in healthy adults; however, it is frequently isolated from non-stool samples in hospitalised patients.

Within hospitalised patients, *E. cloacae* is an important opportunistic pathogen that has been responsible for UTIs, BSIs, pneumonia and bronchopulmonary dysplasia in hospitalised neonates. ITU surveillance data demonstrate that within this setting 31% of *Enterobacter* infections were caused by species resistant to common hospital therapies such as third-generation cephalosporin antibiotics. These resistant species have been associated with increased mortality, hospital stays and hospital charges.

An increasing number of outbreaks have been detected associated with *E. cloacae* with mortality rates of 27–61%.

These have been linked to equipment such as contaminated infusions, door knobs, improperly disinfected digital thermometers and contaminated blood gas machines. Outbreaks often continue for months and require interventions such as improvements in hand hygiene practices, admission restriction and ward closures or changes in antibiotic policy to bring them under control. Due to the genetic diversity within the *E. cloacae* complex, it is often difficult to know whether outbreaks are due to a single source or whether the situation is actually due to polyclonal endemic infections from different isolates within the *E. cloacae* complex.

16.3.2.4 *Acinetobacter* Species

Acinetobacter spp. are non-fermentative Gram-negative coccobacilli belonging to the family Moraxellaceae, and with the exception of *Acinetobacter baumannii*, they are widely distributed in soil and water. *A. baumannii* is the main species causing infections in humans, and is frequently identified in healthcare rather than natural environments.

Infections caused by non-*A. baumannii* species are relatively unusual and typically linked to catheter-related sepsis. By contrast, *A. baumannii* is becoming increasingly recognised as the cause of a range of HCAIs, including pneumonia, BSI, wound infections, UTIs and post-neurosurgery meningitis.

Outbreaks often implicate the hospital environment, where *A. baumannii* can survive for long periods on surfaces, resists desiccation and is spread via contaminated hands. Outside of ITUs, burns and high-dependency units experience the highest rates of infection. Such infections are associated with adverse clinical outcomes including: high rates of morbidity and mortality, prolonged hospital stays and substantial healthcare expense.

Infections with antibiotic-resistant *A. baumannii* have been reported, including organisms resistant to all available antimicrobials. In 2017, carbapenem-resistant *Acinetobacter* spp. were estimated to cause 8500 infections in hospitalised patients resulting in 700 deaths (CDC 2019). Risk factors for infection with resistant strains include: prior antibiotic exposure, prior length of stay in an ITU, mechanical ventilation and trauma. Carbapenemase resistance in *A. baumannii* is mainly due to the expression of OXA-β-lactamases, while non-OXA-meditated carbapenemase resistance (the mechanism seen in *Klebsiella* species) is rare.

16.3.2.5 *Pseudomonas aeruginosa*

Pseudomonas aeruginosa are Gram-negative aerobic coccobacilli, which are ubiquitous, inhabiting water, soil, plants and humans. The growth of *P. aeruginosa* in water is not directly linked to the organic content of that water and therefore it can exist in relatively high numbers in the clinical environment, both in water and on moist surfaces such as sinks and taps.

P. aeruginosa can cause a wide range of infections, from minor skin infections associated with hot tub use to causing 10–20% of HCAI including BSIs in some healthcare centres. It is particularly significant in the cystic fibrosis patient population where it can contribute to a steady decline in lung function leading to the requirement for transplantation. Other patients at risk of *P. aeruginosa* infection are neutropenic patients and those with severe burns. The organism can also act to contaminate devices that are left inside the body, such as respiratory equipment and catheters, leading to its reputation for being a significant cause of VAP. Due to an increase in numbers noted following voluntary reporting, *P. aeruginosa* is now included as part of mandatory reporting figures for BSI in England, with 4336 cases recorded for the year 2019/2020.

P. aeruginosa outbreaks have been linked to contaminated tap water and contaminated medical devices and equipment. Outbreaks may be difficult to initially recognise due to infections being transmitted via an intermediate environmental source, and some countries, such as England, have introduced a requirement to test water outlets in high-risk clinical areas, such as neonatal units, in order to support earlier detection. *P. aeruginosa* like *Acinetobacter* species infections are frequently associated with resistance to many commonly used antibiotics when outbreaks are linked to patient rather than environmental sources.

16.3.3 Viruses

Viruses are not considered to have a colonising state, although some viruses, such as herpes viruses, can become latent. This means that in most cases detection of a virus is considered to represent infection. Many viruses have tropisms that lead them to only cause infections in a particular organ or body system, such as the gastrointestinal or respiratory systems. Conversely, some viruses, such as adenovirus, are capable of causing infection across multiple body systems, and so their presentation will vary based on the location of the infection.

Many viral infections are first acquired in childhood and may be associated with prolonged infectivity and increased viral load. It was recently demonstrated that 12.2% of paediatric patients developed HCAI caused by respiratory or gastrointestinal viruses. Within adult populations, certain patient groups, such as the immunocompromised, may also shed high viral loads leading to an increase in transmission risk to others. Therefore, these clinical environments are at particular risk of viral outbreaks.

16.3.3.1 Respiratory Viruses

Respiratory viruses can infect any age group, with viral loads usually higher in primary infection. Severe complications occur more frequently in children, the immunocompromised and the elderly. Respiratory viruses are most commonly transmitted by airborne droplets or nasal secretions. Infections can be situated either in the upper respiratory tract, linked to areas such as the throat, nasopharynx and sinuses, or the lower respiratory tract linked to the lungs. Within temperate climates, such as the UK, many of these viruses are seasonal in their activity and tend to circulate at higher levels during the winter months (Table 16.2). Outbreaks can occur within healthcare facilities when patients are not placed under appropriate isolation precautions to prevent spread and staff do not wear the necessary personal protective equipment (PPE).

Severe acute respiratory syndrome coronavirus 2 (SARS-CoV-2) is a novel RNA virus and member of the family Coronaviridae and genus Betacoronavirus. The virus was first recognised in China in 2019. Coronavirus disease (COVID-19) is the clinical presentation of SARS-CoV-2 and since its recognition has subsequently led to a global pandemic resulting in over 6 million deaths (see Chapter 5).

Presentation was initially frequently characterised by fever, cough and shortness of breath, with some individuals progressing to pneumonia and respiratory failure. New variants have led to variation in clinical presentation with milder symptoms, such as sore throat and rhinorrhoea, often present. Most people infected with SARS-CoV-2 will experience mild to moderate respiratory illness and recover without requiring special treatment. Progression is more common in older people, and those with underlying health conditions, such as cardiovascular disease, diabetes, chronic respiratory disease and cancer. The incubation period of SARS-CoV-2 is up to 14 days with a mean incubation period of 5.1 days until symptom onset. Excretion of the virus can be prolonged in those patients who have severe disease or significant immunosuppression and, therefore, hospitalised patients may represent an ongoing transmission risk in healthcare.

Transmission of SARS-CoV-2 can occur through direct, indirect or close contact with infected people through infected secretions, such as saliva and respiratory secretions or their respiratory droplets. These infected secretions are expelled when an infected person coughs, sneezes, talks or sings. Within healthcare, infectious secretions can also be present as aerosols, which maintain suspension in the air, linked to aerosol-generating procedures (AGPs). This is a primary route of transmission, not only to other patients, but also to HCWs if the correct PPE is not worn and isolation measures not undertaken. Indirect transmission via contact with contaminated objects or surfaces (fomite transmission) is also believed to be possible.

Numerous healthcare-related outbreaks of SARS-CoV-2 have been reported, including both patients and HCWs. Outside of medical facilities, outbreak reports have arisen from crowded indoor spaces, where occupation has exceeded 1 hour, such as restaurants, places of worship, gyms and areas where choir practice has been undertaken. Prevention of outbreaks is linked to improved ventilation, appropriate use of PPE, social distancing and from 2020 access to vaccination.

Table 16.2 Respiratory viruses typically responsible for infection outbreaks.

Virus	Vaccine availability	Transmission characteristics
Influenza A, B, C	Seasonal vaccine based on circulating strains – contains 2 A strains and 1 B	• Influenza A is associated with both outbreaks and pandemics • Influenza A strain types linked to haemagglutinin and neuraminidase combinations, i.e., H1N1 • Influenza B can cause similar presentations to A, but is not linked to pandemics
Parainfluenza 1, 2, 3, 4 (A, B)	No	• Causes up to 60% of childhood croup cases • Type 3 is the most commonly detected
Respiratory syncytial virus (RSV) A, B	No	• Major cause of lower respiratory tract infection in young children, especially in those under 2 years of age • Can cause hospital outbreaks, especially linked to asymptomatic infection of staff
Rhinovirus	No	• Frequent cause of the common cold
Coronavirus: severe acute respiratory syndrome 2 (SARS-CoV-2)	Yes	• Pandemic outbreaks • Transmission by infected secretions and expelled respiratory droplets
Adenovirus	No	• Causes between 2% and 8% of childhood respiratory infections • Can lead to severe disseminated infection in the bone marrow transplant population

16.3.3.2 Gastric Viruses

Viruses account for over half the diarrhoeal episodes that occur globally in infants and young children. They are almost universally transmitted via the faecal–oral route, although with some viruses, such as norovirus, spread can also be linked to inhaled vomitus or via food contamination (Table 16.3). The vast majority of cases are self-limiting, but some individuals, especially those in healthcare, will require additional support such as rehydration. Outbreaks of gastric viruses frequently occur in closed or semi-closed communities, such as schools, cruise ships and within healthcare settings.

Norovirus (formerly known as Norwalk-like virus) belongs to the family Caliciviridae. Norovirus gastroenteritis is typically a mild self-resolving illness with an incubation period of 24–48 hours and a symptomatic period of 12–60 hours, although the duration can be longer in children, the immunocompromised and the elderly. It is the single most common cause of gastroenteritis with an estimated 21 million cases annually worldwide. Globally, norovirus infection has been estimated to total $4.2 billion in direct health system costs and to reach $60.3 billion in societal costs per year (Bartsch et al. 2016). For the NHS, direct health system costs are accrued through lost bed days, cancelled operations and staff absence.

Patients with norovirus infection can excrete viral loads of 10^8 viral copies per gram in stools, and projectile vomiting is associated with 3×10^7 virus particles emitted as an aerosol. Symptoms start with sudden onset nausea, followed by projectile vomiting and watery diarrhoea. Severe cases seen in healthcare can have additional features including gastrointestinal bleeding, protein malnutrition and higher than expected cause-related mortality.

Norovirus outbreaks are seasonal with the peak occurring in the winter months. Norovirus particles retain infectivity on surfaces and are resistant to a variety of disinfectants. Due to this stability and infectivity, environmental contamination has been implicated in successional outbreaks in numerous scenarios; this is purportedly responsible for the 30% transmission rates seen in close contacts of norovirus patients.

Outbreaks are often difficult to control, and management requires rapid identification of cases and isolation of infected patients. Other infection control measures include:

- emphasising the need for handwashing with soap and water both before and after contact with symptomatic patients;
- affected staff remaining off work until 48 hours after their symptoms have resolved;
- restricting staff movements between affected and unaffected patients;
- restricting visitors.

16.3.3.3 Blood-borne Viruses

The major blood-borne viral pathogens associated with healthcare transmission risk are hepatitis B virus (HBV), hepatitis C virus (HCV) and human immunodeficiency virus (HIV).

Outbreaks of blood-borne viruses (BBVs) have occurred in settings from dental clinics to dialysis units, and have included transmission from HCWs to patients, as well as from patients to HCWs.

Aside from outbreaks, BBVs are mainly of concern in healthcare settings where they are linked to exposure prone procedures (EPP) and needle-stick injuries. EPPs include procedures where the worker's gloved hands may be in contact with sharp instruments, needle tips or sharp tissues inside a patient's open body cavity, wound or confined anatomical space, where the hands or fingertips may not be completely visible at all times (PHE 2017).

Table 16.3 Transmission and prevention of gastric viral infections.

Virus	DNA/RNA	Prevention and transmission
Astrovirus	RNA	No vaccine available. Causes outbreaks in children less than 3 years of age. Usually in schools and nurseries
Norovirus	RNA	Single most common cause of gastroenteritis. Cleaning and isolation are key principles in infection control
Rotavirus	RNA	Oral vaccine available, healthcare outbreaks can occur
Adenovirus	DNA	No vaccine available, can cause outbreaks within bone marrow transplant wards
Hepatitis A	DNA	Vaccine available. Epidemics are associated with food and waterborne transmission

Transmission of BBV to HCWs from needles and other sharp medical instruments can occur where the injury involves a sharp that is contaminated with blood or a bodily fluid from a patient. The most significant consequences of such an injury arise from the potential for exposure to hepatitis C, where the estimated seroconversion rate is up to 1.8%. Risk linked to needle-sticks from other BBVs is estimated to be less than 0.5%. The introduction of standard safety precautions aims to reduce the transmission of these viruses, as well as other organisms linked to blood and bodily fluid.

16.3.4 Clinically Relevant Fungi

Fungi are a frequently underestimated cause of HCAI. It is estimated that *Candida* species cause 8% of healthcare-acquired BSIs. Outside of BSIs, *Aspergillus fumigatus* is a rare but significant cause of HCAI, frequently related to ventilation issues or building work near haematology and oncology patients.

In recent years, *Candida auris* has emerged as a significant fungal pathogen linked to HCAI, with outbreaks occurring across five continents within intensive care units and other healthcare settings. Control of *C. auris* requires enhanced IPC measures, such as enhanced cleaning with chlorine-based agents, as well as isolation and modification to patient treatment plans.

16.4 Standard IPC Interventions for the Management and Prevention of HCAI

A combination of different IPC interventions is employed in order to try to reduce the risk of developing an HCAI. The principal components of these are: early identification of carriage/infection; patient isolation; eradication of carriage if appropriate; improved hand hygiene; environmental control; and good antimicrobial stewardship. All of these interventions aim to control the spread of organisms, thereby reducing the risk of individual patient acquisition or endogenous infection; they have been shown to be useful in ending outbreaks.

16.4.1 Standard Precautions

Standard precautions form the standard package of care that should be utilised with all patients to protect staff and reduce the risk of transmission of HCAI. These were initially referred to as universal precautions and were a way of reducing the risk of BBVs and those infections linked to bodily secretions. Standard precautions, as defined by the CDC, include:

- hand hygiene;
- use of PPE (e.g., gloves, masks, eyewear) when appropriate for the task;
- respiratory hygiene/cough etiquette;
- sharps safety (engineering and work practice controls);
- safe injection practices (i.e., aseptic technique for parenteral medications);
- sterile instruments and devices;
- clean and disinfected environmental surfaces.

16.4.2 Hand Hygiene

Hand hygiene is considered one of the most efficient and cost-effective ways of preventing cross-transmission of microorganisms, by removing contaminants from the hands of HCWs. HCWs contaminate their hands by touching both the environment and patients during routine care activities, and thus if hand hygiene practices are suboptimal then microbial transmission can occur. Effective hand hygiene includes the application of adequate amounts of hand hygiene agent, be that soap or alcohol gel, adequate duration of hand cleansing with suitable mechanical action, coverage of all hand surfaces and adequate drying.

A methodology for prompting hand hygiene at critical points was developed to support the undertaking of hand hygiene within clinical areas. The 'Clean Care is Safer Care' initiative was launched in 2005 by the WHO with the aim of reducing HCAI, and a consensus guideline on hand hygiene was published in 2009, which outlined the WHO 'Five Moments for Hand Hygiene' (WHO 2009). The WHO campaign highlights the five opportunities (and requirements) for hand hygiene:

- before touching a patient;
- before clean/aseptic procedures;
- after body fluid exposure/risk;
- after touching a patient;
- after touching patient surroundings.

The placement of alcohol gel and sinks is a key factor in their use and there must be access within each patient bed-space to adequate hand hygiene facilities, as well as at ward entrances. When auditing hand hygiene, a compliance rate of 90% for 200 observations is commonly used for determining compliance with guidance.

Where appropriate, the use of alcohol gel instead of handwashing may be preferable, as it results in less damage to hands, saves time and for most bacteria and viruses is as efficacious. Alcohol gel solutions containing 70–80% alcohol are required within healthcare environments. Education linked to the use of alcohol gel is key, however, as it should only be used on visibly clean hands. It should not be employed when caring for patients with diarrhoea or suspected/confirmed norovirus or *C. difficile* infection, as these organisms remain viable after exposure to alcohol, so cleaning hands with soap and water in these circumstances is essential.

16.4.3 Infection Precautions (Contact Precaution and Droplet Precautions)

The principle behind contact precautions is that they represent a group of procedures that reduce the risk of transmission of infection through direct and indirect patient contact. They include the use of PPE (masks, gloves, gowns/aprons and eye protection), usually in addition to the use of single rooms for the isolation of patients, to provide a physical barrier. These are applied in addition to the standard precautions outlined in Section 16.4.1.

Contact precautions require HCWs to adhere to hand hygiene upon entering and exiting patient rooms as well as prior to donning, and after removal, of PPE. They also require staff to either use patient-designated equipment or to undertake equipment cleaning between patients. For droplet and aerosol precautions, masks are worn in addition to other items of PPE, especially when undertaking aerosol-generating procures. However, evidence has shown that mask use alone does not prevent viral transmission and that additional eye protection must be used when undertaking AGPs. Incorrect mask removal can present a contamination risk to the HCW's face as well as gloves, and so education on the use of PPE is also required.

16.4.4 Isolation Precautions

Isolation precautions are used to disrupt the chain of transmission by separating infectious patients from those who are neither colonised nor infected. The most effective form of isolation is the use of private rooms where, along with geographical isolation, staff are also cohorted (see Section 16.4.5) to deal with either infected or uninfected patients. In practice, separation of staff is seldom operated outside of outbreak scenarios. In some units where it is not possible to place patients in rooms with physical separation, they are isolated in virtual cubicles where contact precautions are followed and separation is supported by additional measures, such as floor markings. Within the NHS, three quarters of patient isolation requirements are due to either MRSA or *C. difficile* infection. Failure to isolate patients can arise because all single rooms are taken up by patients for non-infectious reasons, no specialist isolation rooms are available or because specific patient factors, such as dependency requirements, apply.

In addition to physical separation, the use of single rooms permits the use of engineering controls to help prevent transmission of airborne/droplet HCAI. These engineering controls include the use of mechanical ventilation, which refers to the process of introducing and distributing outdoor and properly treated air into a building or room. The amount of air circulated per hour in relation to the room volume is the ventilation rate (in air changes per hour). The rate of air change affects the dilution of infectious agents within isolation rooms as well as generating air movement within a physical space to reduce transmission risk.

16.4.5 Cohorting

In many hospitals, the number of single rooms available for patient isolation is limited. The best use of the available rooms should be made for those with infections, but where the capacity of single rooms is exceeded by the number of cases of infection, it may then be necessary and appropriate for patients with the same infection to be nursed together in a cohort ward, or bay area where they can be physically separated from other ward areas. It is common practice when cohorting is undertaken that patients are nursed with dedicated staff who do not move between the cohort ward and other clinical areas (i.e., cohorting may apply to nursing staff as well as patients).

16.4.6 Cleaning and Disinfection

Cleaning of all surfaces should aim to remove epidemiologically important pathogens. Most countries have national guidelines that determine standards for cleanliness, usually based upon the principle of visible cleanliness. Local guidelines for the cleaning of surfaces within hospitals need to take into account parameters that are relevant to the prevention of transmission of HCAI; these include factors such as ward type (likelihood of patients being carriers, for instance), expected frequency of hand contact with surfaces, susceptibility of the patient population and the presence of potential non-patient sources of microorganisms, such as water outlets.

The length of time an organism can survive on a surface is important for determining HCAI risk. The longer an organism can persist, the longer it can present a risk, and the greater the microbial population present, the greater the chance of survival and reaching a susceptible host (Table 16.4). Survival can be due to the organism being recalcitrant to cleaning, i.e., norovirus, or due to an intrinsic resistance to desiccation, i.e., *Klebsiella* species in biofilm. Even if environmental survival is poor, low residual levels for some highly infectious organisms may mean that they are still present in sufficient numbers to cause infection.

Table 16.4 Length of survival of common nosocomial pathogens on surfaces and associated infectious dose, where known.

Organism	Infectious dose and route (where known)	Duration of survival on surfaces
Staphylococcus aureus	<15 colony-forming units (CFU) or 10^6 CFU (skin and oral dose, respectively)	7 days–>1 year
Clostridioides difficile	1 CFU (in mouse models)	5 months
Vancomycin-resistant enterococci	No experimental evidence	5 days–4 months
Klebsiella spp.	No experimental evidence	<1 hour–30 months
E. coli	10 CFU (oral dose)	<1 hour–16 months
Acinetobacter spp.	10^5 CFU (mouse wound model)	3 days–5 months
Pseudomonas aeruginosa	10^8 CFU (oral dose)	6 hours–16 months
Adenovirus	<150 viral copies (intranasal dose)	7 days–3 months
Norovirus	10–100 viral copies (oral dose)	Norovirus (including feline *calicivirus*) 8 hours–14 days
SARS-associated coronavirus	Estimated 10^2–10^3 viral copies (intranasal dose)	4 hours–3 days

Source: Drawn principally from Weinstein and Hota (2004), Kramer et al. (2006), Schmid-Hempel and Frank (2007), Otter et al. (2011) and Karimzadeh et al. (2021).

16.4.7 Active Surveillance

Active surveillance of patients in order to detect 'silent' colonisation with nosocomial pathogens is championed in both the UK and the USA for specific microorganisms. Active screening is based upon the concept that for control of the target organism (usually antibiotic-resistant) early identification and isolation of infected or colonised patients is key, with asymptomatic carriage being a potential reservoir for ongoing transmission. Active surveillance includes taking samples, such as admission screens, in order to support early identification of the carriage of resistant organisms and relevant IPC interventions, such as isolation.

16.4.8 Clinical Protocol-driven Responses

There are two main reasons why patients are at risk of developing an HCAI: their underlying medical condition making them vulnerable to infections, and the treatment and clinical interventions they are subjected to. These interventions often include invasive procedures that bypass the normal defences of the skin and urinary and respiratory tracts (see Section 16.2). It is essential, therefore, that all clinical staff exercise due care and attention when performing these procedures.

Clinical protocols support the correct implementation of clinical interventions and provide a framework around which audit tools can be designed to support ongoing monitoring. To this end, an approach to clinical practice which has commonly become known as 'care bundles' is employed, although within the UK the term 'high-impact intervention (HII)' is also used.

These bundles are care protocols set out in a simple bullet-point format highlighting the five or six essential elements needed to minimise the infection risk associated with each individual aseptic procedure. The aim is for each element to be performed correctly on every occasion and the care bundle/HII incorporates a simple audit tool for self-assessment or peer assessment on a frequent and regular basis to check the performance of the clinical staff undertaking those procedures.

16.4.9 Antimicrobial Stewardship

AMR is a global issue and is linked to public health. Many HCAIs are caused by organisms which are considered to be antimicrobially resistant, commonly possessing one of two features:

- they tend to be resistant to more than one group of antibiotics;
- they may become prevalent due to selection pressures from antibiotic usage in healthcare environments.

Some organisms associated with HCAI, such as *C. difficile*, are not linked to a particular resistance phenotype; however, the majority of organisms acknowledged to increase risk of poor outcomes are linked to AMR. These AMR organisms are associated with higher clinical risk, as the presence of resistance frequently leads to difficulty in treating any resulting infection and impacts on wider patient management, such as patients being placed at the end of surgical lists.

Good antibiotic stewardship is one important way to manage risk linked to selective pressures within healthcare environments. Many HCAIs caused by antibiotic-resistant bacteria flourish under the selective pressure of antibiotic use. Since many of those bacteria are resistant to several classes of antibiotic, even the use of individual agents can lead to genetic selection for bacteria resistant to a wide range of antibiotics. Furthermore, many of the resistance genes are carried on transferable genetic elements that can pass among bacterial populations, particularly in a selective environment such as a hospital (see Chapter 13).

All healthcare organisations should have antibiotic prescribing protocols to promote and audit good stewardship. In the UK, the 'Start Smart, then Focus' programme (PHE 2015) places the emphasis on only prescribing antimicrobials when there is evidence of infection and to document why and when they are commenced. It also includes a requirement to review antibiotic therapy at 48–72 hours with the object of making one of the following decisions, which should also be documented:

- stop antibiotic therapy;
- switch from intravenous (IV) to oral medication;
- change the antibiotic (on the basis of culture results);
- continue with the current antibiotic regimen;
- consider outpatient antimicrobial therapy (OPAT).

An antimicrobial policy should be present that contains information needed to support decision making, alongside guidance for the prophylactic use of antibiotics. An auditing programme should be in operation to monitor compliance. For an extended treatment of antimicrobial stewardship, see Chapter 15.

16.5 Impact of the Clinical Setting on Infection Prevention and Control

The clinical setting impacts on both the risk of HCAI and the IPC interventions that are required. In community and paediatric healthcare settings, the risk profiles are often different, both in terms of organisms present and the common exposure/transmission routes, and so the response to an outbreak needs to consider this.

As healthcare develops, there is an increasing focus on the delivery of a wider variety of care in primary and community settings, thereby impacting on the factors contributing to the risk of HCAI developing. Standard interventions for HCAI may be more restricted in community healthcare settings where isolation and cleaning will be affected by the infrastructure in which the care is delivered. The nature of the patient may also be different, along with the exposure-to-risk period. For example, if the care is being undertaken in a care home, the long-term nature of that care means that opportunity for cumulative exposure may be high. The impact of interventions on patient well-being, such as isolation, may also be higher if experienced in the long term. Therefore, in community settings, the risk–benefit analysis for both individuals and the wider setting is key to ensure interventions are not only effective but also appropriate for those impacted.

One particular setting which may need specific risk assessment is that linked to paediatric care due to the diverse needs and susceptibilities of these patients. HCAIs among children differ from those observed in adult populations, by both the sites and patterns of distribution. Children have an increased risk of infection from sites such as femoral lines, due to nappy wearing. They will also have other breaches of barrier that are not present in adults, such as the presence of umbilical lines in neonates. Children interact closely with their environment, through toys and other objects, and so environmental contamination poses an increased risk. They also utilise shared ward areas more frequently than adult patients and, due to the movement of both patients and their families through hospital environments, it is postulated that they are much more likely to be involved in person-to-person transmission of infection.

16.5.1 Outbreaks and IPC Interventions

In order to monitor and evaluate the effectiveness of IPC measures, rapid identification of potential cases of HCAI is essential. Identification of cases based on laboratory results is referred to as case-based surveillance. Cases can also be identified through direct reporting, often by clinical staff, linked to events happening on the ward. This could include incidents such as HCWs or patients vomiting, indicating a potential norovirus outbreak. This is referred to as event-based surveillance. Finally, with the increasing utilisation of electronic patient records and automated data recording, potential transmission events may be identified through data analysis using statistical tools, i.e., trend analysis. This is often useful in identification of potential outbreaks where indirect sources of transmission are implicated, i.e., environmentally mediated outbreaks.

For all outbreak types, a common feature of the definition is that the observed number of cases exceeds the number expected for a given time and place. One commonly utilised definition of an outbreak is two or more cases linked in person, place and time. This works for the majority of cases within healthcare but not all. For some organisms such as a hospital-acquired *Listeria monocytogenes* or other reportable infections, a single case would be investigated as a possible outbreak with appropriate follow-up undertaken.

16.5.1.1 Definition of Transmission and Exposure

Once a prospective case has been identified, a risk assessment is undertaken, both to determine whether the case is an HCAI and to calculate the risk to others who have been potentially exposed. This risk assessment needs to address both patient and microorganism factors, including:

- route of organism transmission (contact, airborne, droplet, or waterborne);
- patient microorganism load (often higher for viruses than bacteria);
- potential for environmental persistence;
- infectious dose of the organism (including the duration of exposure before infection, i.e., 15 minutes in a room for someone immune-competent with chickenpox);
- patient status: colonised or infected;
- patient susceptibility (immunocompetent or immunocompromised);
- time to onset of infection (community vs hospital-acquired);
- endogenous vs exogenous source of infection;
- surveillance information available (was the sample taken in response to symptoms or as part of an active screening programme);
- is there any environmental surveillance information available (for example, water-testing results);
- patient management considerations (whether the organism is resistant to antibiotics, therefore requiring altered management for that patient and others exposed, or prophylaxis is required).

An assessment is then made to determine if this case forms part of an outbreak. Organism typing linked to clinical surveillance is key in order to provide further information to establish an understanding of transmission chains and cases of HCAI. There is no standard definition to assess when patient-to-patient transmission has occurred; however, cross-transmission of bacteria is suspected when isolates are found to be of identical species and have the same antibiotic-sensitivity pattern. Viral cross-transmission is suspected based on location and time, although increasingly genetic sequencing is being applied to help support transmission assessments.

A number of additional interventions are considered if the transmission is thought to be part of an outbreak. This includes actions to identify further cases in order to determine the extent of the outbreak, as well as actions undertaken to limit further spread.

16.5.1.2 Source Control

Responsive screening is undertaken in response to possible cross-contamination or outbreak events. It supports the understanding of source control, considering where the microorganisms may have come from and any drivers of ongoing transmission. By contrast, active screening is undertaken in specific groups, i.e., surgical patients, to assist early identification of organisms for improved patient management and to identify possible reservoirs for ongoing transmission.

Within healthcare, responsive screening usually involves screening patients who have been identified as exposed in order to detect colonisation or asymptomatic infection. It can also involve screening of patients and the environment to identify sources. This can include screening care personnel, equipment, medical devices or the wider healthcare environment. Within community and public health settings, responsive screening is usually referred to as contact tracing. Contact tracing is undertaken not only to identify the source of any outbreak, but also to identify those exposed in order to prevent further transmission and to commence treatment if required.

Once a source has been identified along with any additional cases, further interventions for source control are frequently required. These include the standard IPC interventions (Section 16.4.1), including isolation and appropriate PPE precautions. Isolation as part of source control extends the requirement of isolation to those patients who have been exposed and may therefore be in the incubation period. Exposed patients will often be moved into single rooms or cohorted together to prevent further cases if infection or colonisation develops.

Outbreaks can also require specific changes to cleaning regimens. This can include the substitution of cleaning agent for cases of norovirus and *C. difficile*, which require disinfection with a chlorine-based agent due to the susceptibility profile of the organisms. Enhanced cleaning regimens may also be required for shared ward areas or as part of discharge cleaning to manage environmental loading and prevent ongoing transmission.

16.6 Measuring Impact and Success

The audit of any implemented IPC protocol is necessary to ensure a continued high level of IPC practice and compliance and also to support targeted education.

There should be regular audits as part of an annual programme that includes: hand hygiene compliance, adherence to antibiotic prescribing guidelines, environmental cleanliness, isolation compliance and the implementation of the clinical protocols in the care bundles/HIIs. The results of these audits should be reviewed in a timely manner at all levels of management in the health and social care organisations in order that those implementing the protocols have ownership of the procedures and their effective application. Performance management at all levels depends upon a combination of the data from surveillance of the infections and audit of the clinical practice.

Local audit is also supported by national interventions, for example, by mandating reporting of HCAI organisms. This enables both local monitoring and also public health surveillance to support ongoing improvement and learning between centres. One example of the success of this approach is to be found in the legislation and national infection control interventions introduced within England in an effort to decrease rates of MRSA infection within hospitals. These interventions included targeted screening of at-risk patients in 2006 and active surveillance of all patients in 2010, activities which were introduced in recognition that the spread of MRSA presented a significant threat to public health. This combined approach led to a reduction in rates of MRSA infection by 85% between April 2003 and March 2011.

16.7 Professional Support for Infection Prevention and Control

Infection prevention and control are the responsibility of all staff working in a healthcare environment, whether in clinical, managerial or support roles. However, it is also an area that requires the leadership and expertise of practitioners specifically trained in infection prevention and control. All healthcare and social care organisations should have access to such expertise and should have an IPC team and committee to deliver the expert service and support for the staff of all the clinical and social care units. The IPC team in hospitals should generally comprise nursing, medical and pharmaceutical professionals with specific training and expertise in medical microbiology, HCAI prevention and control and in antimicrobial prescribing. The team has an important role in outbreak investigation and management, but, most importantly, also provides the guidance and support necessary for effective IPC throughout the organisation.

Finally, the commitment of senior management to making infection prevention and control a high priority sets the culture for a healthcare or social care organisation. Management should ensure monitoring of surveillance and audit data at all levels of the organisation ('from board to ward') and ensure that all staff recognise their respective responsibilities and play their part. This helps generate a culture of pride in delivery of a quality service, essential for successful IPC.

References

Bartsch, S.M., Lopman, B.A., Ozawa, S. et al. (2016). Global economic burden of norovirus gastroenteritis. *PLoS One* 11 (4): e0151219.

Centers for Disease Control (2019). *Antibiotic Resistance Threats in the United States*. Atlanta: Centers for Disease Control.

Horan, T.C., Andrus, M. and Dudeck, M.A. (2008). CDC/NHSN surveillance definition of health care–associated infection and criteria for specific types of infections in the acute care setting. *Am. J. Infect. Control* 36 (5): 309–332.

Karimzadeh, S., Bhopal, R. and Nguyen Tien, H. (2021). Review of infective dose, routes of transmission and outcomes of COVID-19 caused by the SARS-COV-2: comparison with other respiratory viruses. *Epidemiol. Infect.* 149: E96.

Kramer, A., Schwebke, I. and Kampf, G. (2006). How long do nosocomial pathogens persist on inanimate surfaces? A systematic review. *BMC Infect. Dis.* 6 (1): 130.

National Institute for Health and Care Excellence (2014). *Healthcare-Associated Infections: Prevention and Control. Public Health Guideline [PH36]* 11 November 2011 update. London: National Institute for Health and Care Excellence.

Otter, J.A., Yezli, S. and French, G.L. (2011). The role played by contaminated surfaces in the transmission of nosocomial pathogens. *Infect. Control Hosp. Epidemiol.* 32 (7): 687–699.

Public Health England (2015). *Antimicrobial Stewardship: Start Smart - Then Focus*. 17 November 2011, update. London: PHE.

Public Health England (2017). *BBVs in Healthcare Workers: Health Clearance and Management*, vol. 16. London: PHE.

Schmid-Hempel, P. and Frank, S.A. (2007). Pathogenesis, virulence and infective dose. *PLoS Pathog.* 3 (10): e147.

Weinstein, R.A. and Hota, B. (2004). Contamination, disinfection, and cross-colonization: are hospital surfaces reservoirs for nosocomial infection? *Clin. Infect. Dis.* 39 (8): 1182–1189.

World Health Organization (2009). *WHO Guidelines on Hand Hygiene in Health Care.* Geneva: World Health Organisation.

World Health Organization (2016). *Guidelines on Core Components of Infection Prevention and Control Programmes at the National and Acute Health Care Facility Level.* Geneva: World Health Organization.

Further Reading

Department of Health (2012). *Health and Social Care Act 2008 – Code of Practice for the Prevention and Control of Healthcare Associated Infections.* London: Department of Health.

Hansen, S., Schwab, F., Zingg, W. et al. (2018). Process and outcome indicators for infection control and prevention in European acute care hospitals in 2011 to 2012 - results of the PROHIBIT study. *Euro. Surveill.* 23 (21): 1700513.

Mitchell, B.G., Hall, L., White, N. et al. (2019). An environmental cleaning bundle and health-care-associated infections in hospitals (REACH): a multicentre, randomized clinical trial. *Lancet Infect. Dis.* 19 (4): 410–418.

National Audit Office (2009). *Reducing Healthcare Associated Infections in Hospitals in England.* HC 560 Session 2008-2009, 12 June 2009. London: The Stationery Office.

National Institute for Health and Care Excellence (2011). *Healthcare-Associated Infections: Prevention and Control. Public Health Guideline [PH36].* 11 November 2011. London: National Institute for Health and Care Excellence.

National Institute for Health and Care Excellence (2017). *Healthcare-Associated Infections: Prevention and Control in Primary and Community Care. Clinical Guideline [CG139]* 28 March 2012. London: National Institute for Health and Care Excellence.

Pellowe, C., Pratt, R., Loveday, H. et al. (2005). The epic project: updating the evidence base for national evidence-based guidelines for preventing healthcare-associated infections in NHS hospitals in England. A report with recommendations. *J. Hosp. Infect.* 59 (4): 373–374.

Posfay-Barbe, K.M., Zerr, D.M. and Pittet, D. (2008). Infection control in paediatrics. *Lancet Infect. Dis.* 8 (1): 19–31.

Public Health England (2020). *Guidance for Health Clearance of Healthcare Workers (HCWs) and Management of those Infected with Bloodborne Viruses (BBVs) Hepatitis B, Hepatitis C and HIV.* 26 October 2017 update. London: PHE.

Part 5

Contamination and Contamination Control

17

Microbial Spoilage, Infection Risk and Contamination Control

Rosamund M. Baird

Former Visiting Senior Lecturer, School of Pharmacy and Pharmacology, University of Bath, Bath, UK. Now Sherborne, Dorset, UK

CONTENTS

Hugo and Russell's Pharmaceutical Microbiology, Ninth Edition. Edited by Brendan F. Gilmore and Stephen P. Denyer.

Companion website: https://www.wiley.com/go/HugoandRussells9e

17.1 Introduction

Pharmaceutical products used in the prevention, treatment and diagnosis of disease contain a wide variety of ingredients, often in quite complex physicochemical states. Such products must not only meet current good pharmaceutical manufacturing practice requirements for quality, safety and efficacy, but also must be stable and sufficiently attractive to be acceptable to patients. Products made in the pharmaceutical industry today must meet high microbiological specifications; that is, if not sterile, they are expected to have no more than a minimal microbial population at the time of product release.

Nevertheless, from time to time a few rogue products with an unacceptable level and type of contamination will occasionally escape the quality assurance net. The consequences of such contamination may be serious and far-reaching on several accounts, particularly if contaminants have had the opportunity to multiply to high levels. First, the product may be spoiled, rendering it unfit for use through chemical and physicochemical deterioration of the formulation. Spoilage and subsequent wastage of individual batches usually result in major financial problems for the manufacturer through direct loss of faulty product. Secondly, the threat of litigation and the unwanted, damaging publicity of recalls may have serious economic implications for the manufacturer. Thirdly, inadvertent use of contaminated products may present a potential health hazard to patients, perhaps resulting in outbreaks of medicament-related infections, and ironically therefore contributing to the spread of disease. Most commonly, heavy contamination of product with opportunist pathogens, such as *Pseudomonas* spp., has resulted in the spread of nosocomial (hospital-acquired) infections in compromised patients; less frequently, low levels of contamination with pathogenic organisms, such as *Salmonella*, have attracted considerable attention, as have products contaminated with toxic microbial metabolites, such as mycotoxins in herbal medicines. The consequences of microbial contamination in pharmaceutical products are discussed in more detail below.

17.2 Spoilage: Chemical and Physicochemical Deterioration of Pharmaceuticals

Microorganisms form a major part of the natural recycling processes for biological matter in the environment. As such, they possess a wide variety of degradative capabilities, which they are able to exert under relatively mild physicochemical conditions. Mixed natural communities are often far more effective cooperative biodeteriogens than the individual species alone, and sequences of attack on complex substrates occur where initial attack by one group of microorganisms renders them susceptible to further deterioration by secondary, and subsequent, microorganisms. Under suitable environmental selection pressures, novel degradative pathways may emerge with the capability to attack newly introduced synthetic chemicals (xenobiotics). However, the rates of degradation of materials released into the environment can vary greatly, from half-lives of hours (phenol) to months ('hard' detergents) to years (halogenated pesticides).

The overall rate of deterioration of a chemical depends on: its molecular structure; the physicochemical properties of a particular environment; the type and quantity of microbes present; and whether the metabolites produced can serve as sources of usable energy and precursors for the biosynthesis of cellular components, and hence the creation of more microorganisms.

Pharmaceutical formulations may be considered as specialised microenvironments and their susceptibility to microbial attack can be assessed using conventional ecological criteria. Some naturally occurring ingredients are particularly sensitive to attack, and a number of synthetic components, such as modern surfactants, have been deliberately constructed to be readily degraded after disposal into the environment. Crude vegetable and animal drug extracts often contain a wide assortment of microbial nutrients besides the therapeutic agents. This, combined with frequently conducive and unstable physicochemical characteristics, leaves many formulations with a high potential for microbial attack unless steps are taken to minimise it.

17.2.1 Pharmaceutical Ingredients Susceptible to Microbial Attack

- *Therapeutic agents:* Through spoilage, active drug constituents may be metabolised to less potent or chemically inactive forms. Under laboratory conditions, it has been shown that a variety of microorganisms can metabolise a wide assortment of drugs, resulting in loss of activity. Materials as diverse as alkaloids (morphine, strychnine, atropine), analgesics (aspirin, paracetamol), thalidomide (still used in the treatment of some forms of cancer), barbiturates, steroid esters and mandelic acid can be metabolised and serve as substrates for growth. Indeed, the use of microorganisms to carry out subtle transformations on steroid molecules forms the basis of the commercial production of potent therapeutic steroidal agents (see Chapter 25). In practice, reports of drug destruction in medicines are less frequent. There have, however, been some notable exceptions: the metabolism of atropine in eye drops by contaminating fungi; inactivation of penicillin injections by β-lactamase-producing bacteria (see Chapters 11 and 13); steroid metabolism in damp tablets and creams by fungi; microbial hydrolysis of aspirin in suspension by esterase-producing bacteria; and chloramphenicol deactivation in an oral medicine by a chloramphenicol acetylase-producing contaminant.
- *Surface-active agents:*
  Anionic surfactants, such as the alkali metal and amine soaps of fatty acids, are generally stable because of the slightly alkaline pH of the formulations, although readily degraded once diluted into sewage. Alkyl and alkylbenzene sulphonates and sulphate esters are metabolised by ω-oxidation of their terminal methyl groups followed by sequential β-oxidation of the alkyl chains and fission of the aromatic rings. The presence of chain branching involves additional α-oxidative processes. Generally, ease of degradation decreases with increasing chain length and complexity of branching of the alkyl chain.

  Non-ionic surfactants, such as alkyl polyoxyethylene alcohol emulsifiers, are readily metabolised by a wide variety of microorganisms. Increasing chain lengths and branching again decrease ease of attack. Alkylphenol polyoxyethylene alcohols are similarly attacked, but are significantly more resistant. Lipolytic cleavage of the fatty acids from sorbitan esters, polysorbates and sucrose esters is often followed by degradation of the cyclic nuclei, producing numerous small molecules readily utilisable for microbial growth. Ampholytic surfactants, based on phosphatides, betaines and alkylamino-substituted amino acids, are an increasingly important group of surfactants and are generally reported to be reasonably biodegradable.

  The *cationic surfactants* used as antiseptics and preservatives in pharmaceutical applications are usually only slowly degraded at high dilution in sewage. Pseudomonads have been found growing readily in quaternary ammonium antiseptic solutions, largely at the expense of other ingredients such as buffering materials, although some metabolism of the surfactant has also been observed.
- *Organic polymers:* Many of the thickening and suspending agents used in pharmaceutical formulations are subject to microbial depolymerisation by specific classes of extracellular enzymes, yielding nutritive fragments and monomers. Examples of such enzymes, with their substrates in parentheses, are: amylases (starches), pectinases (pectins), cellulases (carboxymethylcelluloses, but not alkylcelluloses), uronidases (polyuronides such as in tragacanth and acacia), dextranases (dextrans) and proteases (proteins). Agar (a complex polysaccharide) is an example of a relatively inert polymer and, as such, is used as a support for solidifying microbiological culture media. The lower-molecular-weight polyethylene glycols are readily degraded by sequential oxidation of the hydrocarbon chain, but the larger congeners are rather more recalcitrant. Synthetic packaging polymers such as nylon, polystyrene and polyester are extremely resistant to attack, although cellophane (modified cellulose) is susceptible under some humid conditions.
- *Humectants:* Low-molecular-weight materials such as glycerol and sorbitol are included in some products to reduce water loss and may be readily metabolised unless present in high concentrations (see Section 17.2.3.3).
- *Fats and oils:* These hydrophobic materials are usually attacked extensively when dispersed in aqueous formulations such as oil-in-water emulsions, aided by the high solubility of oxygen in many oils. Fungal attack has been reported in condensed moisture films on the surface of oils in bulk, or where water droplets have contaminated the bulk oil phase. Lipolytic rupture of triglycerides liberates glycerol and fatty acids, the latter often then undergoing β-oxidation of the alkyl chains with the subsequent production of odoriferous ketones. Although the microbial metabolism of pharmaceutical hydrocarbon oils is rarely reported, this is a problem in engineering and fuel technology when water droplets have accumulated in oil storage tanks and subsequent fungal colonisation has catalysed serious corrosion.
- *Sweetening, flavouring and colouring agents:* Many of the sugars and other sweetening agents used in pharmacy are ready substrates for microbial growth. However, some are used in very high concentrations to reduce water activity in aqueous products and inhibit microbial attack (see Section 17.2.3.3). At one time, a variety of

colouring agents (such as tartrazine and amaranth) and flavouring agents (such as peppermint water) were kept as stock solutions for extemporaneous dispensing purposes, but they frequently supported the growth of *Pseudomonas* spp., including *Pseudomonas aeruginosa*. Such stock solutions should now be preserved, or freshly made as required by dilution of alcoholic solutions which are much less susceptible to microbial attack.

- *Preservatives and disinfectants:* Many preservatives and disinfectants can be metabolised by a wide variety of Gram-negative bacteria, although most commonly at concentrations below their effective 'use' levels. Growth of pseudomonads in stock solutions of quaternary ammonium antiseptics and chlorhexidine has resulted in infection of patients. *Pseudomonas* spp. have metabolised 4-hydroxybenzoate (parabens) ester preservatives contained in eye drops and caused serious eye infections, and have also metabolised the preservatives in oral suspensions and solutions. In selecting suitable preservatives for formulation, a detailed knowledge of the properties of such agents, their susceptibility to contamination and limitations clearly provides invaluable information.

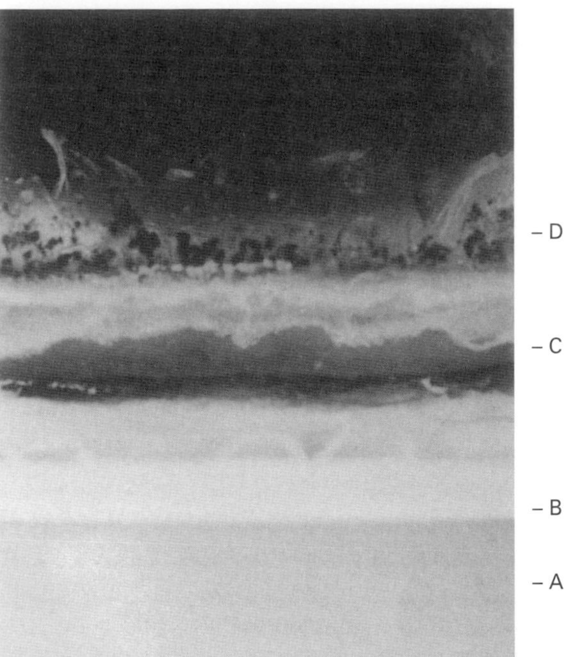

Figure 17.1 Section through an inadequately preserved olive oil, oil-in-water emulsion in an advanced state of microbial spoilage showing: A, discoloured, oil-depleted, aqueous phase; B, oil globule-rich creamed layer; C, coalesced oil layer from 'cracked' emulsion; D, fungal mycelial growth on surface. Also present are a foul taste and evil smell.

17.2.2 Observable Effects of Microbial Attack on Pharmaceutical Products

Microbial contaminants usually need to attack formulation ingredients and create substrates necessary for biosynthesis and energy production before they can replicate to levels where obvious spoilage becomes apparent. Thus, for example, 10^6 microbes will have an overall degradative effect around 10^6 times faster than one cell. However, growth and attack may well be localised in surface moisture films or very unevenly distributed within the bulk of viscous formulations such as creams. Early indications of spoilage are often organoleptic, with the release of unpleasant smelling and tasting metabolites such as 'sour' fatty acids, 'fishy' amines, 'bad eggs', bitter, 'earthy' or sickly tastes and smells. Products may become unappealingly discoloured by microbial pigments of various shades. Thickening and suspending agents such as tragacanth, acacia or carboxymethylcellulose can be depolymerised, resulting in loss of viscosity and sedimentation of suspended ingredients. Alternatively, microbial polymerisation of sugars and surfactant molecules can produce slimy, viscous masses in syrups, shampoos and creams, and fungal growth in creams has produced 'gritty' textures. Changes in product pH can occur depending on whether acidic or basic metabolites are released, and become so modified as to permit secondary attack by microbes previously inhibited by the initial product pH. Gaseous metabolites may be seen as trapped bubbles within viscous formulations. Over time, metabolically-active aerobic microorganisms may consume sufficient oxygen to give rise to a weak vacuum, leading to the partial collapse of sealed containers.

When a complex formulation such as an oil-in-water emulsion is attacked, a gross and progressive spoilage sequence may be observed. Metabolism of surfactants will reduce stability and accelerate 'creaming' of the oil globules. Lipolytic release of fatty acids from oils will lower pH and encourage coalescence of oil globules and 'cracking' of the emulsion. Fatty acids and their ketonic oxidation products will provide a sour taste and unpleasant smell, while bubbles of gaseous metabolites may be visible, trapped in the product, and pigments may discolour it (Figure 17.1).

17.2.3 Factors Affecting Microbial Spoilage of Pharmaceutical Products

By understanding the influence of environmental parameters on microorganisms, it may be possible to manipulate formulations to create conditions which are as unfavourable as possible for growth and spoilage, within the limitations of patient acceptability and therapeutic efficacy. Furthermore, the overall characteristics of a particular formulation will indicate its susceptibility to attack by various classes of microorganisms.

17.2.3.1 Types and Size of Contaminant Inoculum

Successful formulation of products against microbial attack involves an element of prediction. An understanding of where and how the product is to be used and the challenges it must face during its life will enable the formulator to build in as much protection as possible against microbial attack. When failures inevitably occur from time to time, knowledge of the microbial ecology and careful identification of contaminants can be most useful in tracking down the defective steps in the design or production process.

Low levels of contaminants may not cause appreciable spoilage, particularly if they are unable to replicate in a product; however, an unexpected surge in the contaminant bioburden may present an unacceptable challenge to the designed formulation. This could arise if, for example, raw materials were unusually contaminated; there was a lapse in the plant-cleaning protocol; a biofilm detached itself from within supplying pipework; or the product had been grossly misused during administration. Inoculum size alone is not always a reliable indicator of likely spoilage potential. Low levels of aggressive pseudomonads in a weakly preserved solution may pose a greater risk than tablets containing fairly high numbers of fungal and bacterial spores.

When an aggressive microorganism contaminates a medicine, there may be an appreciable lag period before significant spoilage begins, the duration of which decreases disproportionately with increasing contaminant loading. As there is usually a considerable delay between manufacture and administration of factory-made medicines, growth and attack could ensue during this period unless additional steps are taken to prevent it. On the other hand, for extemporaneously dispensed formulations, some control can be provided by specifying short shelf-lives, for example, 2 weeks.

The isolation of a particular microorganism from a markedly spoiled product does not necessarily mean that it was the initiator of the attack. It could be a secondary opportunist contaminant which had overgrown the primary spoilage organism once the physicochemical properties had been favourably modified by the primary spoiler.

17.2.3.2 Nutritional Factors

The simple nutritional requirements and metabolic adaptability of many common spoilage microorganisms enable them to utilise many formulation components as substrates for biosynthesis and growth. The use of crude vegetable or animal products in a formulation provides an additionally nutritious environment. Even demineralised water prepared by good ion-exchange methods will normally contain sufficient nutrients to allow significant growth of many waterborne Gram-negative bacteria such as *Pseudomonas* spp. When such contaminants fail to survive, it is unlikely to be the result of nutrient limitation in the product but due to other, non-supportive, physicochemical or toxic properties.

Acute pathogens require specific growth factors normally associated with the tissues they infect but which are often absent in pharmaceutical formulations. They are thus unlikely to multiply in them, although they may remain viable and infective for an appreciable time in some dry products where the conditions are suitably protective.

17.2.3.3 Moisture Content: Water Activity (A_w)

Microorganisms require readily accessible water in appreciable quantities for growth to occur. By measuring a product's water activity, A_w, it is possible to obtain an estimate of the proportion of uncomplexed water that is available in the formulation to support microbial growth, using the formula

A_w = vapour pressure of formulation/vapour pressure of water under similar conditions.

The greater the solute concentration, the lower is the water activity. With the exception of halophilic bacteria, most microorganisms grow best in dilute solutions (high A_w) and, as solute concentration rises (lowering A_w), growth rates decline until a minimal growth-inhibitory A_w is reached. Limiting A_w values are of the order of 0.95 for Gram-negative rods; 0.9 for staphylococci, micrococci and lactobacilli; and 0.88 for most yeasts. Syrup-fermenting osmotolerant yeasts have spoiled products with A_w levels as low as 0.73, while some filamentous fungi such as *Aspergillus glaucus* can grow at 0.61.

The A_w of aqueous formulations can be lowered to increase resistance to microbial attack by the addition of high concentrations of sugars or polyethylene glycols. However, even Syrup BP (67% sucrose; A_w of 0.86) has occasionally failed to inhibit osmotolerant yeasts and additional preservation may be necessary. With a continuing trend towards the elimination of sucrose from medicines, alternative solutes which are not thought to encourage dental caries such as sorbitol and fructose have been investigated. A_w can also be reduced by drying, although the dry, often hygroscopic medicines (tablets, capsules, powders, vitreous 'glasses') will require suitable packaging to prevent resorption of water and consequent microbial growth (Figure 17.2).

Tablet film coatings are now available which greatly reduce water vapour uptake during storage while allowing ready dissolution in bulk water. These might contribute to increased microbial stability during storage in particularly

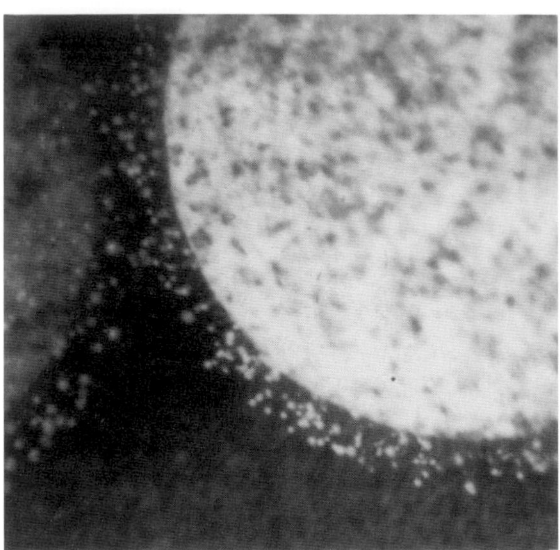

Figure 17.2 Fungal growth on a tablet which has become damp (raised A_w) during storage under humid conditions. Note the sparseness of mycelium, and conidiophores. The contaminant is thought to be a *Penicillium* spp.

humid climates, although suitable foil strip packing may be more effective, albeit more expensive.

Condensed water films can accumulate on the surface of otherwise 'dry' products such as tablets or bulk oils following storage in damp atmospheres with fluctuating temperatures, resulting in sufficiently high localised A_w to initiate fungal growth. Condensation similarly formed on the surface of viscous products such as syrups and creams, or exuded by syneresis from hydrogels, may well permit surface yeast and fungal spoilage.

17.2.3.4 Redox Potential

The ability of microbes to grow in an environment is influenced by their oxidation–reduction balance (redox potential), as they will require compatible terminal electron acceptors to permit their respiratory pathways to function. The redox potential even in fairly viscous emulsions may be quite high because of the appreciable solubility of oxygen in most fats and oils.

17.2.3.5 Storage Temperature

Spoilage of pharmaceuticals could occur potentially over the range of about −20 to 60 °C, although it is much less likely at the extremes. The particular storage temperature may selectively determine the types of microorganisms involved in spoilage. A deep freeze at −20 °C or lower is used for long-term storage of some pharmaceutical raw materials and short-term storage of dispensed total parenteral nutrition (TPN) feeds prepared in hospitals. Reconstituted syrups and multidose eye drop packs are sometimes dispensed with the instruction to 'store in a cool place' such as a domestic fridge (2 to 8 °C), partly to reduce the risk of growth of contaminants inadvertently introduced during use. Conversely, pharmacopoeial-grade Water for Injections should be held at 80 °C or above after distillation and before packing and sterilisation to prevent possible regrowth of Gram-negative bacteria and the release of endotoxins.

17.2.3.6 pH

Extremes of pH prevent microbial attack. Around neutrality, bacterial spoilage is more likely, with reports of pseudomonads and related Gram-negative bacteria growing in antacid mixtures, flavoured mouthwashes and distilled or demineralised water. Above pH 8 (e.g., with soap-based emulsions), spoilage is rare. In products with low pH levels (e.g., fruit-juice-flavoured syrups with a pH 3–4), mould or yeast attack is more likely. Yeasts can metabolise organic acids and raise the pH to levels where secondary bacterial growth can occur. Although the use of low pH adjustment to preserve foodstuffs is well established (e.g., pickling, coleslaw, yoghurt), it is not practicable to make deliberate use of this for medicines.

17.2.3.7 Packaging Design

Packaging can have a major influence on the microbial stability of some formulations in controlling the entry of contaminants during both storage and use. Considerable thought has gone into the design of containers to prevent the ingress of contaminants into medicines for parenteral administration, because of the high risks of infection by this route. Self-sealing rubber closures must be used to prevent microbial entry into multidose injection containers (see Chapter 22) following withdrawals with a hypodermic needle. Wide-mouthed cream jars have now been replaced by narrow nozzles and flexible screw-capped tubes, thereby removing the likelihood of operator-introduced contamination during use of the product. Similarly, hand creams, previously supplied in glass jars, are now packed in closed, disposable dispensers. Where medicines rely on their low A_w to prevent spoilage, packaging such as strip foils must be of water-vapour-proof materials with fully efficient seals. Cardboard outer packaging and labels themselves can become substrates for microbial attack under humid conditions, and preservatives are often included to reduce the risk of damage.

17.2.3.8 Protection of Microorganisms within Pharmaceutical Products

The survival of microorganisms in particular environments is sometimes influenced by the presence of relatively inert materials. Thus, microbes can be more resistant to heat or desiccation in the presence of polymers such as starch, acacia or gelatin. Adsorption on to naturally occurring particulate material may aid establishment and survival in some environments. There is a belief, but limited hard evidence, that the presence of suspended particles such as kaolin, magnesium trisilicate or aluminium hydroxide gel may influence contaminant longevity in those products containing them, and that the presence of some surfactants, suspending agents and proteins can increase the resistance of microorganisms to preservatives, over and above their direct inactivating effect on the preservative itself.

17.3 Hazard to Health

Nowadays, it is well recognised that the inadvertent use of a contaminated pharmaceutical product may also present a potential health hazard to the patient. Although isolated outbreaks of medicament-related infections had been reported since the early part of the twentieth century, it was only in the 1960s and 1970s that the significance of this contamination to the patient was more fully understood.

Inevitably, the infrequent isolation of true pathogens, such as *Salmonella* spp. and the reporting of associated infections following the use of products contaminated with these organisms (tablets with pancreatin and thyroid extract), attracted considerable attention. More often, the isolation of common saprophytic and non-fastidious opportunist contaminants with limited pathogenicity to healthy individuals has presented a significant challenge to compromised patients.

Gram-negative contaminants, particularly *Pseudomonas* spp., which have simple nutritional requirements and can multiply to significant levels in aqueous products, have been held responsible for numerous outbreaks of infection. For example, while the intact cornea is quite resistant to infection, it offers little resistance to pseudomonads and related bacteria when scratched, or damaged by irritant chemicals; loss of sight has frequently occurred following the use of poorly designed ophthalmic solutions which had become contaminated by *P. aeruginosa* and even supported its active growth. Pseudomonads contaminating 'antiseptic' solutions have infected the skin of badly burnt patients, resulting in the failure of skin grafts and subsequent death from Gram-negative septicaemia. Infections of eczematous skin and respiratory infections in neonates have been traced to ointments and creams contaminated with Gram-negative bacteria. Oral mixtures and antacid suspensions can support the growth of Gram-negative bacteria and serious consequences have resulted following their inadvertent administration to patients who were immunocompromised as a result of antineoplastic chemotherapy. Growth of Gram-negative bacteria in bladder-washout solutions has been held responsible for painful infections. In more recent times, *Pseudomonas* contamination of TPN fluids during their aseptic compounding in the hospital pharmacy caused the death of several children in the same hospital.

Fatal viral infections resulting from the use of contaminated human tissue or fluids as components of medicines are well recorded, including the example of HIV infection of haemophiliacs caused by contaminated and inadequately treated factor VIII products, made from pooled human blood. Previously regarded as 'slow viruses', so-called prions, the causative agents responsible for transmissible spongiform encephalopathies, such as Creutzfeldt–Jakob disease (CJD) in humans, are now classed as a distinct group of infectious agents with disturbing properties of resistance. Iatrogenic CJD followed the use of injections of human growth hormone (HGH) derived from human pituitary glands, some of which were infected. Between 1958 and 1985, thousands of children with restricted growth were treated with the hormone and a minority developed the disease. Since then, all HGH produced in the UK has been artificially manufactured.

Pharmaceutical products of widely differing forms are known to be susceptible to contamination with a variety of microorganisms, ranging from true pathogens to a motley collection of opportunist pathogens (Table 17.1). Disinfectants, antiseptics, powders, tablets and other products providing an inhospitable environment to invading contaminants are known to be at risk, as well as products with more nutritious components, such as creams and lotions with carbohydrates, amino acids, vitamins and often appreciable quantities of water.

The outcome of using a contaminated product may vary from patient to patient, depending on the type and degree of contamination and how the product is to be used. Undoubtedly, the most serious effects have been seen with contaminated injected products where generalised bacteraemic shock and in some cases death of patients have been reported. More likely, a wound or sore in broken skin may become locally infected or colonised by the contaminant; this may in turn result in extended hospital bed occupancy, with ensuing economic consequences. It must be stressed, however, that the majority of cases of medicament-related infections are probably not recognised or reported as such. Recognition of these infections presents its own problems. It is a fortunate hospital physician who can, at an early stage, recognise contamination shown as a cluster of infections of rapid onset, such as that following the use of a contaminated intravenous fluid in a hospital ward. The chances of a general practitioner recognising a medicament-related infection of insidious onset, perhaps spread over

Table 17.1 Contaminants found in pharmaceutical products and resulting outcome.

Year	Product	Contaminant and outcome
1907	Plague vaccine	*Clostridium tetani*. Following vaccination,19 patients contracted tetanus
1943	Fluorescein eye drops	*Pseudomonas aeruginosa*. 5 patients developed corneal ulcers
1946	Talcum powder	*Clostridium tetani*. Following use of unsterilised powder, 3 infants died
1948	Serum vaccine	*Staphylococcus aureus*. Death of 3 children in measles vaccination programme
1955	Chloroxylenol disinfectant	*Pseudomonas aeruginosa*. Bladder infections in prostatectomy patients from 'disinfected' urinals
1966	Thyroid tablets	*Salmonella muenchen* and *Salmonella bareilly*. Salmonellosis in 202 patients traced to heavily contaminated (10^6 CFU g^{-1}) raw material, defatted thyroid powder
1966	Antibiotic eye ointment	*Pseudomonas aeruginosa*. Severe eye disorders in 8 patients
1966	Saline solution	*Serratia marcescens*. Urinary tract infections in neonates following use of saline to moisten umbilical stump
1967	Carmine powder	*Salmonella cubana*. Capsules used as faecal markers caused gastrointestinal infections
1967	Hand cream	*Klebsiella pneumoniae*. Outbreak of septicaemia in 6 patients in intensive care unit (ICU)
1969	Peppermint water	*Pseudomonas aeruginosa*. Bowel colonisation of 4 patients
1970	Chlorhexidine–cetrimide antiseptic solution	*Pseudomonas* (now *Burkholderia) cepacia*. Following operations, wound infections in 9 patients
1972	Intravenous fluids	*Pseudomonas, Erwinia* and *Enterobacter* spp. Death of 6 hospital patients, following use of unsterilised intravenous dextrose solution
1972	Pancreatin powder	*Salmonella schwarzengrund* and *Salmonella eimsbuettel*. Infections in 2 children with cystic fibrosis
1977	Contact lens solution	*Serratia* spp. 8 cases of infective keratitis with loss of sight in 2 cases
1982	Iodophor solution	*Pseudomonas aeruginosa* and *Burkholderia cepacia*. Clinical infections from use of antiseptic solution
1984	Thymol mouthwash	*Pseudomonas aeruginosa*. Outbreak of septicaemia
1990	Animal vaccines	*Bovine viral diarrhoea virus*. Live attenuated veterinary vaccine caused possible disease transmission in vaccine recipients
1994	Total parenteral nutrition solution	*Enterobacter cloacae*. Death of 2 children following use of solution prepared in a hospital pharmacy
1997	Miscellaneous herbal medicinal products	*Enterobacter* spp., *Enterococcus faecalis, Clostridium perfringens, Klebsiella pneumonia, Escherichia, Pseudomonas*. Heavy microbial contamination and failure to comply with EP maximum microbial limit of 5×10^5 CFU g^{-1}
1999	Benzalkonium chloride disinfectant	Inoculation of multidose injection vial with *Pseudomonas aeruginosa* via needle puncture after vial septa were wiped with contaminated disinfectant
2004	Influenza vaccine	Gram-negative bacteria, including *Serratia*. A limited number of manufactured lots (4.5 million doses) affected, but all batches quarantined. Manufacturer's licence suspended until approved corrective action taken.
2004	Ultrasound gel	*Burkholderia cepacia*. Outbreak of nosocomial blood infection in 6 patients following transrectal prostate biopsy (isolate found to be a paraben degrader).
2014	Anaesthetic eye drops	*Burkholderia cepacia*. 13 patients developed acute postoperative endophthalmitis following cataract surgery with intraocular lens implantation.
2016	Oral liquid laxative	*Burkholderia cepacia*. 49 confirmed cases of infection, predominantly patients under cancer treatment.

CFU, colony forming units; EP, European Pharmacopoeia

several months, in a diverse group of patients in the community, are much more remote. Once recognised, of course, there is a moral obligation to withdraw immediately the offending product; subsequent investigations of the incident therefore become retrospective.

17.3.1 Microbial Toxins

Gram-negative bacteria contain lipopolysaccharides (endotoxins) in their outer cell membranes (see Chapters 3 and 22); these can remain in an active condition in products even after cell death and some can survive moist heat sterilisation. Although inactive by the oral route, endotoxins can induce a number of physiological effects if they enter the bloodstream via contaminated infusion fluids, even in nanogram quantities, or via diffusion across membranes from contaminated haemodialysis solutions. Such effects may include fever, activation of the cytokine system and endothelial cell damage, all leading to septic and often fatal febrile shock.

The acute bacterial toxins associated with food-poisoning episodes are not commonly reported in pharmaceutical products, although aflatoxin-producing aspergilli have been detected in some vegetable and herbal ingredients, and in samples of starch used for pharmaceutical formulation. However, many of the metabolites of microbial deterioration have quite unpleasant tastes and smell even at low levels, and would deter most patients from using such a medicine.

17.4 Sources and Control of Contamination

17.4.1 In Manufacture

Regardless of whether manufacture takes place in industry or on a smaller scale in the hospital pharmacy, the microbiological quality of the finished product will be determined by the formulation components used, the environment in which they are manufactured and the manufacturing process itself. As discussed in Chapter 22, quality must be built into the product at all stages of the process and not simply inspected at the end of manufacture.

- Raw materials, particularly water and those of natural origin, must be of a high microbiological standard. Water has multiple uses as a constituent of many products and its microbial ecology is of great importance. Four grades of water (potable, purified, highly purified and Water for Injection) are encountered in pharmaceutical production, each with its own microbiological issues, relating to its method and degree of purification (distillation, reverse osmosis, deionisation) and to its storage and distribution (Sandle 2019). Similarly, raw materials of animal origin used in the manufacture of therapeutic agents should be free of microbes and viruses. Bovine serum and trypsin (frequently of porcine origin) are of particular concern to the manufacturing and licensing authorities owing to their potential contamination from the source animal. A 'Certificate of Analysis' showing tests performed and their results should be available. The traceability of raw materials is paramount, particularly if the material is of bovine origin due to the risk from bovine spongiform encephalopathy (BSE). Likewise, materials of herbal origin may contain high numbers of microorganisms, including those of faecal origin, such as *coliforms* and *Salmonella*, and must conform to specifications set by experienced microbiologists in the industry, taking account of the source of the material and working practices used to grow, harvest and prepare them.
- All processing equipment should be subject to planned preventive maintenance and should be properly cleaned after use to prevent cross-contamination between batches.
- Cleaning equipment should be appropriate for the task in hand and should be thoroughly cleaned and properly maintained.
- Manufacture should take place in suitable premises, supplied with filtered air, for which the environmental requirements vary according to the type of product being made.
- Staff involved in manufacture should not only have good health but also a sound knowledge of the importance of personal and production hygiene.
- The end product requires suitable packaging which will protect it from contamination during its shelf-life and is itself free from contamination.

17.4.1.1 Hospital Manufacture

Manufacture in hospital premises raises certain additional problems with regard to contamination control.

Water

Mains water in hospitals is frequently stored in large roof tanks, some of which may be relatively inaccessible and poorly maintained. Water for pharmaceutical manufacture requires some further treatment, usually by distillation, reverse osmosis or deionisation or a combination of these, depending on the intended use of water. Such processes need careful monitoring, as does the microbiological quality of the water after treatment. Storage of water requires particular care, as some Gram-negative opportunist pathogens, notably *Pseudomonas* spp., can survive on traces of organic matter present in treated water and will readily multiply to high numbers at room temperature. Water should therefore be stored at a temperature in excess of 80 °C and circulated in the distribution system at a flow rate of 1–2 m s^{-1} to prevent the build-up of bacterial biofilms in the pipework.

Environment

The microbial flora of the hospital pharmacy environment is a reflection of the general hospital environment and the activities undertaken there. Free-living opportunist pathogens, such as *P. aeruginosa*, can normally be found in wet sites, such as drains, sinks and taps. Cleaning equipment, such as mops, buckets, cloths and scrubbing machines, may be responsible for distributing these organisms around the pharmacy; if stored wet they provide a convenient niche for microbial growth, resulting in heavy contamination of equipment. Contamination levels in the production environment may, however, be minimised by observing good manufacturing practices, by installing heating traps in sink U-bends, thus destroying one of the main reservoirs of contaminants, and by proper maintenance and storage of equipment, including cleaning equipment. Additionally, cleaning of production units by contractors should be carried out to a pharmaceutical specification.

Packaging

Sacking, cardboard, card liners, corks and paper are unsuitable for packaging pharmaceuticals, as they are often heavily contaminated with bacterial or fungal spores. Over time, these have been largely replaced by non-biodegradable plastic materials. In the past, packaging in hospitals was frequently reused for economic reasons. Large numbers of containers were returned to the pharmacy, bringing with them microbial contaminants introduced during use in the wards. Particular problems were encountered with disinfectant solutions where residues of old stock were 'topped up' with fresh supplies, resulting in the issue of contaminated solutions to wards. The practice of refilling reusable disinfectant containers is now strongly discouraged. Furthermore, disinfectants are no longer made up in hospital pharmacies but are purchased ready to use from central supplies.

Another common practice in hospitals was the repackaging of products purchased in bulk into smaller containers. Increased handling of the product inevitably increased the risk of contamination, as shown by one Public Health Laboratory Service Report in 1971 when hospital-repacked items were surveyed and found to be contaminated twice as often as those in the original pack.

17.4.2 In Use

Pharmaceutical manufacturers may justly argue that their responsibility ends with the supply of a well-preserved product of high microbiological standard in a suitable pack and that the subsequent use, or indeed abuse, of the product is of little concern to them. Although much less is known about how products become contaminated during use, their continued use in a contaminated state is clearly undesirable, particularly in hospitals where it could result in the spread of cross-infection. All multidose products are vulnerable to contamination during use. Regardless of whether products are used in hospital or in the community environment, the sources of contamination are the same, but opportunities for observing it are greater in the former. Although the risk of contamination during product use has been much reduced in recent years, primarily through improvements in packaging and changes in nursing and care practices, it is nevertheless salutary to reflect upon past reported case histories.

17.4.2.1 Human Sources

During normal usage, patients may contaminate their medicine with their own microbial flora; subsequent use of such products could result in self-infection (Figure 17.3).

Topical products are considered to be most at risk, as the product will probably be applied by hand, thus introducing contaminants from the resident skin flora of staphylococci, *Micrococcus* spp. and diphtheroids, but also perhaps transient contaminants, such as *Pseudomonas* or *coliforms*, which would normally be removed with effective handwashing. Opportunities for contamination may be reduced by using disposable applicators for topical products or by giving oral products by disposable spoon.

In hospitals, multidose products, once contaminated, may serve as a vehicle of cross-contamination or cross-infection between patients. In the past, zinc-based products packed in large stockpots and used in the treatment and prevention of bedsores in long-stay and geriatric patients were reportedly contaminated during use with *P. aeruginosa* and *Staphylococcus aureus*. If unpreserved, these products permitted multiplication of contaminants, especially if water was present either as part of the formulation, for example in oil/water (o/w) emulsions, or as a film in w/o emulsions which had undergone local cracking, or as a condensed film from atmospheric water. Appreciable numbers of contaminants might then be transferred to other patients when the product was reused. Clearly the

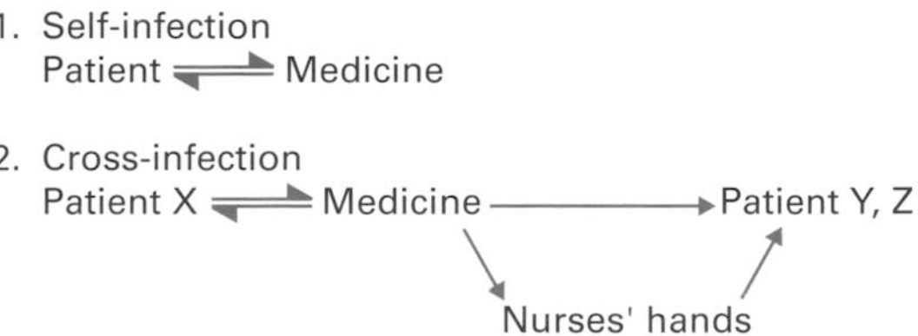

Figure 17.3 Mechanisms of contamination during use of medicinal products.

economics and convenience of using stockpots had to be balanced against the risk of spreading cross-infection between patients and the inevitable increase in length of the patients' stay in hospital. The use of stockpots in hospitals has noticeably declined over the past three decades or so.

A further potential source of contamination in hospitals is the nursing and ancillary staff responsible for medicament administration. During the course of their work, nurses' hands become contaminated with opportunist pathogens which are not part of the normal skin flora but which are easily removed by thorough handwashing and drying. In busy wards, handwashing between attending to patients may be overlooked and contaminants may subsequently be transferred to medicaments during administration. Hand lotions and creams supplied to prevent the chapping of nurses' hands may similarly become contaminated, especially when packaged in multidose containers and left at the side of the handbasin, frequently without lids. Hand lotions and creams should be well preserved and, ideally, packaged in disposable dispensers. Other effective control methods include the supply of products in individual patient's packs and the use of non-touch techniques for medicament administration. The importance of thorough handwashing in the control of hospital cross-infection cannot be overemphasised. In recent years, hospitals have successfully raised the level of awareness on this topic among staff and the general public through widespread publicity and the provision of easily accessible hand disinfection stations at the hospital entrance and at key locations on each ward.

17.4.2.2 Environmental Sources

Small numbers of airborne contaminants may settle in products left open to the atmosphere. Some of these will die during storage, with the rest probably remaining at a static level of about 10^2–10^3 colony-forming units (CFU) per gram or per millilitre. Larger numbers of waterborne contaminants may be accidentally introduced into topical products by wet hands or by a 'splash-back mechanism' if left at the side of a basin. Such contaminants generally have simple nutritional requirements and, following multiplication, levels of contamination have often exceeded 10^6 CFU g^{-1}. In the past, this problem has been encountered particularly when the product was stored in warm hospital wards or in hot steamy bathroom cupboards at home. Products used in hospitals as soap substitutes for bathing patients were particularly at risk and soon not only became contaminated with opportunist pathogens such as *Pseudomonas* spp., but also provided conditions conducive to their multiplication. The problem was compounded by stocks kept in multidose pots for use by several patients in the same ward over an extended period of time.

The indigenous microbial population is quite different in the home from that in hospitals. Pathogenic organisms are found much more frequently in the latter and consequently have been isolated more often from medicines used in hospital. Usually, there are fewer opportunities for contamination in the home, as patients are issued with individual supplies in small quantities.

17.4.2.3 Equipment Sources

Patients and nursing staff may use a range of applicators (pads, sponges, brushes and spatulas) during medicament administration, particularly for topical products. If reused, these easily become contaminated and may be responsible for perpetuating contamination between fresh stocks of product, as has indeed been shown in studies of cosmetic products. Disposable applicators or swabs should therefore always be used.

In hospitals today, a wide variety of complex equipment is used in the course of patient treatment. Humidifiers, incubators, ventilators, resuscitators and other apparatus require proper maintenance and decontamination after use. Chemical disinfectants used for this purpose have in the past, through misuse, become contaminated with opportunist pathogens, such as *P. aeruginosa*, and ironically have contributed to, rather than reduced, the spread of cross-infection in hospital patients. Disinfectants should only be used for their intended purpose and directions for use must be followed at all times.

17.5 The Extent of Microbial Contamination

Most reports of medicament-borne contamination in the literature tend to be anecdotal in nature, referring to a specific product and isolated incident. Little information is available on the overall risk of products becoming contaminated and causing patient infections when subsequently used. Such information is considered invaluable when available not only because it may indicate the effectiveness of existing practices and standards, but also because the value of potential improvements in product quality can be balanced against the inevitable cost of such processes.

17.5.1 In Manufacture

Investigations carried out by the Swedish National Board of Health in 1965 revealed some startling findings on the overall microbiological quality of non-sterile products immediately after manufacture. A wide range of products was routinely found to be contaminated with *Bacillus subtilis*, *Staphylococcus albus* (now known as *Staphylococcus epidermidis*), yeasts and moulds, and in addition large numbers of coliforms were found in a variety of tablets. Furthermore, two nationwide outbreaks of infection in Sweden were subsequently traced to the inadvertent use of contaminated products. Two hundred patients were involved in an outbreak of salmonellosis, caused by thyroid tablets contaminated with *Salmonella bareilly* and *Salmonella muenchen* (now known as *Salmonella enterica* subsp. *enterica* serovar Bareilly and *Salmonella enterica* serovar Muenchen, respectively), and eight patients had severe eye infections following the use of a hydrocortisone eye ointment contaminated with *P. aeruginosa*. The results of this investigation had a profound effect on the manufacture of all medicines; not only were they then used as a yardstick to compare the microbiological quality of non-sterile products made in other countries, but also as a baseline upon which international standards were then to be founded.

Under the UK Medicines Act 1968, pharmaceutical products made in industry were expected to conform to microbiological and chemical quality specifications. The majority of products have since been shown to conform to a high standard, although spot checks have occasionally revealed medicines of unacceptable quality and so have necessitated product recall. By contrast, pharmaceutical products made in hospitals were much less rigorously controlled, as shown by several surveys in the 1970s in which significant numbers of preparations were found to be contaminated with *P. aeruginosa*. In 1974, however, hospital manufacture also came under the terms of the Medicines Act and, as a consequence, considerable improvements were subsequently seen not only in the conditions and standard of manufacture, but also in the chemical and microbiological quality of finished products. Hospital manufacturing operations were later rationalised. Economic constraints caused a critical evaluation of the true cost of these activities. Competitive purchasing from industry in many cases produced cheaper alternatives, and small-scale manufacturing was largely discouraged. Where licensed products were available, National Health Service (NHS) policy dictated that these were to be purchased from a commercial source and not made locally.

Removal of Crown immunity from the NHS in 1991 meant that manufacturing operations in hospitals were then subject to the full licensing provisions of the Medicines Act 1968, that is, hospital pharmacies intending to manufacture were required to obtain a manufacturing licence and to comply fully with current European Commission good pharmaceutical manufacturing practices (GPMP; see Eudralex 2003). Among other requirements, this included the provision of appropriate environmental manufacturing conditions and associated environmental monitoring. Subsequently, the Medicines Control Agency (MCA) issued guidance in 1992 on certain manufacturing exemptions, by virtue of the product batch size or frequency of manufacture. The need for extemporaneous dispensing of 'one-off' special formulae continued in hospital pharmacies, although this work was largely transferred from the dispensing bench to dedicated preparative facilities with appropriate environmental control. Today hospital manufacturing is concentrated on the supply of bespoke products from a regional centre or small-scale specialist manufacture of those items currently unobtainable from industry. Repacking of commercial products into more convenient pack sizes is, however, still common practice.

17.5.2 In Use

Higher rates of contamination are invariably seen in products after opening and use, and, among these, medicines used in hospitals are more likely to be contaminated than those used in the general community. The Public Health Laboratory Service Report of 1971 expressed concern at the overall incidence of contamination in non-sterile products used on hospital wards (327 of 1220 samples) and the proportion of samples found to be heavily contaminated (18% > 10^4 CFU g^{-1} or CFU ml^{-1}). Notably, the presence of *P. aeruginosa* in 2.7% of samples (mainly oral alkaline mixtures) was considered to be highly undesirable.

By contrast, medicines used in the home were not only less often contaminated but also contained lower levels of contaminants and fewer pathogenic organisms. Generally, there were fewer opportunities for contamination here because individual patients used smaller quantities. Medicines in the home may, however, be hoarded and used for extended periods of time. Additionally, storage conditions may be unsuitable and expiry dates ignored; thus, problems other than those of microbial contamination may be seen in the home.

17.6 Factors Determining the Outcome of a Medicament-borne Infection

Although impossible to quantify, the use of contaminated medicines has undoubtedly contributed to the spread of cross-infection in hospitals; undeniably, such nosocomial (hospital-acquired) infections have also extended the length of stay in hospital with concomitant costs. A patient's response to the microbial challenge of a contaminated medicine may be diverse and unpredictable, perhaps with serious consequences. Clinical reactions may not be evident in one patient, yet in another may be indisputable, illustrating one problem in the recognition of medicament-borne infections. Clinical reactions may range from inconvenient local infections of wounds or broken skin, caused possibly from contact with a contaminated cream, to gastrointestinal infections from the ingestion of contaminated oral products, to serious widespread infections such as a bacteraemia or septicaemia, possibly resulting in death, as caused by the administration of contaminated infusion fluids. Undoubtedly, the most serious outbreaks of infection have been seen in the past where contaminated products have been injected directly into the bloodstream of patients whose immunity is already compromised by their underlying disease or therapy.

The outcome of any episode is determined by a combination of several factors, among which the type and degree of microbial contamination, the route of administration and the patient's resistance are of particular importance.

17.6.1 Type and Degree of Microbial Contamination

Microorganisms that contaminate medicines and cause disease in patients may be classified as true pathogens or opportunist pathogens. Pathogenic organisms such as *Clostridium tetani* and *Salmonella* spp. rarely occur in products, but when present cause serious problems. Wound infections and several cases of neonatal death have resulted from use of talcum powder containing *C. tetani*. Outbreaks of salmonellosis have followed the inadvertent ingestion of contaminated thyroid and pancreatic powders. On the other hand, opportunist pathogens such as *P. aeruginosa*, *Klebsiella*, *Serratia* and other free-living organisms are more frequently isolated from medicinal products and, as their name suggests, may be pathogenic if given the opportunity. The main concern with these organisms is that their simple nutritional requirements enable them to survive in a wide range of pharmaceuticals, and thus they tend to be present in high numbers, perhaps in excess of 10^6–10^7 CFU g^{-1} or CFU ml^{-1}. The product itself, however, may show no visible sign of contamination. Opportunist pathogens can survive in disinfectants and antiseptic solutions that are normally used in the control of hospital cross-infection, but which, when contaminated, may even perpetuate the spread of infection. Compromised hospital patients, that is, elderly, neonates, burned, traumatised or immunosuppressed patients, are considered to be particularly at risk from infection with these organisms, whereas healthy patients in the general community have given little cause for concern.

The critical dose of microorganisms that will initiate an infection is largely unknown and varies not only between species but also within a species. Animal and human volunteer studies have indicated that the infecting dose may be reduced significantly in the presence of trauma or foreign bodies or if accompanied by a drug having a local vasoconstrictive action.

17.6.2 Route of Administration

As stated previously, contaminated products injected directly into the bloodstream or instilled into the eye cause the most serious problems. Intrathecal and epidural injections are potentially hazardous procedures. In practice, epidural injections are given through a bacterial filter. Injectable and ophthalmic solutions are often simple solutions and provide Gram-negative opportunist pathogens with sufficient nutrients to multiply during storage; if contaminated, a bioburden of 10^6 CFU as well as the production of endotoxins should be expected. TPN fluids, formulated for individual patients' nutritional requirements, can also provide more than adequate nutritional support for invading contaminants. *P. aeruginosa*, the notorious contaminant of eye drops, has caused serious ophthalmic infections, including the loss of sight in some cases. The problem is compounded when the eye is damaged through the improper use of contact lenses or scratched by fingernails or cosmetic applicators.

The fate of contaminants ingested orally in medicines may be determined by several factors, as is seen with contaminated food. The acidity of the stomach may provide a successful barrier, depending on whether the medicine is taken on an empty or full stomach and also on the gastric emptying time. Contaminants in topical products may cause little harm when deposited on intact skin. Not only does the skin itself provide an excellent mechanical barrier, but few contaminants normally survive in competition with its resident microbial flora. Skin damaged during surgery or trauma or in patients with burns or pressure sores may, however, be rapidly colonised and subsequently infected by opportunist pathogens. Patients treated with topical steroids are also prone to local infections, particularly if contaminated steroid drugs are inadvertently used.

17.6.3 Resistance of the Patient

A patient's resistance is crucial in determining the outcome of a medicament-borne infection. Hospital patients are more exposed and susceptible to infection than those treated in the general community. Neonates, elderly people, diabetics and patients undergoing cancer chemotherapy or traumatised by surgery or accident may have impaired defence mechanisms. People suffering from leukaemia and those treated with immunosuppressants are most vulnerable to infection; there is an undeniable case for providing all medicines in a sterile form for these patients.

17.7 Preservation of Medicines Using Antimicrobial Agents: Basic Principles

17.7.1 Introduction

An antimicrobial 'preservative' may be included in a formulation to minimise the risk of spoilage and preferably to kill low levels of contaminants introduced during storage or repeated use of a multidose container. However, where there is a low risk of contamination, as with tablets, capsules and dry powders, the inclusion of a preservative may be unnecessary. Preservatives should never be added to mask poor manufacturing processes.

The properties of an ideal preservative are well recognised: a broad spectrum of activity and a rapid rate of kill; selectivity in reacting with the contaminants and not the formulation ingredients; non-irritant and non-toxic to the patient; and stable and effective throughout the life of the product.

Unfortunately, the most active antimicrobial agents are often non-selective in action, interacting significantly with formulation ingredients as well as with patients and microorganisms. Having excluded the more toxic, irritant and reactive agents, those remaining generally have only modest antimicrobial efficacy, and no preservatives are now considered sufficiently non-toxic for use in sensitive areas, for example, for injection into central nervous system tissues or for use within the eye. A number of microbiologically effective preservatives used in cosmetics have caused a significant number of cases of contact dermatitis, and are thus precluded from use in pharmaceutical creams. Although a rapid rate of kill may be preferable, this may only be possible for relatively simple aqueous solutions such as eye drops or injections. For physicochemically complex systems such as emulsions and creams, inhibition of growth and a slow rate of killing may be all that can be realistically achieved within a safe concentration range. In order to maximise preservative efficacy, it is essential to have an appreciation of those parameters that influence antimicrobial activity.

17.7.2 Effect of Preservative Concentration, Temperature and Size of Inoculum

Changes in the efficacy of preservatives vary exponentially with changes in concentration. The effect of changes in concentration (concentration exponent, η, see Chapter 19) varies with the type of agent. For example, halving the concentration of phenol ($\eta = 6$) gives a 64-fold (2^6) reduction in killing activity, whereas a similar dilution for chlorhexidine ($\eta = 2$) reduces the activity by only fourfold (2^2). Changes in preservative activity are also seen with changes in product temperature, according to the temperature coefficient, Q_{10}. Thus, a reduction in temperature from 30 °C to 20 °C could result in a significantly reduced rate of kill for *Escherichia coli*, fivefold in the case of phenol ($Q_{10} = 5$) and 45-fold in the case of ethanol ($Q_{10} = 45$). If both temperature and concentration vary concurrently, the situation is more complex; however, it has been suggested that if a 0.1% chlorocresol ($\eta = 6$, $Q_{10} = 5$) solution completely killed a suspension of *E. coli* at 30 °C in 10 minutes, it would require around 90 minutes to achieve a similar effect if stored at 20 °C and if slight overheating during production had resulted in a 10% loss in the chlorocresol concentration (other factors remaining constant).

Preservative molecules are used up as they inactivate microorganisms and as they interact non-specifically with significant quantities of contaminant 'dirt' introduced during use. This will result in a progressive and exponential decline in the efficiency of the remaining preservative. Preservative 'capacity' is a term used to describe the cumulative level of contamination that a preserved formulation can tolerate before becoming so depleted as to become ineffective. This will vary with preservative type and complexity of formulation.

17.7.3 Factors Affecting the 'Availability' of Preservatives

Most preservatives interact in solution to some extent with many of the commonly used formulation ingredients via a number of weak bonding attractions as well as with any contaminants present. Unstable equilibria may form in which only a small proportion of total preservative present is 'available' to inactivate the relatively small microbial mass; the resulting rate of kill may be far slower than might be anticipated from the performance of simple aqueous solutions. However, 'unavailable' preservative may still contribute to the general irritancy of the product. It is commonly believed that where the solute concentrations are very high, and A_w is appreciably reduced, the efficiency of preservatives is often significantly reduced and they may be virtually inactive at very low A_w. The practice of including preservatives in very low A_w products such as tablets and capsules is ill advised, as it only offers minimal protection for the dry tablets; should they become damp, they would be spoiled for other, non-microbial, reasons.

While the most assured route to optimising the efficacy of a preservative agent is to control detrimental influences such as those outlined below, this is not always possible. The concept of the preservative system or 'hurdle technology' has therefore developed where the intrinsic antimicrobial activity of some formulation excipients is used to enhance the overall preservative effect.

17.7.3.1 Effect of Product pH

In the weakly acidic preservatives, activity resides primarily in the unionised molecules and they only have significant efficacy at pH values where ionisation is low. Thus, benzoic and sorbic acids (pK_a = 4.2 and 4.75, respectively) have limited preservative usefulness above pH 5, while the 4(*p*)-hydroxybenzoate (parabens) esters with their non-ionisable ester group and poorly ionisable hydroxyl substituent (pK_a, approximately 8.5) have a moderate protective effect even at neutral pH levels. The activity of quaternary ammonium preservatives and chlorhexidine probably resides with their cations; they are effective in products of neutral pH. Formulation pH can also directly influence the sensitivity of microorganisms to preservatives (see Chapter 19).

17.7.3.2 Efficiency in Multiphase Systems

In a multiphase formulation, such as an oil-in-water emulsion, preservative molecules will distribute themselves in an unstable equilibrium between the bulk aqueous phase and (i) the oil phase by partition, (ii) the surfactant micelles by solubilisation, (iii) polymeric suspending agents and other solutes by competitive displacement of water of solvation, (iv) particulate and container surfaces by adsorption and (v) any microorganisms present. Generally, the overall preservative efficiency can be related to the small proportion of preservative molecules remaining unbound in the bulk aqueous phase, although as this becomes depleted some slow re-equilibration between the components can be anticipated. The loss of neutral molecules into oil and micellar phases may be favoured over ionised species, although considerable variation in distribution is found between different systems.

In view of these major potential reductions in preservative efficacy, considerable effort has been directed to devise equations in which one might substitute variously derived system parameters (such as partition coefficients, surfactant- and polymer-binding constants and oil:water ratios) to obtain estimates of residual preservative levels in aqueous phases. Although some modestly successful predictions have been obtained for very simple laboratory systems, they have proved of limited practical value, as data for many of the required parameters are unavailable for technical-grade ingredients or for the more complex commercial systems.

17.7.3.3 Effect of Container or Packaging

Preservative availability may be appreciably reduced by interaction with packaging materials. Phenolics, for example, will permeate the rubber wads and teats of multidose injection or eye drop containers and also interact with flexible nylon tubes for creams. Quaternary ammonium preservative levels in formulations have been significantly reduced by adsorption on to the surfaces of plastic and glass containers. Volatile preservatives such as chloroform are so readily lost by the routine opening and closing of containers that their usefulness is somewhat restricted to preservation of medicines in sealed, impervious containers during storage, with short in-use lives once opened.

17.8 Quality Assurance and the Control of Microbial Risk in Medicines

17.8.1 Introduction

Manufacturers of medicinal products must comply with the requirements of their marketing authorisation (product licence) and ensure that their products are fit for their intended use in terms of safety, quality and efficacy. A quality management system (QMS) must therefore be in place so that senior management can ensure that the required quality objectives are met through a comprehensively designed and properly implemented system of quality assurance (QA), encompassing both good pharmaceutical manufacturing practice (GPMP) and quality control (QC). QC is that part of GPMP dealing with specifications, documentation and assessing conformance to specification.

QA encompasses, in turn, a scheme of management which embraces all the procedures necessary to provide a high probability that a medicine will conform consistently to a specified description of quality. It includes formulation design, research and development (R&D), GPMP, as well as QC and post-marketing surveillance. As many microorganisms may be hazardous to patients or cause spoilage of formulations under suitable conditions, it is necessary to perform a risk assessment of contamination for each product. At each stage of its anticipated life from raw materials to administration, a risk assessment should be made and strategies should be developed and calculated to reduce the overall risk(s) to acceptably low levels. Such risk assessments are complicated by uncertainties about the exact infective and spoilage hazards likely for many contaminants, and by difficulties in measuring their precise performance in complex systems. As the consequences of product failure and patient harm will inevitably be severe, it is usual for manufacturing companies to make worst-case presumptions and design strategies to cover them fully; lesser problems are also then encompassed. As it must be assumed that all microorganisms may be potentially hazardous for those routes of administration where the likelihood of infection from contaminants is high, then medicines to be given via these routes must be supplied in a sterile form, as is the case with injectable products. It must also be presumed that those administering medicines may not necessarily be highly skilled or motivated in contamination control techniques; additional safeguards to control risks may be included in these situations. This may include detailed information on administration as well as training, in addition to providing a high-quality formulation.

17.8.2 Quality Assurance in Formulation Design and Development

The risk of microbial infection and spoilage arising from microbial contamination during manufacture, storage and use could be eliminated by presenting all medicines in sterile, impervious, single-dosage units. However, the high cost of this strategy restricts its use to situations where there is a high risk of consequent infection from any contaminants. Where the risk is assessed as much lower, less efficient but less expensive strategies are adopted. The high risk of infection by contaminants in parenteral medicines, combined with concerns about the systemic toxicity of preservatives, almost always demands sterile single-dosage units. With eye drops for domestic use the risks are perceived to be lower, and sterile multidose products with preservatives to combat the anticipated in-use contamination are accepted; sterile single-dose units are more common in hospitals where there is an increased risk of infection. Oral and topical routes of administration are generally perceived to present relatively low risks of infection and the emphasis is more on the control of microbial content during manufacture and subsequent protection of the formulation from chemical and physicochemical spoilage.

As part of the design process, it is necessary to include features in the formulation and delivery system that provide as much suitable protection as possible against microbial contamination and spoilage. Owing to potential toxicity and irritancy problems, antimicrobial preservatives should only be considered where there is clear evidence of positive benefit. Manipulation of physicochemical parameters, such as A_w, the elimination of particularly susceptible ingredients (e.g., natural ingredients such as tragacanth powder, used as a thickening agent), the selection of a preservative or the choice of container may individually and collectively contribute significantly to overall medicine stability. For 'dry' dosage forms where their very low A_w provides protection against microbial attack, the moisture vapour properties of packaging materials require careful examination.

Preservatives are intended to offer further protection against environmental microbial contaminants. However, as they are relatively non-specific in their reactivity (see Section 17.7), it is difficult to calculate with any certainty what proportion of preservative added to all but the simplest medicine will be available for inactivating such contamination. Laboratory tests have been devised to challenge the product with an artificial bioburden. Such tests should form part of formulation development and stability trials to ensure that suitable activity is likely to remain throughout the life of the product. They are not normally used in routine manufacturing QC.

Some 'preservative challenge tests' (preservative efficacy tests) add relatively large inocula of various laboratory cultures to aliquots of the product and determine their rate of inactivation by viable counting methods (single-challenge tests), while others reinoculate repeatedly at set intervals, monitoring the efficiency of inactivation until the system fails (multiple-challenge test). This latter technique may give a better estimate of the preservative capacity of the system than the single-challenge approach, but is both time-consuming and expensive. Problems arise when deciding whether the observed performance in such tests gives reliable predictions of real in-use efficacy. Although test organisms should bear some similarity in type and spoilage potential to those met in use, it is known that repeated cultivation on conventional microbiological media (nutrient agar, etc.) frequently results in reduced virulence of strains. Attempts to maintain spoilage activity by inclusion of formulation ingredients in culture media give varied results. Some manufacturers have been able to maintain active spoilage strains by cultivation in unpreserved, or diluted aliquots of, formulations.

The *British Pharmacopoeia* (BP) and the *European Pharmacopoeia* (EP) describe a single-challenge preservative test that routinely uses four test organisms (two bacteria *P. aeruginosa* and *S. aureus* [supplemented with *E. coli* when oral products are tested], a mould *Aspergillus brasiliensis* [formerly *Aspergillus niger*] and a yeast *Candida albicans*), none of which has any significant history of spoilage potential and which are cultivated on conventional media. However, extension of the basic test is recommended in some situations, such as the inclusion of an osmotolerant yeast (*Zygosaccharomyces rouxii*) if it is thought such in-use spoilage might be a problem. Despite its accepted limitations and the cautious indications given as to what the tests might suggest about a formulation, the test does provide some basic but useful indicators of likely in-use stability. UK product licence applications for preserved medicines must demonstrate that the formulation at least meets the preservative efficacy criteria of the *British Pharmacopoeia* or a similar test.

The concept of the D-value (decimal reduction time) as used in sterilisation technology (see Chapter 21) has been applied to the interpretation of challenge testing. Expression of the rate of microbial inactivation in a preserved system in terms of a D-value enables estimation of the nominal time to achieve a prescribed proportionate level of kill. Problems arise, however, when trying to predict the behaviour of very low levels of survivors, and the method has its critics as well as its advocates.

17.8.3 Good Pharmaceutical Manufacturing Practice

GPMP is concerned with the manufacture of medicines, and includes control of ingredients, plant construction, process validation, production and cleaning (see also Chapter 22). Current GPMP (cGPMP) requirements are found in the Medicines and Healthcare Products Regulatory Agency (MHRA) *Rules and Guidance for Pharmaceutical Manufacturers and Distributors*, known as the Orange Guide (MHRA 2022), and its 20 annexes. The recently revised Annex 1 of the EU GMP guide (2022, see Eudralex 2003) reinforces the general guidance for all sterile medicinal products and sterile active substances through adopting the principles of quality risk management (QRM), ensuring that the manufacture of sterile products is subject to special requirements and built upon a robust and scientifically based management system to minimise risks of microbial, particulate and pyrogen contamination, thereby ensuring sterility assurance of the final product. Annex 1 has been prepared in cooperation with the European Medicines Agency, the World Health Organization and the Pharmaceutical Inspection Co-operation Scheme (PIC/S) to maintain global alignment of standards and to provide assurance of quality. Of particular note, the principles of QRM are introduced to allow for the inclusion of new technologies and innovative processes.

With traditional QC, a high reliance has been placed on testing samples of finished products to determine the overall quality of a batch. This practice can, however, result in considerable financial loss if non-compliance is detected only at this late stage, leaving the expensive options of discarding or reworking the batch. Additionally, some microbiological test methods have poor precision and/or accuracy. Validation can be complex or impossible, and interpretation of results can prove difficult. For example, although a sterility assurance level of less than one failure in 10^6 items submitted to a terminal sterilisation process is considered acceptable, conventional 'tests for sterility' for finished products (such as that in the *European Pharmacopoeia*) could not possibly be relied upon to find one damaged but viable microbe within the 10^6 items, regardless of allowing for its cultivation with any precision (see Chapters 21 and 22). Moreover, end-product testing will not prevent and may not even detect the isolated rogue processing failure.

It is now generally accepted that a high assurance of overall product quality can only come from a detailed specification, control and monitoring of *all* the stages that contribute to the manufacturing process. More realistic decisions about conformance to specification can then be made using information from *all* relevant parameters (parametric release method), not just from the results of selective testing of finished products. Thus, a more realistic estimate of the microbial quality of a batch of tablets would be achieved from a knowledge of specific parameters (such as the microbial bioburden of the starting materials, temperature records from granule drying ovens, the moisture level of the dried granules, compaction data, validation records for the foil strip sealing machine and microbial levels in the finished tablets), than from the contaminant content of the finished tablets alone. Similarly, parametric release is now accepted as an operational alternative to routine sterility testing for batch release of some finished sterile products. Through parametric release, the manufacturer can provide assurance that the product is of the stipulated quality, based on the evidence of successful validation of the manufacturing process and review of the documentation on process monitoring carried out during manufacturing. Authorisation for parametric release is given, refused or withdrawn by pharmaceutical assessors, together with GMP inspectors; the requirements are detailed in Annex 17 of the MHRA Orange Guide (MHRA 2022).

It may be necessary to exclude certain undesirable contaminants from starting materials, such as pseudomonads from bulk aluminium hydroxide gel, or to include some form of pre-treatment to reduce their bioburdens by irradiation, such as for ispaghula husk, herbal materials and spices. For biotechnology-derived drugs produced in human or animal tissue culture, considerable efforts are made to exclude cell lines contaminated with latent host viruses. Official guidelines to limit the risk of prion contamination in medicines require bovine-derived ingredients to be obtained from sources where BSE is not endemic. The USA, Australia and New Zealand are recognised as supplying high-quality bovine serum, along with adequate documentation, known as a 'Certificate of Suitability', for each lot used in the manufacturing process. In considering the manufacturing plant and its environs from an ecological and a physiological viewpoint of microorganisms, it is possible not only to identify areas where contaminants may accumulate and even thrive to create hazards for subsequent production batches, but also to manipulate design and operating conditions in order to discourage such colonisation. The facility to clean and dry equipment thoroughly is a very useful deterrent to growth. Design considerations should include the elimination of obscure nooks and crannies (where biofilms may readily become established) and the ability to clean thoroughly in all areas. Many larger items of equipment now have cleaning-in-place (CIP) and sterilisation-in-place (SIP) systems installed to improve decontamination capabilities.

It may be necessary to include intermediate steps within processing to reduce the bioburden and improve the efficiency of lethal sterilisation cycles, or to prevent swamping of the preservative in a non-sterile medicine after manufacture. Some of the newer and fragile biotechnology-derived products may include chromatographic and/or ultrafiltration processing stages to ensure adequate reductions of viral contamination levels rather than conventional sterilisation cycles.

In a validation exercise, it must be demonstrated that each stage of the system is capable of providing the degree of intended efficiency within the limits of variation for which it was designed. Microbial spoilage aspects of process validation might include examination of the cleaning system for its ability to remove deliberately introduced contamination. Chromatographic removal of viral contaminants would be validated by determining the log reduction achievable against a known titre of added viral particles.

17.8.4 Quality Control Procedures

While there is general agreement on the need to control total microbial levels in non-sterile medicines and to exclude certain species that have previously proved troublesome, the precision and accuracy of current methods for counting (or even detecting) some microbes in complex products are poor. Pathogens, present in low numbers, and often damaged by processing, can be very difficult to isolate. Products showing active spoilage can yield surprisingly low viable counts on testing. Although present in high numbers, a particular organism may be neither pathogenic nor the primary spoilage agent, but may be relatively inert, for example, ungerminated spores or a secondary contaminant which has outgrown the initiating spoiler. Unevenly distributed growth in viscous formulations will present serious sampling problems. The type of culture medium (even different batches of the same medium) and conditions of recovery and incubation may significantly influence any viable counts obtained from products (see Chapter 2).

An unresolved problem concerns the timing of sampling. Low levels of pseudomonads shortly after manufacture may not constitute a spoilage hazard if their growth is checked. However, if unchecked, high levels may well initiate spoilage.

The *European Pharmacopoeia* introduced both quantitative and qualitative microbial standards for non-sterile medicines, which became enforceable in some member states. It prescribed varying maximum total microbial levels and exclusion of particular species according to the routes of administration. The *British Pharmacopoeia* also included these tests, but suggested that they should be used to assist in validating GPMP processing procedures and not as conformance standards for routine end-product testing. Thus, for a medicine to be administered orally, the total viable count (TVC) should not be more than 10^3 aerobic bacteria or 10^2 fungi per gram or millilitre of product and there should be an absence of *E. coli*.

Higher levels may be permissible if the product contains raw materials of natural origin, where the TVC should not exceed 10^4 aerobic bacteria, 10^2 fungi and 10^2 bile-tolerant Gram-negative bacteria, with the absence of *E. coli* and *S. aureus* per gram or millilitre and *Salmonella* per 10 gram or millilitre, as specified in the 2021 EP.

Most manufacturers perform periodic tests on their products for total microbial counts and the presence of known problem microorganisms; generally, these are used for in-house confirmation of the continuing efficiency of their cGPMP systems, rather than as conventional end-product conformance tests. Fluctuation in values, or the appearance of specific and unusual species, can warn of defects in procedures and impending problems.

In order to reduce the costs of testing and to shorten quarantine periods, there is considerable interest in automated alternatives to conventional test methods for the detection and determination of microorganisms (see Chapters 2 and 3). Promising methods include electrical impedance, use of fluorescent dyes and epifluorescence and the use of 'vital' stains. Considerable advances in the sensitivity of methods for estimating microbial adenosine triphosphate (ATP) using luciferase now allow the estimation of extremely low bioburdens. The recent development of highly sensitive laser scanning devices for detecting bacteria variously labelled with selective fluorescent probes enables the apparent detection even of single cells.

Endotoxin (pyrogen) levels in parenteral and similar products must be extremely low in order to prevent serious endotoxic shock on administration (see Chapter 22).

Formerly, this was checked by injecting rabbits and noting any febrile response. Most determinations are now performed using the *Limulus* test in which an amoebocyte lysate from the horseshoe crab (*Limulus polyphemus*) reacts specifically with microbial lipopolysaccharides to give a gel and opacity even at very high dilutions. A variant of the test using a chromogenic substrate gives a coloured end point that can be detected spectroscopically. Cell culture tests are available where the ability of endotoxins to induce cytokine release is measured directly.

Sophisticated and very sensitive methods have been developed in the food industry for detecting many other microbial toxins. For example, aflatoxin detection in herbal materials, seed-stuffs and their oils is performed by solvent extraction, adsorption onto columns containing antibodies selective for the toxin and detection by exposure to ultraviolet light.

Although it would be unusual to test for signs of active physicochemical or chemical spoilage of products as part of routine product QC procedures, this may occasionally be necessary in order to examine an incident of anticipated product failure, or during formulation development. Many of the volatile and unpleasant-tasting metabolites generated during active spoilage are readily apparent. Their characterisation by high-performance liquid chromatography or gas chromatography can be used to distinguish microbial spoilage from other, non-biological, deterioration. Spoilage often results in physicochemical changes which can be monitored by conventional methods. Thus, emulsion spoilage may be followed by monitoring changes in creaming rates, pH changes, particle sedimentation and viscosity.

17.8.5 Post-market Surveillance

Despite extensive development and a rigorous adherence to procedures, it is impossible to guarantee that a medicine will never fail under the harsh abuses of real-life conditions. A proper quality-assurance system must include procedures for monitoring in-use performance and for responding to customer complaints. These must be meticulously followed up in great detail in order to decide whether carefully constructed and implemented schemes for product safety require modification to prevent the incident recurring.

17.9 Overview

Prevention is undoubtedly better than cure in minimising the risk of medicament-borne infections. In manufacture, the principles of GPMP are well understood, must be observed and control measures must be built in at all stages of production. Thus, initial stability tests should show that the proposed formulation can withstand an appropriate microbial challenge; raw materials from an authorised supplier should comply with in-house microbial specifications; environmental conditions appropriate to the production process should be subject to regular microbiological monitoring; and, finally, end-product analysis should indicate that the product is microbiologically suitable for its intended use and conforms to accepted in-house and international standards. Any contaminants present in the final product should not present a potential health hazard to the patient, either by virtue of their type or number.

Contamination during use is less easily controlled. Successful measures in the hospital pharmacy have included the packaging of products as individual units, thereby discouraging the use of multidose containers. Unit packaging (one dose per patient) has clear advantages, but economic constraints have limited this practice. Ultimately, the most fruitful approach is through the training and education of patients and hospital staff, so that medicines are used only for their intended purpose. The task of implementing this approach inevitably rests with the clinical and community pharmacists of the future.

References

Eudralex (2003). Directive 2003/94/EC *The Rules Governing Medicinal Products in the European Community, Vol. 4 – Good Manufacturing Practices.* Official Journal of the European Union, Brussels. Most recent revisions can be found on the website of the European Commission at http://ec.europa.eu/health/documents/eudralex/vol-4/index_en.htm

European Pharmacopoeia, 10 (2021) EP Secretariat, Strasbourg.

MHRA (2022). *Rules and Guidance for Pharmaceutical Manufacturers and Distributors*, 11e 'The Orange Guide'. London: Pharmaceutical Press.

Sandle, T. (2019). Microbiology of pharmaceutical grade water. In: *Industrial Pharmaceutical Microbiology: Standards and Controls*, 5e (ed. T. Sandle). Liphook: Euromed Communications.

Further Reading

Alexander, R.G., Wilson, D.A. and Davidson, A.G. (1997). Medicines control agency investigation of the microbial quality of herbal products. *Pharm. J.* 259: 259–261.

Anon. (1994). Two children die after receiving infected TPN solutions. *Pharm. J.* 252: 596.

Baines, A. (2000). Endotoxin testing. In: *Handbook of Microbiological Control: Pharmaceuticals and Medical Devices* (ed. R.M. Baird, N.A. Hodges and S.P. Denyer), 144–167. London: Taylor & Francis.

Baird, R.M. and Shooter, R.A. (1976). *Pseudomonas aeruginosa* infections associated with the use of contaminated medicaments. *Br. Med. J.* ii: 349–350.

Baird, R.M., Brown, W.R.L. and Shooter, R.A. (1976). *Pseudomonas aeruginosa* in hospital pharmacies. *Br. Med. J.* i: 511–512.

Baird, R.M., Elhag, K.M. and Shaw, E.J. (1976). *Pseudomonas thomasii* in a hospital distilled water supply. *J. Med. Microbiol.* 9: 493–495.

Baird, R.M., Hodges, N.A. and Denyer, S.P. (2000). *Handbook of Microbiological Control: Pharmaceuticals and Medical Devices*. London: Taylor & Francis.

Brannan, D.K. (1995). Cosmetic preservation. *J. Soc. Cosmet. Chem.* 46: 199–220.

British Pharmacopoeia (2021). *The Stationary Office*. London.

Denyer, S.P. and Baird, R.M. (2007). *Guide to Microbiological Control in Pharmaceuticals and Medical Devices*, 2e. Boca Raton, FL: CRC Press.

Fraise, A., Maillard, J.-Y. and Sattar, S. (2013). *Principles and Practice of Disinfection, Preservation and Sterilisation*, 5e. Oxford: Blackwell Science.

Gould, G.W. (1989). *Mechanisms of Action of Food Preservation Procedures*. Barking: Elsevier Science Publishers.

Hugo, W.B. (1995). A brief history of heat, chemical and radiation preservation and disinfectants. *Int. Biodeterior. Biodegrad.* 36: 197–217.

Hutchinson, J., Runge, W., Mulvey, M. et al. (2004). *Burkholderia cepacia* infections associated with intrinsically contaminated ultrasound gel: the role of microbial degradation of parabens. *Infect. Control Hosp. Epidemiol.* 25: 291–296.

Kallings, L.O., Ringertz, O., Silverstolpe, L. and Ernerfeldt, F. (1966). Microbiological contamination of medicinal preparations. 1965 Report to the Swedish National Board of Health. *Acta Pharm. Suec.* 3: 219–228.

Kreeft, H.A.J.G., Greiser-Wilke, I., Moennig, V. and Horzinek, M.C. (1990). Attempts to characterise bovine viral diarrhoea virus isolated from cattle after immunization with a contaminated vaccine. *Dtsch. Tierarztl. Wochenschr.* 97: 63–65.

Lalitha, P., Das, M., Purva, P.S. et al. (2014). Postoperative endophthalmitis due to *Burkholderia cepacia* complex from contaminated anaesthetic eye drops. *Br. J. Ophthalmol.* 98: 1498–1502.

Marquez, L., Jones, K.N., Whaley, E.M. et al. (2017). An outbreak of *Burkholderia cepacia* complex infections associated with contaminated liquid Docusate. *Infect. Control Hosp. Epidemiol.* 38: 567–573.

Maurer, I.M. (1985). *Hospital Hygiene*, 3e. London: Edward Arnold.

Meers, P.D., Calder, M.W., Mazhar, M.M. and Lawrie, G.M. (1973). Intravenous infusion of contaminated dextrose solution: the Devonport incident. *Lancet* **ii**: 1189–1192.

Public Health Laboratory Service Working Party Report (1971). Microbial contamination of medicines administered to hospital patients. *Pharm. J.* 207: 96–99.

18

Chemical Disinfectants, Antiseptics and Preservatives

Sean P. Gorman[1] *and Brendan F. Gilmore*[2]

[1] *Emeritus Professor of Pharmaceutical Microbiology, Queen's University Belfast, Belfast, UK*
[2] *Professor of Pharmaceutical Microbiology, School of Pharmacy, Queen's University Belfast, Belfast, UK*

CONTENTS

Hugo and Russell's Pharmaceutical Microbiology, Ninth Edition. Edited by Brendan F. Gilmore and Stephen P. Denyer.

Companion website: https://www.wiley.com/go/HugoandRussells9e

18.1 Introduction

Disinfectants, antiseptics and preservatives are chemical agents that have the ability to destroy, inactivate or inhibit the growth of microorganisms. They play a major role in the control of infection and contamination in medical and health care, and also find widespread use in the management of livestock, the environment, paints and coatings, plastics, pharmaceutical, food and beverage manufacture, textiles, the catering industry and consumer products. The term *biocide* is typically used to describe chemical agents employed to control harmful organisms more broadly; this term is used widely throughout European Union (EU) directives. *Microbicides*, agents specifically used to control microorganisms, fall under this general definition of biocide.

18.1.1 European Union Regulation

Regulation of biocides continues to develop in the European Union and many other countries wherein guidance is defined for both the manufacturers and the users of these products. Between 2000 and 2012, the Biocidal Products Directive (BPD) 98/8/EC and the related directives – Medicinal Products for Human Use Directive 2001/83/EC and the Veterinary Medicinal Products Directive 2001/82/EC – governed the production, marketing and use of non-agricultural products intended for biocidal purposes. Additionally, 'agricultural pesticides' were regulated by the Plant Protection Products Directive 91/414/EC. The BPD regulated biocides are defined as 'active substances and preparations containing one or more active substances, put up in the form in which they are supplied to the user, intended to destroy, deter, render harmless, prevent the action of, or otherwise exert a controlling effect on any harmful organism by chemical or biological means'. The BPD had been transposed into domestic UK law by the Biocidal Products Regulation (BPR) 2001 ([SI 2001/880] as amended). The BPD was superseded by the EU BPR (Regulation (EU) 528/2012), the text of which was adopted in May 2012, entered into force in July 2012 and took effect in member states from September 2013, repealing and replacing the BPD (Directive 98/8/EC). The EU BPR concerns the placing on the market, and the use, of biocidal products intended to protect humans, animals, materials or articles against harmful pests or bacteria, through the action of active substances contained in a biocidal product. The BPR aims to improve the functioning of the biocidal products market within the EU member states, and ensure high levels of protection of human and animal health and the environment, and applies within the European Economic Area (EEA), including Iceland, Liechtenstein and Norway alongside EU member states. The EU BPR aims to harmonise the internal market for biocidal products, introducing several important changes to the previous regulations which include:

- extending the scope of the regime to cover treated articles and materials containing biocides;
- adopting a community authorisation scheme for certain types of products;
- requiring mandatory data-sharing;

Table 18.1 Levels of disinfection attainable when products are used according to manufacturer's instructions.

	Disinfection level		
	Low	**Intermediate**	**High**
Microorganisms killed	Most vegetative bacteria Some viruses Some fungi	Vegetative bacteria including *M. tuberculosis* Most viruses including hepatitis B virus (HBV) Most fungi	All microorganisms unless an extreme challenge or resistance exhibited
Microorganisms surviving	*M. tuberculosis* Bacterial spores Prions	Bacterial spores Prions	Extreme challenge of resistant bacterial spores Prions

- reducing the burden of data collection requirements;
- harmonising fee structures across member states.

The EU BPR defines a treated article as 'any substance, mixture or article which has been treated with, or intentionally incorporates, one or more biocidal products'.

Following the end of the 'transition period' on 31 December 2020, Great Britain no longer participates in the EU scheme for biocidal products regulation. Prior to the United Kingdom's exit from the European Union, the UK Government Health and Safety Executive (HSE) was engaged in negotiations with all EU member states, the European Commission and the European Parliament in the development of a new directly acting EU law, and contributed to the drafting and approval of the EU Biocidal Products Regulation (EU BPR 528/2012). As a result, on leaving the European Union, the existing EU BPR was copied into British law, as the GB Biocidal Products Regulation (GB BPR) 2020. The GB BPR controls biocidal products in Great Britain (England, Scotland and Wales), while the EU BPR controls biocidal products in Northern Ireland. A number of minor differences between GB BPR and the EU BPR exist, which essentially allow GB to make different decisions to the EU, EEA and Switzerland and develop its own programmes for review of existing active substances; however, the core regulatory instruments are largely identical.

18.1.2 Definitions

Some key definitions relevant to chemical microbicides are given below. Other terms used to describe antimicrobial activity are considered in Chapter 19.

18.1.2.1 Disinfectant and Disinfection

Disinfection is the process of removing microorganisms, including pathogens, from the surfaces of inanimate objects. The British Standards Institution (BSI) further defines disinfection as not necessarily killing all microorganisms but reducing them to a level acceptable for a defined purpose, for example, a level that is harmful neither to health nor to the quality of perishable goods. Chemical disinfectants are capable of different levels of action (Table 18.1). The term *high-level disinfection* indicates destruction of all microorganisms, but not necessarily bacterial spores; *intermediate-level disinfection* indicates destruction of all vegetative bacteria including *Mycobacterium tuberculosis,* but may exclude some resistant viruses and fungi and implies little or no sporicidal activity; *low-level disinfection* can destroy most vegetative bacteria, fungi and viruses, but this will not include spores and some of the more resistant microorganisms. Some high-level disinfectants have good sporicidal activity and are described as *liquid chemical sterilants* or *chemosterilants* to indicate that they can effect a complete kill of all microorganisms, as in sterilisation. In defining each of these disinfection levels, the activity and outcome are determined by correct use of the disinfectant product in regard to concentration, time of contact and prevailing environmental conditions as described in subsequent sections of this chapter.

18.1.2.2 Antiseptic and Antisepsis

Antisepsis, a specific type of disinfection, is defined as destruction or inhibition of microorganisms on living tissues having the effect of limiting or preventing the harmful results of infection. It is not a synonym for disinfection. The chemicals used are applied to skin and mucous membranes, so as well as having adequate antimicrobial activity they must not be toxic or irritating for these tissues. Antiseptics are mostly used to reduce the microbial population on the skin before surgery or on the hands to help prevent spread of infection by this route. Sanitisation, a regulated term, refers to the use of disinfectants for reduction, not necessarily elimination, of microorganisms from surfaces to levels considered acceptable or safe as determined by public health regulations. Therefore, sanitisation has a specific meaning with respect to disinfection applications or antisepsis, namely, the removal or inactivation of microorganisms that *pose a threat to public health*. The use of alcohol-based hand sanitisers has become increasingly common globally as an infection control measure during the COVID-19 pandemic. Antiseptics are sometimes formulated as products containing significantly lower concentrations of agents used for disinfection.

18.1.2.3 Preservative and Preservation

Preservatives are included in pharmaceutical and many other types of formulations, both to prevent microbial spoilage of the product and to minimise the risk to the consumer of acquiring an infection when the preparation is administered (see Chapter 17). Preservatives must be able to limit proliferation of microorganisms that may be introduced unavoidably into non-sterile products such as oral and topical medications during their manufacture and use. In sterile products, where multiuse preparations remain available, preservatives should kill any microbial contaminants introduced inadvertently during use. It is essential that a preservative is not toxic in relation to the intended route of administration of the preserved preparation. Preservatives tend to be employed at very low concentrations and consequently levels of antimicrobial action also tend to be of a lower order than for disinfectants or antiseptics. This is illustrated by the British, European and US pharmacopoeial requirements for preservative efficacy where a degree of bactericidal activity is necessary, although this should be obtained within a few hours or over several days of microbial challenge depending on the type of product to be preserved.

18.1.3 Economic Aspects

The international antimicrobial chemical market, particularly in the case of disinfectants, is expected to grow significantly over the coming years, on the basis of concerns about bacterial and other pathogenic threats and the increasing emphasis on hygiene in the home and workplace. In particular, the SARS-CoV-2 pandemic has significantly increased demand for disinfectant and antimicrobial chemicals; this is expected to continue to drive significant growth in the sector, even post pandemic, as consumer and workplace practices with respect to disinfection, sanitisation and hygiene are likely to be altered in the longer term. The global value of the antimicrobial and disinfectant chemical market was estimated at $9.1 billion in 2019 and is projected to increase to $17.1 billion by 2027, representing a combined annual growth rate of 6.7% over this period. Key disinfectant products in use contain aldehydes, iodophors, nitrogen compounds (quaternary ammonium compounds [QACs] and amine compounds), organometallics, organosulphurs, chloroisocyanurates and phenolics. There are around 250 chemicals that have been identified as active components of microbicidal products in the EU.

The aim of this chapter is to introduce the range of chemicals in common use and to indicate their activities and applications.

18.2 Factors Affecting Choice of Antimicrobial Agent

Choice of the most appropriate antimicrobial compound for a particular purpose depends on many factors and the key parameters are described below.

18.2.1 Properties of the Chemical Agent

The process of killing or inhibiting the growth of microorganisms using an antimicrobial agent is basically that of a chemical reaction and the rate and extent of this reaction will be influenced by concentration of agent, temperature, pH and formulation. The significance of these factors on activity is considered in Chapter 19, and is referred to when discussing the individual agents in Section 18.3. Tissue toxicity will influence whether a chemical can be used as an antiseptic or preservative, and this limits the range of agents for these applications or necessitates the use of lower concentrations of that agent. This is discussed further in Section 18.2.5.

18.2.2 Microbiological Challenge

The types of microorganism present and the levels of microbial contamination (the *bioburden*) both have a significant effect on the outcome of treatment. If the bioburden is high, long exposure times and/or higher concentrations of antimicrobial may be required. Microorganisms vary in their sensitivity to the action of chemical agents. Some organisms merit attention either because of their resistance to disinfection (for further discussion, see Chapter 20) or because of their significance in cross-infection or healthcare-associated infections (see Chapter 16). Of particular concern is the significant increase in resistance to disinfectants resulting from microbial growth in the biofilm form rather than free suspension (see Chapter 8). Microbial biofilms form readily on available surfaces, posing a serious problem for hospital infection control committees in advising suitable disinfectants for use in such situations. Recently, the description of dry surface biofilms (dehydrated biofilms which have been shown to exist on dry inanimate surfaces in healthcare, food processing and domiciliary environments) with their demonstrable environmental persistence and significantly elevated tolerance to antimicrobial challenge (even compared with hydrated or wet biofilms) highlights yet another potential challenge to selection of an appropriate disinfectant agent or approach. Dry surface biofilms, as yet, lack a clear or agreed definition in the literature, or standardised test methods, further complicating appropriate disinfectant selection.

The efficacy of an antimicrobial agent must be investigated by appropriate capacity, challenge and in-use tests to ensure that a standard is obtained which is appropriate to the intended use (Chapter 19). In practice, it is not usually possible to know which organisms are present on the articles being treated. Thus, it is necessary to categorise agents according to their antimicrobial activity and for the user to be aware of the level of antimicrobial action required in a particular situation (see Table 18.1).

18.2.2.1 Vegetative Bacteria

At in-use concentrations, chemicals used for disinfection should be capable of killing bacteria and other organisms expected in that environment within a defined contact period. This includes 'problem' organisms such as methicillin-resistant *Staphylococcus aureus* (MRSA), vancomycin-resistant enterococci (VRE) and species of *Listeria*, *Campylobacter* and *Legionella*. Antiseptics and preservatives are also expected to have a broad spectrum of antimicrobial activity, but at their in-use concentrations, after exerting an initial biocidal (killing) effect, their main function may be biostatic (inhibitory). Gram-negative bacilli, which are a major cause of healthcare-associated infections, are often more resistant than Gram-positive species. *Pseudomonas aeruginosa*, an opportunistic pathogen (see also Chapter 7), has gained a reputation as the most resistant of the Gram-negative organisms. However, problems mainly arise when a number of additional factors such as heavily soiled articles or diluted or degraded disinfectant solutions are employed.

18.2.2.2 *Mycobacterium tuberculosis*

M. tuberculosis and other mycobacteria are resistant to many bactericides. Resistance is either (i) intrinsic, mainly due to reduced cellular permeability, or (ii) acquired, due to mutation or the acquisition of plasmids (Chapter 13). Tuberculosis remains an important public health hazard, and indeed the annual number of tuberculosis cases continues to rise in many countries. The greatest risk of acquiring infection is from the undiagnosed patient. Equipment used for respiratory investigations can become contaminated with mycobacteria if the patient is a carrier of this organism. It is important to be able to disinfect the equipment to a safe level to prevent transmission of infection to other patients (Table 18.2).

18.2.2.3 Bacterial Spores

Bacterial spores can exhibit significant resistance to even the most active chemical disinfectant treatment. The majority of disinfectants have no useful sporicidal action in a pharmaceutical context, which relates to disinfection of materials, instruments and environments that are likely to be contaminated by the spore-forming genera *Bacillus, Clostridioides* and *Clostridium*. However, certain aldehydes, halogens and peroxygen compounds display very good activity under controlled conditions and are sometimes used as an alternative to physical methods for sterilisation of heat-sensitive equipment. In these circumstances, correct usage of the agent is of paramount importance, as safety margins are lower in comparison with physical methods of sterilisation (Chapter 21).

Clostridioides difficile is a particularly problematic contaminant in hospital environments, resulting in high levels of morbidity and mortality. In addition to stringent handwashing, meticulous environmental disinfection procedures must be in place, for example, using solutions of 5.25–6.15% sodium hypochlorite for routine disinfection. When high-level disinfection of *C. difficile* is required, 2% glutaraldehyde, 0.55% *o*-phthalaldehyde and 0.35% peracetic acid are effective.

The antibacterial activity of some disinfectants and antiseptics is summarised in Table 18.2.

18.2.2.4 Fungi

The vegetative fungal form is often as sensitive as vegetative bacteria to chemical antimicrobial agents. Fungal spores (conidia and chlamydospores; see Chapter 4) may be more resistant, but this resistance is of much lesser magnitude than that exhibited by bacterial spores. The ability to rapidly destroy pathogenic fungi – such as the important nosocomial pathogen *Candida albicans*, filamentous fungi such as *Trichophyton mentagrophytes* and spores of common spoilage moulds such as *Aspergillus niger* – is put to advantage in many applications of use. Many disinfectants have good activity against these fungi (Table 18.3). In addition, ethanol (70%) is rapidly and reliably active against *Candida* species.

18.2.2.5 Viruses

Susceptibility of viruses to antimicrobial agents can depend on whether or not the viruses possess a lipid envelope. Non-lipid viruses are frequently more resistant to disinfectants and it is also likely that such viruses cannot be readily categorised with respect to their sensitivities to

Table 18.2 Antibacterial activity of commonly used disinfectants and antiseptics.

	Activity against		
Class of compound	**Mycobacteria**	**Bacterial spores**	**General level[a] of antibacterial activity**
Alcohols			
Ethanol/isopropyl	+	–	Intermediate
Aldehydes			
Glutaraldehyde	+	+	High
o-Phthalaldehyde	+	+	High
Formaldehyde	+	+	High
Biguanides			
Chlorhexidine	–	–	Intermediate
Halogens			
Hypochlorite/chloramines	+	+	High
Iodine/iodophor	+	+	Intermediate, problems with *Ps. aeruginosa*
Peroxygens			
Peracetic acid	+	+	High
Hydrogen peroxide	+	+	High
Phenolics			
Clear soluble fluids	+	–	Intermediate
Chloroxylenol	–	–	Low
Bisphenols	–	–	Low, poor against *Ps. aeruginosa*
Quaternary ammonium compounds			
Benzalkonium	–	–	Intermediate
Cetrimide	–	–	Intermediate

[a] Activity expected per manufacturer's instructions and will depend on environmental conditions and bioburden.

Table 18.3 Antifungal activity of disinfectants and antiseptics.

	Time (minutes) to give >99.99% kill[a] of		
Antimicrobial agent	***Aspergillus niger***	***Trichophyton mentagrophytes***	***Candida albicans***
Phenolic (0.36%)	<2	<2	<2
Chlorhexidine gluconate (0.02%, alcoholic)	<2	<2	<2
Iodine (1%, alcoholic)	<2	<2	<2
Povidone-iodine (10%, alcoholic and aqueous)	10	<2	<2
Hypochlorite (0.2%)	10	<2	5
Cetrimide (1%)	<2	20	<2
Chlorhexidine gluconate (0.05%) + cetrimide (0.5%)	20	>20	>2
Chlorhexidine gluconate (0.5%, aqueous)	20	>20	>2

[a] Initial viable counts approximately 1×10^6 colony forming units (CFU) per ml in suspension test.

antimicrobial agents. These viruses, for example, rotaviruses, picornaviruses and adenoviruses (see Chapter 5), are responsible for many healthcare-associated and community-acquired infections and it may be necessary to select an antiseptic or disinfectant to suit specific circumstances. Certain viruses, such as Ebola and Marburg, which cause haemorrhagic fevers, are highly infectious and their safe destruction by disinfectants is of paramount importance. Hepatitis A is an enterovirus considered to be one of the most resistant viruses to disinfection.

There is much concern for the safety of personnel handling articles contaminated with pathogenic viruses such as hepatitis B virus (HBV) and human immunodeficiency virus (HIV). Disinfectants must be able to treat rapidly and reliably accidental spills of blood, body fluids or secretions from HIV-infected patients. Such spills may contain levels of HIV as high as 10^4 infectious units ml^{-1}. Fortunately, HIV (an enveloped virus) is inactivated by most chemicals at in-use concentrations. However, the recommendation is to use high-level disinfectants (see Table 18.2) for decontamination of HIV- or HBV-infected reusable medical equipment. For patient-care areas, cleaning and disinfection with intermediate-level disinfectants are satisfactory. Flooding with a liquid germicide is required only when large spills of cultured or concentrated infectious agents have to be dealt with.

The World Health Organization (WHO), US Centers for Disease Control and Prevention (CDC) and epidemiologists in many countries continue to track outbreaks of influenza, especially in relation to potential epidemic and pandemic situations arising. Influenza pandemics are caused by outbreaks of new influenza A viral variants which are very different to current, or recently circulating, seasonal influenza A viruses. The H1N1 outbreak in 2009–2010 generated considerable concern. As an influenza A virus, however, it is susceptible to a large number of disinfectant products when they are used on hard, non-porous surfaces that may be contaminated. Although limited research has been conducted on the susceptibility of 2009 H1N1 influenza virus to chlorine and other disinfectants in swimming pools and spas, studies have demonstrated that free chlorine levels of 1–3 mg l^{-1} (1–3 ppm) are adequate to disinfect avian H5N1 influenza virus.

The global coronavirus pandemic (COVID-19) has been caused by the transmission of SARS-CoV-2 which, like all other coronaviruses, is an enveloped virus. The fragile outer lipid envelope confers susceptibility to disinfectants. Various studies have reported the environmental stability of SARS-CoV-2 under laboratory conditions, indicating persistence on inanimate surfaces ranging from 24 hours on cardboard, cloth and wood through 48 hours on glass, 96 hours on stainless steel and plastic and up to 7 days on the outer layer of a medical mask. Copper surfaces significantly reduced viral survival to approximately 4 hours. A regularly updated list of disinfectants for use against SARS-CoV-2 ('List N') is maintained by the US Environmental Protection Agency (EPA) and guidance has been provided by the WHO regarding cleaning and disinfection of environmental surfaces. Ethanol at 70–90%, chlorine-based products (hypochlorite at 0.1% [1000 ppm] for environmental disinfection, or 0.5% [5000 ppm] for large blood and body fluid spills) and hydrogen peroxide ≥0.5% are currently recommended disinfectants for inactivation of SARS-CoV-2, although other disinfectants can be considered. The EPA List N comprises a much wider variety of microbicides, covering all major classes of cidal compound, for which manufacturers are filing, or have filed, either a human coronavirus or emerging human pathogen claim (e.g., efficacy claims for those pathogens not identified on the existing product label, but based on previous EPA claims for harder-to-kill viruses).

18.2.2.6 Protozoa

Acanthamoeba spp. can cause acanthamoeba keratitis (see Chapter 6) with associated corneal scarring and loss of vision in wearers of soft contact lenses. The cysts of this protozoan present a particular problem in respect of lens disinfection. The chlorine-generating systems in use are generally inadequate. Both polyaminopropyl biguanide (0.003%), with or without chlorhexidine, and polyhexamethylene biguanide (0.0005%) show activity as an acanthamoebicide in combating levels of 10^3 cysts. Hydrogen-peroxide-based disinfection is considered completely reliable and consistent in producing an acanthamoebicidal effect. More recently, quaternary ammonium compounds and octenidine dihydrochloride have been shown to be highly effective against *Acanthamoeba* trophozoites and cysts at concentrations found in commercially available products and at contact times suitable for hand sanitisation, surface disinfection and topical antisepsis.

18.2.2.7 Prions

Prions are generally considered to be the infectious agents most resistant to chemical disinfectants and sterilisation processes (see Chapters 5, 19, 20 and 21); strictly speaking, however, they are not microorganisms because they neither have cellular structure nor do they contain nucleic acids. As small proteinaceous infectious particles they are a unique class of infectious agent causing spongiform encephalopathies such as bovine spongiform encephalopathy (BSE) in cattle and Creutzfeldt–Jakob disease (CJD) in humans. There is considerable concern about the transmission of these agents from infected animals or patients. Risk of infectivity is highest in brain, spinal cord and eye tissues. Such infected tissues can remain associated with instruments used in surgery creating a risk of transmission; any re-use of equipment must therefore be dependent on effective decontamination and re-sterilisation.

Prions are considered resistant to most disinfectant procedures and some agents, for instance, alcohols, formaldehyde, glutaraldehyde and related products, can 'fix' residual contaminating tissue proteins, thereby protecting prions from subsequent cleaning processes. Medical instruments for disinfection must also not be allowed to dry, since this further increases the difficulty of prion removal. For heat-resistant medical instruments that come into contact with high-infectivity tissues or high-risk contacts, immersion in sodium hydroxide (1 M) or sodium hypochlorite (20,000 ppm available chlorine) for 1 hour has been advised in WHO guidelines to be followed by further treatment including autoclaving, cleaning and routine sterilisation; unfortunately, in many instances these procedures may prove impractical. Alternative approaches have emerged which employ an alkaline detergent or enzyme detergent wash, often at elevated temperature (90 °C) in an automated washer-disinfector, followed by a sterilisation procedure. The favoured procedure is autoclaving at 134–137 °C for periods of up to 18 minutes, sometimes achieved by six successive cycles of 3 minutes duration. Where heat-sensitive equipment, such as endoscopes, are concerned, washing with detergent followed by vapourised hydrogen peroxide gas plasma sterilisation has been proposed. Wherever possible single-use surgical instrumentation is recommended to avoid any need for re-processing.

18.2.3 Intended Application

The intended application of the antimicrobial agent, whether for preservation, antisepsis or disinfection, will influence its selection and also affect its performance. For example, in medicinal preparations, the ingredients in the formulation may antagonise or otherwise attenuate preservative activity (see Chapter 17). The risk to the patient will depend on whether the antimicrobial is in close contact with a break in the skin or mucous membranes or is introduced into a sterile compartment of the body.

In the disinfection of medical instruments, the chemicals used must not adversely affect the materials from which these instruments are constructed, for example, cause corrosion of metals, affect clarity or integrity of lenses or change the texture or mechanical properties of synthetic polymers. Many materials such as fabrics, rubber and plastics are capable of adsorbing certain disinfectants, for example, QACs are adsorbed by fabrics, while phenolics are adsorbed by rubber, the consequence of this being a reduction in the concentration of active compound in the formulation. Furthermore, a disinfectant can only exert its effect if it is in contact with the item being treated. Therefore, access to all parts of an instrument or piece of equipment is essential. For small items, total immersion in the disinfectant must also be ensured.

18.2.4 Environmental Factors

Organic matter can have a drastic effect on antimicrobial capacity either by adsorption or chemical inactivation, thus reducing the concentration of active agent in solution or by acting as a barrier to the penetration of the disinfectant. Blood, body fluids, faeces, pus, milk, food residues or colloidal proteins, even when present in small amounts, all reduce the effectiveness of antimicrobial agents to varying degrees, and some are significantly affected or their activity negated entirely. In their normal habitats, microorganisms have a tendency to adhere to surfaces as aggregates and biofilms and are thus less accessible to the chemical agent. Some organisms are specific to certain environments and their destruction will be of paramount importance in the selection of a suitable agent, for example, *Legionella* in cooling towers and non-potable water supply systems, *Listeria* in the dairy and food industry and HBV on blood-contaminated articles.

Dried organic deposits may inhibit penetration of the chemical agent. Where possible, objects to be disinfected should be thoroughly cleaned. The presence of divalent cations, such as Mg^{2+} and Ca^{2+}, in water can also affect activity of antimicrobial agents, thus water for testing biocidal activity can be made artificially 'hard' by addition of ions (see Chapter 19).

These factors can have very significant effects on activity and are summarised in Table 18.4.

18.2.5 Toxicity of the Agent

In choosing an antimicrobial agent for a particular application, consideration must be given to its toxicity. Increasing concern for health and safety is reflected in the Control of Substances Hazardous to Health (COSHH) Regulations that specify the precautions required in handling toxic or potentially toxic agents. In respect of disinfectants, these regulations affect, particularly, the use of phenolics, formaldehyde and glutaraldehyde. Toxic volatile substances, in general, should be kept in covered containers to reduce the level of exposure to irritant vapour and they should be used with an extractor facility. Limits governing the exposure of individuals to such substances are now listed, for example, 0.7 mg m^{-3} (0.2 ppm) glutaraldehyde for both short- and long-term exposures. Many disinfectants including the aldehydes, glutaraldehyde less so than formaldehyde, may affect the eyes, skin (causing contact dermatitis) and induce

Table 18.4 Properties of commonly used disinfectants and antiseptics.

Class of compound	Effect of organic matter	pH optimum	Toxicity and WEL[a]	Other factors
Alcohols				
Ethanol	Slight		Avoid broken skin, eyes WEL: 1000 ppm/1920 mg m^{-3}, 8 h only	Poor penetration, good cleansing properties, evaporates, flammable
Isopropanol (propan-2-ol)	Slight		WEL: 500 ppm/1250mg m^{-3}, 15 min; 400 ppm/999 mg m^{-3}, 8 h	
Aldehydes				
Glutaraldehyde	Slight	pH 8	Respiratory complaints and contact dermatitis reported Eyes, sensitivity WEL: 0.05 ppm/0.2mg m^{-3}, 15 min and 8 h	Non-corrosive, useful for heat-sensitive instruments Use in well-ventilated area Gloves, goggles and apron worn for preparation
Formaldehyde	Moderate		Respiratory distress, dermatitis WEL: 2 ppm/2.5 mg m^{-3}, 15 min and 8 h	
Biguanides				
Chlorhexidine	Severe	pH 7–8	Avoid contact with eyes and mucous membranes Sensitivity may develop	Incompatible with soap and anionic detergents Inactivated by hard water, some materials and plastic
Chlorine compounds				
Hypochlorite	Severe	Acid/neutral pH	Irritation of skin, eyes and lungs	Corrosive to metals Dichloroisocyanurate likely to produce chlorine gas when used to disinfect acidic urines
Hydrogen peroxide	Slight/moderate	Acid/neutral pH	May irritate skin and mucous membranes WEL: 2 ppm/2.8 mg m^{-3}, 15 min; 1 ppm/1.4 mg m^{-3}, 8 h	May develop high pressure in container
Iodine preparations	Severe	Acid pH	Eye irritation. WEL: 0.1 ppm/1.1 mg m^{-3}, 15 min only	May corrode metals
Phenolics				
Clear soluble fluids	Slight	Acid pH	Protect skin and eyes	Absorbed by rubber/plastic
Black/white fluids	Moderate/severe		Very irritant. Greatly reduced by dilution May irritate skin	
Chloroxylenol	Severe		Irritation of skin and eyes	Absorbed by rubber/plastic
QACs				
Cetrimide	Severe	Alkaline pH	Avoid contact with eyes	Incompatible with soap and anionic detergents
Benzalkonium chloride	Severe	pH 4-10	Avoid respiratory exposure	Absorbed by fabrics, rubber, silicone, some hydrogel contact lens materials

[a] WEL, workplace exposure limit (WELs have now replaced maximum exposure limits, MELs); QAC, quaternary ammonium compound. WELs are concentrations of hazardous substances in the air, averaged over a specified period of time, referred to as a time-weighted average (TWA), and define the upper limits of a substance permitted in the breathing zone of a person. Two time periods are generally used: long-term (8 h) and short-term (15 min). Short-term exposure limits are set to prevent effects such as eye irritation which can occur after only a few minutes contact.
Source: Adapted from HSE (2020).

respiratory distress. Face protection and impermeable nitrile rubber gloves should be worn when using these agents. Table 18.4 lists the toxicity of many of the disinfectants in use, and other concerns of toxicity are described below for individual agents.

The COSHH Regulations specify certain disinfectants that contain active substances not supported under the BPD (the regulatory framework for biocide regulation in the EU between 2000 and 2012, now superseded by the BPR, see Section 18.1.1.) that had to be phased out by 2006. Specified disinfection procedures applied to laboratories in relation to spills and routine use state that certain phenolic agents (including 2,4,6-trichlorophenol and xylenol) can no longer be employed in disinfectant products.

Because of the historically high number of occupational asthma cases caused by glutaraldehyde (an alkylating agent) products in chemical disinfection of endoscopes, a HSE report in 2007 sought alternatives to this agent. The report recommended the preferential use of an oxidising agent such as a chlorine-based or peroxygen-based product rather than a product containing an alkylating agent. However, it was recognised that consideration must be given to incompatibility of disinfectants with endoscope construction materials in some cases (Table 18.5). Although glutaraldehyde is approved by the US Food and Drug Administration (FDA) for cold sterilisation and/or certain high-level disinfection applications, the US EPA has, since 2016, banned its use as an environmental surface disinfectant, due to toxicity concerns.

In all situations where the atmosphere of a workplace is likely to be contaminated by disinfectant, sampling and analysis of the atmosphere may need to be carried out on a periodic basis with a frequency determined by conditions.

Table 18.5 HSE recommendations (2007) for endoscopy disinfection.

Disinfectant agent	COSHH essentials hazard group	COSHH essentials control approach
Chlorine base	A (low hazard)	1 (general ventilation)
Peroxygen	A (low hazard)	1 (general ventilation)
Peracetic acid	C (medium hazard)	3 (containment)
o-Phthalaldehyde	C (medium hazard)	3 (containment)
2% Glutaraldehyde	E (special case)	4 (special case)

HSE, Health and Safety Executive; COSHH, Control of Substances Hazardous to Health. *Source:* Adapted from HSE Research Report 445 (2007).

18.3 Types of Compound

The following section presents, in alphabetical order by chemical grouping, the agents most often employed for disinfection, antisepsis and preservation. This information is summarised in Table 18.6.

18.3.1 Acids and Esters

Antimicrobial activity, within a pharmaceutical context, is generally found only in the organic acids. These are weak acids and will, therefore, dissociate incompletely to give the three entities HA, H^+ and A^- in solution. As the undissociated form, HA, is the active antimicrobial agent, the ionisation constant, K_a, is important and the pK_a of the acid must be considered, especially in formulation of the agent.

18.3.1.1 Benzoic Acid

This is an organic acid, C_6H_5COOH, which is included, alone or in combination with other preservatives, in many pharmaceuticals. Although the compound is often used as the sodium salt, the non-ionised acid, being able to cross the cell membrane, is the active substance. A limitation on its use is imposed by the pH of the final product, as the pK_a of benzoic acid is 4.2 at which pH 50% of the acid is ionised. It is advisable to limit use of the acid to preservation of pharmaceuticals with a maximum final pH of 5.0 and if possible less than 4.0. Concentrations of 0.05–0.1% are suitable for oral preparations. A disadvantage of the compound is the development of resistance by some organisms, in some cases involving metabolism of the acid resulting in complete loss of activity. Benzoic acid also has some use in combination with other agents, salicylic acid for example, in the treatment of superficial fungal infections.

18.3.1.2 Sorbic Acid

This compound is a widely used preservative as the acid or its potassium salt. The pK_a is 4.8 and, as with benzoic acid, activity decreases with increasing pH and ionisation. It is most effective at pH 4 or below. Pharmaceutical products such as gums, mucilages and syrups are usefully preserved with this agent.

18.3.1.3 Sulphur Dioxide, Sulphites and Metabisulphites

Sulphur dioxide has extensive use as a preservative in the food and beverage industries. In a pharmaceutical context, sodium sulphite and metabisulphite or bisulphite have a dual role, acting as preservatives and antioxidants.

Table 18.6 Examples of the main antimicrobial groups as antiseptics, disinfectants and preservatives.

	Antiseptic activity		Disinfectant activity		Preservative activity	
Antimicrobial agent	Concentration	Typical formulation/application	Concentration	Typical formulation/application	Concentration	Typical formulation/application
Acids and esters e.g. benzoic acid, parabens					0.05–0.1% 0.25%	For oral and topical formulations
Alcohols[a] e.g. ethyl or isopropyl	50–90% in water	Skin preparation	50–90% in water	Clean surface preparation		
Aldehydes e.g. glutaraldehyde	10%	Gel for warts	2.0%	Solution for instruments		
Biguanides e.g. chlorhexidine (gluconate, acetate, etc.)[b]	0.02%	Bladder irrigation	0.05%	Clean instrument disinfection (30 min)	0.0025%	Solution for hard contact lenses
	0.2%	Mouthwash			0.01%	Eye drops
	0.5% (in 70% alcohol)	Skin preparation				
	1.0%	Dusting powder, cream, dental gel	0.5% (in 70% alcohol)	Emergency instrument disinfection (2 min)		
	4.0%	Preoperative scrub in surfactant				
Chlorine e.g. hypochlorite	≤0.5% $avCl_2$	Solution for skin and wounds	1– 10%	Solution for surfaces and instruments		
Hydrogen peroxide	1.5%	Stabilized cream	3.0%	Disinfection of soft contact lenses		
	3–6%	Solution for wounds and ulcers, mouthwash				
Iodine compounds e.g. free iodine, povidone-iodine	1.0%	Aqueous or alcoholic (70%) solution	10.0%	Aqueous or alcoholic solution		
	1.0%	Mouthwash				
	2.5%	Dry powder spray				
	7.5%	Scalp and skin cleanser				
	10%	Preoperative scrub, fabric dressing				
Phenolics e.g. clear soluble	0.5%	Dusting powder	1–2%	Solution		
phenolics, chloroxylenol	1.3%	Solution				
	2.0%	Skin cleanser				
QACs e.g. cetyltrimethyl	0.1%	Solution for wounds and burns	1.0%	Instruments (1h)	0.01%	Eye drops
ammonium bromide	0.5%	Cream				
(cetrimide)	1.0%	Skin solution				

[a] Also used in combination with other agents, e.g. chlorhexidine, iodine.
[b] Several forms available having x% chlorhexidine and 10x% cetrimide.
QAC, quaternary ammonium compound

HO—C6H4—COOR

Figure 18.1 *p*-Hydroxybenzoates (R is methyl, ethyl, propyl, butyl or benzyl).

18.3.1.4 Esters of *p*-Hydroxybenzoic Acid (Parabens)

A series of alkyl esters (Figure 18.1) of *p*-hydroxybenzoic acid was originally prepared to overcome the marked pH dependence on activity of the acids. These parabens, the methyl, ethyl, propyl and butyl esters, are less readily ionised, having pK_a values in the range 8–8.5, and exhibit good preservative activity even at pH levels of 7–8, although optimum activity is again displayed in acidic solutions. This broader pH range allows extensive and successful use of the parabens as pharmaceutical preservatives. They are active against a wide range of fungi but are less so against bacteria, especially the pseudomonads which may utilise them as a carbon source. They are frequently used as preservatives of emulsions, creams and lotions where two phases exist. Combinations of esters are most successful for this type of product in that the more water-soluble methyl ester (0.25%) protects the aqueous phase, whereas the propyl or butyl esters (0.02%) give protection to the oil phase. Such combinations are also considered to extend the range of activity. As inactivation of parabens occurs with non-ionic surfactants, due care should be taken in formulation with both materials.

18.3.2 Alcohols

18.3.2.1 Alcohols Used for Disinfection and Antisepsis

The aliphatic alcohols, notably ethanol and isopropanol, are used for disinfection and antisepsis. They are bactericidal against vegetative forms, including *Mycobacterium* species, but are not sporicidal. Overall cidal activity drops sharply below 50% concentration. Alcohols have poor penetration of organic matter and their use is, therefore, restricted to clean conditions. They possess properties such as a cleansing action and volatility, are able to achieve a rapid and large reduction in skin flora and have been widely used for skin preparation before injection or other surgical procedures. The risk of transmission of infection due to poor hand hygiene has been attributed to lack of compliance with handwashing procedures. An alcohol hand-rub offers a rapid, easy-to-use alternative that is more acceptable to personnel and is frequently recommended for routine use. However, the contact time of an alcohol-soaked swab with the skin prior to venepuncture is so brief that it is thought to be of doubtful value.

Ethanol (CH_3CH_2OH) is widely used as a disinfectant and antiseptic. The presence of water is essential for activity; hence, 100% ethanol is relatively ineffective. Concentrations between 60 and 95% are bactericidal and a 70% solution is usually employed for the disinfection of skin, clean instruments or surfaces. At higher concentrations, for example, 90%, ethanol is also active against fungi and most lipid-containing viruses, including HIV, influenza viruses and coronaviruses, though less so against non-lipid-containing viruses. Ethanol is also a popular choice in pharmaceutical preparations and cosmetic products as a solvent and preservative, but it is not recommended for cleaning class II recirculating safety cabinets; ethanol vapours are flammable and the lower explosive limit (LEL) is easily attained. Mixtures with other disinfectants, for example, with formaldehyde ($100\,g\,l^{-1}$), are more effective than alcohol alone.

Isopropyl alcohol (isopropanol, $CH_3.CHOH.CH_3$) has slightly greater bactericidal activity than ethanol but is also about twice as toxic. It is less active against viruses, particularly non-enveloped viruses, and should be considered a limited-spectrum viricide. Used at concentrations of 60–70%, it is an acceptable alternative to ethanol for preoperative skin treatment and is also employed as a preservative for cosmetics.

18.3.2.2 Alcohols as Preservatives

The aryl alcohols and more highly substituted aliphatic alcohols (Figure 18.2) are used mostly as preservatives. These include:

- *Benzyl alcohol* ($C_6H_5CH_2OH$) has antibacterial and weak local anaesthetic properties and is used as an antimicrobial preservative at a concentration of 2%, although its use in cosmetics is restricted.
- *Chlorbutol* (chlorobutanol; trichlorobutanol; trichloro-t-butanol) is typically used at a concentration of 0.5% and is employed as a preservative in injections and eye drops. It is unstable, decomposition occurring at acid pH during autoclaving, while alkaline solutions are unstable at room temperature.
- *Phenylethanol* (phenylethyl alcohol; 2-phenylethanol), having a typical in-use concentration of 0.25–0.5%, is reported to have greater activity against Gram-negative organisms and is usually employed in conjunction with another agent.
- *Phenoxyethanol* (2-phenoxyethanol): typical in-use concentration is 1%. It is more active against *P. aeruginosa* than against other bacteria and is usually combined with other preservatives such as the hydroxybenzoates to broaden the spectrum of antimicrobial activity.

Figure 18.2 Structural formulae of alcohols used in preservation and disinfection: (a) 2-phenylethanol; (b) 2-phenoxyethanol; (c) chlorbutol (trichloro-tert-butanol); (d) bronopol (2-bromo-2-nitropropane-1,3-diol).

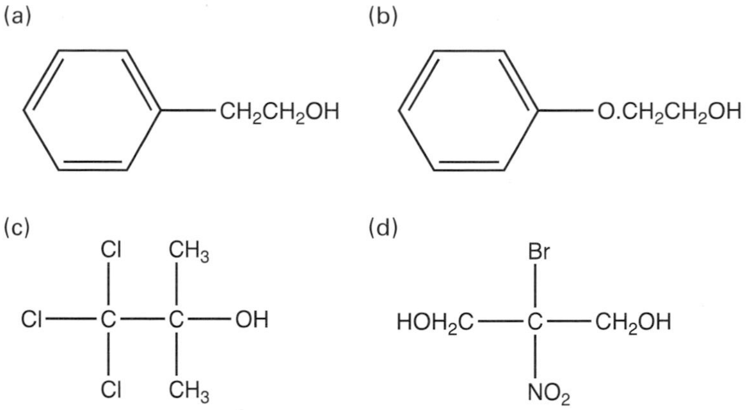

- *Bronopol* (2-bromo-2-nitropropane-1,3-diol): typical in-use concentration is 0.01–0.1%. It has a broad spectrum of antibacterial activity, including *Pseudomonas* species. The main limitation on the use of bronopol is that when exposed to light at alkaline pH, especially if accompanied by an increase in temperature, solutions decompose, turning yellow or brown. A number of decomposition products including formaldehyde are produced. In addition, nitrite ions may be produced and react with any secondary and tertiary amines present forming nitrosamines, which are potentially carcinogenic.

18.3.3 Aldehydes

A number of aldehydes possess broad-spectrum antimicrobial properties, including sporicidal activity. These highly effective microbicides can be employed in appropriate conditions as chemosterilants.

18.3.3.1 Glutaraldehyde

Glutaraldehyde ($CHO(CH_2)_3CHO$) has a broad spectrum of antimicrobial activity and rapid rate of kill, most vegetative bacteria being killed within a minute of exposure, although bacterial spores may require 3 hours or more. The kill rate depends on the intrinsic resistance of spores, which may vary widely. It has the further advantage of not being affected significantly by organic matter. The glutaraldehyde molecule possesses two aldehyde groupings which are highly reactive and their presence is an important component of cidal activity. The monomeric molecule is in equilibrium with polymeric forms, and the physical conditions of temperature and pH have a significant effect on this equilibrium. At a pH of 8, biocidal activity is greatest, but stability is poor due to polymerisation. By contrast, acid solutions are stable but considerably less active, although, as temperature is increased, there is a breakdown in the polymeric forms which exist in acid solutions and a concomitant increase in free, active dialdehyde, resulting in better activity. In practice, glutaraldehyde is generally supplied as an acidic 2% or greater aqueous solution, which is stable on prolonged storage. This is then 'activated' before use by addition of a suitable alkalising agent to bring the pH of the solution to its optimum for activity. The activated solution will have a limited shelf life, of the order of 2 weeks, although more stable formulations are available. Glutaraldehyde is employed mainly for the cold liquid chemical sterilisation of medical and surgical materials that cannot be sterilised by other methods. Endoscopes, including for example arthroscopes, laparascopes, cystoscopes and bronchoscopes, may be decontaminated by glutaraldehyde treatment (see Section 18.2.5 concerning toxicity issues). Times employed in practice for high-level disinfection are often considerably less than the many hours recommended by manufacturers to achieve sterilisation. The contact time for sterilisation can be as long as 10 hours. Times for general disinfection generally range from 20 to 90 minutes at 20 °C depending on formulation and concentration.

18.3.3.2 *Ortho*-phthalaldehyde

Ortho-phthalaldehyde (OPA, 1,2-benzenedicarboxaldehyde) is a relatively recent addition to the aldehyde group of high-level disinfectants, having received FDA approval as a high-level disinfectant in 1999. It exhibits broad-spectrum bactericidal activity, but sporicidal activity requires longer exposure times. This agent has demonstrated excellent mycobactericidal activity with complete kill of *M. tuberculosis* within 12 minutes at room temperature. OPA has several other advantages over glutaraldehyde. It requires no activation and can be readily formulated, is considerably less irritant to the eyes or nasal passages, lacks perceptible odour, has low volatility and has excellent stability over the pH range 3–9. It can be used for disinfection of endoscopes (Table 18.5). *Ortho*-phthalaldehyde exhibits high-level, broad-spectrum virucidal activity, achieving >3 log-reductions against a number of surrogate viruses for hepatitis B and hepatitis C viruses, within 1 minute at a concentration of 0.55%. *Ortho*-phthalaldehyde has also been shown to be active against surrogate coronaviruses, using the quantitative carrier method on stainless-steel coupons. It has been shown to be ineffective in the inactivation of prions.

18.3.3.3 Formaldehyde

Formaldehyde (HCHO) can be used in either the liquid or the gaseous state for disinfection purposes. In the vapour phase, it has been used for decontamination of isolators, safety cabinets and rooms. The combination of formaldehyde vapour with low-temperature steam (LTSF) has been employed for the sterilisation of heat-sensitive items (Chapter 21). Formaldehyde vapour is highly toxic and potentially carcinogenic if inhaled, thus its use must be carefully controlled. It is not very active at temperatures below 20 °C and requires a relative humidity of at least 70%. The agent is not supplied as a gas but either as a solid polymer, paraformaldehyde or a liquid, formalin, which is a 34–38% aqueous solution. The gas is liberated by heating or mixing the solid or liquid with potassium permanganate and water. Formalin, diluted 1:10 to give 4% formaldehyde, may be used for disinfecting surfaces. In general, however, solutions of either aqueous or alcoholic formaldehyde are too irritant for routine application to skin, while poor penetration and a tendency to polymerise on surfaces limit its use as a disinfectant for pharmaceutical purposes.

18.3.3.4 Formaldehyde-releasing Agents

Various formaldehyde condensates have been developed to reduce the irritancy associated with formaldehyde while maintaining activity, and these are described as formaldehyde-releasing agents or masked-formaldehyde compounds.

Noxythiolin (*N*-hydroxy *N*-methylthiourea) is supplied as a dry powder and on aqueous reconstitution slowly releases formaldehyde and *N*-methylthiourea. The compound has extensive antibacterial and antifungal properties and has been used both topically and in accessible body cavities as an irrigation solution and in the treatment of peritonitis.

Taurolidine (bis-(1,1-dioxoperhydro-1,2,4-thiadiazinyl-4) methane) is a condensate of two molecules of the amino acid taurine and three molecules of formaldehyde. It is more stable than noxythiolin in solution and has similar uses.

18.3.4 Biguanides

18.3.4.1 Chlorhexidine

Chlorhexidine is an antimicrobial agent first synthesised in 1954. The chlorhexidine molecule, a bisbiguanide, is symmetrical with a hexamethylene chain linking two biguanide groups, each with a *para*-chlorophenyl radical (Figure 18.3).

Chlorhexidine base is not readily soluble in water; therefore, its freely soluble salts, acetate, gluconate and hydrochloride, are used in formulation. Chlorhexidine exhibits the greatest antibacterial activity at pH 7–8 where it exists exclusively as a dication. The cationic nature of the compound results in activity being reduced by anionic compounds, including alginate and anionic detergents such as sodium lauryl sulphate, due to the formation of insoluble salts. Anions which attenuate or negate the activity of chlorhexidine include bicarbonate, borate, carbonate, chloride, citrate and phosphate, with avoidance of hard water, which can lead to precipitation, recommended. Deionised or distilled water should preferably be used for dilution purposes. Reduction in activity will also occur in the presence of blood, pus and other organic matter. Chlorhexidine has widespread use, in particular as an antiseptic. It has significant antibacterial activity, although Gram-negative bacteria are less sensitive than Gram-positive organisms. A concentration of 0.0005% prevents growth of, for example, *S. aureus*, whereas 0.002% prevents growth of *P. aeruginosa*. Reports of pseudomonad contamination of aqueous chlorhexidine solutions have prompted the inclusion of preservative concentrations of ethanol or isopropanol. Chlorhexidine is ineffective at ambient temperatures against bacterial spores and *M. tuberculosis*. Limited antifungal activity has been demonstrated, which unfortunately restricts its use as a general preservative. Skin sensitivity has occasionally been reported, although, in general, chlorhexidine is well tolerated and non-toxic

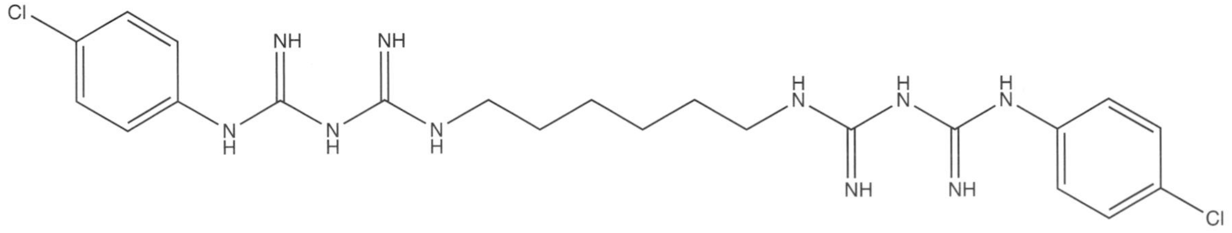

Figure 18.3 Chlorhexidine.

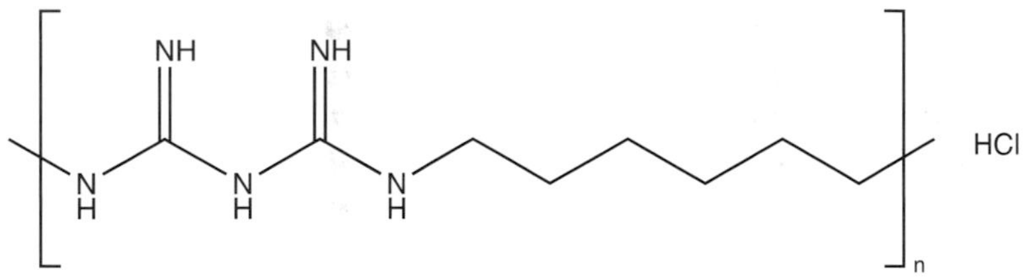

Figure 18.4 Polyhexamethylene biguanide (PHMB).

when applied to skin or mucous membranes and is an important preoperative antiseptic.

18.3.4.2 Polyhexamethylene Biguanides

The antimicrobial activity of the bisbiguanide chlorhexidine exceeds that of monomeric biguanides. This stimulated the development of polymeric biguanides containing repeating biguanide groups linked by hexamethylene chains. One such compound is a commercially available heterodisperse mixture of polyhexamethylene biguanides (PHMB, polyhexanide) having the general formula shown in Figure 18.4.

Within the structure, n varies with a mean value of 5.5. The compound has a broad spectrum of activity against Gram-positive and Gram-negative bacteria and has low toxicity. PHMB is employed as an antimicrobial agent in various ophthalmic products.

18.3.5 Halogens

Chlorine and iodine have been used extensively since their introduction as disinfecting agents in the early nineteenth century. Preparations containing these halogens, such as Dakin's solution and tincture of iodine, were early inclusions in many pharmacopoeias and national formularies. More recent formulations of these elements have improved activity, stability and ease of use.

18.3.5.1 Chlorine

A large number of antimicrobially active chlorine compounds are commercially available, one being liquid chlorine. This is supplied as an amber liquid made by compressing and cooling gaseous chlorine. The terms liquid chlorine and gaseous chlorine refer to elemental chlorine, whereas the word 'chlorine' itself is normally used to signify a mixture of OCl^-, Cl_2, HOCl and other active chlorine compounds in aqueous solution. The potency of chlorine disinfectants is usually expressed in terms of parts per million (ppm) or percentage of available chlorine (avCl).

18.3.5.2 Hypochlorites

Hypochlorites (bleach) are the oldest, and remain the most useful, of the chlorine disinfectants, being readily available, inexpensive and compatible with most anionic and cationic surface-active agents. They exhibit a rapid kill against a wide spectrum of microorganisms, including fungi and viruses. High levels of available chlorine will enable eradication of mycobacteria and bacterial spores. Their disadvantages are that they are corrosive, suffer inactivation by organic matter and can become unstable. Hypochlorites are available as powders or liquids, most frequently as the sodium or potassium salts of hypochlorous acid (HOCl). Sodium hypochlorite exists in solution as follows:

$$NaOCl + H_2O \rightleftharpoons HOCl + NaOH \quad (18.1)$$

Undissociated hypochlorous acid is a strong oxidising agent and its potent antimicrobial activity is dependent on pH as shown:

$$HOCl \rightleftharpoons H^+ + OCl^- \quad (18.2)$$

At low pH, the existence of HOCl is favoured over OCl^- (hypochlorite ion). The relative microbicidal effectiveness of these forms is of the order of 100:1. By lowering the pH of hypochlorite solution, the antimicrobial activity increases to an optimum at about pH 5. However, this is concurrent with a decrease in stability of the solution. This problem may be alleviated by addition of NaOH (see Equation 18.1) in order to maintain a high pH during storage for stability. The absence of buffer allows the pH to be lowered sufficiently for activity on dilution to use-strength. It is preferable to prepare use-dilutions of hypochlorite on a daily basis.

Undiluted bleach stored at room temperature in a closed container has a shelf life of about 6 months. Storage of stock or working solutions of bleach in open containers causes release of chlorine gas, especially at elevated temperatures, and this considerably weakens the antimicrobial activity of the solution.

18.3.5.3 Organic Chlorine Compounds

A number of organic chlorine, or chloramine, compounds are now available for disinfection and antisepsis. These are the *N*-chloro (=*N*—Cl) derivatives of, for example, sulphonamides giving compounds such as chloramine-T and dichloramine-T, and halazone (Figure 18.5), which may be used for the disinfection of contaminated drinking water.

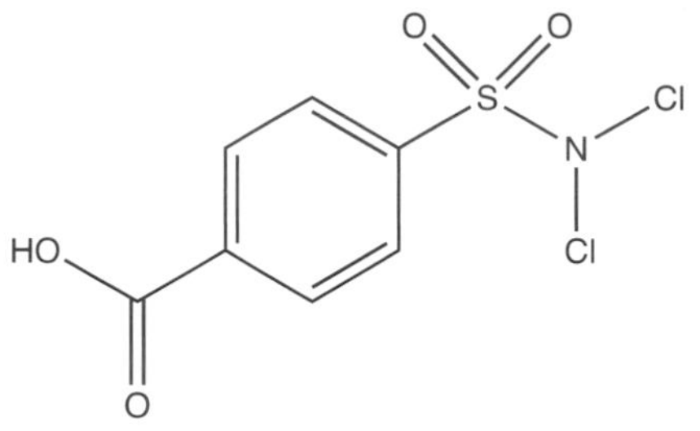

Figure 18.5 Halazone.

A second group of compounds, formed by *N*-chloro derivatisation of heterocyclic compounds containing a nitrogen in the ring, includes the sodium and potassium salts of dichloroisocyanuric acid (e.g., NaDCC). These are available in granule or tablet form and, in contrast to hypochlorite, are very stable on storage if protected from moisture. In water they will give a known chlorine concentration. The antimicrobial activity of the compounds is similar to that of the hypochlorites when acidic conditions of use are maintained. It is, however, important to note that where inadequate ventilation exists, care must be taken not to apply the compound to acidic fluids or large spills of urine in view of the toxic effects of chlorine production. The HSE has set the occupational exposure standard (OES) short-term exposure limit at 1 ppm (see also Section 18.2.5).

18.3.5.4 Chloroform

Chloroform (trichloromethane, CHCl3) has a narrow spectrum of activity, exhibiting bactericidal but not sporicidal action. It has been used extensively as a preservative of pharmaceuticals since the nineteenth century, and appears in many older pharmacopoeias. Marked reductions in concentration may occur through volatilisation from products, resulting in loss of preservative activity and the possibility of microbial growth. As a result of toxicological and stability concerns, the use of chloroform as a preservative in pharmaceutical formulations is now largely obsolete and it is completely banned for use as a preservative in the USA.

18.3.5.5 Iodine

Iodine has a wide spectrum of antimicrobial activity. Gram-negative and Gram-positive organisms, bacterial spores (on extended exposure), mycobacteria, fungi and viruses are all susceptible. The active agent is the elemental iodine molecule, I_2. As elemental iodine is only slightly soluble in water, iodide ions are required for aqueous solutions such as Aqueous Iodine Solution, BP 1988 (Lugol's solution) containing 5% iodine in 10% potassium iodide solution. Iodine (2.5%) may also be dissolved in ethanol (90%) and potassium iodide (2.5%) solution to give Weak Iodine Solution, BP 1988 (iodine tincture).

The antimicrobial activity of iodine is less dependent than chlorine on temperature and pH, although alkaline pH should be avoided. Iodine is also less susceptible to inactivation by organic matter. Disadvantages to the use of iodine in skin antisepsis are staining of skin and fabrics coupled with possible sensitising of skin and mucous membranes.

18.3.5.6 Iodophors

In the 1950s, iodophors (*iodo* meaning iodine and *phor* meaning carrier) were developed, to eliminate the disadvantages of iodine while retaining its antimicrobial activity. These allowed slow release of iodine on demand from the complex formed. Essentially, four generic compounds may be used as the carrier molecule or complexing agent. These give polyoxymer iodophors (i.e., with propylene or ethylene oxide polymers), cationic (quaternary ammonium) surfactant iodophors, non-ionic (ethoxylated) surfactant iodophors and polyvinylpyrrolidone iodophors (PVP-I or povidone-iodine). The non-ionic or cationic surface-active agents act as solubilisers and carriers, combining detergency with antimicrobial activity. The former type of surfactant, especially, produces a stable, efficient formulation, the activity of which is further enhanced by the addition of phosphoric acid or citric acid to give a pH below 5 on use-dilution. The iodine is present in the form of micellar aggregates which disperse on dilution, especially below the critical micelle concentration (cmc) of the surfactant, to liberate free iodine.

When iodine and povidone are combined, a chemical reaction takes place forming a complex between the two. Some of the iodine becomes organically linked to povidone, although the major portion of the complexed iodine is in the form of tri-iodide. Dilution of this iodophor results in a weakening of the iodine linkage to the carrier polymer with concomitant increases in elemental iodine in solution and antimicrobial activity.

The amount of free iodine the solution can generate is termed the 'available iodine'. This acts as a reservoir for active iodine, releasing it when required and therefore largely avoiding the harmful side effects of high iodine concentration. Consequently, when used for antisepsis, iodophors should be allowed to remain on the skin for 2 minutes to obtain full advantage of the sustained-release iodine.

Cadexomer-I_2 is an iodophor similar to povidone-iodine. It is a 2-hydroxymethylene cross-linked (1–4) α-D-glucan carboxymethyl ether containing iodine. The compound is used especially for its absorbent and antiseptic properties in the management of leg ulcers and pressure sores where it is applied in the form of microbeads containing 0.9% iodine.

18.3.6 Heavy Metals

Mercury and silver have antibacterial properties and preparations of these metals were among the earliest used antiseptics; over the years, however, they have been largely replaced by less-toxic compounds. Metallic copper has also been acknowledged historically for its preservative properties, particularly in the form of vessels to transport, and maintain the quality of, water.

18.3.6.1 Silver

Silver enjoyed a renaissance in the late 1990s and early 2000s as an antimicrobial frequently incorporated in urethral catheters for the prevention of device-related infection, and in textiles to control fomite-associated pathogens. However, a recent review of controlled trials found that the use of silver-coated silicone catheters did not offer a significant protective effect against bacteriuria. Silver has found application in a range of hygiene, personal care and healthcare environments. The FDA has issued several sets of guidance on the use of colloidal silver and silver salts in over-the-counter (OTC) drug products and medical devices, and any claims made against such products and devices. Various forms of silver are employed such as colloidal silver, silver halides, silver oxide and combinations such as silver–palladium. A hard surface disinfectant formulation based on silver dihydrogen citrate has been shown to be effective against a wide range of bacteria, fungi and viruses using as little as 30 ppm silver.

18.3.6.2 Copper

Copper alloy surfaces have been shown to exhibit broad antimicrobial action, and in 2008 the EPA recognised the public health benefit of these materials by registering a large number of products. Copper touch surfaces, such as bed rails and trolleys, have been used in a number of healthcare settings as part of a strategy to improve infection control and to delay recolonisation. Antimicrobial copper-oxide-impregnated textiles have found use in clinical settings for such items as bed linen, clothing and towels; impregnated dressings and socks have been shown to reduce infection. The efficacy of copper surfaces in the inactivation of coronaviruses, particularly SARS-CoV-2, has received significant attention during the COVID-19 pandemic, with reports describing the antiviral activity against, and the prevention of transmission of, SARS-CoV-2.

18.3.6.3 Mercurials

The organomercurial derivatives thiomersal (also known as thimerosal) and phenylmercuric nitrate or acetate (PMN or PMA) (Figure 18.6) have been primarily employed as preservatives. Use of both compounds has declined considerably as a result of concerns about mercury toxicity and risk of hypersensitivity or local irritation. They are absorbed from solution by rubber closures and plastic containers to a significant extent. Thiomersal has been used widely in the preservation of bulk formulation vaccines, and during vaccine production, and a number of safety and toxicity concerns have been raised, especially in the use of thiomersal-containing vaccines in infants. However, the WHO has stated that such concerns are theoretical, have been based primarily on toxicity of a related compound, methylmercury, and there is no compelling scientific evidence to support these safety concerns. The WHO continues to recommend the use of vaccines containing thiomersal for global immunisation programmes, as benefits outweigh any theoretical risk. Manufacturers seeking to replace thiomersal in existing vaccines need to provide evidence that change in formulation has no effect on vaccine quality, stability, safety and efficacy, and that a clear rationale exists for replacement. Additionally, a change in formulation could, in some cases, lead to the product being considered a new vaccine and therefore require further clinical trial data.

18.3.7 Hydrogen Peroxide and Peroxygen Compounds

Hydrogen peroxide and peracetic acid are high-level disinfectants as a result of their production of the highly reactive hydroxyl radical. They have the added advantage that their decomposition products are non-toxic and biodegradable. The microbicidal properties of hydrogen

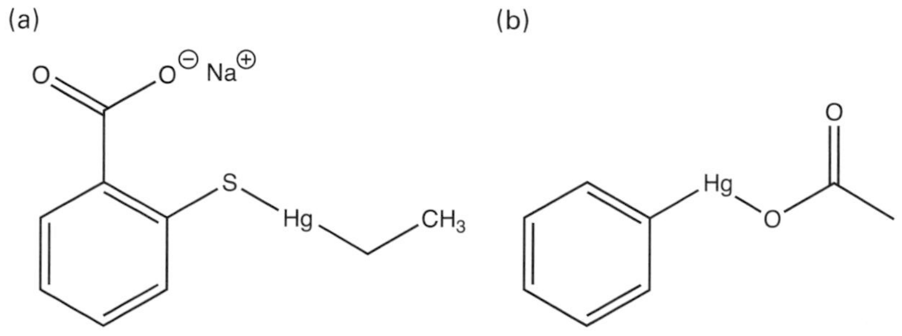

(a) (b)

O O⊖ Na⊕ S Hg CH3 | O Hg O

Figure 18.6 Organomercurials: (a) thiomersal (sodium ethylmercurithiosalicylate); (b) phenylmercuric acetate.

peroxide (H_2O_2) have been known for more than a century, but the use of low concentrations of unstable solutions did little for its reputation. However, stabilised solutions are now available, and because of its unusual properties and antimicrobial activity, hydrogen peroxide has a valuable role for specific applications. Its activity against the protozoan *Acanthamoeba*, which can cause keratitis in contact lens wearers, has made it popular for disinfection of soft contact lenses. Concentrations of 3–6% are effective for general disinfection purposes. At high concentrations (up to 35%) and increased temperature, hydrogen peroxide is sporicidal. Use has been made of this in vapour-phase hydrogen peroxide decontamination of equipment and enclosed spaces (Chapter 21). Hydrogen peroxide (>0.5%), as a cold mist or thermally generated vapour for airborne disinfection, has been widely used throughout the COVID-19 global pandemic, and has been shown to be effective against SARS-CoV-2, as well as bacteria, fungi and bacterial spores.

Peracetic acid (CH_3COOOH) is the peroxide of acetic acid and is a more potent microbicide than hydrogen peroxide, with excellent rapid cidal activity against bacteria, including mycobacteria, fungi, viruses and spores. It can be used in both the liquid and vapour phases and is active in the presence of organic matter. It is finding increasing use at concentrations of 0.2–0.35% as a chemosterilant of medical equipment such as flexible endoscopes. Its disadvantages are that it is corrosive to some metals. It is also highly irritant and must be used in an enclosed system. The combination of hydrogen peroxide and peracetic acid is synergistic and is marketed as a cold sterilant for dialysis machines.

18.3.8 Phenols

Phenols (Figure 18.7) are widely used as disinfectants and preservatives. They have good antimicrobial activity and are rapidly bactericidal but generally are not sporicidal.

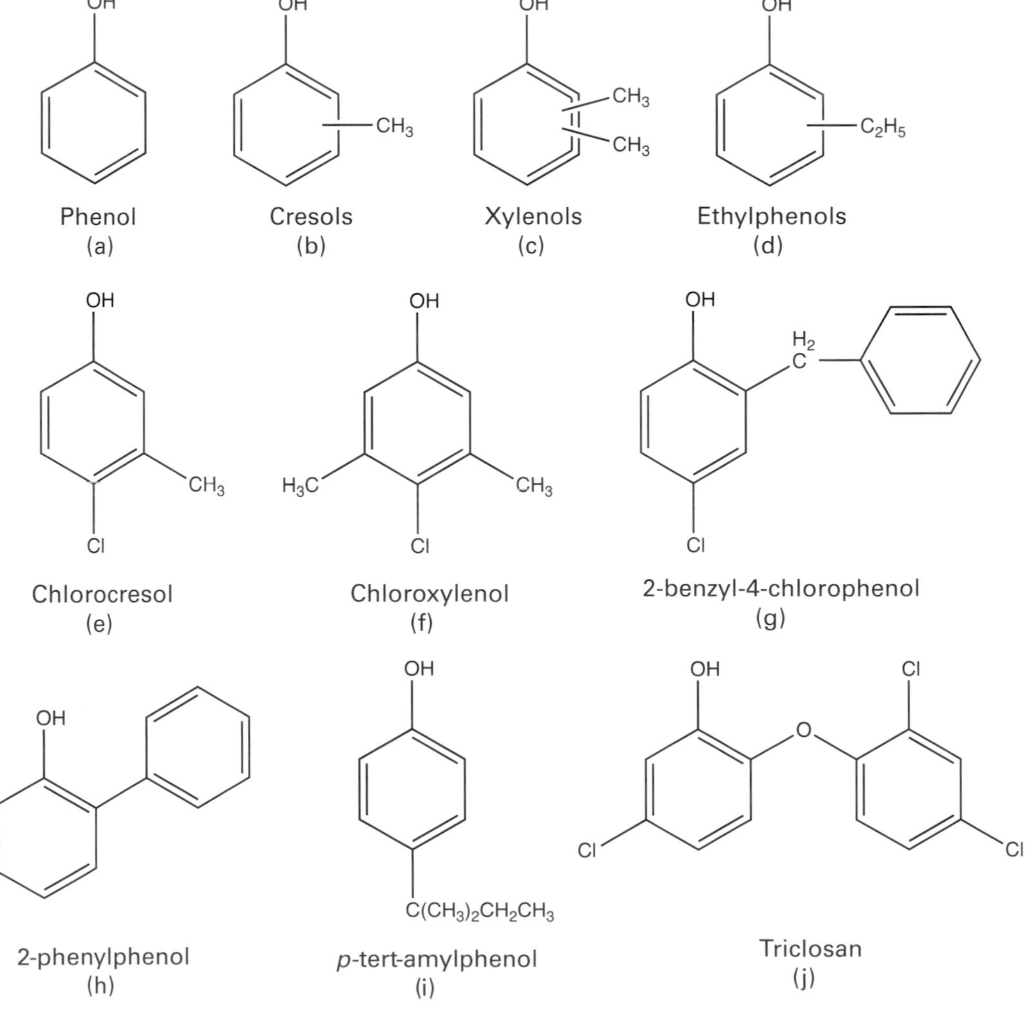

Figure 18.7 (a)–(j) Structures of some common phenols possessing antimicrobial activity.

Their activity is markedly diminished by dilution and is also reduced by organic matter. They are more active at acid pH. Major disadvantages include their caustic effect on skin and tissues, volatility and odour and their systemic toxicity. The more highly substituted phenols are less toxic and can be used as preservatives and antiseptics; however, they are also less active than the simple phenolics, especially against Gram-negative organisms. To improve their poor aqueous solubility, phenolic disinfectants are often formulated with soaps, synthetic detergents and/or solvents.

18.3.8.1 Phenol (Carbolic Acid)

Phenol (Figure 18.7a) no longer plays any significant role as an antibacterial agent. It is largely of historical interest, as it was used by Lister in the 1860s as a surgical antiseptic and has been a standard for comparison with other disinfectants in tests such as the Rideal–Walker test.

18.3.8.2 Clear Soluble Fluids, Black Fluids and White Fluids

Phenols obtained by distillation of coal or petroleum can be separated by fractional distillation according to their boiling point range into phenols, cresols, xylenols and high-boiling-point tar acids. As the boiling point increases, bactericidal activity increases and tissue toxicity decreases, but there is increased inactivation by organic matter and decreased water solubility.

Clear soluble fluids are produced from cresols or xylenols. The preparation known as Lysol (Cresol and Soap Solution BP 1968) is a soap-solubilised formulation of cresol (Figure 18.7b) that has been widely used as a general-purpose disinfectant but has largely been superseded by less irritant phenolics. A higher-boiling-point fraction consisting of xylenols and ethylphenols (Figure 18.7c,d) produces a more active, less corrosive product that retains activity in the presence of organic matter. A variety of proprietary products for general disinfection purposes are available.

Black fluids and white fluids are prepared by solubilising the high-boiling-point tar acids. Black fluids are homogeneous solutions that form an emulsion on dilution with water, whereas white fluids are finely dispersed stable emulsions. Both types of fluid have good bactericidal activity. Preparations are very irritant and corrosive to skin; however, they are relatively inexpensive and are useful for household and general disinfection purposes.

18.3.8.3 Synthetic Phenols

Many derivatives of phenol are now made by a synthetic process. A combination of alkyl or aryl substitution and halogenation of phenolic compounds has produced useful derivatives. Two of the best-known chlorinated derivatives are *p*-chloro-*m*-cresol (chlorocresol, Figure 18.7e), which was frequently employed as a preservative at a concentration of 0.1%, and *p*-chloro-*m*-xylenol (chloroxylenol, Figure 18.7f), which is sometimes used for skin disinfection. Chloroxylenol is sparingly soluble in water and must be solubilised, for example, in a suitable soap solution in conjunction with terpineol or pine oil. Its antimicrobial capacity is weak and is reduced by the presence of organic matter. Other phenol derivatives of note are: 2-benzyl-4-chlorophenol (Figure 18.7g), 2-phenylphenol (Figure 18.7h) and *p*-tert-amylphenol (Figure 18.7i).

18.3.8.4 Bisphenols

Bisphenols are composed of two phenolic groups connected by various linkages. Triclosan (Figure 18.7j) is the most widely used. It has been incorporated into medicated soaps, lotions and solutions and is also included in household products such as plastics and fabrics. There is some concern about bacterial resistance developing to triclosan (see Chapter 20).

18.3.9 Surface-active Agents

Surface-active agents or *surfactants* are classified as anionic, cationic, non-ionic or ampholytic according to the ionisation of the hydrophilic group in the molecule. A hydrophobic, water-repellent group is also present. Within the various classes, a range of detergent and disinfectant activity is found. The anionic and non-ionic surface-active agents, for example, have strong detergent properties but exhibit little or no antimicrobial activity. They can, however, render certain bacterial species more sensitive to some antimicrobial agents, possibly by altering the permeability of the outer envelope. Ampholytic or amphoteric agents can ionise to give anionic, cationic and zwitterionic (positively and negatively charged ions in the same molecule) activities. Consequently, they display both the detergent properties of the anionic surface-active agents and the antimicrobial activity of the cationic agents. They are used quite extensively in Europe for presurgical hand-scrubbing, medical instrument disinfection and floor disinfection in hospitals.

Of the four classes of surface-active agents the cationic compounds play the most important role in an antimicrobial context.

18.3.9.1 Cationic Surface-active Agents

The cationic agents used for their antimicrobial activity all fall within the group known as the QACs (quats or onium ions). These are organically substituted ammonium compounds (Figure 18.8a) where the R substituents are alkyl or heterocyclic radicals to give compounds such as

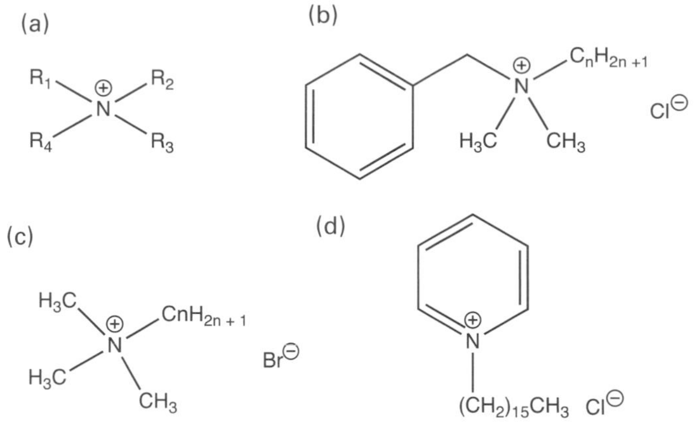

Figure 18.8 Quaternary ammonium compounds (QACs): (a) general structure of QACs; (b) benzalkonium chloride (*n* = 8–18); (c) cetrimide (*n* = 12, 14 or 16); (d) cetylpyridinium chloride.

benzalkonium chloride (Figure 18.8b), cetyltrimethylammonium bromide (cetrimide) (Figure 18.8c) and cetylpyridinium chloride (Figure 18.8d). Inspection of the structures of these compounds (Figure 18.8b,c) indicates that a chain length in the range C_8–C_{18} in at least one of the R substituents is a requirement for good antimicrobial activity. In the pyridinium compounds (Figure 18.8d), three of the four covalent links may be satisfied by the nitrogen in a pyridine ring. Several 'generational' changes have arisen in the development of QACs. Compounds such as alkyldimethylbenzyl ammonium chloride, alkyldimethylethylbenzyl ammonium chloride and didecyldimethylammonium chloride have roles in disinfection where HIV and HBV are present. Polymeric quaternary ammonium salts such as polyquaternium 1 are finding increasing use as preservatives.

The QACs are most effective against microorganisms at neutral or slightly alkaline pH and become virtually inactive below pH 3.5. Not surprisingly, anionic agents greatly reduce the activity of these compounds. Incompatibilities have also been recorded with non-ionic agents, possibly due to the formation of micelles. The presence of organic matter such as serum, faeces and milk will also seriously affect activity.

QACs exhibit greatest activity against Gram-positive bacteria, with a lethal effect observed using concentrations as low as 0.0005%. Gram-negative bacteria are more resistant, requiring a level of 0.0033%, or higher still if *P. aeruginosa* is present. A limited antifungal activity is exhibited and they have no useful sporicidal activity. This relatively narrow spectrum of activity limits the usefulness of the compounds, but as they are generally well tolerated and non-toxic when applied to skin and mucous membranes, they have considerable use in treatment of wounds and abrasions. Benzalkonium chloride and cetrimide are employed extensively in surgery, urology and gynaecology as aqueous and alcoholic solutions and as creams. In many instances, they are used in conjunction with a biguanide disinfectant such as chlorhexidine. The detergent properties of the QACs also provide a useful activity, especially in hospitals, for general environmental cleaning.

Bacterial resistance towards the QACs is now widely acknowledged (see Chapter 20); this risk is best managed by the use of sufficient microbicidal concentrations in circumstances where such levels can be adequately maintained, a useful maxim for all antimicrobial agents.

18.3.10 Other Antimicrobials

The full range of chemicals that can be shown to have antimicrobial properties is beyond the scope of this chapter. The agents included in this section have limited use or are of historic interest.

18.3.10.1 Diamidines

The activity of diamidines is reduced by acid pH and in the presence of blood and serum. Propamidine and dibromopropamidine, as the isethionate salts, have been employed as antimicrobial agents in eye drops (0.1%) for amoebic infection and for topical treatment of minor infections.

18.3.10.2 Dyes

Crystal violet (Gentian violet), brilliant green and malachite green are triphenylmethane dyes used to stain bacteria for microscopic examination. They have a bacteriostatic activity, but are no longer applied topically for the treatment of infections because of carcinogenicity.

The acridine dyes acriflavine and aminacrine have been employed for skin disinfection and treatment of infected wounds or burns, but are slow-acting and mainly bacteriostatic.

18.3.10.3 Quinoline Derivatives

The quinoline derivatives of pharmaceutical interest are little used now. The compound most frequently used is dequalinium chloride, a bisquaternary ammonium derivative of 4-aminoquinaldinium which was formulated as a lozenge for the treatment of oropharyngeal infections.

18.3.11 Antimicrobial Combinations and Systems

There is no ideal disinfectant, antiseptic or preservative. All chemical agents have their limitations in terms of either their antimicrobial activity, resistance to organic matter, stability, incompatibility, irritancy, toxicity or corrosivity. To overcome the limitations of an individual agent, formulations consisting of combinations of agents are available. For example, ethanol and isopropanol have been combined with chlorhexidine, QACs, sodium hypochlorite and iodine to produce more active preparations. The combination of chlorhexidine and cetrimide is also considered to improve activity. QACs and phenols have been combined with glutaraldehyde and formaldehyde so that the same effect can be achieved with lower, less-irritant concentrations of the aldehydes. Some combinations are considered to be synergistic, for example, hydrogen peroxide and peroxygen compounds. Care must be taken in deciding on disinfectant combinations, as the concentration exponents associated with each component of a disinfectant combination will have a considerable effect on the degree of activity (Chapter 19).

Research into the resistance of microbial biofilms provides potential for improving elimination of this problematical microbial mode of growth. Bacteria often use a communication system, quorum sensing (QS), to regulate virulence factor production and the formation of biofilms. Increased understanding of how chemicals can block QS could help provide effective prevention and elimination of biofilm-related infection. The incorporation of antimicrobial agents into materials that form working and contact surfaces or those of medical devices and implants has been positive but much further developmental research is required. Such 'bioactive' surfaces can be formed, for example, by incorporation of silver salts and alloys, biguanides and triclosan, and have the ability to reduce infection arising from microbial adherence and biofilm formation.

Other means are available to potentiate the activity of disinfectants, such as elevated temperature. Ultrasonic energy in combination with suitable disinfectants such as aldehydes and biguanides has been demonstrated to be useful in practice, and ultraviolet radiation increases the activity of hydrogen peroxide. Superoxidised water provides an extremely active disinfectant with a mixture of oxidising species produced from the electrolysis of saline. The main products are hypochlorous acid ($144\,mg\,l^{-1}$) and free chlorine radicals. The antimicrobial activity is rapid against a wide range of microorganisms in the absence of organic matter.

18.4 Disinfection Policies

The aim of a disinfection policy is to control the use of chemicals for disinfection and antisepsis and give guidelines on their use. The preceding descriptions within this chapter of the activities, advantages and disadvantages of the many disinfectants available allow considerable scope for choice and inclusion of agents in a policy to be applied to such areas as industrial plant, walls, ceilings, floors, air, cleaning equipment and laundries and to the extensive range of equipment in contact with hospital patients.

The control of microorganisms is of prime importance in healthcare and industrial environments. Where pharmaceutical products (either sterile or non-sterile) are manufactured, contamination of the product may lead to its deterioration and to infection in the user. In healthcare, there is the additional consideration of patient care, therefore protection from nosocomial (healthcare-associated) infection and prevention of cross-infection must also be covered (Chapter 16). Hospitals will have a disinfection policy and the degree of adherence to, and implementation of, the policy content will require stringent monitoring. A specialised infection prevention and control team or similar, comprising a number of specialised personnel such as the pharmacist, the consultant medical microbiologist and clinical nurse specialist in infection prevention and control and surveillance scientists, should formulate a suitable policy. This core team may usefully be expanded to include, for example, a physician, a surgeon, an epidemiologist, nurse teachers and nurses from several clinical areas, the sterile services manager and the domestic superintendent. This expanded committee will meet regularly to help with the implementation of the policy and reassess its efficiency. Tables 18.2–18.4 indicate the susceptibility of various microorganisms to the range of agents available and Table 18.6 presents examples of the range of formulations available. Although scope exists for choice of disinfectant in many of the areas covered by a policy, in certain instances, specific recommendations are made as to the type, concentration and usage of disinfectant.

Categories of risk (to patients) may usefully be assigned to equipment coming into contact with a patient, dictating the level of decontamination required and degree of concern (Table 18.7). *High-risk* (critical) items have close contact with broken skin or mucous membranes or are those introduced into a sterile area of the body and should, themselves, be sterile; they include instruments, gloves, catheters, syringes and needles. Liquid chemical disinfectants should

Table 18.7 Disinfection approach: classification of equipment according to risk.

Risk level	Examples	Classification	Objective	Decontamination
High risk: critical items	Surgical instruments, implants, catheters	Objects which enter a sterile tissue or system	Sterility – all microorganisms killed including bacterial spores	Thermal or gaseous sterilisation preferable. Chemical sterilisation with aldehyde or peroxygen with extensive contact times
Intermediate risk: semi-critical items	Endoscopes, cystoscopes, respiratory and anaesthesia equipment	Objects in contact with mucous membranes or broken skin	Free of all viable microorganisms except bacterial spores	High-level disinfection with aldehyde or peroxygen; contact times up to 30 min
Low risk: non-critical items	Blood pressure cuffs, food utensils, furniture, floors	Objects in contact with intact skin but not mucous membranes	Some microorganisms remaining	Low-level disinfection using alcohols, chlorine, iodophor, QACs

QAC, quaternary ammonium compound.

only be used if heat or other methods of sterilisation are unsuitable. *Intermediate-risk* (semi-critical) items are in close contact with skin or mucous membranes and disinfection will normally be applied. Endoscopes, respiratory and anaesthetic equipment, wash bowls, bed pans and similar items are included in this category. *Low-risk* (non-critical) items or areas include those detailed earlier such as walls and floors, which are not in close contact with the patient. Cleaning is obviously important with disinfection being required, for example, in the event of contaminated spillage.

References

HSE (2007). *An Evaluation of Chemical Disinfecting Agents Used in Endoscopy Suites in the NHS*, Research Report RR445. Sheffield: Health and Safety Executive.

HSE (2020). *EH40/2005 Workplace Exposure Limits: Containing the List of Workplace Exposure Limits for Use with the Control of Substances Hazardous to Health Regulations 2002 (as Amended)*. Sheffield: Health and Safety Executive.

Further Reading

Alvarado, C.J. and Reichelderfer, M. (2000). APIC guideline for infection prevention and control in flexible endoscopy. *Am. J. Infect. Control* 28: 138–155.

Environmental Protection Agency (US EPA) (2021). *List N: Disinfectants for coronavirus*. https://cfpub.epa.gov/wizards/disinfectants accessed October 2022.

EU Biocidal Products Regulation (2012). *Regulation No. 528/2012 of the European Parliament and of the Council of 22 May 2012 concerning the making available on the market and use of biocidal products*. https://eur-lex.europa.eu/LexUriServ/LexUriServ.do?uri=OJ:L:2012:167:0001:0123:EN:PDF

Filipe, H.A.L., Fiuza, S.M., Henriques, C.A. and Antunes, F.E. (2021). Antiviral and antibacterial activity of hand sanitizer and surface disinfectant formulations. *Int. J. Pharm.* 609: 121139.

Guidance (2021). *Minimise transmission risk of CJD and vCJD in healthcare settings*. Department of Health and Social Care, London. https://www.gov.uk/government/publications/guidance-from-the-acdp-tse-risk-management-subgroup-formerly-tse-working-group (accessed October 2022)

HSE (2021). *Control of Substances Hazardous to Health (COSHH). COSHH Essentials information*. www.hse.gov.uk/coshh/essentials/index.htm

McDonnell, G.E. and Hansen, J.M. (ed.) (2021). *Block's Disinfection, Sterilization, and Preservation*, 6e. Philadelphia, PA: Walters Kluwer.

Nkemngong, C.A., Voorn, M.G., Li, X. et al. (2020). A rapid model for developing dry surface biofilms of *Staphylococcus aureus* and *Pseudomonas aeruginosa* for *in vitro* disinfectant efficacy testing. *Antimicrob. Resist. Infect. Control* 9: 134.

19

Laboratory Evaluation of Antimicrobial Agents

Brendan F. Gilmore[1] *and Sean P. Gorman*[2]

[1] *Professor of Pharmaceutical Microbiology, School of Pharmacy, Queen's University Belfast, Belfast, UK*
[2] *Emeritus Professor of Pharmaceutical Microbiology, Queen's University Belfast, Belfast, UK*

CONTENTS

Hugo and Russell's Pharmaceutical Microbiology, Ninth Edition. Edited by Brendan F. Gilmore and Stephen P. Denyer.

Companion website: https://www.wiley.com/go/HugoandRussells9e

19.1 Introduction

Laboratory evaluation of antimicrobial agents remains a cornerstone of clinical microbiology and antimicrobial/microbicide discovery and development. The establishment of robust and reproducible assays for determining microbial susceptibility to antimicrobial agents is of fundamental importance in the appropriate selection of therapeutic agents and microbicides for use in infection prevention and control, disinfection, preservation and antifouling applications. Such laboratory assays form the basis for high-throughput screening of compounds or biological extracts in the discovery, isolation and development of new antimicrobial drugs and microbicides. Antimicrobial screening assays facilitate identification of antimicrobial agents from various sources and in lead antimicrobial compound optimisation. In the control of human and animal infection, laboratory evaluation of candidate agents yields crucial information which can inform the choice of antimicrobial agent(s) where the causative organism is known or suspected. As the number of microorganisms exhibiting resistance to conventional antimicrobial agents increases, laboratory evaluation of antimicrobial susceptibility is increasingly important for the selection of appropriate therapeutic agents. Evaluation of the potential antimicrobial action and nature of the inhibitory or lethal effects of established and novel therapeutic agents and microbicides are important considerations in the success of therapeutic interventions and infection/contamination control procedures.

Significant concerns that the extensive use of microbicidal agents may be linked to the development of antimicrobial resistance exist (see Chapter 20). Recent concerns regarding significant global public health issues such as the increasing threat of bioterrorism, the prevalence of healthcare-associated infections, avian influenza (H5N1), swine flu (H1N1) and especially the COVID-19 pandemic, caused by the coronavirus SARS-CoV-2, have seen global demand for microbicides and novel biocidal technologies increase dramatically. In addition, the emergence of new infectious agents (e.g., prions) and the increasing transmission rates of significant blood-borne viruses (e.g., HIV, hepatitis B and C), which may readily contaminate medical instruments or the environment, have focused attention on the need for effective and proven disinfecting and sterilising agents.

Finally, increased appreciation of the role played by microbial biofilms in human and animal infectious diseases and their ubiquitous distribution in natural ecosystems have led to the development of novel approaches for the laboratory evaluation of antimicrobial susceptibility of microorganisms growing as surface-adhered sessile populations. These studies have demonstrated that microorganisms in the biofilm mode of growth are phenotypically distinct from their planktonic counterparts and frequently exhibit significantly elevated phenotypic tolerance to antimicrobial challenge (see Chapter 8). This has implications not only for the environmental control of microorganisms but importantly in the selection of appropriate concentrations of antibiotic or microbicide necessary to eradicate them. As such, biofilms may constitute a reservoir of infectious microorganisms which may persist following antimicrobial challenge, especially where antimicrobial selection is based on standard laboratory susceptibility tests on planktonic cultures of microorganisms. Tests for evaluating candidate antimicrobial agents to be used in human and animal medicine as well as environmental microbicides remain significant laboratory considerations.

19.1.1 Definitions

Key terms such as disinfection, preservation, antisepsis and sterilisation are defined in Chapters 18 and 21. A number of other important terms used to describe the antimicrobial activity of agents are also commonly used. A *biocide* may be defined as a chemical or physical agent which kills viable organisms, both pathogenic and nonpathogenic. This broad definition clearly *includes* microoganisms, but is not restricted to them. The term *microbicide* is therefore also used to refer specifically to an agent which kills microorganisms (*germicide* may also be used in this context, but generally refers to pathogenic microorganisms). The terms *bactericidal*, *fungicidal*, *microbicidal* and *viricidal* therefore describe an agent with killing activity against a specific class or classes of organism indicated by the prefix, whereas the terms *bacteriostatic* and *fungistatic* refer to agents which inhibit the growth of bacteria or fungi, respectively (Figure 19.1), but do not necessarily kill them. It should be noted, however, that some microorganisms that appear non-viable and non-cultivable following antimicrobial challenge may be revived by appropriate methods, and that microorganisms incapable of multiplication may retain some metabolic/enzymatic activity. Bacteria also exhibit a stress-induced dormant phenotype, known as the persister phenotype or persisters, whereby they neither grow nor are killed by exogenous stress such as starvation or antimicrobial challenge. This persister phenotype allows members of a population of microbial cells (bacteria, archaea) to survive highly elevated concentrations of antibiotic or antimicrobial agent, and then to resuscitate after the exogenous stressor is removed and more favourable growth conditions return. Recent research has shown that rather than being two distinct stress-induced phenotypes, the viable but non-culturable (VBNC) and persister phenotypes actually describe the same dormant phenotype.

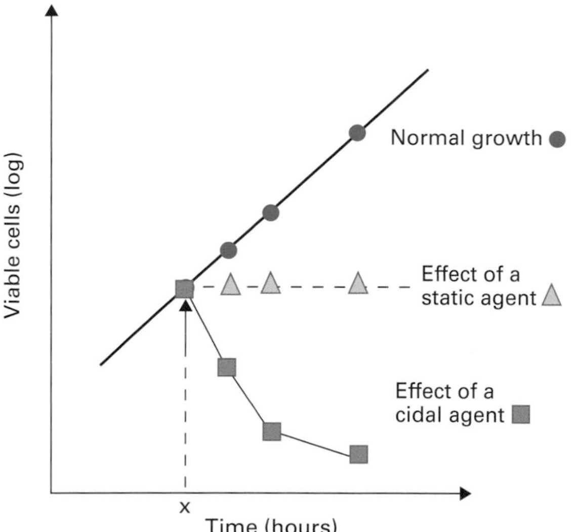

Figure 19.1 Effect on the subsequent microbial growth pattern of inhibitory (static, Δ) or cidal (□) agents added at time X (the normal microbial growth pattern is indicated by the o line).

In the laboratory evaluation of antibacterial agents, the terms *minimum inhibitory concentration* (MIC) and *minimum bactericidal concentration* (MBC) are most commonly used. The British Society for Antimicrobial Chemotherapy (BSAC) guidelines for the determination of minimum inhibitory concentrations define the MIC as the lowest concentration of antimicrobial which will inhibit the visible growth of a microorganism after overnight cultivation, and the MBC as the lowest concentration of antimicrobial that will prevent the recovery and growth of a microorganism after subculture onto antibiotic-free media. Generally, MIC and MBC values are recorded either in milligrams per litre or per millilitre (mg l^{-1} or mg ml^{-1}) or in micrograms per microlitre (μg μl^{-1}). With most cidal antimicrobials, the MIC and MBC are frequently near or equal in value, although with essentially static agents (e.g., tetracycline), the lowest concentration required to kill the microorganism (i.e., the MBC) is invariably many times the MIC and often clinically unachievable without toxicity to the human host. As with microbicides, cidal terms can be applied to studies involving not just bacteria but other microbes, for example, when referring to cidal antifungal agents, the term *minimum fungicidal concentration* (MFC) is used. Recently, thanks to developments in the design of high-throughput laboratory screens for biofilm susceptibility, the *minimum biofilm eradication concentration* (MBEC) can be accurately determined for organisms grown as single- or mixed-species biofilms. The MBEC is the minimum concentration of an antimicrobial agent required to kill a microbial biofilm. For conventional antibiotics and microbicides, the MBEC value may be 1000-fold higher than the MBC for the same planktonic microorganisms. Further studies have shown that often no correlation exists between the MIC and the MBEC, indicating the potential limitations of therapeutic antibiotic selection based on determined MIC values. Analogous to the MIC, the *minimum biofilm inhibitory concentration* (MBIC) is suggested as an additional biofilm susceptibility endpoint parameter, and is defined as the lowest concentration of an antibiotic, or antimicrobial substance, at which there is no time-dependent increase in the number of biofilm cells. However, unlike the MBEC value which is a well-established biofilm susceptibility endpoint parameter, there is a lack of consistency in the literature regarding MBIC determination protocols and definition, with an alternative definition of MBIC as the concentration of antibiotic that displays biofilm inhibition of >90% based on CFU (colony-forming units) or RFU (relative fluorescence units in a resazurin assay) determinations.

The term *tolerance* implies the ability of some bacterial strains to survive (without using or expressing resistance mechanisms), but not grow, at levels of antimicrobial agent that should normally be cidal. This applies particularly to systems employing the cell-wall-active β-lactams and glycopeptides, and to Gram-positive bacteria such as streptococci. Normally, MIC and MBC levels in such tests should be similar (i.e., within one or two doubling dilutions); if the MIC/MBC ratio is 32 or greater, the term tolerance is used. Tolerance may in some way be related to the Eagle phenomenon (paradoxical effect), where increasing concentrations of antimicrobial result in reduced killing rather than the increase in cidal activity expected (see Figure 19.2). Tolerance to elevated antimicrobial challenge concentrations is also a characteristic of microbial biofilm populations. Finally, the term *resistance* has several definitions within the literature; however, it generally refers to the ability of a microorganism to withstand the effects of a harmful chemical agent, with the organism neither killed nor inhibited at concentrations to which the majority of strains of that organism are susceptible. In the case of bacteria, resistance is defined as resistance to an antibiotic or antimicrobial agent that was once capable of treating an infection caused by that bacterial strain. Resistance mechanisms generally involve modification of the normal target of the antimicrobial agent either by mutation, enzymatic changes, target substitution, antibiotic destruction or alteration, antibiotic efflux mechanisms or restricted permeability to antibiotics. Antibiotic-resistance mechanisms are discussed fully in Chapter 13 and those for microbicides in Chapter 20.

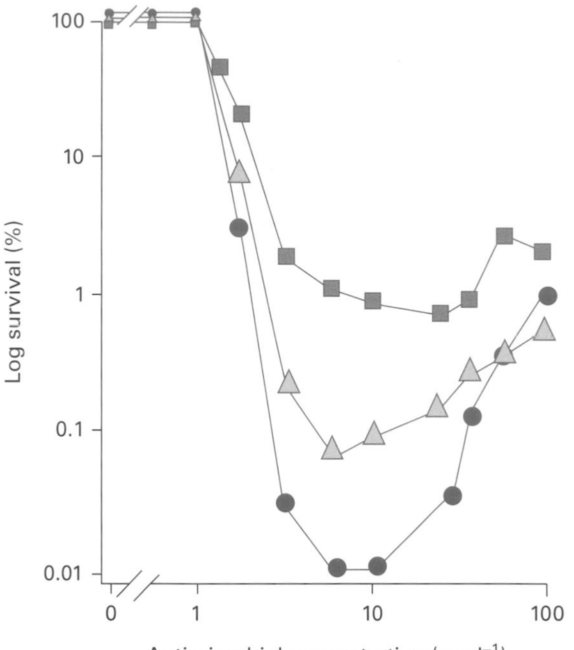

Figure 19.2 Survival of *Enterococcus faecalis* exposed to a fluoroquinolone for 4 hours at 37 °C. Three initial bacterial concentrations were studied, 10^7 CFU ml^{-1} (□); 10^6 CFU ml^{-1} (Δ) and 10^5 CFU ml^{-1} (o). This clearly demonstrates a paradoxical effect (increasing antimicrobial concentrations past a critical level reveal decreased killing), and the effects of increased inoculum densities on subsequent killing. *Source:* Courtesy of Dr. Z. Hashmi.

19.2 Factors Affecting the Antimicrobial Activity of Disinfectants

The activity of antimicrobial agents against a given organism or population of organisms will depend on a number of factors which must be reflected in the tests used to define their efficacy. For example, the activity of a given antimicrobial agent will be affected by the nature of the agent, the characteristics of the challenge organism, the mode of growth of the challenge organism, concentration of the agent, size of the challenge population and duration of exposure of that population to the active agent. Furthermore, environmental/physical conditions (temperature, pH, presence of extraneous organic matter) are also important considerations in modelling the activity of microbicidal agents. Laboratory tests for the evaluation of microbicidal activity must be carefully designed to take into account these factors which may influence significantly the rate of kill within the microbial challenge population. In other words, disinfectant efficacy tests must be designed to mimic likely in-use conditions given their intended applications (those parameters encountered during routine use including surface materials, challenge microorganisms, pH, presence of interfering substances [e.g., divalent cations] and exogenous organic matter [EOM]).

The work of Krönig and Paul in the late 1890s demonstrated that the rate of chemical disinfection was related to both concentration of the chemical agent and the temperature of the system, and that bacteria exposed to a cidal agent do not die simultaneously but in an orderly sequence. This led to various attempts at applying the kinetics of pure chemical reactions (the mechanistic hypothesis of disinfection) to microbe/disinfectant interactions. However, since the inactivation kinetics depend on a large number of defined and undefined variables, such models are often too complicated for routine use. Despite this, the Chick–Watson model (Equation (19.1)), based on first-order reaction kinetics, remains the basic rate law for the examination of disinfection kinetics:

$$\frac{dN}{dT} = -k_0 N \tag{19.1}$$

where N is the number of surviving microbes after time t and k_0 is the disinfection rate constant. The Chick–Watson model may be further refined to account for microbicide concentration (Equation (19.2)):

$$\frac{dN}{dT} = -k_1 C^n N \tag{19.2}$$

where k_1 is the concentration-independent rate constant, C is the microbicide concentration and n is the dilution coefficient. The Chick–Watson model predicts that the number of survivors falls exponentially at a rate governed by the rate constant and the concentration of disinfectant. A general assumption is that the concentration of microbicide remains constant throughout the experiment; however, there are a number of situations when this appears not to be the case (e.g., sequestering) and may result in observed departures from linear reaction kinetics. The factors influencing the antimicrobial activity of disinfectant agents are discussed below.

19.2.1 Innate (Natural) Resistance of Microorganisms

The susceptibility of microorganisms to chemical disinfectants and microbicides exhibits tremendous variation across various classes, species, phenotypes and morphologies. Bacterial endospores and the mycobacteria (e.g., *Mycobacterium tuberculosis*) exhibit the highest innate resistance, while many vegetative bacteria and some viruses appear highly susceptible (see Chapter 18). In addition, microorganisms adhering to surfaces as biofilms or present within other cells (e.g., legionellae within amoebae) may show a marked increase in phenotypic resistance

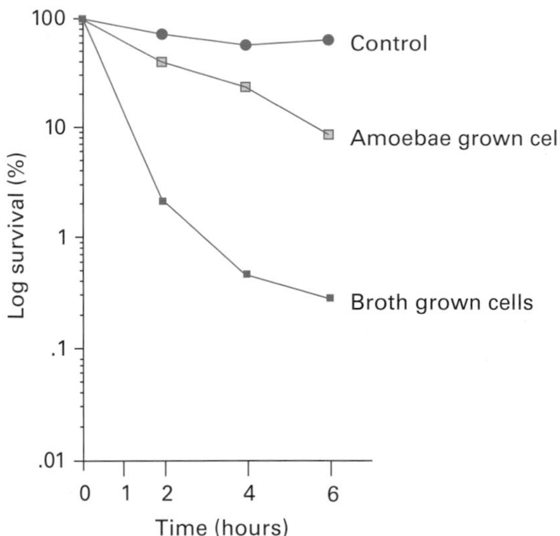

Figure 19.3 Survival of stationary phase broth cultures of *Legionella pneumophila* and amoebae-grown *L. pneumophila* after exposure to 32 mg l^{-1} benzisothiazolone (Proxel) at 35 °C in Ringer's solution; the control has no microbicide present. *Source:* Adapted from Barker et al. (1992).

(or tolerance) to disinfectants and microbicides (Figure 19.3). Therefore, when evaluating new disinfectants, a suitable range of microorganisms and environmental conditions must be included in tests to again mimic in-use conditions rather than optimal laboratory conditions, the results of which may not be reflective of microbicide performance in practice. The European/British Standard suspension test (BS EN 1276:2019) for studies relating to food, industrial, institutional and domestic areas include *Pseudomonas aeruginosa*, *Escherichia coli*, *Staphylococcus aureus* and *Enterococcus hirae* as the challenge organisms to be used in the test. For specific applications, additional strains may be chosen from *Salmonella enterica* serovar Typhimurium, *Lactobacillus brevis* and *Enterobacter cloacae*.

19.2.2 Microbial Density

Many disinfectants require adsorption to the microbial cell surface prior to killing; therefore, dense cell populations or sessile populations may sequester all, or a significant proportion, of the available disinfectant before all cells are affected, thus shielding a proportion of the population from the toxic effects of the chemical agent. Therefore, from a practical point of view, the larger the number of microorganisms present, the longer it takes a disinfectant to bring about complete killing of the population of cells. The implications of pre-disinfection washing and cleaning of objects (which remove most of the microorganisms, as well as extraneous organic material) become obvious. However, when evaluating disinfectants in the laboratory, it must be remembered that unlike sterilisation, kill curves with disinfectants may not be linear and the rate of killing may decrease at lower cell numbers (Figure 19.3). Hence, a 3-log killing may be more rapidly achieved with 10^8 than 10^4 cells. Johnston et al. (2000) demonstrated that even small variations in the initial inoculum size (*S. aureus*) had a dramatic effect on log reductions over time, using a constant concentration of sodium dodecyl sulphate (SDS). The authors argue that the presence of microbes quenches the action of the biocide (self-quenching), since cell and membrane components of lysed bacteria (e.g., emulsifiers such as triacylglycerols and phosphatidylethanolamine) are similar in action to emulsifiers (such as Tween and lecithin) used in standard microbicide quenching/neutralising agents employed in disinfectant tests. However, this may not hold true across all microbicides where similar inoculum size dependency of disinfection is observed (see Russell et al. 1997). Initial bioburden/cell numbers must, therefore, be standardised and accurately quantified in disinfectant efficacy (suspension) tests and agreement reached on the degree of killing required over a stipulated time interval (see Table 19.1).

Table 19.1 Methods of recording viable cells remaining after exposure of an initial population of 1,000,000 (10^6) CFU to a cidal agent.

Viable count remaining (CFU)	Log survival (%)	Log killing	% killing
100,000 (10^5)	10	1-log	90
10,000 (10^4)	1	2-log	99
1000 (10^3)	0.1	3-log	99.9
100 (10^2)	0.01	4-log	99.99
10 (10^1)	0.001	5-log	99.999

19.2.3 Disinfectant Concentration and Exposure Time

The effects of concentration or dilution of the active ingredient on the activity of a disinfectant are of major importance. With the exception of iodophors, the more concentrated a disinfectant, the greater its efficacy and the shorter the exposure time required to destroy the population of microorganisms, that is, there is a direct relationship, frequently exponential, between potency and concentration. Therefore, a graph plotting the $\log_{10}$ of the death time (i.e., the time required to kill a standard inoculum) against the $\log_{10}$ of the concentration is

Table 19.2 Concentration exponents, η, for some disinfectant substances.

Antimicrobial agent	Concentration exponent
Hydrogen peroxide	0.5
Silver nitrate	0.9–1.0
Mercurials	0.03–3.0
Iodine	0.9
Crystal violet	0.9
Chlorhexidine	2
Formaldehyde	1
QACs	0.8–2.5
Acridines	0.7–1.9
Formaldehyde donors	0.8–0.9
Bronopol	0.7
Polymeric biguanides	1.5–1.6
Parabens	2.5
Sorbic acid	2.6–3.2
Potassium laurate	2.3
Benzyl alcohol	2.6–4.6
Aliphatic alcohols	6.0–12.7
Glycol monophenyl ethers	5.8–6.4
Glycol monoalkyl ethers	6.4–15.9
Phenolic agents	4.0–9.9

QAC, quaternary ammonium compound.

typically a straight line, the slope of which is the concentration exponent (η). This is expressed as an equation:

$$\eta = \frac{\left(\text{log death time at concentration } C_2\right) - \left(\text{log death time at concentration } C_1\right)}{\log C_1 - C_2} \tag{19.3}$$

Thus, η can be obtained from experimental data either graphically or by substitution in Equation (19.3) (see Table 19.2).

It is important to note that dilution does not affect the cidal attributes of all disinfectants in a similar manner. For example, mercuric chloride with a concentration exponent of 1 will be reduced by the power of 1 on dilution, and a threefold dilution means the disinfectant activity will be reduced by the value 3^1, that is, to a third of its original potency. Phenol, however, has a concentration exponent of 6, and so a threefold dilution in this case will mean a decrease in activity of 3^6 or 729 times less active than the original concentration. Thus, the likely dilution experienced by the disinfectant agent in use must be given due consideration when selecting an appropriate microbicidal agent for a given application. It should also be remembered that sequestration of the active biocide by organic matter, or an increased bioburden, may also constitute dilution events which need to be considered when evaluating microbicides under in-use conditions.

19.2.4 Physical and Chemical Factors

Known and proven influences on microbicidal efficacy include temperature, pH and mineral content of water ('hardness').

19.2.4.1 Temperature

As with most chemical/biochemical reactions, the cidal activity of most disinfectants increases with an increase in temperature, since temperature is a measure of the kinetic energy within a reaction system. Increasing the kinetic energy of a reaction system increases the rate of reaction by increasing the number of collisions between reactants per unit time. This process is observed up to an optimum temperature, beyond which reaction rates fall again, due to thermal denaturation of some component(s) of the reaction. As the temperature is increased in arithmetical progression, the rate (velocity) of disinfection increases in geometrical progression. Results may be expressed quantitatively by means of a temperature coefficient, either the temperature coefficient per degree rise in temperature (θ), or the coefficient per 10 °C rise (the Q_{10} value). As shown by Koch, working with phenol and anthrax (*Bacillus anthracis*) spores over 120 years ago, raising the temperature of phenol from 20 to 30 °C increased the killing activity by a factor of 4 (the Q_{10} value).

The value of θ may be calculated from the equation:

$$\theta^{(T_1 - T_2)} = t_1 / t_2 \tag{19.4}$$

where t_1 is the extinction time at temperature T_1 °C, and t_2 the extinction at T_2 °C (i.e., $T_1 + 1$ °C).

Q_{10} values may be calculated easily by determining the extinction time at two temperatures differing by exactly 10 °C. Then:

$$Q_{10} = \frac{\text{Time to kill at } T^\circ}{\text{Time to kill at } \left(T + 10\right)^\circ} \tag{19.5}$$

It is also possible to plot the rate of kill against the temperature.

While the value of Q_{10} for chemical- and enzyme-catalysed reactions lies in a narrow range (between 2 and 3), values for disinfectants vary widely, for example, 4 for phenol, 45 for ethanol and almost 300 for ethylene glycol monoethyl ether. Clearly, relating chemical reaction kinetics without qualification to disinfection processes is potentially misleading. Most laboratory tests involving disinfectant-like chemicals are now standardised to 20 °C, that is, around ambient room temperatures.

19.2.4.2 pH

Effects of pH on antimicrobial activity can be complex. As well as directly influencing the survival and rate of growth of the microorganism under test, changes in pH may affect the potency of the agent and its ability to interact with cell surface sites. In many cases (for instance, where the microbicidal agent is an acid or a base), the ionisation state (or degree of ionisation) will depend on the pH. As is the case with some antimicrobials (e.g., phenols, acetic acid, benzoic acid), the non-ionised molecule is the active state (capable of crossing the cell membrane/partitioning) and alkaline pHs which favour the formation of ions of such compounds will decrease the activity. For these microbicidal agents, a knowledge of the molecule's pK_a is important in predicting the pH range over which activity can be observed, since in situations where the pH of the system equals the pK_a of the biocide molecule, ionised and unionised species are in equilibrium. Others, such as glutaraldehyde and quaternary ammonium compounds (QACs), reveal increased cidal activity as the pH rises and are best used under alkaline conditions, possibly due to enhanced interaction with amino groups on microbial biomolecules. The pH also influences the properties of the bacterial cell surface by changing the proportion of anionic groups present and hence altering its interaction with cidal molecules. Since the activity of many disinfectants first requires attachment to cell surfaces, increasing the external pH renders those surfaces more negatively charged and thus enhances the binding of cationic compounds such as chlorhexidine and QACs.

19.2.4.3 Divalent Cations

The presence of divalent cations (e.g., Mg^{2+}, Ca^{2+}), for example, in hard water, has been shown to exert an antagonistic effect on certain microbicides while having an additive effect on the cidal activity of others. Metal ions such as Mg^{2+} and Ca^{2+} may interact with the disinfectant itself to form insoluble precipitates; they can also interact with the microbial cell surface and block disinfectant adsorption sites necessary for activity. Biguanides, such as chlorhexidine, are inactivated by hard water. Hard water should always be employed for laboratory disinfectant and antiseptic evaluations to best reflect the in-use situation; recommended formulae for such tests employing various concentrations of $MgCl_2$ and $CaCl_2$ solutions can be found in the British Standard BS EN 1276:2019.

19.2.5 Presence of Extraneous Organic Material

The presence of extraneous organic material such as blood, serum, pus, faeces or soil is known to affect the cidal activity of many antimicrobial agents. Therefore, it is necessary to determine the likely interaction between organic matter and disinfectants by including this parameter in laboratory evaluations of their activity. In order to simulate 'clean' conditions (i.e., conditions of minimal organic contamination), disinfectants are tested in hard water containing 0.3 g/l bovine serum albumin (BSA), while 3.0 g/l BSA is used to mimic 'dirty' conditions. This standardised method replaces earlier approaches, some of which employed dried human faeces or yeast to mimic the effects of blood, pus or faeces on disinfectant activity. Disinfectants whose activities are particularly attenuated in the presence of organic contaminant include the halogen disinfectants, for example, sodium hypochlorite (where the disinfectant reacts with the organic matter to form inactive complexes), biguanides, phenolic compounds and QACs. The aldehydes (formaldehyde and glutaraldehyde) are largely unaffected by the presence of extraneous organic contaminants. Organic material may also interfere with cidal activity by coating the microbial cell surface blocking adsorption sites necessary for disinfectant activity. For practical purposes and to mirror potential in-use situations, disinfectants should be evaluated under both clean and dirty conditions.

19.3 Evaluation of Liquid Disinfectants

19.3.1 General

Phenol coefficient tests were developed in the early twentieth century when typhoid fever was a significant public health problem and phenolics were regularly used to disinfect contaminated utensils and other inanimate objects. In these tests, alternative disinfecting agents were compared to a phenol standard; details of such tests can be found in earlier editions of this book. As non-phenolic disinfectants became more widely available, however, tests that more closely paralleled the conditions under which disinfectants were being used (e.g., blood spills) and which included a more diverse range of microbial types (e.g., viruses, bacteria, fungi, protozoa) were developed. Evaluation of a disinfectant needs to be based on its ability to kill microbes, that is, its cidal activity, under environmental conditions mimicking as closely as possible real-life situations. As an essential component of each test is a final viability assay, removal or neutralisation of any residual disinfectant (to prevent 'carry-over' toxicity) becomes a significant consideration.

The development of methods to evaluate disinfectant activity in diverse environmental conditions and to determine suitable in-use concentrations/dilutions to be used led to the development by Kelsey, Sykes and Maurer of the so-called *capacity-use dilution test* which measured the ability of a disinfectant at appropriate concentrations to kill successive additions of a bacterial culture. Results were reported simply as pass or fail and not a numerical coefficient. Tests employed disinfectants diluted in hard water (clean conditions) and in hard-water-containing organic material (yeast suspension to simulate dirty conditions), with the final recovery broth containing 3% Tween 80 as a neutraliser. Such tests are applicable for use with a wide variety of disinfectants (see Kelsey and Maurer 1974). Capacity tests mimic the practical situations of housekeeping and instrument disinfection, where surfaces are contaminated, exposed to disinfectant, recontaminated and so forth. The British Standard (BS 6905:1987) method for estimation of disinfectants used in dirty conditions in hospitals by a modification of the original Kelsey–Sykes test is one of the most commonly employed capacity tests in the UK and Europe. In the USA, effectiveness test data for submission to the US Environmental Protection Agency (EPA) for disinfectant claim substantiation must be obtained by methods accepted by the Association of Official Analytical Chemists (AOAC), known collectively as disinfectant efficacy tests (DETs).

The best information concerning the fate of microbes exposed to a disinfectant, however, is obtained by counting the number of viable cells remaining after exposure of a standard suspension of those cells to the disinfectant at known concentration for a given time interval; these are called *suspension tests*. Viable counting is a facile technique used in many branches of pure and applied microbiology (see Chapter 2). Assessment of the number of viable microbes remaining (survivors) after exposure allows the killing or cidal activity of the disinfectant to be expressed in a variety of ways, for example, percentage kill (e.g., 99.999%), as a $\log_{10}$ reduction in numbers (e.g., 5-log killing), or by $\log_{10}$ survival expressed as a percentage. Examples of such outcomes are shown in Table 19.1.

Unfortunately, standardisation of the methodology to be employed in these efficacy tests has proven difficult to obtain, as has consensus on what level of killing represents a satisfactory and/or acceptable result. It must be stressed, however, that unlike tests involving chemotherapeutic agents where the major aim is to establish antimicrobial concentrations that inhibit growth (i.e., MICs), disinfectant tests require determinations of appropriate cidal levels. Levels of killing required over a given time interval tend to vary depending on the regulatory authority concerned. While a 5-log killing of bacteria (starting with 10^6 CFU ml^{-1}) has been suggested for suspension tests, some authorities require a 6-log killing in simulated use tests. With viruses, a 4-log killing tends to be an acceptable result, while with prions it has been recommended that a titre loss of 10^4 prions should be regarded as an indication of appropriate disinfection provided that there has been adequate prior cleaning. With simulated use tests, cleaning followed by appropriate disinfection should result in a prion titre loss of at least 10^7.

19.3.2 Antibacterial Disinfectant Efficacy Tests

Various regulatory authorities in Europe (e.g., European Standard or Norm [EN]; British Standards [BS]; Germany [Deutsche Gesellschaft für Hygiene und Mikrobiologie, DGHM]; France [Association Française de Normalisation, AFNOR]) and North America (e.g., Food and Drug Administration [FDA]; EPA; ASTM International [formerly the American Society for Testing and Materials] and AOAC) have been associated with attempts to produce some form of harmonisation of disinfectant tests. The European Standard methods for disinfectant validation have been widely adopted, however, and serve as a useful illustration of the general approach; they comprise three phases (also referred to as tiers). Phase 1 disinfectant efficacy tests are typically performed at the developmental stage of a disinfectant formulation to determine whether an active agent qualifies for basic disinfectant claims based on effectiveness against specified challenge microorganisms. Two basic Phase 1 tests are described in the EN standard documents EN 1040:2005 (bactericidal activity) and EN1275:2005 (fungicidal/yeasticidal activity). These tests are conducted under laboratory conditions, with no addition of interfering substances, and as such may not be used for efficacy claims, since the tests are not designed to mimic in-use conditions. Phase 2 tests are divided further into Steps 1 and 2 tests where Phase 2, Step 1 tests are quantitative suspension tests which simulate in-use environmental conditions using interfering substances such as BSA; here, EN 13272:2012 and EN 13624:2013 evaluate bactericidal and fungicidal activities, respectively, and EN 14348 describes quantitative suspension tests for mycobactericidal activity. Phase 2, Step 2 tests are carrier tests intended to simulate practical usage conditions, whereby a defined inoculum of the challenge organism is applied to nonporous surfaces (the carrier) and left to air-dry, with the disinfectant being subsequently applied for designated contact times. Interfering substances are included in the test to mimic environmental soiling. Examples of Phase 2, Step 2 standard European methods are EN 14561:2006, 14562:2006 and 14563 quantitative carrier tests for bactericidal, fungicidal/yeasticidal and mycobactericidal activities, respectively; these tests are applied for disinfecting medical instruments (the carrier material).

19.3.2.1 Suspension Tests

While varying to some degree in their methodology, most procedures employ a standard suspension of the microorganism in hard water containing albumin (dirty conditions) and appropriate dilutions of the disinfectant. Tests are carried out at a set temperature (usually around room temperature or 20 °C), and at a selected time interval samples are removed and viable counts are performed following neutralisation of any disinfectant remaining in the sample. Neutralisation or inactivation of residual disinfectant can be carried out by dilution, or by the addition of specific agents (see Table 19.3). Using viable counts, it is possible to calculate the concentration of disinfectant required to kill 99.999% (5-log kill) of the original suspension. Thus, 10 survivors from an original population of 10^6 cells represents a 99.999% or 5-log kill. As bacteria may initially decline in numbers in diluents devoid of additional disinfectant, results from tests incorporating disinfectant-treated cells can be compared with results from simultaneous tests involving a non-disinfectant-containing system (untreated cells). The bactericidal effect B_E can then be expressed as:

$$B_E = \log N_C - \log N_D \quad (19.6)$$

where N_C and N_D represent the final number of CFU ml^{-1} remaining in the control and disinfectant series, respectively.

Unfortunately, viable count procedures assume that one colony develops from one viable cell. Such techniques are, therefore, not ideal for disinfectants (e.g., QACs such as cetrimide) that promote clumping in bacterial suspensions, although the problem may be partially mitigated by adding non-ionic surface-active agents to the diluting fluid. The European Standards EN 13727:2012+A2:2015 and EN 13697:2015 provide detailed test procedures for establishing the cidal activity of chemical disinfectants against microbial suspensions and on surfaces in simulated environmental conditions (carrier test), enabling appropriate efficacy claims to be made for a particular disinfectant.

Table 19.3 Neutralising agents for some antimicrobial agents.

Antimicrobial agent	Neutralising and/or inactivating agent
Alcohols	None (dilution)
Alcohol-based hand gels	Tween 80, saponin, histidine and lecithin
Amoxicillin	β-Lactamase from *Bacillus cereus*[a]
Antibiotics (most)	None (dilution, membrane filtration[b], resin adsorption[c])
Benzoic acid	Dilution or Tween 80[d]
Benzylpenicillin	β-Lactamase from *B. cereus*
Bronopol	Cysteine hydrochloride
Chlorhexidine	Lubrol W[e] and egg lecithin or Tween 80 and lecithin (Letheen)
Formaldehyde	Ammonium ions
Glutaraldehyde	Glycine
Halogens	Sodium thiosulphate
Hexachlorophane	Tween 80
Mercurials	Thioglycolic acid (—SH compounds)
Phenolics	Dilution or Tween 80
QACs	Lubrol W and lecithin or Tween 80 and lecithin (Letheen)
Sulphonamides	*p*-Aminobenzoic acid

[a] Other appropriate enzymes can be considered, e.g., inactivating or modifying enzymes for chloramphenicol and aminoglycosides, respectively.
[b] Filter microorganisms on to membrane, wash, transfer membrane to growth medium.
[c] Resins for the absorption of antibiotics from fluids are available.
[d] Tween 80 (polysorbate 80).
[e] Polyethylene glycol ether W-1.

19.3.2.2 In-use and Simulated Use Tests

Apart from suspension tests, in-use testing of used medical devices and simulated use tests (involving instruments or surfaces deliberately contaminated with an organic load and the appropriate test microorganism) have been incorporated into disinfectant testing protocols. An example is the in-use test first reported by Maurer in 1972. Here, a disinfectant currently in use in which potentially contaminated material (e.g., lavatory brushes, mops) has been placed is tested to see if it contains living microorganisms, and in what numbers. A small volume of fluid is withdrawn from the in-use container, neutralised in a large volume of a suitable diluent and viable counts are performed on the resulting suspension. Two plates are involved in viable count investigations, one of which is incubated for 3 days at 32 °C (rather than 37 °C, as bacteria damaged by disinfectants recover more rapidly at lowered temperatures), and the other for 7 days at room temperature. Growth of one or two colonies per plate can be ignored (a disinfectant is not usually a sterilant), but 10 or more colonies would suggest poor and unsatisfactory cidal action.

Simulated use tests involve deliberate contamination of instruments, inanimate surfaces or even skin surfaces, with a microbial suspension. This may either be under clean conditions or may utilise a diluent containing organic material (e.g., albumin) to simulate dirty conditions. After being left to dry, the contaminated surface is exposed to the test disinfectant for an appropriate time interval. The microbes are then removed (e.g., by rubbing with a sterile swab), resuspended in suitable neutralising medium and assessed for viability as for suspension tests. New products are often compared with a known comparator compound (e.g., 1-minute application of 60% v/v 2-propanol for hand disinfection products – see European Standard EN1500) to show increased efficacy of the novel product.

19.3.2.3 Problematic Bacteria

Mycobacteria are hydrophobic in nature and, as a result, exhibit an increased tendency to clump or aggregate in aqueous media. It may be difficult, therefore, to prepare homogeneous suspensions devoid of undue cell clumping (which may contribute to their resistance to chemical disinfection). As *M. tuberculosis* is very slow-growing, more rapidly growing species such as *Mycobacterium terrae*, *Mycobacterium bovis* or *Mycobacterium smegmatis* can be substituted in tests (as representative of *M. tuberculosis*). Recent global public health concerns regarding the increasing incidences of tuberculosis (including co-infections with HIV) in developing, low and middle-income countries (LMICs) and industrialised nations bring into sharp focus the necessity for representative evaluations of agents with potential tuberculocidal activity. This is particularly true given the high proportion of cases classified as multidrug-resistant tuberculosis (MDR-TB). As a result, specific standard tests have been developed to permit effective evaluation of the mycobactericidal activity of biocides (see Section 19.3.2). Apart from vegetative bacterial cells, bacterial or fungal spores can also be used as the inoculum in tests. In such cases, incubation of culture plates for the final viability determination should be continued for several days to allow for germination and growth.

Compared with suspended (planktonic) cells, bacteria growing on surfaces as biofilms are invariably phenotypically more tolerant to antimicrobial agents. With biofilms, suspension tests can be modified to involve biofilms grown on coupons of an appropriate glass, metal or polymeric substrate, or on the bottom of wells of plastic microtitre plates. After being immersed in, or exposed to, the disinfectant solution for the appropriate time interval, the cells from the biofilm are removed, for example, by sonication, and resuspended in a suitable microbicide-neutralising medium. Viable counts are then performed on the resulting planktonic cells. A reduction in biomass following antimicrobial challenge can also be monitored using a standard crystal-violet-staining technique; however, viable counting permits evaluation of the rate of kill. The Calgary Biofilm Device, discussed in Section 19.9.1, permits the high-throughput screening of antimicrobial agents against biofilms grown on 96 polycarbonate pegs in a 96-well microtitre plate. Finally, some important environmental bacteria survive in nature as intracellular parasites of other microbes, for example, *Legionella pneumophila* within the protozoan *Acanthamoeba polyphaga*. Biocide activity is significantly reduced against intracelluar legionellae (see Figure 19.3) and other intracellular pathogens. Disinfectant tests involving such bacteria should therefore be conducted both on planktonic bacteria and on suspensions involving amoebae-containing bacteria. With the latter, the final bacterial viable counts are performed after suitable lysis of the protozoan host. The legionella/protozoa situation may also be further complicated by the fact that the microbes often occur as intracellular biofilms.

19.3.3 Other Microbe Disinfectant Tests

Suspension-type efficacy tests can also be performed on other microbes (e.g., fungi and viruses) using similar techniques to those described above for bacteria, although significant differences obviously arise in parts of the tests.

19.3.3.1 Antifungal (Fungicidal) Tests

In order for disinfectants to claim fungicidal activity, or for the discovery of novel fungicidal agents, a range of standard tests have been devised. Perhaps the main problem with fungi concerns the question of which morphological form of fungus to use as the inoculum. While unicellular yeasts can be treated in much the same manner as bacteria, whether to use spores (which may be more resistant than the vegetative mycelium) or pieces of hyphae with the filamentous moulds has yet to be fully resolved. Spore suspensions (in saline containing the wetting agent Tween 80) obtained from 7-day-old cultures are presently recommended. The species to be used may be a known environmental strain and likely contaminant, such as *Aspergillus niger* or *Aspergillus brasiliensis*, or a pathogen, such as *Trichophyton mentagrophytes*; other strains such as *Penicillium variabile* are also employed. Clearly, the final selection of organism will vary depending on the perceived use for the disinfectant under test. In general, spore suspensions of at least 10^6 CFU/ml have been recommended. Viable counts are typically performed on a suitable medium (e.g., malt extract agar, Sabouraud dextrose agar) with incubation at 20 °C for 48 hours or longer. European Standard EN 1275:2005 specifies that for fungicidal activity a minimum reduction in viability by a factor of 10^4 within 60 minutes is required; test fungi are *Candida albicans* for yeasticidal activity and *C. albicans* and *A. brasiliensis* for fungicidal activity. Further procedures may be obtained by reference to European Standards EN 1650:1998 (chemical disinfectants and antiseptics used in food, industrial, domestic and institutional areas) and EN 13624:2013 (disinfectants intended for use in the medical area) and also AOAC guidance on the fungicidal activity of disinfectants (955.17).

19.3.3.2 Antiviral (Viricidal) Tests

The evaluation of disinfectants for viricidal activity is a complicated process requiring specialised training and facilities; viruses are obligate intracellular parasites and are therefore incapable of independent growth and replication in artificial culture media. They require some other system employing living host cells. Suggested test viruses include rotavirus, adenovirus, poliovirus, herpes simplex viruses, HIV, vaccinia virus, influenza A virus, pox viruses and papovavirus, although extension of this list to include additional blood-borne viruses, such as hepatitis B and hepatitis C, significant animal pathogens (e.g., foot and mouth disease virus) and SARS-CoV-2 could be argued, given their potential impact on public health or the economy of a nation.

Briefly, the virus is grown in an appropriate cell line that is then mixed with water containing an organic load and the disinfectant under test. After the appropriate time, residual viral infectivity is determined using a tissue culture/plaque assay or other system (e.g., animal host or molecular assay for some specific viral component). Such procedures are costly and time-consuming, and must be appropriately controlled to exclude factors such as disinfectant killing of the cell system or test animal. A reduction of infectivity by a factor of 10^4 has been regarded as evidence of acceptable viricidal activity. The European Standard 14476:2013+A2:2019 specifies the minimum standards for viricidal activity of a chemical disinfectant, and applies to products used in the medical environment, including surface disinfection by spraying, wiping, flooding or other means, textile disinfection, hand sanitiser, hygienic handwashes and instrument disinfection by immersion. For viruses that cannot be grown in the laboratory (e.g., hepatitis B), naturally infected cells/tissues must be used. Further test procedures are detailed in British Standard BS EN 13610:2002 where the viricidal activity of chemical disinfectants used in food and industrial areas is evaluated against bacteriophages. The use of bacteriophage as a model virus in this procedure most likely reflects their ease of growth and survivor enumeration via standard plaque assay on host bacterial lawns grown on solid media.

19.3.3.3 Prion Disinfection Tests

Prions are a unique class of acellular, proteinaceous infectious agent (see Chapter 5), devoid of an agent-specific nucleic acid (DNA or RNA). Infection is associated with the abnormal isoform of a host cellular protein called prion protein (PrP^c). Prions exhibit unusually high resistance to conventional chemical and physical decontamination methods, presenting a unique challenge in infection control. Although numerous published studies on prion inactivation by disinfectants are available in the literature, inconsistencies in methodology make direct comparison difficult. For example, these variations include: strain differences of prion (with respect to sensitivity to thermal and chemical inactivation), prion concentration in tissue homogenate, exposure conditions and determination of log reductions from incubation period assays instead of end-point titrations. Furthermore, since most studies of prion inactivation have been conducted with tissue homogenates, the protective effect of the tissue components may sometimes be significant and thereby contribute to resistance to disinfection. Despite this, a reasonable characterisation of effective and ineffective agents has emerged and is summarised in Table 19.4. Although most disinfectants are inadequate for the elimination of prion infectivity, agents such as sodium hydroxide, a phenolic formulation, guanidine thiocyanate and chlorine have all been shown to have efficacy; further consideration can be found in Chapters 18 and 20.

19.4 Evaluation of Solid Disinfectants

Solid disinfectants usually consist of a disinfectant substance diluted by an inert powder. Phenolic substances adsorbed onto kieselguhr (diatomite) form the basis of many disinfectant powders; another widely used solid disinfectant is sodium dichloroisocyanurate. Other disinfectant or antiseptic powders used in medicine include acriflavine and compounds with antifungal activity such as zinc undecenoate or salicylic acid mixed with talc. These disinfectants may be evaluated by applying them to suitable test organisms growing on a solid agar medium. Discs may be cut from the agar and subcultured for enumeration of survivors. Inhibitory activity is evaluated by dusting the powders onto the surface of seeded agar plates, using the inert diluents as a control. The extent of growth is then observed following incubation.

19.5 Evaluation of Air Disinfectants

The decontamination and disinfection of air are important considerations for both infection and contamination control. A large number of important infectious diseases are spread via microbial contamination of the air. This cross-infection can occur in a variety of situations (hospitals and care facilities, airplanes, public and institutional buildings), while stringent control of air quality with respect to

Table 19.4 Efficacy of chemical agents in prion inactivation.

Ineffective (≤3 log10 reduction within 1 hour)	Effective (>3 log10 reduction within 1 hour at temperature 20–55 °C)
Acetone	Alkaline detergent (specific formulations)
Alcohol, 50–100%	Enzymatic detergent (specific formulation)
Ammonia, 1.0 M	Chlorine >1000 ppm
Alkaline detergent (specific formulations)	Copper, 0.5 mmol/l and H_2O_2, 100 mmol/l
Beta-propiolactone	Guanidine thiocyanate, >3 M
Chlorine dioxide, 50 ppm	Peracetic acid, 0.2%
Ethylene oxide	Phenolic disinfectant (specific formulation), >0.9%
Formaldehyde, 3.7%	QAC (specific formulation)
Glutaraldehyde, 5%	Hydrogen peroxide, 59%
Hydrochloric acid, 1.0 N	SDS, 2% and acetic acid, 1%
Hydrogen peroxide, 0.2–60%	Sodium hydroxide, ≥1 N
Iodine, 2%	Sodium hypochlorite, ≥2% (20,000 ppm) chlorine
Iodophors	Sodium metaperiodate, 0.01 M
Ortho-phthalaldehyde, 0.55%	
Peracetic acid, 0.2–19%	
Phenol/phenolics (concentration variable)	
Potassium permanganate, 0.1–0.8%	
QAC (specific formulation)	
Sodium dodecyl sulphate (SDS), 1–5%	
Sodium deoxycholate, 5%	
Sodium dichloroisocyanurate	
Enzymatic detergent (specific formulations)	
Triton X-100, 1%	
Urea, 4–8 M	

Processes may be listed in both columns (ineffective/effective), due to different testing parameters or testing methods. All experiments conducted without prior cleaning.
Source: Adapted from Rutala and Weber (2010).

airborne contaminants and particulates is critical for contamination control in many aseptic procedures. With the increasing public concern regarding the perceived heightened threat of bioterrorism, and transmission of pandemic viral agents including SARS-CoV-2, effective air disinfection procedures have gained heightened prominence as potential countermeasures to these significant threats to global public health. The microorganisms themselves may be contained in aerosols, including respiratory aerosols, or may occur as airborne particles liberated from some environmental source, for example, agitation of spore-laden bed linen or decaying organic matter. Disinfection of air can be carried out by filtration through high-efficiency particulate air (HEPA) filters, chemical aerosol/vapour/fumigation or by ultraviolet germicidal irradiation (UVGI). Increased airflow can aid the distribution of aerosolised disinfectant, and result in dilution of airborne microorganisms, thus acting as an adjunct to disinfection. Although UVGI disinfectant approaches have demonstrated efficacy against a range of airborne pathogens and contaminating organisms, it is often more practical to use some form of chemical vapour or aerosol to kill them. Formaldehyde vapour is a commonly employed agent for fumigation procedures (not strictly air disinfection), although vapourised hydrogen peroxide is increasingly used as an alternative agent. Due to the potential for formation of carcinogenic bis(chloromethyl) ether when used with hydrochloric acid and chlorine-containing disinfectants, formaldehyde should not be used in the presence of hypochlorites.

The work of Robert Koch in the late 1880s demonstrated that the numbers of viable bacteria present in air can be assessed by simply exposing plates of solid nutrient media to that air. Indeed, this same process is still exploited in environmental monitoring in the form of settle plates. Any bacteria that fall on to the plates after a suitable exposure time can then be detected following an appropriate period of incubation. These gravitational methods are obviously applicable to many microorganisms, but are unsuitable for viruses. However, more meaningful data can be obtained if force rather than gravity is used to collect airborne particles. A stream of air can be directed onto the surface of a nutrient agar plate (surface impaction; slit sampler) or bubbled through an appropriate buffer or culture medium (liquid impingement). Various commercial impactor samplers are available. Filtration sampling, where the air is passed through a porous membrane, which is then cultured, can also be used. For experimental evaluation of potential air disinfectants, bacterial or fungal airborne 'suspensions' can be created in a closed chamber, and then exposed to the disinfectant, which may be in the form of radiation, chemical vapour or aerosol. The airborne microbial population is then sampled at regular intervals using an appropriate forced-air apparatus such as the slit sampler. With viruses, the air can be bubbled through a suitable liquid medium, which is then subjected to some appropriate virological assay system. In all cases, problems arise in producing a suitable airborne microbial 'suspension' and in neutralising residual disinfectant, which may remain in the air.

19.6 Evaluation of Preservatives

Preservatives are widely employed in the cosmetic and pharmaceutical industries as well as in a variety of other manufacturing industries. The addition of preservatives to pharmaceutical formulations to prevent microbial growth and subsequent spoilage, to retard product deterioration and to restrain growth of contaminating microorganisms is commonplace for non-sterile pharmaceutical formulations as well as low-volume aseptically prepared formulations intended for multiple use from one container (see Chapter 17). Indeed, adequate preservation (and validation of effectiveness) is a legal requirement for certain formulations. Effective preservation prevents microbial and, as a consequence, related chemical, physical and aesthetic spoilage that could otherwise render the formulation unacceptable for patient use, therapeutically ineffective or harmful to the patient (due to the presence of toxic metabolites or microbial toxins). The factors which influence the activity of the antimicrobial agent when employed as a preservative are largely those which affect disinfectant activity (described in Section 19.2.4); however, when considering the activity of the agent, the interactions with formulation components (adsorption to suspended particles and oil–water partitioning, for instance; see also Chapter 17) should be considered as additional factors which can potentially attenuate the preservative activity.

While the inhibitory or cidal activity of the preservative chemical can be evaluated using an appropriate *in vitro* test system (see Sections 19.3.2.1 and 19.8.1.2), its continued activity when combined with the other ingredients in the final manufactured product must be established. Problems clearly exist with some products, where partitioning into various phases may result in the absence of preservative in one of the phases, for example, oil-in-water emulsions where the preservative may partition only into the oily phase, allowing any contaminant microorganisms to flourish in the aqueous phase. In addition, one or more of the components may inactivate the preservative. Consequently, suitably designed simulated use challenge tests involving the final product are, therefore, required in addition to direct potency testing of the pure preservative. In the challenge test, the final preserved product is deliberately inoculated with a suitable environmental microorganism which may be fungal (e.g., *C. albicans* or *A. brasiliensis*) or bacterial (e.g., *S. aureus*, *E. coli*, *P. aeruginosa*). For oral preparations with a high sucrose content, the British and European Pharmacopoeias include the osmophilic yeast *Zygosaccharomyces rouxii* as a recommended challenge organism. The subsequent survival (inhibition), death or growth of the inoculum is then assessed using viable count techniques. Different performance criteria are laid down for injectable and ophthalmic preparations, topical preparations and oral liquid preparations in the *British Pharmacopoeia* (Appendix XVI C) and the *European Pharmacopoeia*, which should be consulted for full details of the experimental procedures to be used. The United States Pharmacopeia (USP) specifies an additional category, antacids made with aqueous bases, with less-stringent preservative efficacy acceptance criteria, reflecting the unique challenges of adequately preserving aqueous formulations containing significant proportions (in % w/v) of suspended solids and high concentrations of divalent cations, Mg^{2+}, Ca^{2+} and Al^{3+}. In some instances, the range and/or spectrum of preservation can be extended by using more than one preservative at a time, and a number of synergistic preservative combinations have been described (see also Chapter 20). Thus, a combination of parabens (*p*-hydroxybenzoic acid) with varying water solubilities may protect both the aqueous and oil phases of an emulsion, while a combination of Germall 115 (an imidazolidinyl urea derivative) and parabens results in a preservative system with both antibacterial (Germall 115) and antifungal (parabens) activities.

19.7 Rapid Evaluation Procedures

In most of the tests mentioned above, results are not available until visible microbial growth occurs, at least in the controls. This usually takes 24 hours or more. The potential benefits of rapid antimicrobial susceptibility screening procedures are obvious, particularly in aggressive infections or rapidly progressing nosocomial infections of immunocompromised patients where appropriate antimicrobial selection is critical. To date, only a few rapid methods for detecting microbial viability or growth are presently employed in assessing the efficacy of antimicrobials. For the main, these rapid antimicrobial susceptibility tests (ASTs) have focused on rapid determination of the resistance profile of clinical pathogens, either through genotypic means (looking for the presence of specific resistance genes) or by phenotypic methods (including microscopy-based direct observation of response to antibiotics, or microscopy paired with microfluidics or other optical techniques). These latter approaches include epifluorescent and bioluminescence techniques. The former relies on the fact that when exposed to the vital stain acridine orange and viewed under UV light, viable cells fluoresce green or greenish yellow, while dead cells appear orange. Live/dead staining of sessile bacterial populations has the potential to yield important data with respect to antimicrobial susceptibility, but requires skilled personnel and specialised microscopy equipment.

With tests involving liquid systems, the early growth of viable cells can be assessed by some light-scattering processes; blood culture techniques have classically used the production of CO_2 as an indicator of bacterial metabolism and growth. In addition, the availability of molecular techniques, such as quantitative polymerase chain reaction (PCR), may be useful in demonstrating the presence or growth of microorganisms that are slow or difficult to culture under usual laboratory conditions, for example, viruses. This may obviate the need to neutralise residual disinfectant with some assays.

Rapid colourimetric assays for antimicrobial susceptibility have been developed including the commercially available VITEK2 system (BioMérieux) and colourimetric tests based on the extracellular reduction of tetrazolium salts 2-(2-methoxy-4-nitrophenyl)-3-(4-nitrophenyl)-5-(2,4-disulphophenyl)-2*H*-tetrazolium monosodium (WST-8) and 2,3-bis[2-methoxy-4-nitro-5-sulphophenyl]-2*H*-tetrazolium-5-carboxanilide (XTT). These latter studies have demonstrated the potential for the tetrazolium salts WST-8 and XTT to be used in the rapid, accurate and facile screening of antimicrobial susceptibility and MIC determination in a range of bacteria, including staphylococci, extended β-lactamase-producing clinical isolates (*E. coli*, *Enterococcus faecalis*) and *P. aeruginosa*. Using this method, MIC values in agreement with those obtained using standard methods can be obtained after just 5 hours. The application of matrix-assisted laser desorption ionisation-time-of-flight mass spectrometry (MALDI-TOF MS) has also become commonplace in clinical microbiology, and progress has been made in the use of this powerful technique not only in the rapid identification of clinically significant microorganisms, but in determination of antimicrobial susceptibility/resistance profiles.

In addition, signal amplification techniques employing time-resolved fluorescence or nucleic acid amplification technology (NAAT) have been described; however, the requirement for specific equipment and training, alongside the necessity to compare with real-time phenotypic characterisation, may limit the utility of such techniques in routine clinical microbiology laboratories. In general, however, approaches described in this section for rapid AST are of potential value in the rapid validation of microbicidal/disinfectant activity, but are not currently regarded as, or incorporated into, standard disinfectant methods.

19.8 Evaluation of Potential Chemotherapeutic Antimicrobials

Unlike tests for the evaluation of disinfectants, where determination of cidal activity is of paramount importance, tests involving potential chemotherapeutic agents (antibiotics) invariably have determination of MIC as their main focus. Tests for the bacteriostatic activity of antimicrobial agents are valuable tools in predicting antimicrobial sensitivity/tolerance in individual patient samples and for detection and monitoring of resistant bacteria. However, correlation between MIC and therapeutic outcome is frequently difficult to predict, especially in chronic biofilm-mediated infections. The determination of MIC values must be conducted under standardised conditions, since deviation from standard test conditions can result in considerable variation in data.

19.8.1 Tests for Bacteriostatic Activity

The historical gradient-plate, ditch-plate and cup-plate techniques (see earlier editions of this book) have been replaced by more quantitative techniques such as disc diffusion (Figure 19.4), broth and agar dilution and E-tests (Figure 19.5). All employ chemically defined media (e.g., Mueller–Hinton or Iso-Sensitest) at a pH of 7.2–7.4, and, in the case of solid media, agar plates of defined thickness. Regularly updated guidelines are provided by the Clinical & Laboratory Standards Institute (CLSI) (formerly the National Committee for Clinical Laboratory Standards [NCCLS]) and are widely used in many countries; historically, the British Society for Antimicrobial Chemotherapy

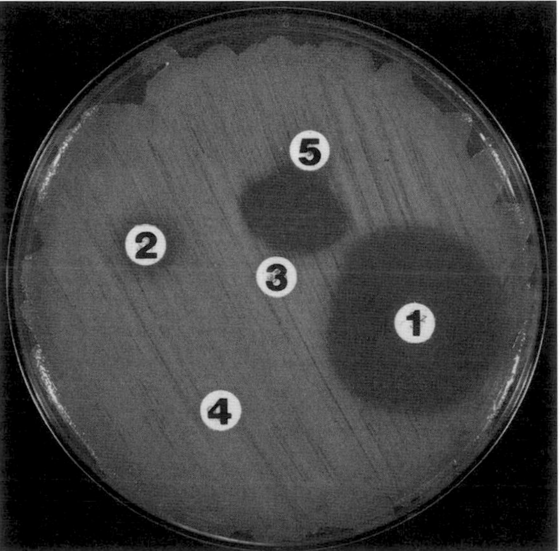

Figure 19.4 Disc test with inhibition zones around two (1, 2) of five discs. The zone around disc 1 is clear and easy to measure, whereas that around disc 2 is indistinct. Although none of the antimicrobials in discs 3, 4 or 5 appear to inhibit the bacterium, synergy (as evidenced by inhibition of growth between the discs) is evident with the antimicrobials in discs 3 and 5. Slight antagonism of the drug in disc 1 by that in disc 3 is evident by the slightly reduced zone of inhibition in proximity to disc 3.

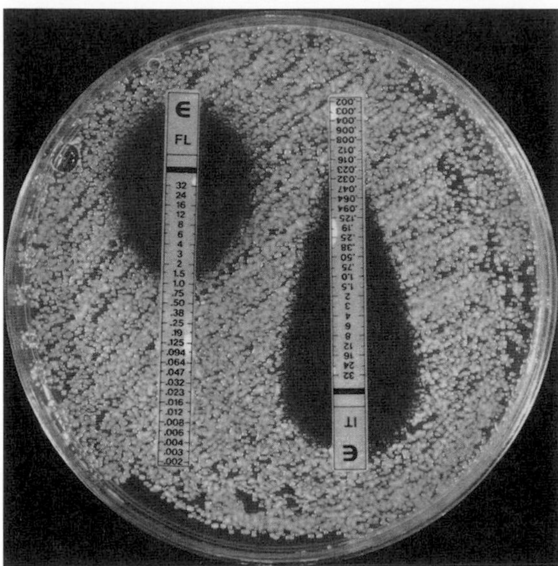

Figure 19.5 E-test on an isolate of *Candida albicans*. Inhibition zone edges are distinct and the MICs for itraconazole (IT) and fluconazole (FL) (0.064 and 1.5 mg l^{-1}, respectively) are easily decipherable.

has produced its own guidelines and testing procedures (e.g., see Howe and Andrews 2012), but has in recent years played an essential role in the European Committee on Antimicrobial Susceptibility Testing (EUCAST) to harmonise break-point data, develop methodology and standardise susceptibility testing throughout Europe.

19.8.1.1 Disc Tests

These are really modifications of the earlier cup- or ditch-plate procedures where filter-paper discs impregnated with the antimicrobial replace the antimicrobial-filled cups or wells. For disc tests, standard suspensions (e.g., 0.5 McFarland standard – this is a measure of the concentration of a microbial population based on optical density) of cells harvested in the log-phase of growth are prepared and inoculated on to the surface of appropriate agar plates to form a lawn. Commercially available filter-paper discs containing known concentrations of antimicrobial agent (it is possible to prepare your own discs for use with novel drugs) are then placed on the dried lawn and the plates are incubated aerobically at 35 °C for 18 hours. The density of bacteria inoculated on to the plate should produce just confluent growth after incubation for that period. Any zone of inhibition occurring around the disc is then measured and, after comparison with known standards, the bacterium under test is identified as susceptible or resistant to that particular antibiotic. For novel agents, these sensitivity parameters are only available after extensive clinical investigations have been correlated with laboratory-generated data. Disc tests are basically qualitative; however, the diameter of the zone of inhibition may be correlated to MIC determination through a linear regression analysis (Figure 19.6).

Although subtle variations of the disc test are used in some countries, the basic principles behind the tests remain similar, and are based on the original work of Bauer and colleagues (Kirby–Bauer method). Some techniques employ a control bacterial isolate on each plate so that comparisons between zone sizes around the test and control bacterium can be ascertained (i.e., a disc potency control). Provided that discs are maintained and handled as recommended by the manufacturer, the value of such controls becomes debatable and probably unnecessary. Control strains of bacteria are available which should have inhibition zones of a given diameter with stipulated antimicrobial discs. Use of such controls endorses the suitability of the methods (e.g., medium, inoculum density, incubation conditions) employed. For slow-growing microorganisms, the incubation period can be extended. Problems arise with disc tests where the inoculum density is inappropriate (e.g., too low, resulting in an indistinct edge to the inhibition zone following incubation), or where the edge is obscured by the sporadic growth of cells within the inhibition zone, that is, the initial inoculum although pure contains cells expressing varying levels of susceptibility – so-called *heterogeneity*. As the distance from the disc increases, there is a logarithmic reduction in the antimicrobial concentration; the result is that small differences in zone diameter with antimicrobials (e.g., vancomycin) which diffuse poorly through solid media may represent significantly different MICs. Possible synergistic or antagonistic combinations of antimicrobials can often be detected using disc tests (Figure 19.4).

19.8.1.2 Dilution Tests

These usually employ liquid media but can be modified to use solid media. Doubling dilutions, usually in the range 0.008–256 mg l^{-1} of the antimicrobial under test, are prepared in a suitable broth medium and an aliquot of log-phase cells is added to each dilution to result in a final cell density of around 5×10^5 CFU ml^{-1}. After incubation at 35 °C for 18 hours, the concentration of antimicrobial contained in the first clear tube is read as the MIC. Needless to say, dilution tests require a number of controls, for example, sterility control, growth control and the simultaneous testing of a bacterial strain with known MIC to show that the dilution series is correct. End points with dilution tests are usually sharp and easily defined, although 'skipped' wells (inhibition in a well with growth either side) and 'trailing' (a gradual reduction in growth over a series of wells) may be encountered. The latter is especially evident with antifungal tests (see below). Nowadays, the dilution

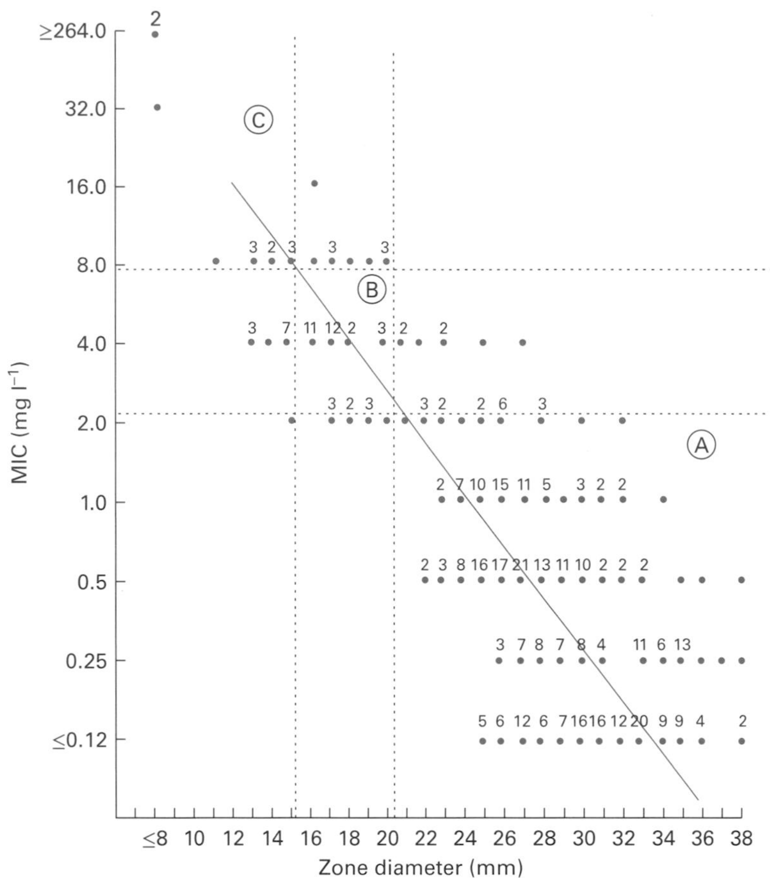

Figure 19.6 A scattergram and regression line analysis correlating zone diameters and MICs. The break points of susceptible (MIC ≤ 2.0 mg l^{-1}, zone diameter ≥ 21 mm) and resistant (MIC ≥ 8.0 mg l^{-1}, zone ≤ 15 mm) bacteria are shown by the dotted lines. For a complete correlation between MICs and zone diameter, all susceptible, intermediate and resistant isolates should fall in boxes A, B and C, respectively. Errors (correlations outside these boxes) occur. *Source:* Courtesy of Dr. Z. Hashmi.

test for established antimicrobials has been simplified by the commercial availability of 96-well microtitre plates which have appropriate antimicrobial dilutions frozen or lyophilised onto wells in the plate. The appropriate antibacterial suspension (in 200–400 μl volumes) is simply added to each well, the plate is incubated as before, and the MIC is read.

Dilution tests can also be carried out using a series of agar plates containing known antimicrobial concentrations. Appropriate bacterial suspensions are inoculated on to each plate and the presence or absence of growth is recorded after suitable incubation. Most clinical laboratories now employ agar dilution break-point testing methods. These are essentially truncated agar dilution MIC tests employing only a small range of antimicrobial concentrations around the critical susceptible/resistant cut-off levels. Many automated identification and sensitivity testing machines now use a liquid (broth) variant of the agar break-point procedure. Similar break-point antimicrobial concentrations are used with thc presence or absence of growth being recorded by some automated procedure (e.g., light-scattering, colour change) after a suitable incubation period.

19.8.1.3 E-tests

Perhaps the most convenient and presently accepted method of determining bacterial MICs, however, is the E (epsilometer)-test. The concept and execution of the E-test are similar to the disc diffusion test except that a linear gradient of lyophilised antimicrobial in twofold dilutions on nylon carrier strips on one side is used instead of the filter-paper impregnated antimicrobial discs. On the other side of the nylon strip are a series of graduated lines and figures denoting MIC values (Figure 19.5). The nylon strips are placed antimicrobial-side down on the freshly prepared bacterial lawn and, after incubation, the MIC is determined by noting where the ellipsoid (pear-shaped) inhibition zone crosses the strip (Figure 19.5). For most microorganisms, there appears to be excellent correlation between dilution and E-test MIC results. As with standard disc diffusion tests, resistant strains may be isolated from within the zone of inhibition.

19.8.1.4 Problematic Bacteria

With some of the emerging antimicrobial-resistant bacterial pathogens, for example, vancomycin-resistant enterococci (VRE), methicillin-resistant *S. aureus* (MRSA), vancomycin-intermediate *S. aureus* (VISA), the standard methodology described above may fail to detect the resistant phenotype. This is due to a variety of factors including heterogeneous expression of resistance (e.g., MRSA, VISA), poor agar diffusion of the antimicrobial (e.g., vancomycin) and slow growth of resistant cells (e.g., VISA). Disc tests are unsuitable for VRE, which should have MICs determined by E-test or dilution techniques. With MRSA, a heavier inoculum should be used in tests and 2–4% additional salt (NaCl) included in the medium with incubation for a full 48 hours. Reducing the incubation temperature to 30 °C may also facilitate detection of the true MIC value. Although 100% of MRSA cells may contain resistance genes, the phenotype may only be evident in a small percentage of cells under the usual conditions employed in sensitivity tests. Expression is enhanced at lower temperatures and at higher salt concentrations. With VISA, MIC determinations require incubation for a full 24 hours or more because of the slower growth rate of resistant cells.

19.8.2 Tests for Bactericidal Activity

MBC testing is required for the evaluation of novel antimicrobials. The MBC is the lowest concentration (in mg l^{-1}) of antimicrobial that results in 99.9% or more killing of the bacterium under test. The 99.9% cut-off is an arbitrary *in vitro* value with 95% confidence limits that has uncertain clinical relevance. MBCs are determined by spreading 0.1 ml (100 µl) volumes of all clear (no growth) tubes from a dilution MIC test onto separate agar plates (residual antimicrobial in the 0.1 ml sample is 'diluted' out over the plate). After incubation at 35 °C overnight (or longer for slow-growing bacteria), the numbers of colonies growing on each plate are recorded. The first concentration of drug that produces <50 colonies after subculture is considered the MBC. This is based on the fact that with MICs, the initial bacterial inoculum should result in about 5×10^5 CFU ml^{-1}. Inhibition, but not killing of this inoculum, should therefore result in the growth of 50,000 bacteria from the 0.1 ml sample. A 99.9% (3-log) kill would result in no more than 50 colonies on the subculture plate. With most modern antibacterial drugs, the concentration that inhibits growth is very close to the concentration that produces death, for example, within one or two dilutions. In general, only MICs are determined for such drugs.

19.8.3 Tests for Fungistatic and Fungicidal Activities

As fungi have become more prominent human pathogens, techniques for investigating the susceptibility of isolates to the growing number of antifungal agents have been developed. These have been largely based on the established bacterial techniques (disc, dilution, E-test) mentioned above, with the proviso that the medium used is different (e.g., use of RPMI 1640 plus 2% dextrose) and that the inoculum density (yeast cells or spores) used is reduced (approximately 10^4 CFU ml^{-1}). With yeast disc and E-tests, a lawn producing just separated/distinct colonies is preferable to confluent growth (see Figure 19.5). Addition of methylene blue (0.5 mg ml^{-1}) to media may improve the clarity of inhibition zone edges. Problems of 'tailing' or 'trailing' in dilution tests, and indistinct inhibition zone edges, are often seen in tests involving azoles and yeasts and appear in some way related to the type of buffer employed in the growth medium. However, their presence has prompted studies into evaluating the use of other techniques as indicators of significant fungistasis, for example, 50% reduction in growth (rather than complete inhibition) as the end point, use of a dye (e.g., Alamar blue) colour change to indicate growth and sterol (ergosterol, a fungal cell wall component) quantitation. Most of these are presently outside the scope of most routine laboratories.

As with MBC estimations, MFC evaluation is an extension of the MIC test. The reference method for broth dilution antifungal susceptibility testing of filamentous fungi is published by the CLSI, as approved standard M38-A2. At the completion of the MIC test (e.g., 72 hours for filamentous fungi), 20 µl are subcultured on to a suitable growth medium from each optically clear microtitre tray well and the growth control well. These plates are then incubated at 35 °C until growth is evident on the growth control subculture (24–48 hours). The MFC is the lowest drug concentration showing no growth or fewer than three colonies per plate to obtain approximately 99–99.5% killing activity.

19.8.4 Evaluation of Possible Synergistic Antimicrobial Combinations

The potential interaction between two antimicrobials can be demonstrated using a variety of laboratory procedures, for example, 'chequerboard' MIC assays where the microorganism is exposed to varying dilutions of each drug alone and in combination, disc diffusion tests (see Figure 19.4) and kinetic kill curve assays. With the former, results can be plotted in the form of a figure called an *isobologram* (see Figure 19.7).

19.8.4.1 Kinetic Kill Curves

In the case of kill curves, the microorganism is inoculated into tubes containing a single concentration of each antimicrobial alone, the same concentrations of each antimicrobial in combination and no antimicrobial – that is, four tubes. All tubes are then incubated and viable counts are performed at regular intervals on each system. With results

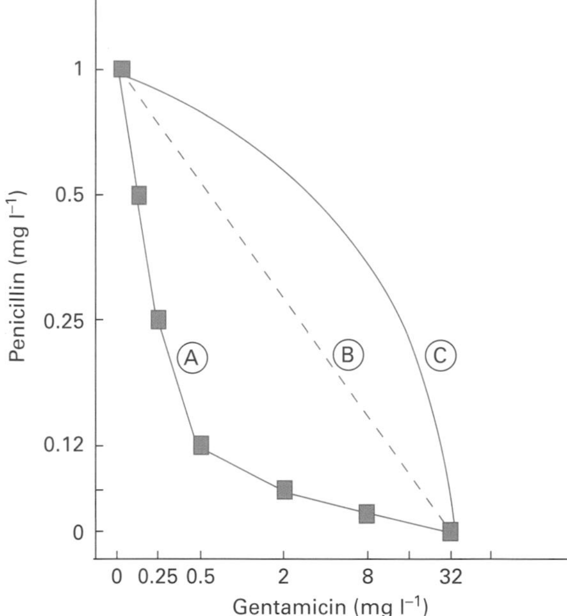

Figure 19.7 Diagrammatic representation of MIC values obtained with two synergistic antimicrobials, penicillin and gentamicin. The resulting graph or isobologram (A) is obtained by linking MIC values for each drug alone and in various dilution combinations. The MIC values for penicillin and gentamicin alone are 1.0 and 32 mg l^{-1}, respectively. The slope of the isobologram for purely additive or antagonistic combinations is shown by B and C, respectively.

plotted on semilogarithmic paper, synergy is defined as a greater than 100-fold increase in killing of the combination compared with either drug alone. Antagonism is defined as at least a 100-fold decrease in killing of the combination when compared with the most active agent alone, while an additive or autonomous combined effect results in a less than 10-fold change from that seen with the most active single drug. Both chemotherapeutic agents and disinfectants are amenable to kill curve assays.

19.9 Tests for Biofilm Susceptibility

As discussed in Chapter 8 and earlier in this chapter, biofilms present an additional challenge to antimicrobial testing, as the biofilm may be tolerant to more than 1000 times the planktonic MIC of that antimicrobial. Antimicrobial testing of biofilms under standardised conditions has really only become established since 1999 and the development of the MBEC assay (Calgary Biofilm Device). Previous techniques for biofilm susceptibility testing suffered from a lack of replicates, as in the case of flow cell technology, or the need for continuous pumping of fluids and bacteria that presented a leakage and contamination risk that was not tolerable in a diagnostic laboratory. Forming biofilms directly in 96-well plates provided replicate numbers, but in this assay system the initial inoculum could not be calculated and the efficacy of treatment was based not on viable cell counts but on a dye absorbance assay that could be measuring a change in extracellular matrix rather than a change in viable bacterial cell number. The MBEC assay placed pegs protruding from the lid of the plate into each well of a 96-well plate. Shear force created by gyration of the plate initiated bacterial adhesion to the peg and subsequent biofilm formation, the density of which could be determined by sonication of the biofilm back into a suspension culture and enumeration of viable cell number by standard plate counts. The peg-borne biofilms could then be used as a biofilm inoculation in a standard 96-well MIC assay, only in this case the susceptibility of a biofilm rather than a planktonic population would be determined. Following antimicrobial exposure bacteria would again be sonicated from the pegs and counted to determine the biofilm MIC (BMIC), biofilm bactericidal concentration (BMBC) and biofilm eradication concentration (MBEC) in a highly standardised and reproducible assay based on existing MIC technology. The MBEC assay forms the basis of ASTM E2799, a standard disinfectant efficacy test method against *P. aeruginosa* biofilms. Mycobacteria and fungi can be assayed using a similar format allowing the biofilm susceptibility of these organisms to be tested.

The increasing interest in biofilm research generally has led to a significant growth in published literature on biofilm experimental methods and assessment of biofilm antimicrobial susceptibility; this has made reproducibility, consistency and method harmonisation a significant challenge. In an attempt to address this critical gap in the biofilm research field, a consortium of leading biofilm researchers has published guidance on reporting experiments involving microbial biofilms (Lourenço et al. 2014). The report defines the minimum information that needs to be specified in conducting a biofilm experiment. This guidance is based around a series of modules covering: sample generation and study design; naturally occurring biofilms and *in vitro*, *ex vivo* and *in vivo* biofilm models; determination of antimicrobial susceptibility; culture- and non-culture-based biofilm assessment including microscopy and flow cytometry methods, spectrophotometric detection methods, 'omics' and molecular methods; statistical assessment; and bioinformatic resources and tools. These minimum information standards are expected to harmonise methods and vocabularies, simplify exchange and comparison of biofilm data between laboratories and decrease the variability of results obtained from biofilm studies.

In parallel, and over the past two decades, a number of published standard biofilm methods have been developed by ASTM International, formerly the American Society for Testing and Materials, including E2196, E2562, E2647, E2799, E2871 and E3321. The overarching standard guide E1427 for selecting test methods to determine the effectiveness of antimicrobial agents and other chemicals for the prevention, inactivation and removal of biofilm provides guidance on the methods used for biofilm formation and measurement, and is a teaching guide for researchers planning studies in biofilm control, enabling further standard method development.

19.9.1 Synergy Biofilm Assays

The reduced susceptibility of biofilms to antimicrobials often results in the effective *in vitro* drug concentration far exceeding a safe or achievable dose. Consequently, combinations of antimicrobial drugs or drugs and other cofactors are frequently proving to be more effective against biofilms than single drug therapies. Synergies in biofilm testing have been defined using formulae based on the American Society for Microbiology standards. The calculation of synergy, as mathematically defined in Harrison et al. (2008), is based on the sum of the fractional bactericidal concentration (FBC) values or FBC indices for each agent in a combination of antimicrobial agents. Therefore, in a two-component assay of agents A and B, synergy would be defined as follows (where the minimum bactericidal concentration for the biofilm is MBC_b):

$$\text{FBC agent A} = \frac{\text{MBC}_\text{b} \text{ of agent A in combination}}{\text{MBC}_\text{b} \text{ of agent A alone}} \tag{19.7}$$

$$\text{FBC agent B} = \frac{\text{MBC}_\text{b} \text{ of agent B in combination}}{\text{MBC}_\text{b} \text{ of agent B alone}} \tag{19.8}$$

$$\sum \text{FBC} = \text{FBC agent A} + \text{FBC agent B} \tag{19.9}$$

As is also the case for planktonic organisms (see above), synergy against biofilms is a much sought-after outcome and its basis may ultimately prove to be a complex interplay between the individual modes of action of antimicrobial agents, their formulation components and the specific survival strategies of the target microbes or microbial systems.

Acknowledgement

The authors gratefully acknowledge Prof Howard Ceri who contributed to this chapter in the previous edition of this book.

References

Barker, J., Brown, M.R.W., Collier, P.J. et al. (1992). Relationship between *Legionella pneumophila* and *Acanthamoeba polyphaga*: physiological status and susceptibility to chemical inactivation. *Appl. Environ. Microbiol.* 58: 2420–2425.

Harrison, J.J., Turner, R.J., Joo, D.A. et al. (2008). Copper and quaternary ammonium cations exert synergistic bactericidal and antibiofilm activity against *Pseudomonas aeruginosa*. *Antimicrob. Agents Chemother.* 52 (8): 2870–2881.

Howe, R.A. and Andrews, J.M. (2012). BSAC standardized disc diffusion susceptibility testing method (version 11). *J. Antimicrob. Chemother.* 67: 2783–2784.

Johnston, M.D., Simons, E.-A. and Lambert, R.J.W. (2000). One explanation for the variability of the bacterial suspension test. *J. Appl. Microbiol.* 88: 237–242.

Kelsey, J.C. and Maurer, I.M. (1974). An improved Kelsey-Sykes test for disinfectants. *Pharm. J.* 30: 528–530.

Lourenço, A., Coenye, T., Goeres, D. et al. (2014). Minimum information about a biofilm experiment (MIABiE): standards for reporting experiments and data on sessile microbial communities living at interfaces. *Pathog. Dis.* 70: 250–256.

Russell, A.D., Furr, J.R. and Maillard, J.-Y. (1997). Microbial susceptibility and resistance to biocides. *ASM News* 63: 481–487.

Rutala, W.A. and Weber, D.J. (2010). Guideline for disinfection and sterilization of prion-contaminated medical instruments. *Infect. Control Hosp Epidemiol.* 31 (2): 107–117.

Further Reading

AOAC Official Methods: 955.17-1955 *Fungicidal Activity of Disinfectants*. Gaithersburg, MD: AOAC International.

Arduino, M.J. and McDonnell, G. (2019). Disinfection and sterilization. In: *Manual of Clinical Microbiology*, 12e (ed. K.C. Carroll, M.A. Pfaller, M.L. Landry, et al.), 224–242. Washington, DC: ASM Press.

ASTM International Standards, Pennsylvania (formerly the American Society for Testing and Materials): E2196,

Standard Test Method for Quantification of Pseudomonas aeruginosa Biofilm Grown with Medium Shear and Continuous Flow Using Rotating Disk Reactor (2002); E2562, a similarly titled method using the CDC biofilm reactor (2007); E2647, employing the drip-flow reactor (2008); E2799, *Standard Test Method for Testing Disinfectant Efficacy against Pseudomonas aeruginosa Biofilm using the MBEC Assay* (2011); E2871, *Standard Test Method for Determining Disinfectant Efficacy Against Biofilm Grown in the CDC Biofilm Reactor Using the Single Tube Method* (2013); and E3321, a standard method for evaluation of urinary catheter biofilm formation (2021).

British Standards: BS 6905:1987, *Method for Estimation of Concentration of Disinfectants Used in 'Dirty' Conditions in Hospitals by the Modified Kelsey Sykes Test;* BS EN 13610:2002, *Chemical Disinfectants. Quantitative Suspension Test for the Evaluation of Virucidal Activity Against Bacteriophages of Chemical Disinfectants Used in Food and Industrial Areas. Test Method and Requirements (Phase 2, Step 1);* BS EN 1276:2019, *Chemical Disinfectants and Antiseptics. Quantitative Suspension Test for the Evaluation of Bactericidal Activity of Chemical Disinfectants Used in Food, Industrial, Domestic and Institutional Areas. Test Method and Requirements (Phase 2, Step 1).* British Standards Institute, London.

British Pharmacopoeia (2021). The Stationery Office, London.

Clinical and Laboratory Standards Institute (2008). *Document M38-A2, Reference Method for Broth Dilution Antifungal Susceptibility Testing of Filamentous Fungi: Approved Standard*, 2e. Philadelphia: CLSI.

European Pharmacopoeia (2021) EP Secretariat, Strasbourg.

European Standards (EN): technical standards drafted and maintained by the European Committee for Standardization (CEN, Brussels). Relevant standards are referenced in the text by their EN number and identified by a date where revised.

Grinshpun, S.A., Buttner, M.P., Mainelis, G. and Willeke, K. (2016). Sampling for airborne microorganisms. In: *Manual of Environmental Microbiology*, 4e (ed. M.V. Yates, C.H. Nakatsu, R.V. Miller and S.D. Pillai), 3.2.2-1–3.2.2-17. Washington, DC: ASM Press.

Kim, J.-S., Chowdhury, N., Yamasaki, R. and Wood, T.K. (2018). Viable but non-culturable and persistence describe the same bacterial stress state. *Environ. Microbiol.* 20 (6): 2038–2048.

Maillard, J.-Y. (2020). Chapter 4, Bacterial resistance to biocides. Part II fundamental principles of activity. In: *Blocks' Disinfection, Sterilization and Preservation*, 6e (ed. G. McDonnell and J. Hansen), 44–67. Philadelphia: Wolters Kluwer.

Noel, D.J., Keevil, C.W. and Wilks, S.A. (2021). Synergism versus Additivity: Defining the Interactions between Common Disinfectants. *mBio* 12 (5): e02281–21.

Procop, G.W., Church, D.L., Hall, G.S. et al. (2017). *Koneman's Color Atlas and Textbook of Diagnostic Microbiology*, 7e. Philadelphia, PA: Lippincott, Williams & Wilkins.

20

Microbicides: Mode of Action and Resistance

Stephen P. Denyer[1] *and Jean-Yves Maillard*[2]

[1] *Emeritus Professor of Pharmacy, Universities of Brighton and Sussex, Brighton, UK*
[2] *Professor of Pharmaceutical Microbiology, School of Pharmacy and Pharmaceutical Sciences, Cardiff University, Cardiff, UK*

CONTENTS

20.1 Introduction

The group of non-antibiotic agents which comprises antiseptics, disinfectants, chemical sterilants and preservatives (often collectively called either microbicides or biocides) has a long history of use for preventing or controlling infection in healthcare and for reducing spoilage in many other applications. These agents have frequently been classified as non-specific protoplasmic poisons contrasting them with antibiotics which are considered to have specific sites of action. Such a broad generalisation is, however, far from the true position.

Hugo and Russell's Pharmaceutical Microbiology, Ninth Edition. Edited by Brendan F. Gilmore and Stephen P. Denyer.

Companion website: https://www.wiley.com/go/HugoandRussells9e

It is often convenient to consider the modes of action of microbicides in terms of their targets within the bacterial cell, in particular the region of the cell in which their activity is deemed to predominate. Thus, agents have been described variously as cell-wall-active, membrane-active or cytoplasm-active. This characterisation, while having the benefits of simplicity, does not necessarily describe their mechanism of action; this is best classified by effects on functional structures and cellular processes. The range and complexity of the reactions involved will become apparent from this account and Table 20.1, and it is worth emphasising here that many of these substances exhibit concentration-dependent dual or even multiple effects. Generally speaking, where a specific agent is employed in more than one application, a progressive increase in concentration is required in moving from preservative and antiseptic action to disinfection and sterilisation. It is worth noting that these agents are often employed in complex formulations for specific uses (e.g., surface disinfection, skin disinfection) and chosen excipients might have an impact on the overall efficacy of the formulation. More detailed treatments of the subject will be found in the references at the end of this chapter.

20.2 Mechanisms of Interaction

For a chemical to exhibit antimicrobial activity, it usually has to undergo a sequence of events that begins with adsorption on to the microbial cell surface. This initial uptake is a physicochemical phenomenon which can be generally characterised into one of several uptake isotherms (Figure 20.1); it bears a relationship to the concentration exponent (see Chapter 19) which describes the influence of concentration on activity (Table 20.2). In the many cases where the agent has an intracellular site of action, adsorption must be followed by passage through porin channels in Gram-negative cells (see Chapter 3), diffusion across, or into, the lipid-rich cytoplasmic membrane and finally, interaction with proteins, enzymes, nucleic acids or other targets within the cytoplasm. These processes are markedly influenced by the physicochemical characteristics of the microbicide, for example, ionisation constant and lipid solubility, so the wide diversity of structures exhibited by microbicide molecules (see Chapter 18) complicates the prediction of antimicrobial potency and explanation of their mechanisms of action. It is also worth noting that some microbicides are highly reactive with their target sites (e.g., alkylating agents: glutaraldehyde, *ortho*-phthalaldehyde; oxidising agent: hydrogen peroxide), and as such their concentration will be depleted rapidly, hindering their penetration into the target cell. Despite this, it is important to recognise that there is a basis upon which the mode of action might be deduced, because there are certain molecular features of microbicides that are associated with activity against particular cellular targets.

20.3 Antimicrobial Effects

Antimicrobial activity is often strongly influenced by the affinity of the microbicide for structural or molecular components of the cell, and this, in turn, may depend upon the attraction of dissimilar charges or on hydrophobic interactions. Microbicides whose active species is positively charged, for example, quaternary ammonium compounds (QACs) and biguanides, display an affinity for the negative charges of sugar residues on the microbial cell surface or phosphate groups on the membrane(s); adsorption of these microbicides, and thus their antimicrobial activity, is increased as the pH rises and the cell surface becomes more electronegative. Microbicides possessing a long alkyl chain, on the other hand, may integrate into the hydrophobic region of phospholipid molecules within the membrane and so cause membrane disruption and fatal permeability changes. Further examples of structure–activity relationships are afforded by aldehydes, particularly glutaraldehyde, which is an electrophile that is able to react with molecules possessing thiol (SH) or amino groups, for example, proteins. This reaction, too, increases with pH, so aldehydes are more active in alkaline conditions. Microbicides containing heavy metal ions, for example, silver or mercury, also damage or inactivate enzymes and structural proteins by virtue of interactions with thiol groups. A number of phenols and bisphenols incorporate a hydroxyl group that is capable of generating a labile proton, that is, they are weak acids. A weakly acidic nature, when combined with significant lipid solubility, are properties associated with uncoupling agents, that is, those molecules that can disrupt the proton-motive force that is responsible for oxidative phosphorylation in the cell. It is thought that these molecules dissolve in the lipid bilayer of the membrane and act as proton conductors by virtue of their ionisability (Section 20.4.4.2). This property, possessed by microbicides such as phenoxyethanol and fentichlor, results in the failure of many important energy-requiring processes in the cell, including the concentration and retention of sugars and amino acids.

20.4 Mechanisms of Action

In any consideration of mechanism of action, due regard should be given to the initial health of the organism, duration of contact with the microbicide and the concentration

Table 20.1 Primary cellular targets for selected microbicides.

Target site	Microbicide								
	Alcohols	Anilides (TCS, TCC)	Bronopol	Biguanides (chlorhexidine, PHMB)	Ethylene/ propylene oxide	Formaldehyde	Glutaraldehyde	Hexachlorophane	Hydrogen peroxide, peracetic acid
Cell wall						+	+		
Cytoplasmic membrane									
Action on membrane potentials		+						+	
Action on membrane-associated enzymes					++		++		+
Electron transport chain								+	
Adenosine triphosphatase				+					
Enzymes with thiol groups			+		+		++		+
Action on general membrane integrity	+	+		+					
Cytoplasm									
General denaturation/ coagulation	+++			+++			++	+++	
Ribosomes									+
Nucleic acids					+				+
Thiol groups			+		+		+		+
Amino groups					+	++	+		+

(Continued)

Table 20.1 (Continued)

Target site	Microbicide								
	Hypochlorites, chlorine-releasers	Isothiazolones	Mercury II salts, organic mercurials	*Ortho*-phthalaldehyde	Parabens	Phenols	β-propiolactone	QACs	Silver salts
Cell wall	+		+			+			
Cytoplasmic membrane									
Action on membrane potentials					+	+			
Action on membrane-associated enzymes	+			++					
Electron transport chain									
Adenosine triphosphatase									
Enzymes with thiol groups	+	+	+	++			+		+
Action on general membrane integrity					+	++		+	
Cytoplasm									
General denaturation/coagulation			+++	+++		+++		+++	+++
Ribosomes			+						
Nucleic acids	+						+		
Thiol groups	+		+	++			+		+
Amino groups	+			+					

Crosses, indicating activity, which appear in several rows for a given compound, demonstrate the multiple actions for the compound concerned. This activity is nearly always concentration-dependent, and the number of crosses indicates the order of concentration at which the effect is elicited, that is, +, elicited at low concentrations, +++, elicited at high concentrations. QACs, quaternary ammonium compounds; PHMB, polyhexamethylene biguanides; TCS, tetrachlorosalicylanilide; TCC, trichlorocarbanilide.

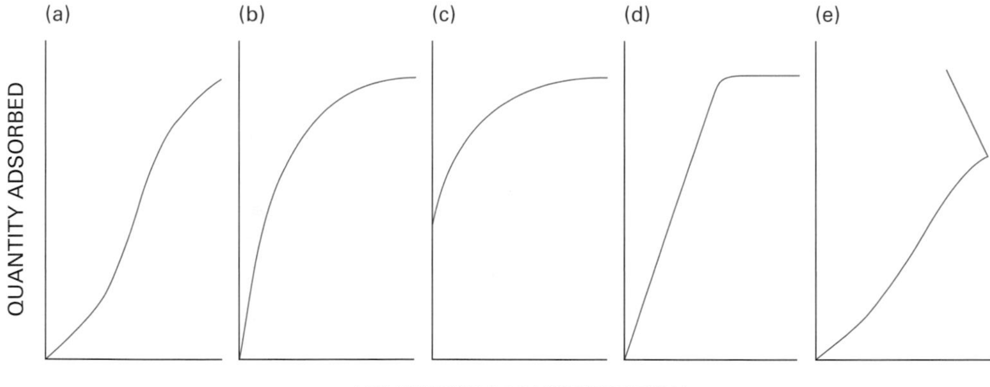

Figure 20.1 Typical uptake isotherms associated with the initial microbicide–bacterium interaction. (a) S-shape, cooperative sorption occurs as applied microbicide concentration increases; (b) L-shape, Langmuir uptake with microbicide molecules orientated at a fixed number of binding sites; (c) H-shape, special form of the L-shape isotherm indicative of high-affinity uptake; (d) C-shape, constant partition of microbicide from solution until bacterial surface is fully saturated; (e) Z-shape, enhanced uptake following breakdown in cell structure at a critical applied microbicide concentration.

Table 20.2 Relationship between microbicide concentration exponent, uptake isotherm and mechanism of interaction.

Concentration exponent	Predominant uptake isotherm	Type of interaction
<2.0	H or L-shape	Strong chemical or ionic bonding with target site, frequently promoting cytoplasm leakage or membrane disruption; uptake limited by binding sites available. Typical examples include QACs and chlorhexidine
2.0–4.0	S-shape	Initial microbicide uptake enhanced by cooperative adsorption, often with specific orientation of adsorbed molecules. Represented by a mixed group of microbicides typically exercising both chemical and physical effects on cellular components; examples include some phenols and lipophilic acids
>4.0	C, S or Z-shape	Weakly physical interaction, often with partition into lipophilic components of the cell envelope; a plateau in uptake can be reached when the envelope is fully saturated, although new sorption sites may be generated with some microbicides at a critical applied concentration (Z shape). Typical examples include phenols and 2-phenoxyethanol which are active as membrane disruptors and proton conductors

of microbicide employed. Antibacterial effects may progress from early, sublethal events to multiple lesions of bactericidal consequence. Figure 20.2 identifies events in order of severity, but should not be interpreted as defining the normal progression of cell injury. As disclosed in the following sections, the microbicide interaction may induce particular lesions over others; this will most certainly be in a concentration-dependent manner.

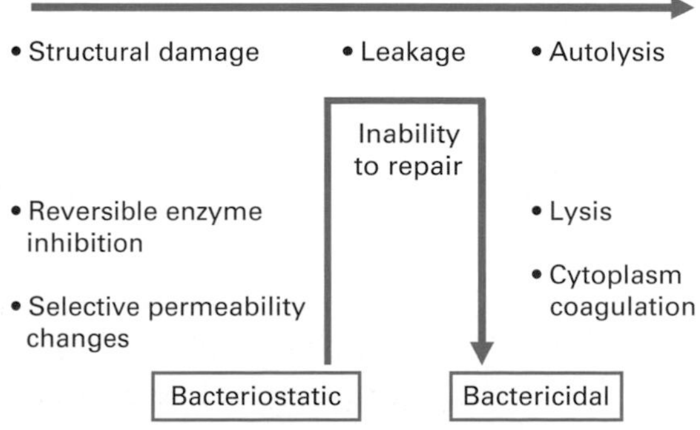

Figure 20.2 Antibacterial events: progression from bacteriostatic to bactericidal lesions.

20.4.1 Oxidation Reactions

Microbicides with oxidising (electron-withdrawing) ability are widely used as disinfectants and chemical sterilants, and include the halogens (chlorine, hypochlorites, bromine, iodophors) and peroxygens (hydrogen peroxide, peracetic acid and chlorine dioxide). They can exert specific effects on essential microbial macromolecules causing, variously: strand breakage and adduct formation on DNA and RNA with disruption of replication, transcription and translocation processes; oxidation of, particularly, unsaturated fatty acids leading to loss of membrane fluidity and subsequent reduced functionality of membrane-bound proteins; and specific modifications to amino acid residues, most notably disulphide bonds, leading to changes in protein primary structure and conformation with consequent disruption of structural enzymic functions. An accumulation of these effects can be particularly devastating to the microbial cell.

20.4.2 Cross-linking Reactions

The aldehydes (formaldehyde, glutaraldehyde and *ortho*-phthalaldehyde) and the sterilant alkylating agents (ethylene oxide and propylene oxide) are both highly reactive chemical classes. The alkylating agents exhibit particularly strong reactions with guanine residues causing cross-linking between DNA strands, inhibiting DNA unwinding and RNA translation. The amino, carboxyl, sulphydryl and hydroxyl groups of structural or enzymic proteins are also susceptible to alkylation, causing cross-links between adjacent amino acid chains and also with other amino-acid-containing structures such as peptidoglycan. The aldehydes are generally more specific with greatest effect against the amino groups of surface-exposed lysine or hydroxylysine residues of proteins, again causing extensive cross-linking.

In all instances, progressive cross-linking leads to macromolecule malfunction causing inhibition or arrest of essential cell functions. It is safe to say that there is no single fatal reaction, but that death results from the accumulated effect of many reactions in a manner similar to oxidising agents (Section 20.4.1).

20.4.3 Coagulation

The cross-linking reactions identified in Section 20.4.2 give rise to macromolecule denaturation which can be recognised under electron microscopy as intracellular coagulation. Coagulative effects are not unique to aldehydes and alkylating agents, however, and high concentrations of disinfectants such as chlorhexidine, phenol, ethanol and mercuric salts will also coagulate the cytoplasm. This most likely arises from the precipitation of protein caused by a variety of interactions including ionic and hydrophobic bonding and the disruption of hydrogen bonds.

20.4.4 Disruption of Functional Structures

The integrity and functions of the bacterial cell are dependent upon critical macromolecular structural arrangements including within the cell wall and cytoplasmic membrane (see Chapter 3). A number of microbicides can have a profound effect on these organelles.

20.4.4.1 Cell Wall

This structure is the traditional target for a group of antibiotics which includes the ß-lactams and glycopeptides (see Chapter 11), but a little-noticed report which appeared in 1948 showed that low concentrations of disinfectant substances caused cell wall lysis such that a normally turbid suspension of bacteria became clear. It is thought that these low concentrations of disinfectants cause enzymes whose normal role is to synthesise the cell wall to reverse their role in some way and effect its disruption or lysis. In the original report, these low concentrations of disinfectants (formalin, 0.12%; phenol, 0.32%; mercuric chloride, 0.0008%; sodium hypochlorite, 0.005% and merthiolate, 0.0004%) caused lysis of *Escherichia coli*, streptococci and staphylococci.

Divalent cations, in addition to their role as enzyme cofactors, also stabilise cell wall, membrane and ribosomal structures. In particular, magnesium serves to link the lipopolysaccharide (LPS) of Gram-negative bacteria to the outer membrane. Chelators, particularly ethylenediamine tetraacetic acid (EDTA), have been used to disrupt this link and cause the release of LPS into the medium. The loss of outer membrane integrity and subsequent permeabilisation has been exploited in the potentiation of microbicides, including combinations of EDTA with chloroxylenol, cetrimide, phenylethanol and the parahydroxy benzoic acid esters (see Chapter 18).

20.4.4.2 Cytoplasmic Membrane

The bacterial cytoplasmic membrane consists of an impermeable, negatively charged, fluid phospholipid bilayer incorporating an organised array of membrane-associated proteins. Through the membrane-bound electron transport chain aerobically, or the membrane-bound adenosine triphosphatase (ATPase) anaerobically, the bacterium succeeds in maintaining a transmembrane gradient of electrical potential and pH such that the interior of the cell is negative and alkaline. This *proton motive force*, as it is called, drives a number of energy-requiring functions which include the synthesis of ATP, the coupling of oxidative processes to phosphorylation, a metabolic sequence called *oxidative phosphorylation* and the transport and concentration in the cells of metabolites such as sugars and amino acids. This, put briefly, is the basis of the chemiosmotic theory linking metabolism to energy-requiring processes.

Certain chemical substances have been known for many years to uncouple oxidation from phosphorylation and to inhibit active transport, and for this reason they are named *uncoupling agents*. They are believed to act by partitioning into the membrane and rendering it permeable to protons, hence short-circuiting the potential gradient or proton motive force. Some examples of antibacterial agents which owe at least a part of their activity to this ability are tetrachlorosalicylanilide (TCS), trichlorocarbanilide (TCC), pentachlorophenol, di-(5-chloro-2-hydroxyphenyl) sulphide (fentichlor), 2-phenoxyethanol and lipophilic acids and esters.

The membrane, apart from providing a dynamic link between metabolism and transport, also serves to maintain the pool of metabolites within the cytoplasm. A general increase in membrane permeability brought about by the association and likely insertion of microbicide molecules into the lipid bilayer was recognised early as being one disruptive effect of many disinfectant substances.

Treatment of bacterial cells with appropriate concentrations of such substances as cetrimide and other QACs, chlorhexidine, polyhexamethylene biguanides (PHMB), phenol and hexylresorcinol causes leakage of a group of characteristic intracellular chemical species. The potassium ion, being a small entity, is the first substance to appear when the cytoplasmic membrane is damaged. Amino acids, purines, pyrimidines and pentoses are examples of other substances which will leak from treated cells. If the action of the drug is not prolonged or exerted only in low concentration, the damage may be reversible and leakage may only induce bacteriostasis. There is, however, evidence that a depletion of intracellular potassium caused by membrane damage can lead to the activation of latent ribonucleases and the consequent breakdown of RNA. Several microbicides, including cetrimide and some phenols, are known to cause the release of nucleotides and nucleosides following an autolytic process. This is irreversible and has been proposed as an autocidal (suicide) process, committing the injured cell to death (Denyer and Stewart 1998).

Surface-associated proteins within the membrane fulfil a number of important roles including wall biosynthesis, nutrient transport and respiration. Usually enzymes, these macromolecules are often topologically organised and uniquely exposed to disruption by biocidal agents. Thus, hexachlorophane inhibits the electron transport chain in bacteria, chlorhexidine has been shown to inhibit ATPase and thiol-containing membrane dehydrogenases are highly susceptible to mercury-containing antibacterials, silver, 2-bromo-2-nitropropane-1,3-diol (bronopol) and isothiazolinones.

20.5 Enhancing Activity

Mention has already been made of the use of permeabilising chelators to enhance the penetration of microbicides to their target (Section 20.4.4.1). Much effort has also been expended in the search for synergistic combinations of microbicides which, when added together, will greatly amplify the bactericidal effect. While theoretically possible, and potentially predictable from mechanism of action studies, in practice this effect is elusive; combinations of phenylmercuric acetate with benzalkonium chloride, lipophilic weak acids with fatty alcohols and chlorocresol with phenylethanol have been reported. The most likely route to enhancing activity however lies with optimising microbicide formulations to ensure maximum availability of the active moiety, particularly important in situations of pH-dependency or poor water solubility. In the area of pharmaceutical and cosmetic preservation, constructive use of formulation ingredients, each with some intrinsic antimicrobial activity, has successfully built on the activity of the original preservative agent to create a cumulative bactericidal effect, an approach called 'hurdle technology'.

20.6 Mechanisms of Resistance to Microbicides

Bacterial survival in the presence of microbicides has been reported since the 1950s, most notably with QACs, biguanides and phenolics. It is often associated with improper practices, sometimes leading to reduced microbicide concentration, including deficient manufacturing methods, preservative failure through careless product use or bad formulation design, inappropriate dilution practices and poor product storage. Members of the genus *Pseudomonas* are often the most frequent isolates from contaminated products.

Overall, there has been more documented evidence of bacterial resistance to antiseptics than to disinfectants (Table 20.3). It is worth mentioning that some bacteria surviving in microbicidal formulations have been associated with outbreaks and pseudo-outbreaks of infection (see Chapter 17). Bacterial resistance to all known preservatives was also reported as early as 1998 (Chapman et al. 1998). Recently, much interest has focused on bacteria surviving high-level disinfection, which is usually employed for the disinfection of medical devices. Thus, bacteria surviving exposure to the in-use (high) concentration of highly reactive microbicides (e.g., glutaraldehyde, chlorine dioxide, hydrogen peroxide) have been isolated and studied. In 2009, a large outbreak of atypical mycobacteria in at least 38 hospitals in Brazil was reported.

Table 20.3 Examples of bacterial resistance associated with microbicidal products.

Microbicides	Resistant bacteria
Used for disinfection	
Ethanol	*Bacillus cereus*[a,b]
Glutaraldehyde	*Mycobacterium chelonae*[a], *Methylobacterium mesophilicum*[a], atypical mycobacteria[a]
Formaldehyde	*Pseudomonas aeruginosa*[a], *Stenotrophomonas maltophilia*, *Klebsiella oxytoca*[a]
QAC	*Burkholderia cepacia*[a], *Serratia marcescens*[a], *Achromobacter xylosoxidans*[a], *Pseudomonas aeruginosa*[a]
Phenolics	*Pseudomonas* spp., *Pseudomonas aeruginosa*[a], *Alcaligenes faecalis*, *Serratia marcescens*[a]
Used for antisepsis	
Alcohols	*Bacillus cereus*[a,b], *Burkholderia cepacia*
Chlorhexidine	*Pseudomonas* spp., *Burkholderia cepacia*, *Flavobacterium meningosepticum*, *Serratia marcescens*, *Ralstonia pickettii*[a], *Achromobacter xylosoxidans*
Chlorhexidine with cetrimide	*Pseudomonas multivorans*, *Stenotrophomonas maltophilia*
Benzalkonium chloride	*Pseudomonas* spp.[a], *Achromobacter* spp., *Enterobacter aerogenes*, *Pseudomonas kingii*, *Burkholderia cepacia*[a], *Serratia marcescens*, *Mycobacterium chelonae*, *Mycobacterium abscessus*
Chloroxylenol	*Serratia marcescens*
Povidone-iodine	*Burkholderia cepacia*[a], *Pseudomonas putida*
Poloxamer-iodine	*Pseudomonas aeruginosa*
Triclosan	*Serratia marcescens*

Adapted from Maillard (2020).
[a] Bacteria associated with pseudo-outbreak or outbreak.
[b] Associated with the presence of endospores.

These mycobacteria were traced to endoscope contamination and were resistant to 2% w/v glutaraldehyde and also to the clinical concentration of front-line antibiotics against mycobacteria (Duarte et al. 2009). This was the first time that microbicide resistance was linked to antibiotic resistance, nosocomial infection and a large infection outbreak.

Over the last 20 years, much progress has been made in understanding the mechanisms conferring resistance to microbicides in bacteria. Interestingly, some mechanisms that were thought to occur only with antibiotics have now been described with microbicides.

20.6.1 General Mechanisms

Several mechanisms conferring some level of resistance to microbicide exposure have been documented. Traditionally, mechanisms of resistance have been divided into intrinsic and acquired resistance. *Intrinsic* (or *innate*) *resistance* is a natural property of the bacteria and provides some explanation as to why some bacteria are less susceptible to chemical (e.g., microbicides) and physical (e.g., UV radiation) agents than others. Intrinsic mechanisms often involve a structural difference, for example, a difference in the permeability of the bacterial membrane to microbicides, but also the expression of chromosomal genes such as those encoding for an efflux pump or a degradative enzyme. *Acquired resistance* refers to the acquisition of a new property by the bacteria through chromosomal mutation or genetic transfer; such a property can be the mutation of a target site or the transfer of a gene encoding for an efflux pump or a degradative enzyme. It should be noted that when gene transfer occurs, often several genes present on the same conjugative plasmid or transposon can be transferred to a recipient cell at the same time. In this case, the term *co-resistance* is often used to denote the simultaneous acquisition of a number of genes conferring resistance to a number of antimicrobials, both microbicides and antibiotics.

Bacterial exposure to a microbicide, particularly at a low concentration, will trigger a stress response which may lead to the expression of a number of mechanisms enabling bacterial survival. Thus, resistance often arises from these mechanisms working together to decrease the detrimental concentration of the microbicide to a level that is no longer harmful for the bacterium (Table 20.4). The expression of only one mechanism confers low-level resistance, often measured as an increase in minimum inhibitory concentration (MIC), but rarely high-level

Table 20.4 Possible mechanisms of bacterial resistance to microbicides.

Effect	Mechanisms	Microbicides (examples)
Barrier to penetration	Cell envelope: spore coat; mycobacterial envelope (intrinsic)	QACs, biguanides, phenolics, aldehydes (except *ortho*-phthalaldehyde)
	Outer membrane: lipopolysaccharide; cation content (intrinsic/acquired/environmental)	
	Porins: reduction in number, size (intrinsic/acquired/environmental)	QACs, biguanides
	Peptidoglycan/mycoylarabinogalactan (intrinsic)	Glutaraldehyde, QACs, biguanides, chlorine-releasing agents
	Biofilm: cell population – reduced diffusion	As above, plus oxidising agents
Decreased accumulation	Efflux (intrinsic/acquired)	QACs, phenolics, chlorhexidine, silver
	Degradation/modification of the microbicide (intrinsic/acquired)	Silver, organomercurials, glutaraldehyde, formaldehyde, phenolics, oxidising agents
Adaptation	Modification of targets (acquired)	Triclosan
	Overproduction of targets/amplification (acquired)	Triclosan
Bypass metabolic activity	Increase in pyruvate synthesis and fatty acid production via an altered metabolic pathway (intrinsic/acquired)	Triclosan
Communication	Gene transfer	Possibly all
	Quorum sensing (cell–cell communication in a population)	Unknown
	Extracellular induction components	Triclosan, QACs
Selective pressure	Selection of insusceptible bacteria (changes in a complex population)	All – documented with triclosan, QACs, biguanides, aldehydes, oxidising agents

QACs, quaternary ammonium compounds.

resistance, such as to an in-use concentration, which would be demonstrated by an increase in minimum bactericidal concentration (MBC). In the case of disinfectants, therefore, it is sometimes preferred that the term 'reduced susceptibility' or 'increased tolerance' is used when the failure of disinfection is unlikely because the in-use concentrations greatly exceed the MIC. Finally, a distinction can be made between mechanisms expressed by a single bacterium and the mechanisms of resistance that arise from a community of bacteria such as in bacterial biofilms.

20.6.1.1 Changes in Cell Permeability

The decrease in microbicide penetration arising from changes in cell permeability is well established and has been described with different bacterial genera, notably with Gram-negative bacteria and mycobacteria. It is also the case with bacterial endospores, which are discussed later in this chapter. In Gram-negative bacteria, the outer membrane, and notably the composition of LPS, offers some protection to the cell, by reducing microbicide penetration. The role of LPS has been exemplified by researchers with the use of permeabilising agents and notably ion chelators such as EDTA. EDTA contributes to the removal (loss) of LPS from the outer membrane by scavenging dications involved in the stabilisation of LPS in the membrane (Section 20.4.4.1). By losing LPS, the outer membrane becomes more permeable and microbicides can penetrate better resulting in enhanced activity. A change in the structure of the outer membrane following a change in protein, fatty acid or phospholipid composition has been associated with a decrease in the efficacy of cationic microbicides. In particular, a decrease in the number of porin proteins as a result of microbicide exposure has been associated with high-level resistance to QACs in pseudomonads. Further, changes in membrane lipid composition, membrane proteins and membrane fluidity in response to microbicide exposure have been documented.

In mycobacteria, the lipid-rich outer cell wall (responsible for the waxy appearance of the colonies) and particularly the presence of a mycoylacylarabinogalactan layer and the composition of the arabinogalactan/arabinomannan within the cell wall account for a reduction in microbicide penetration; increasing the permeability of the mycobacterial outer cell wall, for example, with ethambutol, enhances the activity of microbicides and antibiotics.

20.6.1.2 Efflux

Efflux pumps are cross-membrane proteins which pump out various substrates including microbicides and antibiotics. A large number of efflux pumps in bacteria have been identified and have been divided into five main classes depending on their structure and activity: the small multidrug-resistance (SMR) family; the major facilitator superfamily (MFS); the ATP-binding cassette (ABC) family; the resistance-nodulation-division (RND) family; and the multidrug and toxic compound extrusion (MATE) family (Figure 20.3).

The role of efflux pumps is to remove harmful substances across the bacterial membrane, including microbicides (e.g., QACs and phenolics), to levels that are not damaging for the cell. The quantity of antimicrobial pumped out depends upon the number of pumps present, their expression and efficacy. Carriage of efflux pump genes in environmental and hospital isolates has been well documented in recent years. Some studies have shown that high-level resistance can be achieved by efflux, for instance, against the bisphenol triclosan, but usually, the effect is only associated with an increase in MIC.

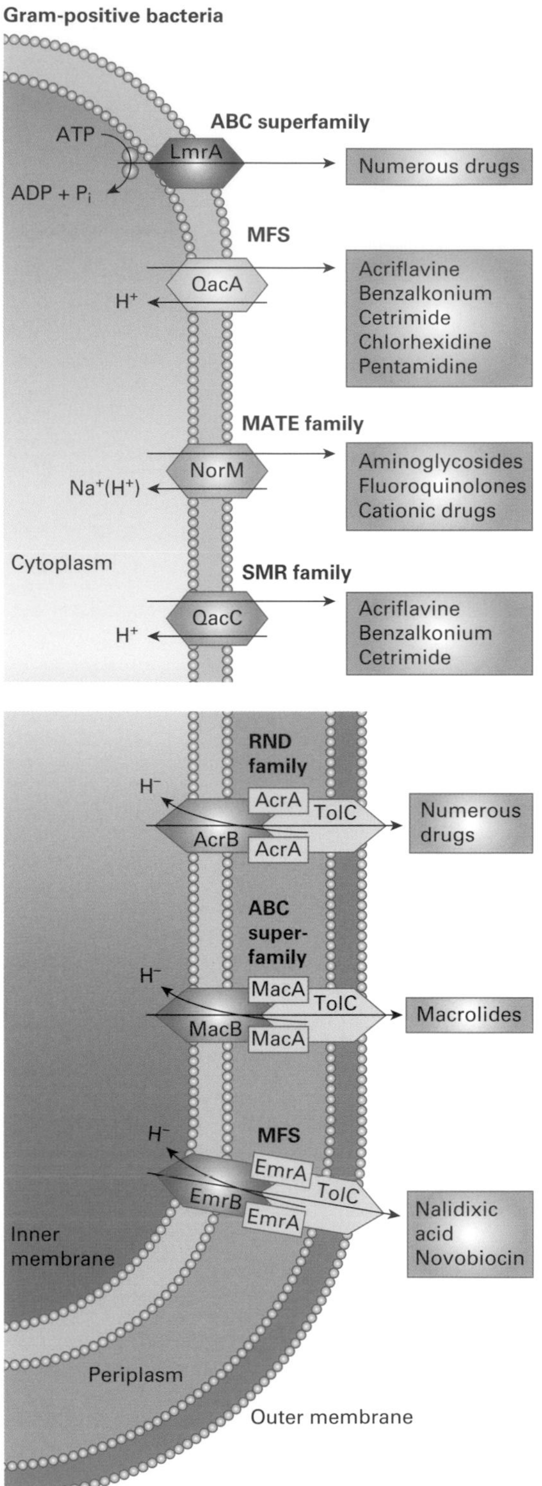

Figure 20.3 Examples of efflux pumps in bacteria. Note the wide range of substrates used by these pumps. *Source:* From Piddock, L.J.V. 2006.

20.6.1.3 Enzymatic Inactivation

Enzymatic degradation plays a role in reducing the harmful concentration of a microbicide and has been observed with aldehydes (e.g., aldehyde dehydrogenase), oxidising agents (e.g., catalases, superoxide dismutase, hydroxyperoxidases), phenolics and parabens. In the case of metallic salts such as silver, the ionic form is reduced to the inactive metal. The role of enzymatic inactivation has not been widely studied, but it is unlikely that a bacterial enzyme alone will contribute to high-level resistance to a microbicide.

20.6.1.4 Modification of Target Site

To date, resistance conferred by the modification of a microbicide target site has only been observed with triclosan. At a low concentration, this bisphenol interacts specifically with a bacterial enoyl-acyl reductase carrier protein, which is involved in the synthesis of fatty acid. Triclosan has been shown to interact with a number of structurally related enzymes in many bacterial genera. A modification of the enzyme confers a low-level resistance to triclosan, although some studies claim that a high-level resistance has been observed. This is unlikely, since at a high concentration triclosan interacts with multiple target sites to bring about a bactericidal effect.

20.6.1.5 Change in Metabolic Pathway

A change in metabolic pathway that confers resistance to a microbicide is a relatively new concept that was thought to occur only with sulphonamides. However, bacterial adaptation to triclosan, as measured by an extended lag phase of growth followed by a normal exponential phase, has been observed in several bacterial genera. The recent use of a microarray in *Salmonella enterica* serovar Typhimurium enabled the identification of a 'triclosan-resistance network' including an alternative pathway to the production of pyruvate and fatty acid. In *Staphylococcus aureus* showing reduced sensitivity to triclosan, a change in lipid composition of the cell membrane was associated with altered expression of various genes involved in fatty acid metabolism. Low-level QAC resistance in *Serratia marcescens* may arise from a change in synthetic or metabolic pathways. Similarly, changes to the metabolome of *E. coli* have been observed following exposure to chlorhexidine.

An alteration in a metabolic pathway is different to an increase or decrease in metabolic activity. Injured bacteria, as a result of an exposure to a microbicide, will die if they are metabolically highly active, as they are unable to repair any accumulating damage effectively. Conversely, an enforced lowered metabolism following microbicide exposure (e.g., growth on a minimal medium following treatment) appears to facilitate bacterial repair and survival. The extended lag phase of growth, so often observed following exposure to a microbicide, has been associated with both the expression of mechanisms leading to a decrease in the damaging concentration of the microbicide and to the operation of repair processes, both ultimately enabling bacteria to resume a normal exponential growth phase.

20.6.2 Induction of Resistance

The induction of antimicrobial resistance in bacteria following microbicide exposure is a relatively recent concern which is particularly pertinent to the increasing number of commercially available products containing a low concentration of a microbicide. This low, often subinhibitory, concentration can induce the expression of resistance mechanisms that can confer bacterial survival to microbicide and/or antibiotic exposure. Low-level resistance as measured by an increase in MIC has often been observed. Prior to the use of genomics, proteomics and metabolomics, induction of resistance in bacteria was observed with an increase in lag phase of growth and a decrease in growth rate, an overexpression of efflux pumps and the production of guanosine 5′-diphosphate 3′-diphosphate (ppGpp). An increase in DNA repair was also associated with an increase in bacterial survival following microbicide exposure.

More recently, a change in the expression of regulons commanding a number of responses, such as a stress response (and repair mechanism), increased efflux, change in membrane composition and a change in metabolic and synthetic pathways, has been recorded following exposure to a low concentration of microbicides. Such a global response is of concern, as it also confers a decreased susceptibility to antibiotics, and recent evidence suggests it might also lead to overexpression of virulence determinants.

Bacterial mutations occur naturally, but they can be driven by stress response mechanisms following exposure to antibiotics. A number of investigations have observed that the mutation rate increases in the presence of an active efflux system. The effect of bacterial mutation in the development of resistance to microbicides has not been widely investigated, with the exception of triclosan. It is also possible that microbicides which interact with the bacterial genome (e.g., dyes, oxidising agents) might produce a higher mutation rate, although this has yet to be documented.

20.6.3 Dissemination of Resistance

Surprisingly, the dissemination of microbicide-resistance mechanisms between bacteria has only recently become a subject of study. The acquisition of new genetic determinants, notably by the process of conjugation, is of concern, as it is often dependent on the presence of large transferable plasmids, and transposons which encode for many genes including bacterial resistance to antibiotics and virulence factors. When several resistance genes are transferred at the same time, the term co-resistance is used. For example, the resistance to the QAC benzalkonium chloride in *S. aureus* has been associated with the presence of plasmids containing *qac*, *bla* and *tet* resistant genes (encoding for efflux pumps and a β-lactamase). A number of mechanisms of resistance such as efflux and degradative enzymes have been documented to be transferred between bacteria. The extent of such dissemination is difficult to measure, although it is thought to readily occur in bacterial communities such as a biofilm.

Equally important to the horizontal transfer of resistance is the maintenance of resistant determinants (plasmids) following the continuous presence of microbicides. Although this issue has not been widely studied, it is of interest with the use of biocidal products which are documented to leave a residual concentration of microbicide on surfaces, antimicrobial-impregnated surfaces, and the continuous presence of microbicides in certain applications, such as drinking-water chlorination.

20.6.4 Bacterial Endospores

The formation of an endospore is a mechanism of bacterial survival when growth conditions are detrimental for the vegetative form. The formation of endospores is a property of only a few bacterial genera, notably *Bacillus* spp. and the *Clostridia*. Such adverse conditions include lack of nutrient but also the presence of microbicides and other detrimental physical and chemical conditions. The spore structure is unique and confers upon the spore high-level resistance to chemical (e.g., microbicides) and physical (e.g., heat) agents. Hence, only a few microbicides, mainly highly reactive ones such as the aldehydes, oxidising agents and chlorine-releasing agents, are sporicidal, while others such as biguanides, QACs and phenolics are only bactericidal against the vegetative bacteria. It should also be noted that extended contact and higher concentrations are required to kill spores compared to their vegetative counterparts; aldehydes such as glutaraldehyde and formaldehyde need a much longer contact time and, in the case of *ortho*-phthalaldehyde, a raised temperature too.

20.6.4.1 Sporulation and Germination

Sporulation, a process in which a bacterial spore develops from a vegetative cell (see Chapter 3), involves seven stages (I–VII); of these, stages IV–VII (cortex and coat development) are the most important in relation to the development of microbicide resistance. Resistance to biocidal agents develops during sporulation and may be an early, intermediate or late/very late event. For example, resistance to chlorhexidine occurs at an intermediate stage, at about the same time as heat resistance, whereas decreasing susceptibility to glutaraldehyde is a very late event.

During germination and/or outgrowth, metabolism and biosynthetic processes increase and cells regain their sensitivity to antibacterial agents. Some inhibitors act at the germination stage (e.g., phenolics, parabens), whereas others such as chlorhexidine and the QACs do not affect germination but inhibit outgrowth. Glutaraldehyde, at low concentrations, is an effective inhibitor of both stages.

20.6.4.2 Spore Structure

The spore structure (see Chapter 3) and the interaction between a microbicide and the spore have been particularly well documented in the genus *Bacillus*. The spore core (protoplast, sometimes referred to as the germ cell) is enclosed within a cell wall which is surrounded by the cortex and several spore coats. Sometimes an exosporium may surround the spore.

The spore core is the target site of sporicides, since it is the location of RNA, DNA, dipicolinic acid (DPA) and most of the essential minerals, such as calcium, potassium, manganese and phosphorus. Also present are substantial amounts of low-molecular-weight basic proteins, the small acid-soluble spore proteins (SASPs) which are rapidly degraded during germination. SASPs, comprising about 10–20% of the protein in the dormant spore, exist in two forms (α/β and γ) and are essential for expression of spore resistance to ultraviolet radiation and also appear to be involved in resistance to some microbicides, for example, hydrogen peroxide. Spores (α^-/β^-) deficient in α-/β-type SASPs are much more peroxide-sensitive than are wild-type (normal) spores. It has been proposed that in wild-type spores DNA is saturated with α-/β-type SASPs and is thus protected from free radical damage.

Bacillus spore coatless mutants and chemically induced coatless spores have illustrated the role of the spore-coat in limiting access of microbicides to the spore core. Further, it is now known that the pressure exerted by the spore cortex on the spore cytoplasmic membrane can help to maintain the essential impermeability of the membrane to many chemicals, potentially adding further protection to the spore core. Finally, the cortex may also act as a barrier to some extent.

20.6.5 Bacterial Biofilms

Bacteria are generally associated with surfaces in a complex community called biofilms (see Chapter 8). Following attachment to a surface, a bacterium will go through a series of metabolic and phenotypic changes, leading to the formation of microcolonies embedded within a matrix of secreted exopolysaccharides. Bacteria in biofilms have been shown to be less susceptible to antibiotics and microbicides than planktonic bacteria. Pre-existing persistent, but not genetically resistant, subpopulations may contribute to this higher tolerance. There are several microbicide-resistance mechanisms, all contributing to a 'biofilm-associated phenotype': reduction in microbicide penetration, reduced bacterial metabolism, quiescence, enzymatic inactivation and efflux (Table 20.5). Environmental biofilms are complex in nature, composed of multiple bacterial species and at times other microorganisms including fungi, protozoa and viruses. Multi-bacterial species biofilms tend to be less susceptible to microbicides than single-species biofilms.

Microbicides have been observed to change the composition of a complex biofilm, composed of different bacterial genera or/and species, thereby contributing to a selection and clonal expansion of the least susceptible species. For example, PHMB, chlorhexidine and Bardac (a QAC) have been shown to select for pseudmonads to the detriment of Gram-positive bacteria. The bisphenol triclosan was shown to reduce the genera diversity of a complex waste drain biofilm and to decrease the overall susceptibility of the remaining population. Recently, dry biofilms have been found associated with dry

Table 20.5 Mechanisms of microbicide resistance in bacterial biofilms.

Resistance mechanisms	Consequence for microbicide action
Establishing a reduced local microbicide concentration	Dilution through a diffusion gradient Non-specific neutralising interaction with cell constituents Lysed bacterial community offering mechanistic inactivation as a result of increased organic load
Enhanced bacterial insusceptibility	Degradation of antimicrobial agent Efflux (more effective against lower concentrations) Early stress-response
Slow growth/metabolism	A local concentration gradient leading to reduced nutrients/O_2 can retard growth rate, mitigating against microbicide injury
Selection for increased resistance	Formation of pockets of surviving bacteria Dormant cells (which regrow rapidly in the presence of exudates released from lysed community)
Acquisition of new resistance determinants	Increased genetic exchange
Intrinsic resistance	Nature of microorganisms present in the consortium (i.e., some being more resistant than others)

Adapted from Maillard and Denyer (2009).

environmental surfaces. These biofilms are particularly resistant to high levels of sodium hypochlorite considerably in excess of in-use concentrations.

20.6.6 Misuse and Abuse of Microbicides

The indiscriminate use of microbicides in an increasing number of applications and, notably, the use or presence of sub-optimal low concentrations has fuelled the debate on emerging bacterial cross-resistance to antibiotics used for human and animal medicine. In recent years, there has been a growing number of examples of clinical or environmental isolates showing a change in susceptibility profile to antibiotics following exposure to microbicides. Indeed, there are now plenty of examples where resistance genes to microbicides and antibiotics can be shown to reside on the same multidrug-resistant plasmids. The likely clinical significance is disputed however and is still largely based on *in vitro* evidence that some mechanisms conferring a decrease in microbicide susceptibility can also lead to resistance to *therapeutic concentrations* of antibiotics. Some of the most common mechanisms involved include expression and over-expression of efflux pumps and changes in cell permeability and metabolism. At present, however, there is no useful rule of thumb to predict cross-resistance between microbicides and antibiotics in bacteria. Nevertheless, there is now sufficient concern to have driven some significant changes in the regulation and use of biocidal products.

20.7 Viricidal Activity of Microbicides

Challenges in establishing robust vaccination strategies and the appearance of viral resistance to antiviral chemotherapy have secured the important role for microbicides to help eliminate or control viral outbreaks. This is particularly pertinent where viral transmission is associated with surfaces. Our understanding of the mechanisms of viricidal action of microbicides remains quite fragmentary, however, with information often extrapolated from data based on testing against bacteria in particular. This approach needs to be interpreted with caution given the fundamental differences in size, structure and chemistry of bacteria and viruses. Viruses present fewer target sites to microbicides than larger and more complex organisms. Furthermore, viruses are not metabolically active, which further reduces the number of targets available to microbicides.

It is generally accepted that viruses can be divided into two groups according to their susceptibility to microbicides (see also Chapter 5). Lipophilic viruses that possess a viral envelope derived from their host (e.g., HIV, herpes simplex virus, influenza virus, coronaviruses) are the most susceptible to microbicides. The hydrophilic viruses comprise all the non-enveloped viruses and differ tremendously in size and structure. Among these, the small non-enveloped viruses such as the picornaviruses (e.g., poliovirus, hepatitis A virus, foot-and-mouth disease virus, norovirus) are often considered to be the least susceptible to microbicide exposure, although some larger viruses such as adenoviruses and rotaviruses can also be quite resilient. Discrepancies in reported viricidal activity often can be traced to the difference in efficacy test methodology used, and notably the lack of an appropriate neutraliser to quench the activity of the microbicides (see Chapter 19). In general terms, where the membrane-active microbicides such as biguanides, phenolics, QACs and alcohols have a good efficacy against enveloped viruses, their activity against non-enveloped viruses is limited; against these pathogens the chemically reactive halogens, peroxides and aldehydes need to be employed (Table 20.6).

One of the biggest challenges for microbicide activity against viruses is that viruses on surfaces are often associated with soiling and fomites. Such an association allows viral survival (most notably for enveloped viruses) on surfaces for long periods of time, as fomites/soiling appear to protect viruses from desiccation. In the absence of satisfactory cleaning, these organic materials can also protect viruses from detrimental chemical agents such as microbicides. Viricidal tests do not always consider viruses embedded in an organic load.

With the exception of certain slow-acting microbicides, virus inactivation generally occurs rapidly or not at all and

Table 20.6 Examples of microbicides used for the control of human pathogenic viruses.

Disinfectant class	Typical use	Activity
Alcohols, e.g., ethanol	• General-purpose disinfection • Used alone or in formulations to potentiate activity of other microbicides	• Acts on envelope and denatures proteins • Not markedly affected by contaminating matter
Aldehydes	• Fumigation (formaldehyde, paraformaldehyde) • Sterilisation or disinfection of medical devices/instruments (glutaraldehyde)	• React readily with proteins; cross-linking reactions • Wide spectrum of activity
Chlorhexidine and PHMB	• In alcoholic solution used as handwash or peri-operative skin preparation	• Act at level of envelope; PHMB binds to protein capsid • Viricidal activity poor in aqueous solution and confined to enveloped viruses
Halogens		
• Sodium hypochlorite or chlorine gas; chlorine dioxide	• General-purpose disinfection, often recommended as the standard for viral pathogens • Water disinfection	• Oxidising agent • Broad-spectrum viricide • Activity affected by presence of reducing agents, temperature and organic matter
• Iodine/iodophore	• Topical antiseptic • Viral inactivation in blood products • Inorganic iodine mostly replaced by polymeric iodophore	• Oxidises thiol groups and unsaturated carbon bonds • Less affected by organic matter than other halogens • Neutralised by reducing agents • Activity improved by addition of alcohol
Peroxides and peracids		
• Hydrogen peroxide	• Stabilised disinfectant/antiseptic preparations • Disinfection of medical implants • Low-temperature vapour sterilisation/decontamination	• Potent oxidant, acting through formation of free radicals
• Peracetic acid	• Surface disinfection • Vapour sterilisation/decontamination in healthcare	• Potent oxidant • Less affected by organic matter than some other disinfectants
Phenolics	• General-purpose germicide	• Enveloped viruses more susceptible • Affected by temperature and organic matter
Quaternary ammonium compounds (QAC)	• Dilute aqueous solutions for topical antisepsis • Hard-surface disinfection • Can be used in alcoholic solution	• Mainly useful against enveloped viruses; non-enveloped viruses are refractory • Readily neutralised by proteins and soap preparations

PHMB, polyhexamethylene biguanides.
Adapted from Maillard et al. (2013).

knowledge of the kinetics of this action is particularly important for effective disinfection. In terms of mechanisms of action, the goal of a viricide should be the destruction of the viral nucleic acid. In reality, very few microbicides have been shown to affect the viral genome; cationic microbicides and alcohols damage the viral envelope (which contains host cell recognition (glyco)protein receptors) releasing an intact viral capsid and genome, although they have been shown to affect the capsid in some instances, but not the viral genome. Microbicides that have been shown to interact and break open the capsid (e.g., chlorine-releasing agents) might not have a damaging effect on the viral nucleic acid. To date, only a few microbicides (mainly oxidising agents) have been observed to damage the viral nucleic acid within the capsid. It has to be accepted, therefore, that viral inactivation by a microbicide does not necessarily imply the complete destruction of a virus, but may often be a consequence of loss of structural functionality or infectivity.

The main mechanism of viral resistance to microbicides is the formation of viral aggregates before or during microbicide exposure. These clumps protect some viruses from the damaging effect of microbicides that fail to penetrate deep within these clumps. Chlorine-releasing agents (e.g., hypochlorite) and PHMB have been shown to produce viral aggregates, limiting their viricidal efficacy. An alteration in virus susceptibility could arise through a morphological change in the viral structure; in this context a change in capsid configuration has been shown to alter the susceptibility of viruses to a lower concentration of microbicides (e.g., glutaraldehyde). Further, repeated exposure to inadequate levels of disinfectant has been shown to produce poliovirus isolates with a decreased susceptibility to chlorine. Finally, multiplicity reactivation, a process aided by clumping that has been observed only *in vitro*, concerns the reassembly of intact viruses that have been structurally damaged by a microbicide intervention, but where the genome remains intact. This process, together with the suggestion that the viral genome of certain viruses (e.g., hepatitis B virus) can remain infectious, emphasises the importance for viricides to destroy the viral nucleic acid.

20.8 Microbicides and Protozoa

The activity of microbicides has been described in a number of amoebae, notably in *Giardia* spp. and *Cryptosporidium* spp., which are major waterborne pathogens (see Chapter 6), and *Acanthamoeba* spp., a pathogen mainly associated with contact lenses and contact lens solutions. Trophozoites (the actively growing form) of *Acanthamoeba* spp. have been shown to be susceptible to low concentrations of chlorhexidine, PHMB, QACs, oxidising agents (hydrogen peroxide, chlorine dioxide, peracetic acid, ozone), chlorine-releasing agents and isothiazolinones. Glutaraldehyde might possess only a poor trophocidal activity. In general, higher concentrations and much longer contact times are needed to achieve a cysticidal activity (e.g., hydrogen peroxide 3% for 4 hours), and the concentration of microbicide (e.g., PHMB, QAC) used for the disinfection of contact lenses might be ineffective against *Acanthamoeba* cysts. Other microbicides such as iodine and bromine and the isothiazolinones have been shown to have no activity against *Acanthamoeba* cysts. It should be noted that differences in inactivation using the same microbicides and parameters have been observed against cysts of different species.

Since most microbicides have a poor cysticidal efficacy at a low concentration, the combination of microbicides or the formulation excipients can become important. For example, a combination of chlorhexidine and thiomersal and/or EDTA has been shown to be cysticidal within 24 hours. QAC cysticidal activity can be improved when combined with tributyltin neodecanoate. A combination of hydrogen peroxide (3%) with catalase and potassium iodide (50 μM) was shown to enhance significantly cysticidal activity against *Acanthamoeba polyphaga*.

The mechanisms of action of microbicides against trophozoites are similar to those observed on bacterial structures. For example, cationic microbicides have been shown to damage the cytoplasmic membrane and to induce pentose leakage in *Acanthamoeba* spp.

Amoebal trophozoites undergo encystation when exposed to detrimental conditions, which include microbicide (e.g., diamidines, chlorhexidine) exposure. Cysts are a dormant form which enable survival for many years in the environment. They are a dehydrated structure with a double wall composed of cellulose and relatively small numbers of proteins. The outer ectocyst wall is composed mainly of protein and lipid-containing materials and the inner endocyst wall contains cellulose.

Encystation is a relatively rapid process that can be divided into three principal stages: induction, during which cellular components are degraded; immature cysts, during which the first cell wall is synthesised; and mature cysts, during which the second cell wall is formed.

The composition and morphological aspects of the cyst wall vary between species and depend upon the composition of the media used during encystation.

The double cyst wall represents a permeability barrier for microbicides (e.g., chlorhexidine, PHMB, diamidines). In addition, the metabolically dormant nature of the cyst might affect the cysticidal activity of microbicides. It is thus not surprising that cysts represent a challenge for

Table 20.7 Susceptibility of different types of microorganisms to microbicides.

Microorganisms[a]	Examples	Comments
Prions	Scrapie, Creutzfeldt–Jakob disease (CJD), new variant CJD	Highly resistant to conventional microbicides due to their proteinaceous nature
Bacterial endospores	*Bacillus* spp., *Geobacillus* spp., *Clostridioides difficile*	*Bacillus* used as biological indicators for sterilisation processes due to their high intrinsic resistance
Protozoal oocysts	Cryptosporidium	Particularly challenging for water disinfection, associated with infection outbreaks
Mycobacteria	*Mycobacterium chelonae*, *Mycobacterium avium intracellulare*, *Mycobacterium tuberculosis*, *Mycobacterium terrae*	Environmental mycobacteria, *M. chelonae* and *Mycobacterium massiliense* might show capacity to develop resistance to repeated microbicide exposure, and might become a challenge for high-level disinfection
Small non-enveloped viruses	Picornaviruses, papillomaviruses	Generally considered the least susceptible viruses to microbicide action
Protozoal cysts	*Giardia* spp., *Acanthamoeba* spp.	Might harbour pathogenic bacteria and thus aid their survival when exposed to microbicides
Fungal spores	*Aspergillus* spp.	There is very little information on microbicide activity against fungal spores
Gram-negative bacteria	*Pseudomonas* spp., *Burkholderia* spp., *Escherichia coli*, *Acinetobacter* spp.	*Pseudomonas* spp. and *Burkholderia* spp. are particularly challenging for preservative systems; pathogenic *E. coli* (e.g., O157) associated with surface contamination often embedded within organic matter
Moulds	*Aspergillus* spp.	Very little information on microbicide activity against moulds. Melanin production likely to be involved in reduced susceptibility of moulds to QACs
Yeasts	*Candida albicans*, *Saccharomyces cerevisiae*	Yeasts usually considered more susceptible than moulds. Overall very little information available on yeast susceptibility to microbicides.
Protozoa	*Acanthamoeba* spp., *Giardia* spp.	Important to control for water disinfection and contact lens disinfection
Large, non-enveloped viruses	Adenoviruses, rotaviruses	Certain rotaviruses more resilient; viruses often associated with soiling
Gram-positive bacteria	Staphylococci, streptococci, enterococci	Less-complex cell walls than Gram-negative bacteria, generally allowing easier microbicide access to target sites
Enveloped viruses	HIV, HSV, influenza, RSV	Viruses on surfaces often associated with fomites

HIV, human immunodeficiency virus; HSV, herpes simplex virus; RSV, respiratory syncytial virus.
[a] Listed in order of resistance to microbicides from high to low.

disinfection (Table 20.7). This is now of particular concern following the recognition that protozoal cysts can protect intracellular bacterial pathogens from disinfection.

20.9 Microbicides and Fungi

Fungi and their spores are a major potential source of contamination in pharmaceutical product preparation and aseptic processing, as they are ubiquitous in the environment. That many pharmaceutically relevant microbicides do have antifungal action, even at relatively low concentrations, is evident from preservative challenge tests (see Chapter 17) which include *Aspergillus brasiliensis* (formerly *niger*) and *Candida albicans* as routine test organisms. The activity of microbicides against fungi has not been widely documented, however (Table 20.7). It is often assumed that the interactions of microbicides with mould and yeast cells can be extrapolated from what is known of the interactions of these agents against bacteria. However, the fungal cell wall is fundamentally different from that of the bacteria and less is known about its capacity to impede the penetration of microbicides. Furthermore, a formulation designed to be bactericidal might not necessarily be fungicidal. The interactions of QACs and biguanides with the fungal cell have been studied to some extent. Available information tentatively links cell wall glucan, wall thickness and consequent relative porosity to the sensitivity of *Saccharomyces cerevisiae* to chlorhexidine. Moulds tend to be less susceptible to microbicides than yeasts, although more evidence is needed, since only a limited number of fungal genera have been investigated.

Fungi have been shown to possess additional mechanisms of resistance to microbicide intervention. The expression of degradative enzymes notably against metallic salts (e.g., copper, mercury) has been documented. In *S. cerevisiae*, the production of hydrogen sulphide combining with heavy metal results in insoluble sulphides which are better tolerated by the microorganism. The expression of formaldehyde dehydrogenase to decrease the effect of formaldehyde has also been reported in *Penicillium* species. The presence of efflux pumps has now been widely reported in fungi, although their role in microbicide resistance has been little investigated.

20.10 Inactivation of Prions

Prions are the cause of transmissible spongiform encephalopathies (see Chapter 5), a group of fatal neurological diseases such as scrapie, Creutzfeldt–Jakob disease (CJD), new variant Creutzfeldt–Jakob disease (vCJD), bovine spongiform encephalopathy (BSE), kuru and Gerstmann–Sträussler–Scheinker syndrome (GSS). It is now widely accepted that prions are an abnormal, protease-resistant form of a normal harmless host protein (PrP). The prion protein undergoes a conformational change from four α-helices to an infectious β-sheet form. These conformational changes cause degeneration of nervous tissue which, under the microscope, exhibits a sponge-like appearance. Prions are found in association with a wide range of tissues and are of particular significance in a pharmaceutical context because of the need to decontaminate surgical or other hospital equipment that has been in contact with such diseased tissue. Prions are very stable in the environment, may form aggregates and are highly resistant to conventional disinfection and sterilisation methodologies (see Chapters 19 and 21).

Prions are considered highly resistant to various types of biocidal product (Table 20.7); this includes strong acids (e.g., 8 M hydrochloric acid for 1 hour), alkylating agents (e.g., glutaraldehyde, β-propiolactone), iodine and iodophors, phenolics, alcohols, oxidising agents in their liquid form (e.g., hydrogen peroxide, peracetic acid) and proteolytic enzymes (see Chapter 19). Mild detergents were also reported inactive, although sodium dodecyl sulphate (SDS) has shown some activity.

Alkali (e.g., 1 M NaOH for 1 hour) is usually effective against prions and as such has been widely used in the laboratory and industrial and clinical environments. However, alkali efficacy might depend on the prion's nature (host), and residual prion infectivity following treatment has been documented. More aggressive treatments combining alkali and gravity-displacement autoclaving at 121 °C for 30 minutes have been used. The use of sodium hypochlorite containing 20,000 ppm of available chlorine for 1 hour has been recommended for use in practice. Sodium dichloroisocyanurate (NaDCC) might not be equally effective against some prion proteins, as some infectivity following treatment has been reported. Hydrogen peroxide in a gaseous form has been shown to be active against prions, although reported efficacy to date depends much on the type of vapourised hydrogen peroxide generator used.

Formulations play an important role in prion decontamination. Complex formulations containing liquid hydrogen peroxide and copper have been shown to be active against prions. The combination of alkali, chelating agents, surfactants and various buffers have been particularly effective, as they combined prion removal from surfaces and prion inactivation. A combination of proteinase K, pronase and SDS has been shown to degrade PrP^{res} material from highly concentrated vCJD-infected brain preparations. Slight changes in formulations might bring a loss of efficacy against prions, however, and new formulations need to be carefully assessed for antiprion activity.

20.11 Conclusion

Microbicides are valuable compounds used in a wide range of applications. They exercise a variety of mechanisms of action, often in multiplicity, which can lead to their successful and widespread application in preservation and disinfection. It should also be noted that microbicides are used in complex formulations where excipients might affect microbicidal efficacy. There is a renewed interest in microbicide use with the rising impact of antibiotic resistance in bacteria and the perceived decline in hygiene standards in healthcare facilities. The number of products commercially available containing a microbicide is increasing, which is a concern when the concentration of a microbicide is sub-optimal. Bacterial resistance to microbicides has now been widely described, with novel mechanisms, such as alterations in a metabolic pathway, still emerging. The use of genomic, proteomic, transcriptomic and metabolomic tools has helped secure a better understanding of the mechanisms involved, but also, and importantly, a better understanding of the induction of resistance as a result of microbicide exposure. Resistant bacteria can be readily isolated from clinical settings. The efficacy of a microbicidal product can be hampered by a number of external factors such as level of soiling, type of surface, temperature and contact time, not forgetting the nature of the target microorganism. The lack of understanding of these factors combined with inappropriate in-use concentrations of a microbicide in certain applications (e.g., antimicrobial surfaces, impregnated textiles) might be conducive not only to the selection of emerging microbial resistance to microbicides but also to antibiotics. The concentration of a microbicide is paramount for its lethal activity.

References

Chapman, J.S., Diehl, M.A. and Fearnside, K.B. (1998). Preservative tolerance and resistance. *Int. J. Cosmet. Sci.* 20: 31–39.

Denyer, S.P. and Stewart, G.S.A.B. (1998). Mechanisms of action of disinfectants. *Int. Biodeterior. Biodegrad.* 41: 261–268.

Duarte, R.S., Lourenco, M.C.S., Fonseca, L.D. et al. (2009). Epidemic of postsurgical infections caused by *Mycobacterium massiliense*. *J. Clin. Microbiol.* 47: 2149–2155.

Maillard, J.-Y. (2020). Chapter 4, Bacterial resistance to biocides. Part II fundamental principles of activity. In *Blocks' Disinfection, Sterilization and Preservation*, 6e. (ed. G. McDonnell and J. Hansen), 44–67. Philadelphia: Wolters Kluwer.

Maillard, J.-Y. and Denyer, S.P. (2009). Emerging bacterial resistance following biocide exposure: should we be concerned? *Chim. Oggi* 27: 26–28.

Maillard, J.-Y., Sattar, S. and Pinto, P. (2013). Chapter 9, Virucidal activity of microbicides. In: *Principles and Practice of Disinfection, Preservation and Sterilization*, 5e (ed. A.P. Fraise, J.-Y. Maillard and S. Sattar), 178–207. Oxford: Blackwell Science.

Piddock, L.J.V. (2006). Multidrug resistance efflux pumps—not just for resistance. *Nat. Rev. Microbiol.* 4: 629–636.

Further Reading

Buffet-Bataillon, S., Tattevin, P., Maillard, J.-Y. et al. (2016). Efflux pump induction by quaternary ammonium compounds and fluoroquinolone resistance in bacteria. *Future Microbiol.* 11 (1): 81–92.

Denyer, S.P. and Hugo, W.B. (1991). *Mechanisms of Action of Chemical Biocides: Their Study and Exploitation*. Society for Applied Bacteriology Technical Series No. 27. Oxford: Blackwell Scientific.

Elsmore, R. and Wright, S. (2016). The authorization of biocidal products under the BPR. *Chim. Oggi* 34: 51–54.

Fraise, A., Maillard, J.-Y. and Sattar, S. (2013). *Russell, Hugo & Ayliffe's Principles and Practice of Disinfection, Preservation and Sterilization*, 5e. Oxford: Blackwell Science.

Leggett, M.J., McDonnell, G., Denyer, S.P. et al. (2012). Bacterial spore structures and their protective role in biocide resistance. *J. Appl. Microbiol.* 113: 485–498.

Maillard, J.-Y. (2007). Bacterial resistance to biocides in the healthcare environment: shall we be concerned? *J. Hosp. Infect.* 65 (suppl 2): 60–72.

Maillard, J.-Y. (2018). Resistance of bacteria to biocides. *Microbiol. Spectr.* 6 (2): ARBA-0006-2017.

Maillard, J.-Y., Bloomfield, S., Rosado Coelho, S.J. et al. (2013). Does microbicide use in consumer products promote antimicrobial resistance? A critical review and recommendations for a cohesive approach to risk assessment. *Microb. Drug Resist.* 19: 344–354.

McDonnell, G.E. (2017). *Antisepsis, Disinfection, and Sterilization: Types, Action, and Resistance*, 2e. Washington: ASM Press.

Webber, M.A., Coldham, N.G., Woodward, M.J. and Piddock, L.J.V. (2008). Proteomic analysis of triclosan resistance in *Salmonella enterica* serovar Typhimurium. *J. Antimicrob. Chemother.* 62: 92–97.

21

Sterilisation Procedures and Sterility Assurance

Alistair K. Brown[1] *and Stephen P. Denyer*[2]

[1]*Lecturer in Molecular Microbiology, Institute of Biosciences, Newcastle University, Newcastle upon Tyne, UK*
[2]*Emeritus Professor of Pharmacy, Universities of Brighton and Sussex, Brighton, UK*

CONTENTS

Hugo and Russell's Pharmaceutical Microbiology, Ninth Edition. Edited by Brendan F. Gilmore and Stephen P. Denyer.

Companion website: https://www.wiley.com/go/HugoandRussells9e

21.1 Introduction

Sterilisation is an essential stage in the processing of any materials destined for parenteral administration, or for contact with broken skin, mucosal surfaces or internal organs, where the threat of infection exists (see Chapter 22). Additionally, the sterilisation of microbiological materials, soiled dressings and other contaminated items following use is essential to minimise the associated health hazard with these articles and reduce potential cross contamination.

Sterilisation procedures involve the use of biocidal agents or the physical removal of contaminating microorganisms from a product or preparation with the objective of killing or eliminating all microorganisms. The process of sterilisation may involve elevated temperature, reactive gas, irradiation or filtration through a microorganism-proof filter. The success of the process depends upon the suitability of the chosen treatment conditions, for example, temperature and duration of exposure. It is however critical to take into consideration that all items to be sterilised may be adversely affected by the process applied and thus present a potential risk of product damage. For a pharmaceutical preparation, this may result in reduced therapeutic efficacy, stability or patient acceptability. Therefore, in selecting any sterilisation process, there is a need to achieve a balance between the maximum acceptable risk of failing to achieve sterility and the maximum level of product damage that is acceptable. Knowledge of the sterilant properties, the characteristics of the product to be sterilised and the nature of the likely contaminants are all essential in the preparation of sterile pharmaceutical products. With these key criteria fully understood, a suitable sterilisation process can be selected to ensure maximum microbial kill/removal with minimum product deterioration.

21.2 Sensitivity of Microorganisms

The pattern of resistance of microorganisms to biocidal sterilisation processes is largely independent of the type of agent employed whether it is heat, radiation or gas. Vegetative forms of bacteria and fungi, along with the larger viruses, are more susceptible to sterilisation processes than small viruses and spores (bacterial or fungal). During the validation of sterilisation processes (see Section 21.12.3), the choice of reference organism is of the utmost importance. The organism of choice must be the most suitable to resist the process, usually selected from the most durable bacterial endospores; *Geobacillus stearothermophilus* is generally utilised for moist heat, strains of *Bacillus atrophaeus* (formerly *Bacillus subtilis var. niger*) for dry heat and gaseous sterilisation and *Bacillus pumilus* for ionising radiation.

When considering the level of treatment necessary to achieve sterility, it is advantageous that knowledge of the type and total number of microorganisms present in a product is available; this will then inform a reliable selection of treatment. However, without this information, it is usually assumed that organisms within the product are no more resistant than the reference endospores or than known specific resistant product isolates. A sterilisation process may thus be developed without a full microbiological background to the product, instead being based on the ability to deal with a 'worst case' scenario. This is indeed the situation for official sterilisation methods, which must be capable of general application in many production situations. Modern pharmacopoeial recommendations have been derived from careful analysis of experimental data on bacterial endospore survival following treatments with heat, ionising radiation or gas, and therefore give the most informed choice available.

The agents responsible for spongiform encephalopathies (prions; proteinaceous infectious particles, see Chapters 5, 19 and 20) require further consideration due to their exceptional degrees of resistance to many lethal agents. These infectious agents, causing conditions such as bovine spongiform encephalopathy (BSE) and Creutzfeldt–Jakob disease (CJD), can be present in bovine products exploited in pharmaceutical preparations. Some work has even cast doubt on the adequacy of the process of 18-minute exposure to steam at 134–138 °C which has been recommended for the destruction of prions (and which far exceeds the lethal treatment required to achieve adequate destruction of endospores). Combinations of chemical and heat treatments have proven more effective with chlorine, guanidine thiocyanate and sodium hydroxide demonstrating a greater than 4-log reduction in prion titre. Chlorine in combination with heat has perhaps provided the most consistent prion inactivation outcome, but even this has shown variable efficacy. Studies have also revealed that sterilising agents such as formaldehyde can actually enhance the resistance of prions, for example, where pre-treatment of scrapie-infected brain tissue with formaldehyde abolished the inactivating effect of autoclaving, emphasising the need to select the correct sterilisation process based on careful experimentation.

21.2.1 Survivor Curves

Populations of microorganisms generally lose their viability in an exponential fashion when exposed to killing processes independent of the initial number of organisms. Survivor curves are a graphical representation of the logarithm of the fraction of survivors plotted against the exposure time or dose (Figure 21.1). Of the three typical survival curves obtained, all have a portion of linear decline which may be continuous (A), or may be modified by an initial shoulder of resistance to the treatment (B) or by a reduced rate of kill at low survivor levels (C). Furthermore, a short activation phase, represented by an initial increase in viable count, may be seen during the heat treatment of certain bacterial endospores. Survivor curves have been employed predominantly in the examination of heat sterilisation processes, but can be realistically applied to any biocidal process.

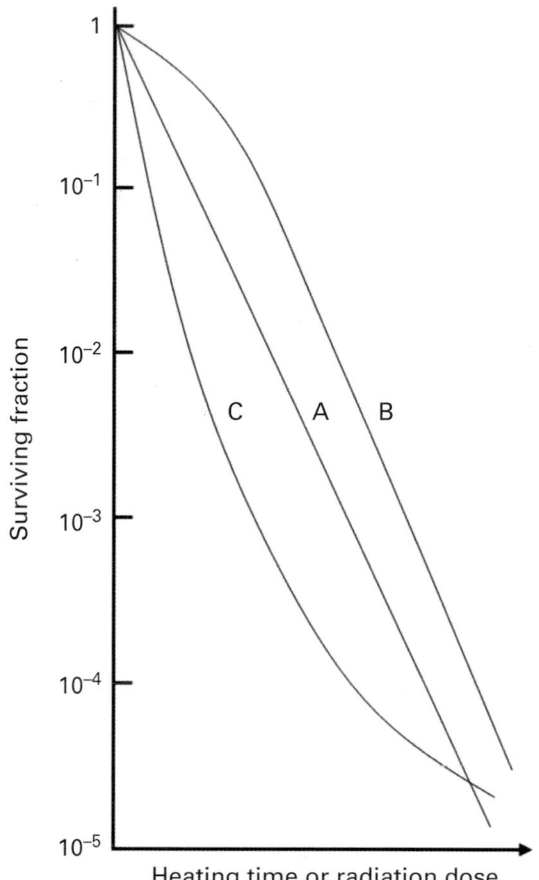

Figure 21.1 Typical survivor curves for bacterial endospores exposed to moist heat or gamma radiation.

21.2.2 Expressions of Resistance

21.2.2.1 *D*-value

The ability of an organism to resist a sterilising agent can be described by means of the *D*-value. For heat and radiation treatments, this is defined as the time taken at a fixed temperature or the radiation dose required to achieve a 90% reduction in viable cells (i.e., a 1-log [tenfold] reduction in survivors; Figure 21.2a). The calculation of the *D*-value assumes a linear survivor curve (A in Figure 21.1), and therefore must be corrected to allow for any deviation from linearity. Some typical *D*-values for resistant bacterial endospores are given in Table 21.1.

21.2.2.2 *z*-value

The *D*-value only denotes the resistance of a microorganism at a particular temperature. The influence of temperature changes on the thermal resistance of a microorganism is represented by the relationship between temperature and log *D*-value, leading to the expression of a *z*-value, representing the increase in temperature needed to reduce the *D*-value of an organism by 90% (i.e., a 1-log [tenfold] reduction; Figure 21.2b). For endospores used as biological indicators (BIs) for moist heat (*G. stearothermophilus*) and dry heat (*B. atrophaeus*) sterilisation processes, mean *z*-values are given as 10 °C and 22 °C, respectively. The *z*-value is not truly independent of temperature but may be considered essentially constant over the temperature ranges used in heat sterilisation processes.

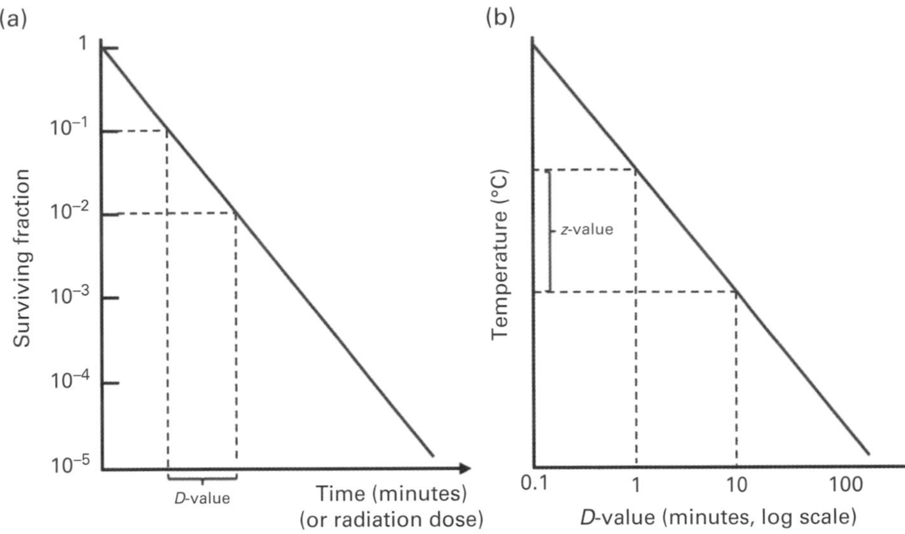

Figure 21.2 Determination of: (a) *D*-value; (b) *z*-value.

Table 21.1 Inactivation factors (IF) for selected sterilisation protocols and their corresponding biological indicator organisms.

Sterilisation protocol	Organism	Typical *D*-value	Log IF
Moist heat (121 °C for 15 min)	*G. stearothermophilus*	1.5 min	10
Dry heat (160 °C for 2 h)	*B. atrophaeus*	3 min	40
Irradiation (25 kGy)	*B. pumilus*	1.9 kGy	13.2

21.2.3 Sterility Assurance

The term 'sterile', in a microbiological context, denotes that no surviving organisms are present in the product. Consequently, there are no degrees of sterility; an item is either sterile or it is not. Therefore, for a product to be considered sterile, no levels of contamination may be considered as negligible, insignificant or acceptable. From the survivor curves presented (Figure 21.1), the elimination of viable microorganisms from a product is a time-dependent process and will be influenced by the rate and duration of biocidal action and the initial microbial contamination level. True sterility, represented by zero survivors, can only be achieved after an infinite exposure period or radiation dose. It is therefore illogical to claim, or expect, that a sterilisation procedure will guarantee absolute sterility (see also Chapter 22).

The likelihood of a product being produced free of microorganisms is best expressed in terms of the probability of an organism surviving the treatment process, a likelihood which is not associated with the absolute term 'sterile'. This approach gives rise to the concept of 'sterility assurance' or a microbial safety index which gives a numerical value to the probability of a single surviving organism remaining in a processed product. For pharmaceutical products, the most frequently applied standard is that the probability, post sterilisation, of a non-sterile unit is no more than 1 in 1 million units processed (i.e., $\leq 10^{-6}$). The sterilisation protocol necessary to achieve this with any given organism of known *D*-value can be established from the inactivation factor (IF) which may be defined as:

$$\text{IF} = 10^{t/D}$$

where t is the contact time (for a heat or gaseous sterilisation process) or dose (for ionising radiation) and D is the *D*-value appropriate to the process employed.

Therefore, for an initial burden of 10^2 endospores, an inactivation factor of 10^8 will be needed to give the required sterility assurance of 10^{-6} (Figure 21.3). The sterilisation process will therefore need to produce sufficient lethality to achieve an 8-log cycle reduction in viable organisms; this will require exposure of the product to eight times the *D*-value of the reference organism (8*D*). Typical production practice assumes that the contaminant will have the same resistance as the relevant biological indicator spores unless full microbiological data are available to indicate otherwise. The inactivation factors associated with certain

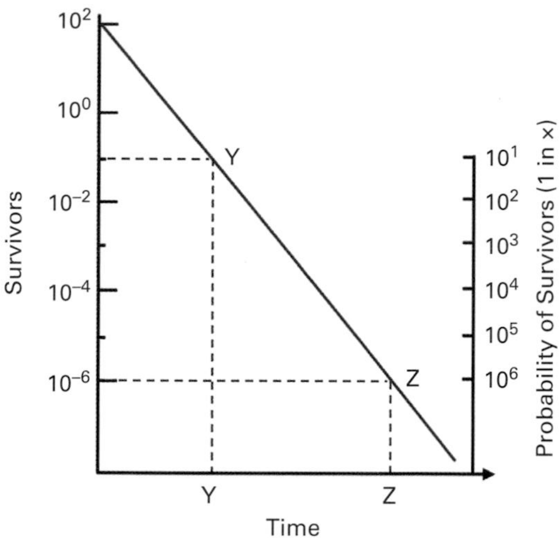

Figure 21.3 Sterility assurance. At Y, there is (literally) 10^{-1} bacterium in one bottle, i.e., in 10 loads of single containers, there would be a 1 in 10 chance that one load would be positive. Likewise, at Z, there is (literally) 10^{-6} bacterium in one bottle, i.e., in 1 million (10^6) loads of single containers, there is a 1 in 1 million chance that one load would be positive.

sterilisation protocols and their biological indicator organisms are given in Table 21.1.

21.3 Sterilisation Methods

Sterilisation process selection should always be considered a compromise between achieving good antimicrobial activity and maintaining product stability. It must, therefore, be validated against a suitable organism and its efficacy continually monitored during use. A limit will nevertheless exist as to the type and size of microbial challenge that can be controlled by the process without significant loss of sterility assurance. Therefore, sterilisation must not be seen as an alternative to good manufacturing practice (GMP), but must be considered as only the final stage in a programme of microbiological control. The *European Pharmacopoeia* recognises five methods for the sterilisation of pharmaceutical products: (i) steam sterilisation (heating in an autoclave); (ii) dry heat; (iii) ionising radiation; (iv) gaseous sterilisation; and (v) filtration. In addition, other approaches involving steam and formaldehyde and ultraviolet (UV) light have evolved for use in certain situations. Each method has several possible permutations of exposure conditions, but experience and product stability requirements have generally served to limit this choice. Nevertheless, it should be remembered that even the recommended methods and regimens do not necessarily demonstrate equivalent biocidal potential (see Table 21.1, for instance), but simply offer alternative strategies for application to a wide variety of product types. Thus, each process should be validated in its application to demonstrate that the minimum required level of sterility assurance can be achieved (Sections 21.2.3 and 21.9).

The factors governing the successful use of these sterilising methods will be covered in the subsequent sections, and their application in pharmaceutical and medical production will be considered. Methods for monitoring the efficacy of these processes are discussed in Section 21.12.

21.4 Heat Sterilisation

Heat is the most reliable and widely used means of sterilisation, with the antimicrobial activity being attributed to the destruction of proteins (e.g., enzymes, glycopeptides, storage and structural proteins) and other essential cellular components. These lethal events proceed most rapidly in a fully hydrated state, therefore requiring a lower heat input (temperature and time). Under high humidity conditions, denaturation and hydrolysis reactions predominate, rather than in the dry state where oxidative changes take place. This method of sterilisation is limited to thermostable products, but can be applied to both moisture-sensitive and moisture-resistant items for which dry (160–180 °C) and moist (121–134 °C) heat sterilisation procedures are respectively used. Where thermal degradation of a product requires consideration, it can usually be minimised by selecting the higher temperature range, as the shorter exposure times employed generally result in a lower fractional degradation.

21.4.1 Sterilisation Processes

In any heat sterilisation process, the articles to be treated must first be raised to sterilisation temperature in an initial heating-up stage. In the traditional approach, timing for the process (the holding time) then begins. It has been recognised, however, that during both the heating-up and cooling-down stages of a sterilisation cycle (Figure 21.4), the product is held at an elevated temperature and these stages may thus contribute to the overall biocidal potential of the process.

A method has been devised to convert all the temperature–time combinations occurring during the heating, sterilising and cooling stages of a moist heat sterilisation cycle (sometimes called autoclaving) to the equivalent time at 121 °C. This involves following the temperature profile of a load, integrating the heat input (as a measure of lethality) and converting it to the equivalent time at the standard temperature of 121 °C. This approach enables the quantification of the overall lethality of any process and is defined as the

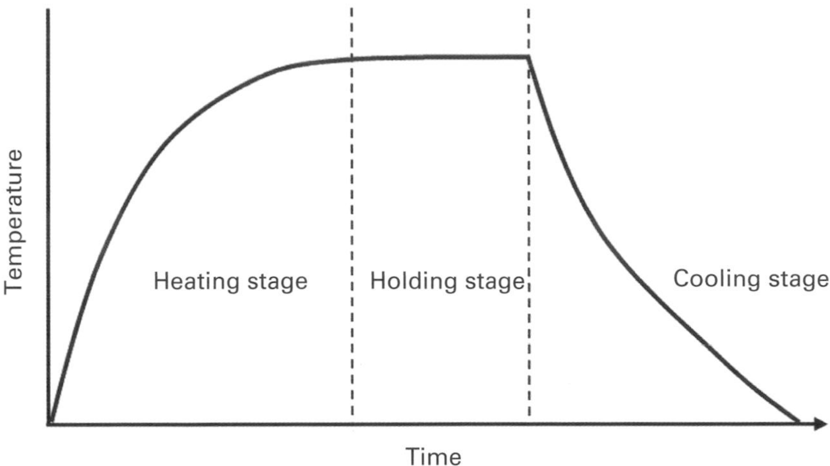

Figure 21.4 Typical temperature profile of a heat sterilisation process.

F-value; this expresses heat treatment at any temperature as equal to that of a standard number of minutes at 121 °C.

For example, if a moist heat sterilisation process has an *F*-value of *x*, then it has the same lethal effect on a given organism as heating at 121 °C for *x* minutes, irrespective of the actual temperature employed or of any fluctuations in the heating process due to heating and cooling stages. The *F*-value of a process will vary according to the moist-heat resistance of the reference organism; when the reference spore is that of *G. stearothermophilus* with a *z*-value of 10 °C, then the *F*-value is known as the F_0-value.

The relationship between *F*- and *D*-values enables the calculation of the probable number of survivors in a load following heat treatment, using the following equation:

$$F = D\left(\log N_0 - \log N\right)$$

where *D* is the *D*-value at 121 °C, and N_0 and *N* represent, respectively, the initial and final numbers of viable cells per unit volume.

The *F*-value concept has evolved from the food industry and principally relates to the sterilisation of articles by moist heat because it permits calculation of the extent to which the heating and cooling phases contribute to the overall killing effect of the autoclaving cycle. The *F*-value enables a sterilisation process to be individually developed for a particular product so that sterility assurance can be achieved in autoclaving cycles in which the traditional pharmacopoeial recommendation of 15 minutes at 121 °C is not attainable. The holding time may be reduced below 15 minutes if there is a substantial killing effect during the heating and cooling phases, and an adequate cycle can be achieved even if the 'target' temperature of 121 °C is not reached.

Thus, *F*-values offer both a means by which alternative sterilising cycles can be compared in terms of their microbial killing efficiency and a mechanism by which over-processing of marginally thermolabile products can be reduced without compromising sterility assurance. Cycles below a holding temperature of 110 °C with an $F_0 < 8$ minutes should not be considered as sterilising cycles, but may be suitable heat treatments to supplement an aseptic process. The F_0 value of a saturated steam sterilisation process is defined by pharmacopoeias as the lethality expressed in terms of the equivalent time in minutes at a temperature of 121 °C delivered by the process to the product in its final container with reference to microorganisms possessing a theoretical *z*-value of 10 °C. F_0 values may be calculated either from the area under the curve of a plot of autoclave temperature against time constructed using special chart paper on which the temperature scale is modified to account for the progressively greater lethality of higher temperatures, or by use of the equation:

$$F_0 = \Delta t \sum 10^{(T-121)/z}$$

where Δt is the time interval between temperature measurements, *T* is the product temperature at time *t* and *z* is (assumed to be) 10 °C.

Therefore, if temperatures were recorded from a thermocouple at 1-minute intervals, then $\Delta t = 1.00$, and a temperature of, for example, 115 °C maintained for 1 minute would give an F_0 value of 1 minute $\times\ 10^{(115-121)/10}$, which is equal to 0.25 minutes. These calculations would be performed as part of the batch records during production as part of the sterility assurance process. Application of the *F*-value concept has been largely restricted to steam sterilisation processes, although there is a less frequently employed but direct parallel in dry heat sterilisation (see Section 21.4.3).

Table 21.2 Pressure–temperature relationships and antimicrobial efficacies of alternative steam sterilisation cycles.

Temperature (°C)	Holding time (min)	Steam pressure		Inactivation factor[a] (decimal reductions)
		(kPa)	(psi)	
115	30	69	10	5
121	15	103	15	10
126	10	138	20	21
134	3	207	30	40

[a] Calculated for a spore suspension having a D_{121} of 1.5 minutes and a z-value of 10 °C.

21.4.2 Moist Heat Sterilisation

Moist heat has been recognised as an efficient biocidal agent from the early days of bacteriology, when it was principally developed for the sterilisation of culture media. It is now the application of choice when processing thermostable products and devices. In the pharmaceutical and medical sectors, it is used in the sterilisation of dressings, sheets, surgical and diagnostic equipment, containers and closures, and aqueous injections, ophthalmic preparations and irrigation fluids (see Chapter 22), in addition to the processing of soiled and contaminated items.

Sterilisation by moist heat usually employs steam at temperatures in the range 121–134 °C, and while alternative strategies are available for the processing of products unstable at these high temperatures, they rarely offer the same degree of sterility assurance and should be avoided if possible. The elevated temperatures generally associated with moist heat sterilisation methods can only be achieved by the generation of steam under pressure (Table 21.2).

The most commonly employed standard temperature/time cycles for bottled fluids and porous loads (e.g., surgical dressings) are 121 °C for 15 minutes and 134 °C for 3 minutes, respectively. Not only do high-temperature–short time cycles often result in lower fractional degradation, they also afford the advantage of achieving higher levels of sterility assurance due to greater IF (Table 21.2). Before the publication of the 1988 *British Pharmacopoeia*, the 115 °C for 30-minute cycle was considered an acceptable alternative to 121 °C for 15 minutes, but it is no longer considered sufficient to give the desired sterility assurance levels for products which may contain significant concentrations of thermophilic spores.

21.4.2.1 Steam as a Sterilising Agent

To act as an efficient sterilising agent, steam should be able to provide moisture and heat efficiently to the article to be sterilised. This is most effectively done using saturated steam, which is steam in thermal equilibrium with the water from which it is derived, that is, steam on the phase boundary (Figure 21.5). Under these circumstances, contact with a cooler surface causes condensation and contraction, drawing in fresh steam and leading to the immediate release of the latent heat, which represents approximately 80% of the total heat energy. In this way, heat and moisture are imparted rapidly to articles being sterilised and dry porous loads are quickly penetrated by the steam.

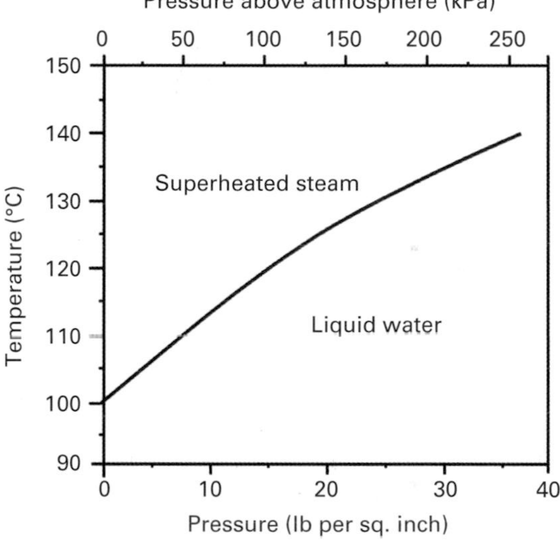

Figure 21.5 Pressure–temperature diagram for water at the phase boundary.

Steam for sterilisation can either be generated within the steriliser, as with portable bench or 'instrument and utensil' sterilisers, in which case it is constantly in contact with water and is known as 'wet' steam, or can be supplied under pressure (350–400 kPa) from a separate boiler as 'dry' saturated steam with no entrained water droplets. The killing potential of 'wet' steam is the same as that of 'dry' saturated steam at the same temperature, but it is more likely to soak a porous load, creating physical difficulties for further steam penetration. Thus, major industrial and hospital sterilisers are usually supplied with 'dry' saturated steam and attention is paid to the removal of entrained

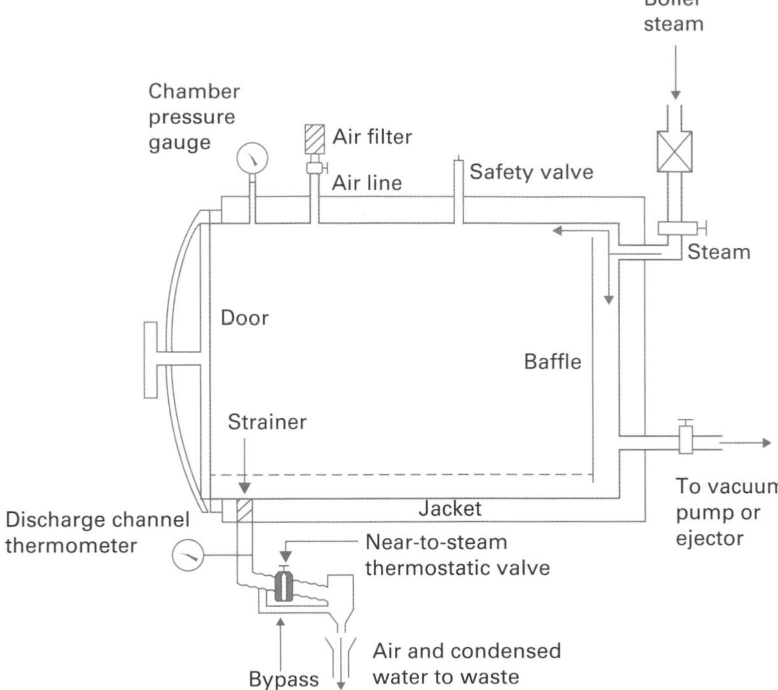

Figure 21.6 Main constructional features of a large-scale steam steriliser (autoclave).

water droplets within the supply line to prevent introduction of a water 'fog' into the steriliser.

Increasing the temperature of 'dry' saturated steam at the phase boundary in the absence of entrained moisture will result in the relative humidity or degree of saturation being reduced and as a result the steam becomes superheated (Figure 21.5). This can arise in a number of ways, for example, by overheating the steam jacket (see Section 21.4.2.2), using too dry a steam supply, excessive pressure reduction during passage of steam from the boiler to the steriliser chamber, and the evolution of heat of hydration when steaming overdried cotton fabrics. The behaviour of superheated steam is not dissimilar to hot air, as condensation and release of latent heat will not occur unless the steam is cooled to the phase boundary temperature. It therefore proves to be an inefficient sterilising agent and, although a small degree of transient superheating can be tolerated, a maximum acceptable level of 5 °C superheat is set, that is, the temperature of the steam is never greater than 5 °C above the phase boundary temperature at that pressure.

The relationship between temperature and pressure holds true only in the presence of pure steam; contamination with air contributes to a partial pressure but not to the temperature of the steam. In the presence of air, the temperature achieved will reflect the contribution made by the steam only and will be lower than that normally attributed to the total pressure recorded. Additional steam will raise the temperature, but residual air surrounding articles may delay heat penetration. Large accumulations of air may collect at the bottom of the steriliser resulting in the complete alteration of the thermal profile of the steriliser chamber. Therefore, efficient air removal is a major objective in boiler-fed steam steriliser design and operation.

21.4.2.2 Steriliser Design and Operation

Steam sterilisers, commonly known as *autoclaves*, are stainless-steel vessels designed to withstand the steam pressures employed during the process.

Portable small sterilisers generally have internal electric heaters to produce steam and are used for pilot or laboratory-scale sterilisation and for the treatment of instruments and utensils. Large-scale sterilisers are routinely used in hospitals and industry, operating on 'dry' saturated steam from a separate boiler (Figure 21.6).

There are two main types of large steriliser, those designed for use with porous loads (i.e., dressings) and generally operated at a minimum temperature of 134 °C, and those designed as bottled fluid sterilisers employing a minimum temperature of 121 °C. The operational stages are common to both and can be summarised as air removal and steam admission, heating-up and exposure, and drying/cooling. Many designs exist and, in this section, only general design features will be considered. Fuller treatments of steriliser design and operation can be found in the relevant Department of Health technical memorandums (DH 2014, 2016a, b).

General Design Features Steam sterilisers are constructed with either cylindrical or rectangular chambers, with capacities ranging from 400 to 800 L. They can be sealed by either a single door or by doors at both ends (to allow through passage of processed materials into sterile areas, see Chapter 22). Safety locking mechanisms secure the doors during sterilisation to prevent opening when the chamber is under pressure and until the chamber has cooled to a preset temperature, 50–80 °C.

In larger sterilisers, the chamber can be surrounded by a steam jacket, this affords a more uniform heating of the autoclave chamber and therefore promotes a more constant temperature throughout the contents. The same jacket can also be filled with water at the end of the cycle to facilitate cooling and thus reduce the overall cycle time. The chamber floor slopes towards a discharge channel through which air and condensate can be removed (Figure 21.6). Temperature is monitored within the opening of the discharge channel and by thermocouples in dummy packages; jacket and chamber pressures are followed using pressure gauges. In hospitals and industry, it is common practice to operate sterilisers on an automatic cycle, where each stage of the operation is controlled by a timer responding to temperature- or pressure-sensing devices.

The operational stages of large sterilisers are as follows and directly relate to Figure 21.6.

1) *Air removal and steam admission:* Air can be removed from steam sterilisers either by downward displacement with steam, evacuation or a combination of both. In a downward displacement steriliser, the heavier cool air is forced out of the discharge channel by incoming hot steam. This has the benefit of warming the contents during air removal, which aids the heating process. It finds widest application in the sterilisation of bottled fluids where bottle breakage may occur under the combined stresses of evacuation and high temperature. This technique of air removal is unsatisfactory for air-retentive loads (i.e., dressings), and mechanical evacuation of the air is essential before the admission of steam. This can be achieved via extreme pressure levels (e.g., 2.5 kPa) or through a period of pulsed evacuation and steam admission, the latter approach improving air extraction from dressing packages. After evacuation, steam penetration into the load is very rapid and heating-up is almost instantaneous. It is accepted that packaging and loading of articles within a steriliser must be organised so as to facilitate air removal.

   During the sterilisation process, small pockets of trapped air may be released, especially from packages, and this air must be removed. Porous load autoclaves achieve this with a near-to-steam thermostatic valve incorporated in the discharge channel. The valve operates on the principle of expandable bellows containing a volatile liquid which vapourises at the temperature of saturated steam thereby closing the valve, and condenses on the passage of a cooler air–steam mixture, thus reopening the valve and discharging the air. Condensate generated during the sterilisation process can also be removed by this device. Small quantities of air will not, however, lower the temperature sufficiently to operate the valve and so a continual light flow of steam is maintained through a bypass around the device to flush away residual air.

   It is common practice to package sterile fluids, especially intravenous fluids, in flexible plastic containers. During sterilisation, these can develop a considerable internal pressure in the airspace above the fluid and it is therefore necessary to maintain a proportion of air within the sterilising chamber to produce sufficient overpressure to prevent these containers from bursting (air ballasting). In sterilisers modified or designed to process this type of product, air removal is therefore unnecessary, but special attention must be paid to the prevention of air 'layering' within the chamber. This is overcome by the inclusion of a fan or through a continuous spray of hot water within the chamber to mix the air and steam. Air ballasting can also be employed to prevent bottle breakage due to the extreme pressures and temperature.
2) *Heating-up and exposure:* When the steriliser reaches its operating temperature and pressure, the sterilisation stage begins. The duration of exposure may include a heating-up time in addition to the holding time and this will normally be established using thermocouples in dummy articles.
3) *Drying or cooling:* Dressing packs and other porous loads may become dampened during the sterilisation process and must be dried before removal from the chamber. This is achieved by steam exhaust and application of a vacuum, often assisted by heat from the steam-filled jacket if fitted. After drying, atmospheric pressure within the chamber is restored by admission of sterile filtered air.

For bottled fluids, the final stage of the sterilisation process is cooling, and this needs to be achieved as rapidly as possible to minimise thermal degradation of the product and to reduce processing time. In some sterilisers, this is achieved by circulating water in the jacket that surrounds the chamber or by spray-cooling with retained condensate delivered to the surface of the load by nozzles fitted into the roof of the steriliser chamber. This is often accompanied by the introduction of filtered, compressed air to minimise container breakage due to high internal pressures. Containers must not be removed from the steriliser until the internal pressure has dropped to a safe level, usually indicated by a temperature of 50–80 °C. Occasionally, spray-cooling water may be a source of bacterial contamination and its microbiological quality must be carefully monitored.

21.4.3 Dry Heat Sterilisation

The lethal effects of dry heat on microorganisms are due largely to oxidative processes, which are less effective than the hydrolytic damage which results from exposure to steam. Thus, dry heat sterilisation usually employs higher temperatures (160–180 °C) and requires exposure times of up to 2 hours depending on the temperature employed.

Bacterial endospores are again much more tolerant than vegetative cells and their recorded resistance varies significantly depending on their degree of dryness. In many early studies on dry heat resistance of spores, their water content was not adequately controlled, so conflicting data arose regarding the exposure conditions necessary to achieve effective sterilisation. This was partly responsible for variations in recommended exposure temperatures and times in different pharmacopoeias.

Dry heat applications are generally restricted to glassware and metal surgical instruments (where its good penetrability and non-corrosive nature are of benefit), non-aqueous thermostable liquids and thermostable powders. In practice, the range of materials that are actually subjected to dry heat sterilisation is quite limited and consists largely of items used in hospitals or dental surgeries. The main industrial application of this sterilisation process is for glass bottles which are to be filled aseptically. This affords not only an adequate sterility assurance level but also aids the destruction of bacterial endotoxins (products of Gram-negative bacteria, also known as pyrogens, which cause fever when injected into the body). These are difficult to eliminate by other means, and therefore for the depyrogenation of glass, temperatures of approximately 250 °C are used.

The *F*-value concept that was developed for steam sterilisation processes has an equivalent in dry heat sterilisation, although its application has been limited throughout the industry. The F_H designation describes the lethality of a dry heat process in terms of the equivalent number of minutes exposure at 170 °C, and in this case a *z*-value of 20 °C has been found empirically to be appropriate for calculation purposes; this contrasts with the value of 10 °C which is typically employed to describe moist-heat resistance.

21.4.3.1 Steriliser Design

Dry heat sterilisation is usually carried out in a hot-air oven which comprises an insulated polished stainless-steel chamber, with a usual capacity of up to 250 L, surrounded by an outer case containing electric heaters located in positions to prevent cool spots developing inside the chamber. A fan is fitted to the rear of the oven to provide circulating air, thus ensuring more rapid equilibration of temperature. Shelves within the chamber are perforated to allow good airflow. Thermocouples can be used to monitor the temperature of both the oven air and articles contained within. A fixed temperature sensor connected to a chart or digital recorder provides a permanent record of the sterilisation cycle. Appropriate door-locking controls are integrated to prevent interruption of a sterilisation cycle once begun.

Recent steriliser developments have led to the use of dry heat sterilising tunnels where heat transfer is achieved by infrared irradiation or by forced convection in filtered laminar airflow tunnels. Items to be sterilised are placed on a conveyor belt and pass through a high-temperature zone (250–300+ °C) over a period of several minutes.

21.4.3.2 Steriliser Operation

Articles to be sterilised must be wrapped or enclosed in containers of sufficient strength and integrity to provide good post-sterilisation protection against contamination. Suitable materials are paper, cardboard tubes or aluminium containers. Container design must ensure that heat penetration is assisted in order to shorten the heating-up stage; this can be achieved by using narrow containers with dull, non-reflecting surfaces. In a hot-air oven, heat is delivered to articles principally by radiation and convection; thus, they must be carefully arranged within the chamber to avoid obscuring centrally placed articles from wall radiation or by impeding airflow. During operation it is essential that the temperature variation within the chamber should not exceed ±5 °C of the recorded temperature. Heating-up times, which may be as long as 4 hours for articles with poor heat-conducting properties, can be reduced by preheating the oven before loading. Following sterilisation, the chamber temperature is usually allowed to fall to around 40 °C before removal of sterilised articles; this can be accelerated by the use of forced cooling with filtered air injection.

21.5 Gaseous Sterilisation

A variety of chemically reactive agents have been considered for use as sterilising gases, either in the true gaseous phase or in the vapour form as a mixture of liquid and gas; these include chlorine dioxide, ethylene oxide, formaldehyde, hydrogen peroxide, nitrogen dioxide, ozone, peracetic acid and propylene oxide. Of these, three have become established in use: ethylene oxide [$(CH_2)_2O$] and formaldehyde (methanal, H.CHO), which both possess broad-spectrum microbicidal activity, and, particularly for the specialist sterilisation of medical devices, vapourised hydrogen peroxide (VHP, H_2O_2). All are surface sterilisers and their applications include the sterilisation of reusable surgical instruments, certain medical, diagnostic and electrical equipment, containers and, in some instances, the surface sterilisation of powders. Gaseous sterilisation processes using ethylene oxide are the most widely used, with VHP now surpassing formaldehyde.

Ethylene oxide treatment can be considered as an alternative to radiation sterilisation in the commercial production of disposable medical devices (see Chapter 22). Gaseous techniques, while capable of providing the necessary levels of sterility assurance, are generally reserved for temperature-sensitive products and items. To ensure adequate sterility, sufficient penetration of product packaging by gas and moisture is essential.

The mechanism of antimicrobial action of the two alkylating gases is assumed to be through reaction with sulphydryl, amino, hydroxyl and carboxyl groups on proteins and imino groups of nucleic acids. Formaldehyde further acts to cross-link with amino and imino groups of proteins and nucleic acids to form protein–protein and protein–nucleic acid aggregates, but it does not react with free double-stranded DNA. Hydrogen peroxide is an oxidising agent, reacting strongly with the thiol groups of many biomolecules within the cell wall and cytoplasmic membrane. It is most active in its vapourised form, penetrating and denaturing three-dimensional protein structures and oxidising lipids; it is likely to owe some of its activity to hydroxyl free radical reactions, particularly in the vapour phase.

At the concentrations employed in sterilisation protocols, type A survivor curves (Figure 21.1) generally predominate for ethylene oxide and formaldehyde with the lethality of these gases then increasing in a non-uniform manner with increased concentration, exposure temperature and humidity. For this reason, sterilisation protocols have generally been established by an empirical approach using a standard product load containing suitable biological indicator test strips (Section 21.12.3). Concentration ranges (given as weight of gas per unit chamber volume) are usually of the order of 800–1200 mg l^{-1} for ethylene oxide and 15–100 mg l^{-1} for formaldehyde, with operating temperatures in the region of 45–63 °C and 70–75 °C, respectively. Even at the higher concentrations and temperatures, the sterilisation processes are lengthy and therefore unsuitable for the resterilisation of high-turnover articles. Further delays occur because of the need to remove toxic residues of the gases before release of the items for use. In the case of VHP, an operating concentration of 1–2 mg l^{-1} of hydrogen peroxide vapour in a typical temperature range of 30–60 °C is used. There is evidence of more complex biphasic type B or C survivor curves (Figure 21.1) with VHP; this necessitates an investigation of the inactivation kinetics with a biological indicator in the steriliser system as a whole before a validation approach and suitable process parameters can be determined.

As alkylating agents, both ethylene oxide and formaldehyde are potentially mutagenic and carcinogenic (as is the ethylene chlorohydrin that results from ethylene oxide reaction with chlorine); they also produce symptoms of acute toxicity including irritation of the skin, conjunctiva and nasal mucosa. Consequently, strict control of their atmospheric concentrations and of their volatile by-products is necessary, and safe working protocols are required to protect personnel. Hydrogen peroxide is an irritant but is not classified as carcinogenic, and VHP is not known to leave toxic residues. Table 21.3 summarises some comparative advantages afforded by ethylene oxide, low-temperature steam and formaldehyde (LTSF) and VHP processes.

21.5.1 Ethylene Oxide

Ethylene oxide gas is highly explosive in mixtures of greater than 3.6% v/v in air; in order to reduce this explosion hazard, it is supplied for sterilisation purposes as a 10% mix with carbon dioxide, or as an 8.6% mixture with HFC-124 (2-chloro-1,1,1,2-tetrafluoroethane), which has replaced fluorinated hydrocarbons (freons). Alternatively, pure ethylene oxide gas can be used below atmospheric pressure in steriliser chambers from which all air has been removed. The safe delivery of 100% ethylene oxide requires that at least 97% of the air must be removed from the chamber. The most common methods for accomplishing this are by using a vacuum pump or by performing a series of partial evacuations followed by a series of nitrogen injections.

The efficacy of ethylene oxide treatment depends on achieving a suitable concentration in each article. This is assisted greatly by the penetrating powers of the gas, which diffuses readily into many packaging materials including rubber, plastics, fabric and paper. This is not without its drawbacks, however, since the level of ethylene oxide in a steriliser will decrease due to absorption during the process and the treated articles must undergo a desorption stage to remove toxic residues. Desorption can be allowed to occur naturally on open shelves, in which case complete desorption may take many days, for example, for materials such as PVC, or special forced-aeration cabinets where flowing,

Table 21.3 Relative merits of ethylene oxide, low-temperature steam and formaldehyde (LTSF) and vapourised hydrogen peroxide (VHP) processes.

Advantages of ethylene oxide	Advantages of LTSF	Advantages of VHP
Wide international regulatory acceptance	Less hazardous than ethylene oxide because formaldehyde is not flammable and is more readily detected by smell	May be safely maintained in a chamber environment
Slower to form solid polymers (with the potential to block pipes, etc.) than formaldehyde	The gas is obtained readily from aqueous solution (formalin) which is a more convenient source than gas in cylinders	Hydrogen peroxide readily vapourised from cartridges under vacuum at low temperatures
Cycle times shorter than LTSF		Generally comparable or shorter cycle times than ethylene oxide
Better gas penetration into plastics and rubber than LTSF		Vacuum aids penetration into topologically complex products
With long exposure times it is possible to sterilise at ambient temperatures		Gas efficiently and quickly removed from chamber post sterilisation
Very low incidence of product deterioration		Compatible with a wide range of polymeric materials

heated air assists gas removal, reducing desorption times to between 2 and 24 hours.

Organisms are more resistant to ethylene oxide treatment in a dried state, as are those protected from the gas by inclusion in crystalline or dried organic deposits. Thus, a further condition to be satisfied in ethylene oxide sterilisation is attainment of a minimum level of moisture in the immediate product environment. This requires a steriliser humidity of 30–70% and frequently a preconditioning of the load to relative humidities of more than 50%.

21.5.1.1 Steriliser Design and Operation

An ethylene oxide steriliser consists of a leakproof and explosion-proof steel chamber, with an optional hot-water jacket to provide a uniform chamber temperature; steriliser capacities range from benchtop at 300–600 L to large industrial-scale sterilisers which may exceed 30,000 L capacity. Successful operation of the steriliser requires removal of air from the chamber by evacuation, humidification and conditioning of the load by passage of sub-atmospheric-pressure steam followed by a further evacuation period and the admission of preheated vapourised ethylene oxide from external pressurised canisters or single-charge cartridges. Variations in conditions throughout the steriliser chamber are minimised using forced gas circulation. Packaging materials must be air-, steam- and gas-permeable to permit sterilisation to be achieved within individual articles in the load. Absorption of ethylene oxide by the contents is compensated for by the introduction of excess gas at the beginning or by the addition of more gas as the pressure drops during the sterilisation process. Addition of water to maintain appropriate relative humidity may also be a requirement of the process due to moisture absorption.

After treatment, the gases are evacuated either directly to the outside atmosphere or through a special exhaust system. Filtered, sterile air is then admitted either for a repeat of the vacuum/air cycle or for air purging until the chamber is opened. In this way, safe removal of the ethylene oxide is achieved, reducing the toxic hazard to the operator. Sterilised articles are removed directly from the chamber and arranged for desorption for the appropriate period of time as stated above (Section 21.5.1). The operation of an ethylene oxide steriliser should be monitored and controlled automatically. A typical operating cycle for pure ethylene oxide gas is shown in Figure 21.7.

21.5.2 Formaldehyde

Formaldehyde gas for use in sterilisation is produced by heating formalin (37% w/v aqueous solution of formaldehyde) to a temperature of 70–75 °C with steam, leading to the process known as LTSF. Formaldehyde has a similar toxicity to ethylene oxide and although absorption to materials appears to be lower, similar desorption routines are recommended. The major disadvantage of formaldehyde is its low penetrative power, limiting the packaging materials that can be employed to primarily paper and cotton fabric.

21.5.2.1 Steriliser Design and Operation

An LTSF steriliser is designed to operate with sub-atmospheric-pressure steam. Air is removed by evacuation and steam is admitted to the chamber to allow heating of the load and to assist in air removal. The sterilisation period

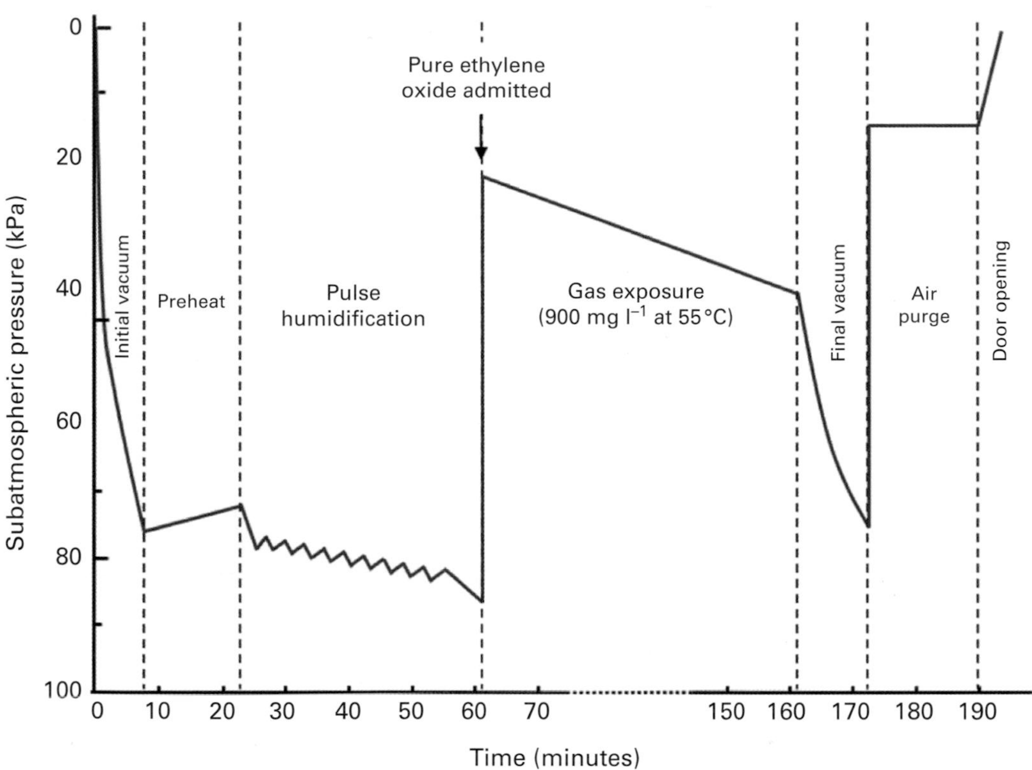

Figure 21.7 Typical operating cycle for pure ethylene oxide gas.

starts with the release of formaldehyde by vapourisation from formalin (in a vapouriser with a steam jacket) and continues through either a simple holding stage or through a series of pulsed evacuations and steam and formaldehyde admission cycles. The chamber temperature is maintained by a thermostatically controlled water jacket with steam and condensate being removed via a drain channel and an evacuated condenser. At the end of the treatment period, formaldehyde vapour is expelled by steam flushing and the load is dried by alternating stages of evacuation and admission of sterile, filtered air. A typical pulsed cycle of operation is shown in Figure 21.8.

21.5.3 Peroxygen Compounds

Hydrogen peroxide (H_2O_2) and peracetic acid (CH_3CO_3H) are used as highly effective oxidising agents to kill microorganisms (see Chapters 18 and 20); both agents have found application in the chemical sterilisation of medical, surgical and dental instruments. When vapourised in contained environments, they will sterilise all surfaces with which they come into contact. This has been exploited, particularly in the case of hydrogen peroxide, for both decontamination and sterilisation purposes. Under atmospheric conditions, one of the main applications for VHP is in environmental disinfection. Commercial VHP processes, using hand-held, portable or integrated devices to create a disinfecting 'fog', are now widely employed in the decontamination of isolators, laminar airflow cabinets, clean rooms, pharmaceutical manufacturing facilities and vacant hospital wards. However, it is the vacuum-based processes that have been developed for the sterilisation of such items as temperature-sensitive medical devices, containers and delivery systems that concern us in this chapter and are detailed below.

VHP is typically used at much lower concentrations than liquid peroxide due to the enhanced biocidal activity of the vapour form. Its efficacy against a wide range of organisms, including endospores, is a distinct advantage, but despite increasing use its mechanism of microbicidal activity is still not fully understood. Hydrogen peroxide leaves little residue on packaging and sterilised items with VHP methods demonstrating low toxicity while spontaneously breaking down into completely harmless by-products. It is axiomatic that any packaging must allow for adequate diffusion of sterilant to the article to be sterilised. While compatible with many plastics and metals, VHP is not suited for use with cellulosic packaging materials (e.g., cardboard or paper) which absorb hydrogen peroxide to the extent that sterilisation is compromised.

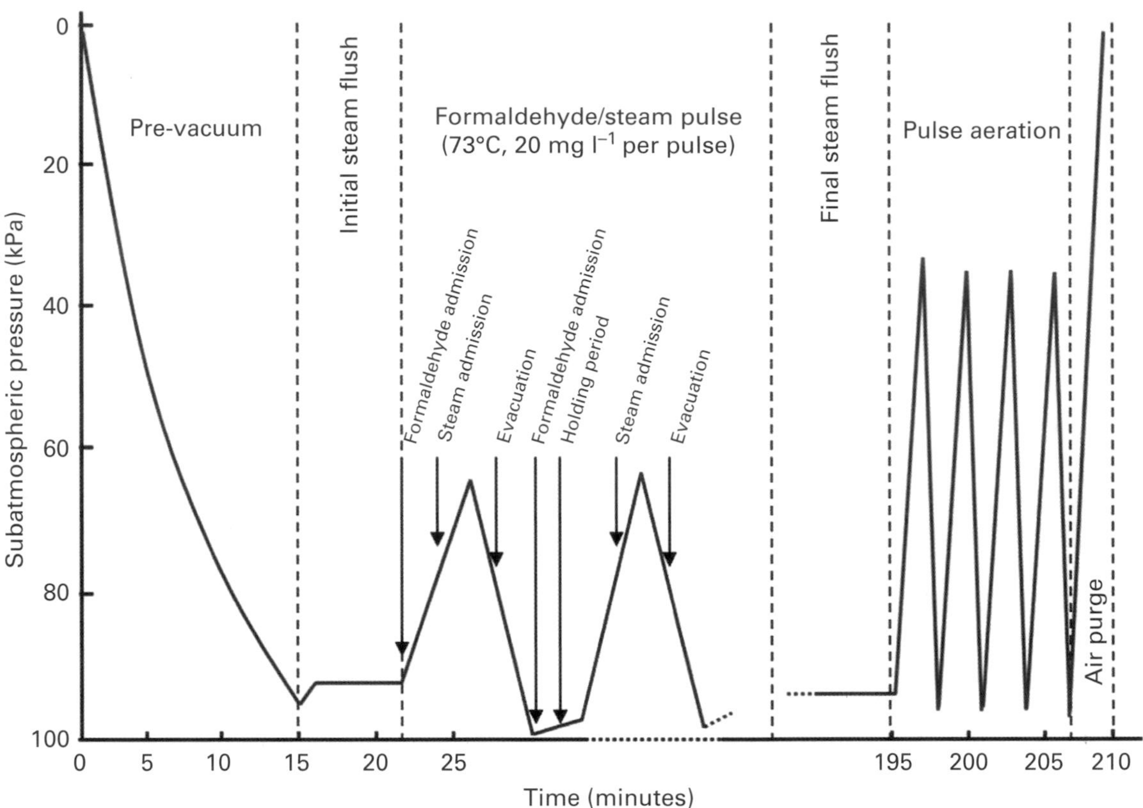

Figure 21.8 Typical operating cycle for low-temperature steam and formaldehyde treatment.

21.5.3.1 VHP Steriliser Design and Operation

A typical VHP steriliser has a capacity of between 900 and 9000 L and is designed to function at sub-atmospheric pressure. While there are variations in the commercial sterilisers available, all operate in a similar manner. In the first stage of the process, air and initial humidity are removed by evacuation to create a deep vacuum within the chamber (the conditioning phase). This assists in drawing aqueous hydrogen peroxide solution (30–35% w/v) from a disposable cartridge through a high-temperature vapouriser into the sterilisation chamber, sometimes in a pulsatile manner, in order to achieve its optimum holding concentration of 1–2 mg l^{-1}. Maintaining this deep vacuum ensures continued air removal which would otherwise impede or slow vapour penetration to surfaces, particularly important in the case of lumen devices. The VHP process operates at a relatively low temperature (often less than 50 °C) under vacuum (most typically between 1 and 10 mbar [0.1–1 kPa]) at a relative humidity of 85–90% with a rapid cycle time of 30–45 minutes, producing only environmentally safe by-products. The chamber temperature is maintained by a thermostatically controlled water jacket with vapour and condensate being removed via a drain channel and an evacuated condenser. At the end of the treatment period, evacuation and admission of sterile, filtered air (aeration phase) ensure sterility and safe operation of the machinery by workers; this phase affects the cycle time greatly, as it is directly proportional to the airflows within the machine and may take from a few minutes to several hours. A typical VHP cycle of operation is shown in Figure 21.9; overall, the processing time is usually less than 6 hours depending on product type, packaging materials, load size and configuration.

In a variation to this approach (see also Section 21.8.2), sterilisers have been designed whereby the hydrogen peroxide admitted to the sterilisation chamber is subsequently excited into a low-temperature plasma state by a radiofrequency-generated electrical field. This is believed to add to the overall microbicidal action of the vapourised hydrogen peroxide by its disassociation into free radicals of higher energy state. When the plasma energy is terminated, the free radicals recombine as oxygen and water vapour.

21.6 Radiation Sterilisation

Several types of radiation find a sterilising application in the manufacture of pharmaceutical and medical products, principal among which are accelerated electrons (particulate radiation), X-rays, gamma rays and UV light

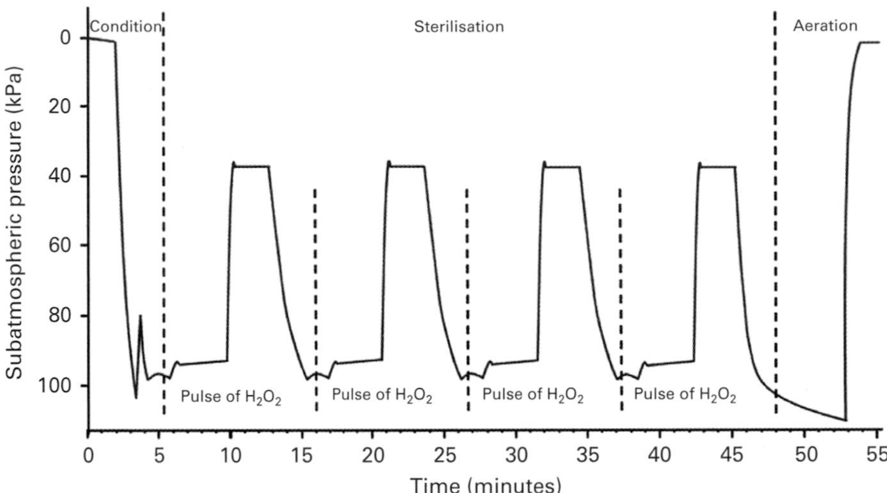

Figure 21.9 Typical operating cycle for vapourised hydrogen peroxide sterilisation.

(electromagnetic radiations). The major target for these radiations is believed to be microbial DNA, with damage occurring as a consequence of ionisation and free-radical production (gamma rays, X-rays and electrons) or excitation (UV light). This latter process is less damaging and less lethal than ionisation, and so UV irradiation is not as efficient a sterilisation method as electron, X-ray or gamma irradiation. Vegetative bacteria generally prove to be the most sensitive to irradiation (with notable exceptions, e.g., *Deinococcus* [*Micrococcus*] *radiodurans*), followed by moulds and yeasts, with bacterial endospores and viruses the most resistant (except in the case of UV light, where fungal spores prove to be most resistant). The extent of DNA damage required to lead to cell death can vary and this, together with the ability to repair the damage, determines the resistance of the organism to radiation. With ionising radiations (gamma ray, X-ray and accelerated electrons), microbial resistance decreases with the presence of moisture or dissolved oxygen (as a result of increased free-radical production) and also with elevated temperatures.

Radiation sterilisation with high-energy gamma rays, X-rays or accelerated electrons has proved to be a useful method in the industrial sterilisation of heat-sensitive products, being employed to a similar extent as ethylene oxide. However, undesirable changes can occur in irradiated preparations, especially those in aqueous solution where radiolysis of water contributes to the damaging processes. Additionally, certain glass and plastic (e.g., polypropylene, polytetrafluoroethylene [PTFE]) materials used for packaging or for medical devices can also suffer damage. Thus, radiation sterilisation is generally applied to articles in the dried state; these include surgical instruments, sutures, prostheses, unit-dose ointments, plastic syringes and dry pharmaceutical products. With these radiations, destruction of a microbial population follows the classic survivor curves (see Figure 21.1), and a *D*-value, given as a radiation dose, can be established for standard bacterial spores (e.g., *B. pumilus*) permitting a suitable sterilising dose to be calculated. In the UK, it is usual to apply a dose of 25 kGy (2.5 Mrad) for pharmaceutical and medical products, although lower doses are employed in the USA and Canada.

UV light, with its lower energy, causes less damage to microbial DNA. This, coupled with its poor penetrability of normal packaging materials, renders UV light unsuitable for sterilisation of pharmaceutical dosage forms. It does find applications, however, in the sterilisation of air, for the surface sterilisation of aseptic work areas, and for the treatment of manufacturing-grade water.

Microwave irradiation has potential as a sterilisation process, generating localised heat as its primary sterilising action, but there is a significant drawback to its use. While the energy transfer is immediate, it can vary throughout the microwave chamber leading to uneven heating of the load. Nevertheless, microwave irradiation sterilisers have been successfully employed in the sterilisation of ampoules, for creating aseptic access ports in bioreactors, in the disposal of clinical waste and for patient-operated disinfection of soft contact lenses.

21.6.1 Steriliser Design and Operation

21.6.1.1 Gamma Ray Sterilisers

Gamma rays for sterilisation are usually derived from a cobalt-60 (^{60}Co) source (caesium-137, ^{137}Cs, may also be used), with a half-life of 5.25 years, which on disintegration emits radiation at two energy levels of 1.33 and 1.17 MeV. The isotope is held as pellets packed in metal rods, each rod carefully arranged within the source and containing up to 20 kCi (7.4×10^{11} kBq) of activity; these rods are replaced or rearranged as the activity of the source either drops or becomes unevenly distributed. A typical ^{60}Co installation may contain up to 1 MCi (3.7×10^{13} kBq) of activity. For safety reasons, this source is housed within a reinforced concrete building with 2-m thick walls, and is stored in a sunken water-filled tank until required for use. Control devices operate to ensure that the source is raised only when the chamber is locked and is immediately lowered if a malfunction occurs. Articles being sterilised are passed through the irradiation chamber on a conveyor belt or monorail system and move around the raised source, the rate of passage regulating the dose absorbed (Figure 21.10).

Radiation monitors are continually employed to detect any radiation leakage during operation or storage, and additionally to confirm a return to satisfactory background levels within the sterilisation chamber following operation. The dose delivered is dependent upon source strength and exposure period, with incubation times typically up to 20 hours. The difference in radiation susceptibilities of microbial cells and humans may be gauged from the fact that a lethal human dose would be delivered by an exposure of seconds or minutes.

21.6.1.2 Electron Accelerators

Less extensively used than gamma irradiation, two types of electron accelerator machine exist: the electrostatic accelerator and the microwave linear accelerator, producing electrons with maximum energies of 5 and 10 MeV, respectively. Although higher energies would achieve better penetration into the product, there is a risk of induced radiation and so they are not used. In an electrostatic accelerator, a high-energy electron beam is generated by accelerating electrons from a hot filament down an evacuated tube under high potential difference. Microwave linear accelerators use this same mechanism for electron generation, but additional energy is imparted in a pulsed manner by a travelling microwave synchronised with the electron flow. Articles for treatment are generally limited to small packs and are arranged on horizontal conveyor belts, usually for irradiation from one side but sometimes from both. The sterilising dose is delivered more rapidly in an electron accelerator than in a ^{60}Co plant, with exposure times for sterilisation usually amounting to only a few seconds or minutes. Varying extents of shielding, depending upon the size of the accelerator, are necessary to protect operators from X-rays generated by the bremsstrahlung (German: 'braking radiation') effect.

21.6.1.3 X-ray Irradiation

As noted above, the rapid deceleration of high-energy electrons, when focussed on a metal of high atomic number, can generate X-rays (photons) with electromagnetic energy of the same order as gamma rays but with a wider energy spectrum. This phenomenon has been exploited for sterilisation by the development of electron accelerators to deliver a concentrated X-ray beam which can be used to successfully irradiate items rotated within that beam. Improved dose uniformity, good penetration and shorter exposure time make X-ray irradiation a viable alternative to gamma for a wide variety of healthcare products including medical devices, combination drug/device products and tissue-based and biological products. Sterilisation by X-ray irradiation is used to a similar extent as electron beam processes.

21.6.1.4 Ultraviolet Irradiation

The optimum wavelength for UV sterilisation is around 260 nm. A suitable source for UV light in this region is a mercury lamp giving peak emission levels at 254 nm. These sources are generally ceiling-/wall-mounted for air disinfection, or fixed to vessels for water treatment. Operators present in an irradiated room should wear appropriate protective clothing and eye protection.

21.7 Filtration Sterilisation

Filtration is unique among sterilisation processes in that it removes, rather than destroys, microorganisms. Additionally, it is capable of preventing the passage of both viable and nonviable particles and can thus be used for both the clarification and sterilisation of liquids and gases. The principal application of sterilising-grade filters is in the treatment of heat-sensitive injections and ophthalmic solutions, biological products and air and other gases for supply to aseptic areas (see Chapter 22).

Filters may also be employed in industrial applications where venting systems are required, for example, on fermenters, centrifuges, autoclaves and freeze-driers. Certain types of filter (membrane filters) have an important role in sterility testing, where they can be employed to trap and concentrate contaminating organisms from solutions under test. The resulting filters are then placed on a solid nutrient medium or in a liquid medium and incubated to encourage colony growth or turbidity (Section 21.13.1).

The major mechanisms of filtration are sieving, adsorption and capture within the matrix of the filter material. Of these, only sieving can be regarded as absolute, as it ensures the exclusion of all particles above a defined size. It is generally accepted that synthetic membrane filters, derived from cellulose esters or other polymeric materials (PTFE, polyvinylidene fluoride [PVDF] and polyethersulphone [PES]), act principally as sieve filters; while fibrous pads, sintered glass and sintered ceramic products can be

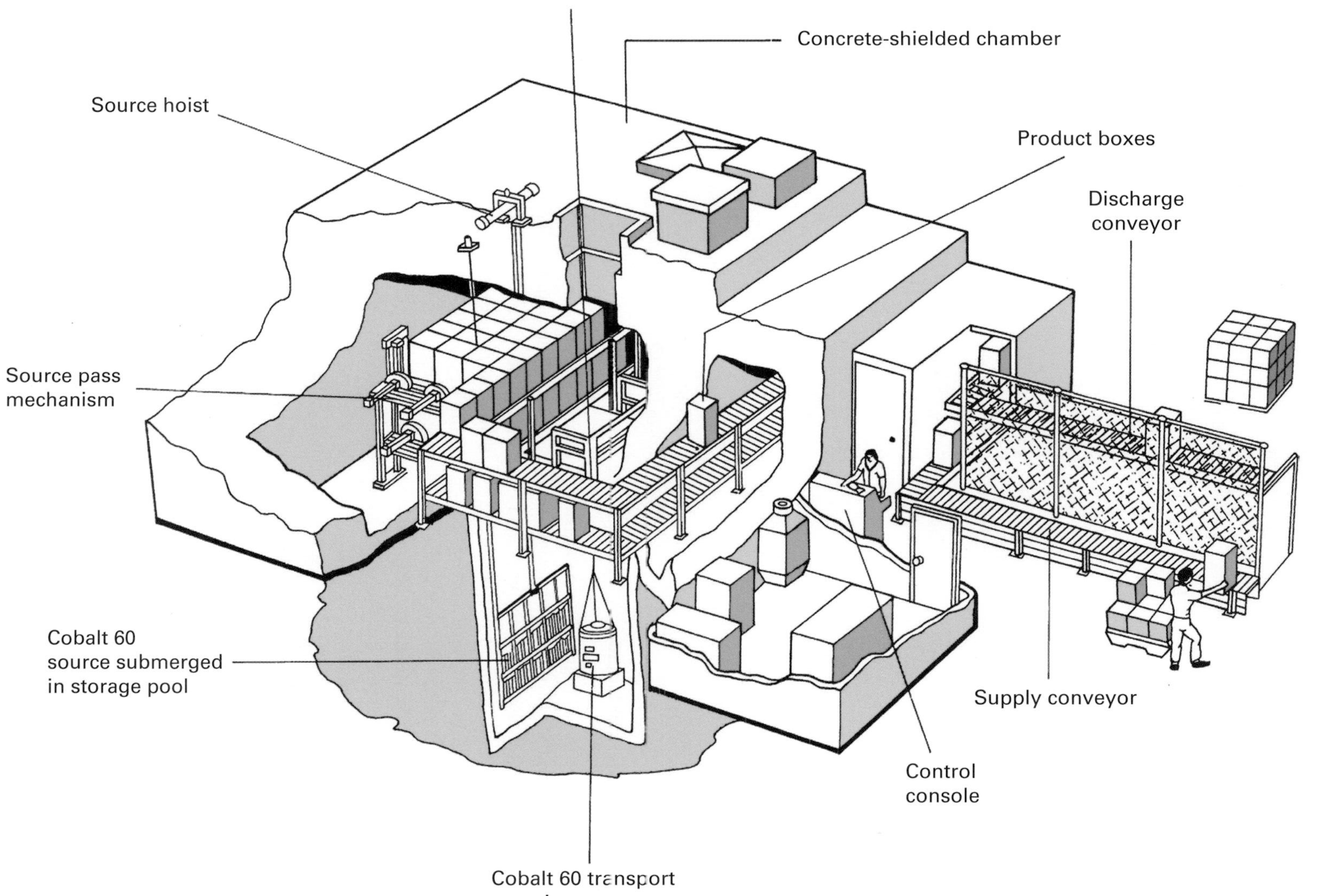

Figure 21.10 Diagram of a typical cobalt-60 irradiation plant.

Table 21.4 Some characteristics of membrane and depth filters.

Characteristic	Membrane filter	Depth filter
Absolute retention of microorganisms greater than rated pore size	+	–
Rapid rate of filtration	+	–
High dirt-handling capacity	–	+
Grow-through of microorganisms	Unlikely	+
Shedding of filter components	–	+
Fluid retention	–	+
Solute adsorption	–	+
Good chemical stability	Depends on membrane	+
Good sterilisation characteristics	+	+

+, applicable; –, not applicable.

regarded as depth filters relying on mechanisms of adsorption and entrapment. Some of the characteristics of filter media are summarised in Table 21.4. The potential hazard of microbial multiplication within a depth filter and subsequent contamination of the filtrate (microbial grow-through) should be recognised.

21.7.1 Filtration Sterilisation of Liquids

In the processing of liquids, a high microorganism removal efficiency is required for filtration to be a viable alternative to other sterilisation methods. For this reason, membrane filters of 0.2–0.22 μm nominal pore diameter are predominantly used, while sintered filters are employed only in restricted circumstances, that is, for the processing of corrosive liquids, viscous fluids or organic solvents. It may be tempting to assume that the pore size is the major determinant of filtration efficiency and two filters of 0.2 μm pore diameter from different manufacturers will behave similarly. This is not so, because, in addition to the sieving effect, trapping within the filter matrix, adsorption and charge effects all contribute significantly towards the removal of particles. Consequently, the thickness of the membrane, its charge and the complex geometry of the channels are all factors which can make the performance of one filter far superior to that of another. As with other sterilisation processes, the major criterion by which filters should be compared is their titre reduction values, that is, the ratio of the number of organisms challenging a filter under defined conditions to the number penetrating it. In all cases, the filter medium employed must be sterilisable, ideally by steam treatment. In the case of membrane filters, this may be for single use only, or, in the case of larger industrial filters, a small, fixed number of resterilisations; sintered filters may be resterilised many times. Filtration sterilisation is an aseptic process and careful monitoring of filter integrity is necessary as well as final product sterility testing (Section 21.13.2.3).

Membrane filters, in the form of discs, can be assembled into pressure-operated filter holders for syringe mounting and in-line use or vacuum filtration tower devices. Filtration under pressure is generally considered most suitable, as filling at high flow rates directly into the final containers is possible without problems of foaming, solvent evaporation or air leaks. To increase the filtration area, and hence process volumes, several filter discs can be used in parallel in multiple-plate filtration systems, or, alternatively, membrane filters can be fabricated into plain or pleated cylinders and installed in cartridges. Membrane filters are often used in combination with a coarse-grade fibreglass depth pre-filter to improve their dirt-handling capacity.

21.7.2 Filtration Sterilisation of Gases

The principal application for filtration sterilisation of gases is in the provision of sterile air to aseptic manufacturing suites (see Chapter 22), hospital isolation units and some operating theatres. Filters employed generally consist of pleated sheets of glass microfibres separated and supported by an aluminium framework; these are employed in ducts, wall or ceiling panels, overhead canopies or laminar airflow cabinets. These high-efficiency particulate air (HEPA) filters can remove up to 99.997% of particles more than 0.3 μm in diameter and thus are acting as depth filters. In practice, their microorganism-removal efficiency is rather better, as the majority of bacteria are found associated with dust particles and only the larger fungal spores are found in the free state. Air is forced through HEPA filters by blower fans, and pre-filters are used to remove larger particles to extend the lifetime of the HEPA filter. The operational efficiency and integrity of a HEPA filter can be monitored by pressure differential and airflow rate measurements, and dioctyl phthalate (DOP) smoke particle penetration tests.

Other applications of filters include: sterilisation of venting or displacement air in tissue and microbiological culture (carbon filters and hydrophobic membrane filters); decontamination of air in mechanical ventilators (glass fibre filters); treatment of exhausted air from microbiological safety cabinets (HEPA filters); and the clarification and sterilisation of medical gases (glass wool depth filters and hydrophobic membrane filters).

21.8 Newer Sterilisation Technologies

Heat is the means of terminal sterilisation that is preferred by the regulatory authorities because of its relative simplicity and the high sterility assurance that it affords. However, a significant number of traditional pharmaceutical products and many recently developed biotechnology products are damaged by heat, as are many polymer-based medical devices and surgical implants; for such products, alternative sterilisation processes must be adopted. While radiation is a viable option for many dry materials, radiation-induced damage is common in aqueous drug solutions, and gaseous methods are also inappropriate for liquids. Aseptic manufacture from individually sterilised ingredients is a suitable solution to the problem of making sterile thermolabile products, but it affords a lower degree of sterility assurance than steam sterilisation and is both time-consuming and expensive. For these reasons, alternative sterilisation strategies have been developed in recent years. Two processes that have progressed to the stage of commercial exploitation are those employing high-intensity light and low-temperature plasma. It must be stressed, however, that although the need to develop alternative strategies for the terminal sterilisation of protein- or nucleic-acid-containing biotechnology products is one of the stimuli for the investigation of new methods in general, these particular processes are unsuitable for such products.

21.8.1 High-intensity Light

UV light has long been known to have the potential to kill all types of microorganisms, but its penetrating power is so poor that it has found practical application only in the decontamination of air (e.g., in laminar-flow workstations and operating theatres), shallow layers of water and surfaces. UV light does not penetrate metal at all, nor glass to any useful degree, but it will penetrate those polymers that do not contain unsaturated bonds or aromatic groups (e.g., polyethylene and polypropylene, but not polystyrene, polycarbonate or polyvinyl chloride). High-intensity light pulse (HILP) sterilisation is a non-thermal technology which uses short (100–400 μs) high-power pulses of broad-spectrum (200–1100 nm) light and has been used to inactivate bacteria (vegetative cells and spores), yeasts, moulds and even viruses. It is based on the generation of short flashes of broad-wavelength light from a xenon lamp that has an intensity almost 100,000 times that of the sun; approximately 25% of the flash is UV light. The mode of action of HILP on microorganisms is similar to the action of the UV-C part of the light spectrum that causes thymine dimerisation in the DNA chain preventing replication and ultimately leading to cell death. HILP has been reported to result in a 0.5–8 $\log^{10}$ CFU ml^{-1} bacterial reduction, but this activity is dependent on the energy delivered through each flash, the distance between multiple lamps and the targeted microorganism. The increased sterilisation efficiency of HILP compared to continuous UV-C may be attributed to its comparatively higher penetration depth and emission power. Regulated pulsed-light delivery is essential to minimise any possible damaging effects of the high peak power on treated products. While pulsed light has been employed in the food industry for the past 20 years, it has been little used with pharmaceutical preparations. Where it is employed in pharmaceutical production, it is predominately exploited in the sterilisation of water and as a means of terminal sterilisation for injectables in UV-transmitting plastic ampoules in a blow–fill–seal operation. Although pulsed light is unlikely to be useful for coloured solutions or those that contain solutes with a high UV absorbance, it is likely that the procedure will be readily applicable not only to water but to some simple solutions of organic molecules, for example, dextrose–saline injection.

21.8.2 Low-temperature Plasma

Plasma is a gas or vapour that has been subjected to an electrical or magnetic field which causes a substantial proportion of the molecules to become ionised. It is thus composed of a cloud of neutral species, ions and electrons in which the numbers of positive and negatively charged particles are equal. Plasma may be generated from many substances but those from chlorine, glutaraldehyde and hydrogen peroxide have been shown to possess the greatest antimicrobial activity.

Low-temperature plasma is a method of sterilisation that is applicable to most of the items and materials for which ethylene oxide is used, that is, principally medical devices excluding drugs; it cannot be used to sterilise liquids, powders and certain fabrics. Commercial plasma sterilisers, which have been available since the early 1990s, typically consist of a sterilisation chamber of 40–160 L (Figure 21.11); this is evacuated, and then filled with hydrogen peroxide vapour which is subsequently converted to a plasma by application of an electric field. An alternative commercial plasma steriliser utilises alternating cycles of peracetic acid vapour and plasma containing oxygen, hydrogen and an inert carrier gas. The cycle times are typically from 60 to 90 minutes and the operating temperatures are less than 50 °C. Major benefits of plasma sterilisation include elimination of the requirement to remove toxic gases at the end

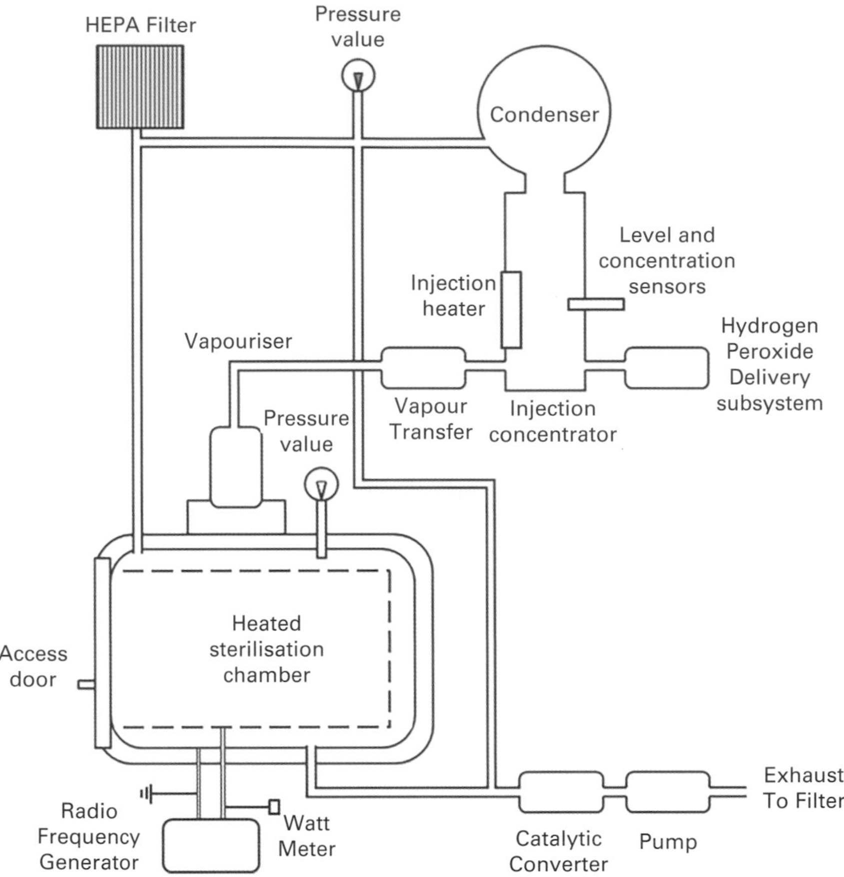

Figure 21.11 Main features of a large-scale low-temperature plasma steriliser.

of the cycle (in contrast to ethylene oxide and LTSF processes); there is also no requirement for the treated device to be aired to remove residual gas, and there is no significant corrosion or reduction in sharpness of exposed surgical instruments.

21.9 Sterilisation Control and Sterility Assurance

To be labelled 'sterile', a product must be free of viable microorganisms. To achieve this, the product, and/or its ingredients, must undergo a sterilisation process of sufficient microbicidal capacity to ensure a minimum level of sterility assurance. It is essential that the required conditions for sterilisation be achieved and maintained through every operation of the steriliser. Some examples of typical conditions employed in sterilisation are shown in Table 21.5.

The quality control of sterile products historically consisted largely, or in some cases, even exclusively, of a sterility test at the end of the manufacturing process. However, a growing awareness of the limitations of sterility tests in terms of their ability to detect low concentrations of microorganisms has resulted in a shift in emphasis from a dependence on end-testing to a situation in which the conferment of the status 'sterile' results from the attainment of satisfactory quality standards throughout the whole manufacturing process. Therefore, the quality is 'assured' by a combination of process monitoring and performance criteria; these may be considered under four headings:

- Bioburden determinations (Section 21.10).
- Environmental monitoring (Section 21.11).
- Validation and in-process monitoring of sterilisation procedures (Section 21.12).
- Sterility testing (Section 21.13).

In well-understood and well-characterised sterilisation processes (e.g., heat and irradiation), where physical measurements may be accurately made, sterility can be assured by ensuring that the manufacturing process as a whole conforms to the established protocols for the first three of the above criteria. In this case, the process has

Table 21.5 Examples of typical conditions employed in the sterilisation of pharmaceutical and medical products.

Sterilisation method	Typical conditions
Moist heat (autoclaving)	121 °C for 15 min
	134 °C for 3 min
Dry heat	160 °C for 120 min
	170 °C for 60 min
	180 °C for 30 min
Ethylene oxide	Gas concentration: 600–1200 mg l^{-1}
	45–63 °C
	30–70% relative humidity
	1–4 h sterilising time
Low-temperature steam and formaldehyde	Gas concentration: 15–100 mg l^{-1}
	Steam admission to 73 °C
	40–180 min sterilising time depending on type of process
Peracetic acid	Concentration 3.5% w/v
	450 °C vapourisation temperature
	Duration dependent on chamber size and local validation
Hydrogen peroxide	Concentration 30–35% w/v
	120 °C vapourisation temperature
	Duration dependent on chamber size and local validation
Low-temperature plasma	35% w/v hydrogen peroxide
	28–40 °C
	60–90 min
Irradiation (Gamma rays or accelerated electrons)	25 kGy (2.5 Mrad) dose
Filtration	≤0.22 µm pore size, sterile membrane filter

satisfied the required parameters thereby permitting parametric release (i.e., release based on process data) of the product without recourse to a sterility test (see Chapter 22).

21.10 Bioburden Determinations

The term *bioburden* is used to describe the concentration of microorganisms in a material; this may be either a total number of organisms per millilitre or per gram, regardless of type, or a breakdown into such categories as aerobic bacteria or yeasts and moulds. Bioburden determinations are normally undertaken by the supplier of the raw material, ensuring that the material supplied conforms to the agreed specification. Additional checks may be made by the recipient where sterility is an essential factor. The maximum permitted concentrations of contaminants may be those specified in various pharmacopoeias or the levels established by the manufacturer during product development.

The level of sterility assurance achieved in a terminally sterilised product is dependent upon the design of the sterilisation process itself and the initial bioburden immediately prior to sterilisation (see Chapter 22). The expenditure on high-quality raw materials is not, in itself, a strategy that will ensure that the product has an acceptably low bioburden immediately prior to sterilisation. It is necessary to ensure that the opportunities for microbial contamination during the manufacturing process are restricted and that any organisms present do not find themselves in conditions favourable to growth. It is for this reason that manufacturing processes are designed to utilise adverse temperatures, extreme pH and organic solvent exposures in order to prevent an increase in the microbial bioburden. Water is the most common, and potentially most significant, source of contamination in the manufactured product and therefore the maintenance of water at elevated temperatures is commonly employed. This strategy limits the growth of organisms such as *Pseudomonas* spp. which can proliferate during storage, even in distilled or deionised water. These types of precautions ensure that chemically synthesised raw materials have bioburdens that are generally much lower than those found in 'natural' products of animal, vegetable or mineral origin.

21.11 Environmental Monitoring

The levels of microbial contamination in the manufacturing areas (see Chapter 22) are monitored on a regular basis to confirm that the numbers do not exceed specified limits. The concentrations of bacteria and of yeasts/moulds in the atmosphere may be determined either by use of 'settle plates' (Petri dishes of suitable media exposed for fixed periods, on which the colonies are counted after incubation) or by use of air samplers which cause a known volume of air to be passed over an agar surface. Similarly, the contamination on surfaces, including manufacturing equipment, may be measured using swabs or contact plates (also known as replicate organism detection and counting [RODAC] plates) which are specially designed Petri dishes slightly over-filled with agar, which, when set, projects very slightly above the plastic wall of the dish. This permits the plate to be inverted on to or against any solid surface, thereby allowing transfer of organisms from the surface on to the agar.

Less commonly, environmental monitoring can extend also to the operators in the manufacturing area whose clothing, for example, gloves or face masks, may be sampled in order to estimate the levels and types of organisms that may arise as product contaminants from those sources.

21.12 Validation and In-process Monitoring of Sterilisation Procedures

In simple terms, validation of a process means demonstrating that a procedure will consistently produce the results that it is intended to. Thus, and with respect to sterile products, validation would be necessary for each of the individual aspects of the manufacturing process. This includes the environmental monitoring, raw materials quality assessment, the sterilisation process itself and the sterility testing procedure. Of these, it is the sterilisation process that is likely to be subject to the most detailed and complex validation procedures. A typical validation procedure for a steam sterilisation process is likely to incorporate most, or all, of the following features:

- calibration and testing of all the physical instruments used to monitor the process, e.g., thermocouples, pressure gauges and timers;
- production of evidence that the steam is of the desired quality (e.g., that the chamber temperature is that expected for pure steam at the measured pressure);
- conduct of leak tests and steam penetration tests using both an empty chamber and a chamber filled with the product to be sterilised in the intended load conformation;
- use of biological indicators either alone or in combination with bioburden organisms to demonstrate that the sterilisation cycle is capable of producing an acceptable level of sterility assurance under 'worst case' conditions;
- production of data to demonstrate repeatability of the 'worst case' conditions sterilisation cycle (typically for triplicate runs);
- testing of software associated with parametric and operational monitoring;
- comprehensive documentation of all of these aspects.

There are different approaches to the demonstration of adequate sterility assurance in steam sterilisation depending upon the thermostability of the product and knowledge of the pre-sterilisation bioburden. Where the product is known to be stable, an overkill approach may be adopted in which biological indicators (Section 21.12.3) containing 10^6 test organisms are inactivated in half the proposed exposure time (thus achieving a 12-log reduction and a sterility assurance level of 10^{-6} in the full exposure period). For a marginally thermostable product, the cycle could be validated on the basis of measurements of the 'worst case' bioburden level and the heat resistance of the known bioburden organisms; such an approach would necessitate rigorous control of the bioburden during routine manufacturing. In the UK, biological indicators are used primarily in validation rather than routine monitoring of heat sterilisation processes, although their use in routine manufacturing may be required in other countries. Chemical indicators of sterilisation (Section 21.12.2) are more convenient to use than biological indicators, but as they provide no direct measure of the efficacy of the process in terms of microbial killing, they are considered to be less useful and in particular instances no longer routinely used. Physical measurements of temperature, pressure, time, relative humidity, etc., are of such fundamental importance to the assurance of sterility that records of these parameters are required to be retained for each batch of sterilised product.

21.12.1 Physical Indicators

In heat sterilisation processes, a temperature record is made of each sterilisation cycle with both dry- and moist heat (i.e., autoclave) sterilisers; this chart/digital record forms part of the batch documentation and is compared against a master temperature record (MTR). It is recommended that the temperature be taken at the coolest part of the loaded steriliser. Further information on heat distribution and penetration within a steriliser can be gained by the use of thermocouples placed at selected sites in the chamber or inserted directly into test packs or bottles. For gaseous sterilisation procedures, elevated temperatures are monitored for each sterilisation cycle by temperature probes, and routine leak tests are performed to ensure gas-tight seals as well as pressure and humidity measurements being recorded. Gas concentration is measured independently of pressure rise, often by reference to weight of gas used. In radiation sterilisation, a plastic (often Perspex) dosimeter which gradually darkens in proportion to the radiation absorbed gives an accurate measure of the radiation dose and is considered to be the best technique currently available for following the radiosterilisation process.

A bubble point pressure test is used to determine the pore size of sterilising filters and may also be used to check the integrity of certain types of filter devices (membrane and sintered glass; Section 21.7) immediately after use. The principle of the test is that the wet filter in its assembled unit is subjected to an increasing air or nitrogen gas pressure. The pressure difference recorded when the first bubble of gas breaks away from the filter is related to the maximum pore size. When the gas pressure is further increased slowly, there is a general surge of bubbles over the entire surface. This pressure difference is related to the mean pore size. A pressure differential below the expected value would signify a damaged or faulty filter. A modification to this test for membrane filters involves measuring the diffusion of gas through a wet filter at pressures below the bubble point pressure (diffusion rate test); a faster diffusion rate than expected would again indicate a loss of filter integrity. In addition, a filter is considered ineffective when an unusually rapid rate of filtration occurs.

Efficiency testing of HEPA filters used for the supply of sterile air to aseptic workplaces (see Chapter 22) is achieved by the generation of upstream DOP or sodium chloride particles of known dimension followed by detection in downstream filtered air. Retention efficiency is recorded as the percentage of particles removed under defined test conditions.

21.12.2 Chemical Indicators

Chemical monitoring of a sterilisation process is based on the ability of heat, steam, sterilant gases and ionising radiation to alter the chemical and/or physical characteristics of a variety of chemical substances. Ideally, this change should take place only when satisfactory conditions for sterilisation prevail, thus confirming completion of a successful sterilisation cycle. In practice, however, the ideal indicator response is not always achieved and so a necessary distinction is made between (i) those chemical indicators which integrate several sterilisation parameters (i.e., temperature, time and saturated steam) and closely approach the ideal and (ii) those which measure only one parameter and consequently can only be used to distinguish processed from unprocessed articles. For example, indicators which rely on the melting of a chemical substance show that the temperature has been attained but not necessarily maintained.

Chemical indicators generally undergo melting or a colour change, the relationship of this change to the sterilisation process being largely influenced by the design of the test device (Table 21.6). It must be remembered, however, that changes do not necessarily correspond to microbiological sterility and consequently the devices should never be employed as sole indicators in a sterilisation process. Nevertheless, when included in strategically placed containers or packages, chemical indicators are valuable monitors of the conditions prevailing at the coolest or most inaccessible areas of a steriliser. The International Organization for Standardization (ISO) standard 11140-1:2014 classifies chemical indicators for autoclaves and sterilisers as:

Class I: process indicators
Class II: specific-use indicators
Class III: single-variable indicators
Class IV: multi-variable indicators
Class V: integrating indicators (integrators)
Class VI: emulating indicators (cycle verification indicators)

Class I indicators differentiate processed from non-processed items in response to one or more critical process variables, for instance, temperature and time. Usually these are in the form of peel-back pouches or chemical indicator tape. Bowie–Dick Class II indicators are used in specific tests or procedures to evaluate steriliser performance; in particular, they evaluate air removal from the steriliser during the procedure. Class III indicators react to a single critical process variable (i.e., temperature or time). Temperature-specific indicators are designed to reveal the attainment of a specific minimum temperature at a specific location within the steriliser chamber or load. This class is not sensitive to other sterilisation parameters, such as time or sterilant. The multi-parameter indicators, Class IV, react to two or more critical variables in the sterilisation cycle; these criteria are established dependent on the equipment being used. Multi-parameter indicators are much more accurate by design, as they provide an integrated response to all the parameters needed to achieve sterilisation, either by a specified colour change or migration along a wick to indicate pass or fail. The Class V indicators are designed to react to all critical parameters over a specified range of sterilisation cycles. The stated values are those required to achieve a stated inactivation by referring to a stated test organism with stated D and, if applicable, z-values. Finally, the Class VI indicators also evaluate all critical variables for a specified sterilisation cycle. Typically, these indicators are placed in the pack, pouch or container and respond to all critical process parameters. An indicated pass verifies exposure to the conditions required for sterilisation of the product.

21.12.3 Biological Indicators

BIs used in thermal, chemical and radiation sterilisation processes consist of standardised bacterial spore samples prepared as suspensions in water or culture medium or as spores dried on paper, aluminium or plastic carriers. For steriliser validation purposes, they are usually placed in dummy packs located at strategic sites in the steriliser. Alternatively, for gaseous sterilisation, these may also be placed within a tubular helix device. After the sterilisation process, the aqueous suspensions or spores on carriers are

Table 21.6 Examples of chemical indicators that have been used for monitoring sterilisation processes.

Sterilisation method	Principle	Device	Indicator class	Parameter(s) monitored
Heat				
Autoclaving or dry heat	Temperature-sensitive coloured solution	Sealed tubes partly filled with a solution which changes colour at elevated temperatures; rate of colour change is proportional to temperature, e.g., Browne's tubes	I, IV	Temperature, time
Dry heat only	Temperature-sensitive chemical	Usually a temperature-sensitive white wax concealing a black marked or printed (paper) surface; at a predetermined temperature the wax rapidly melts, exposing the background mark(s) over time.	I, IV	Temperature, time
Heating in an autoclave only	Steam-sensitive chemical	Usually an organic chemical in a printing ink base impregnated into a carrier material. A combination of moisture and heat produces a darkening of the ink, e.g., autoclave tape. Devices of this sort can be used within dressings packs to confirm adequate removal of air and penetration of saturated steam (Bowie–Dick test)	II	Saturated steam
	Capillary principle (e.g., Thermalog steam chemical integrator)	Consists of a blue dye in a waxy pellet, the melting point of which is depressed in the presence of saturated steam. At autoclaving temperatures, and in the continued presence of steam, the pellet melts and dye travels along a paper wick forming a blue band, the length of which is dependent upon both exposure time and temperature	IV, V	Temperature, saturated steam, time
Gaseous sterilisation				
Ethylene oxide (EO)	Reactive chemical	Indicator paper impregnated with a reactive chemical which undergoes a distinct colour change on reaction with EO in the presence of heat and moisture. With some devices, rate of colour development varies with temperature and EO concentration	I	Gas concentration, temperature, time (selected devices). NB a minimum relative humidity (RH) is required for device to function
	Capillary principle (e.g., Thermalog EO chemical integrator)	Based on the same 'migration along wick' principle as the Thermalog steam chemical integrator. Optimum response in a cycle of 600 mg l^{-1} EO, temperature 54 °C, RH 50%	IV, V	Gas concentration, temperature, time (selected cycles)
Low-temperature steam and formaldehyde	Reactive chemical	Indicator paper impregnated with a formaldehyde-, steam- and temperature-sensitive reactive chemical which changes colour during the sterilisation process	I, IV	Temperature, time (selected cycles)
Vapourised hydrogen peroxide	Reactive chemical	Indicator strip impregnated with a hydrogen peroxide-sensitive reactive chemical which undergoes a graded colour change when exposed to sterilisation conditions	I	Gas concentration, temperature and time (selected cycles)
Radiation sterilisation				
	Radiochromic chemical	Plastic devices impregnated with radiosensitive chemicals which undergo colour changes at relatively low radiation doses	I	Only indicate exposure to radiation
	Dosimeter device	Acidified ferric ammonium sulphate or ceric sulphate solutions respond to irradiation by dose-related changes in their optical density	V	Accurately measure radiation doses

Table 21.7 Biological indicators (BIs) recommended by the *European Pharmacopoeia* for monitoring sterilisation processes.

Sterilisation process	Species	Inoculum size	*D*-value
Steam sterilisation (121 °C)	*Geobacillus stearothermophilus* ATCC[a] 7953	$>5\times10^5$	1.5–4.5 min
Dry heat (160 °C)	*Bacillus atrophaeus* ATCC 9372	$>1\times10^5$	1–3 min
Hydrogen peroxide (VHP) and peracetic acid	*Geobacillus stearothermophilus* ATCC 7953	$>5\times10^5$	–
Ethylene oxide (EO)	*Bacillus atrophaeus* ATCC 9372	$>5\times10^5$	2.6–4.5 min at 54 °C, 60% relative humidity and 600 mg l^{-1} EO
Formaldehyde	*Bacillus atrophaeus* ATCC 9372	$>5\times10^5$	–
Ionising radiation	*Bacillus pumilus* ATCC 27.142	$>1\times10^7$	1.9 kGy

[a] American Type Culture Collection (ATCC).

aseptically transferred to an appropriate nutrient medium, which is then incubated and periodically examined for signs of growth. Spores of *G. stearothermophilus* in sealed ampoules of culture medium are used for steam sterilisation monitoring, and these may be incubated directly at 55 °C; this eliminates the need for an aseptic transfer. Aseptic transfers are also avoided by the use of self-contained units where the spore strip and nutrient medium are present in the same device ready for mixing after use.

The bacterial species to be used in a BI must be selected carefully, as it must be non-pathogenic and should possess above-average resistance to the particular sterilisation process. Resistance is defined by a spore destruction curve obtained via test exposure to the sterilisation process; recommended BI spores and their decimal reduction times (*D*-values; Section 21.2.2.1) are shown in Table 21.7. Care must be taken in the preparation and storage of BIs to ensure a standardised response to sterilisation processes. While certainly offering the most direct method of monitoring sterilisation processes, it should be realised that BIs may be less reliable monitors than physical methods and they are not recommended for routine use, except in the case of gaseous sterilisation. Additionally, there is a need to maintain the resistance characteristics of the BI which can be lost on repeated laboratory subculture.

The long-standing criticism of BIs is that the incubation period required in order to confirm a satisfactory sterilisation process imposes an undesirable delay on the release of the product. This problem has been overcome for steam sterilisation by using a detection system in which a spore enzyme, α-glucosidase (reflective of spore viability), converts a non-fluorescent substrate into a fluorescent product in as little as 1 hour.

Filtration sterilisation requires a different approach from biological monitoring, the test effectively measuring the ability of a filter to produce a sterile filtrate from a culture of a suitable organism. For this purpose, *Serratia marcescens*, a Gram-negative rod-shaped bacterium (minimum dimension 0.5 μm), has been used for filters of 0.45 μm pore size, and a more rigorous test involving *Brevundimonas diminuta* ATCC 19146 (formerly *Pseudomonas diminuta*) having a minimum dimension of 0.3 μm is applied to filters of 0.22 μm pore size and *Acholeplasma laidlawii* is applied to filters of 0.1 μm pore size. The 0.22 μm pore size filters are defined as those capable of completely removing *B. diminuta* from suspension. This test uses a realistic inoculum level of *B. diminuta* of 10^7 cells cm^{-2} of filter area. The extent of the passage of this organism through membrane filters is enhanced by increasing the filtration pressure. Consequently, successful sterile filtration depends markedly upon the challenge conditions. Such tests are used as part of the filter quality assurance process, and a user's initial validation procedure. They are not employed as a test of filter performance in use.

21.13 Sterility Testing

A sterility test is essentially a test which assesses whether a sterilised pharmaceutical or medical product is free from contaminating microorganisms by incubation of either the whole or a part of that product with a nutrient medium. It therefore becomes a destructive test and is of questionable suitability for testing large, expensive or delicate products or equipment. Furthermore, by its very nature it is a statistical process in which part of a batch is sampled and the chance of the batch being passed for use then depends on the sample passing the sterility test. Random sampling should therefore be applied to products that have been processed and filled aseptically. With products sterilised in their final containers, however, samples should be taken from the potentially coolest or least sterilant-accessible part of the batch.

Limitations are inherent in any procedure intended to demonstrate a negative, and as the sterility test is intended to demonstrate that no viable organisms are present, failure to detect them could simply be a consequence of the use of unsuitable media or inappropriate culture conditions. To demonstrate that no organisms are present, it would be necessary to use a universal culture medium suitable for the growth of every possible contaminant and to incubate the sample under an infinite variety of conditions. Clearly, no such medium or combination of media is available and in practice only media capable of supporting non-fastidious bacteria, yeasts and moulds are employed. Furthermore, in pharmacopoeial tests, no attempt is made to detect viruses, which, on a size basis, are the organisms most likely to pass through a sterilising filter. Nevertheless, the sterility test does have an important application in monitoring the microbiological quality of filter-sterilised, aseptically filled products and does offer a final check on terminally sterilised articles. In the UK, test procedures laid down by the *European Pharmacopoeia* remain applicable and must be followed; this provides details of the sample sizes to be adopted in particular cases.

21.13.1 Sterility Testing Methods

Three alternative methods are available when conducting sterility tests according to the *European Pharmacopoeia*: direct inoculation, membrane filtration and addition of concentrated culture medium. When undertaking sterility tests, it is necessary to conduct control tests that confirm the adequacy of the testing facilities by sampling of air and surfaces in addition to carrying out tests using samples 'known' to be sterile (negative controls). In practice, this means samples that have been subjected to a very reliable sterilisation process, for example, radiation, or samples that have been subjected to repeat sterilisation procedures. In order to minimise the risk of introducing contaminants from the surroundings or from the operator during the test itself, testing must be carried out under conditions of strict asepsis, for example, under laminar airflow; isolators are often employed which physically separate the operator from the materials under test.

The culture media employed in sterility tests should previously have been assessed for nutritive (growth-supporting) properties and a lack of toxicity using specified organisms. It must be remembered that any survivors of a sterilisation process may be impaired and thus must be given the best possible conditions for growth.

21.13.1.1 Direct Inoculation

The direct inoculation method involves introducing test samples directly into nutrient media. The *European Pharmacopoeia* recommends two media: (i) fluid mercaptoacetate medium (also known as fluid thioglycolate medium), which contains glucose and sodium mercaptoacetate (sodium thioglycolate) and is particularly suitable for the cultivation of anaerobic organisms (incubation temperature 30–35 °C); and (ii) soyabean casein digest medium (also known as tryptone soya broth), which will support the growth of both aerobic bacteria (incubation temperature 30–35 °C) and fungi (incubation temperature 20–25 °C). Limits are placed upon the ratio of the weight or volume of added sample relative to the volume of culture medium so as to avoid reducing the nutrient properties of the medium or creating unfavourably high osmotic pressures within it. Other media may be used provided that they can be shown to be suitable alternatives or if the identification of specific organisms is required. For example:

- MacConkey agar, which is a selective and differential medium for the detection of coliforms and enteric pathogens according to the *European Pharmacopoeia* (agar medium H).
- The *Harmonised European Pharmacopoeia* proposes reinforced Columbia agar medium containing gentamicin sulphate (20 mg l^{-1}) as a selective enrichment media for Clostridia.
- Cetrimide agar is used in the isolation and identification of *Pseudomonas aeruginosa*. Cetrimide is a quaternary ammonium compound (see Chapter 18) that inhibits the growth of a wide range of Gram-positive and some Gram-negative microorganisms.
- Mannitol salt agar is used to isolate pathogenic staphylococci, selectively inhibiting the growth of most other bacteria as a consequence of its high salt concentration. Pathogenic strains of staphylococci (coagulase-positive staphylococci) produce yellow colonies with yellow zones. Non-pathogenic staphylococci usually produce small red colonies with no colour change to the surrounding medium.
- Xylose lysine deoxycholate agar is used for the isolation and differentiation of enteric pathogens, e.g., Salmonella, which can reduce sodium thiosulphate producing hydrogen sulphide which creates a complex with ferric ammonium citrate giving black or black-centred colonies.
- Sabouraud dextrose agar is used to cultivate yeasts, moulds and aciduric microorganisms as designated by the *European Pharmacopoeia*. Dextrose is fermented

providing carbon and energy. The high dextrose concentration and acidic pH make this medium selective for fungi. Modification with cycloheximide, penicillin and streptomycin additions aids selection from heavily contaminated sources.

21.13.1.2 Membrane Filtration

Membrane filtration is the sterility testing technique recommended by most pharmacopoeias and, consequently, is the method by which most products are examined. The method involves filtration of fluids through a sterile membrane filter (pore size $\leq 0.45\,\mu m$) and any microorganism present will be retained on the surface of the filter membrane. After washing *in situ*, the filter is divided aseptically and portions are transferred to suitable culture media (such as those above) which are then incubated at the appropriate temperature for the required period of time. Water-soluble solids can be dissolved in a suitable diluent and processed in this way, and oil-soluble products may be dissolved in a suitable solvent, for example, isopropyl myristate, before filtering.

21.13.1.3 Addition of Concentrated Culture Medium

The concentrated culture medium sterility test is a highly sensitive method for detecting low levels of contamination in intravenous infusion fluids. A concentrated culture medium is added to the fluid in its original container, so that the resultant mixture is equivalent to single strength culture medium; this enables the sampling of the entire volume.

21.13.2 Antimicrobial Agents

Where an antimicrobial agent comprises the product or forms part of the product, for example, as a preservative, its activity must be nullified in some way during sterility testing so that an inhibitory action in preventing the growth of any contaminating microorganisms is overcome. This is achieved by specific inactivation, dilution or membrane filtration.

21.13.2.1 Specific Inactivation

An appropriate inactivating (neutralising) agent (Table 21.8) is incorporated into the culture medium. The inactivating agent must be non-toxic to microorganisms, as must any product resulting from an interaction of the inactivator and the antimicrobial agent.

Although Table 21.8 lists only benzylpenicillin and ampicillin as being inactivated by β-lactamase (from *Bacillus cereus*), other β-lactams may also be hydrolysed by β-lactamases. Other antibiotic-inactivating enzymes are also known (see Chapter 13) and have been considered as possible inactivating agents, for example, chloramphenicol acetyl-transferase (inactivates chloramphenicol) and enzymes that modify aminoglycoside antibiotics (acetyltransferases, nucleotidyltransferases or phosphotransferases which catalyse modifications at hydroxyl or amine groups of the 2-deoxystreptamine nucleus or the sugar moieties).

Table 21.8 Inactivating agents (neutralising agents).

Inhibitory agents	Inactivating agents
Phenols, cresols	None (dilution)
Alcohols	None (dilution)
Parabens	Dilution and Tween
Mercury compounds	Sulphydryl-containing compounds
Quaternary ammonium compounds	Lecithin + Lubrol W; Lecithin + Tween (Letheen)
Benzylpenicillin[a], ampicillin	β-Lactamase from *Bacillus cereus*
Other antibiotics[a]	None (membrane filtration)
Sulphonamides	*p*-Aminobenzoic acid

[a] See text.

21.13.2.2 Dilution

The antimicrobial agent is diluted in the culture medium to a level at which it ceases to have any activity, for example, phenols, cresols and alcohols (see Chapter 19). This method applies to substances with a high dilution coefficient, η, and may be accompanied by specific inactivation (Table 21.8).

21.13.2.3 Membrane Filtration

This method has traditionally been used to overcome the activity of antibiotics for which there are no inactivating agents, although it could be extended to cover other products if necessary, including preservatives if no specific or effective inactivators are available. Basically, a solution of the product is filtered through a hydrophobic-edged membrane filter that will retain any contaminating microorganisms. The membrane is washed *in situ* to remove any traces of antibiotic adhering to the membrane and is then transferred to appropriate culture media as outlined in Section 21.13.1.2.

21.13.3 Positive Controls

It is essential to show that microorganisms will actually grow under the conditions of the test. For this reason, positive controls must be carried out; in these, the ability of small numbers of suitable microorganisms to grow in media in the presence of the sample is assessed. The microorganism used for positive control tests with a product containing or comprising an antimicrobial agent must, if at all possible, be sensitive to that agent, so that growth of the organism indicates a satisfactory inactivation, dilution or removal of the agent. The *European Pharmacopoeia* suggests the use of designated strains of *Staphylococcus aureus* ATCC 6538, *B. subtilis* ATCC 6633, *P. aeruginosa* ATCC 9027, *Escherichia coli* ATCC 8739 and *Salmonella enterica subsp. enterica serovar Typhimurium* ATCC 14028 as appropriate aerobic organisms, *Clostridium sporogenes* ATCC 11437 as an anaerobe and *Candida albicans* ATCC 10231 or *Aspergillus brasiliensis* ATCC 16404 (formerly *Aspergillus niger*) as fungi. A positive control (medium with added test sample) and a negative control (medium without the test sample) are inoculated simultaneously, and the rate and extent of growth arising in each should be similar. However, the negative control without the test sample is, in effect, exactly the same as the growth promotion control that is also described in the test procedure, so, for the organisms concerned, it is not necessary to do both.

All the controls may be conducted either before, or in parallel with, the test itself, providing that the same batches of media are used for both. If the controls are carried out in parallel with the tests and one of the controls gives an unexpected result, the test for sterility may be declared invalid, and, when the problem is resolved, the test may be repeated.

21.13.4 Specific Cases

Specific details of the sterility testing of parenteral products, ophthalmic and other non-injectable preparations and surgical sutures will be found in the *European Pharmacopoeia*. These procedures cannot conveniently be applied to items such as surgical dressings and medical devices because they are too big. In such cases, the most convenient approach is to immerse the whole object in culture medium in a sterile flexible bag, but care must be taken to ensure that the liquid penetrates to all parts and surfaces of the material.

21.13.5 Sampling

A sterility test attempts to infer the state (sterile or non-sterile) of a batch from the results of an examination of part of a batch, and is therefore a statistical procedure. Suppose that p represents the proportion of contaminated containers in a batch and q the proportion of uncontaminated containers, then, $p+q=1$ or $q=1-p$.

Example:

If a sample of two items is taken from a large batch containing 10% contaminated containers, then the probability of a single item taken at random being contaminated (p) is

$$p = 0.1(\text{where}\,10\% = 0.1)$$

whereas the probability of such an item being uncontaminated (q) is given by

$$q = 1 - p = 0.9$$

The probability of both items being contaminated is given by

$$p^2 = 0.01$$

and of both items being uncontaminated by

$$q^2 = (1-p)^2 = 0.81$$

The probability of obtaining one contaminated item and one non-contaminated item is

$$1 - (0.01 + 0.81) = 0.18 = 2pq$$

In a sterility test involving a sample size of n containers, the probability P of obtaining n consecutive 'steriles' is given by

$$q^n = (1-p)^n$$

The *European Pharmacopoeia* states for batches of greater than 500 items that the sample size required is 20. Values for various levels of p (i.e., the proportion of contaminated containers in a batch) with a constant sample size are given in Table 21.9, which shows that the test cannot detect low levels of contamination. Similarly, if different sample sizes are employed (also based on $(1-p)^n$), it can be shown that as the sample size increases, the probability of the batch being passed as sterile decreases.

It is clear that a sterility test can only show that a proportion of the products in a batch is sterile. The correct conclusion to be drawn from a satisfactory test result is that the batch has passed the sterility test, but this is not a guarantee that the entire batch is sterile.

21.13.6 Retests

Under certain circumstances, a sterility test may require repeating, but the only justification for a second iteration of testing is unequivocal evidence that the first test was invalid; a retest cannot be viewed as a second opportunity

Table 21.9 Sampling in sterility testing.

	Contaminated items in batch (%)					
	0.1	**1**	**5**	**10**	**20**	**50**
p	0.001	0.01	0.05	0.1	0.2	0.5
q	0.999	0.99	0.95	0.9	0.8	0.5
Probability (P), of drawing 20 consecutive sterile items[a]	0.98	0.82	0.36	0.12	0.012	<0.00001

[a] Calculated from $P = (1 - p)^{20} = q^{20}$; 20 is the sample size required by the *European Pharmacopoeia* for batches of >500 items.

for the batch to pass when it has failed the first time. Circumstances that may justify a retest would include, for example, failure of the air filtration system in the testing facility which might have permitted airborne contaminants to enter the product or media during testing, non-sterility of the media used for testing, or evidence that contamination arose during testing from the operating personnel or a source other than the sample being tested.

21.13.7 The Role of Sterility Testing

The techniques discussed in this chapter comprise an attempt to achieve, as far as possible, the continuous monitoring of a particular sterilisation process. The sterility test on its own provides no guarantee as to the sterility of a batch; however, it is an additional check that will detect gross failure, and continued compliance with the test does give confidence as to the efficacy of a sterilisation or aseptic process and this can contribute to sterility assurance. Failure to carry out a sterility test where required, despite the major criticism of its inability to detect other than gross contamination, may have important legal and moral consequences.

References

DH (2014). *Health Technical Memorandum. Decontamination HTMs*. London: Department of Health.

DH (2016a). *Health Technical Memorandum. Decontamination of Surgical Instruments (HTM 01-01)*. London: Department of Health.

DH (2016b). *Health Technical Memorandum. Decontamination of Linen for Health and Social Care (HTM 01-04)*. London: Department of Health.

ISO 11140-1:2014 (2014). *Sterilization of Health Care Products – Chemical Indicators – Part 1: General Requirements*. Geneva: International Organization for Standardization.

Further Reading

Baird, R.M., Hodges, N.A. and Denyer, S.P. (2000). *Handbook of Microbiological Quality Control: Pharmaceuticals and Medical Devices*. London: Taylor & Francis.

British Pharmacopoeia (2021). The Stationery Office, London. (The most recent edition should be consulted).

Denyer, S.P. and Baird, R.M. (2007). *Guide to Microbiological Control in Pharmaceuticals and Medical Devices*, 2e. London: CRC Press.

EDQM (2020). Chapter 5.8 Pharmacopoeial harmonisation. In: *European Pharmacopoeia*, 10e. Strasbourg: Council of Europe.

European Pharmacopoeia, 10. (2021) Council of Europe, Strasbourg. (This pharmacopoeia consists of volumes and supplements. The most recent should be consulted.)

Fraise, A.P., Maillard, J.-Y. and Sattar, S.A. (2013). *Russell, Hugo and Ayliffe's Principles and Practice of Disinfection, Preservation and Sterilization*, 5e. Oxford: Wiley-Blackwell.

McEvoy, B. and Rowan, N.J. (2019). Terminal sterilization of medical devices using vaporised hydrogen peroxide: a review of current methods and emerging opportunities. *J. Appl. Microbiol.* 127: 1403–1420.

MHRA (2022). *The Green Guide: Rules and Guidance for Pharmaceutical Distributors*, 5e. London: Pharmaceutical Press.

Sandle, T. (2013). *Sterility, Sterilisation and Sterility Assurance for Pharmaceuticals*. Cambridge: Woodhead Publishing Ltd.

Zhdanov, A.E., Pahomov, I.M., Ulybin, A.I. and Borisov, V.I. (2020). Low temperature plasma vacuum sterilization of medical devices by using SterAcidAgent®: description and distinctive characteristics. In: *BIODEVICES 2020 - 13th International Conference on Biomedical Electronics and Devices, Proceedings; Part of 13th International Joint Conference on Biomedical Engineering Systems and Technologies, BIOSTEC 2020* (ed. Y. Xuesong, A. Fred and H. Gamboa), 86–93.

Part 6

Pharmaceutical Production

22

Sterile Pharmaceutical Products and Principles of Good Manufacturing Practice

Tim Sandle

Head of Compliance and Quality Risk Management, Bio Products Laboratory, Elstree, UK

CONTENTS

Hugo and Russell's Pharmaceutical Microbiology, Ninth Edition. Edited by Brendan F. Gilmore and Stephen P. Denyer.

Companion website: https://www.wiley.com/go/HugoandRussells9e

22.1 Introduction

Injections, infusions and pharmaceutical forms for application to eyes and mucous membranes must meet the requirement to be sterile; this is also the case for a range of medical devices. Sterility is important, since these products generally breach or compromise host defences exposing the patient to infection from contaminating microorganisms (see Chapter 17). A large proportion of sterile pharmaceutical preparations are given by injection (see Section 22.5). Products administered by injection are often called parenteral products, deriving from the Greek and meaning any route other than through the gut. Thus, certain medicines such as peptides, proteins and many chemotherapeutic agents which would be inactivated in the gastrointestinal tract are given parenterally.

Achieving sterility is not straightforward, whether the product is produced by terminal sterilisation (see Chapter 21) or by assembly from sterile ingredients in a clean environment (aseptic processing). The development and production of sterile medicinal products, whether in large-scale pharmaceutical processing or small-scale biotechnology, as medicines made on a named-patient basis prepared within a hospital pharmacy or involving the processing of sterilised components, are arguably the most difficult and complex facets of the preparation of pharmaceutical medicines. This is not necessarily due to any intrinsic formulation complexities in the products themselves but because those medicines, due to their route of administration, are required to be sterile at the point they are administered to the patient. It is not possible to determine to what extent compromised sterility would affect an individual patient. This is because people are individually unique in relation to form and physiology; it is also because the context of administration and treatment will vary widely between individuals. Nonetheless, a contaminated product, especially one administered intravenously (via a vein) or intrathecally (via the brain or the spinal cord), is likely to cause harm or even death.

In addition to the medicinal product, the various components required for the production, safe transport, storage and use of sterile products are equally as important. These items also need to be sterile when required for aseptic processing post-sterile filtration, whether they are large stainless-steel mixing vessels subjected to steam sterilisation using an autoclave, product packaging, or ready-assembled sterile disposable kits, sterilised using radiation or gas. For other parts of pharmaceutical manufacturing, 'sanitised' equipment (of a low bioburden, typically <10 organisms per square centimetre of surface) is used. A further area to which sterilisation applies is to medical devices. These cover a wide spectrum of items including instruments, apparatus, implants and *in vitro* reagents; all articles designed to diagnose, prevent or treat disease or other conditions.

Each of these various elements which combine to create a sterile product or item relates to the industrial process of sterile manufacturing. Sterile manufacturing itself is a continuum that stretches from development to manufacturing, to finished product, to marketing and distribution and to the utilisation of drugs and biologicals in hospitals, as well as in patients' homes. Although the terms 'sterile manufacture' and 'aseptic manufacturing' are widespread, there is no generic approach to the manufacture of sterile products. Each plant or process will differ in relation to the technologies, products and process steps employed. What governs the manufacture and distribution of sterile pharmaceutical products, however, is the requirements of good manufacturing practice (GMP) and the necessity for having a robust sterility assurance system and contamination control strategy in place (MHRA, 2022). The focal point of GMP is for a product to be produced which is sterile, under controlled conditions, and where there is no risk of contamination until the contents of the outer packaging are intentionally breached.

22.2 Defining Sterility

Before discussing sterile products, it is important to develop an understanding of 'sterility'. Sterility is a transitory and unnatural condition, given the abundance of microorganisms in the environment, including the manufacturing environment which has its own flora but is also at risk from microbial ingress. Sterility can be defined as 'the absence of all viable microorganisms'. Under this definition something would be deemed sterile only when there is a *complete* absence of viable microorganisms (but not necessarily dead cells or microbial by-products). Sterility is an absolute term; there is no partial level of sterility.

Developing 'the absence of viable microorganisms' concept further, how should viability be defined? Viability is itself a difficult concept and microbiologists periodically debate the issue of whether or not 'dead means dead'. Our understanding of viability is also limited by what we can see, and to see microorganisms is still very reliant upon the use of growth media (see Chapter 3); as it stands it is easier to demonstrate that a microorganism is dead than it is to demonstrate that it is alive. It has been estimated that only a very small proportion of microorganisms are culturable using established collection methods, agars and incubation conditions. Indeed, successful culture is entirely dependent upon sophisticated, artificial simulation of natural habitats which closely and necessarily reproduce the natural environment of a microorganism. Therefore, within the manufacturing environment for pharmaceuticals and medical devices it is probable that a diverse spectrum of microorganisms exists, many of which may not be recoverable or culturable on traditional laboratory growth media. Under sub-optimal conditions microorganisms may therefore resort to a state often described as 'viable but non-culturable' (VBNC) or alternatively as 'active but non-culturable' (ABNC). In these states, bacterial cells maintain certain features of viable cells, such as cellular integrity and measurable metabolic activity, yet will not culture.

This notion of viability has implications for the monitoring of the environment (which impacts especially on aseptic filling), assessing the bioburden of a load prior to sterilisation, assessing the microbial content of a product prior to final filtration and for the limitations of the sterility test (see Chapter 21). These uncertainties over viability require that greater emphasis is placed upon sterilisation processes that are consistent, reproducible and which have a degree of 'overkill' built into them, coupled with environmental and personnel controls.

With sterility, no distinction is made between those microorganisms which are known to be causative agents of specific diseases and those which are not normally pathogenic. Any type of microorganism may cause infection and illness if given the opportunity. Microorganisms that are frequently found on humans or animals or in their immediate environment are often assumed to be harmless because they are not associated with a specific disease. This assumption becomes invalid however once the body's antimicrobial defence barriers are breached. Almost any microorganism, even those which have not evolved to be especially invasive, may be opportunistic pathogens, particularly in weak or debilitated patients who are ill-equipped to resist infection (see Chapter 17).

22.3 Sterilisation Methods

The state of sterility is achieved through some form of sterilisation process. Sterilisation is the application of a physical or chemical procedure to destroy microbial life, including bacterial endospores (see Chapter 21). This is unlike disinfection, which refers to the targeted reduction of a microbial population by destruction or inactivation (see Chapter 18). Importantly, the process of sterilisation refers to microorganisms that are 'viable', historically those that are culturable. Significantly, it does not refer to the absence of microbial by-products. By-products include toxins which may cause harm, such as endotoxins, exotoxins or enterotoxins (see Chapter 3). These can be released by microorganisms as the function of their normal metabolism or when they die, and several toxins are resistant to many processes of sterilisation. Of these microbial by-products, the greatest risk to pharmaceutical processing is from endotoxins, often called pyrogens. Since such toxins can cause harm such as fever and multiple organ failure, it is required that sterile products are also free of those toxins and the definition of a sterile parenteral product extends to the product being apyrogenic. Pharmacopoeial limit tests for pyrogens exist, with the most common method employing a coagulation assay based on the *Limulus* amoebocyte lysate (LAL) test.

Although there are a wide variety of mechanisms and processes by which a pharmaceutical or a medical device might be rendered free from microorganisms (that is sterile), they can be grouped into three main categories of sterilisation. These are:

- Physical removal: the complete removal of all microorganisms to achieve a physical absence of microorganisms (such as filtration).
- Physical alteration: changing or deforming the physical cellular or biochemical architecture of a microorganism, including physical destruction or complete disintegration.
- Inactivation: the permanent disruption of critical biochemical and physiological functions, thereby neutralising that microorganism's potential or propensity (whether active or latent) to generate an infection. For complete assurance of inactivation, the microorganism must to all intents and purposes be 'killed' with no residual metabolic activity.

Each of the three fundamental mechanisms results in the same end goal, a medicine or medical device that when employed does not cause infection.

From these important concepts, the primary methods of sterilisation emerge and consist of the following four main approaches:

- high temperature sterilisation (by dry heat or moist heat [steam under pressure]);
- chemical sterilisation (such as gassing using ethylene oxide);
- filtration;
- radiation sterilisation (such as gamma irradiation).

For a detailed treatment of sterilisation methods, see Chapter 21.

All forms of sterilisation can have negative effects on a wide variety of packaging materials (and sometimes on the item or product itself). These effects can vary from material to material and between the different packaging components. Sterilisation can affect polymers, seal strength, label and box adhesion, corrugated and paperboard strength and material colour. The selection of the sterilisation method is therefore of considerable importance.

22.3.1 Factors Affecting Sterilisation

There are a number of factors which affect the success or otherwise of a sterilisation process, which are briefly discussed below.

22.3.1.1 Number and Location of Microorganisms

All other conditions remaining constant, the greater the number of microorganisms present (the bioburden; see Chapter 21), the longer a sterilisation process is required to run. Reducing the number of microorganisms that must be inactivated through meticulous cleaning and disinfection, or by assembling components within classified cleanrooms, increases the margin of safety when the sterilisation process is applied.

In terms of the location of microorganisms, aggregated or clumped microbial cells are more difficult to inactivate than mono-dispersed cells. Microorganisms may also be protected from poorly penetrating sterilisation methods by the production of thick masses of cells and extracellular materials, or biofilms (see Chapter 8). Furthermore, items which have crevices, joints and channels are more difficult to sterilise than those with flat surfaces because penetration of the sterilising agent to all parts of the object is more difficult.

22.3.1.2 Microbial Quality of Starting Materials

The microbial quality of raw materials (including active ingredients and excipients) will present a source of contamination that can prove difficult to remove or to inactivate, particularly when the organisms become bound to product matrices. The selection of materials of good microbiological quality is therefore essential in the management of contamination levels in both formulated products prior to sterilisation and the manufacturing environment. Ingredients of natural origin often carry the highest and most varied bioburden and must be carefully sourced and stored; synthetic raw materials are usually free from all but incidental microbial contamination. Acceptable microbial levels for starting materials are presented in pharmacopoeias and tested using the Microbial Limits Test (harmonised between the European, US and Japanese pharmacopoeias). Bioburden levels are typically not more than 100 or 1000 colony-forming units (CFU) per gram or millilitre, although specific monographs may require different acceptance criteria. In addition to microbial levels, tests to show the absence of certain pathogens (termed 'objectionable microorganisms' in the compendia) may be required according to the material type.

22.3.1.3 Innate Resistance of Microorganisms

Microorganisms vary greatly in their resistance to sterilisation processes. Intrinsic resistance mechanisms in microorganisms vary, with bacterial endospores generally being the most resistant to destruction. Endospores are formed as a mechanism of survival by some vegetative cells in response to adverse environmental signals that indicate a limiting factor for vegetative growth, such as exhaustion of an essential nutrient (for example, species of *Bacillus*; see Chapter 3). Such spores, which exhibit no signs of life ('cryptobiotic'), are highly resistant to environmental stresses such as high temperature (some endospores can be boiled for hours and retain their viability), irradiation, strong acids and disinfectants. Spores can retain viability indefinitely and may germinate back into vegetative cells when the environmental stress is relieved.

Implicit in all sterilisation strategies is the consideration that the most resistant microbial sub-population controls the sterilisation time. That is, to destroy the most resistant types of microorganisms (bacterial spores), the user needs to employ exposure times and a concentration or dose necessary to achieve complete destruction; this is the principle behind using biological indicators to validate a sterilisation method (see Chapter 21).

22.3.1.4 Physical and Chemical Factors

Several physical and chemical factors influence the outcome of a sterilisation process, especially temperature and relative humidity. For example, relative humidity is the single most important factor influencing the activity of gaseous sterilants, such as ethylene oxide, chlorine dioxide and formaldehyde (together with decontamination agents like hydrogen peroxide). It is axiomatic that achieving a certain temperature is critical for the operation of an autoclave and dry heat sterilisation.

22.3.1.5 Organic and Inorganic Matter

Organic matter, such as protein, can interfere with the antimicrobial activity of sterilisation processes by reacting with certain sterilants, thereby reducing the amount available to exercise their sterilising effect. Further, inorganic contaminants can afford physical protection to microorganisms, thereby limiting the potential effectiveness of a sterilisation process.

22.3.1.6 Duration of Exposure

Items must be exposed to the sterilisation process for an appropriate period of time. Most sterilisation processes have minimum cycle times, established during validation runs.

22.3.1.7 Storage

All sterile items should be stored in an area and manner whereby the packs or containers will be protected from dust, dirt, moisture, animals and insects. The shelf life of a sterilised product depends on the following factors:

- quality of the wrapper or container;
- number of times a package is handled before use;
- number of people who have handled the package;
- whether the package is stored on open or closed shelves;
- condition of storage area (e.g., humidity and cleanliness);
- use of plastic dust covers and method of sealing.

22.4 Demonstrating Sterility

The evidence that something is sterile can only be considered in terms of probability; absolute sterility could only theoretically be proved by testing every single item produced (and with technology that will give an undisputable result). No technique currently exists to prove 'sterility' beyond all reasonable doubt (even with the advent of rapid and alternative microbiological methods for the sterility test). Furthermore, the act of testing destroys the very item that is required for administration to the patient, so sterility cannot be proven empirically. Hence, any concept of sterility or sterilisation must recognise that all that can be ascertained is the probabilistic lack of presence of microorganisms rather than an absolute absence of microorganisms.

Therefore, the concept of what constitutes 'sterile' is measured as an assurance of the likelihood of sterility ('sterility assurance', see Section 22.7 and Chapter 21) or with reference to specific sterilisation processes, in terms of the probability of sterility for each item to be sterilised (the 'sterility assurance level', when applied to terminal sterilisation processes; see Section 22.8). In neither case can sterility be absolutely proven through testing. Certainly, a sterility test is incapable of proving sterility (see Chapter 21), even setting aside the uncertainties inherent in representative sampling. This is because:

- microorganisms could be present but undetectable simply because they are not being incubated in their preferred environment, and
- microorganisms could be present but undetectable because their existence has never been discovered.

With terminal sterilisation processes, the probability of a successful sterilisation can be considered in relation to items which can be processed without the sterilisation conditions causing deleterious effects. Probability is assessed in relation to a concept called the sterility assurance level (SAL). Importantly, the SAL concept cannot be applied to aseptically filled products.

SALs are used to estimate the microbial population that was destroyed by the sterilisation process, assuming microorganisms are destroyed in a linear manner. The SAL is demonstrated through validation using innocuous bacterial endospores (biological indicators, see Chapter 21). The assumption is that the inactivation of such highly resistant microorganisms encompasses all less-resistant organisms, including most pathogens. The SAL is normally expressed as 10^{-n}. For example, if the probability of a spore surviving were one in one million, the SAL would be 10^{-6}. The SAL is a fraction of one and therefore carries a negative exponent (so that six-log reduction is written as 10^{-6} rather than 10^{6}); it is additionally important to note that SAL refers to individual items of product and not to a batch of product. Each log reduction (10^{-1}) represents a 90% reduction in microbial population; this is referred to as the D-value (see also Chapter 21). Specifically, for sterilisation processes, the D-value (or decimal reduction time) is the time required, at a given condition (typically temperature) to achieve one log reduction, that is, to kill 90% of the target microorganisms. Thus, a process shown to achieve a '6-log reduction' (10^{-6}) will theoretically reduce a population from a million microorganisms (10^{6}) to one (10^{0}).

The same logic can apply to containers as to microorganisms. For example, a SAL of 10^{-6} when applied to a batch of containers expresses the probability of residual contamination (microbial survival), that is, there is one chance in 10^{6} that any particular container out of 10^{6} containers would theoretically not be sterilised by the process. In pharmaceuticals and healthcare, sterilisers are typically operated so that the theoretical log reduction is greater than 10^{-6} (often 10^{-12} log reduction is sought). This is to address the concern that the bioburden could be present in more than one container. Importantly, the SAL is not an expression of sterility but rather one defined as the probability of an item being non-sterile after it has been exposed to a validated terminal sterilisation process.

This theoretical reduction in microbial population also assumes:

- a single species of microorganism present on or in each product;
- there is a homogenous microbial population;
- the population has a mono-disperse distribution in/on the product to be sterilised, that is, there is no clumping;
- the exclusion of multi-nucleate spores (e.g., ascospores) and multi-nucleate microorganisms (e.g. fungi).

Most sterilisation processes introduce the concept of 'overkill', that is, seeking a SAL of greater than 10^{-6}, often one of 10^{-12}. Because it is not possible to prepare biological indicators with populations much above 10^{6}, the SAL is assessed mathematically using the linear destruction characteristics of microorganisms (see Chapter 21) and by assessing time and temperature exposure.

22.5 Types of Sterile Product

Parenteral drug delivery systems and many medicinal products, such as dressings and sutures, must be sterile in order to avoid the possibilities of microbial infection occurring as a result of their use. Sterility is also important for any material or instrument likely to contact broken skin or internal organs. Although pathogenic bacteria, fungi or viruses pose the most obvious danger to a patient, it should be also realised that microorganisms usually regarded as non-pathogenic and which inadvertently gain access to body cavities in sufficient numbers may cause a severe, possibly fatal infection. Consequently, injections, ophthalmic preparations, irrigation fluids, dialysis solutions, sutures and ligatures, implants and certain surgical dressings, as well as instruments necessary for their use or administration, must be presented in a sterile condition. This section summarises the features of some of the more common sterile products.

22.5.1 Injections

The most obviously recognised sterile pharmaceutical preparations are injections. These vary from very small volume antigenic products such as vaccines to large volume, total parenteral nutrition (TPN) products. Injections may be aqueous solutions, oily solutions (because of poor aqueous solubility or the necessity for a prolongation of drug activity), aqueous suspensions or oily suspensions. They may be aseptically produced or terminally sterilised in their final containers (see Section 22.8). Those drugs that are unstable in solution may be presented as a freeze-dried (lyophilised) powder. The choice of final packaging should not determine the method of sterilisation.

22.5.1.1 Formulation Considerations

An injection must be manufactured under conditions that result in a sterile product containing the minimum possible levels of particles and pyrogenic substances (see Section 22.15). Its formulation and packaging must maintain physical and chemical stability throughout the production process, the intended shelf life and during administration. Many injections are formulated as aqueous solutions, with Water for Injection (WFI) (see Section 22.5.1.5) as the vehicle. Most injections are prepared in single-dose form and this is mandatory for certain routes, for example, spinal injections where the intrathecal route is used, and large-volume intravenous infusions. Multiple-dose injections may require the inclusion of a suitable preservative to prevent contamination following the removal of each dose. Injections used for several routes, including the intrathecal and intracardiac routes, must not contain a preservative because of the potential for long-term harm to the patient.

22.5.1.2 Intravenous Infusions

Intravenous infusions consist of large-volume injections or 'drips' (500 ml or more) that are infused at various rates (50–500 ml h^{-1}) into the venous system. They are generally sterilised in an autoclave. Examples include isotonic solutions of sodium chloride or glucose that are used to maintain fluid and electrolyte balance, for the replacement of extracellular body fluids (e.g., after surgery or prolonged periods of fluid loss), as a supplementary energy source or as a vehicle for drugs. Other important examples are blood products, which are collected and processed in sterile containers, and plasma substitutes such as dextrans (see Chapter 25) and degraded gelatin.

Intravenous Additives

A common hospital practice is to add drugs to infusions immediately before administration. Regularly used additives include potassium chloride, lidocaine (lignocaine), heparin, certain vitamins and antibiotics. Potentially, this can be a hazardous practice; for instance, drug incompatibilities or physical instability may arise. Apart from these problems, if the addition is not carried out under strict aseptic conditions, the fluid can become contaminated with microorganisms during the procedure.

Another approach is to provide an intravenous drug additive service where the drug is added in a controlled environment to a small volume (50–100 ml) infusion in a collapsible plastic container and either used within a short period of time or the preparation stored in a freezer. If stored frozen, the infusion can be removed when required and thawed rapidly in a microwave oven. Many antibiotics are stable for several months when stored in minibags at −20 °C and are unaffected by the thawing process; some, for example, ampicillin, degrade even when frozen.

Total Parenteral Nutrition

TPN is the use of mixtures of amino acids, vitamins, electrolytes, trace elements and an energy source (glucose and fat) in the long-term feeding of patients who are unconscious or unable to take food. All or most of the ingredients to feed a patient for one day are combined aseptically in one large (3 l capacity) collapsible plastic bag, the contents of which are infused over a 12–24-hour period. Transfer of amino acid, glucose and electrolyte infusions, and the addition of vitamins and trace elements, must be carried out with great care under aseptic conditions to avoid microbial contamination. These solutions often provide good growth conditions for bacteria and moulds. Fats are administered as oil-in-water emulsions comprising small droplets of a suitable vegetable oil (e.g., soya bean) emulsified with egg lecithin and sterilised by autoclaving. In many cases, the fat emulsion is added to the 3 l bag.

22.5.1.3 Small-volume Injections

This category includes single-dose injections, usually of 1–2 ml but as large as 50 ml, dispensed in borosilicate glass or plastic (polyethylene or polypropylene) ampoules, sometimes even in pre-assembled syringes; this category includes injections for dental and local anaesthesia. Less frequently, multiple-dose glass vials of 5–25 ml capacity, stoppered with a rubber closure through which a hypodermic needle can be inserted, are used, for example, in the case of insulins and vaccines. The closure is designed to reseal after withdrawal of the needle. It is unwise to include too many doses in a multiple-dose container because of the risk of microbial contamination during repeated use. Preservatives must be added to injections in multiple-dose containers to prevent contamination during withdrawal of successive doses. However, preservatives may not be used in injections in which the total volume to be injected at one time exceeds 15 ml and there is an absolute prohibition on the inclusion of preservatives in intra-arterial, intracardiac, intrathecal or subarachnoid, intracisternal and peridural injections, and various ophthalmic injections.

Small-volume Oily Injections

Certain small-volume injections are available where the drug is dissolved in a viscous oil because it is insoluble in water and therefore a non-aqueous solvent is used. In addition, drugs in non-aqueous solvents provide a depot effect, for example, for hormones. The intramuscular route of injection must be used. The vehicle may be a metabolisable fixed oil such as arachis oil or sesame oil (but not a mineral oil) or an ester, such as ethyl oleate, which is also capable of being metabolised. The latter is less viscous and therefore easier to administer, but the depot effect is of shorter duration. The drug is normally dissolved in the oil, filtered under pressure and distributed into ampoules. After sealing, the ampoules are sterilised by dry heat.

22.5.1.4 Freeze-dried Products

In brief, freeze-drying (lyophilisation) consists of preparing the drug solution (with buffers and cryoprotectants), filtering through a bacteria-proof filter, dispensing into containers, removing water by sublimation in a freeze-drier, then capping and closing the containers. It is a batch manufacture process, of relatively long duration, and is used frequently for drugs of poor stability. Products are reconstituted into solution with a sterile diluent immediately prior to injection.

Many biotechnology products are freeze-dried. β-lactam antibiotics are frequently manufactured in this way as sterile bulks which may then be compounded with other sterile ingredients and dispensed into unit-dose containers, or even dispensed directly into unit-dose containers.

22.5.1.5 Water for Injection

Water used for parenteral products, often as a diluent or vehicle during administration, is known as WFI; it must be sterile and virtually apyrogenic with a specification of <0.25 endotoxin units per millilitre (in practice, WFI contains no detectable endotoxin). WFI can be produced by distillation or by reverse osmosis, with distillation being a more low-risk method (distillation separates out endotoxin and water molecules by molecular weight; reverse osmosis works on the basis of size exclusion under pressure, with a risk arising from endotoxin passing through should there be biofilm formation on the filter membrane).

WFI may also be used at various stages in sterile production, either as part of the product (i.e., diluent or vehicle) or for cleaning and rinsing activities in aseptic environments. In the production environment, WFI made on site can be used immediately for the preparation of injections provided it is sterilised within 4 hours of water collection. Alternatively, the water can be kept at a temperature above 65 °C (typically 80 °C) to prevent bacterial growth with consequent pyrogen production.

22.5.2 Non-injectable Sterile Fluids

There are many other types of solution in a sterile form, for use particularly in hospitals.

22.5.2.1 Non-injectable Water

This is sterile water, not necessarily of injectable water standards, which is used widely during surgical procedures for wound irrigation, moistening of tissues, washing of surgeons' gloves and instruments during use and, when warmed, as a haemostat. Isotonic saline may also be used. Topical water (as it is often called) is prepared in 500 ml and 1 l polyethylene or polypropylene containers with a wide neck and tear-off cap to allow for ease of pouring.

22.5.2.2 Urological (Bladder) Irrigation Solutions

These are used for rinsing of the urinary tract to aid tissue integrity and cleanliness during or after surgery. Either water or glycine solution is used, the latter eliminating the risk of intravascular haemolysis when electrosurgical instruments are used. These are sterile solutions produced in collapsible or semi-rigid plastic containers of up to 3 l capacity.

22.5.2.3 Peritoneal Dialysis Solutions

Peritoneal dialysis solutions are admitted into the peritoneal cavity as a means of removing accumulated waste or toxic products following renal failure or poisoning. They contain electrolytes and glucose (1.4–7% w/v) to provide a solution equivalent to potassium-free extracellular fluid; lactate or acetate is added as a source of bicarbonate ions. Slightly hypertonic solutions are usually employed to avoid increasing the water content of the intravascular compartment. A more hypertonic solution containing a higher glucose concentration is used to achieve a more rapid removal of water.

22.5.2.4 Inhaler Solutions

In cases of severe asthmatic attacks, bronchodilators and steroids for direct delivery to the lungs may be needed in large doses. This is achieved by direct inhalation via a nebuliser device; this converts a liquid into a mist or fine spray. The drug is diluted in small volumes of WFI before loading into the reservoir of the machine. This vehicle must be sterile and preservative-free and is therefore prepared as a terminally sterilised unit dose in polyethylene nebules.

22.5.3 Ophthalmic Preparations

22.5.3.1 Formulation Considerations

Medication intended for instillation on to the surface of the eye is formulated in aqueous solution as eye drops or lotion or in an oily base as an ointment. Because of the possibility of eye infection occurring, particularly after abrasion or damage to the corneal surface, all ophthalmic preparations must be sterile. As there is a very poor blood supply to the anterior chamber, defence against microbial invasion is minimal; furthermore, it appears to provide a particularly good environment for growth of bacteria.

Another type of sterile ophthalmic product is the contact lens solution. However, unlike the other types, this is not used for medication purposes but merely as a wetting, cleaning and/or soaking preparation for contact lenses.

22.5.3.2 Eye Drops

Eye drops are presented for use in (i) sterile single-dose plastic sachets containing 0.3–0.5 ml of liquid, (ii) multiple-dose amber fluted eye dropper bottles including the rubber teat as part of the closed container or supplied separately, or (iii) plastic bottles with integral dropper. A breakable seal indicates that the dropper or cap has not been removed prior to initial use. Although a standard design of bottle is used in hospitals, many proprietary products are manufactured in plastic bottles designed to improve safety and care of use. The maximum volume in each container is limited to 10 ml. Because of the likelihood of microbial contamination of eye dropper bottles during use (arising from repeated opening or contact of the dropper with infected eye tissue or the hands of the patient), it is essential to protect the product with a preservative. Eye drops for surgical theatre use should be supplied in single-dose containers.

Thermostable eye drops and lotions are sterilised at 121 °C for 15 minutes. For thermolabile drugs, filtration sterilisation followed by aseptic filling into sterile containers is necessary. Eye drops in plastic bottles are prepared aseptically.

22.5.3.3 Eye Lotions

Eye lotions are isotonic solutions used for washing or bathing the eyes. They are sterilised by autoclaving in relatively large volume containers (100 ml or greater) of coloured fluted glass with a rubber closure and screw cap, or packed in plastic containers with a screw cap or tear-off seal.

22.5.3.4 Eye Ointments

Eye ointments are prepared in a semi-solid base, for example, Simple Eye Ointment BP, which consists of yellow soft paraffin (8 parts), liquid paraffin (1 part) and wool fat (1 part). The base is filtered when molten to remove particles and sterilised at 160 °C for 2 hours. The drug is incorporated prior to sterilisation if heat-stable, or added aseptically to the sterile base. Finally, the product is aseptically packed in clear sterile aluminium or plastic tubes.

22.5.3.5 Contact Lens Solutions

Most contact lenses are worn for optical reasons as an alternative to spectacles. Contact lenses are of two types: hard lenses, which are hydrophobic, and soft lenses, which may be either hydrophilic or hydrophobic. The surfaces of lenses must be wetted before use and contact-lens-wetting solutions are used for this purpose. Hard, and more especially, soft lenses become heavily contaminated with protein material during use and therefore must be cleaned before disinfection. Contact lenses are potential causes of eye infection and, consequently, microorganisms should be removed before the lens is again inserted into the eye. Contact lens wetting, soaking and cleaning solutions must be sterile.

22.5.4 Dressings

Dressings and surgical materials are used widely in medicine, both as a means of protecting and providing comfort for wounds and for many associated activities such as cleaning and swabbing. They may be used on areas of broken skin. If there is a potential danger of infection arising from the use of a dressing, then it must be sterile. For instance, sterile dressings must be used on all open wounds, both surgical and traumatic, on burns and during and after catheterisation at a site of injection. It is also important to appreciate that sterile dressings must be packaged in such a way that they can be applied to the wound aseptically.

22.5.5 Implants

Implants are small, sterile cylinders of drug, inserted beneath the skin or into muscle tissue to provide slow absorption and prolonged action therapy. This is principally based on the fact that such drugs, invariably hormones, are almost insoluble in water and yet the implant provides a rate of dissolution sufficient for a therapeutic effect. Implants are manufactured from the pure drug made into tablet form by compression or fusion. No other ingredient can be included because this may be insoluble or toxic, or, most importantly, may influence the rate of drug release. Copolymers such as polylactic acid/polyglycolic acid may be used as the implant matrix to provide a controlled rate of drug delivery.

Compression of sterile drugs must be conducted under aseptic conditions using sterile machine parts and materials. The manufacture of heat-stable sterile implants by fusion does not require pre-sterilised ingredients or aseptic processing. The surface of implants must be sterile and protected by suitable packaging.

22.5.6 Absorbable Haemostats

The reduction of blood loss during or after surgical procedures where suturing or a ligature is either impractical or impossible can often be accomplished by the use of sterile, absorbable haemostats. These consist of a soft pad of solid material packed around and over the wound that can be left *in situ* and absorbed by body tissues over a period of time, usually up to 6 weeks. The principal mechanism of action of these is their ability to encourage platelet fracture because of their fibrous or rough surfaces, and to act as a matrix for complete blood clotting. Four products commonly used are oxidised cellulose, absorbable gelatin sponge, human fibrin foam and calcium alginate.

22.5.7 Surgical Ligatures and Sutures

The use of strands of material to tie off blood or other vessels (ligature) and to stitch wounds (suture) is an essential part of surgery. Both absorbable and non-absorbable materials are available for this purpose.

Sterilised surgical catgut consists of absorbable strands of collagen derived from mammalian tissue, particularly (despite its name) the intestines of sheep. Because of its source, it is particularly prone to bacterial contamination, and even anaerobic spores may be found in such material. It is best sterilised by gamma irradiation post-wrapping.

Sutures and ligatures are also made from many materials not absorbed by the body tissues. These consist of uniform strands of metal or organic material, for example, nylon, silk and polypropylene, that will not cause any tissue reactions and are capable of being sterilised. Depending on the physical stability of each material, they are preferably sterilised by autoclaving or gamma radiation. They are packed in single-dose sachets, either dry or surrounded by a preserving fluid with or without a bactericide.

22.5.8 Instruments and Equipment

The method chosen for sterilisation of instruments depends on the nature of the components and the design of the item. The wide range of instruments that may be required in a sterile condition includes syringes (glass or plastic disposable), needles, infusion administration sets, metal surgical instruments (e.g., scalpels, scissors, forceps), rubber gloves and catheters. Relatively complicated equipment such as pressure transducers, pacemakers, kidney dialysis equipment, incubators and aerosol machine parts may also be sterilised. Artificial joints and other orthopaedic implants could also be included in the vast range of items required in a sterile condition in modern medical practice. The choice of method depends largely on the physical stability of the items and the appropriate technique in particular situations. For instance, neonate incubators necessitate a chemical method of sterilisation. On the other hand, even delicate instruments such as pressure transducers are now available that can withstand autoclaving.

22.5.9 General Considerations

Taken more generally, sterile products can cover a very wide range of pharmaceutical and medicinal applications including:

- therapeutic products – containing conventional organic/inorganic drugs;
- biological products – prepared from biological sources, such as vaccines;
- diagnostic agents – dyes and X-ray materials;
- allergenic extracts – for the diagnosis and treatment of allergies;
- radio-pharmaceutical products – for the diagnosis and treatment of diseases;
- genetically manufactured/biotechnology products – including various peptides and monoclonal antibodies.

There are three requirements for sterile products, as determined by European (including UK) and Food and Drug Administration (FDA) regulations. These are:

1) All preparations must be sterile. This normally means a parametric assessment (see Section 22.15.1) of a terminal sterilisation process or passing the sterility test for aseptically filled products.
2) All injectable pharmaceutical preparations and implantable devices must be pyrogen-free or what is termed 'apyrogenic'. This normally means having a level of bacterial endotoxin below a threshold that can elicit a pyrogenic response.
3) All products are clear and practically particle-free (when examined by the unaided eye).

Sterile products can also be grouped in relation to the way in which they are treated (or not) after being filled into the final container (be that a bag, vial or syringe). The distinction is between products that can be terminally sterilised in their final container and those which cannot due to the effect of the sterilisation process upon the product. For example, some protein-based products cannot be subjected to heat. Products which cannot be subjected to terminal sterilisation are aseptically filled and rely on pre-sterilisation of the components and bulk product before being aseptically filled within a cleanroom. For these processes, there are different, and higher, levels of risk.

22.6 Good Manufacturing Practices for Sterile Products

GMP standards for sterile product manufacture have been adopted by many countries and organisations across the world and have more points of commonality than difference. At the simplest level, GMPs are a legal codification of quality principles applied in the manufacturing and testing of pharmaceutical products (e.g., MHRA 2022). GMP is about ensuring that quality is built into the organisation and the processes involved in the manufacture of medicinal products. Important points shared by all GMP systems are summarised in Table 22.1.

GMP is controlled and proven through documentation. When undertaking any process during manufacture, there must be detailed, written procedures in place, and for each activity, from production to laboratory testing, each step must be written down or captured in an electronic record.

22.6.1 Regulatory Framework

The main standards and guidelines for sterile product manufacturing are outlined below. Compliance is ensured by national inspectorates, which may operate on behalf of the regulators and licensing authorities.

Food and Drug Administration: FDA documentation is divided between US laws, as contained in the Code of Federal Regulations (CFR), and inspectorate guidance documents. The CFRs applicable to sterile manufacturing are under Title 21 (Food and Drugs). Contained in Chapter I of

Table 22.1 Key features which apply to all GMP systems.

Feature	Objectives
Manufacturing processes	Clearly defined and controlled to ensure consistency and compliance with specifications and acceptance criteria; changes to be evaluated and validated
Quality by design	Facility and equipment designed for the correct purpose from the start
Validation	All critical processes, including methods and systems used, and equipment must be validated against pre-determined specifications and acceptance criteria
Documentation	Fully documented procedures in place and followed; records must be kept, including personnel involved
Personnel	Establish training programme; full compliance with, and operation of, hygiene principles
Maintenance	Applies to premises and equipment
Quality	Built into the product life cycle (from initial development until product is discontinued) and assessed by regular internal and customer audits. In addition, pharmaceutical manufacturers are subject to periodic independent inspections by regulatory agencies.

Title 21 are parts 200 and 300, which are regulations pertaining to pharmaceuticals. In particular:

- Current Good Manufacturing Practice (cGMP) regulations (Code of Federal Regulations, Sections CFR 210 and 211).

The FDA inspection guides are non-binding documents designed as reference material for investigators and other FDA personnel.

There are two FDA drug inspectorates: the Center for Biologics Evaluation and Research (CBER) and the other located in the Center for Drug Evaluation and Research (CDER). CBER functions to protect and enhance the public's health through the regulation of biologicals and related products, including blood and blood products, vaccines, allergenics, and emerging technologies such as human cells, tissues and cellular and gene therapies. CDER is in place to ensure that all prescription and non-prescription drugs marketed in the United States are safe and effective. CDER evaluates all new drugs before they are sold and monitors drugs on the market to ensure that they continue to meet the standards of purity, potency and quality.

European Good Manufacturing Practices: European GMP relates to European Commission Directive 2003/94/EC which describes principles and guidelines of GMP in respect of medicinal products for human use and investigational medicinal products for human use. European GMP is set out within:

- EudraLex: 'The Rules Governing Medicinal Products in the European Community, Annex 1', published by the European Commission.

European GMP is overseen by the European Medicines Agency (EMA) and enforced by national inspection agencies (for example, in the UK this is the Medicines and Healthcare Products Regulatory Agency).

Pharmaceutical Inspection Convention and the Pharmaceutical Inspection Co-operation Scheme (PIC/S): The PIC/S exists to provide for active and constructive co-operation in the field of GMP. The purpose of the PIC/S is to facilitate the networking between participating authorities and for the exchange of information and experience between GMP inspectors.

The PIC/S publishes a range of documents; like FDA inspection guides these are aimed at aiding inspectors and an understanding of these by the manufacturer can be beneficial.

World Health Organization (WHO): The WHO is a specialised agency of the United Nations that acts as a coordinating authority on international public health. The WHO enforces similar requirements to the European Union's GMP (EU GMP).

International Organization for Standardization (ISO): The ISO publishes a number of standards of relevance to pharmaceutical manufacture. The standard for cleanrooms, ISO 14644, is of particular importance and is referenced both in EU GMP and the FDA Sterile Drug Products guide. A second, ISO 14698, is in two parts and refers to important aspects of biocontamination control in cleanrooms and associated controlled environments. In 2020, an equivalent European standard was issued as EN 17141.

There are a host of other relevant ISO standards pertaining to pharmaceutical manufacture, ranging from high-efficiency particulate air (HEPA) filter standards to irradiation guidance.

International Council for Harmonisation of Technical Requirements for Pharmaceuticals for Human Use (ICH): The ICH publishes quality and GMP documentation. ICH guidance is applicable to those countries and trade groupings that are signatories to the ICH (including the EU, UK, Japan and the USA.). The ICH has produced a number of guidelines relating to the quality of medicines. These include:

- Q7 'Good Manufacturing Practice for Active Pharmaceutical Ingredients';
- Q8 'Pharmaceutical Development';
- Q9 'Quality Risk Management';
- Q10 'Note for Guidance on Pharmaceutical Quality System';
- Q11 'Development and Manufacture of Drug Substances (Chemical Entities and Biotechnological/Biological Entities), Step 3'.

These are either separately adopted or, in the case of EU/UK GMP, embedded in relevant annexes.

In addition to the documents described above, inspectors anticipate that sterile manufacturers will be aware of and keep up-to-date with cGMP. This is a term to describe the evolution of GMPs in-between the update of regulatory guidelines. Some pertinent GMP examples and current GMP focal points are discussed at different points throughout this chapter.

22.6.2 In-process Controls and Quality Control (QC)

The quality of a production process can be followed by the operation of in-process controls. These comprise any test on a product, the environment or the equipment that is used during the manufacturing process. An example of this is testing that an autoclave is functioning correctly. QC is that part of GMP concerned with sampling, specifications and testing, as well as the organisation, documentation and release procedures which ensure that the necessary and relevant tests are carried out, and that materials are not released for use, nor products released for sale or supply, until their quality has been judged satisfactory. For sterile products, QC includes testing for sterility and pyrogens (see Section 22.16 and Chapter 21). '*The Rules and Guidance for Pharmaceutical Manufacturers and Distributors*' states that QC personnel should not be confined to laboratory operations, but must be involved in all decisions which may affect the quality of the product. The independence of QC from production is considered fundamental to the satisfactory operation of QC.

22.7 Sterility Assurance and the Manufacture of Sterile Products

The manufacture of sterile products involves the philosophy and application of sterility assurance. Sterility assurance, as a broad term, refers to the principle of protecting a sterile product throughout its manufacturing life in relation to controls and practices. It is not synonymous with the sterility assurance level, although the reduction of the two concepts is, unfortunately, too common. The term 'sterility assurance' is a combination of two words with the following definitions:

- sterility – state of being free from viable microorganisms; and
- assurance – a positive declaration intended to give confidence.

As suggested above, the term sterility assurance extends beyond the specifically applied 'sterility assurance level', since it concerns a holistic overview of all aspects of the pharmaceutical process. Sterility assurance is applied for both terminally sterilised and aseptically filled products, seeking to introduce the appropriate level of controls to minimise the possibility of an unsterile product. Importantly, all of the physical or mechanical treatments of the sterilised product, its components and its assembly need to be carefully controlled. However, achieving adequate sterility assurance cannot be easily quantified. For terminally sterilised products, there is reliance upon the SAL; for aseptically filled products, the greater emphasis is upon environmental controls (as discussed below) and periodic process simulation tests ('media fills', see Section 22.13).

Reflecting the holistic nature of the concept, sterility assurance embraces the wider aspects of GMP which are designed to protect the product from contamination at all stages of manufacturing (from incoming raw materials through to finished products), plus associated testing and monitoring, and thus it forms an integral part of the quality-assurance system. This concept extends to the use of clean-air devices (such as restricted access barrier systems or isolators) and cleanrooms (of the appropriate classification), containers and closures, product-sterilising filtration (the use of a 0.22-μm filter, see Chapter 21) and the use of sterilised or depyrogenated components, together with appropriate personnel behaviours and gowning.

It is necessary to recognise, however, that sterility assurance cannot be directly assessed for aseptic processing; this is because:

- Sterility testing is severely limited by sample size and microbial recovery.
- Environmental monitoring suffers from inadequate recovery and limited sample size. Furthermore, it is not a direct assessment of the product. This means that the absence of microorganisms in an environmental sample is not confirmation of asepsis, yet neither is recovery of contamination necessarily indicative of product contamination.
- Process simulation demonstrates maximum contamination rates in an individual exercise. These do not directly relate to production runs.

22.8 Terminal Sterilisation and Aseptic Processing

It is not surprising that concerns about patient risk have prompted a regulatory preference for the use of terminal sterilisation. The use of microbiologically effective sterilisation processes on finished formulations in their final container is favoured because of their antimicrobial effectiveness (as demonstrated by the SAL, see Section 22.4) and the resulting certainty of outcome, together with good sterilisation process repeatability. However, the potentially deleterious effects of these sterilisation processes on the product and/or primary package have limited their application in terms of the range of products that can be processed. A wider range of sterile products, including most biologicals, are manufactured by aseptic processing because that approach to sterile product manufacturing is less physicochemically impactful on both the formulated active pharmaceutical ingredient and the primary packaging which serves as a contamination barrier.

This requirement to favour terminal sterilisation is set out in the EMA document 'Sterilisation of the medicinal product, active substance, excipient and primary container' and in the FDA guidance on aseptic manufacturing. Both items of guidance require the manufacturer to make the case why terminal sterilisation cannot be undertaken. Where aseptic processing is selected, a series of control measures are required to show that the aseptic process is time-controlled, particularly in elements such as filter exposure, product hold and filling run time.

Terminal sterilisation: Terminal sterilisation involves filling and sealing product containers under high-quality environmental conditions, although the environmental controls need not be equivalent to aseptically filled products. This means that most products that are to be terminally sterilised may be filled in an EU GMP Grade C/ISO 14644 Class 8 cleanroom area (see Section 22.9). Products are filled and sealed in this type of environment to minimise the microbiological content of the in-process product and to help ensure that the subsequent sterilisation process is successful. It is accepted that the product, container and closure will probably have a low bioburden, but they are not sterile prior to the sterilisation process starting. The product in its final container is then subjected to a terminal sterilisation process such as moist or dry heat, a penetrating gas (like ethylene oxide) or to gamma or electron beam irradiation. As a terminally sterilised drug product, each product unit undergoes a single sterilisation process in a sealed container. The assumption is that the bioburden within the product can be eliminated by the sterilisation process selected.

Terminal sterilisation is also performed for certain components used in the manufacture of aseptically filled products (such as vessels for holding product, sterile filters and container closures). For glassware used in aseptic processing, this is required to have undergone depyrogenation, the destruction of endotoxins by the application of dry heat, commonly 250 °C exposure for 30 minutes. Also relevant to aseptic processing is the removal of endotoxin from container closures through rinsing or washing with pyrogen-free water before sterilisation; this may be undertaken either by the closure manufacturer or the pharmaceutical manufacturer.

The validation of any terminal sterilisation process requires careful planning, and this includes selection of the loads (pre-defined configurations of items to be sterilised). For the validation or qualification approach, different strategies can be adopted. One such approach, which tends to be adopted with early phases of product development, is one that avoids the qualification of every load. Here, a matrix design (bracketing) approach is often adopted, where 'worst case' combinations for all of the intended loads can be selected. The matrix approach uses a philosophy which allows for the testing of a subset of the intended loads to validate the entire range of loads, in lieu of testing each load in the matrix.

Pyrogens and endotoxins are difficult to remove from products once present and it is easier to keep components relatively endotoxin-free rather than to remove them from the final product.

Aseptic processing: Aseptic manufacture is used in cases where the drug substance or medicinal product/device is unstable when subjected to heat (thus, sterilisation in the final container closure system is not possible) or where heat would cause packaging degradation; this would also apply if the product or packaging were sensitive to any alternative form of terminal sterilisation process. Aseptic processing is arguably the most difficult type of sterile operation because the end product cannot be terminally sterilised and therefore there are far greater contamination risks during formulation and filling. With aseptic processing, there is always a degree of uncertainty, particularly because of the risk posed by personnel to the environment in which filling takes place (although this risk can be reduced through the use of barrier technology, see Section 22.11).

A useful definition of aseptic processing is provided in ISO 13408-1 Aseptic Processing of Healthcare Products, Part 1: 'General requirements: aseptic processing – handling of sterile product, containers and/or devices in a controlled environment', in which the air supply, materials, equipment and personnel need to meet a series of controls to maintain sterility. The definition has an additional note which states, 'This includes sterilization by membrane filtration which cannot be separated from the subsequent aseptic process'.

22.9 Cleanrooms and Facility Design

Cleanrooms are highly controlled environments where the air quality needs to ensure that the essential standards of cleanliness required for the manufacture of pharmaceutical and healthcare products are met. In addition, cleanrooms need to be designed so they can be easily cleaned, disinfected and maintained. Design aspects should be considered from the outset; GMP expectations are for 'quality by design' principles to be fundamental in cleanroom construction. These environments are of critical importance to the manufacture of sterile products, with even stricter requirements for cleanroom cleanliness in place for aseptic processing.

The importance of cleanrooms is demonstrated with the aseptic manufacture of a pharmaceutical preparation, where the dosage form and the individual components of the containment systems are sterilised separately and then the whole presentation is brought together by methods which ensure that the existing sterility is not compromised. Sterility of the product is normally achieved through sterile filtration of the bulk solution using a sterilising-grade filter (see Chapter 21). This is undertaken in an EU GMP Grade C/ISO 14644 Class 8 cleanroom environment (see Section 22.9.4). The container and closure are also subject to sterilisation methods separately. The sterilised bulk product is filled into the containers, stoppered and sealed under aseptic conditions (under EU GMP Grade A/ISO 14644 Class 5 air quality) within an EU GMP Grade B/ISO 14644 Class 7 cleanroom, unless filling is undertaken within an isolator system (here, an EU GMP Grade C/ISO 14644 Class 8 cleanroom environment is normally selected as the environment housing the isolator).

22.9.1 Design of Premises

Sterile production should be carried out in a purpose-built unit separated from other manufacturing areas and thoroughfares. The unit should be designed to encourage separation of each stage of production, but should ensure a safe and organised workflow. A plan of such a facility is shown in Figure 22.1. Sterilised products held in quarantine pending sterility test results (see Chapter 21) must be kept separate from those awaiting sterilisation.

22.9.2 Internal Surfaces, Fittings and Floors

Particulate, as well as microbial, contamination must be minimised. To this end, all surfaces must be smooth and impervious in order to: (i) prevent accumulation of dust or other particulate matter; and (ii) permit easily repeated cleaning and disinfection. Smooth rounded coving should be used where the wall meets the floor and the ceiling. Surface materials should be compatible with the cleaning and disinfection agents deployed.

Suitable flooring may be provided by welded sheets of polyvinyl chloride (PVC); cracks and open joints which might harbour dirt and microorganisms must be avoided. The preferred surfaces for walls are plastic, epoxy-coated plaster, plastic fibreglass or glass-reinforced polyester. Often the final finish for the floor, wall and ceiling is achieved using continuous welded PVC sheeting. False ceilings should be adequately sealed to prevent contamination from the space above. Use should be made of well-sealed glass panels, especially in dividing walls, to ensure good visibility and allow satisfactory supervision. Doors and windows should be flush with the walls. Windows should not be openable.

Internal fittings such as cupboards, drawers and shelves should be kept to a minimum. They must be sited where they do not interfere with the airflow of the filtered air supply. Stainless steel or laminated plastic are the preferred materials for such fittings. Stainless steel trolleys may be used to transport equipment and materials within the clean and aseptic areas, but must remain confined to their respective units. Equipment must be designed so that it may be easily cleaned and sterilised or disinfected.

An important step towards achieving microbial control within a cleanroom is the use of defined cleaning techniques, together with the application of detergents and disinfectants according to a specified schedule; regular microbiological monitoring is performed to confirm the efficacy of these procedures (see Section 22.15). The objective of cleaning and disinfection is to achieve appropriate microbiological cleanliness levels for the class of cleanroom for an appropriate period of time. This involves the application of detergents (which 'clean') and disinfectants (which inactivate or destroy microorganisms, depending upon the type of disinfectant). Cleaning agents, such as alkaline detergents and ionic and non-ionic surfactants, are deployed to remove 'soil' from a surface. The removal of soil is an important step prior to the application of a disinfectant, for the greater the degree of soiling remaining on a surface, the lesser the effectiveness of disinfection. Disinfectant types include clear soluble phenolics for interior services and fittings and alcohols for working surfaces; chlorine-based agents are less commonly used because of their corrosive potential on some materials (see Chapter 18). Under EU and UK GMP, two disinfectants must be used in rotation, with the disinfectants having different modes of action to reduce the risk of the emergence of resistant strains (see Chapter 20). One of the disinfectants should be a sporicide, or alternatively the application of a sporicide should form a regular part of the facility disinfection strategy. Regulations also require the disinfectants used to be qualified against representative materials used in the facility, by conducting surface coupon disinfectant efficacy studies where acceptance of the disinfectant is based on achieving a two- or three-log reduction of the microbial challenge populations.

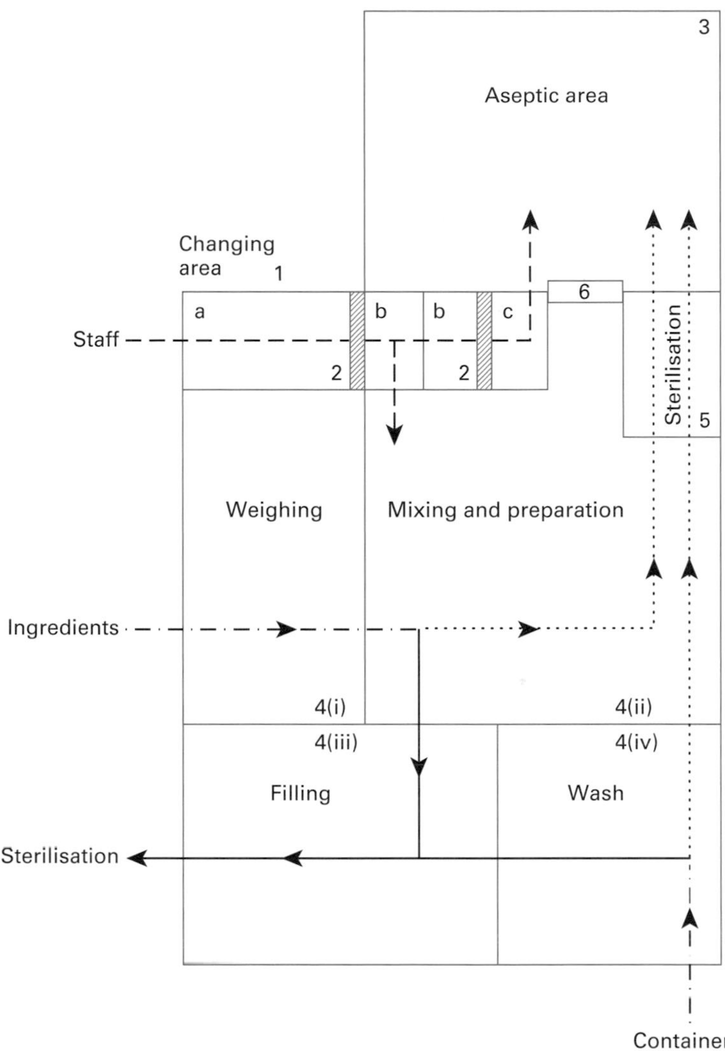

Figure 22.1 Example of a diagrammatic representation of the layout and workflow of a small-scale sterile product manufacturing unit. **1**, the changing area in this example is built on the black (a)–grey (b)–white (c) principle; passage into the clean area is through a and b, whereas entry to the aseptic area is first through a and b followed by c. **2**, dividing step-over sill. **3**, for details of aseptic area requirements, see text; a laminar airflow workstation would be included in this area. **4i–4iv**, these areas are clean areas. In filling rooms for terminally sterilised products, care should be exercised to protect containers from airborne contamination. The final rinse point (i.e., where the containers are finally washed) should be sited as near as possible to the filling point. **5**, articles which are to be transferred directly to the aseptic area from elsewhere must be sterilised by passage through a double-ended steriliser. Solutions manufactured in the clean area may be brought into the aseptic area through a sterilising-grade membrane filter. **6**, double-doored hatchway through which pre-sterilised articles may be passed into the aseptic area. Note: inspection, holding and final packaging areas have been omitted. Direction of workflow: —— → ——, for terminally sterilised products; ··· → ···, for aseptically prepared products; – · → · –, shared stages of preparation.

22.9.3 Services

Clean and aseptic areas must be adequately illuminated; lights are best housed in translucent panels set in a false ceiling. Electrical switches and sockets must be flush with the wall or fitted outside. When required, gases should be pumped in from outside the unit and sterile-filtered if they come into contact with product or vials. Pipes and ducts, if they must be brought into the clean area, must be sealed through the walls. Additionally, in order to prevent dust accumulation, pipes and ducts must be boxed in or readily cleanable. Alternatively, they may be sited above false ceilings.

Sinks should be of stainless steel with no overflow, and water must be of at least purified quality (water supplies are not permitted in aseptic processing areas). Wherever possible, drains should be avoided. If installed they must be fitted with effective, readily cleanable traps and with air breaks to prevent backflow. Any floor channels should be open, shallow and cleanable and connected to drains outside the area; they should be monitored microbiologically. Sinks and drains should be excluded from aseptic areas except where radiopharmaceuticals are being processed when sinks are a requirement.

22.9.4 Air Supply

Cleanrooms are classified in terms of air cleanliness, as assessed by measuring particle concentration per cubic metre. 'Particle' in the context of a cleanroom is a general term for sub-visible matter. An airborne particle refers to particles suspended in air. Air contains a variety of different particles of a range of different sizes; these include particles of dust, dirt, skin and microorganisms. The function of a cleanroom is to reduce the number of airborne particles to a level commensurate to that cleanroom classification. An ISO Class 5/EU GMP Grade A clean air space, for

Table 22.2 Air quality for cleanrooms.

Grade	At rest		In operation	
	Maximum permitted number of particles m^{-3} equal to above			
	0.5 μm	5 μm	0.5 μm	5 μm
A	3520	20	3520	20
B	3520	29	352,000	2900
C	352,000	2900	3,520,000	29,000
D	3,520,000	29,000	Not defined	

Table 22.3 Operations carried out in the various grades of air.

Grade	Examples of operations
For terminally sterilised products	
A	Filling of products, when unusually at risk
B	Background environment to Grade A preparation areas
C	Preparation of solutions, when unusually at risk
	Filling of products at lower risk
D	Preparation of solutions and components for subsequent filling
For aseptic processes	
A	Aseptic preparation and filling
B	Background environment to Grade A preparation areas when not in an isolator
C	Preparation of solutions to be filtered; background support areas for aseptic processing where isolators are used
D	Cleaning of equipment; handling of components after washing

instance, is designed not to allow more than 100 particles (0.5 μm or larger) per cubic foot of air (equivalent to 3520 particles per cubic metre). To put this into context, an office building contains from 500,000 to 1,000,000 particles (0.5 μm or larger) per cubic foot of air (equivalent to between 17.5 and 35 million particles per cubic metre). An important sub-class of particles are viable particles (where people are present a proportion of particles will be viable, although the precise ratio of viable to non-viable varies). Air quality according to the EU GMP classification system is summarised in Table 22.2.

To achieve the stringent standards required for biocontamination control, high fresh-air exchange rates (a minimum of 20 changes per hour are usual in clean and aseptic rooms), extensive air filtering (through HEPA filters), and temperature and humidity control are all required. In addition, protection from uncontrolled ingress of external ambient air is needed, and this is achieved by creating a positive pressure differential between the cleanroom and its surroundings, with the highest pressure in the most critical rooms. Through these measures, cleanrooms can provide appropriately controlled environments for both sterile and non-sterile pharmaceutical manufacturing. An additional air-control requirement is for a local zone of protection to be in place for aseptic processing environments, which requires maintenance and demonstration of local unidirectional airflow to protect the operation (the ISO Class 5/EU GMP Grade A zone).

While regulatory expectations have the ultimate focus of patient safety for air quality, there are some differences between regulators (at least with terminology). A key difference between inspectorate bodies is with cleanroom classification and categorisation. For the FDA, the ISO 14644 (Part 1, 2015) standard of cleanroom classification is used. ISO 14644 is a general standard covering all industries that use cleanrooms (from electronics to pharmaceuticals), of which Part 1 addresses cleanroom classification. In Europe, a grading system, A to D, specified in the EU GMP guide is used for normal cleanroom operation. For routine assessments, both EU and FDA standards require particles of a cut-off size of ≥0.5 μm to be measured. However, a difference between the two regulators is the additional EU GMP expectation to measure particles of a cut-off size of ≥5.0 μm (where larger particles, potentially indicating skin detritus, can be detected; see Table 22.2 above). There are also differences between the EU and ISO standards in relation to the operational state of the cleanrooms with and without personnel present. The WHO uses the same grading system as Europe in its GMP guidelines. The EU GMP grades of air required for typical manufacturing activities are summarised in Table 22.3.

With facility design in general, care is required to avoid cross-contamination (such as avoiding clean equipment being moved at the same time as dirty equipment and ensuring that personnel movement is controlled). Information to support bi-directional flow can be obtained from cleanroom recovery studies where the time taken for particulates to return to an acceptable level is noted. This provides information about the 'rest' time required, following an activity going in one direction being completed and before an activity in the reverse direction commences. The design or layout of an area (see Section 22.9.1) should promote the orderly handling of materials and equipment, the prevention of mix-ups and the prevention of contamination of equipment or product by substances, previously manufactured products, personnel or environmental conditions.

22.10 Operating Principles for Aseptic Processing

There are some broad expectations for aseptic processing; these are:

- The process should be designed and justified based on a comprehensive risk assessment.
- Wherever product or components are exposed, the environment must be a Grade A zone (this includes wrapped sterilised equipment to be loaded into a filling machine or isolator).
- Any equipment surfaces which contact product or components shall be sterile. This includes such items as filling pipework, pumps, needles, stopper containers and forceps used to handle fallen vials.
- Precautions should be taken to minimise the risk of contamination arising from humans; these can range from full gowning through to the operation of barrier systems or the use of isolators and advanced processes.
- To reduce the risk of ingress of particulates, both viable and non-viable, the principle of 'first air' should be followed. 'First air' is air which has passed from the HEPA filter to the critical point where product is exposed in a unidirectional manner without previously contacting any other surface and hence is free of any contaminants.
- Airflows within the Grade A area should be designed to sweep any generated particles away from critical points. The suitability of such airflows should be demonstrated by airflow visualisation studies.
- Aseptic techniques are required for all actions undertaken and any interventions made in the aseptic processing zone.
- Interventions into the aseptic process should be eliminated where possible or otherwise minimised. This can involve the use of sterilise-in-place systems or single-use components to limit aseptic connections at start-up and process optimisation to prevent product jams and defective units. Importantly, while interventions can be risk-assessed, there is no such thing as a low-risk intervention.
- All personnel involved must understand the principles of aseptic processing in order to have a full appreciation of the risks and the consequences of their actions. A GMP expectation is that all staff working with sterile products have a basic understanding of microbiology and contamination control.

Over the last 20 years, engineering and manufacturing technology designed to assist aseptic processing has evolved considerably. In the context of pharmaceutical products and medical devices, blow–fill–seal (BFS), pre-filled syringe filling, restricted access barrier systems (RABS) and isolator technologies represent the main developments (see Section 22.11). Aseptic processes that exclude human intervention (such as robotics or barrier systems) are at a considerably lower risk of breaching asepsis than operations which consist of filling machines operating under unidirectional airflow devices where there is a need for periodic human intervention. Where isolator systems are employed, the background environment for the cleanroom can even be at EU GMP Grade C/ISO 14644 Class 8, based on an appropriate risk assessment. There are additional risk considerations for isolators in that the decontamination procedures used should be validated to ensure full exposure of all isolator surfaces to the chemical agent.

22.10.1 Sterile Filtration

Sterile filtration using membrane filters is a critical step in aseptic processing and is essential for the removal of particulate and microbial contaminants from liquids, air and gases. Microorganism removal is required in order to achieve either a sterile filtrate or, if the drug product is later terminally sterilised, to reduce the bioburden challenge and particularly the numbers of Gram-negative bacteria which might otherwise generate elevated levels of pyrogenic endotoxin.

There is a multitude of filter designs and configurations utilised within the biopharmaceutical industry (see Chapter 21). These include those of a sheet or modular (lenticular) depth filter type for prefiltration and analytical flat filter membranes for microbial sampling and evaluation, but, most commonly, filter cartridges, which either contain depth filter fleeces or filter membranes. Filter membranes are available in a large variety of polymers, which have optimal properties for a wide variety of applications. Unfortunately, no single filter type can satisfy all applications and needs.

Factors affecting microbial retention and hence filter efficiency during a manufacturing operation include:

- Product chemical nature and formulation.
- Pore-size rating and membrane material which determine filter capacity (sterilising grade filters require a pore size of not greater than 0.22 μm, whereas bioburden reduction filters are rated 0.45 μm).
- pH, viscosity, osmolality, surface tension and temperature (these can influence the filtration process and cause blockages, if out of range).
- Differential pressure (to avoid pressure drops across the filter).
- Product flow rate/unit surface area (the product must flow evenly across the membrane in order to capture any organisms present, a slowdown of the flow rate could indicate blockage).

- Upstream bioburden quantity and composition (filters will only work against a given bioburden range, therefore assessing the expected microbial challenge to the filter is important).
- Throughput (volume) of the product being filtered (a filter will only continue to be effective in relation to a given volume of liquid).
- Product hold time (a maximum time is required to avoid any microorganisms present from growing significantly).
- Filter flush volume (filter wetting) and product flush (the wettability of a membrane is tied to the chemical properties of the membrane surface; before product is presented to the membrane, the membrane must be wetted with either a flush fluid or product to be discarded).

For in-process testing, for each batch of product filtered, the maximum acceptable bioburden prior to final sterile filtration must be 10 CFU 100 ml^{-1} (this relates to the bacterial filter efficiency rating and ensures the filter will be able to capture organisms from high volumes of product without blocking). If this requirement cannot be met (based on process understanding), it is necessary to use a prefiltration step through a bacteria-retentive filter and then to confirm an acceptable microbial challenge.

22.10.2 Managing Aseptic Assembly, Connections and Interventions

Any manufacturing process is likely to involve interventions such as the assembly of equipment and materials, connections and in-process transfers and retrieval of dropped containers; each element carries a risk to the microbiological integrity of the product and so must be managed. The ideal mitigation is removal of the intervention completely, for example, the use of sterilise-in-place technologies to eliminate the need for aseptic connections. Interventions represent an increased level of risk and appropriate control and monitoring are required. Where an intervention cannot be completely eliminated, its frequency should be reduced and its performance optimised by the development and use of appropriate tools. The input of experienced process operators in designing these mitigations is essential.

Once an intervention has been optimised, it should be demonstrated that performing the activity does not affect air flows significantly. First air must not be interrupted and there should be no turbulence created which could prevent the effective removal of any particles generated by the intervention or which could entrain extraneous particles and carry them towards the process. This is usually carried out by airflow visualisation studies (smoke studies).

The use of RABS and isolators significantly reduces the risk posed during human interventions, but the principle should still be applied.

22.10.3 Transfer of Materials into and out of Aseptic Processing Areas

EU GMP requires that 'Components, containers, equipment and any other article required in a clean area where aseptic work takes place should be sterilised and passed into the area through double-ended sterilisers sealed into the wall, or by a procedure which achieves the same objective of not introducing contamination'. While this appears a relatively straightforward requirement, there are relatively few applications where materials can be sterilised and passed directly into a Grade A filling zone without any intermediate transfers. This section discusses some points to consider in the transfer of materials.

Dry heat tunnel sterilisers are very effective in processing glass primary containers into Grade A zones. Containers pass through the tunnel on a moving belt and enter the Grade A zone directly. The overpressure in the Grade A zone and the design of the airflow in the tunnel ensure that air moves counter to the product flow, thereby maintaining the integrity of the Grade A zone during transfer. As the process is continuous, no intervention is required to unload containers.

Steam sterilisers are often used to sterilise filling equipment, filters and many other items used in the clean area. It is usually impractical for such a steriliser to open directly into a Grade A zone due to the potential release of moisture and particles. Sterilisers are often located to open into a Grade B support area where operators can carry out unloading. The challenge then is unloading the steriliser, protecting the sterilised items during transfer and subsequently introducing them to the Grade A zone. It is expected that the unloading door of the steriliser is protected by a flow of unidirectional HEPA filtered air to minimise the risk of contamination of the sterilised items. Items are usually double- or triple-wrapped in layers of protective material or placed in specially designed transfer containers.

Where dry heat or steam sterilisation is not possible, items can be sterilised by other means such as ethylene oxide gas or gamma irradiation. These processes are remote from the aseptic processing area and, as they require items to be transported to that area, consideration should be given to outer protective layers and transfer routes through the support areas to the aseptic processing area. The outer protective layers, which are for storage and transfer through to the aseptic processing area, can take a number of different forms ranging from multiple layers of sterilisation grade paper wrapping, through purpose-made multilayer packaging such as that used for tubs of syringes, to sterilisation bags with special docking systems. As mentioned earlier, items entering the Grade A zone must remain sterile and their transfer must not introduce contamination into the Grade A zone.

Connections made to the Grade A zone are required to maintain the sterility of the materials and to protect that zone. This is achieved by one of the following:

- *Transfer hatch:* Interlocking doors and the pressure differential between Grade A and B zones maintain an outward airflow which protects the Grade A zone from ingress of airborne contaminants. The outer layer of packaging is removed, as material is placed into the hatch and a bio-decontamination process is carried out to ensure that the inner package remains sterile. The inner packaging is removed in the Grade A zone. Transfer hatch operations range from simple manual processes using spray and wipe disinfection to automated systems with vapour phase decontamination.
- *Conveyor system:* In some large-scale industrial applications, electron beam systems have been used to decontaminate the outside of syringe tubs as they pass into an automated lid-removal unit
- *Sterilisation bags with docking system:* Items such as vial stoppers are sterilised in flexible bags which have an alpha–beta port which allows the bag to be docked directly to the wall of an isolator or RABS. The alpha–beta system is designed in such a way that the outer non-sterile surfaces of both units lock together and then open to provide a sterile pathway for the discharge of the stoppers.
- *Transfer isolators:* Materials are loaded into the transfer isolator which can then be internally bio-decontaminated and locked onto an isolator or RABS in a similar manner to the bags described above. Transfer isolators can also be used to connect directly to sterilisers and then transfer materials to an isolator or RABS.

22.11 Minimising Human Intervention

It is widely accepted that people present the greatest source of microbial contamination around an aseptic process, irrespective of the level of training and use of protective clothing. Simply standing still people generate hundreds of thousands of particles many of which carry microbes. It is recognised, therefore, that increasing the separation between the human operator and the process reduces the risk of contamination during processing. While open processing and simple barriers are still used by some manufacturers, the general expectation is that automated processes, RABS or isolator technologies are used.

22.11.1 Blow–Fill–Seal Technology

BFS technology is a specialised type of aseptic filling, one at a theoretically lower contamination risk compared with conventional aseptic filling. BFS is an automated process where plastic containers are formed, filled and sealed in a continuous operation without human intervention. This is performed in an aseptic enclosed area inside a specialised machine. The technology can be used to aseptically manufacture certain pharmaceutical liquid dosage forms, for example, ophthalmic preparations. Typically, the plastic containers are formed of polyethylene and polypropylene, the latter, having greater thermostability, being often used to form containers which are then further sterilised by autoclaving.

BFS operations are undertaken under EU GMP Grade A/ISO 14644 Class 5 conditions with the background environment at EU GMP Grade C/ISO 14644 Class 8. Where BFS equipment is used for the production of products that are terminally sterilised, the operation can be carried out within an EU GMP Grade D/ISO 14644 Class 9 background environment if appropriately risk-assessed.

22.11.2 Restricted Access Barrier Systems

A RABS involves the use of a barrier around the Grade A zone, and glove ports are present by which all manual aseptic activities are carried out. The Grade A zone is still protected by a unidirectional flow of filtered air and the area surrounding the barrier is required to be Grade B. As the operators are located in a Grade B area, full aseptic gowning is required. Historically, RABS has represented the next step in the evolution of the traditional cleanroom approach to aseptic processing. RABS are operated with dedicated HEPA airflow to the unit. So-called closed design RABS have exhaust air ducted away. Alternatively, systems exist where air is exhausted from the base of the unit into the surrounding Grade B zone. This is called an open-design RABS.

In closed-operation RABS, the protective barriers are not opened during processing. All intervention is carried out through glove ports. In open-operation RABS, certain operations, for example, addition of stoppers to a stopper feed system, might require the opening of the barrier. Such an intervention is from the Grade B zone and requires the same levels of control as would be required for a traditional process without barriers. It does obviously present a greater risk than a closed RABS process.

22.11.3 Isolators

Isolators are superior to cleanrooms in that the contamination risk is reduced through the construction of a barrier between the critical area (sometimes called the 'micro-environment') and the outside environment. Isolators provide a sealed physical barrier to the ingress of contamination during operation (this is unlike a RABS, which uses a combination of barriers and airflow and may not be physically sealed during operation). While the interior of the isolator is required to meet Grade A standards, there is no requirement for the isolator to be located in a Grade B area. EU GMP Annex 1 specifies at least a Grade D background, although many pharmaceutical manufacturers use Grade C. This also means that operators are not gowned to Grade A/B standards; this assists comfortable working.

During set-up, isolators may be open to the environment (Grade D or Grade C) and so a validated bio-decontamination of all surfaces is required. This must include the surfaces of the isolator itself and also of any materials and equipment placed into the isolator before closing up the system. Bio-decontamination is usually carried out by a gaseous disinfection process such as with hydrogen peroxide vapour. A 6-log reduction in a spore challenge is considered to demonstrate effective bio-decontamination.

Isolators rely on the integrity of the physical barrier to protect the aseptic process and so frequent integrity testing is required. Requirements for this vary between different isolator applications such as small-scale sterility testing, pharmacy compounding, negative pressure isolators used to contain hazardous materials and larger-scale complex systems for pharmaceutical manufacturing processes. The test pressures and limits used for initial set-up and those used for routine monitoring may also vary to account for variations in temperature between tests. The integrity of isolator gloves must be monitored on a frequent basis. This is usually accomplished by a programme of regular visual inspection before, during and after use and routine physical integrity testing. It should be noted that the pressures typically used to test the isolator system (two or three times the operating pressure of the isolator, typically 150–200 pa) are inadequate to detect small holes in gloves. Significantly higher pressures of around 500 Pa are required.

Transfer of materials into and out of the isolator is a major risk area. In order to ensure that all materials entering the Grade A zone are sterilised and the isolator remains physically closed during operation, transfer isolators are often fixed to the processing isolator. Sterilised wrapped materials are loaded into the transfer isolator and surface decontaminated as described in Section 22.10.3. Following bio-decontamination, the connection between the transfer isolator and the processing isolator can be opened.

22.11.4 Single-use Sterile Disposable Technology

In recent years, there have been a number of advances in single-use sterile disposable technologies, which have helped to both reduce the risk of contamination and to streamline process operations. The majority of these technological developments are oriented towards the manufacture of sterile products, particularly aseptically filled products.

Among the earliest to find use were disposable filter capsule devices, which can filter small volumes without the need for filter housings and their associated cleaning needs. Single-use sterile bags are now available to replace glass bottles, plastic carboys or stainless-steel containers for small-volume storage and the transport of biological solutions and of growth media. A more recent development has been disposable mixing systems which can be connected to capsule membrane filters and a holding bag (in a two- or three-dimensional design). These interconnected disposable systems have a considerable advantage in that they are supplied ready to use as sterilised components. Other developments include specialised tubing, single-use ion-exchange membrane chromatography devices, single-use mixers and bioreactors, connection devices and sampling receptacles.

Aseptic connectors have proved to be one of the most useful types of single-use technologies. These devices allow a connection between components to be performed in an environment that does not require unidirectional airflow cabinets or other capital equipment to maintain sterility. This principle allows liquid sterile products to be transferred simply and safely, in a totally closed and automated process, towards or from contained areas via small-scale rapid transfer ports. These devices shorten the time required for the connection and can remove the requirement to undertake the connection under Grade A/ISO Class 5 air.

Single-use items are typically sterilised using gamma irradiation. Ethylene oxide gas remains an alternative sterilisation process, although this is not, as yet, used to the same extent as radiation. The sterilisation cycles are designed to achieve a SAL of 10^{-6}. Gamma irradiation is adopted largely because the radiation dose can be selected to limit degradation of the material from which the device is constructed, primarily plastic.

The advantages of single-use technology to the industry in particular can be summarised as: eliminating the need for cleaning, thereby reducing the overall use of cleaning chemicals; removing the requirement to perform in-house sterilisation (typically by autoclaving) for many components; assisting with storage requirements; lowering process downtime; and increasing process flexibility, thereby reducing risks of cross-contamination. There are inevitably a number of validation steps which need to be undertaken before such technology is adopted by a pharmaceutical manufacturer. In particular, these include checking for any leachables or extractables which might contaminate the product when it comes into contact with the single-use device during processing. Notwithstanding, these disposable single-use sterile items offer increased sterility assurance while affording pharmaceutical organisations the opportunity to move away from equipment which needs to be cleaned and sterilised and from consumables which are recycled or pose a risk with their transfer into cleanrooms.

22.12 Personnel

The major source of microbial contamination within cleanrooms is from personnel; this is unsurprising given our understanding of the human skin microbiome and the evidence gathered from cleanroom environments. Studies indicate that a human will shed approximately 1000 million skin cells per day and that around 10% of the skin shed is expected to harbour microorganisms.

The threat of contamination comes not only from production staff, but also from others present in process areas such as cleaning staff and engineers. It is therefore important that all personnel entering cleanrooms have been suitably trained in how to behave and how to adopt appropriate gowning procedures. Further training should be provided on the principles of good hygiene and in relation to a basic understanding of microbiology.

It is essential that:

- Personnel must receive initial and periodic formal training in GMP, aseptic processing, the principles of contamination control, aseptic gowning and on those job-specific tasks that they must perform.
- Where appropriate, personnel should be initially and periodically thereafter assessed for their proficiency in gowning.
- Personnel should be initially and periodically assessed for their proficiency in aseptic technique. Specific training should also be provided for those individuals performing the initial set-up of the equipment prior to the aseptic process.
- Personnel should conform to the highest standards of aseptic technique at all times even when working with a closed RABS or isolator.
- The gloved hands of personnel are periodically monitored using finger dab agar plates.
- Personnel should be monitored upon each departure from the aseptic core by taking contact plates from selected cleanroom suit locations.
- Glove port gauntlets are assessed microbiologically and by pressure integrity test units.
- Gown materials should be cleaned in specialised laundry facilities, and sterilised using validated methods.
- Gloves on enclosures should be replaced periodically, sterilised and integrity-tested.
- When conducting interventions, personnel should refrain from directly touching product contact surfaces; instead, sterile tools, captive to the filling area, should be used. Tools should always be employed in the execution of an intervention even within an enclosure.

Clothing worn in a clean area must be made from non-shedding fibres; polyester is a suitable fabric. Airborne contamination, both microbial and particulate, is reduced when trouser suits, close-fitting at the neck, wrists and ankles, are worn. Clean suits should be provided once a day, but fresh headwear, overshoes and powder-free gloves are necessary for each working session.

In aseptic areas, the operative must wear sterile protective headwear totally enclosing hair and beard, full-face goggles, powder-free rubber or plastic gloves (often two pairs are worn), a non-fibre-shedding face mask (to prevent the release of droplets) and footwear. A suitable garment is a one- or two-piece trouser suit. Fresh sterile clothing should be provided each time a person enters an aseptic area.

Cleanroom clothing can reduce shedding of $\geq$0.5-μm-size particles by 50%, with a ninefold reduction of particles $\geq$5.0 μm in size which will lead to a corresponding reduction in microbial release given the proportion of these particles that will be carrying microorganisms. However, to achieve this level of reduction, gowns must be processed, stored and donned/worn correctly. The use of cleanroom clothing alone is not sufficient, however, and operators must also observe appropriate hygiene standards, including defined hand and arm washing procedures, and adopt appropriate working behaviours to control microbial levels.

22.13 Media Simulation Trials

The effectiveness of an aseptic process in preventing contamination of previously sterilised components can be established by simulation. In this approach, microbiological growth medium is substituted for product solution and the numbers of contaminated units which arise when an aseptic process is simulated can be determined following incubation of the medium. The GMP expectation is that no units become contaminated.

Media simulation trials are designed by assessing the key risk factors involved in aseptic processing. Considerations include:

- Identifying and evaluating the steps and interventions that can potentially compromise the sterility of the product.
- Defining possible corrective actions used to mitigate the risks identified above.

- Determining and justifying the 'worst case' scenarios (for instance, extremes of line speed, container size, duration of fill, number and type of interventions) to be used during process simulation.
- Identifying the critical process parameters and thus the most suitable control/monitoring plan and related acceptance criteria.
- Improving the overall process understanding and thus the decision-making process in case of deviations.

At least three consecutive separate successful runs are necessary for initial production line qualification. This is applicable also for revalidation following major changes to the equipment/process/product-contact components, or whenever there are doubts about the ability of the aseptic process to exclude contamination (including extended shutdowns, anomalous trends in environmental monitoring and sterility test failures). For routine re-qualification, one run per line with a semi-annual frequency (twice a year) is the GMP expectation.

Ideally, the most accurate simulation would mimic precisely the commercial production process in terms of batch size and total duration of aseptic operations. In practice, and considering that production batch sizes can easily reach values of several hundreds of thousand units, it is permissible to use other simulation models based on processing time but not necessarily the same number of units, provided that the study design addresses all the potential risks of contamination occurring during commercial production.

As far as the size of run is concerned, the FDA guidance states that 'a generally acceptable starting point for run size is in the range of 5,000 to 10,000 units'; the EU GMP recommendations are similar. In practice, for commercial products with production runs usually much bigger than 10,000 units, it could be difficult to justify that a simulation run smaller than 10,000 units can be considered representative of the actual process. Moreover, the run size must be large enough to allow the simulation of all the manipulations and interventions occurring during the commercial process. The following are examples of risk factors to be considered when establishing the process simulation run size:

- Maximum batch size filled on the line to be validated.
- Type of filling process used (isolator-based, highly automated or manually intensive).
- Overall duration of the commercial filling operation (single shift, multiple shifts or a multiple-day campaign).
- Number of typical and atypical interventions occurring during a filling run.
- Sterile filter qualification (the filling run should not exceed the validated duration of filter use).

For conventional filling lines where contamination originating from personnel is greatest, the risk is usually higher at the end of filling, both due to the potential build-up of environmental bioburden during the operation and to operator fatigue. It is axiomatic, therefore, that operator fatigue should be factored into the study design. Where interventions are performed, each operator needs to qualify in at least one media fill per year practising at least one intervention.

From a practical point of view, the most difficult problem is often how to combine a duration equal or close to the longest commercial process with a media fill run usually much smaller than the actual product batch size. Assuming that the filling line is generally not designed to run much slower than its 'standard' speed (in any case it would not be representative of the actual filling conditions), there are several options for combining a long duration with a small batch size. These include:

- Fill the containers alternately with sterile media and WFI (or just leave units empty instead of filling with WFI). Media fill should then take place at the beginning of the filling operations (immediately after the line set-up), during/after manipulations/interventions and at the end of filling.
- Perform the process simulation at the end of a production run for a defined number of vials, with a new set-up of the line, but without performing any room/line cleaning/sanitisation operation in between and with the same personnel (worst case).
- Perform the process simulation running the line intermittently (for example, 10 minutes every hour up to the total duration of the commercial process), taking care to include operations such as line set-up and all the planned interventions. During the idle time, the personnel remain in the filling suite.
- For filling campaigns, fill the media containers before and after the filling of the maximum number of product (or placebo) batches allowed in the campaign (initial validation) or at the end of a full campaign (periodical revalidation).

When a defined filling duration has been validated by media fill, this time frame should not be exceeded during routine production. Any excursion from the validated filling duration should be exceptional and should be investigated as a deviation, considering especially the number and kind of interventions performed in respect to the ones simulated during the media fill runs. If this situation should arise, the appropriateness of releasing for use those units filled in the time frame exceeding the validated one should be determined by the investigation.

22.14 Quality Risk Management

The application of risk assessment to all stages in the production of a sterile pharmaceutical or medical product is essential. Irrespective of the type of sterile manufacturing process, the primary design objective is to avoid the contamination of the product by microorganisms or microbial by-products (such as endotoxins). There are several ways in which this risk can be minimised, and any such measures require a complete understanding of the most common sources of contamination (see also Chapter 17). These are:

- *Air:* Air is not a natural environment for microbial growth (it is too dry and absent of nutrients), but microorganisms such as *Bacillus*, *Clostridium/Clostridiodes*, *Staphylococcus*, *Penicillium* and *Aspergillus* can survive. To guard against this, products and sterile components must be protected with filtered air supplied at sufficient volume.
- *Facilities:* Inadequately sanitised facilities pose a contamination risk. Furthermore, poorly maintained buildings also present a risk such as potential fungal contamination from damp or inadequate seals. The design of buildings and the disinfection regime are thus of critical importance.
- *Water:* The presence of water in cleanrooms should be avoided except WFI where it is part of the production process. Water, particularly potable or if left standing, can support microbial growth and therefore can become a vector for contamination and a reservoir for pyrogens.
- *Incoming materials:* Incoming materials, either as raw materials (which will contain a level of bioburden) or packaged materials or components, present a contamination risk if they are not properly controlled. Paper and cardboard sources in particular present a potential risk.
- *Personnel:* People are the primary source of contamination within cleanrooms, generating a substantial particulate burden from everyday activities such as breathing, talking and body movements. Many of these particles will be carrying microorganisms.

In the context of cleanroom procedures, risks relate to:

- the concentration, type and source of microorganisms;
- the areas where product is exposed;
- the ease by which microorganisms can be dispersed and the possibility of these entering the product.

These factors should be borne in mind when designing different processes and when selecting appropriate technology.

In terms of formalising the assessment of risks, risk assessment involves identifying risk scenarios. In relation to cleanroom and clean air design for sterile products manufacture, this should ideally be a prospective exercise rather than a reaction to a failure (although much can be learned from documenting and understanding past mistakes). This prospective process involves determining what might go wrong in the system and all the associated consequences and likelihoods. To achieve this, some kind of risk assessment tool is required such as Hazard Analysis and Critical Control Points (HACCP) and Failure Modes and Effects Analysis (FMEA). Both analyse the discrete stages in any process, with the former identifying critical steps and their management and the latter judging levels of acceptable risk. Major GMPs refer to the document 'ICH Q9: Quality Risk Management', for the process of designing, executing documenting and managing risk assessments.

22.15 Environmental Monitoring

Environmental monitoring involves the collection of data relating to the numbers or incidents of microorganisms present on surfaces, in the air and liberated from people, and hence provides important information about the state of the environment within which sterile products are produced. In addition, non-viable particle counting, a physical test, is undertaken in conjunction with viable monitoring because of the relationship between high numbers of airborne particles and microorganisms.

These activities are undertaken using a range of different air and surface counting methods:

- Active air sampling: volumetric air sampler.
- Passive air sampling: microbiological media settle plates from which to culture microorganisms.
- Surface samples: contact (replicate organism detection and counting [RODAC]) plates based on microbiological media and swabs.
- Personnel samples: finger culture plates and gown plates.
- Assessment of airborne particle counts using optical particle counters. A particle counter is a device which draws air in using a pump operating at a controlled flow rate. The air is passed into a sensor area and through a light beam created by a laser diode. The amount of light reflected from each particle is measured electronically (as an electronic pulse). The larger the particle, the larger the amount of reflected light (the greater the amplitude of the light pulse). This allows the particle counter to 'count' the number of particles in a given volume of air (as the number of light pulses) and to assess the size of the particles counted.

There are some emerging rapid microbiological methods, such as spectrophotometric particle counters, which can differentiate between inert and biological particles, although these methods remain in their infancy and it is difficult to correlate readings with microbial numbers.

Environmental monitoring is not the same as environmental control. Environmental control is concerned with the design measures necessary to maintain environments within the required operating parameters. Such parameters include: temperature, relative humidity, air velocity, unidirectional air flow, HEPA filtration and pressure differentials between rooms of different classification. Environmental monitoring does, however, relate to environmental control in that monitoring can indicate a failure of a control and it is sensible, from a risk-based perspective, to target monitoring where control is weakest. This can be particularly useful when monitoring is tied to a specific event during the processing of a sterile product, such as when an intervention is performed in the Grade A/ISO Class 5 area.

In constructing an environmental monitoring programme, it is important to be aware of the limitations of monitoring. The methods deployed, for example, are highly variable in terms of collection efficiency. Furthermore, the culture media selected, and the incubation parameters chosen, will only detect those microorganisms which can grow under the particular set of conditions adopted. The approach taken, therefore, is either to use separate growth media for bacteria and fungi (such as tryptone soya agar and Sabouraud dextrose agar incubated at 30–35 °C and 20–25 °C, respectively) or just one medium which is subject to a dual incubation strategy (typically, tryptone soya agar at 20–25 °C followed by 30–35 °C; where this order of incubation is necessary in order to ensure that fungi are recovered).

A further limitation is the timing of when samples are taken. Monitoring only provides a 'snapshot' of one particular moment in time and this may or may not reflect conditions throughout the process. It follows that individual environmental monitoring results are rarely significant (with the exception of the continual monitoring of aseptic processing batches where some samples can relate to specific events). Thus, the most important aspect of environmental monitoring is the examination of trends over time.

Effective environmental monitoring should be based around a structured environmental monitoring programme (Table 22.4).

For aseptic filling, the regulatory expectation is that monitoring should be continuous. For other cleanrooms outside of the aseptic area, the level of monitoring should be based on the level of risk; for instance, processing areas where there is open product would be monitored more frequently than operations where processing is closed. Although the optimal sites for monitoring should be preselected, this is not always possible. Sometimes what appear to be the most appropriate locations for sampling activities should not be sampled because the very act of sampling could cause contamination (such as with an aseptic filling line). Instead, locations close by should be assessed and post-activity sampling carried out.

Table 22.4 Essential features included in an environmental monitoring programme.

Aspect	Features
Monitoring methods	Selection of method; choice of culture media and incubation conditions; identification of any unique measures required, for example, anaerobic monitoring
Sampling	Determine stages in the operation from where samples are taken; selection and mapping of sampling sites; decide frequency and duration of monitoring; prepare method statements describing how samples are taken and handled, including processing and incubation of samples
Responsibilities	Clear designation of responsibilities, including who takes samples
Analysis	Setting alert and action levels; data analysis, including trending
Investigations	Investigative responses when results exceed action levels; determination of corrective and preventative actions

Some important principles to take into consideration when looking at the elements of the environmental monitoring regime are:

- Monitoring of any type must not subject the product to increased risk of contamination. No monitoring is preferable to monitoring that increases the risk of contamination for sterile materials.
- Environmental monitoring activities must be recognised as interventional activities and are subject to similar constraints and expectations (including detailed procedures) as any other intervention.
- Monitoring must be recognised as being subject to adventitious contamination pre and post sampling that is unrelated to the environment, material or surface being sampled. In advanced aseptic operations, methods to minimise that potential may need to go beyond what are employed in the monitoring of conventional occupied cleanrooms. Given the limitations of environmental monitoring, the act of monitoring should neither be over-emphasised nor should the resulting data be subject to over-interpretation.
- Viable monitoring should not be considered an 'in-process sterility test' regardless of whether the sample is taken in an enclosure or from a so-called 'critical'

product contact surface. Environmental monitoring is not a secondary test for sterility assurance; that is, a role it is scientifically incapable of fulfilling.

- Environmental monitoring results should not be considered as 'proof' of either sterility or non-sterility. The absence or presence of microorganisms in an environmental sample is neither confirmation of asepsis nor is it indicative of process inadequacy.
- It must be recognised that microbial monitoring can never recover all microorganisms present in an environment, nor on a surface. Significant excursions from the routine microbial profile within the enclosure and background environments should be investigated.
- Detection of low numbers of microorganisms in occupied cleanrooms should be considered a rare, but not unusual, event.

22.16 Release of Sterile Products

In order to be able to release sterile medicinal products for use, they are required to be prepared in a manner compliant with sterility assurance at an acceptable level; that is, tested for sterility (some terminally sterilised products can be released parametrically), tested for pyrogenicity and tested for particulates, where applicable.

22.16.1 Assessments of Sterility

Sterility test: The standard means to assess the sterility of medicinal products is the sterility test. Recognising the limitations inherent in this test (see Chapter 21), parametric release is often used instead for medicinal products that can be terminally sterilised. However, for aseptically filled products, the sterility test remains mandatory. This pharmacopoeial test for sterility has been traditionally growth-based (using microbiological culture media), but more recently considerable development effort is being put into rapid sterility test methods which avoid culture; at the time of writing, these are not widespread.

Parametric release: Products that can be terminally sterilised can be subject to parametric release without undertaking finished product sterility testing. The European Organization for Quality defines parametric release as: 'A system of release that gives the assurance that the product is of the intended quality based on information collected during the manufacturing process and on the compliance with specific GMP requirements related to Parametric Release'. Importantly, the manufacturer must demonstrate the capability of the sterilisation agent to penetrate to all relevant parts of the product.

Parametric release assumes that a robust sterility assurance system is in place, consisting of:

- Good product design.
- The manufacturer having knowledge of and control of the microbiological condition of starting materials and process aids (e.g., gases and lubricants).
- Good control of the contamination risks inherent in the process of manufacture in order to avoid the ingress of microorganisms and their multiplication in the product. This is usually accomplished by cleaning and sanitation of product-contact surfaces, prevention of aerial contamination by handling in cleanrooms or in isolators, use of process control time limits and, if applicable, filtration.
- Systems for the prevention of mix-up between sterile and non-sterile product streams.
- Maintenance of product integrity.
- A robust and consistent sterilisation process.
- The totality of a quality system that contains the sterility assurance system, for example, change control, training, written procedures, release checks, planned preventative maintenance, failure mode analysis, prevention of human error, validation and calibration.

22.16.2 Assessments of Pyrogenicity

Pyrogens, such as endotoxin from Gram-negative bacteria, can occur independently of viable microorganisms (see Chapter 3). High levels of endotoxin can be found in pharmaceutical facilities as a result of the use of large volumes of water in processing and production. Pyrogens are a major safety concern in parenterally administered drugs and specific maximum limits apply.

Traditionally, pyrogenicity was assessed using a rabbit pyrogen test. This has been replaced by tests for bacterial endotoxin (where it has been identified that endotoxin is the primary pyrogen of concern) or by a more general test for pyrogens, such as the monocyte activation test (MAT). Endotoxin is assayed using the *Limulus* amoebocyte lysate test (or an equivalent test using a recombinant lysate). This is an established and relatively mature test and one which can be applied to the examination of water and to most types of finished products. The MAT is based on the human fever reaction and thus most closely reflects the human situation. If there is pyrogen contamination, the endogenous pyrogen interleukin-1 is released, which is then determined by enzyme-linked immunosorbent assay (ELISA).

22.16.3 Visible Particulates

Each container of liquid parenteral product is required to be inspected for evidence of visible particles, and any containers which are seen to be contaminated must be rejected. In addition, containers are also examined for cracks, misplaced seals and any other flaws. These are material issues which could compromise the integrity of a container and therefore the sterility of its contents. In large-scale production, these checks are frequently automated, but at smaller scale staff are often tasked with the inspection. These staff must be fully trained to be able to detect different particles (or microbial growth) and will require frequent eye tests.

22.17 Summary

Sterile products are an essential part of modern medicine, and are growing in their variety, complexity and use. They present a high risk in their manufacture and use, mainly because the route of administration circumvents the body's natural defences and the patient may already be in a weakened state. Sterility is therefore essential, but, while an absolute term, it is a condition that is difficult to prove and thus it can only really be understood in terms of risk and probability. Ensuring sterility requires an appreciation of how microorganisms can survive within processing environments; the design of these environments and the adoption of GMPs are fundamental to controlling any contamination risk.

For terminally sterilised products and associated sterilisation processes, the sterility assurance concept is useful. This concept cannot, however, be applied to aseptic filling and instead there is a strong reliance upon environmental controls. Since sterility is a transitory condition, assurances need to extend to the product primary and secondary packaging and the way that product is transported to the patient to ensure the integrity of that condition.

In the end, sterile products are taken by a patient on the basis of trust, trust that the product is of a satisfactory standard, and the onus must rest on the pharmaceutical manufacturer to produce a product worthy of that trust.

Acknowledgements

The contribution of Professor J. L. Ford and colleagues who prepared the chapters on sterile products and good manufacturing practice in previous editions of this book is gratefully acknowledged.

Reference

MHRA (2022). *Rules and Guidance for Pharmaceutical Manufacturers and Distributors, 11 (The Orange Guide).* London: Pharmaceutical Press.

Further Reading

Akers, M.J. (2010). Introduction, scope, and history of sterile products. In: *Sterile Drug Products* (ed. M.J. Akers), 1–5. London: Informa Healthcare.

Agalloco, J. (2007). Steam sterilisation-in-place technology and validation. In: *Validation of Pharmaceutical Processes*, 3e (ed. J.P. Agalloco and F.J. Carleton), 202–221. USA: CRC Press.

Agalloco, J. and Akers, J. (2010). The myth called sterility. *Pharm. Technol.* 34 (3) Supplement: S44–S45.

Agalloco, J. (2011). Process selection for sterile products. In: *Microbiology and Sterility Assurance in Pharmaceuticals and Medical Devices* (ed. M.R. Saghee, T. Sandle and E.C. Tidswell), 603–614. New Delhi: Business Horizons.

Bancroft, R. (2013). Sterility assurance: concepts, methods and problems. In: *Principles and Practice of Disinfection, Preservation and Sterilization*, 5e (ed. A.P. Fraise, J.-Y. Maillard and S.A. Sattar), 408–417. Oxford: Wiley-Blackwell.

De Vecchi, F. (2014). Environmental control systems used in parenteral facilities. In: *Environmental Monitoring: A Comprehensive Handbook*, vol. *1* (ed. J. Moldenhauer), 33–80. USA: PDA / DHI.

EN 17141:2020 (2020). *Cleanrooms and Associated Controlled Environments. Biocontamination Control*. London: BSI.

European Medicines Agency (2009). *Guideline on real time release testing (formerly Guideline on parametric release), EMA/CHMP/QWP/811210/2009-Rev1, 2009*. EMA, Amsterdam.

European Medicines Agency (2015). *Guideline on the Sterilisation of the Medicinal Product, Active Substance, Excipient and Primary Container, EMA/CHMP/CVMP/QWP/850374/2015*. EMA, Amsterdam. https://www.ema.

europa.eu/en/documents/scientificguidelineguideline-sterilisation-medicinal-product-activesubstance- excipient-primary-container_en.pdf

FDA (2004). *Guidance for Industry. Sterile Drug Products Produced by Aseptic Processing – Current Good Manufacturing Practice*. Maryland, USA: US Food and Drug Administration.

ICH (2005) *Q9: Quality risk management. International Conference on Harmonization of Technical Requirements for Registration of Pharmaceuticals for Human Use*. ICH, Geneva.

ISO 14698-1 & 2 (2003). *Part 1 - Cleanrooms and Associated Controlled Environments- Biocontamination Control - General Principles and Methods and Part 2 – Evaluation and Interpretation of Biocontamination Data*. Geneva: ISO.

ISO (2008). *ISO 13408-1 : 2008, Including Amendment 1 : 2013 Aseptic Processing of Health Care Products - Part 1 General Requirements*. Geneva: ISO.

ISO (2015). *ISO 14644-1 : 2015, Cleanrooms and Associated Controlled Environments – Part 1: Classification of Air Cleanliness by Particle Concentration*. Geneva: ISO.

Kaeberlein, T., Lewis, K. and Epstein, S.S. (2002). Isolating 'uncultivable' microorganisms in pure culture in a simulated natural environment. *Science* 296: 1127–1129.

Mehmood, M. (2014). Sterility assurance level and aseptic manufacturing process in pharmaceuticals. *Int. J. Pharm. Res. All Sci.* 3 (4): 10–15.

Mosley, G. (2008). Sterility assurance level (SAL) - the term and its definition continues to cause confusion in the industry. *PMF Newsletter* 14 (5): 3.

PHSS (2014). *Technical Monograph 20 – Bio-Contamination. Bio-Contamination Characterisation, Control, Monitoring and Deviation Management in Controlled/GMP Classified Areas*. Swindon, UK: PHSS.

Prabu, S.L., Suriyaprakash, T.N.K., Ruckmani, K. and Thirumurugan, R. (2017). GMP in pharma manufacturing – description of GMP as related to air-handling units and prevention of contamination and implementation of GMP regulatory requirements. In: *Developments in Surface Contamination and Cleaning: Types of Contamination and Contamination Resources* (ed. R. Kohli and K.L. Mittal), 85–123. USA: Elsevier.

Sandle, T. and Saghee, M.R. (2011). Some considerations for the implementation of disposable technology and single-use systems in biopharmaceuticals. *J. Commer. Biotechnol.* 17 (4): 319–329.

Sandle, T. (2011a). A review of cleanroom microflora: types, trends, and patterns. *PDA J. Pharm. Sci. Technol.* 65 (4): 392–403.

Sandle, T. (2011b). Risk Management in Pharmaceutical Microbiology. In: *Microbiology and Sterility Assurance in Pharmaceuticals and Medical Devices* (ed. M.R. Saghee, T. Sandle and E.C. Tidswell), 553–588. New Delhi: Business Horizons.

Sandle, T. (2012). Environmental monitoring: a practical approach. In: *Environmental Monitoring: A Comprehensive Handbook*, vol. 6 (ed. J. Moldenhauer), 29–54. River Grove, USA: PDA/DHI.

Sandle, T. (2013a). *Sterility Testing of Pharmaceutical Products*, 1–6. River Grove, USA: PDA / DHI.

Sandle, T. (2013b). *Sterility, Sterilisation and Sterility Assurance for Pharmaceuticals: Technology, Validation and Current Regulations*, 1–2. Cambridge, UK: Woodhead Publishing Ltd.

Sandle, T. (2013c). Contamination control risk assessment. In: *Contamination Control in Healthcare Product Manufacturing*, vol. 1 (ed. R.E. Masden and J. Moldenhauer), 423–474. River Grove, USA: DHI Publishing.

Sandle, T. (2014). The risk of *Bacillus cereus* to pharmaceutical manufacturing. *Am. Pharm. Rev.* 17 (6): 1–5.

Tidswell, E. (2011). Sterility. In: *Microbiology and Sterility Assurance in Pharmaceuticals and Medical Devices* (ed. M.R. Saghee, T. Sandle and E.C. Tidswell), 589–602. New Delhi: Business Horizons.

Whitman, W., Coleman, D. and Wiebe, W. (1998). Prokaryotes: the unseen majority. *Proc. Natl. Acad. Sci. U. S. A.* 95 (12): 6578–6583.

WHO (2007). *Quality Assurance of Pharmaceuticals: A Compendium of Guidelines and Related Materials*, 2e, vol. 2. *Good Manufacturing Practices and Inspection*. Geneva: WHO Library.

23

The Manufacture and Quality Control of Immunological Products

Tim Sandle

Head of Compliance and Quality Risk Management, Bio Products Laboratory, Elstree, UK

CONTENTS

Hugo and Russell's Pharmaceutical Microbiology, Ninth Edition. Edited by Brendan F. Gilmore and Stephen P. Denyer.

Companion website: https://www.wiley.com/go/HugoandRussells9e

23.1 Introduction

Immunological products comprise a group of pharmaceutical preparations of varied composition but with a common pharmacological purpose: the modification of the immune status of the recipient, either to provide immunity to infectious disease, or in the case of *in vivo* diagnostics to provoke an indication of immune status usually signifying previous exposure to the sensitising agent. The immunological products that are currently available are of the following types: vaccines; *in vivo* diagnostics; immune sera; human immunoglobulins; monoclonal antibodies; and antibody-targeted therapeutics and diagnostics. For the purpose of this chapter, cell-biology-derived immunomodifiers with a non-specific action, for example, cytokines or chemokines, are not included.

Vaccines are by far the most important immunological products. They have enabled the control or eradication of numerous infectious diseases affecting humans and their domesticated animals. For example, the systematic application of smallpox vaccine, deployed under the aegis of the World Health Organization (WHO), achieved the eradication of one of the most devastating infections (Stewart and Devlin 2006). Similarly, the universal application of poliomyelitis vaccine has brought poliomyelitis to the verge of eradication. Diphtheria, tetanus, pertussis (whooping cough), measles and rubella vaccines have been applied worldwide through national or United Nations International Children's Emergency Fund (UNICEF)-sponsored healthcare programmes and have virtually eliminated these diseases in those countries in which there have been the resources and the will to deploy them effectively. Vaccines that provide protection against many other infections are available for use in appropriate circumstances. Some, such as hepatitis B and conjugate vaccines against *Haemophilus influenzae* type b (Hib), meningococci and pneumococci, have had a huge impact on morbidity and mortality wherever they have been applied (Kayser and Razman 2021).

The range of disorders that may be prevented or treated by vaccines has enlarged considerably beyond infectious diseases. The SARS-CoV-2 global pandemic, which began in 2019 (see Chapter 5), signalled the extent that vaccine technology had advanced with several different forms of vaccine (such as RNA, adenovirus and inactivated virus; Chapter 10) brought to market within 6 months to a year of initial development to provide a level of protection against COVID-19 (Subbarao 2021). Vaccines are currently undergoing evaluation for several other purposes including therapy of cancer (aside from the vaccine against the oncogenic human papillomavirus [HPV]), prevention of allergies, desensitisation of allergic patients, fertility control and treatment of addictions.

In vivo diagnostics such as tuberculins, mallein, histoplasmin, coccidioidin and brucellin are used to demonstrate an immune response, and hence previous exposure, to specific pathogens as an aid to diagnosis. Allergen skin test diagnostics are used to indicate sensitisation to materials of biological origin that may be present in the environment or in specific products. Others, such as the Schick test (diphtheria) toxin, are used to detect the presence of protective immunity. Because of their clinical and pharmaceutical limitations, the trend has been to phase out these preparations, and tuberculins (as purified protein derivative [PPD]) are now by far the most important of this group.

Immune sera, which were once very widely used in the prophylaxis and treatment of many infections, have more limited use today. Vaccines and antibiotics have superseded some and lack of proven therapeutic benefit has caused others to be relegated to immunological history. However, some still play an important role in the management of specific conditions. Thus, diphtheria and botulinum antitoxins prepared in horses remain the only specific treatments for diphtheria and botulism, respectively. Equine tetanus antitoxin is still used as an effective prophylactic in some parts of the world, although largely replaced by human tetanus immunoglobulin in developed countries. Similarly, antivenoms (antivenins) prepared in horses, sheep, goats or other animals against the venom of snakes, spiders, scorpions and marine invertebrates still provide the only effective treatment for venomous bites and stings and are important therapeutic agents in some parts of the world.

Human immunoglobulins have important but limited uses, for example, in the prophylaxis of hepatitis A, hepatitis B, tetanus and varicella-zoster. Additional specific immunoglobulins against diphtheria and botulism toxins are under development and vaccinia immunoglobulin may be reintroduced. Monoclonal antibodies to bacterial endotoxin, to cytokines involved in the pathogenesis of septic shock and to specific infectious agents have been developed and evaluated clinically, but after two decades of research these have yet to enter into general use (Brandenburg et al. 2021). Monoclonal antibodies against specific cell receptors have undergone a rapid development and are employed successfully in cancer therapy and are under development for treatment of autoimmune disease (see Chapter 9). Immune sera and human immunoglobulins depend for their protective effects on their content of antibodies derived, in the case of immune sera, from immunised animals, and, in the case of immunoglobulins, from humans who have been immunised or who have high antibody titres as a consequence of prior infection. The form of immunity conferred is known as passive immunity and is achieved immediately, but is limited in its duration to the time that protective levels of antibodies remain in the circulation (see Chapter 10).

Vaccines achieve their protective effects by stimulating the immune system of the recipient to produce T-cells and/or antibodies that impede the attachment of infectious agents, promote their destruction or neutralise their toxins. This form of protection, known as *active immunity*, develops over the course of days following infection and in the case of many vaccines develops adequately only after two or three doses of vaccine have been given at intervals of days or weeks. Once established, this immunity can last for years, but it may need to be reinforced by booster doses of vaccine given at relatively long intervals. The immunogenicity of some vaccines can be improved by formulating them with *adjuvants*. A heterogeneous group of substances, adjuvants are included in vaccines to improve the immune response and to reduce the number of doses required to achieve a protective effect. Aluminium hydroxide gel (hydrated aluminium oxide) and aluminium phosphate are most generally used in human vaccines; recently, monophosphoryl lipid A and cytosine phosphoguanine have been employed (CDC 2020). A much wider range of substances including oily emulsions, saponin, immune-stimulating complexes (ISCOMs), monophosphoryl lipid A and the 5′-C-phosphate-G-3′ (CpG) motif contained in oligodeoxynucleotide (CpG-ODN) are used in veterinary vaccines.

Different types of infectious agents require preferential mobilisation of different arms of the immune response. For example, toxigenic bacterial infections require the production of toxin-neutralising antibodies, whereas intracellular bacterial infections such as tuberculosis require cell-mediated responses involving mixed T-lymphocytes and activated macrophages; many viral infections will require neutralising antibody and cytotoxic T-cell responses for effective protection. Achieving the appropriate response can be difficult and, in the past, it has had to be approached empirically. This is why most successful viral vaccines have been based on live attenuated strains, which simulate natural infection. Non-living vaccines have been effective against many bacterial infections, but markedly less so against those requiring sustained cell-mediated responses. The development of more selective vaccine adjuvants and delivery systems promises to put the future process of vaccine design on a more rational basis.

A property common to vaccines, immune sera and human immunoglobulins is their high specificity of action. Usually each provides immunity to only one infection, although in some cases cross-protection can occur, for example, bacillus Calmette–Guérin (BCG) protects against the species of bacteria that cause tuberculosis and leprosy. Where it is necessary to protect against more than one type of agent, monospecific preparations can be combined. For example, botulism antitoxin usually covers types A, B and E; meningococcal polysaccharide vaccine may cover groups A, C, W125 and Y; and pneumococcal polysaccharide vaccine usually covers 23 serotypes. Heterologous preparations may also be combined as in measles/mumps/rubella and diphtheria/tetanus/pertussis vaccines. With the increasing number of vaccines for infants and young children, the trend is to produce more complex combinations, such as diphtheria/tetanus/pertussis/hepatitis B/inactivated polio/Hib vaccine, to minimise the number of injections. The possible additive or interactive effects of the various components on the immune system have raised concerns about the safety of such combinations. While some evidence of reduced responses to certain components has been obtained, there is little to support suggestions of serious adverse effects from current combinations.

In addition to the three main types of immunological products that are widely available, more specialised preparations include: synthetic peptide immune response modifiers such as those used to block T-cell responses in multiple sclerosis; monoclonal antibodies for cancer therapy or diagnosis; and hybrid toxins containing a bacterial or plant toxin subunit attached to an antibody or human cell receptor-binding protein, and also intended mainly for cancer therapy. These have rather limited applications and, for the most part, are designed to suppress or exploit the specificity of immune responses rather than to stimulate them.

Principles of immunity are discussed in Chapter 9, and Chapter 10 describes a vaccination and immunisation programme.

23.2 Vaccines

The vaccines currently used for the prevention of infectious diseases of humans are all derived, directly or indirectly, from pathogenic microorganisms. The basis of most vaccine manufacture thus consists of procedures which produce from infectious agents, their components or their products, immunogenic preparations that are devoid of pathogenic properties, but which, nonetheless, can still induce a protective response in their recipients. The methods that are used in vaccine manufacture are constrained by technical limitations, cost, problems of delivery to the recipient/patient, by regulatory issues and, most of all, by the biological properties of the pathogens from which vaccines are derived. Those vaccines currently in use in conventional immunisation programmes are of several readily distinguishable types.

23.2.1 Types of Vaccines

23.2.1.1 Live Vaccines

These are preparations of live bacteria, viruses or other agents which, when administered by an appropriate route, cause subclinical or mild infections. In the course of such an infection, the components of the microorganisms in the vaccine evoke an immune response which provides protection against the more serious natural disease. Live vaccines have a long history, dating from the development of smallpox vaccine. Initially, material from mild cases of smallpox was used for inoculation. This process of 'variolation' was hazardous and could produce fatalities and secondary smallpox cases. A much safer alternative was introduced in 1796 by the Gloucestershire physician Edward Jenner, following observations made by Benjamin Jesty, a local farmer, that an attack of the mild condition known as cowpox (probably a rodent pox) protected milkmaids from smallpox during epidemics of this dreaded disease. For many years, the cowpox vaccine was propagated by serial transfer from person to person and at some point evolved into a distinctive virus, vaccinia, with some features of both cowpox and smallpox viruses but quite probably derived from a now extinct poxvirus. Vaccinia was eventually used to eradicate smallpox. Its significance was that it could stimulate a high degree of immunity to smallpox while producing only a localised infection in the recipient.

The natural occurrence of cross-protective organisms of low pathogenicity seems to be a rare event and attenuated strains have usually had to be selected by laboratory manipulation. Thus, the BCG strain of *Mycobacterium bovis,* used to protect against human tuberculosis caused by the related species *Mycobacterium tuberculosis*, was produced by many sequential subcultures on ox bile medium. This process resulted in deletion of many genes present in virulent *M. bovis*, including some essential for pathogenicity. Similarly, treatment of a virulent strain of *Salmonella enterica* serovar Typhi with nitrosoguanidine, which produced multiple mutations, gave rise to the live attenuated typhoid vaccine strain Ty21A. More recently developed attenuated strains of *S. enterica* serovar Typhi and *Vibrio cholerae* have been selected by directed mutagenesis processes which can produce defined mutations in specific genes.

Perhaps surprisingly, nearly all of the most successful attenuated viral vaccine strains in current use were produced by empirical methods long before the genetic basis of pathogenesis by the specific pathogen was understood. Thus, attenuated strains of polio virus for use as a live, oral vaccine (Sabin) were selected by growth of viruses isolated from human cases under culture conditions that did not permit replication of neuropathogenic virus. Comparable procedures were used to select the attenuated virus strains that are currently used in live measles, mumps, rubella and yellow fever vaccines. A more recent approach has been to use genetic reassortants (from the mixing of genes between two organisms to make a new genetic sequence) to produce live rotavirus vaccines.

Now, attenuated strains of pathogens can be obtained by deliberate selective modification of genes responsible for encoding factors determining pathogenesis, such as toxins or immunomodulators, or metabolites essential for *in vivo* growth. Live vaccine strains can also be genetically modified by incorporating genes that encode protective antigens of other infectious agents (these are sometimes referred to as 'chimeric vaccines'). Few of these vaccines have met regulatory approval (one example is a chimeric antigen receptor [CAR] to treat relapsed non-Hodgkin lymphoma), although there are several under evaluation, for example, for vaccination against malaria, Zika, dengue, and tuberculosis.

23.2.1.2 Inactivated (Killed) Vaccines

Inactivated (or killed) vaccines are suspensions of bacteria, viruses or other pathogenic agents that have been killed/inactivated by heat or by disinfectants such as phenol, ethanol and formaldehyde. Killed microorganisms obviously cannot replicate and cause an infection and so it is necessary for each dose of an inactivated vaccine to contain sufficient antigenic material to stimulate a protective immune response. Inactivated vaccines therefore usually have to be relatively concentrated suspensions. In addition, careful control of the culture conditions and the inactivation process is essential to maintain consistency. Even so, such preparations are often rather poorly protective, possibly because of partial destruction of protective antigens during the killing/inactivation process or inadequate expression of these during *in vitro* culture. At the same time, because they contain all components of the microorganism, they can be somewhat toxic. It is thus often necessary to divide the total amount of vaccine that is needed to induce protection into several doses that are given at intervals of a few days or weeks. Such a course of vaccination takes advantage of the enhanced 'secondary' response that occurs when a vaccine is administered to an individual person whose immune system has been sensitised ('primed') by a previous dose of the same vaccine. The best-known inactivated vaccines are whooping cough (pertussis), typhoid, cholera, plague, inactivated polio vaccine (Salk type) and rabies vaccine. The trend now is for these rather crude preparations to be phased out and replaced by better-defined subunit vaccines containing only relevant protective antigens, for example, acellular pertussis and typhoid Vi polysaccharide vaccines.

23.2.1.3 Toxoid Vaccines

Toxoid vaccines are preparations derived from the toxins that are secreted by certain species of bacteria. In the manufacture of such vaccines, the toxin is separated from the bacteria and treated chemically to eliminate toxicity without eliminating immunogenicity, a process termed 'toxoiding'. Toxoids are often subject to variable composition depending on the detoxifying agent and method used, and on whether these processes are applied before or after purification.

A variety of reagents have been used for toxoiding, but by far the most widely employed and generally successful has been formaldehyde. Under carefully controlled conditions, this reacts preferentially with the amino groups of proteins, although many other functional groups potentially may be affected. Ideally, the toxoided protein will be rendered non-toxic, but will retain its immunogenicity. The treated toxins are sometimes referred to as formol toxoids.

Toxoid vaccines are very effective in the prevention of those diseases such as diphtheria, tetanus, botulism and clostridial infections of farm animals, in which the infecting bacteria produce disease through the toxic effects of secreted proteins which enzymically modify essential cellular components. Many of the clostridial toxins are lytic enzymes with very specific substrates such as neural proteins. Detoxification is also required for the pertussis toxin component of acellular pertussis vaccines.

Anthrax adsorbed vaccine is not toxoided but relies on the use of culture conditions that favour production of the protective antigen (binding and internalisation factor) rather than the lethal factor (protease) and oedema factor (adenyl cyclase) components of the toxin. Selective adsorption to aluminium hydroxide or phosphate also slows release of residual toxin.

23.2.1.4 Bacterial Cell Component Vaccines

Rather than use whole cells, which may contain undesirable and potentially reactogenic components such as lipopolysaccharide endotoxins, a more precise strategy is to prepare vaccines from purified protective components. These are of two main types, proteins and capsular polysaccharides. Often more than one component may be needed to ensure protection against the full range of prevalent serotypes. The potential advantage of such vaccines is that they evoke an immune response only to the component, or components, in the vaccine and thus induce a response that is more specific and effective. At the same time, the amount of unnecessary material in the vaccine is reduced and with it the likelihood of adverse reaction. Vaccines that have been based on one or more capsular polysaccharides include: Hib vaccine; the *Neisseria meningitidis* ACWY vaccines; the 23-valent pneumococcal polysaccharide vaccine; and the typhoid Vi vaccine. These have the disadvantage that they are T-cell-independent antigens and thus do not evoke immunological memory or effective protective responses in the very young. This problem can be overcome by chemically coupling the polysaccharides to T-cell-dependent protein carriers.

The pertussis vaccine is another example where, traditionally, whole bacterial cells have been used, but recent developments have led to an acellular pertussis vaccine that may contain detoxified toxin, either alone or combined with several other bacterial antigens.

23.2.1.5 Conjugate Vaccines

The performance of certain types of antigen that give weak or inappropriate immune responses can often be improved by chemically conjugating them to more immunogenic carriers. Among others, polysaccharide–protein, peptide–protein, protein–protein, lipid–protein and alkaloid–protein conjugate vaccines may be prepared in this way. These have a wide range of applications, including prevention of infection, tumour therapy, fertility control and treatment of addictions. This approach has been very successful against infections caused by bacteria that produce polysaccharide capsules. The latter are T-independent antigens and induce weak responses without immunological memory. They are particularly ineffective in the very young.

23.2.1.6 Viral Subunit Vaccines

Three viral subunit vaccines are widely available, two influenza vaccines and a hepatitis B vaccine. The influenza vaccines are prepared by treating intact influenza virus particles from embryonated hens' eggs infected with influenza virus with a surface-active agent such as a non-ionic detergent. This disrupts the virus particles, releasing the virus subunits. The two types that are required in the vaccine, haemagglutinin and neuraminidase, can be recovered and concentrated by centrifugation methods. The hepatitis B vaccine was, at one time, prepared from hepatitis B surface antigen (HbsAg) obtained from the blood of carriers of hepatitis B virus. This very constrained source of antigen has been replaced by production in yeast or mammalian cells that have been genetically engineered to express HbsAg during fermentation. The HPV vaccines for prevention of genital warts and cervical cancer also contain recombinant viral proteins.

23.2.2 The Seed Lot System

The starting point for the production of all microbial vaccines is the isolation of the appropriate infectious agent. Such isolates have usually been derived from human infections and in some cases have yielded strains suitable for vaccine production very readily; in other instances, however, a great deal of manipulation and selection in the laboratory have been needed before a suitable strain has been obtained. For example, bacterial strains may need to be selected for high toxin yield or production of abundant capsular polysaccharide; viral strains may need to be selected for stable attenuation or good growth in cell cultures.

Once a suitable strain is available, the practice is to grow, often from a single viable unit, a substantial volume of culture which is distributed in small amounts in a large number of ampoules and then stored at −70 °C or below, or freeze-dried. This is the original seed lot. From this seed lot, one or more ampoules are used to generate the working seed from which a limited number of batches of vaccine are generated. These are first examined exhaustively in laboratory and animal tests and then, if found to be satisfactory, tested for safety and efficacy in clinical trials. Satisfactory results in the clinical trials validate the seed lot as the material from which batches of vaccine for routine use can subsequently be produced.

It is important that the full history of the seed is known, including the nature of the culture media used to propagate the strain since isolation. If at all possible, media prepared from animal products should be avoided. If this is not practicable, media components must be from sources certified free of transmissible spongiform encephalopathy (TSE) agents (prions; see Chapter 5).

23.2.3 Production of the Bacteria and the Cellular Components of Bacterial Vaccines

The bacteria and cellular components needed for the manufacture of most bacterial vaccines are prepared in laboratory media by well-established fermentation methods. The end product of the fermentation, the harvest, is processed to provide a concentrated and purified bulk lot of vaccine component that may be conveniently stored for long periods or even sold to other manufacturers prior to further processing. It is important that the materials, equipment, facilities and working practices are of a standard acceptable for the manufacture of pharmaceutical products. The requirements for this are defined as good manufacturing practice (GMP; see Chapter 22).

23.2.4 Fermentation

The production of a bacterial vaccine batch begins with the recovery of the bacterial seed contained in an ampoule of the seed lot stored at −70 °C or below, or freeze-dried. The resuscitated bacteria are first cultivated through one or more passages in preproduction media. Then, when the bacteria have multiplied sufficiently, they are used to inoculate a batch of production medium. Again, all media used must be from sources certified free of TSEs. Wherever possible, medium components of animal origin, especially human and ruminant, should be avoided.

The production medium is usually contained in a large fermenter, the contents of which are continuously stirred. Usually, the pH and the oxidation/reduction potential of the medium are monitored and adjusted throughout the growth period to provide conditions that will ensure the greatest bacterial yield. In the case of rapidly growing bacteria the maximum yield is obtained after about a day, but in the case of bacteria that grow slowly, for example, *M. bovis* BCG, the maximum yield may not be reached before 2 weeks. At the end of the growth period, the contents of the fermenter, which are known as the *harvest*, are ready for the next stage in the production of the vaccine

23.2.4.1 Processing of Bacterial Harvests

The harvest is a very complex mixture of bacterial cells, metabolic products and exhausted medium. In the case of a live attenuated vaccine, it should be innocuous, and all that is necessary is for the bacteria to be separated and resuspended under aseptic conditions in an appropriate diluent, possibly for freeze-drying. In a vaccine made from a virulent strain of pathogen, the harvest may be intensely dangerous and great care is necessary in the subsequent processing. Adequate containment will be required, and for class 3 pathogens such as *S. enterica* serovar Typhi or *Yersinia pestis* or bulk production of bacterial toxins, dedicated facilities that will provide complete protection for the operators and the environment are essential.

- *Inactivation/killing:* This is the process by which heat and disinfectants are used to render the live bacteria in the culture non-viable and harmless. Heat and/or formalin or thiomersal are used to kill the cells of *Bordetella pertussis* used to make whole-cell pertussis vaccines, whereas phenol was used to kill the *V. cholerae* and the *S. enterica* serovar Typhi cells used in the now obsolete whole-cell cholera and typhoid vaccines.
- *Separation:* The process by which the bacterial cells are separated from the culture fluid and soluble products. Centrifugation using either a batch or continuous

flow process, or ultrafiltration, is commonly used. Precipitation of the cells by reducing the pH has been employed as an alternative. In the case of vaccines prepared from cells, the supernatant fluid is discarded, and the cells are resuspended in a saline diluent; where vaccines are made from a constituent of the supernatant fluid, the cells are discarded.

- *Fractionation:* This is the process by which components are extracted from bacterial cells or from the medium in which the bacteria are grown and obtained in a purified form. The polysaccharide antigens of *N. meningitidis* are usually separated from the bacterial cells by treatment with hexadecyltrimethylammonium bromide followed by extraction with calcium chloride and selective precipitation with ethanol. Those of *Streptococcus pneumoniae* are usually extracted with sodium deoxycholate, deproteinised and then fractionally precipitated with ethanol. The purity of an extracted material may be improved by resolubilisation in a suitable solvent and reprecipitation. These procedures are often supplemented with filtration through membranes or ultrafilters with specific molecular size cut-off points. After purification, a component may be freeze-dried, stored indefinitely at low temperature and, as required, incorporated into a vaccine in precisely weighed amounts at the blending stage.
- *Detoxification:* The process by which bacterial toxins are converted to harmless toxoids. Formaldehyde is used to detoxify the toxins of *Corynebacterium diphtheriae*, *Clostridium botulinum* and *Clostridium tetani*. The detoxification may be performed either on the whole culture in the fermenter or on the purified toxin after fractionation. Traditionally, the former approach has been adopted, as it is much safer for the operator. However, the latter gives a purer product. The pertussis toxin used in acellular vaccines may be detoxified with formaldehyde, glutaraldehyde or both, hydrogen peroxide or tetranitromethane. In the case of genetically detoxified pertussis toxin, a treatment with a low concentration of formaldehyde is still performed to stabilise the protein.
- *Further processing:* This may include physical or chemical treatments to modify the product. For example, polysaccharides may be further fractionated to produce material of a narrow molecular size specification. They may then be activated and conjugated to carrier proteins to produce glycoconjugate vaccines. Further purification may be required to eliminate unwanted reactants and by-products. These processes must be done under conditions that minimise extraneous microbial contamination. If sterility is not achievable, then strict bioburden limits are imposed.
- *Adsorption:* This describes the adsorption of the components of a vaccine on to a mineral adjuvant or carrier (aluminium hydroxide or aluminium phosphate; rarely calcium phosphate). Their effect is to increase the immunogenicity and decrease the toxicity, local and systemic, of a vaccine. Diphtheria vaccine, tetanus vaccine, diphtheria/tetanus vaccine and diphtheria/tetanus/pertussis (whole-cell or acellular) vaccine are generally prepared as adsorbed vaccines.
- *Conjugation:* The linking of a vaccine component that induces an inadequate immune response with a vaccine component that induces a good immune response. For example, the immunogenicity for infants of the capsular polysaccharide of *H. influenzae* type b is greatly enhanced by the conjugation of the polysaccharide with diphtheria or tetanus toxoid, or with the outer-membrane protein of *N. meningitidis*. More recently, in attempts to improve efficacy, protein carriers that themselves induce a protective immune response against the pathogen have been conjugated to the capsular polysaccharide, for example, Panton–Valentine leucocidin conjugated to *Staphylococcus aureus* capsular polysaccharide.

23.2.5 Production of the Viruses and the Components of Viral Vaccines

Viruses replicate only in living cells, so the first viral vaccines were necessarily made in animals: smallpox vaccine in the dermis of calves and sheep, and rabies vaccines in the spinal cords of rabbits and brains of mice. Such methods are no longer used in advanced vaccine production; the only intact animal hosts that are still used are embryonated hens' eggs. Almost all the virus that is needed for viral vaccine production is obtained from cell cultures infected with virus of the appropriate strain.

23.2.5.1 Growth of Viruses

Embryonated hens' eggs are still the most convenient hosts for growth of the viruses that are needed for influenza and yellow fever vaccines, although cell-based and synthetic recombinant methods are also employed for influenza vaccine production. Influenza viruses accumulate in high titre in the allantoic fluid of the eggs, and yellow fever virus accumulates in the nervous system of the embryos. A few bacterial vaccines, for example, against rickettsial and chlamydial agents, are also prepared in embryonated eggs. It is important to use eggs from disease-free flocks and emphasis is placed on screening the latter for various avian viruses. The allantoic fluid or embryos must be harvested under conditions that minimise extraneous microbial contamination.

Where cell cultures are used for virus production, they must be of known origin, obtained from validated sources and shown to be free of extraneous agents. The media used in their production should not contain components of human or animal origin, unless the latter are from TSE-free sources.

23.2.5.2 Processing of Viral Harvests

The processing of the virus-containing material from infected embryonated eggs may take one of several forms. In the case of influenza vaccines, the allantoic fluid is centrifuged to provide a concentrated and partially purified suspension of virus. This concentrate is treated with organic solvent or detergent to split the virus into its components when split virion or surface antigen vaccines are prepared. The chick embryos used in the production of yellow fever vaccine are homogenised in sterile water to provide a virus-containing pulp. Centrifugation then precipitates most of the embryonic debris and leaves much of the yellow fever virus in an aqueous suspension. Further purification can then be performed as required.

Cell cultures provide infected fluids that contain little debris and can generally be satisfactorily clarified by filtration. Because most viral vaccines made from cell cultures consist of live attenuated virus, there is no inactivation stage in their manufacture. There are, however, two important exceptions: inactivated poliomyelitis virus vaccine is inactivated with dilute formaldehyde or β-propiolactone and rabies vaccine is inactivated with β-propiolactone. The preparation of these inactivated vaccines also involves a concentration stage – by adsorption and elution of the virus in the case of poliomyelitis vaccine and by ultrafiltration in the case of rabies vaccine. When processing is complete, the bulk materials may be stored until needed for blending into final vaccine. Because of the lability of many viruses, however, it is necessary to store most purified materials at temperatures of −70 °C.

23.2.6 Blending

Blending is the process in which the various components of a vaccine are mixed to form a final bulk. It is undertaken in a large, closed vessel fitted with a stirrer and ports for the addition of constituents and withdrawal of the final blend. When bacterial vaccines are blended, the active constituents usually need to be greatly diluted and the vessel is first charged with the diluents, usually containing a preservative. Thiomersal has been widely used in the past, but is now being phased out and replaced by phenoxyethanol or alternatives. A single-component final bulk is made by adding bacterial suspension, bacterial component or concentrated toxoid in such quantity that it is at the required concentration in the final product. A multiple-component final bulk of a combined vaccine is made by adding each required component in sequence. When viral vaccines are blended, the need to maintain adequate antigenicity or infectivity may preclude dilution, and tissue culture fluids, or concentrates made from them, are often used undiluted or, in the case of multicomponent vaccines, merely diluted one with another. After thorough mixing, a final bulk may be divided into a number of moderate-sized volumes to facilitate handling.

23.2.7 Filling and Drying

As vaccine is required to meet orders, bulk vaccine is distributed into single-dose ampoules or into multidose vials as necessary. Vaccines that are aseptically filled as liquids are sealed and capped in their containers, whereas vaccines that are provided as dried preparations are freeze-dried before sealing.

Single-component bacterial vaccines are listed in Table 23.1. For each vaccine, notes are provided of the basic material from which the vaccine is made, the salient production processes and tests for potency and for safety. The multicomponent vaccines that are made by blending together two or more of the single-component vaccines are required to meet the potency and safety requirements for each of the single components that they contain. The best known of the combined bacterial vaccines is the adsorbed diphtheria, tetanus and pertussis vaccine (DTPer/Vac/Ads) that is used to immunise infants, and the adsorbed diphtheria and tetanus vaccine (DT/Vac/Ads) that is used to reinforce the immunity of school entrants. The trend is to produce increasingly complex combinations, and heptavalent and octavalent preparations are now available.

Single-component viral vaccines are listed in Table 23.2, with notes similar to those provided with the bacterial vaccines. The only combined viral vaccine that is widely used is the measles, mumps and rubella vaccine (MMR Vac). In a sense, however, both the inactivated (Salk) poliovaccine (Pol/Vac [inactivated]) and the live (Sabin) poliovaccine (Pol/Vac [oral]) are combined vaccines in that they are both mixtures of virus of each of the three serotypes of poliovirus. Influenza vaccines, too, are combined vaccines in that they usually contain components from several virus strains, usually from two strains of influenza A and one strain of influenza B.

23.2.8 Quality Control

The quality control of vaccines is intended to provide assurances of both the probable efficacy and the safety of every

Table 23.1 Bacterial vaccines used for the prevention of infectious disease in humans and typical features of their production.

Vaccine	Source material	Processing	Potency assay	Safety tests
Anthrax[a]	Medium from cultures of *Bacillus anthracis*	**1** Separation of cells from medium **2** Filtration of supernatant **3** Adsorption of protective antigen complex to aluminium adjuvant	3 + 3 quantal assay in guinea pigs using challenge with *B. anthracis*	Exclusion of live *B. anthracis* and of anthrax toxins
BCG[b]	Cultures of live BCG cells in liquid or on solid media	**1** Bacteria centrifuged from medium **2** Resuspension in stabiliser solution **3** Freeze-drying	Viable count; induction of sensitivity to tuberculin in guinea pigs	Exclusion of virulent mycobacteria; excessive dermal reactivity Exclusion of extraneous microorganisms
Diphtheria (adsorbed)[b]	Cultures of *C. diphtheriae* in liquid medium	**1** Separation and concentration of toxin **2** Conversion of toxin to toxoid **3** Adsorption of toxoid to adjuvant	3 + 3 quantal assay in guinea pigs using intradermal challenge with diphtheria toxin or serological assay for antitoxin	Inoculation of guinea pigs to exclude untoxoided toxin Toxin assay in Vero cell cultures
Haemophilus influenzae type b conjugate[b]	Cultures of *H. influenzae* type b Protein carrier (tetanus/ diphtheria toxoid, CRM 197)	**1** Separation of capsular polysaccharide **2** Size selection **3** Activation and conjugation with a protein carrier **4** Purification **5** Filtration	Estimation of capsular polysaccharide content and molecular size, free polysaccharide	Absence of unreacted intermediates Endotoxin assay Sterility
Neisseria meningitidis types A, C, W135, Y conjugate[a]	Cultures of *N. meningitidis* of serotypes A, C, W135, Y Carrier protein; tetanus/ diphtheria toxoid, CRM 197	**1** Precipitation with hexadecyltrimethylammonium bromide **2** Solubilisation and purification **3** Size selection **4** Activation and conjugation **5** Purification **6** Blending **7** Freeze-drying	Estimation of capsular polysaccharide content and molecular size, free polysaccharide	Absence of unreacted intermediates Endotoxin assay Sterility
Pneumococcal polysaccharide conjugate[b]	Cultures of selected serotypes of *S. pneumoniae* Carrier protein; tetanus toxoid, CRM 197, *H. influenzae* OMP	**1** Precipitation of extracted polysaccharides with ethanol **2** Size restriction **3** Activation and conjugation to carrier protein **4** Purification **5** Blending **6** Filtration	Physicochemical/immunoassay of polysaccharides, molecular size distribution, free saccharide	Absence of unreacted intermediates Absence of pyrogens Sterility

Tetanus (adsorbed)[b]	Cultures of *C. tetani* in liquid medium	**1** Conversion of toxin to toxoid **2** Separation and purification of toxoid **3** Adsorption to adjuvant	3 + 3 quantal assay in mice using subcutaneous challenge with tetanus toxin or measurement of serological response	Inoculation of guinea-pigs to exclude presence of untoxoided toxin Sterility
Typhoid Vi capsular polysaccharide antigen[a]	Cultures of *S. typhi* grown in liquid medium	Extraction of capsular antigen	Estimation of capsular antigen and molecular size	Endotoxin assay Sterility
Typhoid live vaccine[a]	Cultures of *S. typhi* strain Ty21A	Encapsulation	Estimation of content of live bacteria	Absence of live enteric pathogens
Whooping cough (pertussis) whole cell[b]	Cultures of *B. pertussis* grown in liquid or on solid media	**1** Harvest **2** Killing with heat, thiomersal or formalin **3** Resuspension **4** Blending **5** Adsorption	3 + 3 quantal assay in mice using intracerebral challenge with live *B. pertussis*	Estimation of bacteria to limit content to 20×10^9 per human dose Weight gain test in mice to exclude excess toxicity Pertussis toxin assay Endotoxin assay Sterility
Whooping cough (pertussis) (acellular)[b]	Cultures of *B. pertussis*	**1** Harvest **2** Extraction, detoxification and blending of cell components (pertussis toxin, filamentous haemagglutinin, pertactin, fimbriae) **3** Adsorption to adjuvant	Immunogenicity assay (product specific) or modified quantal assay using intracerebral challenge with live *B. pertussis*	Specific toxin and endotoxin assays Sterility

Diphtheria and pertussis vaccines are seldom used as single-component vaccines but as components of diphtheria/tetanus vaccines and diphtheria/tetanus/pertussis vaccines. Combined diphtheria/tetanus/pertussis/Hib and diphtheria/tetanus/pertussis/Hep B vaccines with or without inactivated polio vaccine are available.
Bacterial vaccines of restricted availability include anthrax, botulism, cholera, plague, Q fever, typhus and tularaemia vaccines.
[a] Vaccines used to provide additional protection when circumstances indicate a need.
[b] Vaccines used in conventional immunisation schedules.

Table 23.2 Viral vaccines used for the prevention of infectious diseases in humans and typical features of their production.

Vaccine	Source material	Processing	Potency assay	Safety tests
Hepatitis A[a]	Human diploid cells infected with hepatitis A virus	**1** Separation of virus from cells **2** Inactivation with formaldehyde **3** Adsorption to aluminium hydroxide gel	Assay of antigen content by ELISA	Inoculation of cell cultures to exclude presence of live virus
Hepatitis B[a]	Yeast cells genetically modified to express surface antigen	**1** Separation of HbsAg from yeast cells **2** Adsorption to aluminium hydroxide gel	Immunogenicity assay or HbsAg assay by ELISA	Test for presence of yeast DNA
Influenza (split virion)[a]	Allantoic fluid from embryonated hens' eggs infected with influenza viruses A and B	**1** Harvest of viruses **2** Disruption with surface-active agent or solvent **3** Blending of components of different serotypes	Assay of haemagglutinin content by single radial diffusion	Inoculation of embryonated hens' eggs to exclude live virus
Influenza (surface antigen)[a]	Allantoic fluid from embryonated hens' eggs infected with influenza viruses A and B	**1** Inactivation and disruption **2** Separation of haemagglutinin and neuraminidase **3** Blending of haemagglutinins and neuraminidase of different serotypes	Assay of haemagglutinin content by single radial diffusion	Inoculation of embryonated hens' eggs to exclude live virus
Measles[b]	Chick embryo cell cultures infected with attenuated measles virus	**1** Clarification **2** Freeze-drying	Infectivity titration in cell cultures	Tests to exclude presence of extraneous viruses
Mumps[b]	Chick embryo cell cultures infected with attenuated mumps virus	**1** Clarification **2** Freeze-drying	Infectivity titration in cell cultures	Tests to exclude presence of extraneous viruses
Poliomyelitis (inactivated)	Human diploid cell cultures infected with each of the three serotypes of poliovirus	**1** Clarification **2** Inactivation with formaldehyde **3** Concentration **4** Blending of virus of each serotype	Estimation of D antigen content	Inoculation of cell cultures and monkey or transgenic mouse spinal cords to exclude live virus
Poliomyelitis (live or oral)[b] (Sabin type)	Cell cultures infected with attenuated poliovirus of each of the three serotypes	**1** Clarification **2** Blending with β-propiolactone	Infectivity titration in cell cultures	Neurovirulence test in monkeys or transgenic mice
Rubella[b] (German measles)	Human diploid cell cultures infected with rabies virus	**1** Clarification **2** Blending with stabiliser **3** Freeze-drying	Infectivity titration in cell cultures	Tests to exclude presence of extraneous viruses
Varicella[a]	Human diploid cell cultures infected with attenuated varicella virus	**1** Clarification **2** Freeze-drying	Infectivity titration in cell cultures	Tests to exclude presence of extraneous viruses
Yellow fever[a]	Aqueous homogenate of chick embryos infected with attenuated yellow fever virus 17D	**1** Centrifugation to remove cell debris **2** Freeze-drying	Infectivity titration in cell cultures by plaque assay	Tests to exclude extraneous viruses

Viral vaccines of restricted application include Congo–Crimean haemorrhagic fever vaccine (for which there is no approved vaccine), dengue fever vaccine, Japanese encephalitis B vaccine, rabies vaccine, smallpox vaccine, tick-borne encephalitis vaccine and Venezuelan equine encephalitis vaccine.

ELISA, enzyme-linked immunosorbent assay.

[a] Vaccines used to provide additional protection when circumstances indicate a need.

[b] Vaccines used in conventional immunisation programmes. Measles, mumps and rubella vaccines are generally administered in the form of a combined measles/mumps/rubella vaccine (MMR vaccine).

batch of every product. It is achieved in three ways: (i) in-process control; (ii) final product control and (iii) requirements that for each product the starting materials, intermediates, final product and processing methods are consistent.

The results of all quality control tests must be recorded in detail and authorised by a qualified person, as, in those countries in which the manufacture of vaccines is regulated by law, they are part of the evidence on which control authorities judge the acceptability or otherwise of each batch of each preparation.

23.2.8.1 In-process Control

In-process quality control is the control exercised over starting materials and intermediates. Its importance stems from the opportunities that it provides for the examination of a product at the stages in its manufacture at which testing is most likely to provide the most meaningful information. Regulatory agencies stipulate many in-process controls supplemented by end-product testing. Numerous examples of in-process control exist for various types of vaccine, but three demonstrate the principle.

The quality control of both diphtheria and tetanus vaccines requires that the products are tested for the presence of free toxin, that is, for specific toxicity due to inadequate detoxification with formaldehyde, at the final product stage. By this stage, however, the toxoid concentrates used in the preparation of the vaccines have been much diluted and, as the volume of vaccine that can be inoculated into the test animals (guinea pigs) is limited, the tests are relatively insensitive. In-process control, however, provides for tests on the undiluted concentrates and thus increases the sensitivity of the method at least 100-fold.

An example from virus vaccine manufacture is the titration, prior to inactivation, of the infectivity of the pools of live poliovirus used to make inactivated poliomyelitis vaccine. Adequate infectivity of the virus from the tissue cultures is an indicator of the adequate virus content of the starting material and, as infectivity is destroyed in the inactivation process, there is no possibility of performing such an assay after formaldehyde treatment.

A more general example from virus vaccine production is the rigorous examination of tissue cultures to exclude contamination with infectious agents from the source animal or, in the cases of human diploid cells or cells from continuous cell lines, to detect cells with abnormal characteristics. Monkey kidney cell cultures are tested for simian herpes B virus, simian virus 40, mycoplasma and tubercle bacilli. Cultures of human diploid cells and continuous line cells are subjected to detailed karyological examination (examination of chromosomes by microscopy) to ensure that the cells have not undergone any changes likely to impair the quality of a vaccine or lead to adverse effects.

23.2.8.2 Final Product Control

Assays

Vaccines containing inactivated microorganisms or their by-products are generally tested for potency in assays in which the amount of the vaccine that is required to protect animals from a defined challenge dose of the appropriate pathogen, or its product, is compared with the amount of a standard vaccine that is required to provide the same protection. The usual format of the test is the 3 + 3 dose quantal assay that is used to estimate the potency of whole-cell pertussis vaccine (British Pharmacopoeia 2020). Three logarithmic serial doses of the test vaccine and 3 of the standard vaccine are made and each is used to inoculate a group of 16 mice. In the case of both the test vaccine and the standard, the middle dose is chosen on the basis of experience, so that it is sufficient to induce a protective response in about 50% of the animals to which it is given. Each lower dose may then be expected to protect less than 50% of the mice to which it is given and each higher dose to protect more than 50% of the animals. Fourteen days later all of the mice are inoculated ('challenged') with a suitable virulent *B. pertussis* strain and, after a further 14 days, the number of mice surviving in each of the 6 groups is counted. The number of survivors in each group is used to calculate the potency of the test vaccine relative to the potency of the standard vaccine by the statistical method of probit analysis (Finney 1971; as used for analysing the relationship between a stimulus (dose) and the quantal (all or nothing) response). The potency of the test vaccine may be expressed as a percentage of the potency of the standard vaccine. However, as the standard vaccine will have an assigned potency in international units (IU), it is more usual to express the potency of the test vaccine in similar units. Tests similar to that used to estimate the potency of pertussis vaccine are prescribed for the potency determinations of diphtheria vaccine and tetanus vaccines. In these cases, the respective bacterial toxins are used as the challenge material (British Pharmacopoeia 2020). Tests that do not involve challenge but involve titration of the antitoxin response *in vitro*, for example, by enzyme-linked immunosorbent assay (ELISA), are now being adopted.

Vaccines containing live microorganisms are generally tested for potency by determining their content of viable particles. In the case of the most widely used live bacterial vaccine, BCG vaccine, dilutions of vaccine are prepared in a medium which inhibits clumping of cells, and fixed volumes are dropped on to solid media capable of supporting mycobacterial growth. After a fortnight, the colonies generated by the drops are counted and the live count of the undiluted vaccine is calculated. The potency of live viral vaccines is estimated in much the same way except that a substrate of living cells is used. Dilutions of vaccine are inoculated on to tissue culture monolayers in Petri dishes or in plastic trays, and the infective particle count of the vaccine is calculated from the infectivity of the dilutions as indicated by plaque formation, cytopathic effect, haemadsorption or other effect and the dilution factor involved.

Safety Tests

Because many vaccines are derived from basic materials of intense pathogenicity – the lethal dose of tetanus toxin for a mouse is estimated to be 3×10^{-2} ng, for instance – safety testing is of paramount importance. Effective testing provides a guarantee of the safety of each batch of every product and most vaccines in the final container must pass one or more safety tests as prescribed in a pharmacopoeial monograph. This generality does not absolve a manufacturer from the need to perform in-process tests as required, but it is relaxed for those preparations that have a final formulation that makes safety tests on the final product either impractical or meaningless.

Bacterial vaccines are regulated by relatively simple safety tests. Those vaccines composed of killed bacteria or bacterial products must be shown to be completely free from the living microorganisms used in the production process. Inoculation of appropriate bacteriological media with the final product provides an assurance that all organisms have been killed. Those vaccines prepared from toxins, for example, diphtheria and tetanus toxoids, require in addition a test system capable of revealing inadequately detoxified toxins; this can be done by inoculation of guinea pigs, which are exquisitely sensitive to both diphtheria and tetanus toxins. A test for sensitisation of mice to the lethal effects of histamine is used to detect active pertussis toxin in pertussis vaccines. An improved non-lethal method is also available. The trend is to replace *in vivo* assays by cell culture methods where possible, but these do not always emulate *in vivo* effects. Inoculation of guinea pigs is also used to exclude the presence of abnormally virulent organisms in BCG vaccine. Molecular genetic methods, such as nucleic acid amplification to probe for genes specific to virulent strains, can assist with vaccine development and quality control. Viral vaccines can present problems of safety testing far more complex than those experienced with most bacterial vaccines. With inactivated viral vaccines, the potential hazards are those due to incomplete virus inactivation and the consequent presence of residual live virus in the preparation. The tests used to detect such live virus consist of the inoculation of susceptible tissue cultures and of susceptible animals. The cultures are examined for cytopathic effects, and the animals for symptoms of disease and histological evidence of infection at autopsy. This test is of particular importance in inactivated poliomyelitis vaccines, the vaccine being injected intraspinally into monkeys or mice transgenic for the poliovirus receptor. At autopsy, sections of brain and spinal cord are examined microscopically for any histological lesions that are indicative of proliferating poliovirus.

With attenuated viral vaccines, the potential hazards are those associated with reversion of the virus during production to a degree of virulence capable of causing disease in recipients. To a large extent, this possibility is controlled by very careful selection of a stable seed but, especially with live attenuated poliomyelitis vaccine, it is usual to compare the neurovirulence of the vaccine with that of a vaccine known to be safe in field use. The technique involves the intraspinal inoculation of monkeys with both the reference vaccine and the test vaccine followed by comparison of the neurological lesions and symptoms, if any, that are caused. If the vaccine causes abnormalities in excess of those caused by the reference, it fails the test. A modification of this test which uses transgenic mice instead of monkeys is now available. An *in vitro* method (mutational analysis by polymerase chain reaction and restriction enzyme cleavage [MAPREC] test) which relies on detecting RNA sequences specific to virulent virus has also been developed. A widespread problem with safety testing of live viral vaccines is that the host specificity of many viruses limits the availability of suitable animal models.

Tests of General Application

In addition to the tests designed to estimate the potency and to exclude the hazards peculiar to each vaccine, there are a number of tests of more general application. These relatively simple tests are as follows.

- *Sterility:* In general, vaccines are required to be sterile. The exceptions to this requirement are smallpox vaccine made from the dermis of animals and bacterial vaccines such as BCG, Ty21A and tularaemia vaccine, which consist of living but attenuated strains. These have a bioburden limit which defines the number of permissible microorganisms but excludes pathogens. WHO recommendations and pharmacopoeial monographs stipulate, for vaccine batches of different size, the numbers of containers that must be tested and found to be sterile. The preferred method of sterility testing is membrane filtration, as this technique permits the testing of large volumes without dilution of the test media. The test system must be capable of detecting aerobic and anaerobic bacteria and fungi (see Chapter 21).

- *Freedom from abnormal or general toxicity:* The purpose of this simple test is to exclude the presence in a final container of a highly toxic contaminant. Five mice of 17–22 g and two guinea pigs of 250–350 g are inoculated with one human dose or 1.0 ml, whichever is less, of the test preparation. All must survive for 7 days without signs of illness. Current pharmacopoeial monographs usually no longer require this test if another *in vivo* test has been performed on the product; it ceased to be used within the European Union from 2020.
- *Pyrogenicity or endotoxin content:* The type of pyrogen test required is dependent upon the regulatory agency. Where the risk is primarily bacterial endotoxin, either the Limulus amoebocyte lysate (LAL) test or an alternative endotoxin method is used. LAL uses *Limulus polyphemus* amoebocyte lysate or a recombinant equivalent. Where a more general test for pyrogens is required, the traditional method was the rabbit test. In many regions, including the European Union, the rabbit test has been replaced by the monocyte activation test (see Chapter 22).
- *Presence of aluminium and calcium:* The quantity of aluminium in vaccines containing aluminium hydroxide or aluminium phosphate as an adjuvant is limited to 1.25 mg per dose and it is usually estimated complexometrically. The quantity of calcium is limited to 1.3 mg per dose and is usually estimated by atomic absorption spectrometry.
- *Free formaldehyde:* Inactivation of bacterial toxins with formaldehyde may lead to the presence of small amounts of free formaldehyde in the final product. The concentration, as estimated by colour development with acetylacetone, must not exceed 0.02%.
- *Phenol concentration:* When phenol is used to preserve a vaccine, its concentration must not exceed 0.25% w/v or, in the case of some vaccines, 0.5% w/v. Phenol is usually estimated by the colour reaction with aminophenazone and hexacyanoferrate.
- *pH:* The potentiometric determination of pH is made by measuring the potential difference between two appropriate electrodes immersed in the solution to be examined: one of these electrodes is sensitive to hydrogen ions and the other is the reference electrode. The pH apparatus is calibrated with the buffer solution of potassium hydrogen phthalate and one other buffer solution of different pH. The pH in the test sample should comply with the limits approved for the particular products.
- *Osmolality:* Osmolality is a practical means of giving an overall measure of the contribution of the various solutes present in a solution to the osmotic pressure of the solution. Osmolality is determined by measurement of the depression of freezing point of the test sample using appropriate apparatus. The osmolality of the test sample should comply with the limits approved for the particular products, for example, a minimum of 240 mOsmol/kg.

23.2.8.3 Newer Vaccine Developments

The previous sections have largely been a description of long-established quality-assurance processes for mature vaccine technologies. Advances in molecular biology have now widened the options in vaccine design, however, and these include DNA, mRNA, viral vector and recombinant protein vaccine platforms (see Chapter 10).

Developments in these areas have been accelerated by recent infectious threats, for example, Ebola, but particularly by the COVID-19 pandemic, which has required emergency-use approval by regulators with very short timescales to production and distribution. These newer technologies require additional or alternative approaches to quality control and evaluation, and a consensus on these methods has yet to appear (World Health Organization 2020; Knezevic et al. 2021). By way of example, however, Table 23.3 identifies some of the key elements associated with mRNA vaccine quality assurance.

Table 23.3 Major quality control considerations for mRNA vaccines.

Vaccine component	Key considerations of quality
Raw nucleic acid material	Quality of the transcription enzymes, nucleotides and linear DNA templates used in production of the mRNA
mRNA drug substance	mRNA antigen coding sequence identification; any additional protein coding sequences; purity, with sequence lengths being a critical parameter; percentage 5′ capped and polyadenylated
Nanoparticle delivery system	Purity of lipid; amount of RNA encapsulated; size distribution of particles; surface charge; stability
Final product	Identity; stability, particularly thermal stability; potency *in vitro* and *in vivo*; endotoxin levels; sterility; abnormal toxicity; process-related impurities

23.3 *In Vivo* Diagnostics

23.3.1 Preparation

The most widely used of these are the tuberculins employed to detect sensitisation by mycobacterial proteins and hence the possible presence of infection. These are prepared by growing approved strains of *M. tuberculosis* (or *M. bovis* or *Mycobacterium avium* in preparations intended for veterinary use) in a protein-free medium for several weeks. The culture is then steamed for a prolonged period to kill surviving bacteria and to facilitate release of tuberculoproteins from the cells. The culture supernatant is recovered by centrifugation and further concentrated by evaporation and sterile filtered to make a product known as 'old tuberculin'. The crude material may then be standardised against a reference preparation by titration in the skin of guinea pigs sensitised to *M. tuberculosis*. In practice, further purification is usually performed by precipitation with trichloroacetic acid or other protein precipitant to produce PPD, which is standardised by *in vivo* assay. Concentrated preparations containing 100,000 IU/ml are used to formulate working strengths such as 1000, 100 and 10 IU/ml. These have to be diluted in a medium containing a Tween surfactant to reduce adsorption to glass. The concentrated material can be used for intradermal testing by a multineedle device such as in the Heaf or Tine tuberculin skin test methods.

23.3.2 Quality Control

Apart from standardisation of potency, which also serves as an identity test, the tuberculin material must be checked for sterility and for the absence of viable mycobacteria. Because of their slow growth, the latter may not be detected by conventional sterility tests and it is usual to perform check tests by guinea-pig inoculation, or by prolonged culture on Lowenstein–Jensen medium. The product is also checked for absence of reactogenicity in unsensitised guinea pigs and if required by the regulatory authority, for abnormal toxicity.

Analogous intradermal test reagents such as mallein, histoplasmin and coccidioidin, are produced by similar methods. Their use has declined, however, as they, like the tuberculin test, detect previous exposure and sensitisation to the antigens of the agent but not necessarily active infection.

23.4 Immune Sera

23.4.1 Preparation

Immune sera are preparations derived from the blood of animals, usually horses, but mules, donkeys, sheep or goats are also used. The animals must be in good health, free of infections and obtained from sources free of transmissible spongiform encephalopathies, and kept under veterinary supervision. To prepare an immune serum, horses or other animals are injected with a sequence of spaced doses of an antigen until a trial blood sample shows that the injections have induced a high titre of antibody to the injected antigen. An adjuvant may be used if required. A large volume of blood is then removed by venepuncture and collected into a vessel containing sufficient citrate solution to prevent clotting. The blood cells are allowed to settle, and the supernatant plasma is drawn off. Alternatively, the blood can be mechanically defibrinated. The crude plasma can be sterilised by filtration and dispensed for use, but it is preferable to fractionate it to separate the immune globulin. This is done by fractional precipitation of the plasma by the addition of ammonium sulphate. The globulin fraction is recovered and treated with pepsin to yield a refined immune product containing the Fab fragment. This refined globulin contains no more than a trace of the albumin and other proteins that were present in the plasma. It is less antigenic, has a longer half-life in the circulation and is less likely to provoke anaphylaxis or serum sickness than whole serum or crude globulin. The antibody content of the refined product is determined by specific assay; the product is diluted to the required concentration and transferred into ampoules. Two or more monovalent immune sera may be blended together to provide a multivalent immune serum.

23.4.2 Quality Control

The quality of immune sera is controlled by potency tests and by conventional tests for safety and sterility. The potency tests have a common design in that, in the case of all immune sera, the potency is estimated by comparing the amount of the product that is required to neutralise an effect of a homologous toxin with the amount of a standard preparation that is required to achieve the same effect. Serial dilutions of the immune serum and of a standard preparation are made and to each is added a constant amount of the homologous antigen. Each mixture is then inoculated into a group of animals, usually guinea pigs or mice, and the dilutions of the immune serum and of the standard, which neutralise the effects of toxin, are noted. As the potencies of the standard preparations are expressed in IU, the potencies of the immune sera are determined in corresponding units per millilitre (British Pharmacopoeia 2020). The quality of globulin fractions is usually monitored by gel electrophoresis to detect contaminating proteins and uncleaved immunoglobulin, and by size-exclusion high-performance liquid

Table 23.4 Immune sera used in the prevention or treatment of infections in humans.

Immunoserum	Potency assay method	Potency requirement
Botulinum antitoxin	Neutralisation of the lethal effects of botulinum toxins A, B and E in mice. Similar assays can also be used to titrate the activity of monoclonal antibodies which can include activity against types A–G	500 IU ml^{-1} type A 500 IU ml^{-1} type B 50 IU ml^{-1} type E
Diphtheria antitoxin	Neutralisation of the erythrogenic effect of diphtheria toxin in the skin of guinea pigs The activity of the sera can also be titrated by ELISA or by neutralisation of toxin activity in Vero cell cultures	1000 IU ml^{-1} if prepared in other species
Tetanus antitoxin	Neutralisation of the paralytic effect of tetanus toxin in mice The antitoxin activity can also be titrated by ELISA	1000 IU ml^{-1} for prophylaxis 3000 IU ml^{-1} for treatment

In each of the assays of potency, the amount of the immune serum and the amount of a corresponding standard antitoxin that are required to neutralise the effects of a defined dose of the corresponding toxin are determined. The two determined amounts and the assigned unitage of the standard antitoxin are then used to calculate the potency of the immune serum in international units (IU).

chromatography to detect aggregates and small fragments. The immune sera are also tested for contaminating viruses by inoculation on to cell cultures capable of detecting a wide range of viruses relevant to the particular product.

Table 23.4 lists the immune sera for which there is currently a demand, or a potential need, and indicates their required potencies and the salient features of the potency assay methods.

23.5 Human Immunoglobulins

23.5.1 Source Material

Human immunoglobulins are preparations of the immunoglobulins, principally immunoglobulin G (IgG) subclasses, that are present in human blood. They are derived from the plasma of donated blood and from plasma obtained by plasmapheresis. Normal immunoglobulin, that is immunoglobulin that has relatively low titres of antibodies representative of those present in the population at large, is prepared from pools of plasma obtained from not fewer than 1000 individuals. Specific immunoglobulins, that is immunoglobulins with a high titre of a particular antibody, are usually prepared from smaller pools of plasma obtained from individuals who have suffered recent infections or who have undergone recent immunisation and who thus have a high titre of a particular antibody. Each contribution of plasma to a pool is tested for the presence of hepatitis B surface antigen (HBsAg), for antibodies to HIV 1 and 2 and for antibodies to hepatitis C virus in order to identify, and to exclude from a pool, any plasma capable of transmitting infection from donor to recipient. The solvent detergent process, one of the methods used to inactivate enveloped viruses, uses treatment with a combination of tributyl phosphate and octoxinol 10; these reagents are subsequently removed by oil extraction or by solid phase extraction (Zuercher et al. 2019).

23.5.2 Fractionation

The immunoglobulins are obtained from the plasma pools by fractionation methods that are based on ethanol precipitation in the cold with rigorous control of protein concentration, pH and ionic strength. Some of the fractionation steps may contribute to the safety of immunoglobulins by inactivating or removing contaminating viruses that have not been detected by tests on the blood donations. Additional viral inactivation steps are in place, such as nanofiltration. The immunoglobulins may be presented either as a freeze-dried or a liquid preparation at a concentration that is at least 10 times that in the initial pooled plasma. Glycine may be added as a stabiliser. Multidose preparations contain an antimicrobial preservative, but single-dose preparations do not (Zuercher et al. 2019).

23.5.3 Quality Control

The quality control of immunoglobulins includes potency tests and conventional tests for safety, endotoxin and sterility. The potency tests consist of toxin or virus neutralisation tests that parallel those used for the potency assay of immune sera, except that for in-process control of some immunoglobulins wider use is made of *in vitro* assays. In addition to the safety and sterility tests, total protein is determined by nitrogen estimations, the protein composition by sodium dodecyl sulphate (SDS)–polyacrylamide gel electrophoresis (PAGE) and molecular size by

Table 23.5 Immunoglobulins used in the prevention and treatment of infections in humans.

Immunoglobulins	Potency assay method	Potency requirement
Normal	Neutralisation tests in cell cultures or in animals, or *in vitro* ELISA estimations	Measurable amounts of one bacterial antibody and of one viral antibody for which there are international standards
Hepatitis B	Radioimmunoassay or enzyme immunoassay	Not less than 100 IU ml^{-1}
Measles	Neutralisation of the infectivity of measles virus for cell cultures	Not less than 50 IU ml^{-1}
Rabies	Neutralisation of the infectivity of rabies virus for mice	Not less than 150 IU ml^{-1}
Tetanus	Neutralisation of the paralytic effect of tetanus toxin in mice ELISA estimation of antitoxin	Not less than 50 IU ml^{-1}
Varicella-zoster	ELISA in parallel with a standard varicella-zoster immunoglobulin	Not less than 100 IU ml^{-1}

In each of the assays of potency, the amount of the immunoglobulin and the amount of a corresponding standard preparation that are required to neutralise the infectivity or other biological activity of a defined amount of virus or to neutralise a defined amount of a bacterial toxin are determined. The two determined amounts and the assigned unitage of the standard preparation are then used to calculate the potency of the immunoglobulins in international units (IU). ELISA, enzyme-linked immunosorbent assay.

high-performance liquid chromatography. The presence of immunoglobulins derived from species other than humans is excluded by precipitin tests. Table 23.5 lists six human immunoglobulins and their requisite potencies and indicates the methods by which the potencies are determined.

23.6 Monoclonal Antibodies

23.6.1 Preparation

Monoclonal antibodies are immunoglobulins or a fragment of an immunoglobulin, with defined specificity, produced by a single clone of cells (see Chapter 9). They can be obtained from immortalised B-lymphocytes that are cloned and expanded as continuous cell lines (murine and human monoclonal antibodies) or from rDNA-engineered mammalian or bacterial cell lines (engineered monoclonal antibodies). Production of monoclonal antibodies is based on a seed lot system using a master cell bank and a working cell bank derived from the cloned cells. Two approaches are currently in use: single harvest (production at finite passage level) and multiple harvest (continuous-culture production). In the first method, the cells are cultivated up to a defined maximum number of passages or population doublings (in accordance with the stability of the cell line). In the second method, cells are continuously cultivated for a defined period (in accordance with the stability of the system and production consistency). In this case, monitoring is necessary throughout the life of the culture; the required frequency and type of monitoring will depend on the nature of the production system. Bulk harvests can be made by pooling individual harvests before purification. The purification process to remove unwanted host-cell-derived proteins, nucleic acids and carbohydrates is also designed to remove and/or inactivate non-enveloped and enveloped viruses and other impurities.

23.6.2 Quality Control

The quality of therapeutic monoclonal antibodies is controlled by rigorous characterisation of the products using chemical and biological methods. The final product should be tested for bioburden (including screening for mycoplasmas) and bacterial endotoxins, with purity, integrity and potency assessed by suitable analytical methods and compared to a reference preparation. Similarly, the identity test can be done by suitable methods comparing the product with the reference preparation. Molecular size distribution can be determined by size-exclusion chromatography. Depending on the nature of the monoclonal antibody, its microheterogeneity and isoforms, a number of different tests can be used to demonstrate molecular identity and structural integrity. These tests may include peptide mapping, isoelectric focusing, ion exchange chromatography, hydrophobic interaction chromatography, oligosaccharide mapping, monosaccharide content and mass spectrometry. The purity can be examined by SDS–polyacrylamide gel electrophoresis under reducing and non-reducing conditions or capillary electrophoresis. For monoclonal antibodies with specific antimicrobial activity, an appropriate assay is performed to determine the level of this activity. Monoclonal antibodies have been developed for post-exposure prophylaxis of anthrax (anti-protective antigen), botulism (anti-toxins A–G) and plague (anti-V antigen).

23.7 Acknowledgements

The earlier contribution of Michael Corbel and Dorothy Xing, who established this chapter in the previous two editions, is gratefully acknowledged.

References

Brandenburg, K., Schromm, A., Weindl, G. et al. (2021). An update on endotoxin neutralization strategies in Gram-negative bacterial infections. *Expert Rev. Anti Infect. Ther.* 19 (4): 495–517.

British Pharmacopoeia (2020). London: The Stationery Office.

CDC (2020). Adjuvants and Vaccines, US Centers for Disease Control and Prevention. https://www.cdc.gov/vaccinesafety/concerns/adjuvants.html

Finney, D.J. (1971). *Probit Analysis*. London: Cambridge University Press.

Kayser, V. and Razman, I. (2021). Vaccines and vaccination: history and emerging issues. *Hum. Vaccin. Immunother.* 17 (12): 5255–5268..

Knezevic, I., Liu, M.A., Peden, K. et al. (2021). Development of mRNA vaccines: scientific and regulatory issues. *Vaccine* 9: 81. https://doi.org/10.3390/vaccines9020081.

Stewart, A. and Devlin, P. (2006). The history of the smallpox vaccine. *J. Infect.* 52 (5): 329–334.

Subbarao, K. (2021). The success of SARS-CoV-2 vaccines and challenges ahead. *Cell Host Microbe* 29 (7): 1111–1123.

WHO (2020). Evaluation of the quality, safety and efficacy of RNA-based prophylactic vaccines for infectious diseases: regulatory considerations WHO/RNA/DRAFT/22DECEMBER2020 https://www.who.int/docs/default-source/biologicals/ecbs/reg-considerations-on-rna-vaccines_1st-draft_pc_tz_22122020.pdf?sfvrsn=c13e1e20_3 (Accessed October 2022).

Zuercher, A.W., Berger, M., Bolli, R. et al. (2019). Plasma-Derived Immunoglobulins. In: *Nijkamp and Parnham's Principles of Immunopharmacology* (ed. M. Parnham, F. Nijkamp and A. Rossi), 327–368. Cham: Springer https://doi.org/10.1007/978-3-030-10811-3_20.

Further Reading

British National Formulary 83 (2022) British Medical Association and Pharmaceutical Press, London. (This publication contains a useful section on immunological products. New editions appear twice yearly. Also available from http://bnf.org/bnf/index.htm)

Plotkin, S.A. and Fantini, B. (ed.) (1996). *Vaccinia, Vaccination, Vaccinology – Jenner, Pasteur and Their Successors*. Paris: Elsevier.

Plotkin, S.A., Orenstein, W.A., Offit, P.A. and Edwards, K.M. (ed.) (2018). *Vaccines*, 7e. Amsterdam: Elsevier.

Powell, M.F. and Newman, M.J. (1995). *Vaccine Design. The Subunit and Adjuvant Approach*. New York: Plenum Press.

24

Recombinant DNA Technology

Miguel Cámara[1] *and Stephan Heeb*[2]

[1] *Professor of Molecular Microbiology and Co-Director of the National Biofilms Innovation Centre, School of Life Sciences, Biodiscovery Institute, University of Nottingham, Nottingham, UK*
[2] *Assistant Professor in Molecular Microbiology, School of Life Sciences, University of Nottingham, Nottingham, UK*

CONTENTS

Hugo and Russell's Pharmaceutical Microbiology, Ninth Edition. Edited by Brendan F. Gilmore and Stephen P. Denyer.

Companion website: https://www.wiley.com/go/HugoandRussells9e

24.1 Introduction: Biotechnology in the Pharmaceutical Sciences

The rapid developments in biotechnology and the applications of genetic engineering to practical human problems have allowed the advancement of pharmaceutical biotechnology at a staggering pace. Furthermore, the release of the human genome sequence has also been key for the identification of human genetic diseases and the design of revolutionary approaches for their treatment.

Genetic engineering involves altering DNA molecules outside an organism, making the resultant DNA molecules function in living cells. Many of these cells have been genetically engineered to produce substances that are medically useful to humans. Pharmaceutical biotechnology involves the use of living organisms such as microorganisms to create new pharmaceutical products, or safer and more effective versions of conventionally produced pharmaceuticals, more cost-effectively.

Since the manufacture of the first recombinant pharmaceutical, insulin, there has been a burst in the generation of new recombinant drugs, some of which will be covered later on in this chapter. Furthermore, the use of recombinant DNA technology has spread further allowing the development of not only subunit vaccines, such as the one used in the prevention of hepatitis B, but also attenuated vaccines, vector vaccines and DNA or RNA vaccines. One of pharmaceutical biotechnology's great potentials lies in gene therapy, which consists in the modification of the genetic material of living cells to prevent, control or cure disease. It encompasses repairing or replacing defective genes and for example making tumours more susceptible to other kinds of treatment.

This chapter aims to describe some essential genetic manipulation techniques and to illustrate, with some key examples, their use for the generation of recombinant pharmaceutical drugs. Applications of recombinant DNA techniques in the diagnosis of diseases will also be covered.

24.2 Enabling Techniques

To understand how recombinant pharmaceuticals are manufactured, we first need to review some of the essential DNA manipulation techniques used to generate these products. We will start by looking at ways to cut and join fragments of DNA and then examine step-by-step how these techniques can be exploited to clone and express genes from eukaryotic and prokaryotic cells.

24.2.1 Cutting and Joining DNA Molecules

DNA is made up of four bases (A, adenine; G, guanine; C, cytosine; and, T, thymine); it can be isolated from any type of cell and fragmented using restriction endonucleases. These are enzymes produced by microorganisms which cut foreign DNA and can restrict the proliferation of infecting viruses. Some of these enzymes cut at specific points known as 'restriction sites' which are palindromic sequences (complementary sequences with identical nucleotide sequences when read in the 5′ to 3′ direction) of various lengths. For example, *Eco*RI (*Escherichia coli* restriction enzyme I) has specificity for the sequence GAATTC and hydrolyses the G—A phosphodiester bond. Enzymes which recognise and cut at restriction sites of 4–8 base pairs (bp) are particularly useful, as the probability of a site appearing in a random DNA fragment is inversely proportional to its length.

There are two different types of DNA ends that can be generated using restriction enzymes: cohesive or sticky and blunt ends (Table 24.1). DNA fragments obtained by restriction enzyme digestion can be covalently joined together using the enzyme DNA ligase. There is a limitation, however, with regard to the type of ends this enzyme is able to bond together. Only blunt ends generated by some restriction enzymes (e.g., *Dra*I and *Eco*RV) or compatible sticky ends generated by either the same restriction enzymes (e.g., *Eco*RI) or by enzymes that generate complementary overhanging ends (e.g., *Sau*3AI and *Bam*HI) will be bonded by the DNA ligase (Table 24.1).

24.2.2 Cloning Vectors

Genes present in DNA fragments that have been excised with restriction endonucleases can be maintained (replicated) and expressed by inserting them (cloning) into vectors after ligation. These cloning vectors are of different types and are relatively small DNA molecules that have the ability to self-replicate in a host cell. The main types of vectors used for gene cloning are plasmids, cosmids and bacteriophages, which are normally used according to the size of the DNA fragments that need to be cloned.

24.2.2.1 Cloning of Small Fragments of DNA

To allow the cloning of small DNA fragments, plasmids of generally up to 10 kb (1 kilobase (kb) = 1000 base pairs (bp)) are the main vectors of choice.

Plasmids

Plasmids are circular extrachromosomal DNA molecules that replicate independently within cells using their own origin of replication. There are a number of features generally found in plasmids used as cloning vectors:

Antibiotic resistance markers: These are genes coding for proteins that confer resistance to specific antibiotics.

Table 24.1 Restriction enzymes and the compatibility of digested ends for ligation.

Restriction enzyme	Restriction site	Digested ends	Compatibility for ligase	Ligation products
*Sau*3A	5′-**GATC**-3′ 3′-**CTAG**-5′	*Sticky* 5′- **GATC**-3′ 3′-**CTAG** −5′		5′-GATCC-3′ 3′-**CTAG**G-5′
			Compatible	
*Bam*HI	5′-GGATCC-3′ 3′-CCTAGG-5′	*Sticky* 5′-G GATCC-3′ 3′-CCTAG G-5′		5′-G**GATC**-3′ 3′-CCTAG-5′
			Incompatible	
*Eco*RI	5′-**GAATTC**-3′ 3′-**CTTAAG**-5′	*Sticky* 5′-**G** **AATTC**-3′ 3′-**CTTAA** **G**-5′		5′-**G**AATTC-3′ 3′-**CTTAAG**-5′
			Compatible	
*Eco*RI	5′-GAATTC-3′ 3′-CTTAAG-5′	*Sticky* 5′-G AATTC-3′ 3′-CTTAA G-5′		5′-G**AATTC**-3′ 3′-CTTAA**G**-5′
			Incompatible	
*Dra*I	5′-**TTTAAA**-3′ 3′-**AAATTT**-5′	*Blunt* 5′-**TTT** **AAA**-3′ 3′-**AAA** **TTT**-5′		5′-**TTT**ATC-3′ 3′-**AAA**TAG-5′
			Compatible	
*Eco*RV	5′-GATATC-3′ 3′-CTATAG-5′	*Blunt* 5′-GAT ATC-3′ 3′-CTA TAG-5′		5′-GAT**AAA**-3′ 3′-CTA**TTT**-5′

These markers therefore allow the selection of hosts carrying the plasmids.

*Multiple cloning sites (*MCS*):* These are stretches of DNA designed to contain a number of unique different restriction sites, providing a choice of possible restriction enzymes to be used for the cloning of DNA fragments.

Origin of replication: Required for plasmid replication in a specific host. These DNA sequences also determine the number of copies at which the plasmid will replicate, from just one to several hundred per cell. Plasmids having more than one host-specific origin of replication are known as shuttle vectors.

Insertional inactivation markers: These facilitate the selection of recombinant from non-recombinant plasmids. The most commonly used is the *lacZ* gene coding for β-galactosidase. This enzyme cleaves 5-bromo-4-chloro-3-indolyl-β-D-galactopyranoside (X-Gal), an artificial substrate that mimics galactose, which results in the generation of an insoluble blue product. Insertion of a recombinant DNA fragment in *lacZ* will result in the disruption of β-galactosidase production and the inability to cleave X-Gal. Hence, colonies from bacteria carrying an intact *lacZ* gene, that is, from non-recombinant plasmids, appear blue on agar plates containing X-Gal. By contrast, those with a successful insertion in *lacZ*, that is, harbouring recombinant plasmids, appear white.

Figure 24.1 shows all these features in a simplified diagram of the cloning vector pUC18.

An ideal plasmid for cloning should have a small size (2–10 kb), be conjugation-defective, that is, non-self-mobilisable from cell to cell, and produce a selectable phenotype in host cells. It should also contain a large multiple cloning site and replicate at a high copy number (>10 copies per cell).

24.2.2.2 Cloning of Large Fragments of DNA

Sometimes there is a need to clone large fragments of DNA, for example, for the isolation of complete gene clusters. An example would be the cloning of large eukaryotic genes or genes required for the synthesis of a certain molecule. Sometimes, the synthesis of a compound requires more than 10 different genes and these are frequently organised in operons co-transcribed in a single messenger RNA (mRNA) molecule. To enable the cloning of large genes or full-length operons, vectors such as bacteriophages, cosmids or bacterial artificial chromosomes (BACs) need to be used.

Bacteriophages

The most popular has been the *E. coli* λ (lambda) bacteriophage, which is composed of a tubular protein tail and a protein head packed with approximately 50 kb of

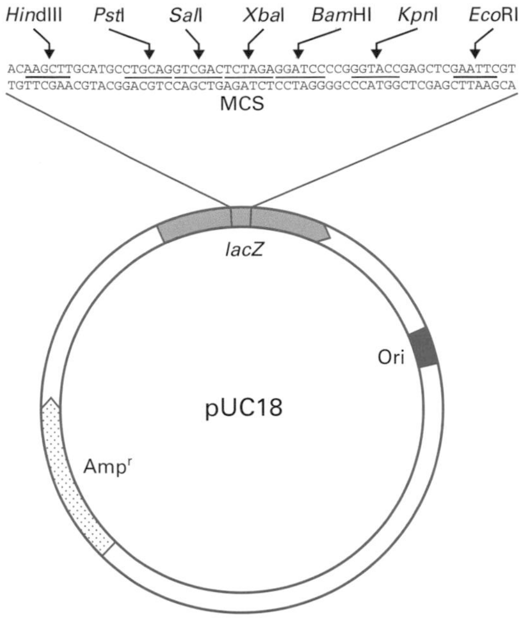

Figure 24.1 Simplified diagram of the plasmid pUC18. *lacZ* represents the insertional inactivation marker coding for β-galactosidase activity. A multiple cloning site (MCS) is present within the *lacZ* gene allowing the cloning of DNA fragments. 'Ori' represents the origin of replication which, in this case, is functional in *Escherichia coli* and Amp^r represents an ampicillin-resistance marker.

double-stranded DNA (Figure 24.2). After injection of the viral DNA into *E. coli*, bacteriophage λ can multiply and enter a lytic cycle leading to the lysis of the host cell and the subsequent release of a large number of phage particles. Alternatively, injection of the DNA can lead to a lysogenic cycle in which the phage DNA is integrated into the *E. coli* chromosome where it is maintained until the environmental conditions change and is then excised, entering a lytic cycle. Out of the 50 kb that make the λ bacteriophage less than half are essential for its propagation and therefore around 20 kb can be replaced by recombinant DNA, hence their name λ replacement vectors. For this reason, these are very useful vectors for the generation of genomic libraries. DNA in λ bacteriophages contain at each end small single-stranded complementary DNA fragments called λ cohesive ends (λ*cos* ends). Recombinant phages can be assembled in a test tube into phage-like particles by enzymes which recognise and process the λ*cos* ends, provided that they are 35–45 kb apart. These enzymes as well as the head and tails required for the assembly process are commercially available as part of *in vitro* packaging kits. The *in vitro* packaging results in the formation of recombinant phages that can be transduced to *E. coli* cells. Transduced *E. coli* will be identified by the formation of lysis plaques in agar plates seeded with a mixture of *E. coli* and recombinant λ bacteriophages.

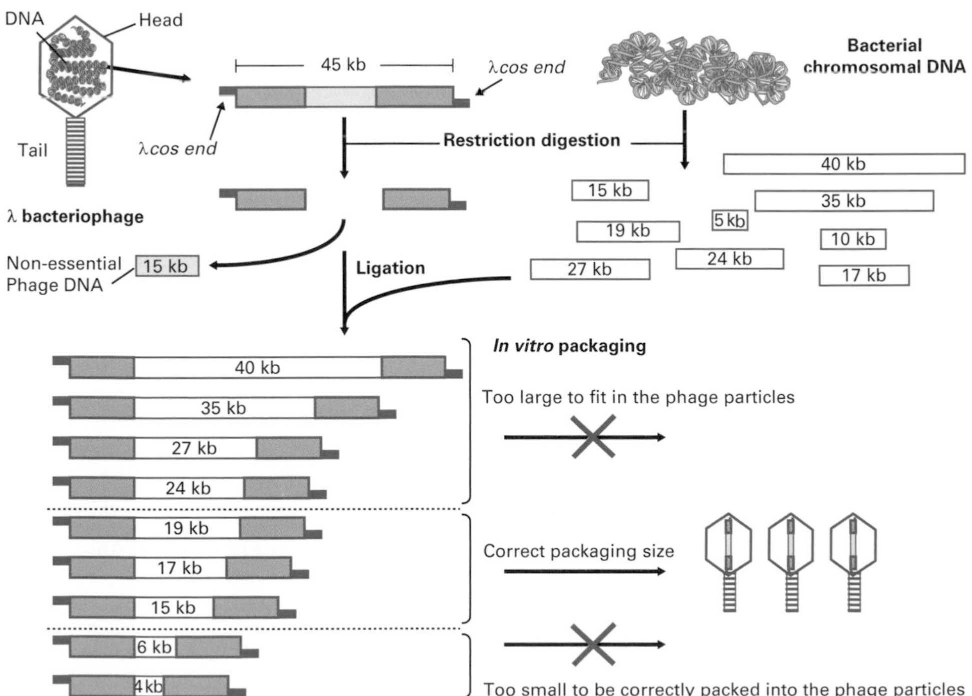

Figure 24.2 Cloning of DNA into λ replacement vectors. The DNA from the λ bacteriophage can be purified from the phage particles and digested with restriction enzymes to remove an internal fragment of around 15 kb which is not required for the life cycle of the bacteriophage. This fragment can be replaced with other fragments of DNA such as those coming from digested bacterial chromosomal DNA. As the λ bacteriophage can only pack DNA fragments flanked by λ*cos* ends which are 35–45 kb apart, any recombinant fragments larger or smaller than that will not be successfully packed.

Cosmids and Fosmids

Cosmids are plasmids maintained in *E. coli* that have been engineered to carry λ*cos* sequences. This allows their packaging *in vitro* into λ phage particles to be transduced into *E. coli* cells for replication. Once inside the bacterial host, the cosmid DNA is circularised by the joining of the λ*cos* ends and thereafter it replicates as a normal plasmid. This implies that the cloned DNA will be available as *E. coli* colonies and not as plaques like with the λ bacteriophages. As less DNA is required for plasmid than for bacteriophage replication, cosmids can carry up to 40 kb of cloned DNA still enabling the packaging into λ phage particles.

Eukaryotic and more particularly mammalian genomic DNA rich in multiple repeated elements can be subject to deletions and rearrangements when cloned in standard multi-copy cosmids and replicated in bacteria. The occurrence of these unwanted modifications can be reduced by using special cosmids in which the multi-copy origin of replication has been replaced by the single-copy origin of replication from the *E. coli* F′ factor. These cloning vectors are known as *fosmids*.

Bacterial Artificial Chromosomes

Although cosmids and fosmids enable the cloning of relatively large DNA fragments, the amount of DNA that can be packed into a λ bacteriophage head is limited to around 50 kb. To clone even larger DNA fragments, cloning vectors derived from the single-copy *E. coli* F′ factor, similar to the fosmids, have been designed. In this case, the λ*cos* ends are absent or not used for packaging and instead the recombinant plasmids are introduced directly into the *E. coli* cells by transformation. This allows the cloning of DNA fragments of several hundred kb resulting in what are then called bacterial artificial chromosomes.

24.2.3 Introduction of Vector into Hosts

For the expression and maintenance of recombinant genes, the recombinant vectors harbouring them need to be introduced into suitable hosts. The four main methods used to achieve this are transformation, electroporation, conjugation and transduction.

Transformation is the direct incorporation of DNA into host cells. Bacteria such as *E. coli* can be primed to take up recombinant plasmid DNA by treatment with ice-cold calcium chloride until they reach a 'competent' state. These cells are then mixed with the recombinant plasmid and exposed briefly to a heat shock of 42 °C which causes them to take up the DNA.

Electroporation is the most efficient way of introducing DNA not only into bacteria but also into eukaryotic cells. This technique is based on the induction of free DNA uptake by the cells after subjecting them to a strong electric field.

In some cases, *conjugation* can be used as a natural route for transmission of plasmid DNA from a donor cell to a recipient cell by direct contact through cell–cell junctions. Only plasmid cloning vectors containing conjugative elements can be transferred by conjugation. This procedure requires direct contact between the donor and the recipient cell. Conjugation is not as frequently used as electroporation, as most plasmid vectors used for the cloning of recombinant DNA lack conjugative functions, preventing these plasmids from being passed to other cells inadvertently.

Finally, in *transduction* (prokaryotes) and *transfection* (eukaryotes), the transfer of recombinant non-viral DNA to a cell is achieved by a virus. This is the method of choice for the introduction of recombinant λ bacteriophages, cosmids and fosmids into *E. coli* cells.

24.2.4 Construction of Genomic Libraries

Before we study how genomic libraries are made, we first need to understand the differences between the genetic organisation in eukaryotic and prokaryotic cells. Bacterial genes are uninterrupted sequences of nucleotides encoding the genetic information required for the synthesis of a protein. These genes can sometimes be co-transcribed with adjacent genes of related function into the same mRNA molecule. This set of co-transcribed genes is called an operon (Figure 24.3). The mRNA in bacteria does not generally need to be processed before translation, and transcription and translation occur simultaneously.

By contrast, genes from eukaryotic cells contain non-coding sequences called introns and coding sequences called exons. The former are removed after transcription by a process called 'splicing' that occurs in the nucleus of the cell. In addition, the mRNA is subjected to further processing involving the addition of a methylated guanine (M_7Gppp) called CAP on its 5′ end, required for translation, and a poly-adenine tail on its 3′ end (Figure 24.3). Mature mRNA is then exported from the nucleus into the cytoplasm, where it is translated into proteins. Eukaryotic genes appear to be transcribed individually, as operons have not been described in eukaryotes.

To enable the cloning and isolation of a specific gene(s) from a cell, several steps are required. The first consists of choosing the source of genetic material, which, in prokaryotic cells, is normally the chromosomal DNA. By contrast, in eukaryotic cells this is more often the mature mRNA, as it is not interrupted by introns and consequently codes for complete, active proteins. The second step consists of the preparation of the purified DNA or RNA for cloning. This step is more straightforward when using prokaryotic DNA (Section 24.2.4.1) than eukaryotic RNA (Section 24.2.4.2). The result will be the construction of a collection of cloned

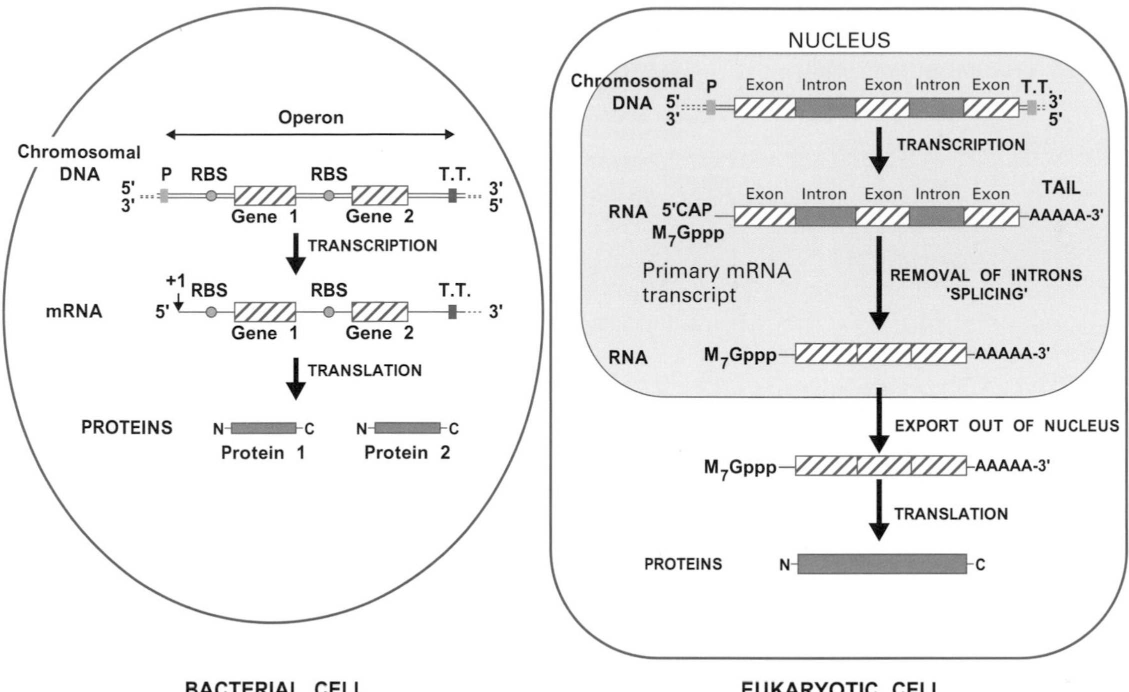

Figure 24.3 Genetic organisation in prokaryotes and eukaryotes. In prokaryotes (the bacterial cell in this figure), genes can sometimes be grouped in operons and hence transcribed together in a single molecule of mRNA. In these organisms, the whole process of transcription and translation takes place simultaneously in the cytoplasm. By contrast, in eukaryotes, genes are organised in single transcriptional units incorporating introns. Upon transcription in the nucleus, eukaryotic mRNA is firstly modified by the addition of a CAP (methylated guanine) and a poly(A) tail and then by the splicing out of the introns. The mature mRNA is then exported into the cytoplasm where it is translated into proteins. P, promoter; T.T., transcriptional terminator; RBS, ribosome binding site.

DNA fragments propagated in bacteria that is called the genomic library. This library should ideally contain representatives of every sequence in the chromosome of a prokaryotic cell and every expressed gene in the case of a eukaryotic cell. The final step consists of the screening of the recombinant clones to identify the required gene(s).

24.2.4.1 Prokaryotic Gene Libraries: Shotgun Cloning

The construction of a prokaryotic gene library can be achieved by a technique called 'shotgun cloning' (Figure 24.4). This involves the purification and partial digestion of the genomic (chromosomal) DNA from a prokaryotic organism with restriction endonucleases to produce a random mixture of fragments of different sizes. Chromosomal DNA can also be mechanically sheared and in this case the extremities must be repaired and made blunt with DNA polymerase in the presence of deoxynucleotides (dNTPs). These fragments are then fractionated into different sizes and ligated into a cloning vector appropriately digested. The recombinant vectors are then transformed, in the case of plasmids, or transfected, in the case of bacteriophages and cosmids, into the host cell of choice. The resulting genomic library can then be screened for the presence of the recombinant gene of interest by a number of methods (see Section 24.2.5).

24.2.4.2 Eukaryotic cDNA Gene Libraries

The shotgun approach cannot be applied for the construction of eukaryotic gene libraries due to the presence of introns in the DNA, which prevents the direct cloning of functional genes from digested chromosomal DNA. Instead mature mRNA from the cytoplasm of cells expressing the desired gene is used as the source of genetic material. For example, to make a genomic library containing the insulin gene, RNA from pancreatic cells expressing this gene will have to be isolated. Remember that cells show distinct differentiation in different tissues and only express a low percentage of the whole genome according to their role in the tissue of which they form part. Consequently, it will not be possible to purify RNA coding for insulin from, for example, cells of the pituitary gland. Therefore, the cells expressing the gene of interest will have to be isolated first, and then their mRNA purified. As mentioned earlier, virtually every eukaryotic mRNA has on its 3′ end a poly-adenine tail. This provides a convenient way to isolate mature mRNA from total cellular RNA, the majority of which (98%) is ribosomal RNA (rRNA) and transfer RNA (tRNA). The total RNA purified from a cell can be passed through an affinity column packed with cellulose linked to deoxythymidine oligonucleotides [oligo(dT)]. As the total RNA passes through the column, only the mRNA molecules

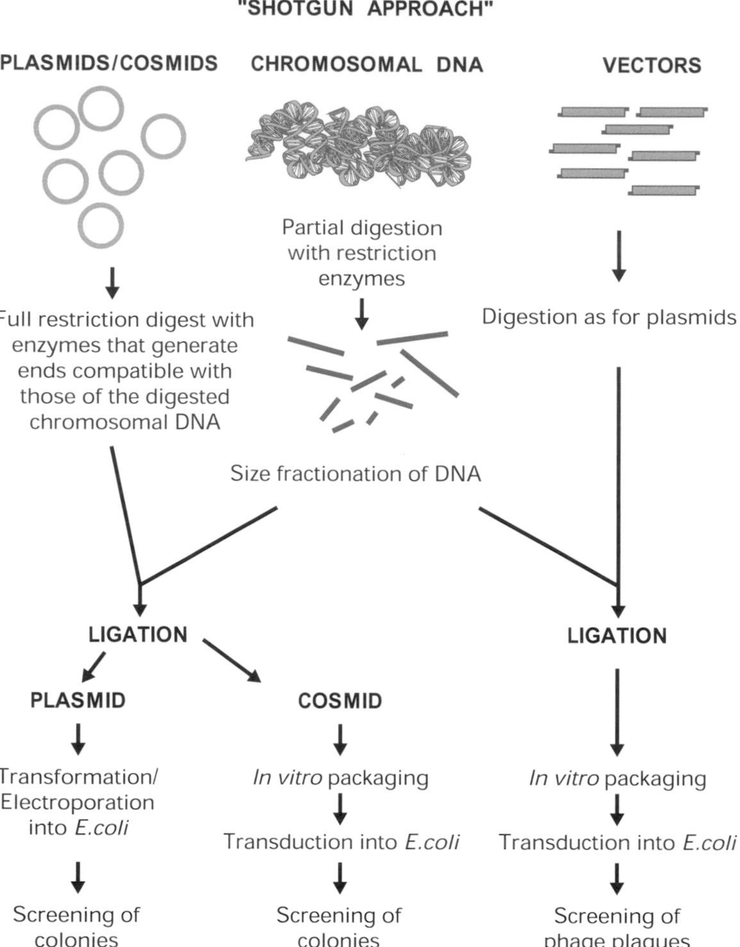

Figure 24.4 Construction of prokaryotic genomic libraries by shotgun cloning. The shotgun approach for the construction of genomic libraries involves the purification and digestion of chromosomal DNA from the prokaryotic organisms, followed by the cloning into a digested suitable vector using DNA ligase. The recombinant vector is then introduced into the host cell using the appropriate method and then the colonies or plaques are screened for the presence of the recombinant gene of interest.

which have poly-adenine tails will bind to the oligo(dT), while the rest will flow through the column to be discarded. The purified mRNA then has to be converted into double-stranded cDNA (complementary DNA) to enable its cloning into a suitable vector.

Synthesis and Cloning of cDNA

There are generally two main strategies used for the synthesis of cDNA from mRNA called the replacement synthesis and the primer–adaptor synthesis. For both strategies, the first-strand cDNA synthesis is based on the priming of the mRNA with an oligo(dT) which anneals to the poly(A) tail of the mRNA molecule and, consequently, with the action of the enzyme reverse transcriptase and in the presence of dNTPs, the synthesis of the first cDNA strand takes place. This results in the formation of a mRNA/cDNA heteroduplex hybrid. The second stage is different for the two strategies mentioned. The most commonly used is the replacement synthesis, which is based on the use of ribonuclease H (RNase H), an enzyme that cleaves the RNA moiety of RNA/DNA hybrids and has $5' \rightarrow 3'$ and $3' \rightarrow 5'$ exonuclease activities. This results in partial digestion of the RNA in both directions. The resulting RNA fragments can serve as primers for DNA synthesis using DNA polymerase I. This enzyme, with its $5' \rightarrow 3'$ exonuclease and polymerase activities, will fill the nicks and effectively remove the RNA primers. The cDNA fragments synthesised will be joined using DNA ligase. This method causes the loss of some nucleotides at the 5′ end of the mRNA, including the CAP region.

The primer–adaptor method for the synthesis of the second strand of cDNA starts with the removal of the RNA strand from the mRNA/cDNA hybrid, by treatment with alkali. This is followed by the addition of a poly(C) tail to the 3′ end of the DNA strand using an enzyme called terminal transferase. This enables the hybridisation of a complementary poly(G) primer that will be the starting point for the synthesis of the second cDNA strand by the DNA polymerase (Figure 24.5). This method, in contrast to the replacement synthesis, generates cDNA molecules with a complete 5’ CAP region. However, it requires more steps and the terminal transferase step is difficult to control.

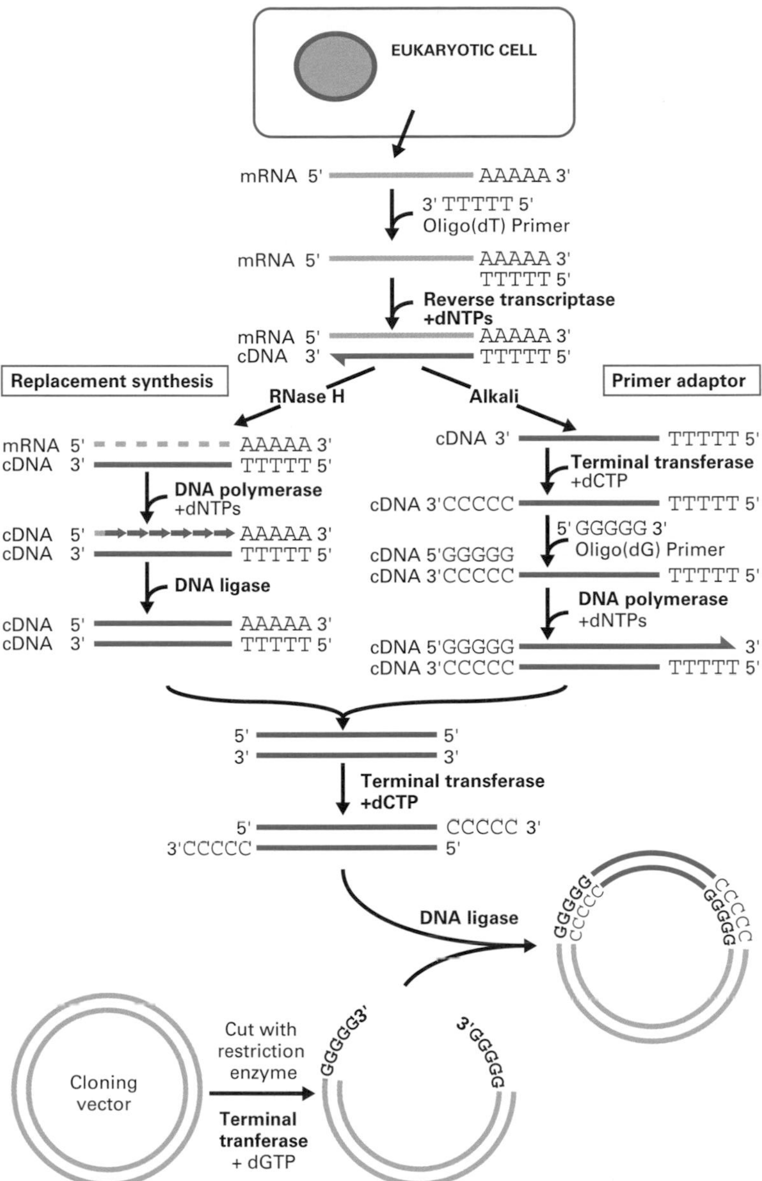

Figure 24.5 Synthesis and cloning of complementary DNA (cDNA). Cloning of eukaryotic genes involves the isolation of mRNA from the cytoplasm of the cells expressing the gene of interest. To allow the cloning of the mRNA, the synthesis of double-stranded cDNA is first required. This involves the synthesis of the first cDNA strand by reverse transcriptase using an oligo(dT) primer. To generate the second strand of cDNA, there are two main methods. The replacement synthesis method involves the generation of nicks in the mRNA strand by the RNase H enzyme followed by the synthesis of the complementary strand, using the RNA fragments generated by the RNase H as primers, by the DNA polymerase. The DNA fragments generated are then joined together by the DNA ligase. By contrast, the primer–adaptor method requires the degradation of the mRNA strand by alkali followed by the addition of a poly(C) tail at the 3′ end of the cDNA strand by the terminal transferase. For the synthesis of the second strand of cDNA, addition of an oligo(dG) primer and DNA polymerase are required. The double-stranded cDNA generated by either method can be cloned into any vector upon addition of poly(C) sticky ends by the terminal transferase, provided that the vector has complementary poly(G) ends created by this enzyme. dNTPs, deoxynucleotides.

Finally, the cloning of the resulting cDNA is aided by the addition of a poly(C) tail at the 3′ ends of the cDNA fragments using terminal transferase and the ligation of these to a linearised vector containing a complementary poly(G) tail also generated by the terminal transferase.

24.2.4.3 Comparison between Libraries

There are a number of points to take into consideration when choosing a strategy to generate a genomic library. The larger the insert size, the lower the number of clones required to have full representation of an entire genome. To reduce the number of recombinant clones to be screened before the gene of interest is identified, cosmids, λ bacteriophages or BACs should be used, as they can take larger DNA inserts. Furthermore, if we want to isolate a large DNA fragment containing, for example, all the genes required for the biosynthesis of an antibiotic, plasmid libraries might not be the right choice. By contrast, if we are trying to isolate a single gene and the extent of the screening is not a problem, plasmid libraries are ideal, as they reduce the subcloning steps required to single out the gene of interest. Table 24.2 shows a comparison between the insert sizes taken by different vectors, their hosts and the genomic libraries for which they can be suitable.

24.2.5 Screening of Genomic Libraries

Once the genomic library has been generated, it is necessary to screen for the gene of interest within thousands of

Table 24.2 Comparison of vectors used for the construction of genomic libraries.

Vector	Insert size (kb)	Host	Cloning method suitability
Plasmid	<10	Specified by origin of replication present on the plasmid	Shotgun cloning cDNA cloning
λ Bacteriophages (replacement only)	7–22	*E. coli*	Shotgun cloning
Cosmids and fosmids	25–45	*E. coli*	Shotgun cloning
BACs	Up to 750	*E. coli*	Shotgun cloning

BACs, bacterial artificial chromosomes

recombinant clones. The choice of screening method will very much depend on the availability of reagents and the information on the target gene to be isolated.

24.2.5.1 Hybridisation Screening

This technique is used when some of the DNA sequence for the gene screened for is known, or when a fragment of this gene is available from a previous cloning. Alternatively, a DNA fragment from a closely related gene can be used as a probe for the isolation of the gene of interest. The hybridisation technique requires plating the library on a set of agar plates to generate a replica, on nitrocellulose or nylon membranes, of the plaques or colonies, each containing a different recombinant DNA fragment. This process transfers a portion of each plaque or colony to the membranes and is done in such a way that the pattern of plaques/colonies on the original plate is maintained on the filters. The membranes are then hybridised with a radio-labelled DNA probe containing part of the sequence to be isolated from the library. The probe will only bind/hybridise to the recombinant clones containing that sequence. After this process, the membranes are exposed to X-ray film (autoradiography). The presence of dark spots on the films represents the location of colonies containing the target gene. By orienting the film with the original agar plate, the colony/plaque carrying the complementary sequence can be identified and the desired clone isolated. An alternative to the use of radio-isotopes for the probes resides in the use of nucleotides labelled with a molecule such as digoxigenin (DIG). In that case, detection of the hybridised probes is performed with anti-DIG antibodies conjugated to an enzyme such as alkaline phosphatase, which reacts with a substrate to produce chemiluminescence.

24.2.5.2 Immunological Screening

This technique is used when we need to isolate a gene coding for a protein for which there are antibodies available. The success of this technique relies on the expression of the gene of interest, as it requires the synthesis of the target protein from the target recombinant gene. The screening steps are similar to those used for the hybridisation screening with the difference that the membranes containing portions of plaques or colonies have to be incubated with the antibodies that will recognise the target protein. This antibody, called the primary antibody, will bind tightly to those colonies/plaques containing the recombinant gene of interest, provided that the protein encoded by this gene has been synthesised. The position of the bound antibody is revealed by incubating the membranes with a labelled antibody (secondary antibody) that recognises the primary antibody. There are different types of labels for antibodies, all of which can easily be detected.

24.2.5.3 Protein Activity Screening

This type of screening is limited to proteins that have a specific activity that can easily be identified within a large population of recombinant clones. Needless to say, to detect a protein activity, the gene coding for this protein must be expressed and an active protein must be produced. Understanding of this technique can be helped by illustrating this screening with an example. Suppose we want to isolate a gene coding for a bacterial haemolytic toxin from a genomic library, then, as we know that this toxin lyses red blood cells, we could plate the library on plates containing agar mixed with blood. Those colonies/plaques producing the haemolytic toxin could easily be identified by the presence of a haemolytic halo around them resulting from the action of the toxin on the red blood cells.

24.2.6 Optimising Expression of Recombinant Genes

The primary objective of pharmaceutical companies involved in the production of recombinant drugs is the maximal expression of recombinant genes to generate large quantities of these drugs. Unfortunately, the cloning of a gene into a vector does not ensure that it will be properly expressed. Therefore, to improve expression of a cloned gene, the different stages that lead to the synthesis of the protein have to be optimised. This is achieved by the use of so-called *expression vectors* (Figure 24.6).

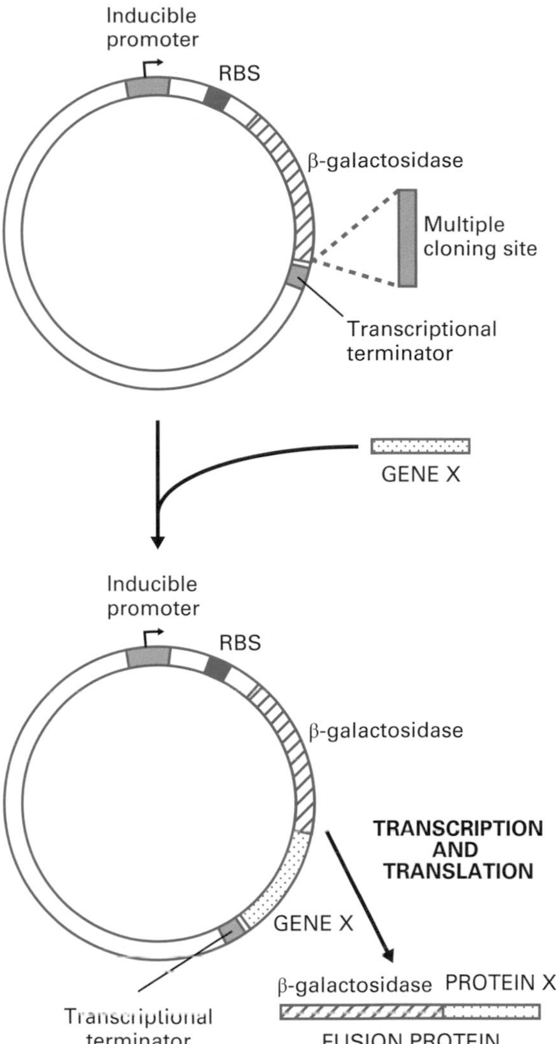

Figure 24.6 Expression vectors and the generation of fusion proteins. Expression vectors have optimised all the signals required for transcription (inducible promoter and transcriptional terminator) and for translation (ribosome-binding site). Some of them carry the gene for β-galactosidase with a multiple cloning site that allows the insertion of small genes for the generation of fusion proteins.

Some expression vectors have been designed to produce large quantities of protein in specific cell hosts. For example, the *bacmids* are shuttle expression vectors derived from a baculovirus double-stranded DNA circular genome and are used to transfect insect cells in order to produce large quantities of a recombinant protein in fermenters.

24.2.6.1 Optimising Transcription

To optimise transcription, it must be ensured that the recombinant gene is placed after a promoter (Figure 24.6) that will be recognised by the RNA polymerase of the host cell where the gene is going to be expressed. Two types of promoters can be used: (i) *constitutive promoters*, which are active all the time, and (ii) *inducible promoters*, where transcription is turned off during culture growth and turned on for example upon the addition of an inducing molecule to the culture, usually shortly before harvesting, when high numbers of bacteria are present in the culture. Inducible promoters are very useful when expressing foreign genes coding for proteins toxic to the bacterial hosts, as their premature expression could lead to growth impairments and consequently low yields of recombinant protein.

Furthermore, to ensure that transcription finishes after the 3′ end of the recombinant gene, a transcriptional terminator (Figure 24.6) must be placed just downstream of this gene.

24.2.6.2 Optimising Translation

A key feature that determines whether a gene is going to be efficiently translated by a certain host is the nucleotide sequence of the ribosome-binding site (RBS), located upstream of the gene (Figure 24.6), which needs to be efficiently recognised by the ribosomes of this host. In addition, the distance between the RBS and the translation 'start' codon needs to be optimal to enable the right interactions between the mRNA and the ribosomes to start the protein synthesis. There are commercially available vectors carrying sequences for RBSs and translation start codons which are optimally recognised by the ribosomes of the host cells, ensuring that any recombinant genes cloned after the start codon will be maximally translated.

Small proteins are frequently susceptible to proteolytic degradation when produced in a foreign host. This degradation can be avoided by expressing their genes fused to that of a larger protein. This is normally achieved by cloning the small gene downstream of a gene coding for a protein such as β-galactosidase. To obtain the fusion protein (Figure 24.6), it is essential to ensure that the reading frame is conserved and that no translation stop codons are present between the β-galactosidase and the target gene, enabling the ribosomes to read through. Usefully, affinity columns that will bind the fused polypeptides are available, which facilitates the purification of the recombinant protein by affinity chromatography.

24.2.6.3 Post-translational Modifications

Although high levels of protein production may be achieved by optimising transcription and translation of a gene, the obtained protein may still need to undergo post-translational modifications before it is active. Some of these modifications include correct disulphide bond formation, proteolytic cleavage of a precursor, glycosylation and additions to amino acids such as phosphorylation,

Table 24.3 Comparison of different hosts used for the expression of recombinant genes.

Hosts	Advantages	Disadvantages
Prokaryotic hosts		
Escherichia coli	Easy to grow in large-scale volumes Transcriptional and translational control well known Successfully used in the manufacture of insulin, interferon and human somatotropin	Difficult to achieve export of some proteins into growth medium Degradation of small proteins by proteases Unable to undertake most post-translational modifications, e.g., glycosylation Many proteins retained in the cytoplasm as insoluble aggregates
Bacilli *Bacillus subtilis* *Bacillus brevis*	Many proteins can be exported into growth medium Easy to grow in large-scale volumes	Regulation of gene expression not very well known Lack of high-level expression vectors Unable to carry out most post-translational modifications, e.g., glycosylation
Eukaryotic hosts		
Yeasts *Saccharomyces cerevisiae* *Pichia pastoris* *Hansenula polymorpha*	Easy to grow in large-scale volumes Efficient protein glycosylation Good export of heterologous proteins into growth medium Wide range of high-level expression systems available Recombinant proteins do not form insoluble aggregates in the cytoplasm	Gene expression can be difficult to control Sometimes fails to achieve accurate post-translational modification of recombinant proteins
Insect cells *Spodoptera frugiperda*	High expression levels Free of virus or prion-type agents pathogenic to mammals Can produce accurate glycosylation	Difficult to scale up High mannose glycosylation of the wanted proteins can make them undesirably immunogenic
Mammalian cells	Precise post-translational modification of human proteins Good expression systems available High stability of recombinant proteins	Gene regulation not well known Low protein secretion levels Can harbour infectious agents such as viruses Difficult to scale up
Transgenic animals	Precise post-transcriptional modifications Easy to generate large amount of recombinant protein, e.g., one goat can generate 1 kg of recombinant protein in milk per year Relatively inexpensive	Risk of contamination with infectious agents Products can sometimes be unstable

acetylation, sulphation and acylation. Unfortunately, the practical *E. coli* host, in which most recombinant proteins are produced, does not possess the same type of cellular machinery required for these modifications. Recently, *Campylobacter jejuni* has been found to possess a eukaryotic-like system for protein glycosylation and efforts are being made to genetically engineer *E. coli* strains to perform the adequate glycosylation of recombinant proteins as do mammalian cells. Hence, it is essential to select a suitable host for the expression of the target gene that can carry out the required post-translational modifications that will enable the synthesis of large amounts of a biologically authentic product. Table 24.3 shows a comparison of a selection of hosts currently used for the production of recombinant proteins.

24.2.7 Amplifying DNA: the Polymerase Chain Reaction

This is an extremely simple and powerful technique that was perfected by Kary Mullis in the mid-1980s and has revolutionised many studies in molecular biology, currently having applications ranging from forensic studies to the development of new recombinant drugs. This technique allows the generation of large amounts of copies of a specified DNA sequence from a single DNA molecule without the need for cloning.

The polymerase chain reaction (PCR) exploits certain characteristics of DNA replication, as it uses single-stranded DNA as a template for the synthesis of complementary new strands in a 5′ to 3′ direction. The single-stranded DNA templates can be generated by heating double-stranded

DNA above 90 °C. DNA polymerase synthesises double-stranded DNA by extending the complementary strand of a template. Hence, the DNA polymerase can be directed to synthesise a specific region of DNA by using a synthetic, complementary oligonucleotide primer that will anneal to the template when the temperature is lowered. The PCR reaction uses a special DNA polymerase (*Taq* DNA polymerase from the thermophilic bacterium *Thermus aquaticus*) that can withstand temperatures above 100 °C and which has an optimal activity at 72 °C, which has the advantage of reducing non-specific primer annealing that may occur at lower temperatures.

In PCR, both strands of a target DNA serve simultaneously as templates upon the addition of a pair of primers, one for each strand of DNA. A typical PCR amplification is shown in Figure 24.7. Every PCR cycle is normally repeated up to 30 times. The net result of a PCR is that, at the end of n cycles, it will generate 2^n double-stranded DNA copies of a single DNA fragment located between the two primers.

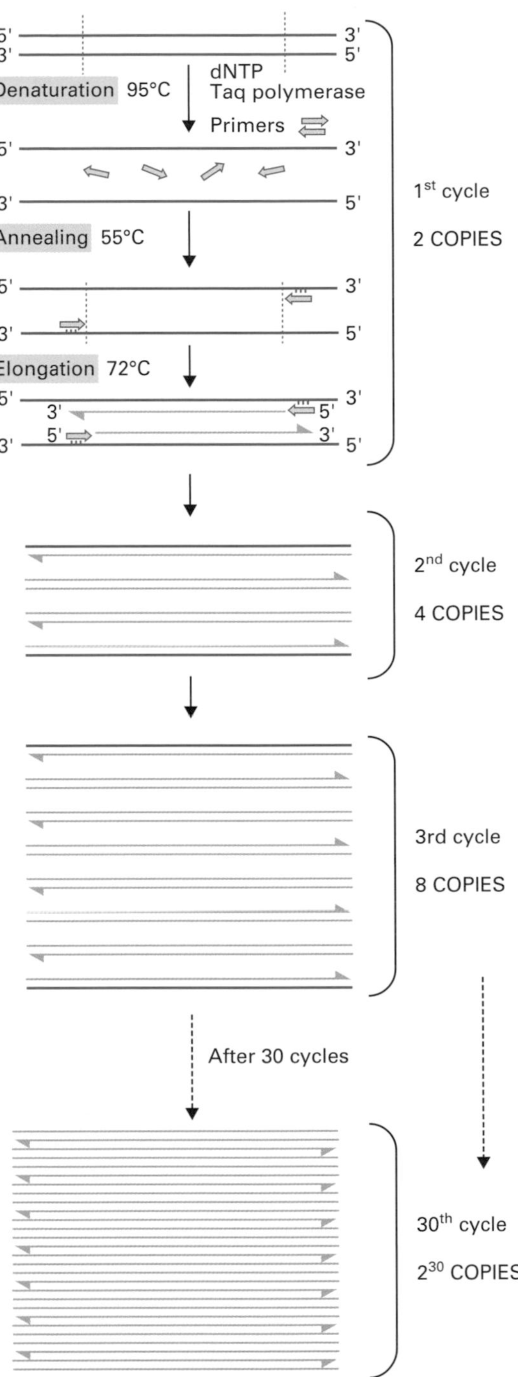

Figure 24.7 The polymerase chain reaction (PCR). A single PCR reaction involves the following steps. (1) Denaturation of the target double-stranded DNA by heating at 95 °C and addition of an excess of two oligonucleotide primers, each complementary to a different strand of the target sequence, Taq DNA polymerase and deoxynucleotides (dNTPs). (2) Annealing of the primers to the DNA strands by decreasing the temperature to 55 °C. (3) Elongation (or synthesis) of the new strand of DNA by the Taq DNA polymerase after increasing the temperature to 72 °C. This cycle can be repeated up to 30 times. In each cycle, the number of DNA copies is doubled; hence, at the end of a PCR reaction, there could be 2^{30} copies of an original target DNA molecule.

24.2.7.1 Advantages and Limitations of PCR

There are some obvious advantages of using PCR. The main one is specificity, as it allows, using the appropriate primers, the amplification of specific DNA fragments from a population of different cells. It is also a very rapid technique, as it only takes a few hours to amplify a fragment of DNA compared with days using conventional cloning methods. An important feature of PCR is its versatility, as it allows the incorporation of mismatches on the 5′ end of the primers provided that the 3′ end has perfect complementarity with the targeted strand. This can be exploited to add restriction sites to enable subsequent cloning of the amplified DNA, or introducing specific mutations into genes. Furthermore, the equipment used for PCR is relatively inexpensive and allows the analysis of a large number of samples at one time. Finally, PCR does not require purified template DNA and can amplify genes from whole cells or tissue samples.

However, there are also a number of limitations to the use of PCR. The designing of primers for this technique requires some knowledge of the DNA sequence to be amplified. Although there are new genetically engineered DNA polymerases that can synthesise large fragments of DNA, there are still some restrictions with regard to the maximum length of DNA that can be amplified. Ideally, fragments of 0.1–3 kb can be easily amplified, although this technique, under the appropriate conditions, would amplify larger fragments (up to 20 kb). In addition, the slightest sample contamination can lead to false positive results, which can have detrimental effects when this technique is used in diagnostics. Finally, sometimes there is a risk of non-specific amplification when the primers anneal to sequences similar to the targets, leading to the amplification of the wrong DNA.

24.2.7.2 Clinical Applications of PCR

The development of PCR has revolutionised not only basic research but also different areas of medicine. Table 24.4 shows a list of some of the most important clinical applications of PCR. These types of analysis were practically impossible without PCR owing to the large quantity of samples that needed handling, the amount of time required to obtain results or the lack of sensitivity of the available tests.

Table 24.4 Clinical applications of PCR.

Application	Examples
Diagnostics of inherited diseases	Cystic fibrosis
	Drug-metabolising enzyme defects
	Duchenne muscular dystrophy
	Fragile X syndrome
	Haemophilia B
	Hereditary thrombophilia
	Kennedy's disease
	Lesch–Nyhan syndrome
	Myeloid leukaemias and various cancers
	Tay–Sachs disease
Infectious disease screening	Adenovirus
	Bacillus anthracis
	Borrelia spp. (Lyme disease)
	Chlamydia trachomatis
	Cytomegalovirus
	Hepatitis B and hepatitis C virus
	Herpes virus
	Human immunodeficiency virus
	Human papillomavirus
	Influenza A and B
	Severe acute respiratory syndrome coronavirus 2 (SARS-CoV-2)
	Measles virus
	Mycobacterium tuberculosis
	Mycoplasma genitalium and *Trichomonas vaginalis*
	Neisseria gonorrhoeae
	Yersinia pestis
Forensic examination	Identification of criminals from samples of blood, tissue, hair, etc.
Prenatal screening	Batten's disease
	β-Thalassaemia
	Duchenne muscular dystrophy
	Haemophilia
	Sex determination
	Sickle cell anaemia
Human leucocyte antigen (HLA) subtyping	Prevention of insulin-dependent diabetes mellitus
Susceptibility to cardiovascular disease	Mutations in gene coding for angiotensin-converting enzyme (ACE)
	Mutation in the angiotensinogen gene
	Mutation in the apolipoprotein CII gene
	Mutation in the low-density lipoprotein receptor
Susceptibility to cancer	Neoplastic disease
	Lymph node metastasis in melanoma
	Acute promyelocytic leukaemia
	Thyroid cancer
	Bladder, breast and colorectal cancers
	Non-Hodgkin lymphoma

24.2.8 Genome Editing Using CRISPR–Cas9 Endonuclease

24.2.8.1 General Principle

Bacteria have evolved different mechanisms to protect themselves against spreading potentially deleterious mobile genetic elements such as infective bacteriophages. The use of restriction enzymes like those routinely used in the laboratory to cut DNA *in vitro* at specific sites is one such mechanism, cutting incoming foreign DNA. Bacteria protect their own DNA from being cut in error by their own restriction enzymes through methylation at specific sites with a modification system employing enzymes called methylases. Thus, when exogenous DNA is taken up from different strains or species, it generally doesn't have the appropriate protective methylation and hence gets digested by the endogenous restriction enzymes as a defence mechanism. In addition to the restriction–modification systems, many bacteria have additionally evolved an adaptive protection mechanism against recurrent incoming mobile genetic elements in what is akin to an acquired immune system. This is a sophisticated mechanism that involves dedicated RNAs and several proteins, although the overall principle which is useful in biotechnology is relatively simple (Figure 24.8); here, small 20-base-pair fragments of previously invading DNA from bacteriophage are incorporated into the bacterial chromosomes leaving a record of past infections. These DNA fragments, originally termed 'spacers', are inserted next to clustered regularly interspaced short palindromic repeats (CRISPR) that are constantly co-transcribed into a CRISPR RNA (crRNA). When an external mobile genetic element that has a sequence complementary to the spacer (called then the protospacer) enters the bacterial cell on a repeat occasion, Cas9, a protein with endonuclease activity, makes cuts within that genetic element thereby disabling its replicative capability. This involves an additional RNA termed the trans-activating tracrRNA, which has complementarity to the crRNA and interacts with the Cas9 protein to guide the endonuclease with high specificity towards its 20-bp target DNA, where it performs a double-stranded cut. In this way, bacterial cells are protected against bacteriophages which carry genomic sequences that are complementary to the spacer RNAs incorporated in the system during a past infection.

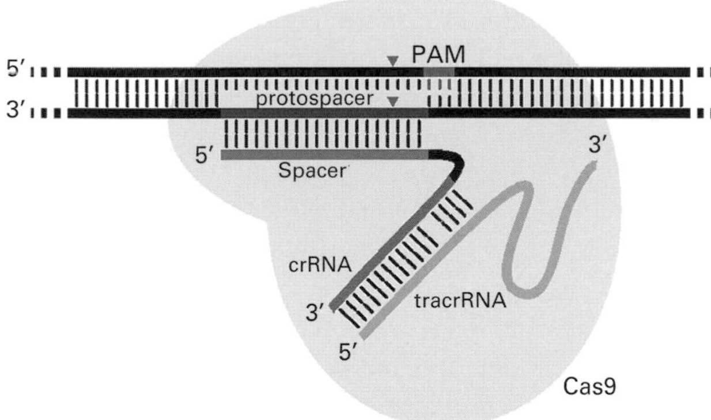

Figure 24.8 General principle of the CRISPR–Cas9 endonuclease system. The Cas9 endonuclease (grey shadow) is guided by two CRISPR RNA molecules, the targeting crRNA and the trans-activating tracrRNA. Both these RNAs have a region of complementarity and anneal to direct the endonuclease towards a 20-nucleotide protospacer region in the targeted DNA that is complementary to the spacer region. The only constraint for the endonuclease to perform a double-stranded cut in the DNA (at the triangles) is the essential presence of a short protospacer adjacent motif (PAM) that varies depending on the bacterial species from which the Cas9 enzyme originates. The crRNA and the tracrRNA can be transcribed *in vivo* from different promoters, or they can be engineered to be transcribed as a single, chimeric guide RNA (gRNA).

This genetic editing system has been engineered to allow the generation of double-strand breaks in DNA at specific places *in vivo*, instead of *in vitro* with purified DNA, and with high specificity. The additional advantage over the classic site-specific restriction enzymes described earlier is that this system can be targeted towards desired sites in the chromosome. Dedicated vectors that express genes encoding different Cas9 endonucleases and transcribe the tracrRNA and engineered crRNA separately or jointly are now commercially available, with a number of possible variations. For example, one of the limitations of using a Cas9 endonuclease from a particular organism is the requirement for a specific short protospacer adjacent motif (PAM). The Cas9 endonuclease from *Streptococcus pyogenes*, one of the most commonly used, requires the sequence NGG (with N being any nucleotide) immediately downstream of the targeted protospacer sequence to perform the double-stranded cuts. Hence, vectors producing Cas9 endonucleases from different bacteria and with different PAM requirements are commercially available to circumvent this limitation and expand the possibilities. Vectors to facilitate the insertion of spacer sequences and that transcribe the tracrRNA and engineered crRNA as a single 'guide RNA' (gRNA) are also available, with the advantage of reducing the number of elements required to achieve an efficient and well-targeted endonuclease activity.

24.2.8.2 Chromosomal DNA Deletions, Insertions and Allelic Replacements

Relatively large chromosomal deletions, as long as essential genes are not removed, can be achieved by simultaneously targeting the CRISPR–Cas9 endonuclease to two sites flanking the deletion to be made (Figure 24.9). After the double-stranded DNA cuts have been made, the DNA-repair machinery of the cell will join the resulting extremities by non-homologous end-joining (NHEJ, Figure 24.9), with a high probability of losing the fragment cut out. This can sometimes lead to the repair machinery deleting further DNA than initially intended, in a rather uncontrolled way. To circumvent this, double-stranded DNA having complementarity to the ends to be joined can be introduced into the cells at the time of inducing the CRISPR–Cas9 cuts; DNA repair recombinases will then use the DNA provided to repair both ends by homology-directed repair (HDR, Figure 24.9). The DNA with homology arms provided can be made to internally carry a functional gene, like an antibiotic-resistance marker to facilitate the selection of successful recombinants, or if a gene was deleted, a replacement with a different allele can be carried out.

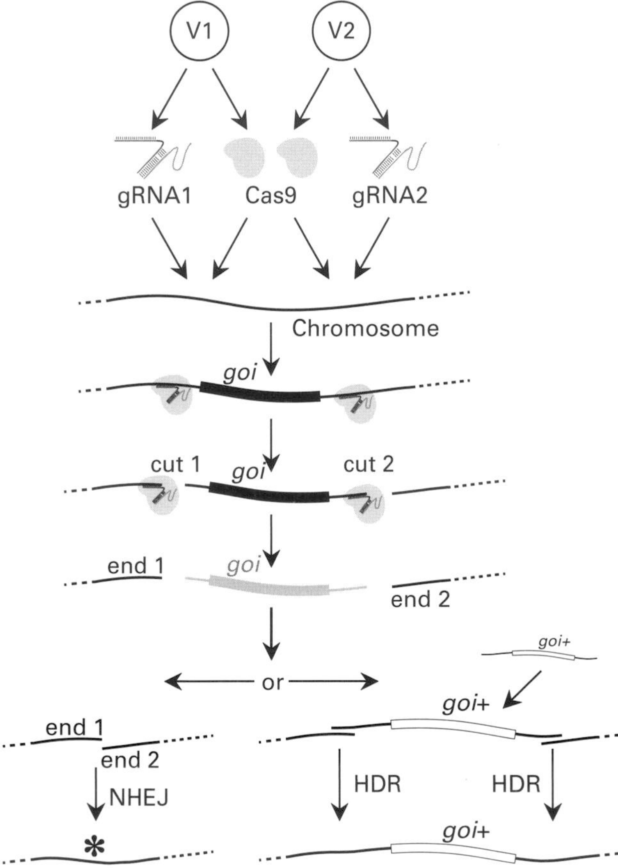

Figure 24.9 Genome editing *in vivo* using CRISPR–Cas9. The CRISPR–Cas9 endonuclease system is engineered to target two sites in the genome, flanking a region that is to be deleted, or replaced by a different DNA fragment. In this example, two vectors are introduced in the targeted cells, V1 transcribing gRNA1 which is targeted towards one site at one side of the chromosomal gene of interest (*goi*), and V2 transcribing the other gRNA2 targeting the second site, at the other side of *goi*. Both vectors can also encode the Cas9 endonuclease, which after interacting with the two gRNAs binds to the corresponding target sites and operates two double-stranded cuts. Once the double strand cuts happen, the small excised fragment is subsequently degraded and lost. From this point, the DNA repair machinery of the cell will perform a non-homologous end-joining (NHEJ) between the two ends, resulting ultimately in the deletion of *goi* and the creation of a molecular scar (*). However, if a DNA fragment having at its extremities regions of homology to the ends is provided at the time of cutting, homology-directed repair (HDR) can happen, providing a directed way to perform the repair and enabling the possibility to introduce alternative DNA and genes (e.g., *goi+*) between the ends.

24.2.8.3 Applications of CRISPR–Cas9 to Biotechnology and the Clinic

Using CRISPR–Cas9 as a tool to genetically engineer microorganisms is hard to justify in species for which numerous and efficient tools have already been developed. Additionally, many bacteria appear to lack the NHEJ mechanism, implying that additional DNA fragments have to be provided to carry out HDR. However, for species for which genetic engineering tools have not yet been developed, or in species where classical methods are long and inefficient, the CRISPR–Cas9 system offers a very attractive solution. This has been the case for example to improve the production of antimycin and candicidin in *Streptomyces albus*, or the production of oxytetracycline in *Streptomyces rimosus*, to enhance the production of the anti-diabetes drug acarbose in *Actinoplanes* spp., or to generate new exopolysaccharides in *Paenibacillus polymyxa*. The discovery of genes required for the production of new antimicrobials such as formicamycins from *Streptomyces formicae*, showdomycin in *Streptomyces showdoensis* or novel polyketides in *Streptomyces viridochromogenes* has also been greatly facilitated by the use of CRISPR–Cas9. NHEJ and HDR DNA-repair mechanisms are almost universal, making the CRISPR–Cas9 approach potentially usable in all living organisms, including in eukaryotes, and potentially, in the near future, in humans. In the laboratory, different approaches to treat various types of cancers, or cure genetic defects like those causing cystic fibrosis, have already generated excellent results using CRISPR–Cas9 approaches *ex vivo*, so this technology appears to have a promising future.

24.3 Biotechnology in the Pharmaceutical Industry

One of the first and most important commercial applications of genetic engineering was the introduction of genes coding for clinically important proteins into bacteria. Because bacterial cells are cheap to grow on a large scale in fermenters, they can synthesise vast amounts of protein from the recombinant genes they carry. This results in a significant reduction in cost and an increase in the availability of these proteins. There are currently a large number of important recombinant drugs available on the market, examples of which are provided in Table 24.5. This section will cover the genetic manipulation strategies used to produce some of the better known of these drugs.

24.3.1 Recombinant Human Insulin

Recombinant human insulin, used for the treatment of diabetes, was the first drug produced using genetic engineering in 1982. Before this, animals and notably pigs and cattle were the only non-human sources of insulin. Animal insulin differs slightly from the human form and, consequently, it can potentially elicit an immune response against it in humans making it ineffective. Importantly also, the use of recombinant human insulin prevents the risks arising from potential contamination of animal insulin with other hormones or viruses. To understand how insulin is produced using recombinant DNA techniques, we first need to review its structure. Figure 24.10 illustrates how insulin is initially synthesised as preproinsulin, a single polypeptide which is processed during export into proinsulin and finally into active insulin, once proteolytic cleavage of the connecting sequence for the two A and B insulin chains has occurred. These two chains remain joined through disulphide bonds.

Currently, different approaches are employed to produce recombinant insulin, one of which is shown in Figure 24.10. Firstly, two DNA fragments coding for the A or the B insulin chains are synthesised chemically. Each of these synthetic fragments is then individually inserted into a plasmid after the *E. coli* gene coding for β-galactosidase. This enables this bacterium to produce large fusion proteins with the insulin chains tacked onto the end of the β-galactosidase enzyme. These fusion proteins can then be purified from bacterial extracts and the insulin chains released upon treatment with cyanogen bromide, which cleaves peptide bonds following methionine residues. As methionine was inserted at the boundaries between the β-galactosidase and the insulin chains, and there is no methionine present internally within the insulin molecule, treatment with cyanogen bromide results in the cleavage of intact insulin chains from the fusion proteins. The purified A and B insulin chains can be mixed and reconstituted into an active insulin molecule. Currently there are also other methods used to produce recombinant insulin which are based on the generation of single β-galactosidase fusions to the full-length insulin gene containing the coding sequences for both A and B chains. These alternative methods can simplify the manufacture of this drug.

24.3.2 Recombinant Somatostatin

Somatostatin, also known as the 'antigrowth hormone', modulates the action of the growth hormone and is frequently used to treat acromegaly (uncontrolled bone growth). Being a very small peptide, the gene coding for it can be easily chemically synthesised and cloned into a suitable expression vector. As *E. coli* tends to degrade small peptides, the generation of a β-galactosidase–somatostatin fusion protein prevents this degradation. Furthermore, as with insulin, the absence of methionine residues in the somatostatin amino acid sequence allows the insertion of a methionine codon in the junction between β-galactosidase and the somatostatin gene. This enables the subsequent cleavage with cyanogen bromide of the recombinant hormone purified from *E. coli*. The strategy used to generate recombinant somatostatin is shown in Figure 24.11.

24.3.3 Recombinant Somatotropin

Somatotropin, also known as the 'human growth hormone' (hGH), consists of 191 amino acids; hGH is produced in the pituitary gland and regulates growth and development. Regular injections of hGH are given to children with dwarfism caused by the lack of this hormone so that they can reach near normal heights. In this case, unlike insulin, animal-derived hormones are ineffective and only the human protein works. Because of continuous shortages of pituitaries from human cadavers, the production of recombinant hGH has been imperative. Furthermore, the infection of children with fatal viruses from cadavers has been an additional reason for moving away from this source of hormone. When recombinant hGH was first produced, the gene for the hGH, which is 573-bp long, was found in practice to be too large to be synthetically produced to generate the recombinant hormone in the manner that was achieved with insulin and somatostatin. Two alternative practical approaches for generating recombinant hGH were therefore used, one of which resulted in the formation of this hormone with an added methionine at the *N*-terminus; Figure 24.12 shows these two strategies.

Initially, the coding region for hGH was isolated from a cDNA library. The DNA fragment coding for the mammalian signal peptide can then be excised by a restriction enzyme that also removes the first 24 codons of the mature protein. A chemically synthesised DNA fragment containing a methionine codon, to enable translation in *E. coli*, followed by these first 24 codons was therefore ligated to the DNA fragment coding for the remaining amino acids

Table 24.5 Examples of some commercial clinically important recombinant proteins.

Protein	Size/structure	Commercial names/company	Expression host	Application
Human insulin	Two peptide chains: A = 21 amino acids B = 30 amino acids	Humulin (Eli Lilly) Humalog (Eli Lilly) Novolin (Novo Nordisk)	*E. coli*	Treatment of diabetes mellitus
Human somatotropin	191 amino acids	Protropin (Genentech) Genotropin (Pharmacia & Upjohn) Humatrope (Eli Lilly) Nutropin (Genetech) Biotropin (Bio-Technology General)	*E. coli*	Treatment of human growth hormone deficiency in children
Interferon α_{2a} and α_{2b}	166 amino acids	Roferon A (Hoffmann-La Roche) Actimmune (Genentech)	*E. coli*	Treatment of various cancers and viral diseases
Interferon γ_{1b}	143 amino acids – glycosylated	Actimmune (Genentech)	*E. coli*	Treatment of chronic granulomatous disease
Tissue plasminogen activator	530 amino acids – glycosylated	Activase (Genentech)	*E. coli* Yeast Animal cells	Treatment of acute myocardial infarction and pulmonary embolism
Interleukin-2	133 amino acids	Proleukin (Chiron Corporation)	*E. coli* Animal cells	Treatment of kidney carcinoma and metastatic melanoma
Human serum albumin	582 amino acids with 17 disulphide bridges	Albutein (Alpha Therapeutic Corporation)	Yeast	Treatment of hypovolaemic shock Adjunct in haemodialysis
Factor VIII	2332 amino acids – glycosylated	Recombinate (Hyland Immuno) Kogenate (Bayer) ReFacto (Wyeth)	Mammalian cells	Treatment of haemophilia
Factor IX	415 amino acids – glycosylated	BeneFIX (Hyland Immuno)	Mammalian cells	Treatment of haemophilia B
Erythropoietin	166 amino acids – glycosylated	Eprex (Janssen-Cilag) NeoRecormon (Roche)	Mammalian cells	Treatment of anaemia associated with dialysis and azidothymidine (AZT) treatment of AIDS
Hepatitis B surface antigen	Monomer consisting of 226 amino acids	Engerix B (SmithKline Beecham) HB-Vax II (Aventis Pasteur)	Yeast Mammalian cells	Vaccination
Influenza virus hemagglutinin	547 amino acids glycosylated monomer	FluBlok (Protein Sciences Corporation)	Insect cells	Vaccination
SARS-CoV-2 spike glycoprotein	Full-length, 1273 amino acids	NVX-CoV2373 (Novavax)	Insect cells	Vaccination
	Modified mRNA (modRNA) encoding engineered spike protein	Comirnaty (Pfizer–BioNTech) Spikevax (Moderna)	*in vitro* transcription from DNA assembled in *E. coli*	Vaccination, translation of the modRNA happens in human cells

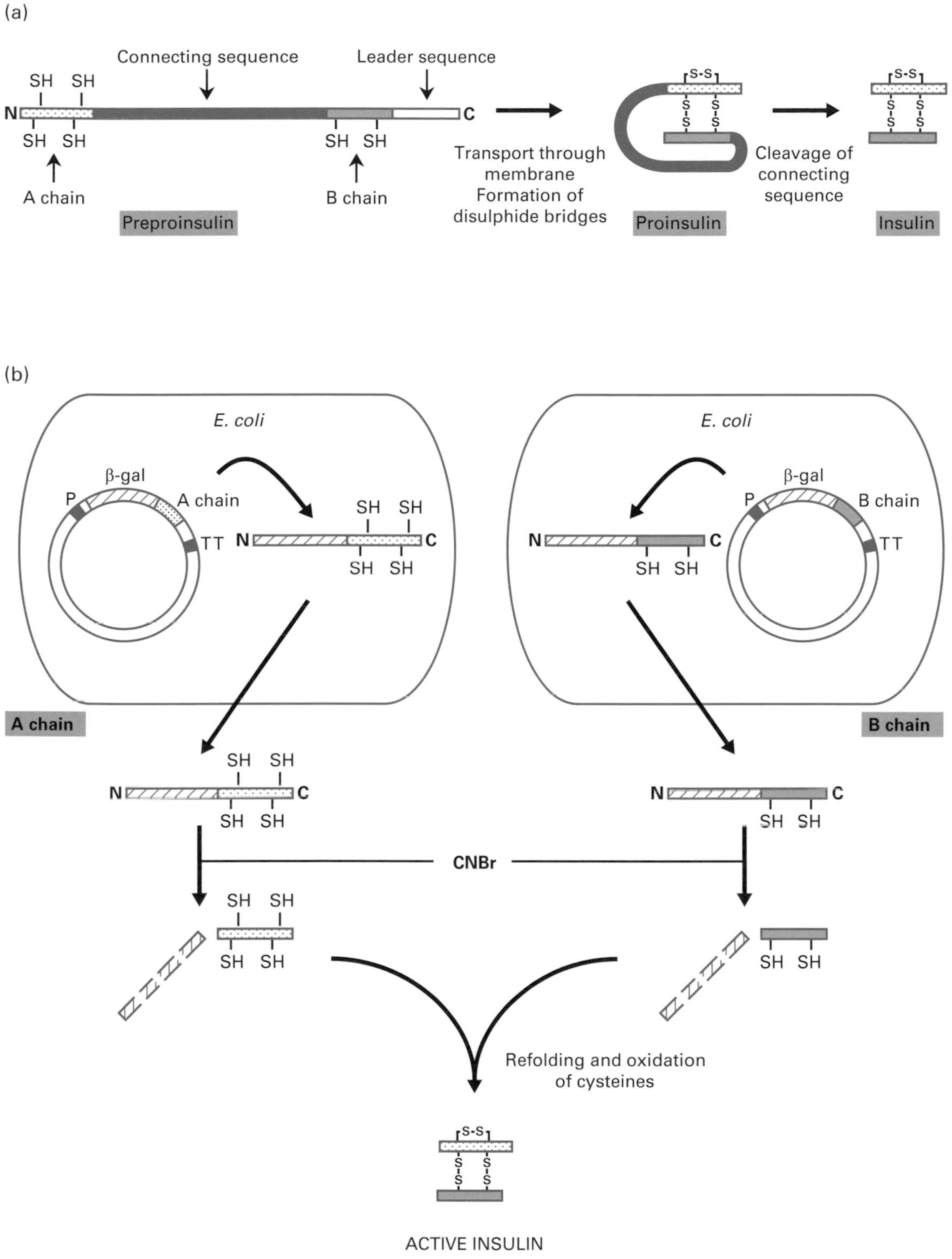

(a)

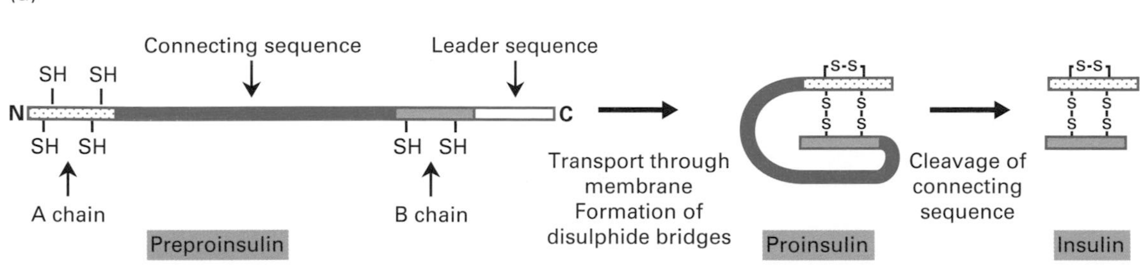

(b)

Figure 24.10 Production of recombinant insulin. (a) Insulin consists of two polypeptide chains (chains A and B). It is initially synthesised as part of a larger peptide called *preproinsulin*. The transport across the cell membrane of preproinsulin results in the cleavage of the signal peptide and the formation of disulphide bridges to generate *proinsulin*. Finally, the connecting peptide is cleaved generating the mature insulin. (b) One of the strategies used to make recombinant insulin comprises the cloning of the DNA fragment coding for the A chain and the B chain into two separate expression vectors as β-galactosidase (β-gal) fusions in *E. coli*. The fusion proteins are then purified and the insulin is cleaved with cyanogen bromide (CNBr) after a methionine incorporated at the β-galactosidase and insulin junction. The presence of several methionines in the β-galactosidase results in multiple cleavage of this molecule by CNBr. Finally, the resulting insulin A and B chains are refolded and the cysteines are oxidised for the generation of the active insulin.

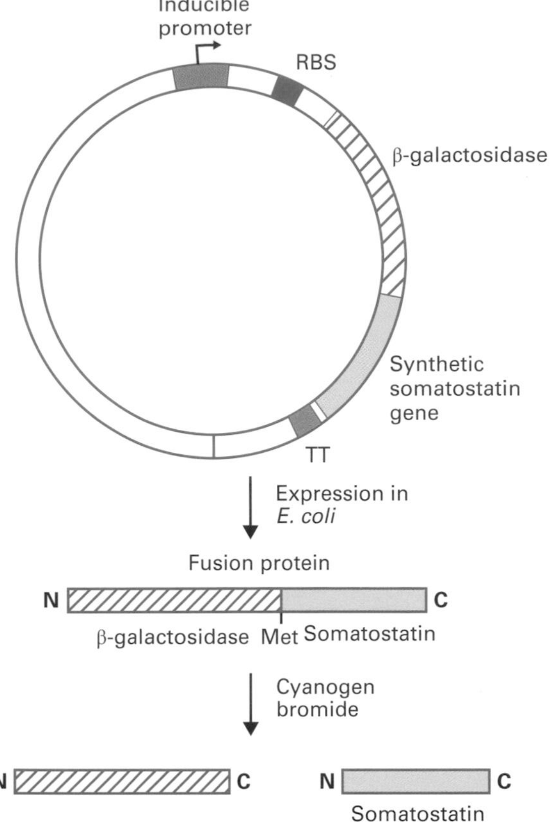

Figure 24.11 Production of recombinant somatostatin. The small size of somatostatin allows the chemical synthesis of the gene coding for it. This gene can be cloned into an expression vector and fused to the β-galactosidase gene. The fusion protein generated in *E. coli* is then purified and the somatostatin polypeptide is released by treatment with cyanogen bromide. RBS, ribosome-binding site; TT, transcriptional terminator; Met, methionine.

24–191 of the hGH (Figure 24.12a). The resulting DNA was cloned into an expression vector and transformed into *E. coli* where the recombinant hGH accumulated in the cytoplasm. The recombinant hormone can be isolated from bacterial cell extracts and, in contrast to the non-recombinant protein, carries a methionine residue at the *N*-terminus.

Figure 24.12b shows an alternative method consisting of the replacement of the mammalian signal peptide for a secretion signal peptide functional in bacteria. This enables the purification of the recombinant hGH from the periplasm of the bacterial cell, reducing the difficulties associated with the purification of recombinant proteins from the cytoplasm. To achieve this, once the mammalian signal peptide has been removed as above, a synthetic DNA molecule containing the missing 24 codons of the hGH, without an added methionine codon, is ligated to the DNA fragment coding for the 24–191 remaining residues. The resulting DNA molecule is then inserted in an expression vector that codes for a bacterial signal peptide in fusion with the hGH gene. Once transformed into *E. coli*, the recombinant hGH is produced and the signal sequence will target the protein for secretion into the periplasmic space where it will accumulate. The periplasmic proteases release the signal peptide, leaving hGH without additional amino acids. The protein can then be easily purified from the periplasmic space after release by hypotonic disruption of the outer membrane.

Progress made over the years on the techniques used to manufacture synthetic DNA enables now the production of much larger DNA fragments, simplifying the cloning steps required to generate large recombinant proteins.

24.3.4 Recombinant Hepatitis B Vaccine

Before the development of recombinant DNA technology, there were two main strategies employed for vaccine production: the generation of *inactivated vaccines* consisting of chemically killed derivatives of the infectious agent, and *attenuated vaccines*, which are altered viruses and bacteria that are avirulent and can no longer cause disease (see Chapter 10). However, these first-generation vaccines can be potentially dangerous, as they could be contaminated with infectious organisms or might revert to a virulent form. To avoid these problems, recombinant DNA technology has enabled the production of *subunit vaccines* consisting solely of immunogenic surface proteins which can elicit immune responses without the risk of infection.

The hepatitis B virus (HBV) vaccine was the first successful subunit vaccine developed. This virus infects the liver and can cause serious damage. It has a surface antigen HBsAg which is found in the blood of infected patients and has been shown to elicit a significant immune response. The gene coding for this antigen has been isolated from the virus and cloned into a vector that allows it to be highly expressed in yeast cells. Figure 24.13 shows the widely employed strategy currently used for the production of the second-generation HBV vaccine. In this case, since the 3.2-kb genomic sequence of the HBV virus is known, the gene coding for the HBsAg has been directly cloned into a shuttle expression vector that replicates in both *E. coli* for the genetic manipulation steps and in yeasts such as *Saccharomyces cerevisiae* for the production of the recombinant antigen. Transcription of the gene encoding HBsAg is driven from a strong yeast promoter and is stopped by a transcriptional terminator present in the vector. The vector also has a leucine biosynthesis marker for selection in yeasts and a tetracycline resistance marker for selection in bacteria. The yeast harbouring this plasmid can grow in

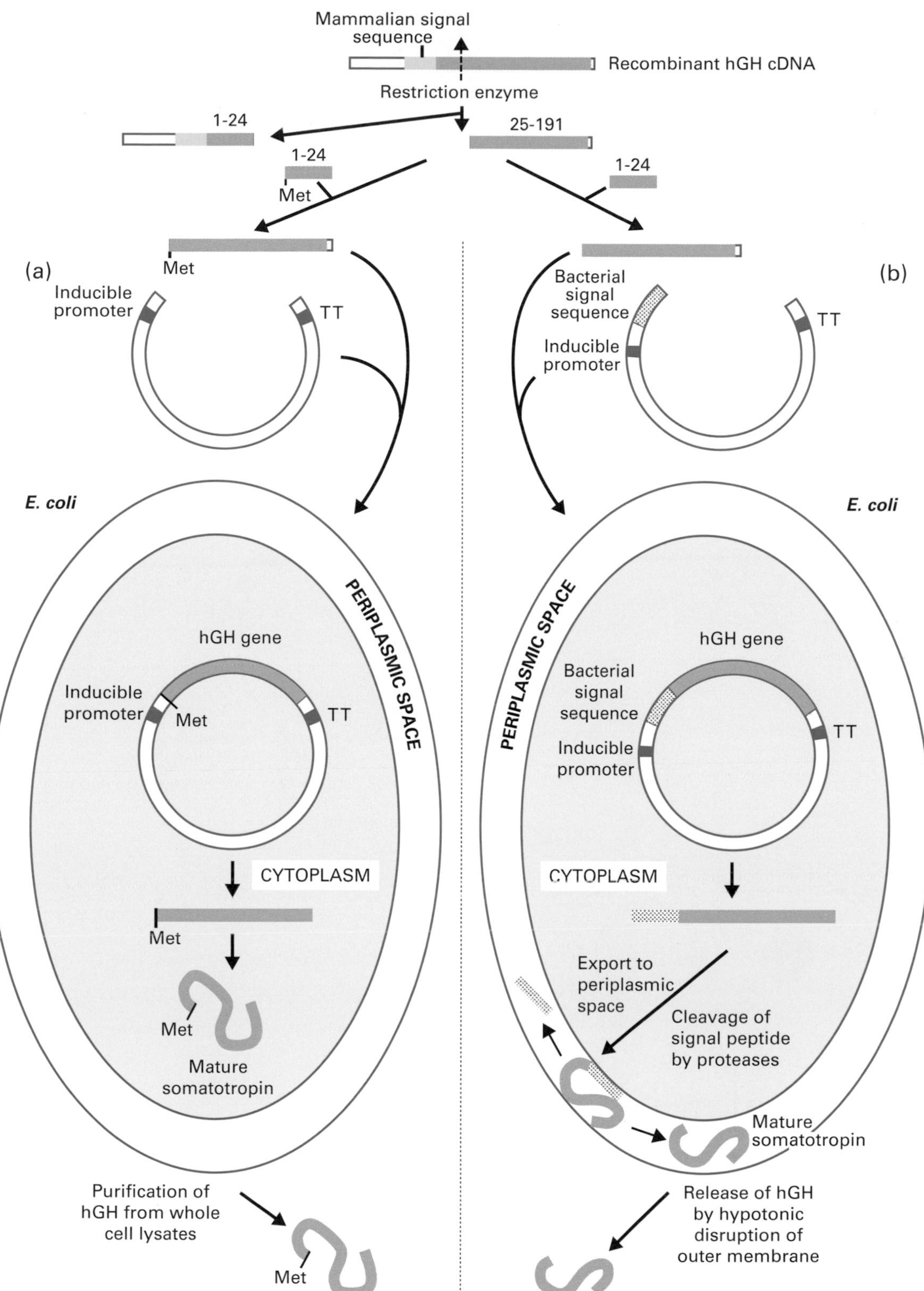

Figure 24.12 Two strategies to produce recombinant human growth hormone (hGH). These two strategies use as the starting material the recombinant cDNA for hGH which contains the mammalian signal sequence required for the secretion of this protein from mammalian cells. This signal peptide is first removed using a restriction enzyme that cleaves after the nucleotides coding for the first 24 amino acids of the hGH. From this stage, two strategies can be followed. (a) A chemically synthesised fragment containing the genetic information for the first 24 amino acids of the hGH, plus a methionine codon in the 5′ end, is ligated to the remaining cDNA fragment coding for amino acids 25–191 and introduced into an expression vector. The hGH produced from this vector in *E. coli* accumulates in the cytoplasm and is extracted from whole-cell lysates. (b) A chemically synthesised fragment also containing the genetic information for the first 24 amino acids of the hGH, but without an added methionine codon, is ligated to the remaining cDNA fragment and cloned into an expression vector immediately after the sequence for a bacterial signal peptide. Consequently, when produced in *E. coli*, the hGH is tagged on its *N*-terminus with this signal peptide that drives the export of this protein to the periplasm. Once in the periplasm, the signal peptide is cleaved by proteases and the mature hGH can be released and purified upon hypotonic disruption of the outer membrane. cDNA, complementary DNA; TT, transcriptional terminator; Met, methionine.

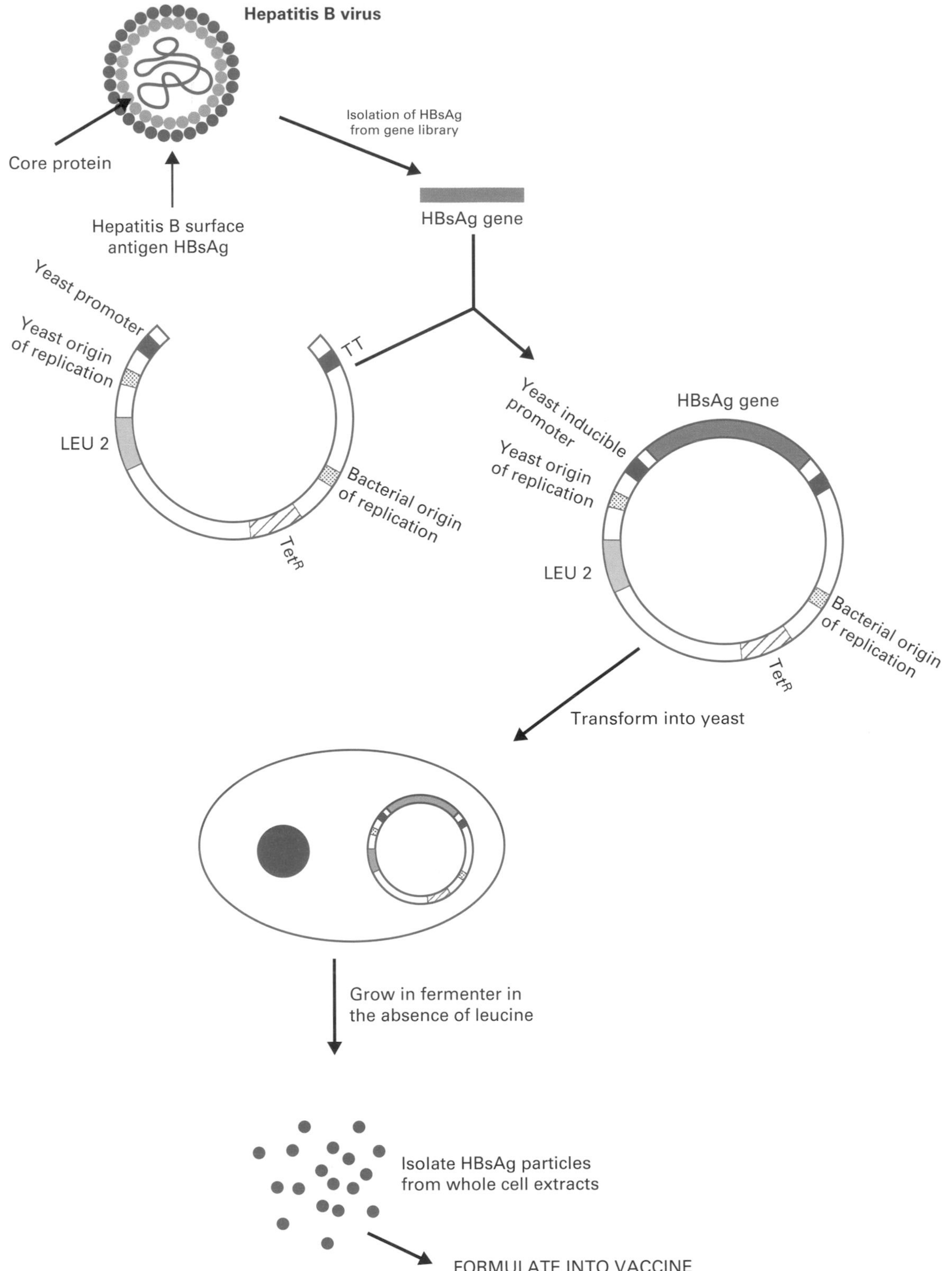

Figure 24.13 Production of hepatitis B subunit vaccine. The gene for the hepatitis B surface antigen (HBsAg) was isolated from a genomic library and cloned into a shuttle vector that promotes high expression levels of this gene in yeast cells. The presence of a leucine biosynthesis (LEU2) marker allows the selection of yeasts containing this plasmid by growing them in the absence of leucine. Recombinant yeast cells producing the HBsAg are grown in large fermenters and the antigen is purified from whole-cell extracts for further formulation into the hepatitis B subunit vaccine. TT, transcriptional terminator; Tet^R, tetracycline resistance marker.

fermenters in the absence of leucine, generating large amounts of the antigen that can be subsequently extracted from the cells.

24.3.5 Recombinant Influenza and Coronavirus Vaccines

Influenza virus types A, B and C cause flu in mammals and birds. The influenza virus type A has been the cause of several pandemics in the past causing the deaths of millions of people. Its 13.6-kb genome consists of 8 single-stranded linear RNA molecules that code for 11 proteins. Due to the segmented nature of its genome, alleles can easily be swapped between different influenza virus strains during the co-infection of a host. This makes the virus extremely adaptable and able to escape the immune system by rapidly acquiring novel combinations of its immunogenic proteins. Two of these proteins are located on the surface of the viral particles and define their antigenicity: a hemagglutinin (H or HA) and a neuraminidase (N or NA). To date, there are 18 different H antigens (H1 to H18) and 11 different N antigens (N1 to N11) known, thus the influenza A viruses are classified accordingly as H1N1 (*swine flu* or *Spanish flu*), H5N1 (*bird flu*) and H7N7 (*horse flu*), for example. *Seasonal flu* recurs annually and since 2003 it is caused mostly by variants of the H3N2, H1N1 and influenza B viruses, the exact types changing over time alongside developing acquired resistances throughout the human population by exposure and vaccinations. Therefore, the evolving prevalence of the different serotypes is constantly being monitored with the aim of anticipating the serotype composition of potential pandemic influenza viruses. Due to the short time frame between the identification of a novel strain and the need for a vaccine against it, recombinant biotechnology is essential. As the hemagglutinin is the most rapidly evolving gene product and is crucial for viral attachment and evasion from the immune system, recombinant influenza virus vaccines are developed using the gene coding this protein. To achieve this, firstly the RNA is converted into double-stranded cDNA, cloned and then sequenced. This allows the complete identification and genotyping of the virus. Secondly, the gene coding for the hemagglutinin is subcloned into a bacmid expression vector and the recombinant glycoprotein (rHA) is produced in large quantities by transfecting *Spodoptera frugiperda* insect cells growing in fermenters as for the hepatitis B vaccine.

The severe acute respiratory syndrome coronavirus 2 (SARS-CoV-2) appeared towards the end of 2019 and caused a global pandemic (COVID-19) that infected millions across the world in less than a year and caused more than six million reported deaths (see Chapter 5). Very rapidly, bacmids similar to those developed to produce influenza viruses were engineered to express the SARS-CoV-2 spike protein gene in insects and produce vaccines against this new virus. At the same time, a new technology based on the production of modified mRNA (modRNA) was used for the first time to produce the antigenic spike protein of the virus directly in the human body (see Chapter 10). For this, the sequence to be transcribed into modRNA, consisting of the protein to be displayed and additional stabilisation and expression sequences, is constructed in a plasmid. The plasmid DNA is then purified from *E. coli*, linearised with an appropriate restriction enzyme and transcribed *in vitro* with T7 RNA polymerase in the presence of artificial nucleotides that substitute for natural ones: for example, N^1-methylpseudouridine and 5-methylcytosine are incorporated during the *in vitro* transcription in place of the usual uridine (alternative base to thymine in RNA) and cytosine, respectively. These substitutions, which do not affect translation into protein, have been found to reduce the immunogenicity and increase the stability of the resulting modRNA when injected intramuscularly. The modRNA is finally embedded into liposomal nanoparticles that enhance its uptake by muscle cells; after being internalised in the cytoplasm it is translated into the desired spike protein which ends up being exposed on the surface of the cells, thereby inducing the desired immune response.

24.3.6 Production of Recombinant Antibiotics

A large number of the antibiotics currently in use have been isolated, at least in template form, from the Gram-positive soil bacterium *Streptomyces*, with many other microorganisms also being used as sources for antibiotics. The biosynthesis of an antibiotic can sometimes utilise 10–30 separate enzyme-catalysed reactions, which makes the cloning of all the genes coding for these enzymes very difficult. A strategy used to isolate the complete set of antibiotic biosynthetic genes consists of the transformation of a recombinant gene library from an organism producing the antibiotic into a mutant strain of the same organism which is incapable of its production. The transformants can then be screened for the production of the antibiotic by plating them onto agar plates that have been seeded with a sensitive bacterium. The appearance of halos of growth inhibition around the recombinant colonies indicates the successful cloning of the antibiotic biosynthetic gene cluster. This strategy was successfully employed for the cloning and production of the antibiotic undecylprodigiosin from *Streptomyces coelicolor* as illustrated in Figure 24.14.

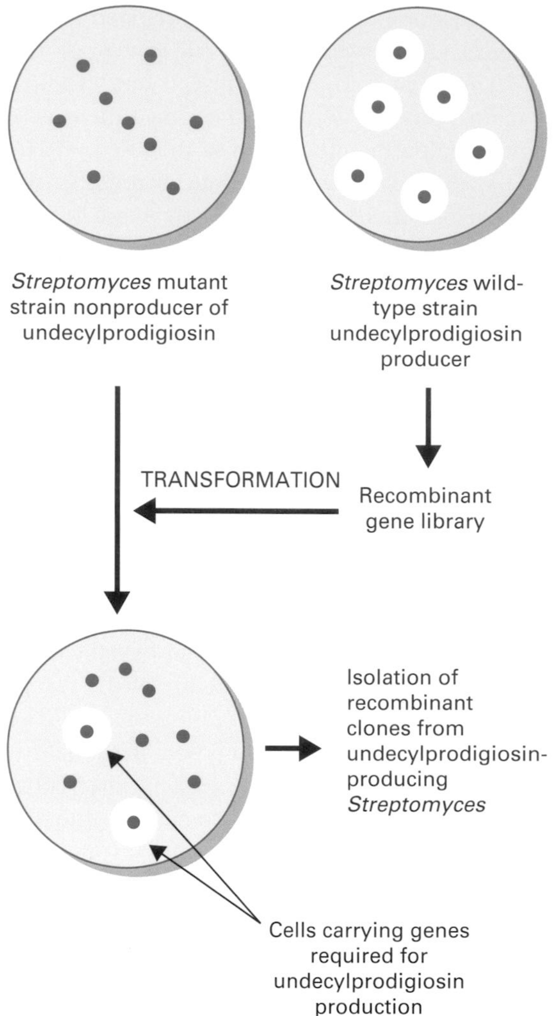

Figure 24.14 Isolation of genes responsible for antibiotic production. For the isolation of the genes required for undecylprodigiosin biosynthesis, a *Streptomyces* strain, unable to make this antibiotic, was transformed with a genomic library from a *Streptomyces* undecylprodigiosin-producing strain. The resulting cells were plated onto agar seeded with a bacterium sensitive to undecylprodigiosin. The recombinant genes required for undecylprodigiosin biosynthesis could be isolated from colonies showing a halo of cell lysis around them resulting from the production of this antibiotic.

In some instances, recombinant DNA technology has been successfully used to generate novel antibiotics by introducing in the same organism the genes responsible for the synthesis of two closely related antibiotics. By cross-feeding antibiotic precursors between two similar metabolic pathways, novel antibiotics can be generated. This strategy has been very successful in the cross-fertilisation of antibiotic pathways between different *Streptomyces* spp.

24.4 New Diagnostics Using Recombinant DNA Technology

For many years, clinical diagnostic laboratories had limitations in the detection of pathogenic bacteria and parasites due to the necessity for their culture prior to identification of these agents; this proved to be a lengthy procedure detrimental to timely diagnosis. In addition, many inherited genetic disorders could not be identified owing to the lack of appropriate techniques and the unavailability of the human genome sequence. The rapid developments in molecular biology have enabled modern medicine to overcome some of these problems. Currently, a good diagnostic test must be *specific* for a target molecule, *sensitive* enough to detect minute levels of that molecule, *rapid* and technically *simple*.

This section will introduce some molecular diagnostic techniques, based on the detection of specific nucleic acid sequences, currently used in the clinic.

24.4.1 Diagnosis of Infectious Diseases

Each pathogenic microorganism contains genetic material that distinguishes it from its host and from other microorganisms. This specific material constitutes a signature that allows the identification of a particular microorganism from a complex mixed population. In the diagnosis of infectious diseases, identification of specific sequences from microbial pathogens will allow appropriate treatment at an early stage as well as prevention of the spread of disease.

The two main techniques used for the diagnosis of infectious disease targeting nucleic acids are hybridisation and PCR-based amplification. There are currently hundreds of approved primers and probes specific for the detection of infectious diseases; Table 24.6 shows just a few examples.

24.4.1.1 DNA Hybridisation Techniques

Nucleic acid hybridisation is based on the precise nucleotide base pairing and hydrogen bonding between one strand of nucleotides and a complementary nucleotide sequence. Any diagnostic nucleic acid hybridisation consists of three essential elements: a DNA probe, the target DNA and the signal detection system. Recent developments in detection systems and improvements in safety have enabled the use of highly sensitive non-radioactive methods. Figure 24.15 illustrates the general steps required for DNA hybridisation using chemiluminescent-based detection. This non-radioactive approach achieves signal amplification by enzymatic conversion of a chemiluminescent substrate. Firstly, DNA from the biological sample

Table 24.6 Examples of infectious diseases currently identified by PCR.

Disease	Causative pathogen
AIDS	Human immunodeficiency virus
Anthrax	*Bacillus anthracis*
Chagas disease	*Trypanosoma cruzi*
Chlamydia	*Chlamydia trachomatis*
Common cold	Adenovirus
Dengue fever	Dengue virus
Food poisoning	*Salmonella typhi*, *Entercoccus faecium*, Enterovirus
Gastritis	*Campylobacter intestinalis*
Gastroenteritis	Enterotoxigenic *Escherichia coli*
Gonorrhoea	*Neisseria gonorrhoeae*
Hepatitis	Hepatitis virus
Herpes	Herpes simplex virus
Hospital-acquired diarrhoea	*Clostridioides difficile*
Malaria	*Plasmodium falciparum*
Plague	*Yersinia pestis*
Q fever	*Coxiella burnetii*
Respiratory failure	*Legionella pneumophila*, influenza virus, coronavirus
Tuberculosis	*Mycobacterium tuberculosis*
Tularemia	*Francisella tularensis*
Whooping cough	*Bordetella pertussis*

including the target DNA from the pathogen to be identified needs to be extracted. A diagnostic biotin-labelled probe is then mixed with the target DNA bound to a membrane support. The hybridised probe is then incubated with streptavidin, which has multiple sites that avidly bind biotin. Subsequent incubation with biotin conjugated to alkaline phosphatase results in the enzymatic labelling of the bound streptavidin. Finally, addition of a special substrate for the alkaline phosphatase results in the conversion of this substrate into a product which emits light and which can be detected after exposure to X-ray films or by using sensitive imaging cameras.

The procedure described above can also be scaled down, automated and redesigned to use thousands of sequence-specific probes at once in what are called *microarrays*. In this case, non-labelled DNA probes are synthesised and minute droplets are spotted at high density onto glass slides where they will remain bound. The DNA from the biological sample is then labelled at the extremities with a fluorescent dye and after denaturation into single strands it is allowed to anneal with the probes bound on the slide. After washing, any labelled DNA fragments which annealed to specific probes are visualised by illuminating the slide with light of the appropriate wavelength to cause the dyes to fluoresce. As microarrays can carry thousands of probes per cm^2, this is performed by automated scanning devices and dedicated software which identifies the probes producing positive signals. This technique allows the screening at once of a very large number of pathogens or defined genetic markers.

24.4.1.2 PCR Amplification Using Fluorescent Primers

As in many other fields, PCR has brought a revolutionary change in nucleic-acid-based diagnosis. In a clinical setting, PCR has many desirable features such as the sensitivity to work with tiny amounts of DNA samples from blood or tissue to achieve a specific and significant amplification of target sequences. Furthermore, the rapidity of this process, as explained previously in this chapter, provides a significant advantage in the early diagnosis and treatment of infectious diseases.

A PCR fluorescence-based technique has been used successfully in the diagnosis of infectious diseases. In this case, the PCR aimed at detecting the desired specific DNA from the infectious microorganism is performed in the presence of a non-fluorescent 'probe' primer containing a fluorogen molecule attached to its 5′ end that will anneal between the two amplifying primers. When the DNA polymerase extends one of the primers and encounters the annealed probe, its 5′ exonuclease activity degrades it and releases its fluorogen-tagged nucleotide, which then becomes fluorescent. The resulting increase in specific fluorescence in the reaction is then measured at each cycle and is interpreted as the presence of target DNA. The earlier the fluorescence is detected in the PCR cycle, the more target DNA there is in the sample. This simple approach is extremely sensitive and has become the gold standard for the rapid testing of large numbers of samples.

The procedure can also be applied to detect specific RNAs, for example, to detect RNA viruses. In this case, the extracted RNA has to be converted first to double-stranded cDNA with reverse transcriptase before the PCR amplification. The procedure is then called reverse transcriptase PCR or RT-PCR.

24.4.2 Diagnosis of Genetic Disorders

The use of new diagnostic techniques has allowed individuals to discover whether they or their offspring are at risk of suffering from specific inherited diseases. DNA analysis using PCR has been used for the identification of carriers

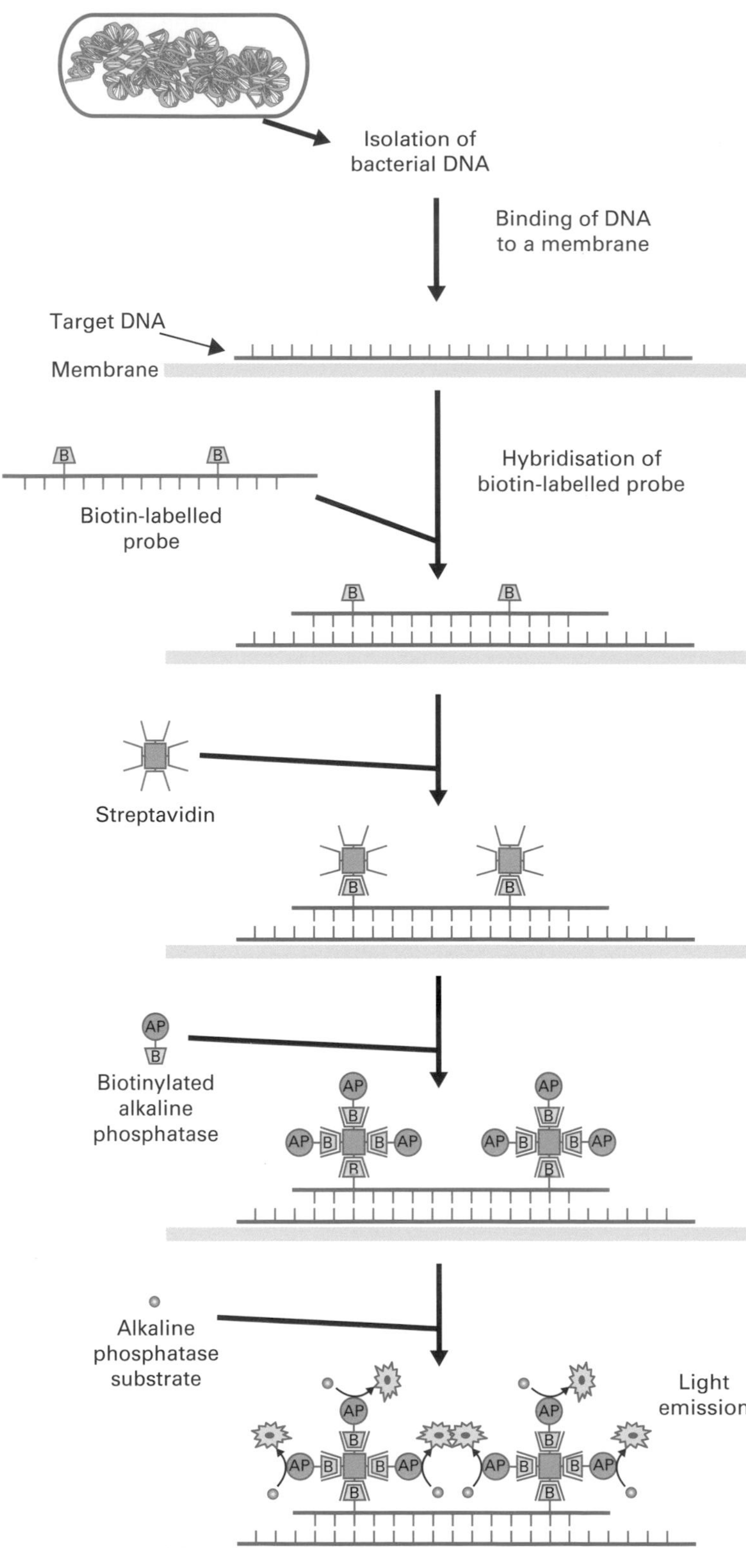

Figure 24.15 Diagnosis using DNA hybridisation with biotin-labelled probes. The DNA from the pathogen to be identified is first purified and bound to a membrane. The membrane is then incubated with a diagnostic biotinylated probe. The biotin from the probe will be recognised by streptavidin which has several biotin-recognition sites. Subsequent incubation with biotin-labelled alkaline phosphatase results in the recognition of the bound streptavidin. As several molecules of biotin-labelled alkaline phosphatase will bind to a single streptavidin molecule, incubation of the membranes with chemiluminescence substrate for this enzyme will lead to an amplified reaction and the generation of light-emitting products.

Table 24.7 Some of the inherited human diseases currently diagnosed by PCR.

α_1-Antitrypsin deficiency	Fabry disease	Maple syrup urine disease
Adenosine deaminase deficiency	Familial hypercholesterolaemia	Phenylketonuria
β- and δ-thalassaemia	Fragile X syndrome	Retinoblastoma
Cancer, various predispositions	Gaucher's disease	Severe combined immunodeficiency disorder
Coagulation factor dysfunctions	Haemophilia A and B	Sickle cell anaemia
Cystic fibrosis	Hereditary thrombophilia	Tay–Sachs disease
Drug-metabolising enzyme defects	Lesch–Nyhan syndrome	Von Willebrand disease

of hereditary disorders, for prenatal diagnosis of deleterious genetic conditions and for the early diagnosis of these disorders before the manifestation of any symptoms. Table 24.7 shows some examples of genetic human disorders that are currently identified by PCR.

The increasing repertoire of genetic disorders that are being catalogued and the development of new methods to modify genes (e.g., using CRISPR–Cas9, Section 24.2.8.3) or to produce desired proteins *in vivo* within human cells (modRNA, Section 24.3.5) will enable future recombinant DNA technology breakthroughs in the development of successful gene therapies against many chronic and acute conditions.

Further Reading

Behera, B.K. (2020). *Biopharmaceuticals: Challenges and Opportunities*, 1e. Boca Raton, FL: CRC Press Taylor & Francis Group.

Crommelin, D.J.A., Sindelar, R.D. and Meibohm, B. (2019). *Pharmaceutical Biotechnology*, 5e. Cham: Springer.

Glick, B.R. and Patten, C.L. (2017). *Molecular Biotechnology: Principles & Applications of Recombinant DNA*, 5e. Washington, DC: American Society for Microbiology Press.

Groves, M.J. (2019). *Pharmaceutical Biotechnology*, 2e. Boca Raton, FL: CRC Press Taylor & Francis Group.

Ho, R.J.Y. and Gibaldi, M. (2013). *Biotechnology and Biopharmaceuticals: Transforming Proteins and Genes into Drugs*, 2e. New York: John Wiley & Sons Ltd.

Hofmann, A. and Clokie, S. (2018). *Wilson and Walker's Principles and Techniques of Biochemistry and Molecular Biology*, 8e. Cambridge University Press.

Madigan, M.T., Bender, K.S., Buckley, D.H. et al. (2017). *Brock Biology of Microorganisms*, 15e. NJ: Pearson Education.

Nelson, D.L. and Cox, M.M. (2021). *Lehninger Principles of Biochemistry*, 8e. New York: W.H. Freeman.

Patra, J.K., Shukla, A.C. and Das, G. (2020). *Advances in Pharmaceutical Biotechnology*, 1e. Singapore: Springer.

Patrinos, G., Ansorge, W. and Danielson, P.B. (2017). *Molecular Diagnostics*, 3e. San Diego, CA: Elsevier Science.

Primrose, S.B. and Twyman, R. (2006). *Principles of Gene Manipulation and Genomics*, 7e. Oxford: Blackwell Publishing Ltd.

Silva, A.C., Moreira, J.N., Sousa Lobo, J.M. and Almeida, H. (2020). *Current Applications of Pharmaceutical Biotechnology*, 1e. Cham: Springer.

Watson, J.D. (2007). *Recombinant DNA: Genes and Genomes, a Short Course*, 3e. New York: W.H. Freeman.

Part 7

Current Trends and New Directions

25

The Wider Contribution of Microbiology to the Pharmaceutical Sciences

Mathew W. Smith[1], James C. Birchall[2], and Sion A. Coulman[3]

[1] *Reader, School of Pharmacy and Pharmaceutical Sciences, Cardiff University, Cardiff, UK*
[2] *Professor of Pharmaceutical Sciences, School of Pharmacy and Pharmaceutical Sciences, Cardiff University, Cardiff, UK*
[3] *Senior Lecturer, School of Pharmacy and Pharmaceutical Sciences, Cardiff University, Cardiff, UK*

CONTENTS

Hugo and Russell's Pharmaceutical Microbiology, Ninth Edition. Edited by Brendan F. Gilmore and Stephen P. Denyer.

Companion website: https://www.wiley.com/go/HugoandRussells9e

25.1 Introduction

There has long been a tendency, particularly in the medical and pharmaceutical fields, to regard microbes as harmful entities to be destroyed. However, as will be described in this chapter, the exploitation of microorganisms and their products has assumed an increasingly prominent role in the diagnosis, treatment and prevention of human diseases. Non-medical uses are also of significance, for example, the use of bacterial spores (*Bacillus thuringiensis*) and viruses (baculoviruses) to control insect pests, the fungus *Sclerotinia sclerotiorum* to kill some common weeds and improved varieties of *Trichoderma harzianum* to protect crops against fungal infections, and these will also be explored.

25.1.1 Early Treatment of Human Disease

The earliest uses of microorganisms to treat human disease can be traced to the belief that the formation of pus in some way drained off noxious humours responsible for systemic diseases. Although the spontaneous appearance of pus in their patients' wounds satisfied most physicians, deliberate contamination of wounds was also practised. Bizarre concoctions of bacteria such as 'ointment of pigs', 'dung' and 'herb sclerata' were particularly favoured during the Middle Ages. Early Central European and South American civilisations cultivated various fungi for application to wounds. In the nineteenth century, sophisticated concepts of microbial antagonism were developed following Pasteur's experiments demonstrating inhibition of anthrax bacteria by 'common bacteria' simultaneously introduced into the same culture medium. Patients suffering with diseases such as diphtheria, tuberculosis and syphilis were treated by deliberate infection with what were then thought to be harmless bacteria such as staphylococci, *Escherichia coli* and lactobacilli. Following their discovery in the early part of the last century, bacterial viruses (bacteriophages) were considered as potential antibacterial agents – an idea that soon fell into disuse but has recently been revived (Chapter 26).

25.1.2 Present-day Exploitation

Some of the most important and widespread uses of microorganisms in the pharmaceutical sciences are in the production of antibiotics and vaccines and the use of microorganisms in the recombinant DNA industry. These are described in Chapters 11, 23 and 24. However, there are a variety of other medicinal agents derived from microorganisms including vitamins, amino acids, dextrans, iron-chelating agents and enzymes. Microorganisms as whole or their subcellular fractions, in suspension or immobilised in an inert matrix, are employed in a variety of assays. Microorganisms have also been used in the pharmaceutical industry to achieve specific modifications of complex drug molecules such as steroids, in situations where synthetic routes are difficult and expensive to carry out, and more recently microorganisms have been employed as platforms for the discovery of novel therapeutic peptides and proteins.

25.2 Pharmaceuticals Produced by Microorganisms

25.2.1 Dextrans

Dextrans are polysaccharides produced by lactic acid bacteria, in particular members of the genus *Leuconostoc* (e.g., *Leuconostoc dextranicus* and *Leuconostoc mesenteroides*), following growth on sucrose. These sugar polymers first came to the attention of industrial microbiologists in sugar refineries where large gummy masses of dextran clogged pipelines. Dextran is essentially a glucose polymer consisting of (1–6)-α-links of high but variable molecular weight (15,000–20,000,000; Figure 25.1). Growth of the dextran-producing strain is carried out in large fermenters using media with a low nitrogen but high carbohydrate content. The average molecular weight of the dextrans produced will vary with the strain used. This is important,

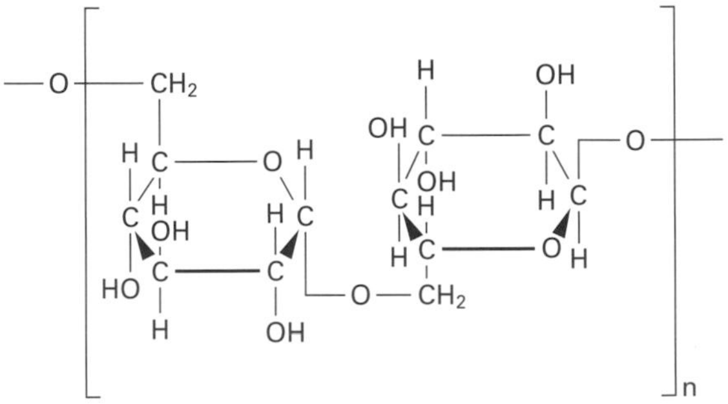

Figure 25.1 Structure of dextran showing (1–6)-α-linkage.

since the laboratory or clinical utility of the dextran is dependent on a defined molecular weight. Two main methods are employed for obtaining dextrans of a suitable molecular weight. The first involves acid hydrolysis of very-high-molecular-weight polymers, while the second uses small preformed dextrans as templates for the polymerisation process. These templates are added to the culture fluid to produce dextrans of shorter chain length. Once formed, dextrans of the required molecular weight are obtained by precipitation with organic solvents prior to formulation.

Dextrans are produced commercially for use as plasma substitutes (plasma expanders), which can be administered by intravenous injection to maintain or restore the blood volume, and for application to ulcerated wounds or to burns where they form a hydrophilic layer that absorbs fluid exudates.

A summary of the properties of the different types of dextrans available is presented in Table 25.1. Dextrans for clinical use as plasma expanders require a molecular weight between 40,000 and 300,000. Polymers below 40,000 molecular weight are excreted too rapidly from the kidneys, while those above 300,000 molecular weight are potentially dangerous because of retention in the body. In practice, infusions containing dextrans of average molecular weights of 40,000, 70,000 and 110,000 are commonly encountered.

Iron dextran injection, containing a complex of iron hydroxide with dextrans of average molecular weight between 5000 and 7000, is used for the treatment of iron-deficiency anaemia in situations where oral therapy is either ineffective or impractical. The sodium salt of sulphuric acid esters of dextran, that is, dextran sodium sulphate, has anticoagulant properties comparable with those of heparin and is formulated as an injection for intravenous use.

25.2.2 Vitamins, Amino Acids and Organic Acids

Several chemicals used in medicinal products are produced by fermentation.

25.2.2.1 Vitamins

Vitamin B_2 (riboflavin), one of the B group vitamins, is present in milk, liver, kidneys, cereals and vegetables, and is also synthesised by intestinal flora in carbohydrate-rich diets. Vitamin B_2 deficiency, although rare, is characterised by symptoms that include an inflamed tongue, dermatitis and injury to the bone marrow. In genuine cases of malnutrition, these symptoms will accompany those induced by

Table 25.1 Properties and uses of dextrans.

Type of dextran[a]	Molecular weight (average)	Product	Sterilisation method	Clinical uses
Dextran 40	40,000	10% w/v in 5% w/v glucose injection or 0.9% w/v sodium chloride injection	Autoclave	IV infusion: improves blood flow and tissue function in burns and conditions associated with local ischaemia
Dextran 70	70,000	6% w/v in 5% w/v glucose injection or 0.9% w/v sodium chloride injection	Autoclave	IV: used to produce an expansion of plasma volume in conditions associated with loss of plasma proteins
Dextran 110	110,000	6% w/v in 5% w/v glucose injection or 0.9% w/v sodium chloride injection	Autoclave	IV: as for dextran 70
Iron dextran	5000–7500 (complex with ferric chloride)	Colloidal solution in 0.9% w/v sodium chloride injection	Autoclave	Deep IM or IV (slow infusion): iron-deficiency anaemia (where oral therapy ineffective or impractical)
Dextran sodium sulphate		Powder for preparing solution	Autoclave	Anticoagulant (intravenous use of solution)
Chemically cross-linked dextrans				Water-insoluble: chromatographic techniques (fractionation and purification)

IV, intravenous; IM, intramuscular.
The current *British Pharmacopoeia* and *British National Formulary* should be consulted for further information, including toxic manifestations.
[a] In the USA, dextran injections with average molecular weights of about 75,000 are also available.

other vitamin deficiencies. Riboflavin is produced commercially in significant yields by the moulds *Eremothecium ashbyii* and *Ashbya gossypii* and some bacteria including genetically engineered *Bacillus subtilis* (Table 25.2).

Pernicious anaemia is a fatal disease first reported in 1880, but it was not until 1926 that it was discovered that eating raw liver effected a remission. The 'anti-pernicious' ingredient was subsequently isolated and called vitamin B_{12} or cyanocobalamin. Vitamin B_{12} was initially obtained from liver but during the 1960s it was determined that it could also be obtained as a by-product of microbial metabolism (Table 25.2). Hydroxycobalamin is the form of choice for therapeutic use and can be derived either by chemical transformation of cyanocobalamin or directly as a fermentation product.

Biotin, formerly known as vitamin H, is now regarded as another member of the vitamin B family and is found in similar food types. Biotin acts as an essential cofactor in chemical reactions that maintain normal metabolic function. It is also an essential growth factor for some bacteria. Its chemical structure was established in the early 1940s and a practical, highly stereospecific, chemical synthesis enabled D-biotin, identical to that found in yeasts and other cells, to be produced.

25.2.2.2 Amino Acids

Amino acids find applications as ingredients of infusion solutions for parenteral nutrition and individually for the treatment of specific conditions. They are obtained either by fermentation processes similar to those used for antibiotics or in cell-free extracts employing enzymes isolated from bacteria (Table 25.2). Details of the many and varied processes reported in the literature will be found in the appropriate references in the 'Further Reading' section at the end of the chapter.

Table 25.2 Examples of vitamins, amino acids, antibiotics and organic acids produced by microorganisms.

Pharmaceutical	Producer organism	Use
Vitamins		
Riboflavin (vitamin B_2)	*Eremothecium ashbyii* *Ashbya gossypii* *Bacillus subtilis*	Treatment of vitamin B_2 deficiency disease
Cyanocobalamin (vitamin B_{12})	*Propionibacterium freudenreichii* *Propionibacterium shermanii* *Pseudomonas denitrificans*	Treatment of pernicious anaemia
Amino acids		Supplementation of feeds/food; intravenous infusion fluid constituents
Glutamate	*Corynebacterium glutamicum*	
Lysine	*Brevibacterium flavum*	
Antibiotics[a]		Antibacterial drugs
Benzylpenicillin	*Penicillium notatum* *Penicillium chrysogenum*	
Gentamicin	*Micromonospora purpurea*	
Nystatin	*Streptomyces noursei*	
Organic acids		
Citric acid	*Aspergillus niger*	Effervescent products; sodium citrate used as an anticoagulant; potassium citrate used to treat cystitis
Lactic acid	*Lactobacillus delbrueckii* *Rhizopus oryzae*	Calcium lactate is a convenient source of Ca^{2+} for oral administration; constituent of intraperitoneal dialysis solutions
Gluconic acid	*Gluconobacter suboxydans* *Aspergillus niger*	Calcium gluconate is a source of Ca^{2+} for oral administration; gluconates are used to render bases more soluble, e.g., chlorhexidine gluconate

[a] For further information, see Chapter 11.

25.2.2.3 Organic Acids

Examples of organic acids (citric, lactic, gluconic) produced by microorganisms, together with pharmaceutical and medical uses, are given in Table 25.2. Citric and lactic acids also have widespread uses in the food and drink and plastics industries. Gluconic acid is also used as a metal-chelating agent in, for example, detergent products.

25.2.3 Iron-chelating Agents

The growth of many microorganisms in iron-deficient growth media results in the secretion of low-molecular-weight iron-chelating agents called siderophores, which are usually phenolate or hydroxamate compounds. The therapeutic potential of these compounds has generated considerable interest. Uncomplicated iron deficiency can be treated with oral preparations of iron (II) (ferrous) sulphate, but such treatment is not without hazard and iron salts remain a common cause of poisoning in children. The accidental consumption of around 3 g of ferrous sulphate by a small child leads to acidosis, coma and heart failure, which, if untreated, are fatal. Desferrioxamine B (Figure 25.2), the deferrated form of a siderophore produced by *Streptomyces pilosus*, is a highly effective antidote for the treatment of acute iron poisoning. Desferrioxamine owes its effectiveness both to its high affinity for ferric iron (its binding constant is in excess of 10^{30}) and because the iron–desferrioxamine complex is highly water-soluble and is readily excreted through the kidneys. In haemolytic anaemias such as thalassaemia, desferrioxamine is used together with blood transfusions to maintain normal blood levels of free iron and haemoglobin. Desferrioxamine is prepared as a sterile powder for use as an injection, but it is also administered orally in acute iron poisoning to remove unabsorbed iron from the gut.

Patients with iron overload disorders treated with desferrioxamine may, however, have increased susceptibility to infections. The important role played by iron availability during infections in vertebrate hosts has only been recognised relatively recently. The ability of the host to withhold growth-essential iron from microbial and, indeed, neoplastic invaders while retaining its own access to this metal has led to suggestions that microbial iron chelators or their semisynthetic derivatives may be of use in antimicrobial and anticancer chemotherapy. Preliminary work has shown some encouraging results. The bacterial siderophores parabactin and compound II secreted by *Paracoccus denitrificans* have been shown to inhibit the growth of leukaemia cells in culture and in experimental animals. They also appear capable of inhibiting the replication of RNA viruses. Siderophores such as desferrioxamine may therefore find increasing applications not only in the treatment of iron poisoning and iron-overloaded disease states but also as chemotherapeutic agents.

25.2.4 Enzymes

Several enzymes have important therapeutic, medical or pharmaceutical uses (Table 25.3). In this section, those enzymes used therapeutically will be described.

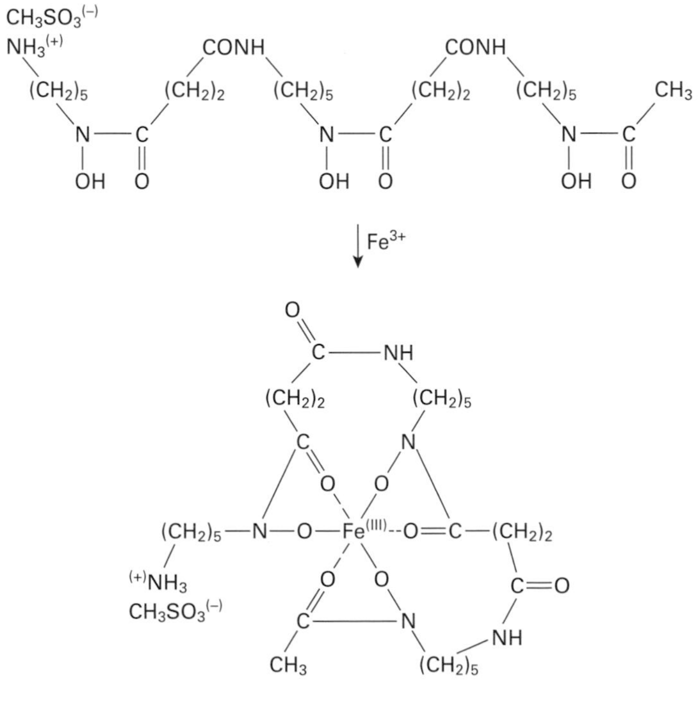

Figure 25.2 Structure of desferrioxamine B and its corresponding iron chelate.

Table 25.3 Clinical uses and other applications of enzymes.

Enzyme	Source	Clinical and/or other use
Streptokinase	Certain streptococcal strains	Liquefying blood clots
Streptodornase	Certain streptococcal strains	Liquefying pus
L-Asparaginase	*Escherichia coli or Erwinia* spp.	Cancer chemotherapy
Neuraminidase	*Vibrio cholerae*	Possible: increase immunogenicity of tumour cells
β-Lactamases	*Bacillus cereus* (or other bacteria, as appropriate)	Sterility testing, treatment of penicillin-induced allergic reaction
Other antibiotic-modifying or antibiotic-inactivating enzymes	Some AGAC-resistant bacteria	Sterility testing, assay
	Some CMP-resistant bacteria	Sterility testing
Glucose oxidase	*Aspergillus niger*	Blood glucose analysis

AGAC, aminoglycoside–aminocyclitol antibiotics (see Chapter 11); CMP, chloramphenicol.

Applications of microbially derived enzymes for antibiotic inactivation in sterility testing and diagnostic assays are discussed in Section 25.5.

25.2.4.1 Streptokinase and Streptodornase

Mammalian blood will clot spontaneously within minutes if allowed to stand, but if left to stand longer the clot begins to dissolve as a result of the action of a proteolytic enzyme called plasmin. Plasmin is normally present as its inactive precursor, plasminogen. Certain strains of streptococci were found to produce a substance that is capable of activating plasminogen (Figure 25.3), a phenomenon that suggested a potential use in liquefying clots, that is, fibrinolysis. This substance, called streptokinase, was isolated and determined to be an enzyme.

Streptokinase is administered by intravenous or intra-arterial infusion in the treatment of thromboembolic disorders, for example, pulmonary embolism, deep vein thrombosis and arterial occlusions. It is also used in emergency medicine for acute myocardial infarction.

A second enzyme, streptodornase, present in streptococcal culture filtrates, was observed to liquefy pus. Streptodornase is a deoxyribonuclease that breaks down deoxyribonucleoprotein and DNA, both constituents of pus, resulting in a reduction in pus viscosity. Streptokinase and streptodornase together have been used to facilitate drainage by liquefying blood clots and/or pus in the chest cavity. The combination can also be applied topically to wounds that have excessive suppuration.

Streptokinase and streptodornase are isolated following growth of non-pathogenic streptococcal producer strains in media containing excess glucose. They are obtained as a crude mixture from the culture filtrate and can be prepared relatively free of each other. They are commercially available as either streptokinase injection or as a combination of streptokinase and streptodornase; streptodornase is not licensed in the UK and newer recombinant agents such as alteplase have largely supplanted their use.

25.2.4.2 L-Asparaginase

L-Asparaginase, an enzyme derived from *E. coli* or *Erwinia chrysanthemi*, converts L-asparagine to aspartic acid and ammonia. In contrast to normal tissue, some tumours have an essential requirement for L-asparagine, and L-asparaginase has therefore been investigated as a selective cancer chemotherapeutic. Although L-asparaginase showed early promise in a variety of experimentally induced tumours, it has primarily found utility in humans for the treatment of acute lymphoblastic leukaemia and occasionally for myeloid leukaemia.

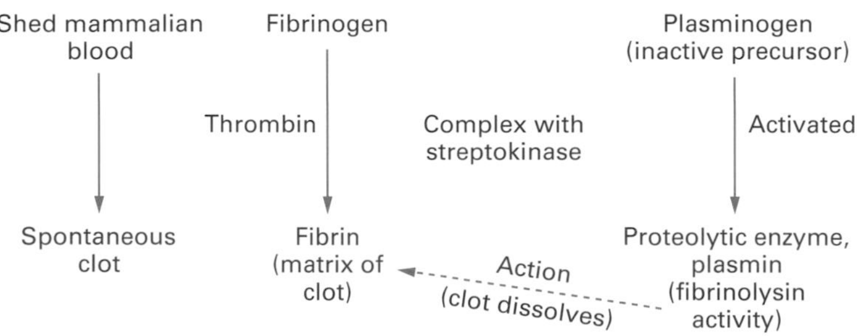

Figure 25.3 Action of streptokinase.

25.2.4.3 Neuraminidase

Many tumours escape immune surveillance through mechanisms including the masking of cell surface antigens by, for example, *N*-acetylneuraminic (sialic) acid residues. Neuraminidase, derived from *Vibrio cholerae*, has been used experimentally to increase the immunogenicity of tumour cells by stripping sialic acid residues from the outer surface of certain tumour cells resulting in presentation of tumour-specific antigens to the host immune system. In laboratory animals, administration of neuraminidase-treated tumour cells was found to be effective against a variety of mouse leukaemias. Preliminary investigations in acute myelocytic leukaemia patients during the 1980s suggested that treatment of tumour cells with neuraminidase in combination with conventional chemotherapy or radiotherapy might increase remission rates. However, despite early promise, broader clinical application has to date not been realised.

25.2.4.4 β-Lactamases

β-Lactamase enzymes, while presenting a considerable therapeutic challenge due to their ability to confer bacterial resistance by inactivating penicillins and cephalosporins (Chapter 13), are nevertheless useful in the sterility testing of certain antibiotics (see Section 25.5.5) and, prior to culture, in inactivating various β-lactams in blood or urine samples in patients undergoing therapy with these drugs. One other important therapeutic application is in the rescue of patients presenting symptoms of a severe allergic reaction following administration of a β-lactamase-sensitive penicillin. In such cases, a highly purified penicillinase obtained from *Bacillus cereus* has been administered either intramuscularly or intravenously and in combination with other supportive measures such as adrenaline and antihistamines.

25.3 Applications of Microorganisms in the Partial Synthesis of Pharmaceuticals

Microorganisms and microbially derived enzymes continue to play a significant role in the production of novel antibiotics. The potential of microorganisms as chemical catalysts, however, was a later development and first realised in the synthesis of industrially important steroids. These reactions assumed increasing importance following the discovery that certain steroids could be formulated as potent therapeutics, for example, hydrocortisone has anti-inflammatory activity, and derivatives of the steroidal sex hormones are useful as oral contraceptive agents. In addition, chiral inversion of non-steroidal anti-inflammatory drugs (NSAIDs) has also been demonstrated, for example, resulting in the formation of optically pure ibuprofen.

25.3.1 Production of Antibiotics

In the antibiotics industry, the hydrolysis of benzylpenicillin to give 6-aminopenicillanic acid by the enzyme penicillin acylase is an important stage in the synthesis of many clinically useful penicillins (Chapter 11). The combination of genetic engineering techniques to produce hybrid microorganisms with significantly higher acylase levels, together with their entrapment in gel matrices, which appears to improve the stability of the hybrids, has resulted in considerable increases in 6-aminopenicillanic acid yields.

A second example is provided by the production by fermentation of cephalosporin C, which is used solely for the subsequent preparation of semisynthetic cephalosporins (Chapter 11).

Furthermore, antibiotics produced by fermentation of various moulds and particularly *Streptomyces* spp. can be utilised by medicinal chemists as starting blocks in the production of what might be more effective antimicrobial compounds.

25.3.2 Steroid Biotransformations

Previously, steroid hormones could only be obtained in small quantities directly from mammals and therefore attempts were made to synthesise them from plant sterols, which can be obtained economically in large quantities. However, adrenocortical steroids are characterised by the presence of an oxygen molecule at position 11 in the steroid nucleus, and although it is relatively easy to hydroxylate a steroidal compound, it is extremely difficult to achieve site-specific hydroxylation, such that many of the routes used for synthesising the desired steroid are lengthy, complex and consequently expensive. This problem was overcome when it was realised that many microorganisms are capable of performing limited oxidations with both stereospecificity and regiospecificity. By simply adding a steroid to growing cultures of the appropriate microorganism, specific site-directed chemical changes can be introduced into the molecule. In 1952, the first commercially employed process involving the conversion of progesterone to 11α-hydroxyprogesterone by the fungus *Rhizopus nigricans* was introduced (Figure 25.4). This reaction is an important stage in the manufacture of cortisone and hydrocortisone from more readily available steroids. Table 25.4 gives several other examples of microbially directed oxidations that have been or are employed in the manufacture of steroidal drugs.

More recently, microorganisms utilised for biotransformation reactions have been immobilised by entrapment in

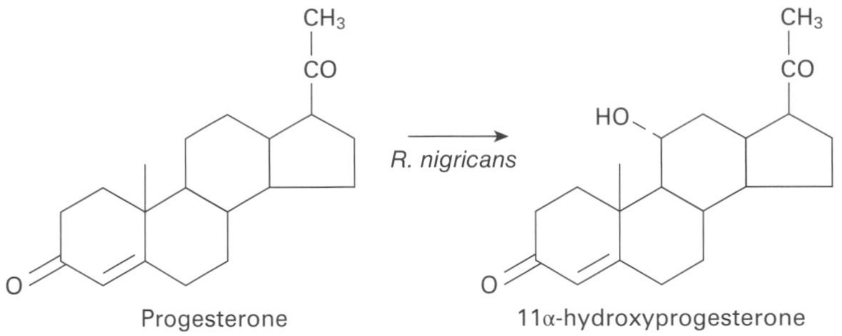

Figure 25.4 Conversion of progesterone to 11α-hydroxyprogesterone by *Rhizopus nigricans*.

Table 25.4 Examples of biological transformations of steroids.

Starting material	Product	Type of reaction
Progesterone	11α-Hydroxyprogesterone	Hydroxylation
Compound S[a]	Hydrocortisone	Hydroxylation
11α-Hydroxyprogesterone	D-11α-Hydroxyprogesterone	Dehydrogenation
Hydrocortisone	Prednisolone	Dehydrogenation
Cortisone	Prednisone	Dehydrogenation

[a] Derived from diosgenin by chemical transformation.

a polymer gel matrix to avoid the often costly and time-consuming enzyme extraction steps that can result in enzyme inactivation. Immobilisation also serves to increase the stability of membrane-associated enzymes that are unstable in the solubilised state, as well as permitting the conversion of water-insoluble compounds such as steroids in two-phase water–organic solvent systems.

25.3.3 Chiral Inversion

Several clinically relevant drugs including salbutamol (a β-adrenoceptor agonist), propranolol (a β-adrenoceptor antagonist) and the 2-arylpropionic acids (NSAIDs) are administered in their racemic form but undergo *in vivo* chiral inversion through metabolic transformations by microorganisms that mimic phase I metabolic processes, that is, functionalisation reactions. For example, the activity of NSAIDs (e.g., ibuprofen) resides almost exclusively in the *S*(+) isomers. However, unidirectional chiral inversion from *R*(−) to *S*(+) (Figure 25.5) occurs *in vivo* over a 3-hour period. The *S*(+) form is a more effective inhibitor of prostaglandin synthesis, and enzymes from some fungal species (e.g., *Verticillium lecanii*) convert a racemic mixture into the *S*(+) isomer *in vitro*. Another example is the biotransformation of ±propranolol to *S*(+) propranolol by *Rhizopus arrhizus* and *Geotrichum candidum* with around 83% efficiency.

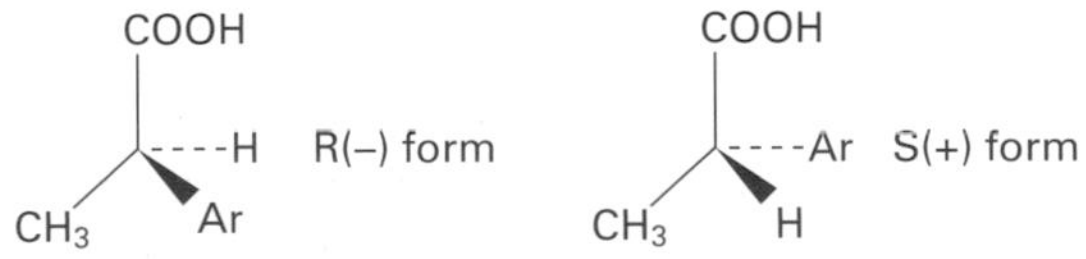

Figure 25.5 Alternative isomeric forms of profens.

25.4 Applications of Microorganisms in the Discovery of Pharmaceuticals

Microbial display platforms expressing recombinant polypeptides (peptides, antibodies, enzymes) on their surface are emerging as invaluable tools for the investigation of protein–protein interactions and can serve as biological combinatorial libraries for the discovery of new therapeutics. To date, three microbial display platforms have been described: phage, bacterial, and yeast displays. All three technologies share the common principle of a direct link between genotype and phenotype affording the identification of the displayed polypeptide by gene sequencing. Of the three technologies described, it is probably phage display that has witnessed the most widespread application.

25.4.1 Phage Display

The filamentous bacteriophage readily accepts relatively large insertions of additional genetic material into its genome, which allows for the display of polypeptides or antibodies as fusions with bacteriophage coat proteins.

Phage libraries containing a repertoire of many billions of viral particles that each display a unique polypeptide sequence or antibody can be subjected to an affinity selection process against a target of interest. Those phage clones that display a polypeptide/antibody that strongly interacts with the target can be recovered and amplified for further rounds of selection before the direct link between genotype and phenotype is exploited to identify the polypeptide/antibody displayed. To date, over 70 antibodies derived in this way have entered clinical trials with more than 10 approved for clinical use. A smaller number of phage-display-derived polypeptides have entered clinical trials or been approved for therapeutic use. For example, DX-88 (Ecallantide, originally Dyax Corp.) is a highly specific and potent inhibitor of kallikrein ($K_i \sim 20$–40 pM) approved for use in the USA in hereditary angioedema. Kallikrein is a key molecule in the regulation of inflammatory and blood clotting processes and plays a role in a number of autoimmune and inflammatory conditions. Romiplostim (Amgen) is an Fc–peptide fusion that acts as an analogue for thrombopoietin and is licensed in the UK for the treatment of chronic immune thrombocytopenic purpura in patients who fail to respond to other treatments including corticosteroids or immunoglobulins.

25.5 Use of Microorganisms and Their Products in Assays

Microorganisms have found widespread uses in bioassays for:

- determining the concentration of compounds (e.g., amino acids, vitamins and some antibiotics) in complex chemical mixtures or in body fluids;
- diagnosing diseases;
- testing chemicals for potential mutagenicity and carcinogenicity;
- monitoring processes involving the use of immobilised enzymes; and
- sterility testing of antibiotics.

25.5.1 Antibiotic Bioassays

Although antibiotics may be assayed by a variety of methods, the following section will only take into consideration microbiological and radioenzymatic assays.

25.5.1.1 Microbiological Assays

In microbiological assays, the response of a growing population of microorganisms to the antimicrobial agent under investigation is measured. The usual methods involve agar diffusion assays in which the drug diffuses into agar seeded with a susceptible microbial population producing a zone of growth inhibition.

In the commonest form of microbiological bioassay used today, samples to be assayed are applied in some form of reservoir (paper disc or well) to a thin layer of agar seeded with indicator organism. The drug diffuses into the medium and after incubation a zone of growth inhibition forms, in this case as a circle around the reservoir. All other factors being constant, the diameter of the zone of inhibition is essentially related to the concentration of antibiotic in the reservoir.

During incubation, the antibiotic diffuses from the reservoir and that part of the microbial population distant to the influence of the antibiotic increases by cell division. The edge of the area of microbial growth is formed when the minimum concentration of antibiotic that will inhibit the growth of the organism on the plate (critical concentration) reaches, for the first time, a population density too great for it to inhibit. The position of the zone edge is thus determined by the initial population density, the growth rate of the organism and the rate of diffusion of the antibiotic.

In situations where the likely concentration range of the tests will lie within a relatively narrow range (e.g., in determining potency of pharmaceutical preparations) and maximal precision is sought, a Latin square design with tests and calibrators at two or three levels of concentration may be used. For example, an 8×8 Latin square can be used to assay three samples and one calibrator, or two samples and two calibrators at two concentrations each (over a twofold or a fourfold range), with a coefficient of variation of around 3%. Using this technique, parallel dose–response lines should be obtained for the calibrators and the tests at the two dilutions (Figure 25.6). Using such a method, potency can be computed or determined from carefully prepared nomograms.

Conventional plate assays require several hours' incubation and consequently the possibility of using rapid microbiological assay methods (see Chapter 3) has been studied. Perhaps the most promising of these uses the firefly luciferase (or similar enzyme) to measure small amounts of adenosine triphosphate (ATP) in a bacterial culture, ATP levels being reduced by the inhibitory action of specific antibiotics. While this may be used to determine antibiotic concentration, it is more likely to be used in antibiotic sensitivity testing.

25.5.1.2 Radioenzymatic (Transferase) Assays

Radioenzymatic assays depend on the fact that bacterial resistance to aminoglycosides, such as gentamicin, tobramycin, amikacin, netilmicin, streptomycin and spectinomycin,

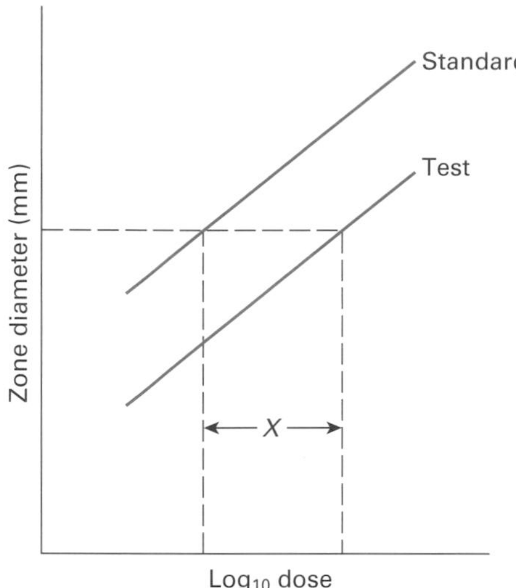

Figure 25.6 Graphical representation of a 2 × 2 assay response. *X* is the horizontal distance between the two lines. The antilog of *X* gives the relative potency of the standard and test.

and chloramphenicol is frequently associated with the presence of specific enzymes (often coded for by transmissible plasmids), which either acetylate, adenylate or phosphorylate the antibiotics, thereby rendering them inactive (Chapter 13). Aminoglycosides may be susceptible to attack by aminoglycoside acetyltransferases (AAC), aminoglycoside adenylyltransferases (AAD)/aminoglycoside nucleotidyl transferases (ANT), or aminoglycoside phosphotransferases (APH). Chloramphenicol is attacked by chloramphenicol acetyltransferases (CAT). Acetyltransferases attack susceptible amino groups and require acetyl coenzyme A, while AAD or APH enzymes attack susceptible hydroxyl groups and require ATP (or another nucleotide triphosphate).

Several AAC and AAD enzymes have been used for assays. The enzyme and the appropriate radio-labelled cofactor ([1-^{14}C] acetyl coenzyme A, or [2-^{3}H] ATP) are used to radiolabel the drug being assayed. The radiolabelled drug is separated from the reaction mixture after the reaction has been allowed to go to completion; the amount of radioactivity extracted is directly proportional to the amount of drug present. Aminoglycosides are usually separated by binding them to phosphocellulose paper, whereas chloramphenicol is usually extracted using an organic solvent.

These types of assays are rapid, taking approximately 2 hours, show good precision and are much more specific than microbiological assays. However, despite the precision and rapidity of radioenzymatic assays, genotypic assays that detect antimicrobial resistance genes or their products are the commercial mainstay for assessing an organism's resistance to antibiotics.

Table 25.5 Some examples of microorganisms that have been used as bioassays for vitamins.

Assay microorganism	Vitamin
Lactobacillus casei	Biotin
Lactobacillus arabinosus	Calcium pantothenate
Lactobacillus leichmannii	Cyanocobalamin
L. casei	Folic acid
Saccharomyces uvarum	Inositol
L. arabinosus	Nicotinic acid
Acetobacter suboxydans	Pantothenol
L. casei	Pyridoxal
Neurospora crassa or Saccharomyces carlsbergensis	Pyridoxine
L. casei	Riboflavin
Lactobacillus viridans	Thiamine

25.5.2 Vitamin and Amino Acid Bioassays

The principle of microbiological bioassays for growth factors such as vitamins and amino acids is quite simple. Unlike antibiotic assays (see Section 25.5.1) that are based on studies of growth inhibition, these assays are based on growth exhibition. All that is required is a culture medium that is nutritionally adequate for the test microorganism in all essential growth factors except the one being assayed. If a range of limiting concentrations of the test substance is added, the growth of the test microorganism will be proportional to the amount added. A calibration curve of concentration of substance being assayed against some parameter of microbial growth, for example, cell dry weight, optical density or acid production, can be plotted. One example of this is the assay for pyridoxine (vitamin B_6), which can be assayed using a pyridoxine-requiring mutant of the mould *Neurospora*. Using elegant study designs, it is possible to assay a variety of different growth factors with a single test organism simply by preparing a basal medium with different growth-limiting nutrients. Table 25.5 summarises some of the vitamin and amino acid microbial bioassays that have found application. In practice, however, high-performance liquid chromatography (HPLC) has replaced bioassays as the method of choice for most amino acids and several B group vitamins; commercially available enzyme-linked immunosorbent assay (ELISA) kits are also employed.

25.5.3 Phenylketonuria Testing

Phenylketonuria (PKU) is an inborn error of metabolism in which the body is unable to convert surplus phenylalanine

(PA) to tyrosine for use in the biosynthesis of, for example, thyroxine, adrenaline and noradrenaline. This results from a deficiency in the liver enzyme phenylalanine 4-monooxygenase (phenylalanine hydroxylase). A secondary metabolic pathway comes into play in which there is a transamination reaction between PA and α-ketoglutaric acid to produce phenylpyruvic acid (PPVA), a ketone and glutamic acid. Overall, PKU may be defined as a genetic defect in PA metabolism such that there are elevated levels of both PA and PPVA in blood and excessive excretion of PPVA (Figure 25.7).

Control of PKU can be achieved simply by resorting to a low-PA-containing diet. However, failure to diagnose PKU will result in cognitive impairment, and thus early diagnosis is essential. In 1968, the UK Medical Research Council Working Party on PKU recommended the adoption of the Guthrie test as a convenient method for screening newborn infants. This assay employs *B. subtilis* as the test organism. In minimal culture medium, growth of this bacterium is inhibited by β-2-thienylalanine (Figure 25.8a) and is competitively reversed in the presence of PA (Figure 25.8b) or PPVA. The use of filter-paper discs impregnated with blood or urine permits the detection of elevated levels of PA and PPVA. The test can be quantified by the measurement of the diameter of the growth zone around the filter-paper disc and comparing it with a calibration curve constructed from known concentrations of PA or PPVA (Figure 25.8c). If positive, the Guthrie test provides presumptive evidence for the presence of PKU which is then confirmed by chemical means. While this bacterial inhibition assay is still in use in laboratories in developing countries, it has been largely superseded in favour of newer

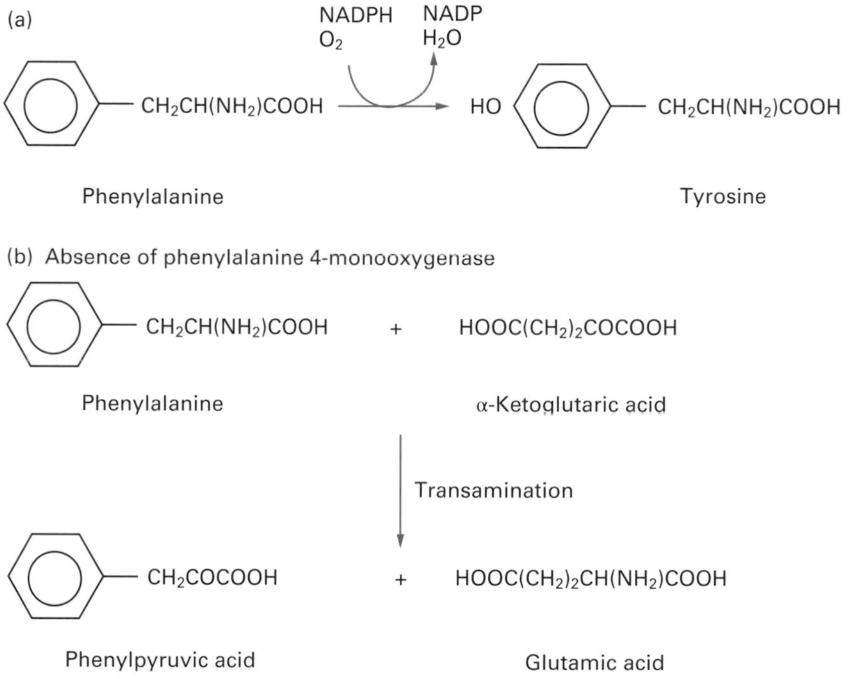

Figure 25.7 (a) Normal metabolism, in which phenylalanine is converted by phenylalanine 4-monooxygenase to tyrosine. (b) Phenylketonuria, in which there is a transamination reaction between phenylalanine and α-ketoglutaric acid. Phenylalanine 4-monooxygenase is absent in about 1 in every 10,000 human beings because of a recessive mutant gene.

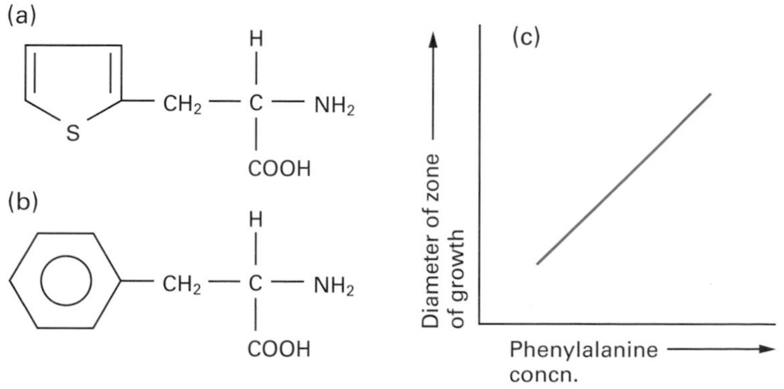

Figure 25.8 (a) β-Thienylalanine. (b) Phenylalanine. (c) Standard curve in Guthrie test.

techniques such as tandem mass spectrometry (MS/MS) that can be used to detect a wider variety of congenital diseases.

25.5.4 Carcinogen and Mutagen Testing

A carcinogen is a substance that causes living tissues to become carcinomatous, that is, to produce a malignant tumour. A mutagen is a chemical (or physical) agent that induces mutation in a human (or other) cell.

Mutagenicity tests are used to screen a wide variety of chemicals for their ability to cause a mutation in the DNA of a cell. Such mutations can occur at either the gene level (a *point mutation*) at individual chromosomes, or at the level of a chromosome set, that is, a change in the number of chromosomes (*aneuploidy*). Some compounds are only mutagenic or carcinogenic after metabolism (often in the liver). This aspect must, therefore, be considered in designing a suitable test method for such agents (see Section 25.5.4.2).

25.5.4.1 Mutations at the Gene Level

Forward mutation refers to mutation of the natural ('wild-type') organism to a more stringent organism. By contrast, reverse (backward) mutation is the return of a mutant strain to the wild-type form, that is, it is a heritable change in a previously mutated gene that restores the original function of that gene.

There are two types of reverse mutation:

- *Frame-shift* – in these mutants, the gene is altered by the addition or deletion of one or more bases so that the triplex reading frame for RNA is modified.
- *Base-pair* – in these mutants, a single base is altered so that the triplex reading frame is again modified.

These principles of reverse mutation are utilised in one important method, the Ames test (Section 25.5.4.2), which is used to detect compounds that act as mutagens or carcinogens (most carcinogens are mutagens).

25.5.4.2 The Ames Test

The Ames test is used to screen a wide variety of chemicals for potential carcinogenicity or conversely for their potential as cancer chemotherapeutic agents. The test enables a large number of compounds to be screened rapidly by examining their ability to induce mutagenesis in several specially constructed bacterial mutants derived from *Salmonella enterica* serovar Typhi. The test strains contain mutations in the histidine operon such that they cannot synthesise the amino acid histidine. Two additional mutations increase further the sensitivity of the system. The first is a defect in their lipopolysaccharide structure (Chapter 3) such that they are in fact deep rough mutants possessing only 2-keto-3-deoxyoctonate (KDO) linked to lipid A. This mutation increases the permeability of the mutants to large hydrophobic molecules. The second mutation concerns a DNA excision repair system, which prevents the organism repairing its damaged DNA following exposure to a mutagen.

The assay method involves treatment of a large population of these mutant tester strains with the test compound. Histidine-requiring mutants are used to detect mutagens capable of causing base-pair substitutions (in some strains) or frame-shift mutations (other strains). This can be carried out by incorporating both the test strain and test compound in molten agar (at 45 °C), which is then poured on to a minimal glucose agar plate. Alternatively, the suspected mutagens can be applied to the surface of the top agar as a liquid or as a few crystals. The medium used for the top agar contains a limited concentration of histidine, which permits the bacteria on the plate to undergo several divisions, since for many mutagens some growth is a necessary prerequisite for mutagenesis to occur. After incubation for 2 days at 37 °C, the number of 'revertant' colonies can be counted and compared with control plates from which the test compound has been omitted. Each revertant colony is assumed to be derived from a cell that has mutated back to the wild-type and thus can now synthesise its own histidine (see Figure 25.9 for a summary).

A further refinement to the Ames test permits screening of agents that require metabolic activation before their mutagenicity or carcinogenicity is apparent. This is achieved by incorporating into the top agar layer, along with the bacteria, homogenates of liver (commonly rat or human) whose activating enzyme systems have been induced by exposure to polychlorinated biphenyl mixtures. This test is sometimes referred to as the *Salmonella*/microsome assay because the fraction of liver homogenate used, called the S9 fraction, contains predominantly liver microsomes.

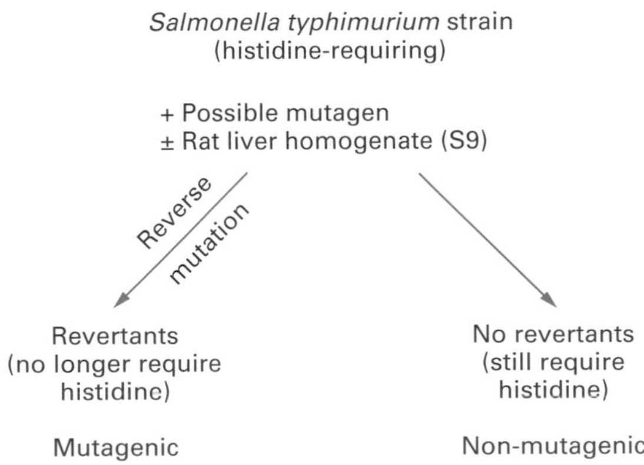

Figure 25.9 Summary of the Ames test.

It is important to realise that this test is flexible and continues to undergo modification and development. One such refinement, the fluctuation method, involves the use of a coloured pH indicator in liquid medium to detect growth of the revertant cells in micro-titre plates (96-well or 384-well), the frequency of mutation being measured as the number of wells that have changed colour compared to controls. This method is comparable to the traditional pour plate method in terms of sensitivity and accuracy, but benefits from reduced sample volume and a simple colourimetric end point; several commercial kits are available.

Almost all the known human carcinogens have been tested by the Ames method and shown to be positive. These include agents such as β-naphthylamine, cigarette smoke condensates, aflatoxin B and vinyl chloride, as well as drugs used in cancer treatment such as adriamycin, daunomycin and mitomycin C. Although the test is not perfect for the prediction of mammalian carcinogenicity or mutagenicity and for making definitive conclusions about potential toxicity or lack of toxicity in humans, it nevertheless provides useful screening information rapidly and cheaply. The Ames test remains an important part of a battery of tests, the others of which are non-microbial in nature, for detecting mutagenicity or carcinogenicity.

25.5.5 Use of Microbial Enzymes in Sterility Testing

Sterile pharmaceutical preparations must be tested for the presence of fungal and bacterial contamination before use (see Chapter 21). If the preparation contains an antibiotic, then it must be removed or inactivated and this is generally achieved by membrane filtration. However, the technique has certain disadvantages including accidental contamination and retention of the antibiotic on the filter followed by subsequent liberation into the nutrient medium.

Enzymatic inactivation of the antibiotic (see also Chapter 13) before testing provides an elegant solution to this problem, for example, using an appropriate β-lactamase to inactivate penicillins and cephalosporins. Other antibiotics that are susceptible to inactivating enzymes are chloramphenicol (by chloramphenicol acetyltransferase) and the aminoglycosides, for example, gentamicin, which can be inactivated by phosphorylation, acetylation or adenylylation.

25.5.6 Immobilised Enzyme Technology

The therapeutic uses of microbially derived enzymes have already been examined (Section 25.2.4). However, enzymes also form the basis of many diagnostic tests used in clinical medicine. For example, glucose oxidase, an enzyme used in blood glucose analysis, is obtained commercially from *Aspergillus niger*. Although the design of glucose blood monitoring test strips has become more refined, the basic principle remains the same. Glucose oxidase is sandwiched between polycarbonate and cellulose acetate membranes. When a pinprick volume of blood is applied, the polycarbonate membrane allows the diffusion of glucose into the sandwich but limits entry of larger molecules thus reducing background contaminants. The enzyme oxidises the glucose, resulting in the formation of hydrogen peroxide. The hydrogen peroxide diffuses through the cellulose membrane where it is measured amperometrically following interaction with a platinum electrode. More recently, several types of implantable glucose oxidase electrodes have been developed for continuous monitoring of blood glucose levels in diabetics. While there are challenges relating to enzyme inactivation *in vivo*, glucose calibration and immune response, several 'continuous glucose monitoring' devices have been approved. Such devices feature a wireless subcutaneous biosensor that continuously samples interstitial fluid to monitor patient glucose levels for up to 14 days. It is likely that biosensors employing immobilised enzymes which are potentially useful for monitoring many substances of clinical importance will become readily available in the not-too-distant future.

25.6 Use of Microorganisms as Models of Mammalian Drug Metabolism

The safety and efficacy of a drug must be exhaustively evaluated before its approval for use in the treatment of human diseases. Investigations of the mechanisms by which a drug is metabolised are extremely valuable, as they potentially provide information on its mode of action, why it exhibits toxicity and how it is distributed, excreted and stored in the body. Traditionally, drug metabolism studies have relied on the use of animal models and, to a lesser extent, liver microsomal preparations, tissue culture and perfused organ systems. Each of these models has certain advantages and disadvantages. Animals in particular are expensive to purchase and maintain, and there is considerable pressure from animal welfare groups to curb the use of animals in scientific research.

The many similarities between certain microbial enzyme systems and mammalian liver enzyme systems have led to the utilisation of various microbial models for the exploration of mammalian drug metabolism. The major advantages of using microorganisms are their ability to produce significant quantities of metabolites that would otherwise be difficult to obtain from animal systems or by chemical synthesis, and the considerable reduction in operating costs compared with animal studies.

Microbial drug metabolism studies are usually carried out by firstly screening a large number of microorganisms for their ability to metabolise a drug substrate. The organism is usually grown in a medium such as peptone glucose in flasks that are shaken to ensure good aeration. Drugs as substrates are generally added after 24 hours of growth and are then sampled for the presence of metabolites at intervals up to 14 days after substrate addition. Once it has been determined that a microorganism can metabolise a drug, the process can be scaled up for the production of large quantities of metabolites for the determination of their structure and biological properties.

As an example of this, the metabolism of the antidepressant drug imipramine can be considered. In mammalian systems, this is metabolised to five major metabolites: 2-hydroxyimipramine, 10-hydroxyimipramine, iminodibenzyl, imipramine-*N*-oxide and desipramine (Figure 25.10).

For microbial metabolism studies, a large number of fungi are screened, from which several are chosen for the preparative scale production of imipramine metabolites. *Cunninghamella blakesleeana* produces the hydroxylated metabolites 2-hydroxyimipramine and 10-hydroxyimipramine; *Aspergillus flavipes* and *Fusarium oxysporum* f. sp. *cepae* yield the *N*-oxide derivative and iminodibenzyl, respectively; while the pharmacologically active metabolite desipramine is produced by *Mucor griseocyanus* together with the 10-hydroxy and *N*-oxide metabolites. By scaling up this procedure, significant quantities of the metabolites that are formed during mammalian metabolism can be obtained.

Microorganisms thus have considerable potential as tools in the study of drug metabolism. Although they cannot completely replace animals, they are extremely useful as predictive models for initial studies.

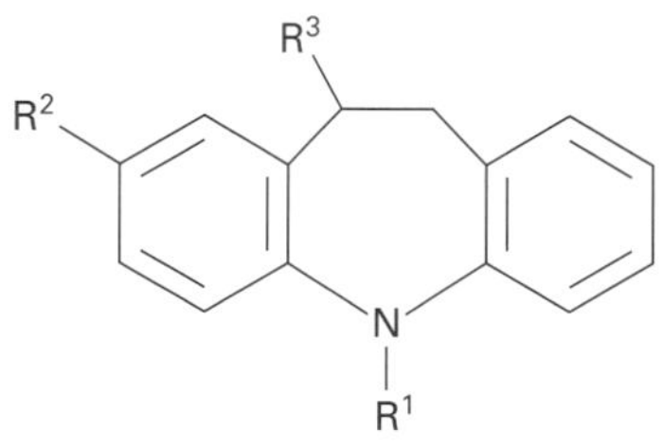

Imipramine	$R^1 = (CH_2)_3N(CH_3)_2$; $R^2 = R^3 = H$
Desipramine	$R^1 = (CH_2)_3NHCH_3$; $R^2 = R^3 = H$
2-hydroxyimipramine	$R^1 = (CH_2)_3N(CH_3)_2$; $R^2 = OH$; $R^3 = H$
10-hydroxyimipramine	$R^1 = (CH_2)_3N(CH_3)_2$; $R^2 = OH$; $R^3 = H$
Iminodibenzyl	$R^1 = R^2 = R^3 = H$
Imipramine-*N*-oxide	$R^1 = (CH_2)_3N(CH_3)_2$; $R^2 = R^3 = H$ (N→O)

Figure 25.10 Structure of imipramine and its metabolites.

25.7 Microorganisms as Therapy

25.7.1 Bacteriophages

In the early 1900s, before the discovery of penicillin, Félix D'Hérelles observed that patients with high titres of bacteriophages in their faeces recovered from dysentery and typhoid fever more rapidly. This paved the way for the commercialisation of bacteriophage preparations for a variety of bacterial infections by, for example, the Société Française de Teintures Inoffensives pour Cheveux (The French Society for Safe Hair Colouring) or L'Oréal as it is known today. Following the advent of modern antibiotic therapy in the 1930s, the science of phage therapy was all but bankrupted, but the emergence of antibiotic resistance has led to a resurgent interest in research and development of phage therapeutics (Chapter 26) and a number of commercial enterprises are involved in the development of clinically relevant phage medicines. Most phages have a specific affinity for only a small group of bacteria, predicated by the interaction of phage components with bacterial surface receptors. Upon interaction, the viral DNA is translocated into the bacterial cell for transcription where lytic or lysogenic replication may occur (Chapter 5). Lytic phages replicate and assemble and then 'burst' from the host cell, resulting in cell death. In the lysogenic life cycle, bacteriophage DNA becomes integrated in the host bacterium's genome. This newly generated material termed a prophage is replicated during cell division. The lysogenic life cycle is shifted to a lytic one when exposed to some external trigger, such as UV radiation.

Lytic phages are in many ways an ideal antibacterial agent. They are target-specific and the existence of more than 1×10^8 species of phage suggests there may be a phage therapeutic for every bacterial species; they kill bacteria rapidly and amplify at the site of infection, and are relatively inexpensive to produce. The US Food and Drug Administration (FDA) recognises that humans ingest vast quantities of phages on a daily basis and tacitly accept that they are safe for oral administration. Indeed, commercial FDA-approved phage food safety products are available to address *Listeria monocytogenes*, *E. coli* O157:H7, Salmonella and Shigella contamination in food.

Phages have been employed therapeutically to treat bacterial infections, particularly in Russia and Georgia, and more recently in the West as last-resort treatment where antibiotics have failed. It is perhaps topical administration that has seen the most interest, however, with the application of cocktails of phage to chronic wounds either as simple suspensions or incorporated into some form of dressing system such as a biodegradable polymer infused with phage and antibiotics. Clinical trials have been progressed for chronic otitis infections, the treatment of infected venous ulcers and in nebulised delivery for treating *Pseudomonas aeruginosa* infection in patients with cystic fibrosis. In 2019, the FDA approved the first US trial for intravenous phage therapy. The systemic administration of phage therapeutics is complicated by a limited knowledge of the pharmacokinetic and pharmacodynamic properties of most phage species, with many early studies indicating that the timing of administration is critical for infection control.

Another therapeutic development has focussed on phage enzymes such as the endolysins employed by bacteriophage to degrade bacterial cell walls and thereby enable the release of phage progeny. These enzymes can be successfully used to lyse Gram-positive bacteria from without and have been shown to be effective in eradicating infections caused by antibiotic-resistant streptococci and *Staphylococcus aureus*.

Recent reports suggest that phages, which are naturally immunostimulatory, may be useful as vaccine delivery vehicles either by vaccinating with phages displaying the antigen or by utilising phages to deliver a DNA expression cassette integrated into the phage genome.

25.7.2 Probiotics

The bacterial microflora that colonises the gastrointestinal (GI) tract is an essential feature of normal human physiology and represents a symbiotic relationship where the bacteria both protect the host against pathogenic microbes and aid in the digestion of food, contributing to the production of essential host nutrients. Under certain conditions (e.g., illness, infection, antibiotic therapy), the bacterial population in the GI tract may be diminished, contributing to disease states. Probiotics are live cultures of 'good' bacteria that are purported to survive transit through the stomach, subsequently colonising the intestinal mucosa and replacing the diminished natural microflora or displacing pathogenic microorganisms. *Bifidobacteria* and *Lactobacillus* spp. are the most commonly encountered probiotic bacteria, primarily because they are reported to survive the harsh environment of the upper GI tract more readily than other species. Of note, *Bifidobacteria* spp. are among the first colonisers of the neonate intestine, as a consequence of both *Bifidobacteria* and prebiotic content in breast milk, and contribute to defence against pathogenic invaders and maturation of the immune system. Probiotics are generally formulated as capsules or as food supplements particularly as dairy products such as yoghurts. Often probiotic formulations are combined with prebiotics – indigestible oligosaccharides that are fermented by anaerobic bacteria in the gut, yielding metabolic substrates that promote probiotic growth.

Probiotics have been investigated for efficacy in a range of conditions that may be associated with diminished bacterial microflora. Several probiotic species including *Lactobacillus* spp. have shown utility in both the prevention and treatment of nosocomial, antibiotic and traveller's diarrhoea. Long-term treatment with *E. coli* Nissle 1917 (>12 months) is reported to be at least equivalent to mesalazine therapy in preventing relapse in ulcerative colitis.

A cautionary note, however: probiotics are increasingly marketed as a 'lifestyle' nutrient to healthy individuals to promote general GI and immune health, despite limited evidence of any significant effect. Nevertheless, research into the benefits of probiotics in both healthy and diseased individuals is ongoing, using recognised and novel probiotic species, and may in the future reap significant reward.

25.7.3 Toxins

25.7.3.1 Botulinum Toxin

In the late nineteenth century, a Belgian professor of microbiology, van Ermengem, conducted a series of experiments to identify the cause of a fatal outbreak of food poisoning, the clinical symptoms of which had been described over a century before by the German physician Justinus Kerner. van Ermengem's endeavours resulted in the identification of botulinum toxin, a potent exotoxin produced by the Gram-positive anaerobic bacterium *Clostridium botulinum*. It is this toxin that is responsible for what is now widely recognised as botulism food poisoning. The symptoms of botulism, which remains a relatively common cause of fatal food poisoning, include GI disturbances, dysphagia, facial paralysis and, depending on the ingested dose, more widespread muscle weakness resulting in possible respiratory paralysis and subsequent death.

In the mid-twentieth century, the work of Burgen and colleagues established that the basic mechanism of action for botulinum toxin is neuromuscular blockade. Now, some 70 years later, we understand that the toxic component of the protein complex is a 150 kDa single-chain polypeptide, consisting of a 100 kDa heavy chain linked to a 50 kDa light chain by a disulphide bridge, which temporarily inhibits acetylcholine release from the presynaptic membrane of cholinergic nerve terminals. Seven different serotypes of the botulinum neurotoxin (A–G) have been identified. The 150 kDa toxic component of these macromolecular protein complexes is relatively homologous, conferring only subtle differences between the mechanisms of action of the serotypes. However, the non-toxic proteins within the bacterium-derived botulinum toxin protein complex also differ, depending on the strain of *C. botulinum*. Botulinum toxin serotypes therefore possess molecular weights between 300 and 900 kDa.

In the late 1970s and 1980s, nanogram quantities of the botulinum toxin were being locally injected, by clinical researchers, into the muscles of human volunteers to induce local paralysis in an attempt to treat various movement disorders. In 1989, after more than a decade of clinical development, the FDA approved the first botulinum toxin therapy. This commercial product contained the botulinum toxin A serotype and was used for the treatment of strabismus, blepharospasm and hemifacial spasm. In 1991, Allergan obtained both the license and the manufacturing facilities to become the sole supplier of botulinum toxin A for clinical therapy and they branded their product Botox.

The number of botulinum toxin A products has since expanded and proprietary products available in the UK currently include Alluzience, Azzalure, Bocouture, Botox, Dysport, Letybo and Xeomin. Different products contain different forms of the toxin, are formulated differently and/or are licensed for different therapeutic indications. For example, Xeomin contains only the 150 kDa light-chain region of the toxin and contains human albumin and sucrose as excipients, whereas Botox contains the 900 kDa macromolecular protein complex and contains human albumin and sodium chloride as excipients. Doses of commercial botulinum toxin A preparations are therefore not interchangeable and specific brands should be prescribed for specific clinical indications. Doses are significantly less than the lethal dose for a human, but systemic side effects of the toxin have been observed, albeit rarely. Clinical administration of the toxin relies on multiple localised injections, often in the secondary care setting, directly into the target tissue. However, the therapeutic effect of botulinum toxin is transient, typically 6–12 months, and patients therefore return for treatment at regular intervals.

In the past three decades, the use of botulinum toxin A in clinical practice has increased almost exponentially and it is now used to treat a diversity of medical conditions. Specific licensed clinical indications in the UK, under specialist use only, include bladder dysfunctions, blepharospasm, chronic sialorrhea, focal spasticity, glabellar and lateral canthal lines, hemifacial spasm, migraine, severe hyperhidrosis and spasmodic torticollis (cervical dystonia). However, it has also been used off-label, by specialists, for other clinical indications related to gastrointestinal disorders, movement disorders, ophthalmic disorders, pain, spasticity, surgical interventions and tendon release in the Ponseti treatment of talipes. The toxin is also renowned for its widespread use in the cosmetic industry. A significant population of patients and cosmetic clients have therefore now been treated with botulinum toxin A, and in general it appears to be a safe and effective addition to the therapeutic armoury. Botulinum toxin type B has also been used therapeutically in humans, but only for limited clinical applications and a relatively small number of patients compared to the botulinum toxin A serotype.

While the clinical use of botulinum toxin is primarily restricted to conditions that are associated with superficial/accessible tissues, to minimise the risk of systemic uptake, there is no doubt that the neurotoxin has emerged as a useful therapeutic entity and has revolutionised the treatment of some refractory clinical conditions such as severe hyperhidrosis.

25.7.3.2 Cholera Toxin

V. cholerae is a bacterial pathogen that colonises the small intestine leading to cholera, an infection characterised by life-threatening acute diarrhoea. Cholera is endemic in developing countries and in areas where hygiene and sanitary conditions are poor, and even with supportive therapy that includes rehydration and restoration of electrolytes, morbidity and mortality rates remain high. An oligomeric protein (87 kDa) secreted by *V. cholerae* was confirmed as the causative agent of cholera in 1963 by Finkelstein and colleagues and has been termed cholera toxin (CT). CT is a member of the superfamily of AB toxins comprising a catalytic heterodimeric A subunit (A1 and A2 chains) and a glycolipid receptor-binding homopentameric B-subunit connected by a disulphide bond. When *V. cholerae* colonises the small intestine, it secretes CT which subsequently interacts, via the B-subunit, with an enterocyte membrane receptor GM1 (monosialotetrahexosylganglioside) localised in lipid rafts. The CT is then internalised into early endosomes and trafficked to the trans-Golgi network, eventually ending up in the endoplasmic reticulum where protein disulphide isomerase dissociates and unfolds the A1 chain from CT. The A1 chain is then translocated by the Sec61 channel into the cytosol where it interacts with proteins that regulate adenylate cyclase (AC) leading to the constitutive activation of AC. This is accompanied by an increase in intracellular cyclic adenosine monophosphate (cAMP) concentration resulting in phosphorylation of the cystic fibrosis transmembrane conductance regulator (CFTR). The net consequence is extracellular secretion of chloride ions into the small intestine, producing an osmotic gradient that draws water into the lumen, resulting in diarrhoea.

CT, despite its pathogenicity, has significant immunological properties and has been proposed as a mucosal adjuvant for subunit vaccines where the toxin is co-administered or complexed with the antigen. Mucosally administered vaccines, that is, oral, nasal, rectal or vaginal, have a number of advantages over the more traditional intravenous vaccines, not least the ability to stimulate mucosal and systemic protection and may perhaps enhance vaccine uptake rates given no needles are involved. The mechanism of adjuvanticity of CT is complex and may not be fully elucidated, but evidence suggests the A-subunit, when administered orally, enhances antigen presentation following complex interactions with mucosal cells and cells of the immune system (see Chapter 9). The role of the B-subunit in adjuvanticity is interesting and it has found safe use in a killed whole-cell monovalent vaccine against cholera in humans. CT-B does not appear to survive transit through the GI tract, but there is growing evidence of autoimmune stimulation following nasal or intravenous administration and therefore the B-subunit may offer utility in the treatment of autoimmune diseases; it has been investigated for its immunotherapeutic potential as an anti-inflammatory in the treatment of Crohn's disease and asthma. A number of preclinical *in vivo* studies have been undertaken to ascertain the effectiveness of CT as a mucosal adjuvant for antigens derived from (for example) *Helicobacter pylori*, influenza, tetanus, HIV and *Streptococcus pneumoniae*, and for the treatment of diabetes mellitus. To date, however, while oral doses of CT elicit strong adjuvanticity, they can also induce severe diarrhoea among other adverse reactions, and they are not well tolerated by patients. To address this, researchers are exploring other administration routes (e.g., nasally administered CT) and efforts to 'detoxify' CT through genetic engineering.

25.8 Insecticides

Like animals, insects are susceptible to infections, which may be caused by viruses, fungi, bacteria or protozoa. The use of microorganisms to spread diseases to particular insect pests offers an attractive method of biological control, particularly in view of the ever-increasing incidence of resistance to chemical insecticides. However, any microorganism used in this way must be highly virulent, specific for the target pest but non-pathogenic to animals, humans or plants. It must be economical to produce, stable on storage and preferably rapidly acting. Bacterial and viral pathogens have so far shown the most promise.

Perhaps the best studied, commercially available insecticidal agent is *B. thuringiensis*. This insect pathogen contains two toxins of major importance. The δ-endotoxin is a Cry protein present inside the bacterial cell as a crystalline inclusion within the spore case. This toxin is primarily active against the larvae of lepidopteran insects (caterpillar pests; moths and butterflies). Its mechanism of action is summarised in Figure 25.11. Commercially available preparations of *B. thuringiensis* are spore–crystal mixtures prepared as dusting powders or spray-on suspensions. They are used primarily to protect commercial crops from destruction by caterpillars and are surprisingly non-toxic to humans and animals. Although such a preparation has a rather narrow spectrum of activity, a variant *B. thuringiensis* strain has been isolated and found to produce a different δ-endotoxin with activity against coleopteran insects (beetles) rather than lepidopteran or dipteran (flies and mosquitoes) insects.

The second *B. thuringiensis* toxin, the β-exotoxin, has a much broader spectrum encompassing the Lepidoptera, Coleoptera and Diptera. It is an adenine nucleotide, probably an ATP analogue that acts by competitively inhibiting enzymes that catalyse the hydrolysis of ATP and

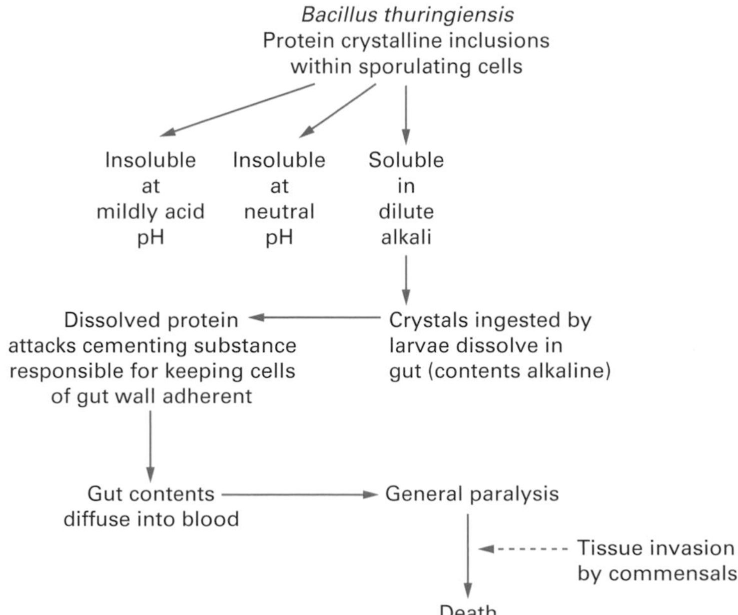

Figure 25.11 Mechanism of action of δ-endotoxin from *B. thuringiensis*.

pyrophosphate. However, this compound is toxic when administered to mammals, so commercial preparations of the *B. thuringiensis* δ-endotoxin are obtained from strains that do not produce the β-exotoxin.

Strains of *Bacillus sphaericus* pathogenic to mosquitoes were isolated in the early 1980s. Strains of this organism with increased toxicity to mosquitoes have been isolated and are licensed as control agents with several commercially available formulations of *B. sphaericus* now available as larvicides.

Other insect pathogens are being evaluated for activity against insects that are vectors for diseases such as sleeping sickness, as well as those that cause damage to crops. Viruses may well have the greatest potential for insect control, as they are host-specific and highly virulent, and one infected insect can release vast numbers of virus particles into the environment. They have already been used with considerable success against the spruce sawfly and pine moth.

25.9 Bioterrorism

Bioterrorism, or biological terrorism, involves the deliberate release of biological agents such as viruses, bacteria and toxins, to intentionally cause terror, illness or death in a target population. In a climate of increasing political instability and radical fundamentalism, there are many concerns over the likelihood of exposure to, and the ability to protect civilians from, such attacks. There are a variety of biological agents that could potentially be used as biological weapons. The US Centers for Disease Control and Prevention (CDC) and the UK Health Security Agency (UKHSA; formerly Public Health England) have defined bioterrorism agents into three categories (A, B and C) based largely on their lethality, ease of transmission and ability to cause panic. Category A agents, that is, those that pose the greatest threat, are *Bacillus anthracis* (anthrax), *C. botulinum* toxin (botulism), *Yersinia pestis* (plague), *Variola major* (smallpox), *Francisella tularensis* (tularemia) and the filovirus (Ebola, Marburg) and arenavirus (Lassa, Machupo) strains that cause viral haemorrhagic fevers. Categories B and C represent agents of generally more moderate morbidity and lower mortality, with category C recognising emerging pathogens with potential for major health impact.

In the event of a biological attack, governmental organisations would invoke a preparedness plan that would include environmental decontamination, for example, hypochlorite solution, and pharmaceutical prophylaxis and/or treatment. Although it is practically, ethically, politically, socially and economically difficult to vaccinate against known bioterror pathogens, it may be possible to stockpile and thereafter disseminate pharmaceutical prophylactics and therapeutics. For example, in the UK, public health agencies would respond with short-term antibiotic cover with, for example, ciprofloxacin or doxycycline (anthrax, plague) or doxycycline/rifampicin or co-trimoxazole (brucella). Botulinum antitoxin would also be provided for treatment of botulism. Clearly, the effectiveness of this plan in preventing illness and death would depend on the ability to detect the threat and respond rapidly.

In the future, the problem may help to provide the solution, as advances in genetic medicine, a science that exploits bacteria and viruses, could produce vaccine platforms that can be efficiently stockpiled to protect susceptible populations against bioweapons.

25.10 Concluding Remarks

Microorganisms are not always the killers they are portrayed to be. In fact, humankind has been remarkably adept at harnessing microbes for a variety of purposes. In many instances, for example, antibiotics by whole or partial synthetic production (Chapter 11) and various forms of vaccines, products have been obtained to turn the tables on infecting organisms. Other products have been used for a variety of purposes (including many non-pharmaceutical or non-medical ones, outside the scope of this chapter). Microorganisms have also been employed for specific assay purposes and different types of chemical transformations, as well as in genetic engineering (Chapter 24). Immobilised microorganisms have now been used with considerable success in the partial synthesis of steroids and antibiotics and in the production of the antiviral nucleoside analogue adenine arabinoside (Chapter 5). In a changing scientific landscape where modern recombinant and molecular technologies are being rapidly adopted, there remains significant scope for the practice of pharmaceutical microbiology and the beneficial harnessing of microbes is likely to continue for many years.

Further Reading

Alfaleh, M.A., Alsaab, H.O., Mahmoud, A.B. et al. (2020). Phage display derived monoclonal antibodies: from bench to bedside. *Front. Immunol.* 11: 1986. https://doi.org/10.3389/fimmu.2020.01986. PMID: 32983137; PMCID: PMC7485114.

Ames, B.N., McCann, J. and Yamasaki, E. (1975). Methods for detecting carcinogens and mutagens with the *Salmonella*/ mammalian microsome mutagenicity test. *Mutat. Res.* 31: 347–364.

Arora, P.A. (2021). *Microbial Products for Health, Environment and Agriculture: 31*. Singapore: Springer.

Atanasov, A.G., Zotchev, S.B., Dirsch, V.M. et al. (2021). Natural products in drug discovery: advances and opportunities. *Nat. Rev. Drug Discov.* 20: 200–116.

Azerad, R. (1999). Microbial models of drug metabolism. *Adv. Biochem. Eng. Biotechnol.* 63: 169–218.

Baltz, R.H., Davies, J.E. and Demain, A.L. (2010). *Manual of Industrial Microbiology and Biotechnology*, 3e. Washington, DC: ASM Press.

Barredo, J.L. (2005). *Microbial Processes and Products*. New York: Humana Press.

Boyer, J.L. and Crystal, R.G. (2006). Genetic medicine strategies to protect against bioterrorism. *Trans. Am. Clin. Climatol. Assoc.* 117: 297–311.

Breeze, A.S. and Simpson, A.M. (1982). An improved method using acetyl-coenzyme A regeneration for the enzymic inactivation of aminoglycosides prior to sterility testing. *J. Appl. Bacteriol.* 53: 277–284.

Burnham, C.A., Leeds, J., Nordmann, P. et al. (2017). Diagnosing antimicrobial resistance. *Nat. Rev. Microbiol.* 15: 697–703. https://doi.org/10.1038/nrmicro.2017.103.

Centers for Disease Control and Prevention Bioterrorism website. http://emergency.cdc.gov/agent/agentlist-category.asp (accessed October 2022).

Chalivendra, S. (2021). Microbial toxins in insect and nematode pest biocontrol. *Int. J. Mol. Sci.* 22 (14): 7657. https://doi.org/10.3390/ijms22147657. PMID: 34299280; PMCID: PMC8303606.

Demain, A.L., Somkuti, G.A., Hunter-Cevera, J.C. and Rossmore, H.W. (1989). *Novel Microbial Products for Medicine and Agriculture*. Amsterdam: Elsevier.

Dolly, J.O. and Aoki, K.R. (2006). The structure and mode of action of different botulinum toxins. *Eur. J. Neurol.* 13 (Suppl 4): 1–9.

Felber, E.S. (2006). Botulinum toxin in primary care medicine. *J. Am. Osteopath. Assoc.* 106 (10): 609–615.

Górski, A., Międzybrodzki, R. and Borysowski, J. (2019). *Phage Therapy: A Practical Approach*. Singapore: Springer.

Guthrie, L. and Kelly, L. (2019). Bringing microbiome-drug interaction research into the clinic. *Lancet* 44: P708–P715.

Health and Safety Executive (2021) The Approved List of biological agents. Advisory Committee on Dangerous Pathogens. www.hse.gov.uk/pubns/misc208.pdf (accessed October 2022).

Hewitt, W. (2004). *Microbiological Assay for Pharmaceutical Analysis*. Boca Raton: Interpharm/CRC.

Hutt, A.J., Kooloobandi, A. and Hanlon, G.W. (1993). Microbial metabolism of 2-arylpropionic acids: chiral inversion of ibuprofen and 2-phenylpropionic acid. *Chirality* 5: 596–601.

Jones, R.L. and Grady, R.W. (1983). Siderophores as antimicrobial agents. *Eur. J. Clin. Microbiol.* 2: 411–413.

Junter, G.A. and Jouenne, T. (2004). Immobilized viable microbial cells: from the process to the proteome: leader or the cart before the horse. *Biotechnol. Adv.* 22 (8): 633–658.

Kier, D.K. (1985). Use of the Ames test in toxicology. *Regul. Toxicol. Pharm.* 5: 59–64.

Kim, S.K., Guevarra, R.B., Kim, Y.T. et al. (2019). Role of probiotics in human gut microbiome-associated diseases. *J. Microbiol. Biotechnol.* 29 (9): 1335–1340. https://doi.org/10.4014/jmb.1906.06064.

Lacey, L. (2007). *Bacillus thuringiensis* serovariety *israelensis* and *Bacillus sphaericus* for mosquito control. *J. Am. Mosq. Control Assoc.* 23: 133–163.

Lim, E.C.H. and Seet, R.C.S. (2007). Editorial: Botulinum toxin, quo vadis? *Med. Hypotheses* 69: 718–723.

Mason, P. (2007). Probiotics: are they worth taking? *Pharm. J.* 278: 373–376.

Miller, M.J., Zhu, H., Xu, Y. et al. (2009). Utilization of microbial iron assimilation processes for the development of new antibiotics and inspiration for the design of new anticancer agents. *Biometals* 22 (1): 61–75.

Oliveira, M., Mason-Buck, G., Ballard, D. et al. (2020). Biowarfare, bioterrorism and biocrime: a historical overview on microbial harmful applications. *Forensic Sci. Int.* 314: 110366. https://doi.org/10.1016/j.forsciint.2020.110366.

Oliver, N.S., Toumazou, C., Cass, A.E. and Johnston, D.G. (2009). Glucose sensors: a review of current and emerging technology. *Diabet. Med.* 26 (3): 197–210.

Pham, J.V., Yilma, M.A. and Feliz, A. (2019). A review of the microbial production of bioactive natural products and biologics. *Front. Microbiol.* 10: 1404.

Poland, G.A., Jacobson, R.M., Tilburt, J. and Nichol, K. (2009). The social, political, ethical and economic aspects of biodefense vaccines. *Vaccine* 27: D23–D27.

Price, J., James, N. and Gale, A. (2008). Botulinum toxin—its form, formulation and pharmacology. *Hosp. Pharm.* 15: 319–328.

Issue on industrial microbiology (1981). *Scientific American*. 245(3): [An excellent series of papers describing the manufacture by microorganisms of products useful to humankind.]

Sikri, N. and Bardia, A. (2007). A history of streptokinase use in acute myocardial infarction. *Tex. Heart Inst. J.* 34 (3): 318–327.

Smith, R.V. and Rosazza, J.P. (1975). Microbial models of mammalian metabolism. *J. Pharm. Sci.* 64: 1737–1759.

Truong, D., Dressler, D., Hallett, M. and Zachary, C. (2014). *Manual of Botulinum Toxin Therapy*, 2e. Cambridge: Cambridge University Press.

Verall, M.S. (1985). *Discovery and Isolation of Microbial Products*. Chichester: Ellis Horwood.

White, L.O. and Reeves, D.S. (1983). Enzymatic assay of aminoglycoside antibiotics. In: *Antibiotics: Assessment of Antimicrobial Activity and Resistance*, Society for Applied Bacteriology Technical Series No. 18 (ed. A.D. Russell and L.B. Quesnel), 199–210. London: Academic Press.

26

Alternative Strategies to Antibiotics: Priorities for Development

Brendan F. Gilmore

Professor of Pharmaceutical Microbiology, School of Pharmacy, Queen's University Belfast, Belfast, UK

CONTENTS

26.1 Introduction

Over the last 80 years, antibiotics have transformed the clinical management of infections and have underpinned the development of modern clinical medicine. The widespread clinical use of antibiotics has reduced both morbidity and mortality associated with (principally) bacterial infections, saving countless lives, and has improved economic productivity and facilitated major advances in surgery and the clinical management of a diverse range of diseases. The discovery of penicillin in 1928, and its development and clinical introduction in the early 1940s, led to what is now widely acknowledged to be the 'golden era' of antibiotic discovery. In the two and half decades that followed, the majority of classes of currently used natural and synthetic antibiotics were discovered, including the aminoglycosides, tetracyclines, chloramphenicol, macrolides, glycopeptides, oxazolidinones, quinolones and the streptogramins (see Figure 26.1).

As a result of this seemingly inexhaustible pipeline of new antibiotics coming to the market during this golden era in drug discovery, the pursuit of virtually all other antibiotic alternatives was abandoned, and the potential for emergence of antibiotic resistance and its consequences, recognised from the very beginning of the antibiotic era, was largely ignored. The rate of new antibiotic discovery declined steeply after this time, despite the introduction of significant numbers of newer synthetic or semi-synthetic compounds derived from already discovered classes of antibiotics; this has left a discovery pipeline that is unable to meet the requirements for new antibiotics in the face of unabated emergence and spread of antibiotic-resistant pathogens. The fluoroquinolones, introduced in the 1970s and 1980s, were the only new class of broad-spectrum antibiotic approved during this period, while only one new class of antibiotic, the narrow-spectrum lipopeptide daptomycin, has made it into clinical practice since. In the face

Hugo and Russell's Pharmaceutical Microbiology, Ninth Edition. Edited by Brendan F. Gilmore and Stephen P. Denyer.

Companion website: https://www.wiley.com/go/HugoandRussells9e

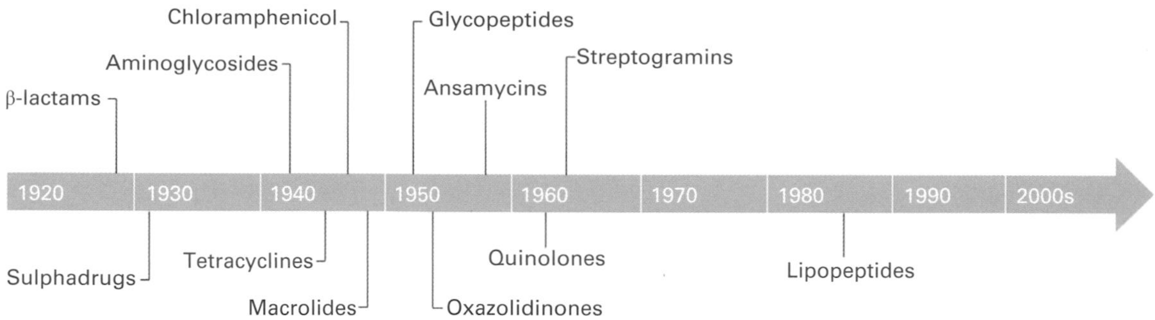

Figure 26.1 The antibiotic discovery timeline. *Source:* Adapted from Lewis (2012).

of rising antibiotic resistance, and an antibiotic discovery pipeline that is critically depleted, attention is only now returning to the potential offered by historical and recently discovered antibiotic alternatives.

Antibiotics have been among the most important, transformative and successful discoveries of the twentieth century. Estimates have indicated that antibiotics add 5–10 years to US life expectancy from birth, while the RAND Corporation estimates that failing to tackle antibiotic resistance, and by extension a lack of access to effective antibiotics, will mean that the world population will be between 11 and 444 million less by 2050 than would otherwise be expected. The O'Neill Review on Antimicrobial Resistance (AMR) (ONeill 2016) predicts 10 million deaths per annum attributable to antibiotic-resistant infections by 2050. The true economic impact of effective antibiotics is multifaceted and thus even more difficult to estimate accurately, but recent estimates suggest that a lack of access to effective antibiotics as a result of antibiotic resistance could cause a fall in global gross domestic product (GDP) of 1.1% in a low-impact AMR scenario, or 3.8% in a high-impact scenario, by 2050. An additional 28.3 million people could fall into extreme poverty by that year, mostly in low-income countries. The O'Neill AMR review predicts a cumulative loss in global economic production of $100 trillion by 2050 due to antibiotic resistance. This demonstrates how highly dependent we have become on antibiotics to maintain public health and economic prosperity globally; the successes attributed to antibiotics may prove temporary, however, if we are unable to discover new antibiotic agents or develop new therapeutic approaches, based on antibiotic alternatives, to treat antibiotic-resistant infections.

Two major issues pose an existential threat to continuation of the antibiotic era: the unceasing rise in the emergence and incidence of antibiotic resistance in the most clinically significant bacterial pathogens (see Chapter 13); and the steady exit or decline in research and development effort by major pharmaceutical companies in the area of antibiotic discovery. The ESKAPE pathogens (*Enterococcus faecium*, *Staphylococcus aureus*, *Klebsiella pneumoniae*, *Acinetobacter baumannii*, *Pseudomonas aeruginosa*, and Enterobacter species) are a group of bacteria which exhibit multiple drug resistance and for which antibiotic development is particularly critical, given their contribution to both morbidity and mortality. Members of the ESKAPE pathogen group, along with clinical *Mycobacterium tuberculosis* strains, some of which are resistant to virtually all available antibiotics, contribute substantially to the significant number of deaths attributable to AMR, estimated at 1.27 million globally in 2019. The emergence and spread of antibiotic resistance are, unfortunately, an inevitable consequence of the anthropogenic use of antibiotics which is widespread and often empirical, leading to inappropriate use and exposure of non-target host bacteria (such as the gut microflora) or environmental microorganisms to non-lethal concentrations of antibiotics. Such exposure drives evolutionary adaptation and resistance development.

The second issue, antibiotic innovation through discovery and design of new antibiotics and the improvement of existing drugs, is more clearly under our control. However, recent decades have witnessed almost all of the major pharma companies exiting the antibiotic innovation field. This is illustrated by the findings of the annual Pew Charitable Trusts report, *Tracking the Global Pipeline of Antibiotics in Development* (2021), which reports that of the 38 companies with antibiotics in clinical development (43 antibiotics in total), only two rank among the top 50 pharmaceutical companies by sales and that 95% of these antibiotics are being developed by small companies (70% of which are pre-revenue, having no products on the market). Indeed, the continued decline in major pharmaceutical industry involvement in antibiotic research and development is mirrored by an annually increasing proportion of pre-revenue companies committed to this work; these companies are much less likely to withstand economic challenges. All in all, the antibiotic pipeline is significantly depleted and less resilient as a result. It is often highlighted that the business case for development of new antibiotics is simply not sustainable, since antibiotics typically have a higher attrition rate at clinical trials (around 60% of drugs entering phase 3 clinical trials are approved, but many lead compounds fail to make it to this stage, with only 14% of antibiotics in phase I likely to gain approval); this attrition contributes to the significant costs (estimated at \$1.4 billion) from first discovery to gaining US Food and Drug Administration (FDA) approval. This is compounded by the fact that antibiotics do not, at the current market costs charged to healthcare providers, make sufficient profit during their patent lifetime to justify the significant financial outlay. The nature of antibiotic prescribing (short courses, sporadically throughout a patient's lifetime) and antibiotic stewardship (responsible and restricted prescribing practices) potentially limit the relative volume of prescribing and demand, and make the development of drugs for chronic, long-term conditions such as diabetes, hypertension and depression much more attractive business prospects.

Against this increasingly familiar background, this chapter examines a range of emerging potential alternative approaches for the treatment and management of bacterial infections, with an emphasis on those approaches which are currently under clinical consideration. It is not the intention to cover antibiotic alternatives in depth, but simply to provide an overview of the current developmental landscape. The reader is directed to 'Further Reading' listed at the end of this chapter, and to other relevant chapters in this edition. Many of the approaches described here have a historical foundation, but their application has been niche, and not subject to rigorous clinical trials, having been supplanted by the availability of effective antibiotics over the past eight decades. Interest in these alternative approaches has experienced a significant upturn, however, both for the reasons described above and as a mechanism to reduce our dependence on antibiotics. While numerous alternative approaches to the treatment of bacterial infections have been proposed, the reality is that many are too specialist, suffer from the same developmental issues as conventional antibiotics or stand little chance of replacing conventional antibiotic therapy. Notwithstanding, a number of antibiotic alternatives might offer a realistic therapeutic option as adjuncts to antibiotics, rather than supplanting their use altogether. In 2016, the Wellcome Trust and UK Department of Health (DoH) jointly commissioned a pipeline portfolio review of alternatives to antibiotics. The working party considered at least 19 different approaches that target the bacteria or the host to treat infection in a manner different to classical antibacterial compounds, and identified those approaches which were most likely to progress to clinical trial and application in the future. The top ten approaches which were deemed to warrant attention were prioritised and placed into two tiers, tier 1 focusing on clinical development and tier 2 on preclinical development in a 5-year time period. Notably, with the exception of antibiofilm peptides, all top-ten approaches had been known for more than 15 years, and there had been little progress towards therapeutic breakthroughs.

A summary of the alternative approaches to antibiotics prioritised by the Wellcome Trust/DoH working party is given in Table 26.1. Importantly, antimicrobial peptides (AMPs) were not included in tier 1 primarily because almost all clinical trial data relate to topical products, while the focus of the Wellcome Trust/DoH review was systemic alternatives to antibiotics. The review, which subsequently informed the work of O'Neill on antimicrobial resistance, concluded that just these priority alternatives alone would require an investment of at least £1.5 billion, spent over the following 10 years, in order to develop a pipeline of translational products which could lead to new products. Additional long-term investment and sustainable funding would then be needed to bring these products into clinical use. In addition to the alternatives described in Table 26.1, a number of other emerging approaches were reviewed and are currently being pursued, including virulence inhibitors (e.g., inhibitors of the *P. aeruginosa* metalloprotease elastase, lasB), immune suppression, antibacterial and anti-resistance nucleic acids, toxin sequestration using liposomes, metal chelation and antibiotic-degrading enzymes to reduce emerging resistance. As yet, none of the identified, prioritised alternatives are at a stage to be brought into clinical use in the near future, and none can be expected to supplant completely the use of antibiotics; clearly parallel investment in the development of both innovative antibiotics and antibiotic alternatives is urgently required.

26.2 Bacteriophage Therapy

Bacteriophages (phages) are viruses which specifically infect and kill bacteria, and have no effect on mammalian cells (see also Chapter 5). In general, phages exhibit highly specific cellular tropism, with a particular phage infecting a given species of bacteria, often in a strain-specific manner. Bacteriophages are the most abundant biological entities on earth, with an estimated 10^{31} bacteriophages on the planet, and phage predation reduces the global population of bacteria by half every 48 hours. Unsurprisingly, this phage predation plays a central role in global processes such as carbon and nutrient cycling in the oceans. Bacteriophages have evolved alongside bacteria for the past 4 billion years, with both bacterial hosts and phages exhibiting mechanisms by which to adapt to their environment.

Table 26.1 Prioritised alternative approaches identified by the Wellcome Trust/DoH working party on alternatives to antibiotics (Czaplewski et al. 2016).

Tier 1 approaches (translational funding to clinical evaluation at phase 2)		**Probable spectrum of activity and initial use**
Antibodies	Antibodies binding to and inactivating a target pathogen, its virulence factors or toxins; widely considered the alternative approach most likely to have major clinical impact. Considered low risk with strong science basis, history of safe use and technically feasible.	Prevent Gram-positive and Gram-negative infections, possibly adjunctive use
Probiotics	Live organisms (also known as live biotherapeutic products [LBPs]) which when administered in adequate amounts produce a health benefit in the host. Mixtures of probiotic bacteria with spores of non-toxigenic *Clostridioides difficile* could provide benefits or improve clinical management of *C. difficile*-associated diarrhoea and antibiotic-associated diarrhoea. Support for basic research into mechanism of action and potential synergy of probiotics with antibiotics or other alternatives could stimulate wider use	Prevent or treat *C. difficile*-associated diarrhoea and antibiotic-associated colitis
Lysins	Phage lysins, enzymes produced by bacteriophages, degrade the cell wall of susceptible bacteria (direct antibacterial effect) or degrade biofilm extracellular matrix, reducing antibiotic tolerance (adjunctive effect) or reducing bacterial bioburden. A focus on lysins active against Gram-negative pathogens should be prioritised	Treat Gram-positive infection
Wild-type bacteriophages	Wild-type bacteriophages infect and kill bacteria, generally highly specific with no activity against non-target microorganisms; they have the potential to replace antibiotics in some scenarios. Viable entities which replicate and potentially evolve during the course of infections are unique in pharmaceutical development. Potential for resistance development (may be circumvented by the use of multiple phages/phage cocktail), rapid elimination and limited action against biofilms may restrict applications	Treat Gram-positive and Gram-negative infections
Engineered bacteriophages	Bacteriophages engineered with new properties for therapeutic applications and with improved spectrum of activity and bioavailability/distribution *in vivo*	Treat Gram-positive and Gram-negative infections
Immune stimulation	Proposed as an adjunct to antibiotic therapy, reliant on appropriate immune response; repurposed drugs considered in the review (e.g., phenyl butyrate and vitamin D to enhance expression of innate antimicrobial peptides deemed feasible). Mechanisms of action not clear, may involve toll-like receptors (TLRs), which once understood would enable more targeted interventions to be designed	Prevent, or provide adjunctive therapy for, Gram-positive and Gram-negative infections
Vaccines	Long-established and emerging technologies, with sustained historical investment in new targets, have potential to substantially reduce incidence of infection and need for antibiotics	Prevention of Gram-positive more than Gram-negative infections

Table 26.1 (Continued)

Tier 2 approaches (strong support for funding while monitoring breakthroughs regarding systemic therapy)		**Probable spectrum of activity and initial use**
Antimicrobial peptides	Advantages include broad spectrum of activity, rapid bactericidal activity, low resistance potential and low immunogenicity. Clinical trial focus to date is primarily on topical applications; early clinical trials have not yet led to therapeutic breakthrough for systemic infections. Important to understand reasons for lack of systemic success (may include bioavailability/pharmacokinetic issues, toxicity, lability to proteases) and how these limitations may be addressed (formulations, incorporation of non-natural amino acids). Topical application (e.g., aerosol/inhalation) could be additive to systemic therapies	Treatment or adjunctive approach for Gram-positive and Gram-negative infections
Host defence peptides and innate defence peptides	Host defence peptides (small, natural peptides) and innate defence peptides (small, synthetic peptides) exhibit indirect antibacterial effect by increasing expression of anti-inflammatory chemokines and cytokines, reducing expression of proinflammatory cytokines. Preclinical assessment and clinical trial validation required; potential for increased side effect profile compared to antimicrobial peptides.	Adjunctive approach for Gram-positive and Gram-negative infections
Antibiofilm peptides	Preclinical identification of peptides capable of reducing initial attachment and inhibiting biofilm formation; potential adjunctive approach to improve conventional antibacterial therapies	Adjunctive approach for Gram-positive and Gram-negative infections

Source: Adapted from Czaplewski et al. (2016).

Since their earliest study in the laboratory, bacterial strains which evolve resistance to a specific bacteriophage have been characterised, indicating a dynamic relationship between host and predator. These studies have led to the discovery of a number of antiviral defence mechanisms in prokaryotes, including: downregulation of phage receptors on the cell surface; the production of exopolysaccharides to limit viral access to receptors; adaptations in the bacterial membrane to prevent injection of viral genetic material; and abortive infections whereby an infected cell undergoes programmed cell death triggered by the presence of phages and controlled by the activation of toxin–anti-toxin systems, membrane depolarisation or inhibition of translation. Incidentally, the discovery of clustered regularly interspaced short palindromic repeat (CRISPR)–Cas systems (discussed in Chapter 24) in bacteria, which provide a mechanism for adaptive immunity against bacteriophages, has revolutionised molecular biology, since the CRISPR–Cas systems of prokaryotes can be adapted to manipulate and edit genomes of both prokaryotes and eukaryotes. This discovery was recognised by the award of the 2020 Nobel Prize in Chemistry.

The structure of a typical bacteriophage is shown in Figure 26.2. The bacteriophage genome is normally double-stranded DNA (dsDNA), and dsDNA-tailed phages, or

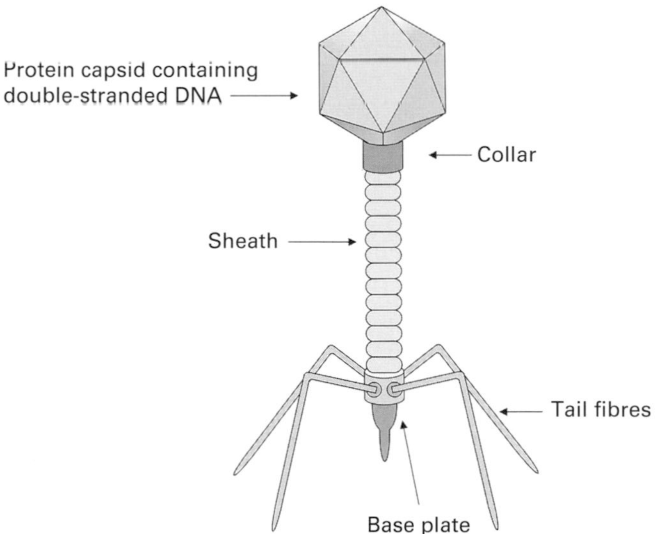

Figure 26.2 Structural features of a typical dsDNA bacteriophage. *Source:* Image courtesy of Dr T. Skvortsov.

Caudovirales, are thought to represent 95% of all known phages. However, single-stranded DNA (ssDNA) phages, such as the *Microviridae*, appear to be prevalent in diverse habitats and are significantly different from dsDNA bacteriophages; furthermore, two families of bacteriophages with RNA genomes have been described. The genome is enclosed within a protein capsid, and the tips of the tail fibres are receptors which recognise and bind to specific viral attachment sites on the bacterial cell surface, initiating infection. When a bacteriophage encounters a host bacterium, it attaches, via the tail fibres, and injects its genome into the cell. Host protein synthesis is then inhibited to make way for the manufacture of early phage proteins, the replication of viral DNA, a synthesis of viral structural proteins and the assembly of new viral particles, or virions. When completed, the host cell, whose metabolic machinery has been devoted entirely to production of virions, contains numerous viral progeny which are liberated from the cell by lysis, under the control of virally encoded enzymes acting on both the cytoplasmic membrane and the cell wall. The newly released viruses are then able to infect other host cells. However, not all phages go through this lytic cycle. Lysogenic phages, by contrast, inject their DNA into host bacterial cells and lytic genes are repressed, and the DNA is then incorporated (or integrated) into the host genome where it remains as a prophage and is replicated with the bacterial genome. In this way, the bacteriophage genome is carried in the bacterial progeny. Such phages are also known as temperate phages, inducing a state of lysogeny in the host. While this may be seen as a form of parasitism, the phenomenon can also be responsible for conferring advantageous characteristics to the host, including toxin production or antimicrobial resistance, due to incorporation of genes carried on the prophage. The prophage can leave the lysogenic life cycle, either spontaneously or via induction (e.g., UV-induced DNA damage) and re-enter the lytic infection cycle.

Bacteriophages were discovered at the beginning of the nineteenth century and were first described by Frederick William Twort (1915) and reported independently by Félix d'Hérelle (1917), who proposed that they were a new type of virus which infected bacteria, which he named bacteriophages. Despite an early lack of understanding of phage biology, their potential for treatment of certain types of infection was recognised, and early successes in the treatment of topical, gastrointestinal (GI) and urinary tract infections were promising indicators that phage therapy would be a valid option in the treatment of bacterial infections. However, toxicity issues associated with endotoxin release and, in particular, the emergence of antibiotics in the 1940s and 1950s caused the use of bacteriophages to decline almost entirely, except in Eastern Europe and the former Soviet Union. Their application for treatment of infections has persisted in these countries to the present day, and accrued experience in their long history of use has helped facilitate renewed interest in these bacterial viruses as potential antibiotic alternatives. In the intervening years, phage biology has been studied extensively in the context of molecular biology and significant advances have been made in the understanding of their fundamental biology, host immunity and genomic manipulation.

Bacteriophages offer a number of potential therapeutic advantages over conventional antibiotics (see also Chapter 5). These include: *specificity* – exquisite species (sometimes strain) specificity has the advantage of targeting a specific pathogen and sparing the host microbiome, and the spectrum of activity can be broadened through use of a mixture or cocktail of phages; *mode of action* enables activity against antibiotic-resistant strains, and although rapid development of phage resistance has been described, this can be avoided through use of phage cocktails; *pharmacokinetics* of bacteriophage are unique compared to conventional antimicrobials, since after administration phage particle numbers increase due to viral replication, which may avoid the necessity for repeat dosing; *formulation* of phages into a wide range of conventional pharmaceutical products has been described allowing oral, topical and parenteral administration; *side effects* – few side effects from bacteriophage therapy have been reported despite a long history of use in humans; however, care must be taken to ensure phages selected for therapeutic application do not carry genes for toxin or virulence factor production, antibiotic resistance or induction of lysogeny; *rapid phage discovery* platforms allow inexpensive discovery of new phages, which may be particularly valuable in low-middle income countries.

Interest in phage therapy has experienced a dramatic increase over the past three decades, primarily due to the realisation that the antibiotic discovery pipeline is currently unable to keep pace with emerging antibiotic resistance, and a number of companies and institutions are investing in phage discovery and therapeutics. The application of bacteriophages in the food industry has already gained FDA approval, with phage cocktails for protection of dairy products against contamination by *Listeria monocytogenes* having been granted GRAS (generally regarded as safe) status (see also Chapter 5). A number of companies are pursuing CRISPR-engineered bacteriophages, for example, for the selective eradication of *Escherichia coli* and *K. pneumoniae* based on carriage of extended-spectrum beta-lactamase and carbapenemase genes in organ transplant and cancer patients, with others under development for *E. coli* (urinary tract infections) and *P. aeruginosa*.

Recently, a number of high-profile compassionate-use phage therapy cases have brought phage therapy to the attention of the public. In 2018, the first dedicated centre for phage therapy in North America, the Center for Innovative Phage Applications and Therapeutics (IPATH), was opened in the University of California San Diego School of Medicine. The opening of this centre marks an important milestone in the development of clinical applications of bacteriophage therapy in the USA, and may address current issues around clinical study design for phage therapy which is slowing the translation of this potentially important alternative approach to antibiosis. In 2017, a personalised bacteriophage-based therapeutic treatment (nine lytic bacteriophages) was successfully used in a 68-year-old diabetic patient with necrotising pancreatitis complicated by multidrug-resistant (MDR) *A. baumannii* infection. The administration of the bacteriophage cocktail intravenously and percutaneously to abscess cavities led to clearance of an otherwise untreatable infection and the patient's return to health. In 2019, a 15-year-old cystic fibrosis patient with disseminated *Mycobacterium abscessus* infection was successfully treated using a well-tolerated, three-phage cocktail (including an engineered lytic phage) administered intravenously, which resulted in clinical improvement, wound closure, substantial resolution of infected skin nodules and no reported adverse effects of phage therapy. Reports of such compassionate-use cases of phage are likely to increase in the near future, which will add much needed momentum to translational activities.

However, there remains a paucity of clinical trial data of sufficient quality or robustness to satisfy Western regulatory bodies, and the most recent clinical studies have been performed under emergency-use approval from the relevant regulatory authorities, which are less stringent in design than the robust, randomised clinical trials to which conventional antibiotic compounds are subject. These types of phase I–III trials are urgently required if the translation of phage therapeutics is to be accelerated from bench to bedside. Additionally, the specificity of phages (widely regarded as a major advantage in avoiding collateral activity against non-target bacteria, thus avoiding microbiome disturbances) leads to products of narrow spectrum which, in order to be successful, will require screening of patients and accurate, rapid point-of-care diagnostics to match phage to pathogen. Despite this, there are encouraging signs that phage therapy may play a greater role in the treatment of bacterial infections in the future.

26.3 Bacteriophage Lysins

Bacteriophage lysins are highly evolved enzymes which lyse the host bacterial cell at the end of the phage life cycle, releasing progeny phage particles. This is achieved through a highly coordinated event whereby phage-encoded *holin* molecules first accumulate in patches in the host bacterial cell membrane subsequently forming holes through which *endolysin* (often referred to as *lysin*) molecules then reach the overlying cell wall. The endolysin binds with high affinity to peptidoglycan, which is then cleaved in the active site of the enzyme. Localised degradation of the cell wall leads to extrusion and externalisation of the cytoplasmic membrane through the cell wall due to the high osmotic pressure of the cytoplasm; this is rapidly followed by cell lysis and release of progeny bacteriophage particles. Endolysins are heat-stable enzymes which have been isolated and purified initially from Gram-positive bacteria, but, more recently, Gram-negative bacteria. Purified lysins achieve rapid lysis of planktonic and biofilm bacteria, and have emerged as one of the most promising antibiotic alternatives in recent years. Interestingly, lysins exhibit a similar specificity to phages, typically showing activity against the species from which they are isolated. This may be an advantage in selective, microbiome-sparing decolonisation and infection control. Of course, they are not self-replicating like bacteriophages, so behave like protein therapeutic drugs. Since they are potentially immunogenic, it was anticipated that antibodies raised as a result of therapeutic use would render subsequent treatments ineffective; however, several studies have shown this not to be the case. Animal studies have revealed that lysins administered systemically exhibit very short half-lives, but are still able to produce satisfactory antimicrobial activity due to their rapid activity. Early work on lysins demonstrated that they are highly effective at clearing streptococci in a mouse model of *Streptococcus pyogenes* pharyngeal colonisation. The first example of the systemic use of lysins was with PlyG, an endolysin for *Bacillus anthracis*, which, when delivered intraperitoneally to a mouse model of *B. anthracis* bacteraemia, saved animals from rapid death.

Currently, the most advanced phage lysin in clinical development is lysin CF-301 (Exebacase®, ContraFect Corporation), which is the first and, to date, only bacteriophage-derived lysin to enter clinical trials in the USA. CF-301 targets *S. aureus* and is being developed for the treatment of *S. aureus* (including methicillin-resistant *S. aureus* [MRSA]) bloodstream infections and endocarditis. It has successfully completed phase I and phase II trials with phase III trials set to commence in 2022/2023. ContraFect is also pursuing CF-370, an engineered phage lysin with potent activity against *P. aeruginosa,* which has uniquely been shown to bypass the *P. aeruginosa* outer membrane. It has also been shown to exhibit excellent activity in the eradication of *P. aeruginosa* biofilms and shows synergy with antibiotics. The development of CF-370 is being supported by the Combating Antibiotic-Resistant Bacteria Biopharmaceutical Accelerator (CARB-X). In general, the application of phage lysins shows significant clinical promise and technical feasibility, making them one of the antibiotic alternatives with greatest therapeutic potential.

26.4 Vaccines and Immunotherapies

26.4.1 Vaccines for Bacterial Infections

Vaccines for the prevention of bacterial and viral diseases have been available for many years, in some cases predating the use of antibiotics (see Chapter 10). The long historical use of vaccines in humans, combined with innovations in molecular biology and the development of completely novel vaccination methods, including mRNA vaccines, continues to innovate the vaccines research and development field, making vaccines a promising alternative to antibiotics. In fact, the use of vaccination in prevention of bacterial infections, particularly MDR community- and healthcare-associated infections, is one of the most important approaches available to substantially reduce the need for conventional antibiotics, and thereby help control antibiotic resistance development. This is exemplified by reference to the pneumococcal vaccine, where the WHO estimates that globally *Streptococcus pneumoniae* infections are responsible for over 14.5 million episodes of pneumococcal disease and 800,000 deaths per annum in children under 5 years of age. Global coverage with the pneumococcal conjugate vaccine would significantly reduce morbidity and prevent the majority of these deaths. In addition, universal coverage by a pneumococcal conjugate vaccine would be expected to reduce by 47% the amount of antibiotics used for *S. pneumoniae* pneumonia cases in these children, equating to a reduction of 11.4 million days of antibiotic use per year.

For many diseases, including whooping cough, diphtheria, tuberculosis (TB), measles and mumps, vaccines remain the most important form of infection prevention and control. Table 26.2 illustrates the range of bacterial vaccines currently available in the UK, with many of these (diphtheria, tetanus, pertussis, meningococcal, *Haemophilus* and bacillus Calmette–Guérin [BCG]) forming integral components of the healthcare programme for the early years of life (see Chapter 10). Indeed, the focus of twenty-first century vaccine development has been directed primarily towards childhood infectious diseases, but is now shifting towards prevention of infections that occur throughout all stages of life. Furthermore, the focus is also on improving current vaccines to increase their efficacy at extremes of age, to

Table 26.2 Examples of currently available vaccines and immunotherapies for bacterial infections (BNF 83 2022).

Microorganism	Indication	Form
Bacillus anthracis	Anthrax	Cell-free vaccine containing purified antigens (adjuvant adsorbed) from a non-encapsulated, attenuated strain of *B. anthracis*
Bordetella pertussis	Whooping cough	Acellular vaccine containing highly purified components of *B. pertussis*
Clostridium tetani	Tetanus	Cell-free purified toxin of *C. tetani* adsorbed on aluminium hydroxide or aluminium phosphate to improve antigenicity. Tetanus immunoglobulin also available
Corynebacterium diphtheriae	Diphtheria	Adsorbed (aluminium hydroxide or aluminium phosphate) toxin of *C. diphtheriae*. Diphtheria antitoxin available for passive immunisation in suspected cases of diphtheria
Clostridium botulinum	Botulism	Polyvalent botulism antitoxin, for post-exposure prophylaxis of botulism
Haemophilus influenzae	Invasive *H. influenzae* type b disease	Capsular polysaccharide of *Haemophilus* type b. Conjugate vaccine (adjuvant adsorbed)
Neisseria meningitidis	Meningitis	Meningococcal group B vaccine (recombinant DNA, adsorbed), meningococcal group C vaccine (capsular polysaccharide meningococcal group C conjugate), tetravalent vaccines covering serogroups A, C, W135 and Y are available
Mycobacterium bovis	Tuberculosis	Bacillus Calmette–Guérin (BCG) vaccine, live-attenuated strain derived from *M. bovis*
Salmonella enterica serovar Typhi	Typhoid	Vi capsular polysaccharide antigen (from *Salmonella typhi*). Live-attenuated *S. typhi* vaccine for oral use
Streptococcus pneumoniae	Pneumococcal infection	Polyvalent capsular antigens. Pneumococcal polysaccharide vaccines (adsorbed)
Vibrio cholerae	Cholera	Oral vaccines containing heat and formaldehyde inactivated whole cell Inaba and Ogawa strains of *V. cholerae* serotype O1 with recombinant cholera toxin-B subunit produced in Inaba strains of *V. cholerae*

increase duration of efficacy and to target pathogens of global public health significance. While detailed discussion of vaccines for viral infections is covered elsewhere in this book (see Chapters 5 and 10), in the context of antibiotic alternatives new advances in vaccine technology, including those developed for prevention of coronavirus disease (COVID)-19, have relevance for future bacterial vaccine development. Importantly also, effective vaccinations for viral diseases such as influenza and more recently COVID-19 can have significant importance in reducing antibiotic use and limiting resistance development because, despite being ineffective for treatment of viral infections, antibiotics are often unnecessarily and inappropriately administered to these patients. This is highlighted by a recent (2021) meta-analysis of antibiotic prescribing in COVID-19 patients in the UK, which showed that approximately 75% of patients hospitalised with COVID-19 received antibiotics, despite only 8% having a bacterial co-infection. New or improved vaccines need to move beyond toxin neutralisation and treatment of invasive disease, to vaccines that can target mucosal infections including tuberculosis, skin and soft tissue infections, urinary tract infections and pneumonia. As older adults are at highest risk of morbidity and mortality associated with bacteraemia and pneumonia, and have been identified as the patient group with the greatest unmet vaccine needs, these populations stand to benefit most from new vaccines. Therefore, it seems likely that new vaccines will be developed for this patient population first, and subsequently extended to all other age groups. In the past century, bacterial vaccines have been a pillar of global infection prevention and public health, and their role is set to expand significantly in this coming century to meet the demands of AMR.

The O'Neill AMR review highlights the four broad categories of vaccine which are likely to be most useful for controlling the rise of AMR infections by protecting individuals from such infections and preventing the overuse of antibiotics, these are: vaccines which prevent community-acquired infections (including diphtheria, tetanus, pneumococcal and *Haemophilus influenzae* type B infections) which may be part of national vaccination and immunisation programmes; vaccines which prevent healthcare-associated infections (primarily the ESKAPE pathogens, *E. coli* [including extra-intestinal pathogenic *E. coli* or ExPEC] and *C. difficile*) which can be used in a more targeted fashion in high-risk populations; vaccines for prevention of viral infections, which can reduce unnecessary antibiotic prescribing in patients who would otherwise contract these infections; and vaccines to prevent infections in farm animals where large quantities of antibiotics are currently used. While vaccines exist for the first category (community-acquired infections), with new candidates in development, vaccines in the second category (healthcare-associated infections), especially the ESKAPE pathogens and *C. difficile*, are currently lacking and those vaccines in development do not provide complete coverage for all pathogens listed. Recent successes in the development of several novel and effective vaccines against severe acute respiratory syndrome-coronavirus-2 (SARS-CoV-2) have highlighted our ability to rapidly deliver ground-breaking vaccine products; this could undoubtedly help address the need for vaccines in the third category (viral infections) and thereby reduce antibiotic consumption in these patients.

26.4.2 Immunotherapies

Immunotherapies are strategies for the management of disease, including infectious diseases, that target or manipulate components of the immune system. The development of immunotherapies, particularly therapeutic monoclonal antibodies (mAbs), for diseases such as cancer, arthritis and inflammatory bowel diseases has proven to be highly successful (see Chapter 9); immunotherapies for infectious diseases (viral, fungal and bacterial) are also under clinical development and show outstanding promise as potential adjuvants or replacements for conventional antibiotics. Immunotherapies are classified as either *passive immunotherapies* which use immune cells, antibodies or recombinant antibody derivatives produced *ex vivo*, or *active immunotherapies* which use virulence factors to trigger components of the host immunological memory, such as T-cells and the humoral response. Aside from vaccines, several additional immunotherapeutic approaches have been successfully used, with a number of approaches in clinical development. This section will provide a brief introduction to emerging (non-vaccine) immunotherapies for bacterial infections.

26.4.2.1 Monoclonal Antibody Therapy

Monoclonal antibodies (mAbs) have been approved for clinical applications since the late 1980s. They exploit the specificity and selectivity of an antibody to its cognate antigen to achieve a number of effects: bind to cell surface receptors and induce a signal cascade resulting in cell death; interfere with normal receptor–ligand interactions necessary to maintain cell viability; recruitment of constituents of cell-mediated immunity (macrophages, monocytes, natural killer cells) to the target cell through recognition of the Fc (fragment crystallisable) region of the antibody; or activation of the complement cascade following binding to the target antigen. Despite a significant early focus on the development of mAbs for *M. tuberculosis* which has to date proven elusive, a number of engineered mAbs have recently advanced to clinical trial for *P. aeruginosa* and *S. aureus* infections. Interestingly, in contrast to antibiotics, a number of the major pharmaceutical companies are actively pursuing mAbs for bacterial infections. AstraZeneca is advancing a bispecific (i.e., having two binding domains which bind two different antigens or epitopes) mAb IgG1 (MEDI3902): this targets both the PcrV protein (a component of the type III secretion system) of *P. aeruginosa* intended to trigger host cell cytotoxicity and the Psl exopolysaccharide (a component of the *P. aeruginosa* extracellular matrix), thereby potentially inhibiting colonisation and surface adherence/biofilm formation. In addition, the same company is conducting phase II trials on a novel long-acting mAb (MEDI4893) targeting alpha toxin for the immunoprophylaxis of *S. aureus* infection.

26.4.2.2 Checkpoint Inhibitors

Immune checkpoints are regulators of the immune system, which protect otherwise healthy, non-target cells from attack by the host immune system. Checkpoint inhibitors use mAbs to disrupt the interaction between immune checkpoint proteins which otherwise interact and send an 'off' signal to T-cells to avoid attack. Checkpoint inhibition has shown exceptional promise in cancer therapy, but, to date, this approach has been restricted to the management of TB in the area of bacterial infections. The application of checkpoint inhibitors for bacterial infection has not yet proceeded to clinical trials, but data from *in vitro* and *in vivo* experiments are promising. During active TB, persistent immune stimulation leads to the expression of inhibitory receptors such as programmed cell death protein 1 (PD-1), cytotoxic T-lymphocyte-associated antigen 4 (CTLA-4), lymphocyte-activation gene 3 (LAG-3) and T-cell immunoglobulin mucin-3 (TIM-3). Inhibition of these inhibitory receptors with their ligands has been shown to improve or restore T-cell function in active TB infections.

26.4.2.3 Other Immunotherapeutic Approaches for Treating Bacterial Infection

A number of other immunotherapeutic approaches for the treatment of bacterial infections are now emerging and are likely to receive significant attention in the coming years as antibiotic alternatives; these include T-cell based immunotherapies, cytokine therapies and antibody–antibiotic conjugates. T-cell-based immunotherapies rely on inducing T-cell activation during infections. In the case of TB infection, unconventional T-cells that are not limited to antigen recognition via the major histocompatibility complex (MHC) and are therefore capable of targeting non-classical antigens are activated and can recognise lipids in the mycobacterial cell wall, inducing cytokine production and mounting an effective immune response to *M. tuberculosis*. A group of unconventional killer T-cells, the invariant natural killer T-cells (iNKT), are being investigated in phase I and phase II clinical trials for TB infections. Similarly, cytokine therapies are also being investigated for the management of active TB infections; for example, recombinant human interleukin-2 (rhIL-2) and granulocyte–macrophage colony-stimulating factor (GM-CSF) are both currently under investigation. Finally, antibody–antibiotic conjugates, whereby a specific antibody targeting a cell-surface structure or component of the extracellular matrix is conjugated to an antibiotic molecule, aim to improve the efficacy of antibiotics through highly specific targeted delivery to the site of infection. This is an attractive approach which could have broad applications in antibiotic delivery to a wide range of pathogens, and several anti-*S. aureus* antibody–drug conjugates targeting cell wall teichoic acids are currently being advanced to phase I trials.

26.5 Probiotics

Probiotics are defined as live microorganisms which, when administered in adequate amounts, confer a health benefit on the (human) host. In order for a microorganism to qualify as a probiotic, therefore, a clinical benefit must be established through appropriately designed and powered clinical studies and the data made available through publication and deposited in an appropriate clinical trials registry which is available to the public. The use of harmless bacteria to replace pathogenic ones (bacteriotherapy) is not a new concept, but there has been significant expansion in both interest and clinical study of probiotics in the past two decades, with numerous products now available for use clinically and by the general public. This has included strongly marketed food additives and probiotic-fortified dairy products promoted for prophylaxis and promotion of a healthy gut microbiota. A recent review of probiotic clinical trials has helped to address the perception that such trials have been heterogenous, of low quality and skewed by bias in their design, and poorly reported in the literature. From published clinical trials, the most commonly studied probiotics were: *Lactobacillus rhamnosus* (strain *L. rhamnosus* GG [LGG]); *Bifidobacterium animalis* ssp. *lactis* BB12; and VSL#3, a mixed probiotic culture comprising 3 different bifidobacteria, 4 lactobacilli and one strain of *Streptococcus thermophilus*. The most frequently used probiotic microorganisms are, for the most part, normal components of the gut microflora, and include representatives from the lactobacilli, lactococci, bifidobacteria, enterococci and streptococci (see Table 26.3). Other bacteria such as

Table 26.3 Microorganisms commonly used as probiotics.

Bacillus subtilis
Bacillus coagulans
Bifidobacterium bifidum
Bifidobacterium animalis (subspecies *lactis)*
Bifidobacterium breve
Bifidobacterium infantis
Bifidobacterium lactis
Bifidobacterium longum
Enterococcus faecium
Escherichia coli Nissle 1917
Lactobacillus acidophilus
Lactobacillus casei immunitas
Lactobacillus delbrueckii ssp. *bulgaricus*
Lactobacillus fermentum
Lactobacillus helveticus
Lactobacillus paracasei ssp. *paracasei 19*
Lactobacillus plantarum
Lactobacillus raffinolactis
Lactobacillus reuteri
Lactobacillus rhamnosus
Lactobacillus salivarius
Leuconostoc spp.
Pediococcus pentosaceus
Streptococcus thermophilus
Saccharomyces boulardii
Saccharomyces cerevisiae

Bacillus species and yeasts such as *Saccharomyces* are also included in probiotic products. Typically, complete strain identification is not reported in over half of the published clinical studies, and dosage information ranges from undisclosed (e.g., a given volume or number of drops of a formulation) to ranges between 10^7 and 10^{11} colony-forming units (CFU) per day (despite a recommendation for appropriate dosage reporting in CFUs). Probiotic products may contain one or two strains of microorganism, but many products are preparations of three or more individual microorganisms and there exists a great diversity of probiotic formulations within the published literature.

The current indications (supported by clinical trial data) for probiotics are equally diverse: for prophylaxis and treatment in adult health (constipation, irritable bowel syndrome, antibiotic-associated diarrhoea [AAD], *Clostridioides difficile*-associated diarrhoea [CDAD], infectious diarrhoea [ID], migraine prevention, adjunctive therapy for *Helicobacter pylori* eradication); women's health (bacterial vaginosis, vulvovaginal candidiasis); and paediatric health (oral health [tonsillitis, laryngitis, dental caries], diarrhoeal diseases, constipation, childhood eczema/atopic dermatitis, common infectious disease [CID] prophylaxis, cow milk protein allergy [CMPA] and necrotising enterocolitis [NEC] in premature or low-birth-weight infants). Recently, there has been a noticeable shift towards clinical trials for non-gastrointestinal conditions, with trials ongoing for probiotic use in communicable diseases, infection and metabolic diseases. This trend marks an expansion of potential applications for probiotics in the prophylaxis and treatment of a diverse range of diseases.

26.5.1 Gastrointestinal Conditions

The majority of probiotic interventions and published studies to date relate to their use in gastrointestinal diseases and digestive system diseases. Probiotic microorganisms are easily formulated into dairy products (yoghurts, yoghurt drinks), but also food supplement powders, or conventional formulations such as tablets or capsules. In order to bring about a probiotic effect, as per the official definition, the probiotic agent must be administered in adequate quantity to bring about the intended clinical benefit. It is estimated that in the GI tract, dosages of somewhere in the region of 10^9–10^{11} CFUs per day are necessary to elicit a probiotic effect. Although the precise mechanisms by which probiotics bring about their intended health benefits are not fully elucidated, a prerequisite property is for those organisms to survive transit through the stomach in sufficient quantity to colonise the gut. Colonisation may be achieved through competition with the resident microflora by the production of antimicrobial peptides, or bacteriocins (see Section 26.6 below).

A significant proportion of probiotic formulations currently available for both adult and paediatric health has been shown to be of benefit in diarrhoeal diseases, irritable bowel and constipation. The use of probiotics has shown significant benefits for premature, low-birth-weight infants at risk of developing NEC. A review of 24 clinical studies employing >5000 patients has shown the safety and efficacy of probiotics in the prevention of this condition, giving a reduction in both morbidity and mortality with no adverse effects.

C. difficile, an anaerobic Gram-positive spore-forming bacillus, is a component of the normal gut microbiome which can, under certain conditions (such as broad-spectrum antibiotic use), overgrow in the GI tract and produce toxins which lead to diarrhoea (*C. difficile*-associated diarrhoea or *C. difficile*-associated colitis). While a number of probiotics claim efficacy in CDAD and AAD, there has been conflicting published data as to the effectiveness of certain probiotics in prevention and treatment of these diarrhoeal conditions. It has been found, however, that probiotic use may reduce the incidence of CDAD in high-risk populations by around 50%, with *Saccharomyces boulardii* shown to be particularly effective. More recent studies have shown that both *Bacillus clausii* and *Lactobacillus reuteri* secrete compounds which are directly inhibitory to *C. difficile*. While faecal microbiota transplantation (FMT) has also been studied for *C. difficile*-associated colitis, with some excellent results leading to its adoption as standard care in some countries, safety issues have arisen (including the first recorded death from the procedure in 2019, due to the transfer of a drug-resistant *E. coli* leading to bacteraemia). Despite this, FMT may prove a useful procedure for the identification of novel probiotic species for treatment and prophylaxis of CDAD in at-risk patients.

26.5.2 Recurrent Vaginitis

Vaginitis is a common condition which may be caused by bacteria or yeasts, most frequently *Candida albicans*, which overgrow and displace the normal microbial flora of the vaginal mucosa. Vaginitis may be effectively treated with probiotics which restore the normal balance of lactobacilli in the vagina. Bacterial vaginosis (BV) is a common infection characterised by an overgrowth of the Gram-negative bacterium *Gardnerella vaginalis*, a normal constituent of the vaginal microbiome, as well as other BV-causing bacteria; there is also a corresponding decrease in normal vaginal lactobacilli and alteration of normal vaginal pH. A number of studies have demonstrated that oral or vaginal administration of probiotics is effective at preventing and treating recurrent bacterial vaginosis. These studies show that several probiotics, including the lactobacilli *Lactobacillus acidophilus*, *L. rhamnosus* and *Lactobacillus fermentum*, are capable of returning the vaginal microbiome to normal following oral or intravaginal administration.

26.6 Antimicrobial Peptides

AMPs are a diverse group of naturally occurring peptides which exhibit antimicrobial activity against a wide range of pathogens, including Gram-positive and Gram-negative bacteria, fungi and viruses. They are typically either linear cationic amphipathic peptides or macrocyclic peptides, usually consisting of 10–50 amino acids. Antimicrobial peptides often exhibit rapid, broad-spectrum activity against a wide variety of bacteria, with more than one mechanism or site of action (multi-hit), making the emergence of resistance less likely than single mechanism of action antibiotics. AMPs, such as LL-37, gramicidin, magainin and the polymyxins (see also Chapter 12), exhibit surprisingly good activity against Gram-negative bacteria, due to their ability to perturb the bacterial outer membrane which often acts as a barrier to numerous antibiotic molecules.

The current global market for peptide drugs (including AMPs) is approximately \$25 billion (around 3% of total global pharmaceutical sales), and is estimated to increase to \$50 billion by 2024. While the major proportion of the peptide drug market is dominated by sales in cancer and metabolic diseases, recent years have observed a shift towards the development of peptides for infectious diseases. Examples of some preclinical and clinically approved-antimicrobial peptides are given below in Table 26.4.

Nevertheless, despite several favourable characteristics of AMPs when compared with antibiotics, a number of barriers to clinical translation exist. Laboratory evaluation of AMP activity may not correlate well with clinical efficacy, since AMP activity is sensitive to environmental parameters including physiological salt conditions which can lead to a reduction in bactericidal activity due to loss of electrostatic interactions with the cell membrane. AMPs may be extensively bound to serum proteins such as albumin, negating their activity *in vivo*, and they may also be susceptible to degradation by both host and bacterial proteases which can limit their application to topical delivery indications. Their cationic nature, alongside susceptibility to proteolytic degradation in the GI tract, can lead to poor oral absorption and bioavailability. Furthermore, the non-specific interaction of antimicrobial peptides with cell membranes can lead to host toxicity, while, in parallel, toxicity due to poor pharmacokinetic clearance of some antimicrobial peptides leading to acute kidney injury has been reported in phase III clinical trials. Despite the perception that AMPs do not induce resistance in bacteria, some examples of resistance due to target modification in the cell membrane or specific enzymatic degradation have been reported, for example, towards nisin, and polymyxins (see *mcr*-1 resistance to colistin, Chapter 13). Therefore, the potential for resistance to AMPs must be given due consideration in their clinical use. Finally, the cost of preparing AMPs by solid-phase peptide synthesis (SPPS) remains high (\$50–\$400 per gram of amino acid) compared to antibiotics (e.g., aminoglycoside production costs \$0.40 per gram), although costs are falling. It has been highlighted that despite the long historical use of antimicrobial peptides for some clinical applications, and the volume of AMPs currently described, these compounds have, in general, a poor track record of translation to the market. Notwithstanding, AMPs are still regarded as a class of compound with high potential as antibiotic alternatives, with a number in advanced clinical development.

Table 26.4 Examples of antimicrobial peptides.

AMP	Discovery	Description	Spectrum of activity	Mechanism	Molecular weight (g mol^{-1})
Nisin A	1928	Polycyclic antibiotic	*E. coli*, Gram-positive bacteria	Depolarisation of cell membrane	3354
Gramicidin S	1944	Polycyclic peptide	*S. aureus*, *E. coli*	Membrane depolarisation/disruption/immunomodulation	1140
Polymyxin B	1947	Cyclic polypeptide	Gram-negative bacteria	Membrane disruption/immunomodulation	1203.5
Polymyxin E (colistin)	1949	Cyclic polypeptide	*A. baumannii*, *K. pneumoniae*	Membrane disruption/immunomodulation	1155
Melittin	1967	α-helical peptide	MRSA	Membrane disruption/immunomodulation	2846.5
Daptomycin	1986	Lipopeptide	*S. aureus*, MRSA, VRE	Membrane depolarisation/disruption/immunomodulation	1619
Magainin	1987	α-helical peptide	*E. coli*	Membrane disruption	2409.9
LL-37	1996	Human cathelicidin	*Enterobacter cloacae*, *K. pneumoniae*, *P. aeruginosa*	Membrane disruption/immunomodulation	4493
Buforin	1996	α-helical peptide	*E. coli*	Membrane disruption/immunomodulation	2434.9
Teixobactin	2015	Cyclic depsipeptide	MRSA, VISA	Disruption of cell wall synthesis	1242.5

MRSA, methicillin-resistant *S. aureus*; VRE, vancomycin-resistant *Enterococcus*; VISA, vancomycin-intermediate *S. aureus*.
Source: Adapted from Koo and Seo (2019) and Dijksteel et al. (2021).

Currently, there are just under 6000 AMPs listed in the data repository of antimicrobial peptides (DRAMP) with 77 in drug development (pre-clinical or clinical stage). To date, however, only colistin (polymyxin E) and daptomycin have gained FDA approval as antibiotics, with nisin, gramicidin and melittin approved for clinical use. Nisin is approved for food preservation and has GRAS status, and is produced by the probiotic bacterium, *Lactococcus lactis*. Gramicidin is a component of Neopsorin (a combination of gramicidin, polymyxin B and the aminoglycoside neomycin) and is used clinically for ophthalmic infections. Polymyxins B and E are in clinical use, and differ by one amino acid only, with polymyxin B indicated for the treatment of ophthalmic and topical infections (in combination with other antimicrobial agents); polymyxin E (colistin) has activity against *P. aeruginosa*, *K. pneumoniae* and *A. baumannii* and is indicated for the treatment of wound and pulmonary infections by intravenous infusion. Melittin, a 26 amino acid alpha-helical peptide isolated from the venom of the European honeybee *Apis mellifera*, exhibits potent anti-inflammatory activity for which it has gained FDA approval. However, recent studies also demonstrate that it possesses broad-spectrum antimicrobial activity and therefore it could be potentially used in this capacity in applications beyond its current approved indications. Several AMPs are in phases I–III trials, and it is expected that significantly more compounds will enter clinical development in the next 5 years. The AMP pipeline appears to be abundant and with a high potential to deliver antibiotic alternatives in the near future.

26.7 Conclusion

The control of bacterial infections with conventional antibiotics has been compromised by the emergence and proliferation of antibiotic-resistant pathogens, a significantly depleted antibiotic discovery pipeline, and an ageing population; such factors together threaten to bring to an end the antibiotic era. In order to avert such a global health crisis, it will be essential to investigate and develop clinical alternatives to antibiotics, alongside rapid point-of-care diagnostics and antimicrobial stewardship programmes. In addition, concerted and sustained funding will be required to advance these alternative approaches to the clinic. It is unrealistic to expect that the alternatives discussed in this chapter will supplant the use of antibiotics entirely; some are niche approaches not suited to widespread clinical application, while others, such as vaccines, antimicrobial peptides and bacteriophage-derived lysins, may prove useful adjuncts to future antibiotic therapies.

Acknowledgements

The contribution of Prof Geoff Hanlon who prepared the chapter on alternative strategies for antimicrobial therapy in the previous edition of this book is gratefully acknowledged.

References

Czaplewski, L., Bax, R., Clokie, M. et al. (2016). Alternatives to antibiotics – a pipeline portfolio review. *Lancet Infect. Dis.* 16: 239–251.

British National Formulary (BNF) 83 *(March 2022 – September 2022)*. London: BMJ Group and Pharmaceutical Press. *(A new volume is published every 6 months and the reader is advised to consult the most recent edition.)*

Dijksteel, G.S., Ulrich, M.M.W., Middelkoop, E. and Boekema, B.K.H.L. (2021). Review: lessons learned from clinical trials using antimicrobial peptides (AMPs). *Front. Microbiol.* 12: 616979.

Koo, H.B. and Seo, J. (2019). Antimicrobial peptides under clinical investigation. *Pept. Sci.* 111: e24122.

Lewis, K. (2012). Recover the lost art of drug discovery. *Nature* 485: 439–440.

ONeill, J. (2016). Tackling drug-resistant infections globally: final report and recommendations. In: *The Review on Antimicrobial Resistance*, 1–80. London: Wellcome Trust and HM Government.

Further Reading

Ahmad, M. and Kahn, A.U. (2019). Global economic impact of antibiotic resistance: a review. *J. Glob. Antimicrob. Resist.* 19: 313–316.

Antimicrobial Resistance Collaborators (2022). Global burden of bacterial antimicrobial resistance in 2019 : a systematic analysis. *Lancet* 399 (10325): 629–655.

Criscuolo, E., Spandini, S., Lamanna, J. et al. (2017). Bacteriophages and Their Immunological Applications against Infectious Threats. *J. Immunol. Res.* 2017: Article 3780697.

Dedrick, R.M., Guerrero-Bustamante, C.A., Garlena, R.A. et al. (2019). Engineered bacteriophages for treatment of a patient with a disseminated drug-resistant *Mycobacterium abscessus*. *Nat. Med.* 25: 730–733.

Dronkers, T.M.G., Ouwehand, A.C. and Rijkers, G.T. (2020). Global analysis of clinical trials with probiotics. *Heliyon* 6: e04467.

Fischetti, V.A. (2008). Bacteriophage lysins as effective antibacterials. *Curr. Opin. Microbiol.* 11: 393–400.

Fischetti, V.A. (2018). Development of phage lysins as novel therapeutics: a historical perspective. *Viruses* 10: 310.

Langford, B.J., So, M., Raybardhan, S. et al. (2021). Antibiotic prescribing in patients with COVID-19: rapid review and meta-analysis. *Clin. Microbiol. Infect.* 27 (4): 520–531.

Mombelli, B. and Gismondo, M.R. (2000). The use of probiotics in medical practice. *Int. J. Antimicrob. Agents* 16: 531–536.

Pendleton, J.N., Gorman, S.P. and Gilmore, B.F. (2013). Clinical relevance of the ESKAPE pathogens. *Expert Rev. Anti Infect. Ther.* 11 (3): 297–308.

Pew Charitable Trusts (2021). Tracking the Global Pipeline of Antibiotics in Development. http://www.pewtrusts.org/en/projects

Poolman, J.T. (2020). Expanding the role of bacterial vaccines into life-course vaccination strategies and prevention of antimicrobial-resistant infections. *NPJ Vaccines* 5: 84.

Ramamurthy, D., Nundalall, T., Cingo, S. et al. (2021). Recent advances in immunotherapies against infectious diseases. *Immunother. Adv.* 1 (1): 1–16.

Sanders, M.E., Merenstein, D.J., Ouwehand, A. et al. (2016). Probiotic use in at-risk populations. *J. Am. Pharm. Assoc.* 56: 680–686.

Schooley, R.T., Biswas, B., Gill, J.J. et al. (2017). Development and use of personalised bacteriophage-based therapeutic cocktails to treat a patient with a disseminated resistant *Acinetobacter baumannii* infection. *Antimicrob. Agents Chemother.* 61 (10): e00954–e00917.

Shi, G., Kang, X., Dong, F. et al. (2022). DRAMP 3.0: an enhanced comprehensive data repository of antimicrobial peptides. *Nucleic Acids Res.* 50: D488–D496.

Index

Note: Page number in *italics* denote figures, those in **bold** denote tables.

Hugo and Russell's Pharmaceutical Microbiology, Ninth Edition. Edited by Brendan F. Gilmore and Stephen P. Denyer.

Companion website: https://www.wiley.com/go/HugoandRussells9e

d

e

f

i

q

r

s

t

U

V